WILLIAM LLEWE

ANABOLICS

9th EDITION

DISCLAIMER: This information was gathered from sources including textbooks, medical journals, and pharmaceutical reports, as well as interviews with athletes, steroid dealers, and medical experts. Neither the author nor publisher assumes any liability for the information presented in this text. This book is not intended to provide medical advice. The purpose of this reference book is only to provide a compendium of information for the reader, for entertainment purposes only. None of the information in this book is meant to be applied. Readers are advised that many of the substances described in this reference book may be prohibited or used only under a physician's care in many jurisdictions. Readers should consult with appropriate medical authorities before using any drug, and the proper legal authorities if unsure of the status of substances described herein. Neither the publisher nor author advocate readers engage in any illegal activities.

Copyright © 2009 and published by Molecular Nutrition, LLC in Jupiter, FL 33458. All rights reserved. None of the content in this publication may be reproduced, stored in a retrieval system, resold, redistributed, or transmitted in any form or by any means (electronic, mechanical, photocopying, recording, or otherwise) without the prior written permission of the publisher. William Llewellyn's ANABOLICS are trademarks used herein under license.

Molecular Nutrition LLC, 5500 Military Trail, Ste. 22-308, Jupiter, FL 33458
www.molecularnutrition.net

Preface

ANABOLICS is a reference manual of drug compounds used to enhance body composition, strength, and/or athletic performance. This book includes an extensive review of the history, global availability, and application of anabolic/androgenic steroids, as well as related performance-enhancing drugs such as human growth hormone, insulin, anti-estrogens, diuretics, reductase inhibitors, and fat loss ("cutting") agents. The core focus of ANABOLICS is to provide a nonbiased and comprehensive review of the current medical science surrounding these drugs, as well as the practical (often nonmedical) protocols in which they are used by bodybuilders and athletes. The effort of this book is always to help readers understand the potential risks of these drugs, in addition to their benefits. ANABOLICS is not intended to promote steroid or other drug use, but is designed to help readers, may they be physicians, patients, or illicit users, better understand these drugs, and make well-informed decisions about them.

The 9th Edition of ANABOLICS took two years to complete, and is the most extensive reworking of this book since it was first released in 2000. This edition is a very important achievement to me personally, as it most closely represents my original vision for a comprehensive reference book. While I am certainly very proud of previous editions, I had always felt there were areas of the book in strong need of revision. A lot has been happening in anabolic science, and unfortunately time-sensitive information about steroid use and availability often took priority during updates over more general areas of information. With the 9th edition, I was finally able to conduct a full front-to-back rebuild of ANABOLICS. This includes an extensive, and I believe extremely important, rewriting of many fundamental sections of this book. I hope it will help readers better understand how steroids can affect the body, both positively and negatively, and perhaps even develop better strategies for minimizing risks.

Regular readers will notice the latest edition includes updates and format changes in the following sections.

Anabolic Overview (Part I):

The steroid Side Effects section has been rewritten. The new expanded section includes an extensive review of the current state of research on the potential health and cosmetic side effects of anabolic/androgenic steroid use. More than 200 medical citations are included.

A new section called Clinical Applications reviews the extensive legitimate medical uses for anabolic/androgenic steroids. Common medical administration protocols are also outlined.

Practical Application (Part II):

The Steroid Cycles and Sample Cycles sections have been rewritten. They now include a return to fundamental steroid use and stacking protocols. Special emphasis is placed on minimizing adverse reactions and health risks with the intelligent assembly of cycles.

A Frequently Asked Questions section has been added to address some of the most basic questions about steroid safety and efficacy.

Safer Use Guidelines have been provided, which outline effective strategies for helping to reduce the short-term and long-term health risks of nonmedical anabolic/androgenic steroid use.

A chapter on Understanding Blood Tests covers one of the most important preventative practices for steroid users, namely examining individual health markers via blood testing. Includes strategies for using a series of basic tests to assess pre-use health status, on-cycle adverse health impact, and post-cycle metabolic recovery.

The Underground Steroids section has been rewritten. Included are a series of testing results on a group of underground steroid products. An analysis of dosage, heavy metal contamination, oil purity, and active pharmaceutical ingredient (API) purity is included, and highlight potential alarming trends in underground steroid quality.

Drug Profiles (Part III):

In addition to updates concerning drug manufacture and global availability in the individual Anabolic/Androgenic Steroid Profiles, the Non-Steroid Profiles have been rewritten. Pertinent information such as product descriptions, structures, side effects, benefits, administration protocols, and availability has been organized in detailed sections so it can be more easily accessed.

A new Cardiovascular Support section has been added, and includes products that can help protect the cardiovascular system from anabolic/androgenic steroid toxicity.

Steroid Availability Tables (Appendix A):

Global steroid manufacturing status has been extensively updated. Many dozens of new steroid preparations have been added, and numerous out of commerce steroids unlikely to be circulating have been removed.

Photographic Database (Appendix B):

The photographic database has been extensively expanded, and includes approximately 3,000 pictures of anabolic/androgenic steroids and other drugs. Nearly one third of all library pictures are new for the 9th edition. Legitimate pharmaceuticals are labeled and grouped by their country of manufacture. The following terms are used to identify the origin of individual drug products, and have changed slightly from previous editions.

Real (or no specification other than country): These are legitimate pharmaceutical products that are distributed in pharmacies or veterinary clinics in the labeled country of origin. Real drugs offer the greatest assurance of product purity and safety, although production standards may vary by country or market (veterinary/human).

Counterfeit (CF): This is an illicit duplicate of a real drug product and/or manufacturer. These items are of unknown quality and safety, often contain substitute or no steroid ingredients, and should never be knowingly consumed.

Export (EX): These are drugs made by registered pharmaceutical companies, but are not licensed for sale in their country of origin. They must be exported. Export products should be made in legitimate pharmaceutical manufacturing facilities, but depending on the region may not be made under the same close government supervision as locally distributed products.

Underground (UG): These products are made from unlicensed illegal manufacturers specifically for sale on the black market. Given the completely unregulated nature of these drugs, they offer little assurance of quality, and are generally not recommended. In some instances the country of origin is identified for an underground product. This specifically indicates the drug may be sold in some domestic pharmacies and/or veterinary clinics, even though it is not legally registered for sale.

Fake: This is an illicitly manufactured drug that purports to be a real pharmaceutical, but bears no relation to an actual product. Fake is a distinction that suggests all forms of the photographed steroid should be considered illegitimate.

NLM: Indicates a drug that is No Longer Manufactured. This distinction is important because when NLM drugs are still found in active black market commerce they usually turn out to be illegitimate.

Glossary:

A glossary has been added, including explanations of some of the more common medical terms used throughout this book.

William Llewellyn's ANABOLICS, 9th ed.

TABLE OF CONTENTS

PART I: ANABOLIC OVERVIEW

An Introduction to Testosterone 5
Direct and Indirect Anabolic Effects 7
Free vs. Bound Testosterone 10
Estrogen Aromatization 12
DHT Conversion 14
Brief History of Anabolic/Androgenic Steroids 15
Synthetic AAS Development 16
Synthetic AAS Chemistry 21
Steroid Nomenclature 26
Clinical Applications 27   * NEW *
Side Effects 33   Updated
Acute Steroid Safety: Studies with Real-World Dosages 54
The Endocrinology of Muscle Growth 56

PART II: PRACTICAL APPLICATION

Steroid Cycles 65   Updated
Sample Steroid Cycles 69   Updated
PCT: Post Cycle Therapy 84   Updated
Injection Protocols 88   Updated
Steroid Frequently Asked Questions 91   * NEW *
Understanding Blood Tests 93   * NEW *
Harm Reduction/Safer Use Guidelines 108   * NEW *
Counterfeit Steroids 111   Updated
Counterfeit Steroid Identification 115   Updated
Country Specifics 117
Underground Steroids 119   Updated
Designer Steroids 124
Anabolic Steroid Possesion and the Law 126   Updated

PART III: DRUG PROFILES

ANABOLIC/ANDROGENIC STEROIDS (Listed by Common Brand)

1-Testosterone (dihydroboldenone) 135
20 AET-1 (testosterone buciclate) 138
Agovirin Depot (testosterone isobutyrate) 141   B-109
Anabol 4-19 (norclostebol acetate) 144
Anabolicum Vister (quinbolone) 146
Anadrol®- 50 (oxymetholone) 149   B-1   Updated
Anadur® (nandrolone hexyloxyphenylpropionate) 154
Anatrofin (stenbolone acetate) 157
Anavar (oxandrolone) 159   B-7   Updated
Andractim® (dihydrotestosterone) 163   B-11
Andriol® (testosterone undecanoate) 166   B-11   Updated

v

William Llewellyn's ANABOLICS, 9th ed.

Androderm® (testosterone)	169	B-13	Updated
AndroGel® (testosterone)	172	B-14	Updated
Andromar Retard (testosterone cyclohexylpropionate)	175		
Andronaq (testosterone suspension)	178	B-107	
Bolfortan (testosterone nicotinate)	182		
Cheque Drops® (mibolerone)	185	B-15	
Danocrine® (danazol)	188		
Deca-Durabolin® (nandrolone decanoate)	190	B-15	Updated
Delatestryl® (testosterone enanthate)	194	B-86	Updated
Depo®-Testosterone (testosterone cypionate)	199	B-79	Updated
Deposterona (testosterone blend)	204	B-30	
Dianabol® (methandrostenolone, methandienone)	207	B-31	Updated
Dimethyltrienolone (dimethyltrienolone)	212		
Dinandrol (nandrolone blend)	215	B-39	
Drive® (boldenone/methylandrostenediol blend)	218	B-40	Updated
Durabolin® (nandrolone phenylpropionate)	220	B-41	Updated
Dynabol® (nandrolone cypionate)	223	B-43	
Dynabolon® (nandrolone undecanoate)	226	B-43	
Emdabol (thiomesterone)	229		
Equilon 100 (boldenone blend)	232	B-43	Updated
Equipoise® (boldenone undecylenate)	235	B-43	Updated
Equitest 200 (testosterone blend)	238	B-51	
Ermalone (mestanolone)	241		
Esiclene® (formebolone, formyldienolone)	244		
Estandron (testosterone/estrogen blend)	247	B-52	
Fherbolico (nandrolone cyclohexylpropionate)	250	B-69	
Finajet (trenbolone acetate)	253	B-111	Updated
Genabol (norbolethone)	257		
Halodrol (chlorodehydromethylandrostenediol)	260		
Halotestin® (fluoxymesterone)	263	B-52	Updated
Havoc (methepitiostane)	267		
Hydroxytest (hydroxytestosterone)	270		
Laurabolin® (nandrolone laurate)	273	B-53	
Libriol (nandrolone/methandriol blend)	276	B-53	
Madol (desoxymethyltestosterone)	278		
Masteron® (drostanolone propionate)	281	B-54	Updated
Megagrisevit-Mono® (clostebol acetate)	284		
MENT (methylnortestosterone acetate)	287		
Metandren (methyltestosterone)	291	B-56	Updated
Methandriol (methylandrostenediol)	294	B-56	Updated
Methosarb (calusterone)	297		
Methyl-1-testosterone (methyldihydroboldenone)	299		
Methyl-D (methyldienolone)	302		
Metribolone (methyltrienolone)	305		
Miotolan® (furazabol)	308		
MOHN (methylhydroxynandrolone)	311		
Myagen (bolasterone)	314		
Nandrabolin (nandrolone/methandriol blend)	317		
Nebido (testosterone undecanoate)	319	B-57	
Neo-Ponden (androisoxazol)	322		
Neodrol (dihydrotestosterone)	325		
Neotest 250 (testosterone decanoate)	327		

Nilevar® (norethandrolone)	330	B-57	
Omnadren® 250 (testosterone blend)	333	B-57	
Orabolin® (ethylestrenol)	336	B-58	
Oral Turinabol (4-chlorodehydromethyltestosterone)	339	B-59	Updated
Oranabol (oxymesterone)	342		
Oreton (testosterone propionate)	345	B-100	Updated
Orgasteron (normethandrolone)	350		
Parabolan® (trenbolone hexahydrobenzylcarbonate)	353	B-59	Updated
Perandren (testosterone phenylacetate)	356		
Primobolan® (methenolone acetate)	359	B-65	Updated
Primobolan® Depot (methenolone enanthate)	362	B-60	Updated
Promagnon (chloromethylandrostenediol)	365		
Prostanozol (demethylstanozolol tetrahydropyranyl)	367		
Proviron® (mesterolone)	369	B-66	Updated
Roxilon (dimethazine)	372		
Roxilon Inject (bolazine caproate)	374		
Spectriol (testosterone/nandrolone/methandriol blend)	376	B-69	
Sten (testosterone cypionate & propionate)	378	B-69	Updated
Steranabol Ritardo (oxabolone cypionate)	381		
Sterandryl Retard (testosterone hexahydrobenzoate)	383		
Striant® (testosterone)	386		
Superdrol (methyldrostanolone)	389		
Sustanon® 100 (testosterone blend)	392		
Sustanon® 250 (testosterone blend)	395	B-69	Updated
Synovex® (testosterone propionate & estradiol)	399	B-78	
Test® 400 (testosterone propionate/cypionate/enanthate)	402	B-78	
Testoderm® (testosterone)	405		
Testolent (testosterone phenylpropionate)	408	B-79	
Testopel® (testosterone)	411		
Testoviron® (testosterone propionate/enanthate blend)	414	B-110	Updated
THG (tetrahydrogestrinone)	418		
Thioderon (mepitiostane)	421		
Trenabol® (trenbolone enanthate)	423	B-115	Updated
Tri-Trenabol 150 (trenbolone blend)	426	B-117	Updated
Tribolin (nandrolone/methandriol blend)	429	B-116	
Triolandren (testosterone blend)	431		
Winstrol® (stanozolol)	434	B-117	Updated

ANABOLIC/ANDROGENIC STEROIDS (Listed by Generic Name)

4-chlorodehydromethyltestosterone (Oral Turinabol)	339	B-59	Updated
androisoxazol (Neo-Ponden)	322		
bolasterone (Myagen)	314		
bolazine caproate (Roxilon Inject)	374		
boldenone blend (Equilon 100)	232	B-43	Updated
boldenone undecylenate (Equipoise®)	235	B-43	Updated
boldenone/methylandrostenediol blend (Drive®)	218	B-40	Updated
calusterone (Methosarb)	297		
chlorodehydromethylandrostenediol (Halodrol)	260		
chloromethylandrostenediol (Promagnon)	365		
clostebol acetate (Megagrisevit-Mono®)	284		
danazol (Danocrine®)	188		

demethylstanozolol tetrahydropyranyl (Prostanozol)	367		
desoxymethyltestosterone (Madol)	278		
dihydroboldenone (1-Testosterone)	135		
dihydrotestosterone (Andractim®)	163	B-11	
dihydrotestosterone (Neodrol)	325		
dimethazine (Roxilon)	372		
dimethyltrienolone (Dimethyltrienolone)	212		
drostanolone propionate (Masteron®)	281	B-54	Updated
ethylestrenol (Orabolin®)	336	B-58	
fluoxymesterone (Halotestin®)	263	B-52	Updated
formebolone, formyldienolone (Esiclene®)	244		
furazabol (Miotolan®)	308		
hydroxytestosterone (Hydroxytest)	270		
mepitiostane (Thioderon)	421		
mestanolone (Ermalone)	241		
mesterolone (Proviron®)	369	B-66	Updated
methandrostenolone, methandienone (Dianabol®)	207	B-31	Updated
methenolone acetate (Primobolan®)	359	B-65	Updated
methenolone enanthate (Primobolan® Depot)	362	B-60	Updated
methepitiostane (Havoc)	267		
methylandrostenediol (Methandriol)	294	B-56	
Methyldienolone (Methyl-D)	302		
methyldihydroboldenone (Methyl-1-testosterone)	299		
methyldrostanolone (Superdrol)	389		
methylhydroxynandrolone (MOHN)	311		
methylnortestosterone acetate (MENT)	287		
methyltestosterone (Metandren)	291	B-56	Updated
methyltrienolone (Metribolone)	305		
mibolerone (Cheque Drops®)	185	B-15	
nandrolone blend (Dinandrol)	215	B-39	
nandrolone cyclohexylpropionate (Fherbolico)	250	B-69	
nandrolone cypionate (Dynabol®)	223	B-43	
nandrolone decanoate (Deca-Durabolin®)	190	B-15	Updated
nandrolone hexyloxyphenylpropionate (Anadur®)	154		
nandrolone laurate (Laurabolin®)	273	B-53	
nandrolone phenylpropionate (Durabolin®)	220	B-41	Updated
nandrolone undecanoate (Dynabolon®)	226	B-43	
nandrolone/methandriol blend (Libriol)	276	B-53	
nandrolone/methandriol blend (Tribolin)	429	B-116	
nandrolone/methandriol blend (Nandrabolin)	317		
norbolethone (Genabol)	257		
norclostebol acetate (Anabol 4-19)	144		
norethandrolone (Nilevar®)	330	B-57	
normethandrolone (Orgasteron)	350		
oxabolone cypionate (Steranabol Ritardo)	381		
oxandrolone (Anavar)	159	B-7	Updated
oxymesterone (Oranabol)	342		
oxymetholone (Anadrol®- 50)	149	B-1	Updated
quinbolone (Anabolicum Vister)	146		
stanozolol (Winstrol®)	434	B-117	Updated
stenbolone acetate (Anatrofin)	157		
testosterone (Androderm®)	169	B-13	Updated

testosterone (AndroGel®)	172	B-14	Updated
testosterone (Striant®)	386		
testosterone (Testoderm®)	405		
testosterone (Testopel®)	411		
testosterone blend (Deposterona)	204	B-30	
testosterone blend (Equitest 200)	238	B-51	
testosterone blend (Omnadren® 250)	333	B-57	
testosterone blend (Sustanon® 100)	392		
testosterone blend (Sustanon® 250)	395	B-69	Updated
testosterone blend (Triolandren)	431		
testosterone buciclate (20 AET-1)	138		
testosterone cyclohexylpropionate (Andromar Retard)	175		
testosterone cypionate & propionate (Sten)	378	B-69	Updated
testosterone cypionate (Depo®-Testosterone)	199	B-79	Updated
testosterone decanoate (Neotest 250)	327		
testosterone enanthate (Delatestryl®)	194	B-86	Updated
testosterone hexahydrobenzoate (Sterandryl Retard)	383		
testosterone isobutyrate (Agovirin Depot)	141	B-109	
testosterone nicotinate (Bolfortan)	182		
testosterone phenylacetate (Perandren)	356		
testosterone phenylpropionate (Testolent)	408	B-79	
testosterone propionate & estradiol (Synovex®)	399	B-78	
testosterone propionate (Oreton)	345	B-100	Updated
testosterone propionate/cypionate/enanthate (Test® 400)	402	B-78	
testosterone propionate/enanthate blend (Testoviron®)	414	B-110	Updated
testosterone suspension (Andronaq)	178	B-107	
testosterone undecanoate (Andriol®)	166	B-11	Updated
testosterone undecanoate (Nebido)	319	B-57	
testosterone/estrogen blend (Estandron)	247	B-52	
testosterone/nandrolone/methandriol blend (Spectriol)	376	B-69	
tetrahydrogestrinone (THG)	418		
thiomesterone (Emdabol)	229		
trenbolone acetate (Finajet)	253	B-111	Updated
trenbolone blend (Tri-Trenabol 150)	426	B-117	Updated
trenbolone enanthate (Trenabol®)	423	B-115	Updated
trenbolone hexahydrobenzylcarbonate (Parabolan®)	353	B-59	Updated

ANABOLIC AGENTS (NON-STEROID)

Arachidonic acid (eicosa-5,8,11,14-enoic acid)	441		
Kynoselen®	444	C-11	Updated
Lutalyse® (diniprost)	446		Updated

ANTI-ACNE

Accutane (isotretinoin)	451		Updated

ANTI-ESTROGENS

Arimidex® (anastrozole)	455	C-1	Updated
Aromasin® (exemestane)	457		Updated
Clomid® (clomiphene citrate)	459	C-3	Updated
Cytadren® (aminoglutethimide)	461	C-4	Updated
Evista (raloxifene)	464		Updated

William Llewellyn's ANABOLICS, 9th ed.

Fareston® (toremifene citrate)	466		Updated
Faslodex® (fulvestrant)	468		Updated
Femara® (letrozole)	470	C-4	Updated
Fertodur® (cyclofenil)	472	C-3	Updated
Lentaron® (formestane)	474	C-11	Updated
Nolvadex® (tamoxifen citrate)	476	C-12	Updated
Teslac® (testolactone)	478		Updated

ANTI-PROLACTIN

Dostinex® (cabergoline)	483		Updated
Parlodel® (bromocriptine mesylate)	485	C-13	Updated

APPETITE STIMULANTS

Periactin (cyproheptadine hydrochloride)	489		Updated

CARDIOVASCULAR SUPPORT

Lipid Stabil™	493		Updated
Lovaza® (omega-3 ethyl esters)	494		Updated

DIURETICS

Aldactone® (spironolactone)	497	C-1	Updated
Dyrenium® (triamterene)	499		Updated
Hydrodiuril® (hydrochlorthiazide)	501		Updated
Lasix® (furosemide)	503	C-11	Updated

ENDURANCE/ERYTHROPOIETIC DRUGS

Aranesp® (darbepoetin alfa)	507		Updated
Epogen® (epoetin alfa)	509	C-4	Updated
Provigil® (modafinil)	511		Updated

FAT LOSS AGENTS – SYMPATHOMIMETICS

Adipex-P (phentermine hydrochloride)	515		Updated
Albuterol (albuterol sulfate)	516		Updated
Clenasma (clenbuterol hydrochloride)	518	C-2	Updated
Ephedrine (ephedrine hydrochloride)	521		Updated
Meridia® (sibutramine hydrochloride monohydrate)	523	C-11	Updated
Zaditen® (ketotifen fumarate)	525	C-14	Updated

FAT LOSS AGENTS – THYROID

Cytomel® (liothyronine sodium)	529	C-4	Updated
Synthroid® (levothyroxine sodium)	531	C-13	Updated

FAT LOSS AGENTS – OTHER

DNP (2,4-dinitrophenol)	535		Updated
Lipostabil N (phosphatidylcholine/sodium deoxycholate)	537	C-11	Updated

GROWTH HORMONES & RELATED

Human Growth Hormone (somatropin)	541	C-5	Updated
Increlex® (mecasermin)	544		Updated
Protropin® (somatrem)	546	C-5	Updated

HYPOGLYCEMICS

Insulin 551   C-10   Updated

LIVER DETOXIFICATION

Essentiale forte N 561   * NEW *
LIV-52® 562   Updated
Liver Stabil™ 563   * NEW *

REDUCTASE INHIBITORS

Avodart® (dutasteride) 567   C-1   Updated
Proscar® (finasteride) 569   C-13   Updated

TANNING AGENTS

Oxsoralen (methoxsalen) 573   Updated
Trisoralen® (trioxsalen) 575   Updated

TESTOSTERONE STIMULATING DRUGS

HCG (human chorionic gonadotropin) 579   C-8

ENDNOTES

GLOSSARY

APPENDIX

DRUG AVAILABILITY TABLES: COUNTRY   A-1   Updated

STEROID PHOTO LIBRARY   B-1   Updated

DRUG PHOTO LIBRARY (NON-STEROID)   C-1   Updated

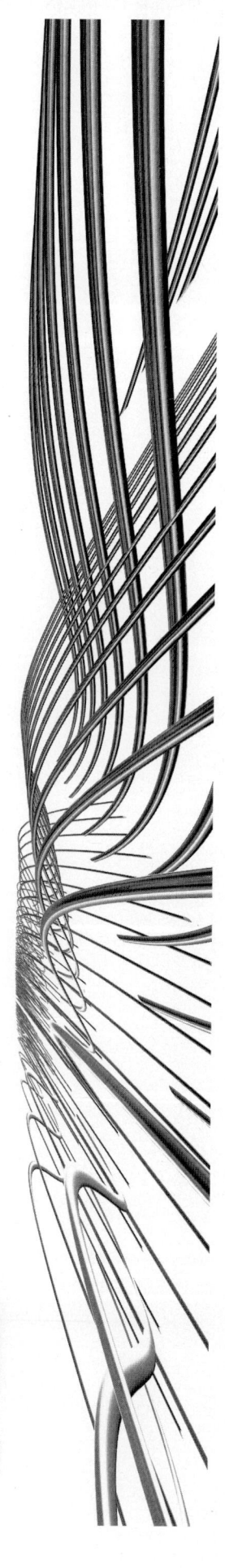

Part I
Anabolic Overview

INTRODUCTION

An Introduction to Testosterone

Anabolic steroids are a class of medications that contain a synthetically manufactured form of the hormone testosterone, or a related compound that is derived from (or similar in structure and action to) this hormone. In order to fully grasp how anabolic steroids work, it is, therefore, important to understand the basic functioning of testosterone.

Testosterone is the primary male sex hormone. It is manufactured by the Leydig's cells in the testes at varying amounts throughout a person's life span. The effects of this hormone become most evident during the time of puberty, when an increased output of testosterone will elicit dramatic physiological changes in the male body. This includes the onset of secondary male characteristics such as a deepened voice, body and facial hair growth, increased oil output by the sebaceous glands, development of sexual organs, maturation of sperm, and an increased libido. Indeed the male reproductive system will not function properly if testosterone levels are not significant. All such effects are considered the masculinizing or "androgenic" properties of this hormone.

Increased testosterone production will also cause growth promoting or "anabolic" changes in the body, including an enhanced rate of protein synthesis (leading to muscle accumulation). Testosterone is the reason males carry more muscle mass than women, as the two sexes have vastly contrasting amounts of this hormone. More specifically, the adult male body will manufacture between 2.5 and 11mg per day[1] while females only produce about 1/4mg. The dominant sex hormone for women is estrogen, which has a significantly different effect on the body. Among other things, a lower androgen and higher estrogen level will cause women to store more body fat, accumulate less muscle tissue, have a shorter stature, and become more apt to bone weakening with age (osteoporosis).

The actual mechanism in which testosterone elicits these changes is somewhat complex. When free in the blood stream, the testosterone molecule is available to interact with various cells in the body. This includes skeletal muscle cells, as well as skin, scalp, kidney, bone, central nervous system, and prostate tissues. Testosterone binds with a cellular target in order to exert its activity, and will, therefore, effect only those body cells that posses the proper hormone receptor site (specifically the androgen receptor). This process can be likened to a lock and key system, with each receptor (lock) only being activated by a particular type of hormone (key). During this interaction, the testosterone molecule will become bound to the intracellular receptor site (located in the cytosol, not on the membrane surface), forming a new "receptor complex." This complex (hormone + receptor site) will then migrate to the cell's nucleus, where it will attach to a specific section of the cell's DNA, referred to as the hormone response element. This will activate the transcription of specific genes, which in the case of a skeletal muscle cell will ultimately cause (among other things) an increase in the synthesis of the two primary contractile proteins, actin and myosin (muscular growth). Carbohydrate storage in muscle tissue may be increased due to androgen action as well.

Once this messaging process is completed, the complex will be released, and the receptor and hormone will disassociate. Both are then free to migrate back into the cytosol for further activity. The testosterone molecule is also free to diffuse back into circulation to interact with other cells. The entire receptor cycle, including hormone binding, receptor-hormone complex migration, gene transcription and subsequent return to cytosol is a slow process, taking hours, not minutes, to complete. For example, in studies using a single injection of nandrolone, it is measured to be 4 to 6 hours before free androgen receptors migrate back to the cytosol after activation. It is also suggested that this cycle includes the splitting and formation of new androgen receptors once returned to cytosol, a possible explanation for the many observations that androgens are integral in the formation of their own receptor sites.[2]

In the kidneys, this same process works to allow androgens to augment erythropoiesis (red blood cell production).[3] It is this effect that leads to an increase in red blood cell concentrations, and possibly increased oxygen transport capacity, during anabolic/androgenic steroid therapy. Many athletes mistakenly assume that oxymetholone and boldenone are unique in this ability, due to specific uses or mentions of this effect in drug literature. In fact, stimulation of erythropoiesis occurs with nearly all anabolic/androgenic steroids, as this effect is simply tied with activation of the androgen receptor in kidney cells. The only real exceptions might be compounds such as dihydrotestosterone and some of its derivatives,[4] which are rapidly broken down upon interaction with the 3alpha-hydroxysteroid dehydrogenase enzymes (kidney tissue has a similar enzyme distribution to muscle tissue, see "anabolic/androgenic dissociation" section), and therefore

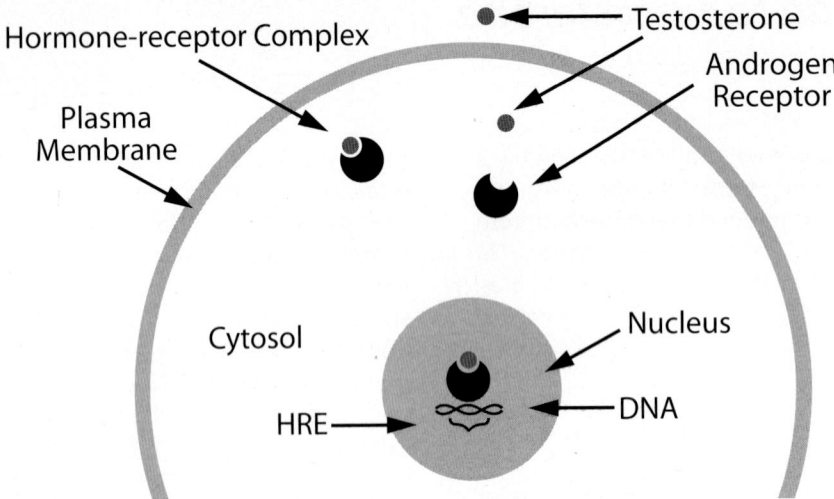

CELLULAR DIAGRAM: Testosterone freely diffuses through the plasma membrane and binds with an intracellular androgen receptor. The hormone-receptor complex then enters the cell nucleus to bind with a specific segment of DNA (the Hormone Response Element), activating the transcription of specific genes.

display low activity in these tissues.

Adipose (fat) tissues are also androgen responsive, and here these hormones support the lipolytic (fat mobilizing) capacity of cells.[5] This may be accomplished by an androgen-tied regulation of beta-adrenergic receptor concentrations or general cellular activity (through adenylate cyclase).[6] We also note that the level of androgens in the body will closely correlate (inversely) with the level of stored body fat. As the level of androgenic hormones drops, typically the deposition of body fat will increase.[7] Likewise as we enhance the androgen level, body fat may be depleted at a more active rate. The ratio of androgen to estrogen action is in fact most important, as estrogen plays a counter role by acting to increase the storage of body fat in many sites of action.[8] Likewise, if one wished to lose fat during steroid use, estrogen levels should be kept low. This is clearly evidenced by the fact that non-aromatizing steroids have always been favored by bodybuilders looking to increase the look of definition and muscularity while aromatizing compounds are typically relegated to bulking phases of training due to their tendency to increase body fat storage. Aromatization is discussed in more detail in a following section (see: Estrogen Aromatization).

As mentioned, testosterone also elicits androgenic activity, which occurs by its activating receptors in what are considered to be androgen responsive tissues (often through prior conversion to dihydrotestosterone. See: DHT Conversion). This includes the sebaceous glands, which are responsible for the secretion of oils in the skin. As the androgen level rises, so does the release of oils. As oil output increases, so does the chance for pores becoming clogged (we can see why acne is such a common side effect of steroid use). The production of body and facial hair is also linked to androgen receptor activation in skin and scalp tissues. This becomes most noticeable as boys mature into puberty, a period when testosterone levels rise rapidly, and androgen activity begins to stimulate the growth of hair on the body and face. Some time later in life, and with the contribution of a genetic predisposition, androgen activity in the scalp may also help to initiate male-pattern hair loss. It is a misconception that dihydrotestosterone is an isolated culprit in the promotion of hair loss, however; as in actuality it is the general activation of the androgen receptor that is to blame (see: DHT Conversion). The functioning of sex glands and libido are also tied to the activity of androgens, as are numerous other regions of the central nervous/neuromuscular system.

Direct and Indirect Anabolic Effects

Although testosterone has been isolated, synthesized, and actively experimented with for many decades now, there is still some debate today as to exactly how steroids affect muscle mass. At this point in time, the primary mode of anabolic action with all anabolic/androgenic steroids is understood to be direct activation of the cellular androgen receptor and increases in protein synthesis. As follows, if we are able to increase our androgen level from an external source by supplementing testosterone or a similar anabolic steroid, we can greatly enhance the rate in which protein is retained by the muscles. This is clearly the primary cause for muscle growth with all anabolic/androgenic steroids. As our hormone levels increase, so does androgen receptor activation, and ultimately the rate of protein synthesis.

But other indirect mechanisms could possibly affect muscle growth outside of the normally understood androgen action on protein synthesis. An indirect mechanism is one that is not brought about by activation of the androgen receptor, but the affect androgens might have on other hormones, or even the release of locally acting hormones or growth promoters inside cells (perhaps mediated by other membrane bound receptors). We must remember also that muscle mass disposition involves not only protein synthesis, but also other factors such as tissue nutrient transport and protein breakdown. We need to look at androgenic interaction with these factors as well to get a complete picture. Concerning the first possibility, we note that studies with testosterone suggest that this hormone does not increase tissue amino acid transport.[9] This fact probably explains the profound synergy bodybuilders have noted in recent years with insulin, a hormone that strongly increases transport of nutrients into muscle cells. But regarding protein breakdown, we do see a second important pathway in which androgens might affect muscle growth.

Anti-Glucocorticoid Effect of Testosterone

Testosterone (and synthetic anabolic/androgenic steroids) may help to increase mass and strength by having an anti-catabolic effect on muscle cells. Considered one of the most important indirect mechanisms of androgen action, these hormones are shown to affect the actions of another type of steroid hormone in the body, glucocorticoids (cortisol is the primary representative of this group).[10] Glucocorticoid hormones actually have the exact opposite effect on the muscle cell than androgens, namely sending an order to release stored protein. This process is referred to as catabolism, and represents a breaking down of muscle tissue. Muscle growth is achieved when the anabolic effects of testosterone are more pronounced overall than the degenerative effects of cortisol. With intense training and a proper diet, the body will typically store more protein than it removes, but this underlying battle is always constant.

When administering anabolic steroids, however, a much higher androgen level can place glucocorticoids at a notable disadvantage. With their effect reduced, fewer cells will be given a message to release protein, and more will be accumulated in the long run. The primarily mechanism believed to bring this effect out is androgen displacement of glucocorticoids bound to the glucocorticoid receptor. In fact, in-vitro studies have supported this notion by demonstrating that testosterone has a very high affinity for this receptor,[11] and further suggesting that some of its anabolic activity is directly mediated through this action.[12] It is also suggested that androgens may indirectly interfere with DNA binding to the glucocorticoid response element.[13] Although the exact underlying mechanism is still in debate, what is clear is that steroid administration inhibits protein breakdown, even in the fasted state, which seems clearly indicative of an anti-catabolic effect.

Testosterone and Creatine

In addition to protein synthesis, a rise in androgen levels should also enhance the synthesis of creatine in skeletal muscle tissues.[14] Creatine, as creatine phosphate (CP), plays a crucial role in the manufacture of ATP (adenosine triphosphate), which is a main store of energy for the muscles. As the muscle cells are stimulated to contract, ATP molecules are broken down into ADP (adenosine diphosphate), which releases energy. The cells will then undergo a process using creatine phosphate to rapidly restore ADP to its original structure, in order to replenish ATP concentrations. During periods of intense activity, however, this process will not be fast enough to compensate and ATP levels will become lowered. This will cause the muscles to become fatigued and less able to effort a strenuous contraction. With increased levels of CP available to the cells, ATP is replenished at an enhanced rate and the muscle is both stronger and more enduring. This effect will account for some portion of the early strength increases seen during steroid therapy. Although perhaps not technically considered an anabolic effect as tissue hypertrophy is not a direct result, androgen support of creatine synthesis is certainly still looked at as a positive and growth-supporting result in the mind of the bodybuilder.

Testosterone and IGF-1

It has also been suggested that there is an indirect mechanism of testosterone action on muscle mass mediated by Insulin-Like Growth Factor. To be more specific, studies note a clear link between androgens and tissue release of,[15] and responsiveness to, this anabolic hormone. For example, it has been demonstrated that increases in IGF-1 receptor concentrations in skeletal muscle are noted when elderly men are given replacement doses of testosterone.[16] In essence, the cells are becoming primed for the actions of IGF-1, by testosterone. Alternately we see marked decreases in IGF-1 receptor protein levels with androgen deficiency in young men. It also appears that androgens are necessary for the local production and function of IGF-1 in skeletal muscle cells, independent of circulating growth hormone, and IGF-1 levels.[17] Since we do know for certain that IGF-1 is at least a minor anabolic hormone in muscle tissue, it seems reasonable to conclude that this factor, at least at some level, is involved in the muscle growth noted with steroid therapy.

Direct and Indirect Steroids?

In looking over the proposed indirect effects of testosterone, and pondering the effectiveness of the synthetic anabolic/androgenic steroids, we must resist the temptation to believe we can categorize steroids as those which directly, and those which indirectly, promote muscle growth. The belief that there are two dichotomous groups or classes of steroids ignores the fact that all commercial steroids promote not only muscle growth but also androgenic effects. There is no complete separation of these traits at this time, making clear that all activate the cellular androgen receptor. I believe the theory behind direct and indirect steroid classifications originated when some noted the low receptor binding affinity of seemingly strong anabolic steroids like oxymetholone and methandrostenolone.[18] If they bind poorly, yet work well, something else must be at work. This type of thinking fails to recognize other factors in the potency of these compounds, such as their long half-lives, estrogenic activity, and weak interaction with restrictive binding proteins (see: Free vs. Bound Testosterone). While there may possibly be differences in the way various compounds could foster growth indirectly, such that advantages might even be found with certain synergistic drug combinations, the primary mode of action with all of these compounds is the androgen receptor. The notion

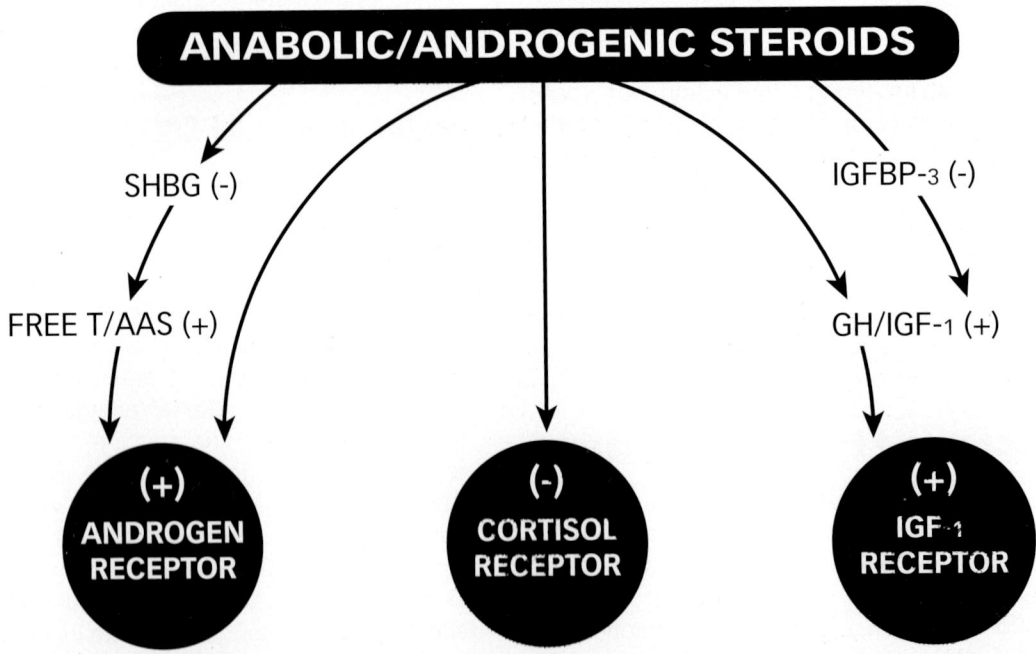

MECHANISM OF ACTION DIAGRAM: The mechanism of anabolic action due to the administration of anabolic/androgenic steroids. AAS causes not only direct stimulation of the androgen receptor, but also supports muscle growth by increasing the levels of free androgens, increasing androgen receptor density, inhibiting corticosteroid action, increasing GH/IGF-1, and suppressing IGF-1 binding proteins.

that steroid X and Y must never be stacked together because they both compete for the same receptor when stimulating growth, while X and Z should be combined because they work via different mechanisms, should likewise not be taken too seriously. Such classifications are based on speculation only, and upon reasonable investigation are clearly invalid.

Free vs. Bound Testosterone

A very small amount of testosterone actually exists in a free state, where interaction with cellular receptors is possible. The majority will be bound to the proteins SHBG (sex hormone binding globulin, also referred to as sex steroid binding globulin and testosterone-estradiol binding globulin) and albumin, which temporarily prevent the hormone from exerting activity. Steroid hormones actually bind much more avidly to SHBG than albumin (with approximately 1,000 times greater affinity), however albumin is present in a level 1,000 times greater than SHBG. Therefore, the activity of both binding proteins in the body is relatively equal. The distribution of testosterone in men is typically 45% of testosterone bound to SHBG, and about 53% bound to albumin. The remaining 2% of the average blood concentration exists in a free, unbound state. In women, the percentage of free testosterone is lower, measured to be approximately 1%. A binding protein called ABP (androgen binding protein) also helps to mediate androgen activity in the reproductive system, although since it is found exclusively in these tissues, it is not relevant to muscle growth.

The level of free testosterone available in the blood is likewise an important factor mediating its activity, as only a small percentage is really active at any given time. It must also be noted that as we alter testosterone to form new anabolic/androgenic steroids, we also typically alter the affinity in which the steroid will bind to plasma proteins. This is an important consideration, as the higher percentage we have of free hormone, the more active the compound should be on a milligram for milligram basis. And the variance can be substantial between different compounds. For example, Proviron® (1-methyl dihydrotestosterone) binds with SHBG many times more avidly than testosterone,[19] while mibolerone (7,17 dimethyl-nandrolone) and bolasterone (7,17 dimethyl-testosterone) show virtually no affinity for this protein at all (clearly the reason these steroids are such potent androgens).

The level of SHBG present in the body is also variable, and can be altered by a number of factors. The most prominent seems to be the concentration of estrogen and thyroid hormones present in the blood. We generally see a reduction in the amount of this plasma binding protein as estrogen and thyroid content decreases, and a rise in SHBG as they increase. A heightened androgen level due to the administration of anabolic/androgenic steroids has also been shown to lower levels of this protein considerably. This is clearly supported by a 1989 German study, which noted a strong tendency for SHBG reduction with the oral anabolic steroid stanozolol (Winstrol®).[20] After only 3 days of administering a daily dose of .2mg/kg body-weight (about 18mg for a 200lb man), SHBG was lowered nearly 50% in normal subjects. Similar results have been obtained with the use of injectable testosterone enanthate; however, milligram for milligram, the effect of stanozolol was much greater in comparison. The form of administration may have been important in reaching this level of response. Although the injectable was not tried in the German study, we can refer to others comparing the effect of oral vs. transdermal estrogen.[21] These show a much greater response in SHBG levels when the drug is given orally. This is perhaps explained by the fact that SHBG is produced in the liver. Therefore, we cannot assume that injectable Winstrol® (or injectable steroids in general) will display the same level of potency in this regard.

Lowering the level of plasma binding proteins is also not the only mechanism that allows for an increased level of free testosterone. Steroids that display a high affinity for these proteins may also increase the level of free testosterone by competing with it for binding. Obviously if testosterone finds it more difficult to locate available plasma proteins in the presence of the additional compound, more will be left in an unbound state. A number of steroids including dihydrotestosterone, Proviron®, and Oral-Turinabol (chlorodehydromethyltestosterone) display a strong tendency for this effect. If the level of free-testosterone can be altered by the use of different anabolic/androgenic steroids, the possibility also exists that one steroid can increase the potency of another through these same mechanisms. For example, Proviron® is a poor anabolic, but its extremely high affinity for SHBG might make it useful by allowing the displacement of other steroids that are more active in these tissues.

We must not let this discussion lead us into thinking that binding proteins serve no valuable function. In fact they play a vital role in the transport and functioning of endogenous androgens. Binding proteins act to protect the steroid against rapid metabolism, ensure a more stable blood hormone concentration, and facilitate an even distribution of hormone to various body organs. The recent discovery of a specific receptor for Sex Hormone-Binding Globulin (SHBG-R) located on the membrane surface of steroid responsive body cells also suggests a much more complicated role for this protein than solely hormone transport. However, it remains clear that manipulating the tendency of a hormone to exist in an unbound state is an effective way to alter drug potency.

Estrogen Aromatization

Testosterone is the primary substrate used in the male body for the synthesis of estrogen (estradiol), the principal female sex hormone. Although the presence of estrogen may seem quite unusual in men, it is structurally very similar to testosterone. With a slight alteration by the enzyme aromatase, estrogen is produced in the male body. Aromatase activity occurs in various regions of the male body, including adipose,[22] liver,[23] gonadal,[24] central nervous system,[25] and skeletal muscle[26] tissues. In the context of the average healthy male, the amount of estrogen produced is generally not very significant to one's body disposition, and may even be beneficial in terms of cholesterol values (See Side Effects: Cardiovascular Disease). However, in larger amounts it does have potential to cause many unwanted effects including water retention, female breast tissue development (gynecomastia), and body fat accumulation. For these reasons, many focus on minimizing the build-up or activity of estrogen in the body with aromatase inhibitors such as Arimidex and Cytadren, or anti-estrogens such as Clomid or Nolvadex, particularly at times when gynecomastia is a worry or the athlete is attempting to increase muscle definition.

We must, however, not be led into thinking that estrogen serves no benefit. It is actually a desirable hormone in many regards. Athletes have known for years that estrogenic steroids are the best mass builders, but it is only recently that we are finally coming to understand the underlying mechanisms why. It appears that reasons go beyond the simple size, weight, and strength increases that one would attribute to estrogen-related water retention, with this hormone actually having a direct effect on the process of anabolism. This is manifest through increases in glucose utilization, growth hormone secretion, and androgen receptor proliferation.

Glucose Utilization and Estrogen

Estrogen may play a very important role in the promotion of an anabolic state by affecting glucose utilization in muscle tissue. This occurs via an altering of the level of available glucose 6-phosphate dehydrogenase, an enzyme directly tied to the use of glucose for muscle tissue growth and recuperation.[27][28] More specifically, G6PD is a vital part of the pentose phosphate pathway, which is integral in determining the rate nucleic acids and lipids are to be synthesized in cells for tissue repair. During the period of regeneration after skeletal muscle damage, levels of G6PD are shown to rise dramatically, which is believed to represent a mechanism for the body to enhance recovery when needed. Surprisingly, we find that estrogen is directly tied to the level of G6PD that is to be made available to cells in this recovery window.

The link between estrogen and G6PD was established in a study demonstrating levels of this dehydrogenase enzyme to rise after administration of testosterone propionate. The investigation further showed that the aromatization of testosterone to estradiol was directly responsible for this increase, and not the androgenic action of this steroid.[29] The non-aromatizable steroids dihydrotestosterone and fluoxymesterone were tested alongside testosterone propionate, but failed to duplicate the effect of testosterone. Furthermore, the positive effect of testosterone propionate was blocked when the aromatase inhibitor 4-hydroxyandrostenedione (formestane) was added, while 17-beta estradiol administration alone caused a similar increase in G6PD to testosterone propionate. The inactive estrogen isomer 17-alpha estradiol, which is unable to bind the estrogen receptor, failed to do anything. Further tests using testosterone propionate and the anti-androgen flutamide showed that this drug also did nothing to block the positive action of testosterone, establishing it as an effect independent of the androgen receptor.

Estrogen and GH/IGF-1

Estrogen may also play an important role in the production of growth hormone and IGF-1. IGF-1 (insulin-like growth factor) is an anabolic hormone released in the liver and various peripheral tissues via the stimulus of growth hormone (See Drug Profiles: Growth Hormone). IGF-1 is responsible for the anabolic activity of growth hormone such as increased nitrogen retention/protein synthesis and cell hyperplasia (proliferation). One of the first studies to bring this issue to our attention looked at the effects of the anti-estrogen tamoxifen on IGF-1 levels, demonstrating it to have a suppressive effect.[30] A second, perhaps more noteworthy, study took place in 1993, which looked at the effects of testosterone replacement therapy on GH and IGF-1 levels alone, and compared them to the effects of testosterone combined again with tamoxifen.[31] When tamoxifen was given, GH and IGF-1 levels were notably suppressed, while both values were elevated with the administration of testosterone enanthate alone. Another study has shown 300 mg of testosterone enanthate weekly to cause a slight IGF-1 increase in normal men. Here the 300 mg of testosterone ester caused an elevation of estradiol levels, which would be expected at such a dose. This was compared to the effect of the same dosage of nandrolone decanoate; however, this steroid failed to produce the same increase. This result is quite interesting, especially when we note that estrogen levels were actually lowered[32] when this steroid was given. Yet another demonstrated that GH and IGF-1 secretion is increased with testosterone administration on males with delayed puberty, while dihydrotestosterone (non-aromatizable) seems to suppress GH and IGF-1 secretion.[33]

Estrogen and the Androgen Receptor

It has also been demonstrated that estrogen can increase the concentration of androgen receptors in certain tissues. This was shown in studies with rats, which looked at the effects of estrogen on cellular androgen receptors in animals that underwent orchiectomy (removal of testes, often done to diminish endogenous androgen production). According to the study, administration of estrogen resulted in a striking 480% increase in methyltrienolone (a potent oral androgen often used to reference receptor binding in studies) binding in the levator ani muscle.[34] The suggested explanation is that estrogen must either be directly stimulating androgen receptor production, or perhaps diminishing the rate of receptor breakdown. Although the growth of the levator ani muscle is commonly used as a reference for the anabolic activity of steroid compounds, it is admittedly a sex organ muscle, and different from skeletal muscle tissue in that it possesses a much higher concentration of androgen receptors. This study, however, did look at the effect of estrogen in fast-twitch skeletal muscle tissues (tibialis anterior and extensor digitorum longus) as well, but did not note the same increase as the levator ani. Although discouraging at first glance, the fact that estrogen can increase androgen receptor binding in any tissue remains an extremely significant finding, especially in light of the fact that we now know androgens to have some positive effects on muscle growth that are mediated outside of muscle tissue.

Estrogen and Fatigue

"Steroid Fatigue" is a common catchphrase these days, and refers to another important function of estrogen in both the male and female body, namely its ability to promote wakefulness and a mentally alert state. Given the common availability of potent third-generation aromatase inhibitors, bodybuilders today are (at times) noticing more extreme estrogen suppression than they had in the past. Often associated with this suppression is fatigue. Under such conditions, the athlete, though on a productive cycle of drugs, may not be able to maximize his or her gains due to an inability to train at full vigor. This effect is sometimes also dubbed "steroid lethargy." The reason is that estrogen plays an important supporting role in the activity of serotonin. Serotonin is one of the body's principle neurotransmitters, vital to mental alertness and the sleep/wake cycle.[35][36] Interference with this neurotransmitter is also associated with chronic fatigue syndrome,[37][38] so we can see how vital it is to fatigue specifically. Estrogen suppression in menopause has also been associated with fatigue,[39] as has the clinical use of newer (more potent) aromatase inhibitors like anastrozole,[40] letrozole,[41] exemestane,[42] and fadrozole[43] in some patients. These things may be important to consider when planning your next cycle. Although not everyone notices this problem when estrogen is low, for those that do, a little testosterone or estrogen can go a long way in correcting this. It is also of note that the use of strictly non-aromatizable steroids sometimes causes this effect as well, likely due to the suppression of natural testosterone production (cutting off the main substrate used by the male body to make estrogen).

Anti-Estrogens and the Athlete

So what does this all mean to the bodybuilder looking to gain optimal size? Basically I think it calls for a cautious approach to the use of estrogen maintenance drugs if mass is the key objective (things change, of course, if we are talking about cutting). Obviously, anti-estrogens should be used if there is a clear need for them due to the onset of estrogenic side effects, or at the very least, the drugs being administered should be substituted for non-estrogenic compounds. Gynecomastia is certainly an unwanted problem for the steroid user, as are noticeable fat mass gains. But if these problems have not presented themselves, the added estrogen due to a cycle of testosterone or Dianabol, for example, might indeed be aiding in the buildup of muscle mass, or keeping you energetic. An individual confident they will notice, or are not prone to getting, estrogenic side effects, may therefore want to hold off using estrogen maintenance drugs so as to achieve the maximum possible gains in tissue mass.

DHT Conversion

As we see from our discussion with estrogen, in considering the physiological effects of any steroid, we must look at all of its active metabolites, and not just the initial compound. This includes not only estrogenic products, but androgenic metabolites as well. With this in mind, it is important to note that the potency of testosterone is considerably increased in many androgen responsive tissues when it converts to dihydrotestosterone. More commonly referred to by the three-letter abbreviation DHT, this hormone is, in fact, measured to be approximately three to four times stronger than testosterone. It is the most potent steroid found naturally in the human body, and important to discuss if we are to understand the full activity of testosterone, as well as other anabolic/androgenic steroids that undergo a similar conversion.

Testosterone is converted to dihydrotestosterone upon interaction with the 5-alpha reductase enzyme. More specifically, this enzyme removes the C4-5 double-bond of testosterone by the addition of two hydrogen atoms to its structure (hence the name di-hydro testosterone). The removal of this bond is important, as in this case it creates a steroid that binds to the androgen receptor much more avidly than its parent steroid. 5-alpha reductase is present in high amounts in tissues of the prostate, skin, scalp, liver, and various regions of the central nervous system, and as such represents a mechanism for the body to increase the potency of testosterone specifically where strong androgenic action is needed. In these areas of the body little testosterone will actually make its way to the receptor without being converted to dihydrotestosterone, making DHT by far the active form of androgen here.

DHT and Androgenic Side Effects

In some regards this local potentiation of testosterone's activity may be unwelcome, as higher androgenic activity in certain tissues may produce a number of undesirable side effects. Acne, for example, is often triggered by dihydrotestosterone activity in the sebaceous glands, and the local formation of dihydrotestosterone in the scalp is typically blamed for triggering male pattern hair loss. You should know that it is a terrible misconception among bodybuilders that dihydrotestosterone is an isolated culprit when it comes to these side effects. All anabolic/androgenic steroids exert their activities, both anabolic and androgenic, through the same cellular androgen receptor. Dihydrotestosterone is no different than any other steroid except that it is a more potent activator of this receptor than most, and can be formed locally in certain androgen-sensitive tissues. All steroids can cause androgenic side effects in direct relation to their affinity for this receptor, and DHT has no known unique ability in this regard.

Benefits of DHT

While a lot of attention is being paid to the negative side effects of the androgen dihydrotestosterone, you should know that there are some known benefits to the strong androgenic activity brought about by this hormone as well. For example, DHT plays an important role in the organization and functioning of the central nervous system. Many neural cells contain active androgen receptors, and it is thought that there may even be a specific importance of dihydrotestosterone in this area of the body. Studies have shown DHT to have a profoundly greater impact in these cells compared to testosterone. More specifically, animal models demonstrated that both testosterone and DHT would result in increased androgen receptor proliferation in neural cells three and seven hours after being administered, however only DHT was able to sustain this increase at the twenty-one hour mark.[44] Although some might contend that this difference is simply due to DHT forming a more stable and lasting complex with the androgen receptor, others suggest that DHT and testosterone might even be affecting neural cells differently, such that the dihydrotestosterone-receptor complex and testosterone-receptor complex might be activating the transcription of different target genes.

The strong interaction between the central nervous system and skeletal muscles, collectively referred to as the neuromuscular system, is of key importance to the athlete. There appears to be little doubt that the ability of the body to adapt to training, and to activate nerve endings in muscle tissue, is reliant on the interactions of the neuromuscular system. Inhibiting the formation of DHT during a testosterone cycle may therefore inadvertently interfere with strength and muscle mass gains. This would explain why bodybuilders commonly report a drop in steroid potency when they add the 5-alpha reductase inhibitor finasteride to a testosterone cycle. Many complain strength and even muscle mass gains slow significantly when this medication is added, which would not make sense if testosterone and androgen receptor activation in muscle tissue were solely responsible for growth. Clearly more is involved, and we cannot look at dihydrotestosterone simply as a side-effect hormone.

Brief History of Anabolic/Androgenic Steroids

While it had been clear for many centuries that the testicles were crucial for the male body to properly develop, it was not until modern times that an understanding of testosterone began to form. The first solid scientific experiments in this area, which eventually led to the discovery and replication of testosterone (and related androgens), were undertaken in the 1800s. During this century a number of animal experiments were published, most of which involved the removal and/or implantation of testicular material from/in a subject. Although very crude in design by today's standards, these studies certainly laid the foundation for the modern field of endocrinology (the study of hormones). By the turn of the century, scientists were able to produce the first experimental androgen injections. These were actualized either through the filtering of large quantities of urine (for active hormones), or by extracting testosterone from animal testicles. Again, the methods were rough but the final results proved to be very enlightening.

Chemists finally synthesized the structure of testosterone in the mid-1930's, sparking a new wave of interest in this hormone. With the medical community paying a tremendous amount of attention to this achievement, the possible therapeutic uses for a readily available synthetic testosterone quickly became an extremely popular focus. Many believed the applications for this type of a medication would be extremely far-reaching, with uses ranging from the maintenance of an androgen deficiency, to that of a good health and well-being treatment for the sickly or elderly. During the infancy of such experimentation, many believed they had crossed paths with a true "fountain of youth."

Dihydrotestosterone and nandrolone, two other naturally occurring steroids, were also isolated and synthesized in the early years of steroid development. To make things even more interesting, scientists soon realized that the androgenic, estrogenic, and anabolic activity of steroid hormones could be adjusted by altering their molecular structure. The goal of many researchers thereafter became to manufacture a steroid with extremely strong anabolic activity, but will display little or no androgenic/estrogenic properties. This could be very beneficial, because side effects will often become pronounced when steroid hormones are administered in supraphysiological amounts. A "pure" anabolic would theoretically allow the patient to receive only the beneficial effects of androgens (lean muscle mass gain, increased energy and recuperation, etc.), regardless of the dosage. Some early success with the creation of new structures convinced many scientists that they were on the right track. Unfortunately none of this progress led researchers their ultimate goal. By the mid-1950's, well over one thousand testosterone, nandrolone, and dihydrotestosterone analogues had been produced, but none proved to be purely anabolic compounds.

The failure to reach this goal was primarily due to an initial flawed understanding of testosterone's action. Scientists had noticed high levels of DHT in certain tissues, and believed this indicated an unusual receptor affinity for this hormone. This led to the belief that the human body had two different androgen receptors. According to this theory, one receptor site would respond only to testosterone (eliciting the beneficial anabolic effects), while the other is activated specifically by the metabolite, dihydrotestosterone. With this understanding, eliminating the conversion of testosterone to DHT was thought capable of solving the problem of androgenic side effects, as these receptors would have little or none of this hormone available for binding. More recently, however, scientists have come to understand that only one type of androgen receptor exists in the human body. It is also accepted that no anabolic/androgenic steroid can possibly be synthesized that would participate only with receptors in tissues related to anabolism. DHT, which was once thought not to bind to the same receptor as testosterone, is now known to do so at approximately three to four times the affinity of its parent, and the unusual recovery of DHT from androgen responsive tissues is now attributed to the distribution characteristics of the 5a-reductase enzyme.

Synthetic AAS Development

In order to develop products that would be effective therapeutically, chemists needed to solve a number of problems with using natural steroid hormones for treatment. For example, oral dosing was a problem, as our basic steroids testosterone, nandrolone, and dihydrotestosterone are ineffective when administered this way. The liver would efficiently break down their structure before reaching circulation, so some form of alteration was required in order for a tablet or capsule to be produced. Our natural steroid hormones also have very short half-lives in the body, so when administered by injection, an extremely frequent and uncomfortable dosing schedule is required if a steady blood level is to be achieved. Therefore, extending steroid activity was a major goal for many chemists during the early years of synthetic AAS development. Scientists also focused on the nagging problems of possible excess estrogenic buildup in the blood, particularly with testosterone, which can become very uncomfortable for patients undergoing therapy.

Methylated Compounds and Oral Dosing

Chemists realized that by replacing the hydrogen atom at the steroid's 17th alpha position with a carbon atom (a process referred to as *alkylation*), its structure would be notably resistant to breakdown by the liver. The carbon atom is typically added in the form of a methyl group (CH3), although we see oral steroids with an added ethyl (C2H5) grouping as well. A steroid with this alteration is commonly described as a C-17 alpha alkylated oral, although the terms methylated or ethylated oral steroid are also used. The alkyl group cannot be removed metabolically, and therefore inhibits reduction of the steroid to its inactive 17-ketosteroid form by occupying one of the necessary carbon bonds. Before long, pharmaceutical companies had utilized this advance (and others) to manufacture an array of effective oral steroids including methyltestosterone, Dianabol, Winstrol®, Anadrol 50®, Halotestin®, Nilevar, Orabolin, and Anavar. The principle drawback to these compounds is that they place a notable amount of stress on the liver, which in some instances can lead to actual damage to this organ.

Because the alkyl group cannot be removed, it mediates the action of the steroid in the body. Methyltestosterone, for example, is not simply an oral equivalent of testosterone, as the added alkylation changes the activity of this steroid considerably. One major change we see is an increased tendency for the steroid to produce estrogenic side effects, despite the fact that it actually lowers the ability of the hormone to interact with aromatase.[45] Apparently with 17-alkylation present on a steroid, aromatization (when possible) produces a more active form of estrogen (typically 17alpha-methyl or 17alpha-ethyl estradiol). These estrogens are more biologically active than estradiol due to their longer half-life and weaker tendency to bind with serum proteins. In some instances, 17alpha-alkylation will also enhance the ability of the initial steroid compound to bind with and activate the estrogen or progesterone receptor.[46] An enhancement of estrogenic properties is also obvious when we look at methandrostenolone, which is an alkylated form of boldenone (Equipoise®), and Nilevar, which is an alkylated form of the mild anabolic nandrolone. Dianabol is clearly more estrogenic than Equipoise®, a drug not noted for producing strong side effects of this nature. The same holds true for the comparison of Nilevar to Deca-Durabolin, a compound that we also know to be extremely mild in this regard.

C17 alpha alkylation also typically lowers the affinity in which the steroid binds to the androgen receptor, as is noted with the weak relative binding affinity of such popular agents as Dianabol and Winstrol (stanozolol). However, since this alteration also greatly prolongs the half-life of a steroid, as well as increases the tendency for it to exist in an unbound state, it creates a more potent anabolic/androgenic agent in both cases. This explains why Dianabol and stanozolol are notably effective in relatively lower weekly doses (often 140 mg weekly will produce notable growth) compared to injectables such as testosterone and nandrolone, which often need to reach doses of 300-400 mg weekly for a similar level of effect.

Non-Alkylated Orals

In an attempt to solve the mentioned problems with liver toxicity we see with c17-alpha alkylated compounds, a number of other orals with different chemical alterations (such as Primobolan®, Proviron®, Andriol̈, and Anabolicum Vister) were created. Primobolan® and Proviron® are alkylated at the one position (methyl), a trait which also slows ketosteroid reduction. Andriol® uses a 17beta carboxylic acid ester (used with injectable compounds, discussed below), however, here the oil-dissolved steroid is sealed in a capsule and is intended for oral administration. This is supposed to promote steroid absorption through intestinal lymphatic ducts, bypassing the first pass through the liver. In addition to 1 methylation, Primobolan® also utilizes a 17 beta ester (acetate) to further protect against reduction to inactive form (here there is no lymphatic system absorption). Anabolicum Vister uses 17beta enol ether linkage to protect the steroid, which is very similar to esterification as the ether breaks off to release a steroid base (boldenone in this case). While all of these types of compounds do not place the same stress on the liver, they are also much less resistant to breakdown than 17 alkylated orals, and are ultimately less active milligram for milligram.

Esters and Injectable Compounds

You may notice that many injectable steroids will list long chemical names like testosterone cypionate and testosterone enanthate, instead of just testosterone. In these cases, the cypionate and enanthate are esters (carboxylic acids) that have been attached to the 17-beta hydroxyl group of the testosterone molecule, which increase the active life span of the steroid preparation. Such alterations will reduce the steroid's level of water solubility, and increase its oil solubility. Once an esterified compound has been injected, it will form a deposit in the muscle tissue (depot) from which it will slowly enter circulation. Generally the larger the ester chain, the more oil soluble the steroid compound will be, and the longer it will take for the full dosage to be released. Once free in circulation, enzymes will quickly remove the ester chain and the parent hormone will be free to exert its activity (while the ester is present the steroid is inert).

There are a wide number of esters, which can provide varying release times, used in medicine today. To compare, an ester like decanoate can extend the release of active parent drug into the blood stream for three to four weeks, while it may only be extended for a few days with an acetate or propionate ester. The use of an ester allows for a much less frequent injection schedule than if using a water-based (straight) testosterone, which is much more comfortable for the patient. We must remember when calculating dosages, that the ester is figured into the steroid's measured weight. 100 mg of testosterone enanthate, therefore, contains much less base hormone than 100 mg of a straight testosterone suspension (in this case it equals 72mg of testosterone). In some instances, an ester may account for roughly 40% or more of the total steroid weight, but the typical measure is somewhere around 15% to 35%. Below are the free base equivalents for several popular steroid compounds.

It is also important to stress the fact that esters do not alter the activity of the parent steroid in any way. They work only to slow its release. It is quite common to hear people speak about the properties of different esters, almost as if they can magically alter a steroid's effectiveness. This is really nonsense. Enanthate is not more powerful than cypionate (perhaps a few extra milligrams of testosterone released per injection, but nothing to note), nor is Sustanon some type of incredible testosterone blend. Personally, I have always considered Sustanon a very poor buy in the face of cheaper 250 mg

100 mg of steroid as:	Approximate Free Equivalent:
Trenbolone acetate	87 mg
Testosterone propionate	83 mg
Testosterone enanthate	72 mg
Testosterone cypionate	70 mg
Testosterone undecanoate	63 mg
Nandrolone phenylpropionate	67 mg
Nandrolone decanoate	64 mg

enanthate ampules. Your muscle cells see only testosterone; ultimately there is no difference. Reports of varying levels of muscle gain, androgenic side effects, water retention, etc. are only issues of timing. Faster-releasing testosterone esters will produce estrogen buildup faster simply because there is more testosterone free in the blood from the start of the cycle. The same is true when we state that Durabolin® is a milder nandrolone for women compared to Deca. It is simply easier to control the blood level with a faster acting drug. Were virilization symptoms to become apparent, hormone levels will drop much faster once we stop administration. This should not be confused with the notion that the nandrolone in Durabolin® acts differently in the body than that released from a shot of Deca-Durabolin®.

It is also worth noting that while the ester is typically hydrolyzed in general circulation, some will be hydrolyzed at the injection site where the steroid depot first contacts blood. This will cause a slightly higher concentration of both free steroid and ester in the muscle where the drug had been administered. On the plus side, this may equate to slightly better growth in this muscle, as more hormone is made available to nearby cells. Many bodybuilders have come to swear by the use of injection sites such as the deltoids, biceps, and triceps, truly believing better growth can be achieved if the steroid is injected directly into these muscles. The negative to this is that the ester itself may be irritating to the tissues at the site of injection once it is broken free. In some instances it can be so caustic that the muscle itself will become swollen and sore due to the presence of the ester, and the user may even suffer a low-grade fever as the body fights off the irritant (the onset of such symptoms typically occurs 24-72 hours after injection). This effect is more common with small chain esters such as propionate and acetate, and can actually make a popular steroid such as Sustanon (which contains testosterone propionate) off-limits for some users who experience too much discomfort to justify using the drug. Longer chain esters such as decanoate and cypionate are typically much less irritating at the site of injection, and therefore are preferred by sensitive individuals.

Anabolic/Androgenic Dissociation

Although never complete, scientists had some success in their quest to separate the androgenic and anabolic properties of testosterone. A number of synthetic anabolic steroids had been developed as a result, with many being notably weaker and stronger than our base androgen. In order to first assess the anabolic and androgenic potential of each newly developed steroid, scientists had generally used rats as a model. To judge androgenic potency the typical procedure involved the post-administration measure (% growth) of the seminal vesicles and ventral prostate. These two tissues will often respond unequally to a given steroid, however, so an average of the two figures is used. Anabolic activity was most commonly determined by measuring the growth of the levator ani, a sex organ (not skeletal) muscle. This tissue may not be the most ideal one to use though, as it contains more androgen receptor than most skeletal muscles (the AR is still less abundant here than in target tissues such as the ventral prostate).[47][48] In integrating both measures, the anabolic index is used, which relates the ratio of anabolic to androgenic response for a given steroid. An anabolic index greater than one indicates a higher tendency for anabolic effect, and therefore classifies the drug as an anabolic steroid. A measure lower than one in turn assesses the steroid as androgenic. There is some variance between experimental results and the actual real world experiences with humans, but (with a few exceptions) designations based on the anabolic index are generally accepted. Below are discussed a few factors that greatly affect anabolic/androgenic dissociation.

Nandrolone and 19-norandrogens

The section of this book dealing with DHT conversion is important, because it helps us understand the anabolic steroid nandrolone and many of its derivatives. Nandrolone is identical to testosterone except it lacks a carbon atom in the 19th position, hence its other given name 19-nortestosterone. Nandrolone is very interesting because it offers the greatest ratio of anabolic to androgenic effect of the three natural steroids (see: Synthetic AAS Chemistry). This is because it is metabolized into a less potent structure (dihydronandrolone) in androgen target tissues with high concentrations of the 5-alpha reductase enzyme, which is the exact opposite of what happens with testosterone. Apparently the removal of the c4-5 double bond, which normally increases the androgen receptor binding capability of testosterone, causes an unusual lowering of this ability with nandrolone. Instead of becoming three to four times more potent, it becomes several times weaker. This is a very desirable trait if you want to target anabolic effects over androgenic. This characteristic also carries over to most synthetic steroids derived from nandrolone, making this an attractive base steroid to use in the synthesis of new, primarily anabolic, steroids.

5-alpha Irreducible Steroids

When we look at the other mild anabolic steroids Primobolan®, Winstrol®, and Anavar, none of which are derived from nandrolone, we see another interesting commonality. These steroids are DHT derivatives that are unaffected by 5alpha-reductase, and therefore become neither weaker nor stronger in androgen responsive target tissues with high concentrations of this enzyme. In essence, they have a very balanced effect between muscle and androgen tissues, making them outwardly less androgenic than testosterone. This is why these steroids are technically classified as anabolics, and are undeniably less troublesome than many other steroids in terms of promoting androgenic side effects. However, if we wanted to look for the absolute least androgenic steroid, the title would still go to nandrolone (or perhaps one of its derivatives). Female bodybuilders should likewise take note that despite the recommendations of others, steroids like Anavar, Winstrol and Primo are not the least risky steroids to use. This is of great importance, as male sex hormones can produce many undesirable and permanent side effects when incorrectly taken by females (See: Side Effects, Virilization).

3-alpha Hydroxysteroid Dehydrogenase

The 3-alpha hydroxysteroid dehydrogenase enzyme is also important, because it can work to reduce the anabolic potency of certain steroids considerably. As follows, not all potent binders of the androgen receptor are, as a rule, great muscle-building drugs, and this enzyme is an important factor. Dihydrotestosterone is a clear example. Just as the body converts testosterone to DHT as a way to potentiate its action in certain tissues (skin, scalp, prostate, etc.), it also has ways of countering the strong activity of DHT, in other tissues where it is unneeded. This is accomplished by the rapid reduction of DHT to its inactive active metabolites, namely androstanediol, before it reaches the androgen receptor. This activity occurs via interaction with the 3-alpha hydroxysteroid dehydrogenase enzyme. This enzyme is present in high concentrations in certain tissues, including skeletal muscle, and DHT is much more open to alteration by it than other steroids that possess a c4-5 double-bond (like testosterone).[49] This causes dihydrotestosterone to be an extremely poor anabolic, despite the fact that it actually exhibits a much higher affinity for the cellular androgen receptor than most other steroids. Were it able to reach the cellular androgen receptor without first being metabolized by 3a-HSD, it certainly would be a formidable muscle-building steroid. Unfortunately this is not the case, explaining why injectable dihydrotestosterone preparations (no longer commercially produced) were never favorite drugs among athletes looking to build mass. This trait is also shared by the currently popular oral androgen Proviron®, which is, in essence, just an oral form of DHT (1-methyl dihydrotestosterone to be specific) and known to be an extremely poor tissue builder.

Anabolics and Potency

One must remember that being classified as an anabolic just means that the steroid is more inclined to produce muscle growth than androgenic side effects. Since both effects are mediated through the same receptor, and growth is not produced by androgen receptor activation in muscle tissue alone (other CNS tissues, for example, are integral to this process as well), we find that a reduction in the androgenic activity of a compound will often coincide with a similar lowering of its muscle-building effectiveness. If we are just looking at overall muscle growth, androgenic steroids (usually potent due to their displaying a high affinity to bind with the androgen receptor in all tissues) are typically much more productive muscle-builders than anabolics, which usually bind with

Compound	Human SHBG	Rabbit Muscle	Rat Muscle	Rat Prostate	Ratio M vs. P
methyltrienolone	<.01	1	1	1	1
dihydrotestosterone	1	.07	<.01	.46	.03
mesterolone	4.4	.21	.08	.25	.32
testosterone	.19	.07	.23	.15	1.53
nandrolone	.01	.20	.24	.60	.4
methyltestosterone	.05	.1	.11	.13	.85
methenolone	.03	.09	.24	.14	1.67
stanozolol	.01	.03	.02	.03	.6
methandrostenolone	.02	.02	.02	.03	.75
fluoxymesterone	<.01	.02	.01	.02	.77
oxymetholone	<.01	<.01	<.01	<.01	1.54
ethylestrenol	<.01	.01	<.01	<.01	2

RBA of various anabolic/androgenic steroids as competitors for human SHBG binding of DHT, and for receptor binding of methyltrienolone in cytosol from rabbit, rat skeletal muscle and prostate. Source: Endocrinology 114(6):2100-06 1984 June, "Relative Binding Affinity of Anabolic-Androgenic Steroids...", Saartok T; Dahlberg E; Gustafsson JA.

lower affinity in many tissues. In fact, with all of the analogues produced throughout the years, the base androgen testosterone is still considered to be one of the most effective bulking agents. The user must simply endure more side effects when acquiring his or her new muscle with this type of drug. Individuals wishing to avoid the stronger steroids will, therefore, make a trade-off, accepting less overall muscle gain in order to run a more comfortable cycle.

RBA Assay:

Another way of evaluating the potential ratio of anabolic to androgenic activity is the practice of comparing the relative binding affinity (RBA) of various steroids for the androgen receptor in rat skeletal muscle versus prostate. When we look at the detailed study published in 1984, we see some recognizable (and expected) trends. Aside from dihydrotestosterone and Proviron® (mesterolone), which undergo rapid enzymatic reduction in muscle tissue to inactive metabolites, the remaining anabolic/androgenic steroids seem to bind with near equal affinity to receptors in both tissues. They seem to be relatively "balanced" in effect. This study also discusses the unique activity of testosterone and nandrolone compounds, which are good substrates for the 5a-reductase enzyme found in androgen target tissues (such as the prostate), and seem to provide the most notable variance between anabolic and androgenic effect in humans due to this local metabolism. When it comes to real-world use in humans, anabolic steroids do not always behave in 100% uniformity with their anabolic and androgenic profiles as determined by animal models, so all such figures need to be taken with a small grain of salt.

Synthetic AAS Chemistry

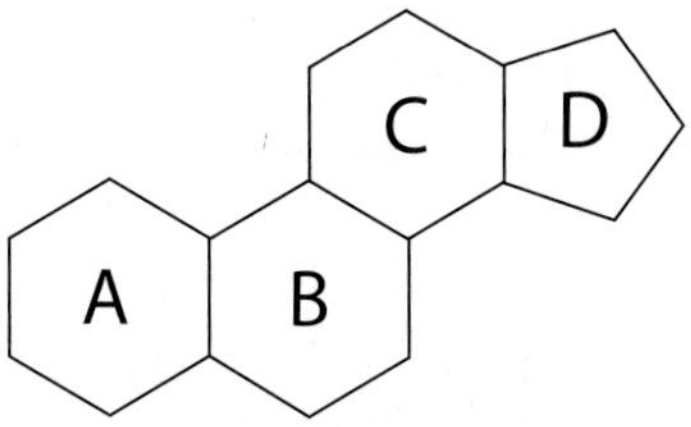

Steran Nucleus
(All natural and synthetic AAS hormones share this base structure)

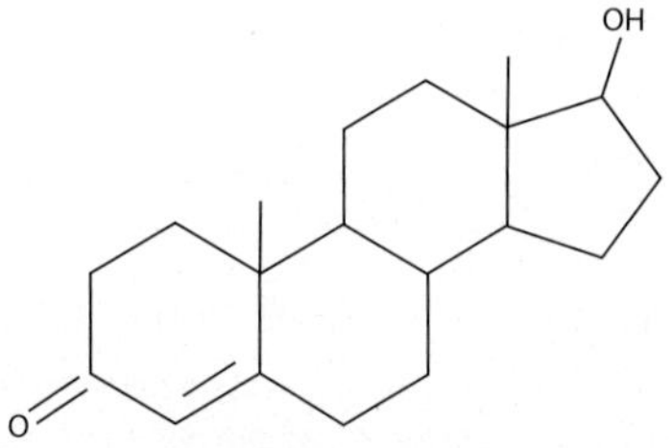

Testosterone

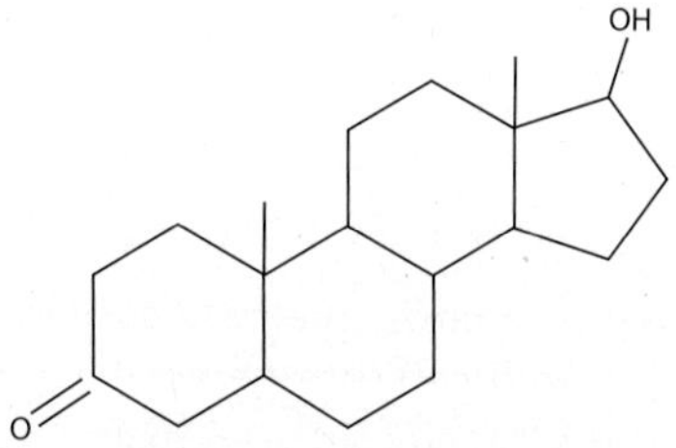

Dihydrotestosterone

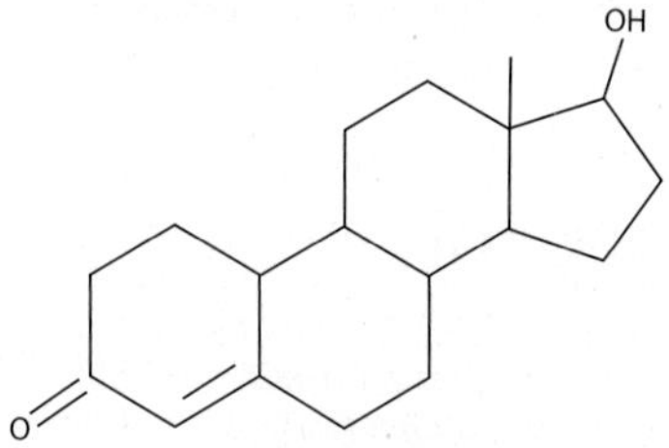

Nandrolone

All anabolic/androgenic steroids are preparations containing one of the above three natural steroid hormones, or chemically altered derivatives thereof. In creating new synthetic compounds, one of the three natural hormones is selected as a starting point, typically due to the possession of particular traits that may be beneficial for the new compound. For instance, of the three natural steroids above, dihydrotestosterone is the only steroid devoid of the possibility of aromatization and 5-alpha reduction. It was likewise a very popular choice in the creation of synthetics that lack estrogenic activity and/or exhibit a more balanced androgenic to anabolic activity ratio. Nandrolone was typically used when even lower androgenic action is desired, due to its weakening upon interaction with the 5-alpha reductase enzyme. Nandrolone also aromatizes much more slowly than testosterone. Testosterone is our most powerful muscle-building hormone, and also exhibits strong androgenic activity due to its conversion to a more potent steroid (dihydrotestosterone) via 5-alpha reductase.

Testosterone derivatives

Boldenone (+c1-2 double bond)

Boldenone is testosterone with an added double-bond between carbon atoms one and two. However, this bond changes the activity of the steroid considerably. First, it dramatically slows aromatization, such that boldenone converts to estradiol at about half the rate of testosterone. Secondly, this bond causes the steroid to be a very poor substrate for the 5-alpha reductase enzyme. The more active 5-alpha reduced metabolite 5alpha-dihydroboldenone is produced only in very small amounts in humans. The hormone instead tends to convert via 5-beta reductase to 5beta-dihydroboldenone (a virtually inactive androgen). This makes it lean towards being an anabolic instead of an androgen, although both traits are still notably apparent with this steroid. The c1-2 double bond also slows the hepatic breakdown of the structure, increasing its resistance to 17-ketosteroid deactivation and its functional half-life and oral bioavailability.

Methyltestosterone (+ 17alpha methyl)

This is the most basic derivative of testosterone, differing only by the added 17-alpha methylation that makes the steroid orally active. Conversion to 17-alpha methylestradiol makes this steroid extremely estrogenic, despite the fact that this alteration actually reduces interaction with the aromatase enzyme.

Methandrostenolone (+c 1-2 double bond; 17-alpha methyl)

In many regards, methandrostenolone is very similar to boldenone, as it too exhibits reduced estrogenic and androgenic activity due to the c1-2 double-bond. However, this steroid does have a reputation of being somewhat estrogenic, owing to the fact that it converts to a highly active form of estrogen (17alpha-methylestradiol See: Methylated Compounds and Oral Dosing). Methandrostenolone is also much more active milligram for milligram, as the 17-alpha methyl group also gives it a longer half-life and allows it to exist in a more free state than its cousin boldenone.

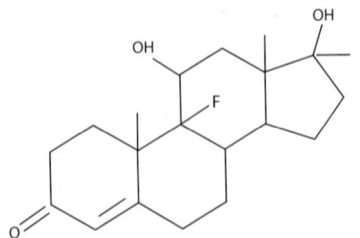

Fluoxymesterone (+11-beta hydroxyl; 9-fluoro; 17-alpha methyl)

Halotestin is a c-17alpha alkylated oral derivative of testosterone. The 11-beta group functions to inhibit aromatization, so there is no estrogen conversion at all with this steroid. It also works to lower the affinity of this steroid toward restrictive serum binding proteins. I have no specific explanation for the function of the 9-fluoro group at this time, however, I can say that it neither blocks aromatization nor 5-alpha reduction. This is supported by the fact that other 9-fluoro steroids have been shown to aromatize, as well as studies showing fluoxymesterone to be an active substrate for the 5-alpha reductase enzyme.

Nandrolone derivatives

Norethandrolone
(+ 17-alpha ethyl)

Norethandrolone is simply nandrolone with an added 17-alpha ethyl group. This alteration is rarely used with anabolic/androgenic steroids, and is much more commonly found with synthetic estrogens and progestins. Although 17-ethylation inhibits 17-ketosteroid reduction just as well as 17-methylation, and therefore allows this steroid to exhibit a similarly high level of oral activity, this group also tends to increase progesterone receptor binding. Norethandrolone is clearly a "troublesome" hormone in terms of water retention, fat gain, and gynecomastia, which may in part be due to its heightened binding to this receptor.

Ethylestrenol
(+17alpha-ethyl; - 3-Keto)

Ethylestrenol is an oral derivative of nandrolone, very similar in structure to norethandrolone. In fact, it differs from this steroid only by the removal of the 3-keto group, which is vital to androgen receptor binding. As such, ethylestrenol is possibly the weakest steroid milligram for milligram ever sold commercially. Any activity this steroid does exhibit is likely from its conversion to norethandrolone, which does seem to occur with some affinity (apparently the 3 oxygen group is metabolically added to this compound without much trouble). This is probably the most interesting trait of ethylestrenol, which is an undistinguished compound otherwise.

Trenbolone
(+ c9-10 double bond; c11-12 double bond)

Although a derivative of nandrolone, the two additional double-bonds present on trenbolone make any similarities to its parent hormone extremely difficult to see. First, the 9-10 bond inhibits aromatization. Nandrolone is very slowly aromatized, however, some estrogen is still produced from this steroid. Not so with trenbolone. The 11-12 bond additionally increases androgen receptor binding. This steroid also does not undergo 5-alpha reduction like nandrolone, and as such does not share the same dissociation between anabolic and androgenic effects (trenbolone is much more androgenic in comparison).

Dihydrotestosterone derivatives

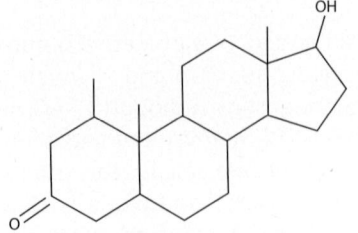

Mesterolone (+ 1-methyl)

Mesterolone is a potent orally active derivative of dihydrotestosterone. Similar to methenolone, it possesses a non-toxic 1-methyl group, which increases its resistance to hepatic breakdown. This alteration does not increase the stability of the 3-keto group however, and as such, this steroid is a poor anabolic like its parent.

Drostanolone (+ 2-methyl)

Drostanolone is simply dihydrotestosterone with an added 2-methyl group. This addition greatly increases the stability of the 3-keto group, vital to androgen binding. As such, the activity of this steroid in muscle tissue is greatly enhanced (see: Anabolic/Androgenic Dissociation).

Oxymetholone (+2 hydroxymethylene; 17alpha-methyl)

Oxymetholone is an orally active derivative of dihydrotestosterone. The 17-methyl group is well understood at this point as we have discussed it with many steroids, however, the 2-hydroxymethylene group is not seen on any other commercial steroid. We do know that this group greatly enhances anabolic potency by increasing the stability of the 3-keto group, and that the configuration of this substituent also appears to allow this steroid to bind and activate the estrogen receptor.

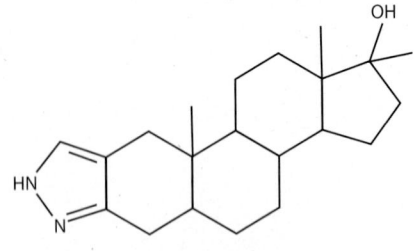

Stanozolol (+ 3,2 pyrazol; 17-alpha methyl)

Stanozolol is a potent anabolic steroid, owing to the fact that the 3-2 pyrazol group creates a stable configuration off the A-ring that allows for androgen receptor binding (this steroid is one of the few that does not possess an actual 3-keto group). As such, it is highly active in muscle tissue, unlike dihydrotestosterone.

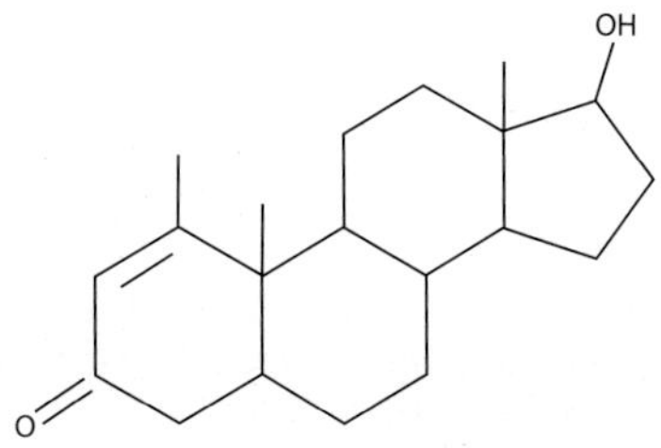

Methenolone
(+ 1-methyl; 1-2 double bond)

Methenolone also is a potent anabolic steroid, due to the fact that the c1-2 double bond increases the stability of the 3-keto group. The 1-methyl group works to increase its oral bioavailability, making methenolone (as methenolone acetate) one of the few orally active non-17-alkylated orals. The c 1-2 bond may also help increase hepatic resistance (slightly) to 17-ketosteroid deactivation as well.

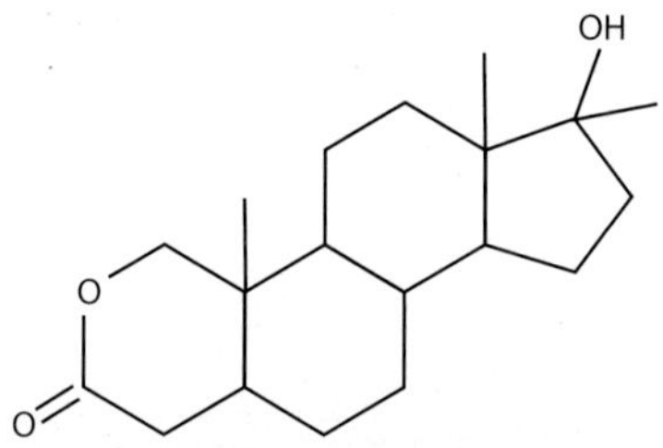

Oxandrolone
(2-oxygen substitution;
17-alpha methyl)

Oxandrolone is an orally active derivative of dihydrotestosterone, due to its 17-methylation. It also differs from DHT by the substitution of its 2-carbon molecule with oxygen. This is the only commercial steroid to carry this group, and further, the only to have a modification to the base carbon structure of the Steran nucleus. The 2-oxo group increases resistance of the 3-keto group to metabolism considerably, making oxandrolone a potent anabolic.

Steroid Nomenclature

Perhaps not obvious at first glance, there is a naming convention in place that was used to create identities for the various anabolic/androgenic steroid hormones. This typically involves forming a root word to convey the structural base of the steroid, and signifying other unique structural characteristics by including appropriate prefixes or suffixes. Below, we will look at the common roots, prefixes, and suffixes used in steroid nomenclature, and identify them, as they are used in the various commercial compound names. As you will see, the adoption of names like nandrolone, methandrostenolone, and ethylestrenol were not as arbitrary as one might imagine. This section is also helpful if you wish to understand the deeper chemical designations for the various substances that one might find in the medical literature, which involve the exclusive use of this terminology (such as is the representation of methandrostenolone as 17b-hydroxy-17a-methylandrosta-1,4-dien-3-one).

Common prefixes and suffixes used in steroid naming:

Structural Property	Prefix	Suffix
Carbonyl (C=O)	oxo-; keto-	-one
Hydroxyl	hydroxy-	-ol
Double Bnd (C=C)		-ene; -en
Methyl	meth-; methyl-	
Ethyl	eth-; ethyl-	

Common roots used in steroid naming:

Androstane	Base carbon structure of dihydrotestosterone (no double-bond)
Androstene	Base carbon structure of or similar to testosterone (one double-bond)
Androstadiene	Base carbon structure similar to methandrostenolone (two double-bonds; di-ene)
Estren; Estra *also: Norandrostene*	Base structure of nandrolone (19-norandrostene) and estrogen

Common Commercial Compound Names:

Name	Taken From	Incorporated Into Name As
Boldenone	[17b-ol, androstadiene, 3-one]	BOL DEN ONE
Ethylestrenol	[17a ethyl, estren, 17b-ol]	ETHYL ESTREN OL
Fluoxymesterone	[9-fluoro, 11b-hydroxyl, 17a-methyl, testosterone, 3-one]	FLU OXY ME STER ONE
Mesterolone	[1-methyl, dihydrotestosterone, 17b-ol, 3-one]	ME STER OL ONE
Methandienone	[17a-methyl, androstadiene, 3-one]	METH ANDIEN ONE
Methandrostenolone	[17a-methyl, androstadiene, 17b-ol, 3-one]	METH ANDROSTEN OL ONE
Methenolone	[1-methyl, c1-2 double bond (en), 17b-ol, 3-one]	METH EN OL ONE
Nandrolone	[norandrostene, 17b-ol, 3-one]	NANDR OL ONE
Norethandrolone	[19-nor, 17a-ethyl, (nor)androstene, 17b-ol, 3-one]	NOR ETH ANDR OL ONE
Oxandrolone	[2-oxy, androstane, 17b-ol, 2-one]	OX ANDR OL ONE
Oxymetholone	[2-hydroxymethylene, 17a-Methyl, 17b-ol, 3-one]	OXY METH OL ONE
Stanozolol	[Stanolone (androstanolone, DHT), 2-pyrazol, 17b-ol]	STANO ZOL OL
Trenbolone	[tri-en, 17b-ol, 3-one]	TREN BOL ONE

Clinical Applications

Anabolic/androgenic steroids are approved for sale by prescription in virtually every pharmaceutical market around the world. Having been applied for many decades to treat a variety of diseased states, today these drugs have a number of well-established medical uses. They have been used to treat most patient populations, including men and women of almost all ages, ranging from children to the elderly. In many instances anabolic/androgenic steroids have proven to be life saving medications, which is a fact easily overlooked with all of the discussion about steroid abuse. This section details some of the most common and accepted medical applications for anabolic/androgenic steroids.

Androgen Replacement Therapy/Hypogonadism

The most widely used medical application for anabolic/androgenic steroids in the world is that of androgen replacement therapy. Also referred to as Hormone Replacement Therapy (HRT) or Testosterone Replacement Therapy (TRT), this therapy involves the supplementation of the primary male hormone testosterone to alleviate symptoms of low hormone levels (clinically referred to as hypogonadism). Patients may be adolescent males suffering from childhood hypogonadism or a specific disorder that causes androgenic hormone disruption, although most of the treated population consists of adult men over the age of 30. In most cases hormone levels have declined in these men as a result of the normal aging process.

The most common complaints associated with low testosterone in adult men include reduced libido, erectile dysfunction, loss of energy, decreased strength and/or endurance, reduced ability to play sports, mood fluctuations, reduced height (bone loss), reduced work performance, memory loss, and muscle loss.[50] When associated with aging, these symptoms are collectively placed under the label of "andropause". In a clinical setting this disorder is referred to as late-onset hypogonadism. Blood testosterone levels below 350ng/dL are usually regarded as clinically significant, although some physicians will use a level as low as 200ng/dL as the threshold for normal. Hypogonadism is, unfortunately, still widely under-diagnosed. Most physicians will also not recommend treatment for low testosterone unless a patient is complaining about symptoms (symptomatic androgen deficiency).

Androgen replacement therapy effectively alleviates most symptoms of low testosterone levels. To begin with, raising testosterone levels above 350ng/dL (the very low end of the normal range) will often restore normal sexual function and libido in men with dysfunctions related to hormone insufficiency. With regard to bone mineral density, hormone replacement therapy is also documented to have a significant positive effect. For example, studies administering 250 mg of testosterone enanthate every 21 days showed a 5% increase in bone mineral density after six months.[51] Over time this may prevent some loss of height and bone strength with aging, and may also reduce the risk of fracture. Hormone replacement therapy also increases red blood cell concentrations (oxygen carrying capacity), improving energy and sense of well-being. Therapy also supports the retention of lean body mass, and improves muscle strength and endurance.

Unlike steroid abuse, hormone replacement therapy in older men may also have benefits with regard to cardiovascular disease risk. For example, studies tend to show hormone replacement as having a positive effect on serum lipids. This includes a reduction in LDL and total cholesterol levels, combined with no significant change in HDL (good) cholesterol levels.[52,53] Testosterone supplementation also reduces midsection obesity, and improves insulin sensitivity and glycemic control.[54] These are important factors in metabolic syndrome, which may also be involved in the progression of atherosclerosis. Additionally, testosterone replacement therapy has been shown to improve the profile of inflammatory markers TNF·, IL-1,, and IL-10.[55] The reduced inflammation may help protect arterial walls from degeneration by plaque and scar tissue. The medical consensus today appears to be that replacement therapy generally does not have a negative effect on cardiovascular disease risk, and may actually decrease certain risk factors for the disease in some patients.

In addition to the normal list of potential side effects, there are a few areas of caution with elderly patients. To begin with, testosterone administration may increase prostate volume and PSA values.[56,57] While this does not appear to be of clinical significance with normal healthy patients, benign prostate hypertrophy and prostate cancer can be stimulated by testosterone. Men with prostate cancer, high PSA values, or breast cancer are generally not prescribed testosterone. Androgen supplementation has also been linked to sleep apnea, which can interfere with the most restful (REM) phase of sleep.[58] The studies have produced conflicting data, however, and the potential relationship remains the subject of much debate.[59] Lastly, testosterone replacement therapy has demonstrated negative, positive, and neutral effects on cognitive functioning in elderly men.[60][61][62] Studies do suggest that the dose can dictate the level of response, with the most positive effects noted when the androgen level reaches the mid- to upper-range of normal, not supraphysiological.[63] Elderly patients with preexisting deficits in cognitive function should have their cognitive performance and blood hormone levels monitored closely during hormone replacement therapy.

Common Treatment Protocols:

Transdermal: Transdermal application is the most commonly prescribed method for supplementing testosterone in the United States and Canada, and is generally the first course of therapy initiated with androgen replacement therapy patients. This method of drug delivery offers a number of advantages to the patient when compared to injection. Since the transdermal application is painless, patient compliance and comfort is increased in comparison. Transdermal application also provides stable day-to-day hormone levels, and does not produce the broad fluctuations usually noticed with injectable testosterone esters. The most common protocol among hormone replacement doctors is to prescribe a dosage of 2.5-10 mg of testosterone per day (approximate absorbed dose). This is applied as a rub-on gel or adhesive transdermal patch that is replaced daily. Note that due to metabolism in the skin, transdermal application of testosterone tends to increase serum dihydrotestosterone (DHT) levels more profoundly than testosterone injection. This may exacerbate androgenic side effects during therapy in some patients, causing some to seek out injectable forms of testosterone as an alternative.

Injection: Testosterone enanthate and testosterone cypionate are the most widely prescribed injectable testosterone drugs in the United States and Canada. In many other markets the blended ester products Sustanon 100 and Sustanon 250 are also commonly prescribed. Injection of one of these testosterone ester products will provide the patient supplemental androgen levels for approximately 2 to 3 weeks after each application. The most common protocol among hormone replacement doctors is to administer 200 mg of testosterone enanthate or cypionate once every 2 to 3 weeks. It is important to remember that testosterone esters will deliver varying levels of testosterone to the body on a day-to-day basis throughout each application window. Levels will be highest the first several days after injection, and will slowly decline to baseline over the following weeks. Physicians are usually encouraged to monitor their patients closely to ensure androgen supplementation is sustaining hormone levels within the normal range (and alleviating symptoms of hypogonadism) throughout the entire therapeutic period. The longer acting injectable testosterone preparation Nebido (testosterone undecanoate) is undergoing review in the U.S., and has already been approved in other markets. This drug requires only 4 to 5 injections per year for most patients.

Oral: Testosterone undecanoate (Andriol) is the only prescription medication that delivers testosterone via an oral capsule. This medication is not approved for sale in the United States, but is a prescription drug in Canada and many other markets around the world. Patient compliance and comfort are high with this form of therapy, as there are no special routines or requirements aside from taking a few capsules each day with meals. Oral testosterone undecanoate is usually given at an initial dosage of 120 to 160 mg per day, which equates to three to four 40 mg capsules. This dosage may be reduced in subsequent weeks to 120 mg per day. The capsules are given in two divided doses per day, which are usually taken with breakfast and dinner. While this form of therapy is highly convenient, serum hormone levels can fluctuate greatly on a day-to-day basis. The amount of fat consumption has a particularly strong impact on hormone bioavailability, and meals providing at least 20 grams of fat are recommended when taking the capsules for maximum absorption. Note that as with transdermal testosterone, oral testosterone undecanoate tends to increase serum dihydrotestosterone (DHT) levels more profoundly than testosterone injections.

Angioedema, Hereditary

Anabolic steroids are commonly prescribed for the treatment of hereditary angioedema, a rare and potentially life-threatening disorder of the immune system. Hereditary angioedema is caused by genetic mutations of blood clotting factors, characterized by a decrease in the level or functioning of the protein C1 esterase inhibitor. This protein controls C1, which is a "complement system" protein that plays an important role in the control of inflammation. Symptoms of hereditary angioedema include an intermittent but rapid swelling of the hands, arms, legs, lips, eyes, tongue, or throat. Swelling may also be noticed in the digestive tract, resulting in abdominal cramping, nausea, or vomiting. In the most serious cases, the patient may notice a swelling of the throat and a blockage of the airway passages, resulting in asphyxiation and sydden death. Many attacks occur without a specific trigger, although stress, trauma, surgery, and dental work are commonly associated with angioedema attacks.

Oral c-17 alpha alkylated anabolic/androgenic steroids have been shown to be a useful form of preventive therapy, stabilizing complement system protein levels and reducing the frequency and severity of angioedema attacks.[64] They are usually administered in a low dose, which is to be taken for long-term support of this disorder. The anabolic steroids that have been most commonly used in the United States for this purpose are stanozolol and danocrine, although historically many other agents have also been prescribed including oxandrolone, methyltestosterone, oxymetholone, fluoxymesterone, and methandrostenolone. The amount of steroid needed can vary depending on the individual, and is usually maintained at the lowest therapeutically effective dosage in an effort to offset undesirable side effects. FDA approved prescribing guidelines for stanozolol recommended an initial dosage of 2 mg three times daily (6 mg per day). This would be slowly adjusted downward to a maintenance level after a positive response was noted, usually to 2 mg given once every 1 to 2 days.

Anemia

As a class of drugs, anabolic/androgenic steroids stimulate the synthesis of erythropoietin in the kidneys, a hormone that supports the manufacture of new red blood cells. By doing this, the administration of steroids tends to increase the red cell count and hematocrit level, making them of tangible therapeutic value for treating certain forms of anemia (a disease characterized by insufficient red blood cell production). Forms of anemia likely to respond to steroid therapy include anemias caused by renal insufficiency, sickle cell anemia, refractory anemias including aplastic anemia, myelofibrosis, myelosclerosis, agnogenic myeloid metaplasia, and anemias caused by malignancy or myelotoxic drugs. The level of response will vary depending on the patient, type of therapy, and form of anemia, but in many cases the management of a normal hematocrit level can be achieved.

In the United States, both oxymetholone (Anadrol 50) and nandrolone decanoate (Deca-Durabolin) are approved by the FDA for the treatment of severe anemia. The guidelines for using oxymetholone with both male and female anemic patients (children and adults) recommend a dosage of 1-2 mg/kg/per day. This would equate to a daily dosage of 75-150 mg for an individual weighing about 160 lbs. Doses as high as 5 mg/kg/day are sometimes necessary to achieve the desired therapeutic response. The guidelines for nandrolone decanoate recommend a dosage of 50-100 mg per week for women and 100-200 mg per week for men. Children (2 to 13 years of age) are recommended a dosage of 25- 50 mg every 3 to 4 weeks.

In recent years, the advent of recombinant erythropoietin as a prescription drug has changed the face of anemia treatment considerably. While anabolic/androgenic steroids still offer therapeutic value here, and are still marketed and sold to treat anemic patients, they are presently regarded as adjunct or fallback medications for use only when therapy with an erythropoietin alone has failed to achieve a desired response. The hematocrit increase from anabolic/androgenic steroids is generally less predictable and positive than the newer erythropoietins, and these drugs also tend to produce very noticeable side effects when given in the levels necessary to stimulate erythropoiesis, especially in women and children. In many instances the risks to therapy strongly outweigh the benefits of anabolic/androgenic steroids, given that there are newer and directly targeted medications available with much lower side effect potential.

Breast Cancer

Anabolic/androgenic steroids are sometimes prescribed to treat beast cancer in postmenopausal women or premenopausal women who have had their ovaries removed. These drugs are of value when the cancer is hormone responsive, which means that its growth can be affected (positively or negatively) by hormonal manipulation. Androgens and estrogens have opposing actions on hormone-responsive tumors, with estrogens supporting the growth of breast cancer tissue and androgens inhibiting it[65]. The supplementation of an anabolic/androgenic steroid can shift the androgen to estrogen balance in a direction that favors a reduction in tumor size, a therapy that has elicited a successful response in a fair number of patients. The masculinizing side effects of steroid therapy can be very pronounced in women, however, so therapy is usually initiated with great caution. An oral androgen such as fluoxymesterone is usually preferred to a slower acting injectable steroid such as nandrolone decanoate as well, as it can be abruptly halted if undesirable side effects become too apparent. Both primarily anabolic agents, however, have been widely prescribed for this purpose.

In recent years the development of newer and more targeted anti-estrogenic drugs such as selective estrogen receptor modulators (SERMs) and aromatase inhibiting drugs have almost completely eliminated the use of anabolic/androgenic steroids for breast cancer treatment. Medicative treatment for breast cancer today usually consists of a SERM like Nolvadex (tamoxifen), which may be used with a strong aromatase inhibitor such as Arimidex (anastrozole) or Femara (exemestane).

Anabolic/androgenic steroids are still made available in the United States and many other nations for treating breast cancer, and are sometimes still applied. They are very much regarded as adjunct or fallback medications, however, for use only when therapy with anti-estrogenic drugs alone has failed to achieve a desired response.

Decreased Fibrinolytic Activity

Anabolic steroids may be prescribed to treat conditions associated with decreased fibrinolytic activity. Fibrinolysis is the process in which a blood clot is broken down and metabolized by the body. It represents a counter to blood coagulation, with the two systems working together to maintain the hemostatic balance. Disorders of the fibrinolytic system are rare, although can be very serious in nature when they do occur. Decreased fibrinolytic activity can result in a shift in blood clotting factors that greatly favor coagulation (hypercoagulability), increasing the risk of a serious cardiovascular event such as thromboembolism, heart attack, or stroke. Oral C-17 alpha alkylated anabolic steroids are recognized to increase fibrinolytic activity, and as a result have been beneficial in many patients suffering from decreased fibrinolytic activity linked to Antithrombin III deficiency or fibrinogen excess.[66][67] Stanozolol has been most commonly used in the United States for this treatment, although similar therapeutic benefits can be seen with many other anabolic steroids. The maintenance dose is tailored to the individual, and is determined with close monitoring of both side effects and changes to blood coagulation parameters. Esterified injectables and oral non-alkylated steroids do not produce the same fibrinolytic response.[68]

Infertility (Male)

In a small percentage of cases, anabolic/androgenic steroids may be prescribed for the treatment of male infertility. When the cause of infertility is low sperm concentration due to Leydig-cell secretion deficiencies, an androgen might be able to alleviate the condition. In such cases the steroid may increase the sperm count, sperm quality and the fructose concentration,[69][70] which can increase the chance of conception. The oral androgen mesterolone (Proviron) is most commonly prescribed for this purpose, although has not been granted FDA approval for sale in the United States. Note that anabolic/androgenic steroids usually reduce male fertility, so the potential for these agents to successfully treat male fertility is limited.

Growth Failure

Anabolic steroids may be prescribed to treat growth failure in children, both with and without growth hormone deficiency. These agents have been shown to have positive effects on both muscle and bone mass. When they are administered before the ends of the long bones (epiphysis) have fused and further linear growth has been halted, their anabolic effects on bone may support an increase in height.[71] This can occur both through direct anabolic action of the steroid on bone cells, and indirectly via the stimulation of growth hormone and IGF-1 release.[72] An anabolic steroid that is non-aromatizable and non-estrogenic is typically used for this purpose, as estrogen is known to cause an acceleration of growth arrest. Anabolic steroid therapy must always be used with caution in pediatric patients, however. In addition to the possibility of common adverse effects, even non-aromatizable steroids may accelerate the rate of epiphysis closure.[73]

In the United States, oxandrolone is the anabolic steroid most widely prescribed for the treatment of growth failure. It is usually given as a supportive medication, used to augment the anabolic effects of human growth hormone therapy. The drug is typically taken for periods of 6-12 months at a time, in an effort to accelerate the growth rate without substantially affecting the rate of epiphysis fusion. A dosage of 2.5 mg per day is often used for this purpose, although this may be adjusted upwards or downwards depending on the patient's sex, age, bodyweight, and sensitivity to adverse effects. When used under optimal conditions, the result may be an enhancement of the growth rate and an increase in total height compared to not initiating therapy. This benefit has been difficult to achieve consistently in clinical studies, however. A number of trials with oxandrolone have failed to produce a statistically significant effect on total height, questioning its ultimate value.[74] The short-term benefits of anabolic steroids on the growth rate, however, remain well supported.

Libido (Female)

The steroid methyltestosterone is approved for prescription sale in the United States and many other markets to improve libido in female menopause patients. Small doses of the drug are typically included in products that also supplement estrogens, the combination aimed at treating the full spectrum of menopause symptoms, including reduced female libido. The dosage used is low compared to those of other clinical applications for methyltestosterone, and will usually amount to no more than 2mg per day.

Osteoporosis

Anabolic steroids increase bone mineral density, and may be prescribed for the treatment of osteoporosis. Benefits of therapy include the stimulation of new bone formation, inhibition of bone resorption (breakdown), and enhancement of calcium absorption.[75][76] These drugs have additionally been shown to reduce bone pain associated with osteoporosis[77], a frequent complication with elderly patients suffering from the condition. Osteoporosis is most common in postmenopausal women, and is usually linked to the changes in hormonal chemistry that are noted later in life. This disorder does occur to a high degree in the elderly of both sexes, however. Osteoporosis can also be caused by the prolonged administration of corticosteroids, which can directly stimulate bone resorption and inhibit new bone growth. This is identified as steroid- or glucocorticoid-induced osteoporosis.

Nandrolone decanoate is the anabolic steroid most commonly prescribed for the treatment of osteoporosis. The drug tends to offer measurable benefits with regard to bone density, and may reduce the likelihood of bone fracture in patients.[78][79] The dosage used to treat postmenopausal women is usually 50 mg once every 3 to 4 weeks. Adverse reactions are common with therapy, however, including virilization symptoms (hoarseness and body/facial hair growth)[80] and unfavorable alterations in serum cholesterol.[81] Therapy appears to be better tolerated in patients above the age of 65, who as a group seem to notice lower adverse effects. Male patients are given a nandrolone decanoate dosage of 50 mg once every 1 to 2 weeks. Therapy for both sexes is usually conducted for at least six months, and may last for one year or longer if necessary. The long therapeutic window is usually required in order to give the drug enough time to measurably effect bone strength.

In the United States, however, the use of an anabolic steroid such as nandrolone decanoate for the direct treatment of osteoporosis is presently viewed as controversial. In spite of substantial clinical data and history supporting the use of steroids for this purpose in the United States, many medical organizations hold the opinion that the potential side effects of steroid therapy are too substantial to justify their benefits with osteoporosis. No agent is presently FDA approved for this purpose. Oxandrolone does remain FDA approved for osteoporosis patients, but for the specific purpose of alleviating bone pain associated with the disease, not for augmenting bone mineral density. Anabolic steroids remain in use for osteoporosis in many other nations, however, and are still prescribed to varying patient populations including men, women, and the elderly.

Turner's and Klinefelter's Syndrome

Anabolic/androgenic steroids may be used to treat certain genetic conditions, most commonly Turner's syndrome in females and Klinefelter's syndrome in males. Both are chromosomal disorders characterized by deviations from the normal XX/XY pairing. They result in (among other health issues) abnormalities in growth, sexual development, and ongoing sexual functioning. Males with Klinefelter's syndrome are sterile, and typically have a rounder (less muscular) physique. They also develop small testicles (microorchidism), and may suffer with gynecomastia. In these patients the supplementation of testosterone (in a similar fashion to that used for androgen replacement therapy) is common, and can help alleviate some of the issues with sexual functioning and body composition. Females with Turner's syndrome will be of short stature, and develop other physical abnormalities including a broad chest, low hairline, low-set ears, and webbed neck. Low doses of a primarily anabolic steroid may be used in adolescent patients as an adjunct to growth hormone therapy to support the linear growth rate. Oxandrolone is the steroid most commonly used in the United States for this purpose, and has been clinically successful at increasing final height when used in dosage of .05-.1 mg/kg per day.[82]

Weight Loss/Muscle Wasting

Anabolic steroids may be administered for the treatment of clinically significant weight loss. Common causes include prolonged corticosteroid therapy, extensive surgery, chronic infections or severe trauma. In a general sense, these agents can be highly useful when a patient is subject to a long hospital stay or period of bed rest, when normal daily muscle stimulation is not present and a significant loss of muscle mass is noticed. Severe burn injuries may also call for the supportive application of anabolic steroids, as this is a type of injury also associated with secondary muscle loss. Anabolic steroids may additionally be prescribed to individuals with weight loss not associated with any known cause. The failure to maintain a healthy (normal) level of body weight for ones' height, and an inability of diet and exercise alone to correct weight loss, are usually the determining factors in recommending such treatment.

The significant loss of lean body mass can present its own set of health issues. Individuals that are chronically underweight may suffer from low energy and a reduced sense of wellness, and are at greater risk of mortality.[83] Severe weight loss during recovery from surgery or illness may also measurably delay or complicate the recovery phase.[84] In the most severe cases, an ability of the patient to maintain acceptable lean body mass can be the key determining factor in recovery. The ability of anabolic steroids to increase protein synthesis makes them among the most accepted agents for the treatment of clinically significant weight loss, provided the patient does not have a health condition or is taking any other medicine that would exclude them from using these drugs. They can positively affect both muscle and bone as well, making them very versatile anabolic agents.

In the United States, oxandrolone is the agent most frequently prescribed for most kinds of clinically significant weight loss. The dosage used for this purpose is typically 10 mg given twice per day (20 mg total), although lower doses may be given in some female, elderly, or younger patients in an effort to avoid undesirable androgenic side effects. The drug is commonly administered for a period of 3 to 4 weeks during the early stages of recovery, although may be given for a longer duration if necessary. Given that the support of constructive protein metabolism is a trait shared by virtually all anabolic steroids, many agents other then oxandrolone are clinically useful for this purpose. In many other regions, agents with a high anabolic-to-androgenic activity ratio are predominantly used for this purpose including stanozolol, nandrolone, methenolone, and methandrostenolone.

Anabolic steroids may also be prescribed to treat more severe cases of muscle wasting. This is a condition characterized by strong ongoing protein catabolism, which means that muscle protein is being predominantly broken down (as opposed to synthesized) in the body, and a progressive loss of weight, strength, and energy is noticed. In a medical setting, severe muscle wasting is referred to as cachexia. Cachexia is not associated with insufficient food intake (dietary malnutrition), but has a metabolic cause than cannot be alleviated with changes in diet. This cause is also usually identified when discussing the condition (ie, cancer cachexia, HIV related cachexia). HIV related muscle wasting is the most common form of cachexia treated with anabolic steroids. The use of these drugs as supportive therapy for cancer cachexia has not been well established, however, and currently the subject of ongoing investigation.

Nandrolone decanoate, oxandrolone, and oxymetholone have been the anabolic steroids most commonly used in the U.S. to treat muscle wasting specifically associated with HIV infection. Although no specific FDA recommendations have been adopted, studies with nandrolone decanoate have shown a dosage of 150 mg every 14 days to have a similar anabolic benefit, and a significantly lower incidence of side effects, as 6 mg (18 IU) of human growth hormone per day.[85] In 2003, oxymetholone was the subject of successful Phase III clinical trials for HIV wasting.[86] The dosage of this study (100-150 mg per day) mirrors those that are most commonly prescribed by physicians. In recent years, however, the discontinuance of nandrolone decanoate on the pharmaceutical market and a perceived higher patient comfort profile in oxandrolone has made oxandrolone the preferred agent for HIV cachexia. The dosage of oxandrolone used may range from 20 mg to 80 mg per day. The most consistent clinical benefits have been seen with a 40 mg and 80 mg daily dose.[87]

Steroid Side Effects

While anabolic/androgenic steroids (AAS) are generally regarded as therapeutic drugs with high safety, their use can also be associated with a number of adverse cosmetic, physical, and psychological effects. Many of these side effects are often apparent during therapeutic-use conditions, although their incidence tends to increase profoundly as the dosages reach supratherapeutic ranges. Virtually everyone that abuses anabolic/androgenic steroids for physique- or performance-enhancing purposes notices some form of adverse effects from their use. According to one study, the exact frequency of tangible side effects in a group of steroid abusers was 96.4%. This shows very clearly that it is far more rare to abuse these drugs and not notice side effects than it is to endure them.[88] In addition to the side effects that anabolic/androgenic steroids can have on various internal systems, there are others which may not be immediately apparent to the user. The following is a summary of the biological systems and reactions effected by AAS use.

Cardiovascular System

The use of anabolic/androgenic steroids in supratherapeutic (and often therapeutic) doses can have a number of adverse effects on the cardiovascular system. This may be noticed in several areas including unfavorable alterations in serum cholesterol, a thickening of ventricular walls, increased blood pressure, and changes in vascular reactivity. In an acute sense these drugs are admittedly very safe. The risk of an otherwise healthy person suffering a heart attack from an isolated steroid cycle is extremely remote. The risk of stroke is also extremely low. When these drugs are abused for long periods, however, their adverse effects on the cardiovascular system are given time to accumulate. An increased chance of early death due to heart attack or stroke is, likewise, a valid risk with long-term steroid abuse. In order to better understand this risk, we must look specifically at how anabolic/androgenic steroids affect the cardiovascular system in several key ways.

Cholesterol/Lipids

Anabolic/androgenic steroids use can adversely affect both HDL (good) and LDL (bad) cholesterol values. The ratio of HDL to LDL cholesterol fractions provides a rough snapshot of the ongoing disposition of plaque in the arteries, either favoring atherogenic or anti-atherogenic actions. The general pattern seen during steroid use is a lowering of HDL concentrations, which is often combined with stable or increased LDL levels. Triglyceride levels may also increase. The shift can be unfavorable in all directions. Note that in some cases, the total cholesterol count will not change significantly. The total cholesterol level can, therefore, give a false representation of uncompromised lipid health. Almost invariably the underlying HDL/LDL ratio will decrease. While this ratio should return to normal following the cessation of steroid intake, plaque deposits in the arteries are more permanent. If unfavorable shifts in lipids are exacerbated by the long-term use of steroidal compounds, significant damage to the cardiovascular system can result.

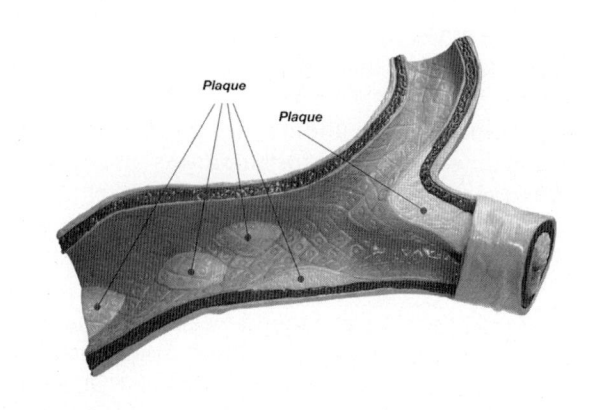

Over time, plaque deposits may begin to narrow and clog arteries.

Anabolic/androgenic steroids are most consistent in their lowering of HDL levels. This adverse effect is mediated through the androgenic stimulation of hepatic lipase, a liver enzyme responsible for the breakdown of HDL (good) cholesterol.[89] With more hepatic lipase activity in the body, the favorable (anti-atherogenic) HDL cholesterol particles are cleared from circulation more quickly, and their levels drop. This is an effect that seems to be very pronounced at even modest supratherapeutic dosage levels. For example, studies with testosterone cypionate noted a 21% drop in HDL cholesterol with a dosage of 300 mg per week.[90] Increasing this dosage to 600 mg did not have any significant additional effect, suggesting that the dosage threshold for strong HDL suppression is fairly low.

Oral steroids, especially c-17 alpha alkylated compounds, are particularly potent at stimulating hepatic lipase and suppressing HDL levels. This is due to first pass concentration and metabolism in the liver. A drug like stanozolol may, therefore, be milder than testosterone with regard to androgenic side effects, but not when it comes to cardiovascular strain. A study comparing the effects of a weekly injection of 200 mg testosterone enanthate to only a 6mg daily oral dose of stanozolol demonstrates the strong difference between these two types of drugs very well.[91] After only six weeks, 6mg of stanozolol was shown to reduce HDL and HDL-2 cholesterol levels by an average of 33 and 71% respectively. HDL levels (mainly the HDL-3 subfraction) were reduced by only 9% in the testosterone group. LDL cholesterol levels also rose 29% with stanozolol, while they dropped 16% with testosterone. Esterified injectable steroids are generally less stressful to the cardiovascular system than oral agents.

It is also important to note that estrogens can have a favorable impact on cholesterol profiles. The aromatization of testosterone to estradiol may, therefore, prevent a more dramatic change in serum cholesterol. A study examined this effect by comparing the lipid changes caused by 280 mg of testosterone enanthate per week, with and without the aromatase inhibitor testolactone.[92] Methyltestosterone was also tested in a third group, at a dose of 20 mg daily, to judge the comparative effect of an oral alkylated steroid. The group using only testosterone enanthate in this study showed a small but not significant decrease in HDL cholesterol values over the course of the 12-week investigation. After only four weeks, however, the group using testosterone plus the aromatase inhibitor displayed an HDL reduction of an average of 25%. The group taking methyltestosterone experienced the strongest HDL reduction in the study, which dropped 35% after four weeks. This group also noticed an unfavorable rise in LDL cholesterol levels.

The potential positive effect of estrogen on cholesterol values also makes the issue of estrogen maintenance something to consider when it comes to health risks. To begin with, one may want to consider whether or not estrogen maintenance drugs are actually necessary in any given circumstance. Are side effects apparent, or is their use a preventative step and perhaps unnecessary? The maintenance drug of choice can also have a measurable impact on cholesterol outcomes. For example, the estrogen receptor antagonist tamoxifen citrate does not seem to exhibit anti-estrogenic effects on cholesterol values, and in fact tends to increase HDL levels in some patients. Many individuals decide to use tamoxifen to combat estrogenic side effects instead of an aromatase inhibitor for this reason, particularly when they are using steroids for longer periods of time, and are concerned about their cumulative cardiovascular side effects.

Enlarged Heart

The human heart is a muscle. It possesses functional androgen receptors, and is growth-responsive to male steroid hormones. This fact partly accounts for men having a larger heart mass on average than women.[93] Physical activity can also have a strong effect on the growth of the heart. Resistance exercise (anaerobic) tends to increase heart size by a thickening of the ventricular wall, usually without an equal expansion of the internal cavity. This is known as concentric remodeling. Endurance (aerobic) athletes, on the other hand, tend to increase heart size via expansion of the internal cavity, without significant thickening of the ventricles (eccentric remodeling). Even with concentric or eccentric remodeling, diastolic function usually remains normal in the athletic heart. The heart muscle is also dynamic. When regular training is removed from a conditioned athlete, the wall thickening and cavity expansion tend to reduce.

Anabolic steroid abusers are at risk for thickening of the left and right ventricular walls,[94] known as ventricular hypertrophy. Hypertrophy of the left ventricle (the main pumping chamber) in particular is extensively documented in anabolic/androgenic steroid abusers.[95] While left ventricular hypertrophy is, again, also found in natural power athletes, substance-abusing athletes tend to have a much more profound wall thickening. They also tend to develop pathological issues related to this thickening, including impaired diastolic function, and ultimately reduced heart efficiency.[96] The level of impairment is closely associated with the dose and duration of steroid abuse. A left ventricle wall exceeding 13mm in thickness is rare naturally, and may be indicative of steroid-abuse or other causes.[97] It may further suggest that pathological left ventricular hypertrophy has developed. Additional testing of such patients is recommended.

Left ventricular hypertrophy (LVH) is an independent predictor of mortality in overweight individuals with high blood pressure.[98] It has also been linked to atrial fibrillation, ventricular arrhythmia, and sudden collapse and death.[99] While LVH in non-steroid-using athletes tends to be without clinical significance, pathological increases in QT dispersion are noticed in steroid abusers with LVH.[100] These changes tend to be similar to the increases in QT dispersion noted in hypertensive patients with LVH.[101] Among other things, this could leave a steroid abusing individual more susceptible to a serious adverse event, including arrhythmia or heart attack. Isolated medical case studies of longtime steroid abusers support an association between LVH and related pathologies including ventricular tachycardia (arrhythmia originating in the left ventricle), left ventricular hypokinesis (weakened contraction of the left ventricle), and decreased ejection fraction (reduced pumping volume and efficiency).[102]

Heart mass can increase or decrease in relation to the current state of anabolic/steroid use, the average dosage, and duration of intake. Likewise, the heart usually begins to reduce in size once anabolic/androgenic steroids are no longer being used. This effect is similar to the way the heart will reduce in size once an athlete no longer follows a rigorous training schedule.[103] Even with this effect, however, some changes in heart muscle size and function caused by the drugs may persist. Studies examining the effects of steroid use and withdrawal on left ventricular hypertrophy noted that athletic subjects who abstained from steroid abuse for at least several years still had a slightly greater degree of concentric left ventricular hypertrophy compared to non-steroid-using athletic controls.[104] The disposition of pathological left ventricular hypertrophy following long-term steroid abuse and then abstinence remains the subject of investigation and debate.

Heart Muscle Damage

Anabolic/androgenic steroid abuse is suspected of producing direct damage to the heart muscle in some cases. Studies exposing heart cell cultures to AAS have reported reduced contractile activity, increased cell fragility, and reduced cellular (mitochondrial) activity, providing some support for a possible direct toxic effect to the heart muscle.[105][106] Furthermore, a number of case reports have found such pathologies as myocardial fibrosis (scar tissue buildup in the heart), myocardial inflammation (inflammation of heart tissue), cardiac steatosis (accumulation of triglycerides inside heart cells), and myocardial necrosis (death of heart tissue) in long-term steroid abusers.[107][108][109][110] A direct link between drug abuse and cardiac pathologies is assumed in these cases, but cannot be proven given the slow nature in which these cardiac pathologies develop, and the influence many other factors (such as diet, exercise, lifestyle, and genetics) can have on them. Individuals remain cautioned about the possibility of cardiac muscle damage with long-term steroid abuse.

Blood Pressure

Anabolic/androgenic steroids may elevate blood pressure. Studies of bodybuilders taking these drugs in supratherapeutic doses have demonstrated increases in both systolic and diastolic blood pressure readings.[111] Another study measured the average blood pressure reading in a group of steroid users to be 140/85, which was compared to 125/80 in weight lifting controls not taking steroids.[112] Hypertension, or consistently high blood pressure at or above 140/90 for either systolic or diastolic measures, has been reported in steroid users,[113] although in most cases the elevations are more modest. Increased blood pressure may be caused by a number of factors, including increased water retention, increased vascular stiffness, and increased hematocrit. Aromatizing or highly estrogenic steroids tend to cause the greatest influences over blood pressure, although elevations cannot be excluded with non-estrogenic anabolic/androgenic steroids. Blood pressure tends to normalize once anabolic/androgenic steroids have been discontinued.

Hematological (Blood Clotting)

Anabolic/androgenic steroids can cause a number of changes in the hematological system that affect blood clotting. This effect can be very variable, however. The therapeutic use of these drugs is known to increase plasmin, antithrombin III, and protein S levels, stimulate fibrinolysis (clot breakdown), and suppress clotting factors II, V, VII, and X.[114][115] These changes all work to reduce clotting ability. Prescribing guidelines for anabolic/androgenic steroids warn of potential increases in prothrombin time, a measure of how long it takes for a blood clot to form.[116] If prothrombin time increases too greatly, healing may be impaired. The effects of anabolic/androgenic steroids on prothrombin time are generally of no clinical significance to healthy individuals using these drugs in therapeutic dosages. Patients taking anticoagulants (blood thinners), however, could be adversely affected by their use.

Conversely, anabolic/androgenic steroid abuse has been linked to increases in blood clotting ability. These drugs can elevate levels of thrombin[117] and C-reactive protein,[118] as well as thromboxane A2 receptor density,[119] which can support platelet aggregation and the formation of blood clots. Studies of steroid users have demonstrated statistically significant increases in platelet aggregation values in some subjects.[120] There are also a growing number of case reports where (sometimes fatal) blood clots, embolisms, and stokes have occurred in steroid abusers.[121][122][123][124][125] Although it has been difficult to conclusively link these events directly to steroid abuse, the adverse effects of anabolic steroids on components of the blood coagulation system are well understood. These serious adverse effects are now regarded as recognized risks of steroid abuse among many that study these drugs.

In therapeutic levels, the anti-thrombic effects of anabolic/androgenic steroids seem to dominate physiology, and decreases in blood clotting ability may be noted. At a certain supratherapeutic dosage point, however, the pro-thrombic changes appear to overtake the anti-thrombic changes, and physiology begins to favor fast and abnormally thick clot formation (hypercoagulability). The exact dosage threshold or conditions required to increase blood clotting has not been determined, and some studies with steroid users taking supraphysiological doses fail to demonstrate increased coagulability.[126] Individuals remain warned of the potential increases in thrombic risk with anabolic/androgenic steroid abuse. Blood clotting tendency should return to the pretreated state after the discontinuance of anabolic/androgenic steroids.

Hematological (Polycythemia)

Anabolic/androgenic steroids stimulate erythropoiesis (red blood cell production). One potential adverse effect of this is polycythemia, or the overproduction of red blood cells. Polycythemia can be reflected in the hematocrit level, or the percentage of blood volume that is made up of red cells. As the hematocrit rises, so too does the viscosity of the blood. If the blood becomes too thick, its ability to circulate becomes impaired. This can greatly increase the risk of serious thrombic event including embolism and stroke. A high hematocrit level is also an independent risk factor for heart disease.[127] The normal hematocrit level in men is 40.7 to 50.3%, and in women it is 36.1 to 44.3% (numbers may vary very slightly depending on the source). For the sake of scale, while a hematocrit of 50% may be normal, a hematocrit of 60% or above is considered critical (life threatening).

Anabolic/steroid administration tends to raise the hematocrit level by several percentage points, sometimes more. As a result, many steroid-using bodybuilders will have hematocrit levels that are above the normal range. For example, one study measured the average hematocrit in a group of steroid abusing competitive bodybuilders to be 55.7%.[128] This level is considered clinically high, and would increase blood viscosity enough to raise the risk of serious cardiovascular event. Although not likely to be an isolated cause, high hematocrit is believed to have been a contributing factor in the deaths of a number of steroid abusers, usually paired with high blood pressure, homocysteine, and/or atherosclerosis. The average hematocrit level in bodybuilders not taking anabolic/androgenic steroids was 45.6%, well within the normal range for healthy adult men.

Many physicians that specialize in hormone replacement therapy consider a hematocrit level of 55% to be an absolute cutoff point. At or above this point, and anabolic/androgenic steroid therapy cannot be continued safely. Drug intake would be ceased at this point until the hematocrit issues have been corrected. Minor elevations in hematocrit may be addressed with phlebotomy. For this, 1 pint of blood may be removed periodically during steroid intake, often every two months. Proper hydration is also important, as dehydration can temporarily cause the hematocrit level to elevate, giving a false positive for polycythemia. The daily intake of aspirin is also commonly advised if the hematocrit is above normal, as this will reduce platelet aggregation, or the tendency for platelets to stick together and form clots. Individuals remain cautioned of the potential cardiovascular danger of high hematocrit levels associated with anabolic/androgenic steroid use.

Homocysteine

Anabolic/androgenic steroids may elevate homocysteine levels. Homocysteine is an intermediary amino acid produced as a byproduct of methionine metabolism. High levels of homocysteine have been linked to elevations in the risk for cardiovascular disease.[129] It is believed to play a direct role in the disease, increasing oxidative stress, including the oxidation of LDL cholesterol, and accelerating atherosclerosis.[130] Elevated levels of homocysteine may also induce vascular cell damage, support platelet aggregation, and increase the likelihood of thrombic event.[131][132][133] The normal range for homocysteine levels in men aged 30 to 59 years is 6.3-11.2umol/L. For women of the same age the average is 4.5-7.9umol/L. Increased risk of heart attack, stroke, or other thrombic event are noted with even modest elevations in homocysteine. According to one study, a homocysteine level exceeding 15umol/L in patients with heart disease is associated with a 24.7% increased likelihood of death within five years.[134]

Androgens stimulate elevations in homocysteine,[135] and men have an approximately 25% higher level on average than women.[136] Anabolic/androgenic steroid abuse has been associated with hyperhomocysteinaemia, or consistent clinically high homocysteine levels.[137] One study found that the average homocysteine concentration in a group of 10 men that had been self-administering anabolic/androgenic steroids (in a cyclic pattern) for 20 years was 13.2 umol/L.[138] Three of these men died of a heart attack during the investigation, and had homocysteine levels between 15umol/L and 18umol/L. The average homocysteine level in bodybuilders who had never taken steroids was 8.7umol/L, while it was 10.4umol/L in previous steroid users (3 months abstinence). One study did show that administering 200 mg of testosterone enanthate (with and without an aromatase inhibitor) for three weeks failed to produce a significant elevation in homocysteine.[139] It is unknown if the moderate dosage, drug type (esterified injectable vs. c17-aa), or short duration of intake were factors in the differing outcome from other studies. Individuals remain warned of the potential for elevations in the homocysteine level with steroid abuse.

Vascular Reactivity

The endothelium is a layer of cells that line the entire circulatory system. These cells are found on the inside of all blood vessels, and help increase or decrease blood flow and pressure by relaxing or constricting the vessels (referred to as vasodilation and vasoconstriction, respectively). These cells also help regulate the passage of materials in and out of blood vessels, and are involved in a number of important vascular processes including blood clotting and new blood vessel formation. Having a more flexible (reactive) endothelium is generally considered desirable for health, and, likewise, the endothelium is often compromised in individuals with cardiovascular disease. Patients with endothelial dysfunction tend to notice greater vasoconstriction, restricted blood flow, higher blood pressure, local inflammation, and reduced circulatory capacity.[140] This may place them at greater risk for heart attack, stroke, or thrombosis (blood clot).

Endothelial cells are androgen responsive, which may partly account for men exhibiting less vascular reactivity than women.[141] Similarly, anabolic/androgenic steroid use has been shown to impair endothelial activity and vascular reactivity. Studies at the University of Innsbruck in Austria compared the level of endothelial dilation in 20 steroid users to a group of control athletes.[142] Those individuals using anabolic steroids noticed slight but measurably impaired vascular dilation and endothelial function. Additional studies at the University of Wales in Cardiff comparing vascular dilation in active, previous, and non-steroid users, also demonstrated anabolic steroids to cause a decline in endothelial-independent vasodilation.[143] These effects leave the steroid user with more relative "stiffness" in the vascular system, which could increase the chance of an adverse cardiovascular event. In both studies, vascular reactivity improved after the discontinuance of anabolic/androgenic steroids.

Proving an Association

Direct links between steroid abuse and individual cases of stroke and heart attack have been difficult to prove. There are a number of things that have made this difficult. For one, cardiovascular disease is very common in men. It also usually takes decades to develop. This makes individual contributing factors (which include many things such as diet, lifestyle, health status, and genetic variables) extremely difficult to isolate. Data concerning the long-term use of steroids in physique- or performance-enhancing doses is also very limited. It would be unethical to conduct a controlled study where participants were given abusive doses of steroids for many years, so the data

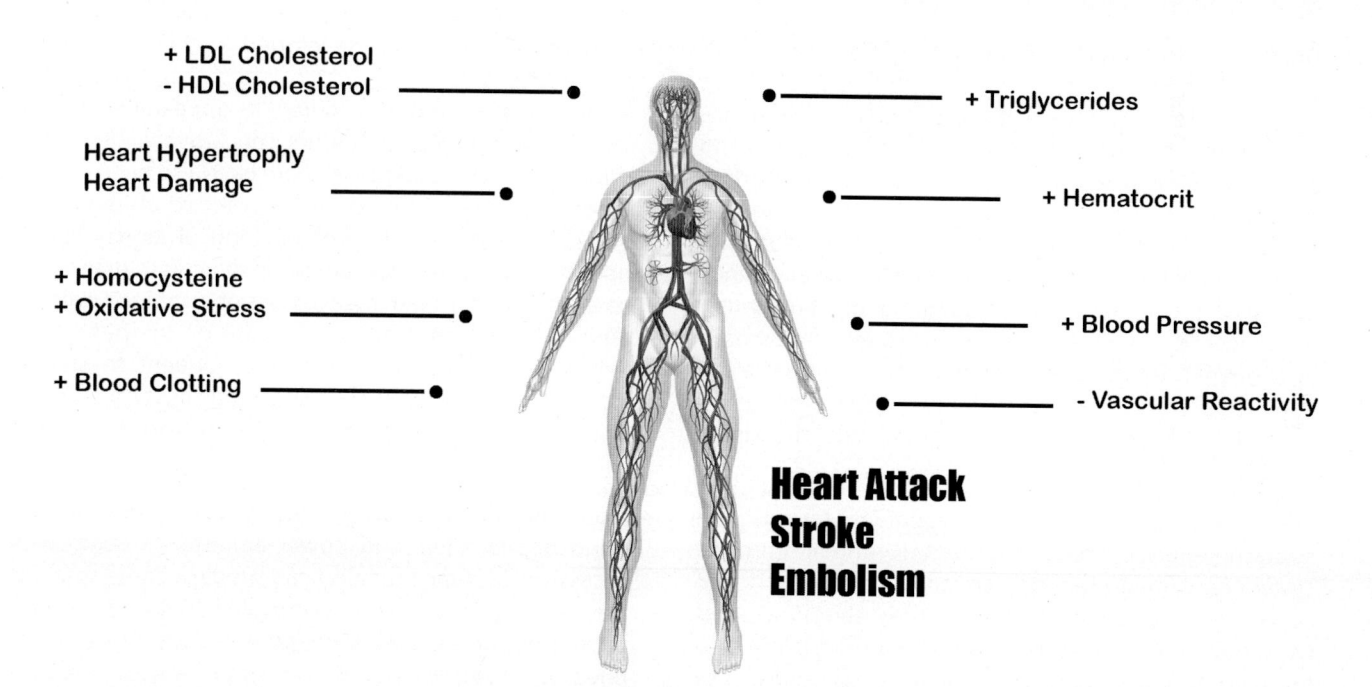

+ LDL Cholesterol
- HDL Cholesterol

Heart Hypertrophy
Heart Damage

+ Homocysteine
+ Oxidative Stress

+ Blood Clotting

+ Triglycerides

+ Hematocrit

+ Blood Pressure

- Vascular Reactivity

**Heart Attack
Stroke
Embolism**

Anabolic/androgenic steroid abuse can produce changes in a number of areas of cardiovascular health that can work together to increase the risk of heart attack, stroke, or embolism.

that is referenced tends to be from case studies. Individual case studies are important, but are usually considered too week to meet the requirements of statistical proof. Still, it would be a mistake to confuse this lack of proven association with proof of nonassociation. The cardiovascular risks of steroid abuse remain well supported by both documented acute changes in cardiovascular markers, and a growing body of case reports of injury or death. There are few medical experts close to the study of these drugs today that would actually deny their risks.

Immune System

The human immune system is responsive to sex hormones. This results in functional differences in immunity between the sexes. Women tend to have a more active immune system compared to men, and are slightly more resistant to bacterial infection and other types of infection.[144] The female immune system is also more prone to developing autoimmune diseases, which may be linked to its higher level of activity.[145] The day-to-day activity of the immune system can also fluctuate throughout the menstrual cycle, further demonstrating the strong influence of sex steroids.[146] The slightly weaker resistance to infection of men appears to be caused by testosterone, which is an immunosuppressive hormone.[147] Androgens may modulate the immune system directly, through their conversion to estrogens,[148] or by modifying glucocorticoid activity.[149]

Anabolic/androgenic steroids have displayed both immunostimulatory and immunosuppressive actions in animal models.[150] Given that these drugs can influence the immune system through a variety of pathways, and anabolic steroids are a fairly diverse class of drugs, their effects on the immune system may vary depending on the particular conditions. When used therapeutically, changes in immune system functioning are usually minor, and have not amounted to strong immunostimulation or immunosuppression. Anabolic/androgenic steroids have also been used safely in many immunocompromised patients, such as those with muscle wasting associated with HIV infection, without any significant change in immune system or viral markers.[151,152]

The use of anabolic/androgenic steroids in supratherapeutic doses may slightly impair immune system functioning, reducing an individual's resistance to certain types of infection. In one study, steroid abusers were shown to have lower serum levels of IgG, IgM, and IgA immunoglobulins (antibodies) compared to bodybuilding controls, consistent with immunosuppression.[153] Although this may logically increase the chance of contracting certain types of illness, a significant increase in the history of illness could not be established in these same steroid abusers. Given the very random nature of illness, however, it may be difficult to establish such a link without extensive study. The effect of hormone manipulation on immunity should also be temporary, and return to a normal state once pre-treated hormonal chemistry is restored. Individuals remain warned of the potential for minor immunosuppression and increased chance of illness with steroid abuse.

Kidneys (Renal System)

Anabolic/androgenic steroids are generally well tolerated by the renal system. These drugs are largely excreted from the body through the kidneys, although there is no inherent strong toxicity in this process. In fact, there are many instances in which these drugs may be used as supportive treatment in patients with compromised kidney function. For example, anabolic steroids have been prescribed to increase the production of red blood cells in patients with anemia related to various forms of kidney disease.[154,155] They have even been used as general anabolic (lean body mass) support, and to treat hypogonadism, in patients undergoing dialysis.[156,157] While care must be taken with such patients, therapy may often be conducted very safely. In otherwise healthy individuals, clinical renal toxicity caused by the short-term administration of anabolic/androgenic steroids is unlikely.

There have been isolated reports of severe kidney damage in steroid abusers. For example, a handful of individuals have developed Wilms' Tumor (nephroblastoma),[158,159] which is a rare form of kidney cancer usually found in children. Its appearance in adult steroid users is suspect, but not conclusive evidence that drugs were the actual cause. There have also been isolated reports of renal cell carcinoma in steroid abusers.[160,161] Since this is the most common form of kidney cancer, however, conclusive links are again difficult to draw. There have additionally been case reports of combined liver and renal failure with steroid abuse.[162,163] In these cases kidney failure may have been subsequent to steroid-induced liver toxicity, as cholestasis (bile duct obstruction) is known to cause acute tubular necrosis and renal failure.[164]

Kidney health should be a concern for long-term steroid-using bodybuilders and power athletes. To begin with, excessive resistance training can produce some strain on the renal system. A condition called rhabdomyolysis is caused by the extreme damage of muscle tissue, which releases myoglobin and a number of nephrotoxic compounds into the blood.[165] In high levels this can damage kidney tissue and even cause renal failure. There have been rare case reports of severe clinical rhabdomyolysis in bodybuilders, both with and without mention of steroid abuse.[166 167 168 169] Steroid use may also cause hypertension, which can lead to kidney damage.[170] While anabolic/androgenic steroids are generally not regarded as direct kidney toxic drugs, they may be used to support a lifestyle and long-term metabolic state characterized by extreme training, heightened daily muscle protein turnover, and elevated blood pressure. Over time this may compromise kidney health. Regular monitoring of kidney function is recommended.

Liver (Hepatic System)

Many oral anabolic/androgenic steroids (or injectable forms of oral steroids) are toxic to the liver (hepatotoxic). These compounds can cause serious and sometimes life-threatening damage when abused, and occasionally even under therapeutic conditions. Those agents commonly associated with clinical hepatotoxicity include (but are not limited to) fluoxymesterone, methandrostenolone, methylandrostenediol, methyltestosterone, norethandrolone, oxymetholone, and stanozolol.[171 172 173 174 175] These steroids all have either an ethyl or methyl group at carbon-17 (c-17alpha alkylation). All c-17alpha alkylated anabolic/androgenic steroids possess some level of hepatotoxicity. Liver strain, as assessed by elevated liver enzymes, has also been reported with non-alkylated esterified injectable steroids including nandrolone decanoate and testosterone enanthate in extremely rare instances.[176 177] These steroids have never been associated with serious hepatic damage, however, and are not regarded as liver toxic.

Alkylation of c-17alpha specifically protects the steroid molecule from metabolism by the enzyme 17beta-hydroxysteroid dehydrogenase (17beta-HSD). This enzyme normally oxidizes a steroid's 17beta-hydroxyl (17beta-ol) group, which must remain intact for the drug to impart any anabolic or androgenic effect. Oxidation of 17-beta-ol is one of the primary pathways of hepatic steroid deactivation. Without protection from this enzyme, very little active drug will survive the first pass through the liver and reach circulation after oral dosing. Alkylation of c-17alpha effectively protects the steroid from 17beta-HSD by occupying a hydrogen bond necessary for the breakdown of 17beta-ol to 17-keto. The compound must be metabolized through other pathways as a result, and immediate hepatic deactivation is prevented. The process allows a very high percentage of the steroid dose to pass into the bloodstream intact, but it also places some strain on the liver in the process.

The exact mechanism of hepatotoxicity induced by alkylated anabolic/androgenic steroids remains unknown, but it is speculated to be due in large part to the natural activity of androgens in the liver. This liver possesses a high concentration of androgen receptors, and is responsive to these hormones.[178] With physiological androgens such as testosterone and dihydrotestosterone, however, only a moderate level of activity is permitted in this organ. This is because the liver is normally very efficient at metabolizing steroids, which mutes their local activity. But with the liver unable to easily deactivate alkylated steroids, however, a far greater level of hepatic androgenic activity is allowed. The concentration of steroid in the liver is also very high after oral administration, as the digestive tract delivers the drug directly to this organ before it can reach circulation. The fact that the most potent steroid ever given to humans on a mg-for-mg basis is also the most liver toxic, also supports a close association between androgenic potency and hepatotoxicity.[179 180]

Early liver toxicity is usually visible in blood test results for hepatic function before physical symptoms or dysfunction develop. This is most likely to include elevations in aminotransferase enzymes AST and ALT, also called serum glutamic-oxalocetic transaminase (SGOT) and serum glutamic pyruvic transaminase (SGPT), respectively. The cholestatic enzymes alkaline phosphatase (ALP) and gamma-glutamyltranspeptidase (GGT) may also be elevated, along with other markers (see: Understanding Blood Tests). Screening for abnormalities in hepatic markers is regarded as the most effective way of preventing liver damage from steroid administration. Should asymptomatic toxicity go unnoticed and without a change in drug intake, it is likely to progress to more severe hepatic strain, injury, or hepatic dysfunction. Immediate cessation of anabolic/androgenic steroid use and a full assessment of liver and full-body health is advised should any signs of unacceptable liver toxicity become apparent.

The most common form of actual liver dysfunction caused by the administration of oral anabolic/androgenic steroids is cholestasis.[181] This describes a condition where the flow of bile becomes decreased, usually because of obstruction of the small bile ducts in the liver (intrahepatic). This causes bile salts and bilirubin to accumulate in the liver and blood instead of being properly excreted thorough the digestive tract. Inflammation (hepatitis) may also be present.[182] Symptoms of cholestasis may include anorexia, malaise, nausea, vomiting, upper abdominal pain, or pruritus (itching). The stool may also change to a clay color (alcholic stool) due to the reduced excretion of bile, and the urine may become amber. Cholestatic jaundice may develop, which is characterized by a yellowing of the skin, eyes, and mucous membranes due to high levels of bilirubin in the blood (hyperbilirubinemia). Intrahepatic cholestasis may also coincide with hepatocellular necrotic lesions (death of liver tissue).

Intrahepatic cholestasis will usually resolve itself without serious injury or medical intervention within several weeks of discontinuing all hepatotoxic steroids. More serious cases may take several months before normal hepatic enzyme levels and functioning are restored. Hepatic lesions are likely to heal over time as well, at least partially. In some cases physicians have initiated supportive treatment with ursodeoxycholic acid (ursodiol), which is a secondary bile salt known to possess hepatoprotective and anti-cholestatic effects, in an effort to hasten recovery.[183] The exact value of using this medication to treat steroid-induced cholestatic jaundice remains unknown, however. The liver is highly resilient, and intrahepatic cholestasis is unlikely to continue degrading after drug discontinuance unless additional pathologies are present.

More serious hepatic complications are rare, but have included peliosis hepatis[184] (blood-filled cysts on the liver), portal hypertension with variceal bleeding[185] (bleeding caused by increased blood pressure in portal vein related to obstructed blood flow), hepatocellular adenoma[186] (non-malignant liver tumor), hepatocellular carcinoma[187] (malignant liver tumor), and hepatic angiosarcoma[188] (aggressive malignant cancer of the lining of blood vessels inside the liver). Some of these pathologies can be very insidious at times, developing quickly and without clear early symptoms. Although many of these potentially life-threatening side effects have often been attributed to very ill patients receiving steroid medications, a growing number of case reports are now involving otherwise healthy young bodybuilders abusing these drugs. Additionally, there are at least two case reports of a previously healthy bodybuilder developing liver cancer after taking high doses of oral anabolic/androgenic steroids, and one confirmed death.[189][190]

Physical

Acne

Androgens stimulate the sebaceous glands in the skin to secrete an oily substance called sebum, which is made of fats and the remnants of dead fat-producing cells. Excess stimulation, as with steroid abuse, may also cause a significant increase in the size of the sebaceous glands.[191] Sebaceous glands are found at the base of the hair follicles in all hair-containing areas of the skin. If the androgen level becomes too high and the sebaceous glands become overactive, the hair follicles may begin to clog with sebum and dead skin cells, resulting in acne.

Acne vulgaris (common acne) is frequent in steroid users, especially when the drugs are taken in supratherapeutic levels. This often includes acne lesions on the face, back, shoulders, and/or chest.

A mild incidence of acne vulgaris is usually addressed with topical over-the-counter acne medications and a rigorous skin cleaning routine that removes excess oil and dirt. More serious acne may develop in sensitive individuals, including acne conglobata (severe acne with connected nodules under the skin) or acne fulminans (highly destructive inflammatory acne). Such incidences may require medical intervention, which usually involves treatment with isotretinoin. Topical anti-androgen drugs are also under investigation for the treatment of severe acne, and have shown a great deal of promise in early trials.[192] Acne is typically resolved with the cessation of steroid use, although the overproduction of sebum may persist until the sebaceous glands have had time to atrophy back to original size. Serious forms of acne may produce lasting scars.

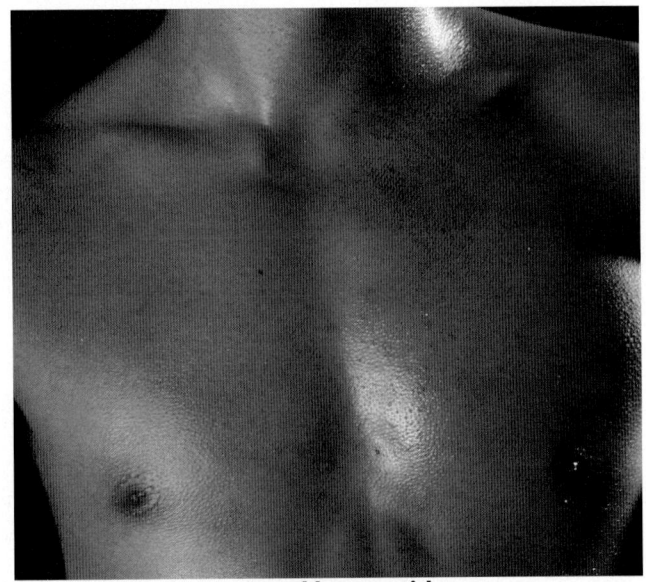

Acne on the chest caused by steroid use.

Hair Loss (Androgenetic Alopecia)

Anabolic/androgenic steroids may contribute to a form of hair loss on the scalp known as androgenetic alopecia (AGA). This disorder is characterized by a progressive miniaturization of hair follicles, and a shortening of the anagen phase of hair growth, under androgen influence. The hair produced by affected follicles will progressively thin, covering the scalp less and less effectively. In men, the baldness produced is usually identified most simply as male pattern. This will initially include a receding hairline (fronto-temporal thinning) and thinning on the crown, areas where androgen receptor concentrations are high.

In women, the balding usually takes on a more diffuse pattern, with thinning throughout the top of the head. Most women with androgenetic alopecia do not have a receding hairline.

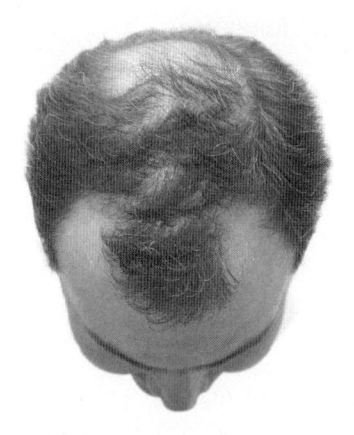

With male AGA, hair loss is most pronounced on the temples and crown.

Androgenetic alopecia is the most common form of hair loss in men and women alike. It is especially common in males, and more than 50% of the population will notice it by the age of 50.[193] As its name signifies, androgenetic alopecia involves the interplay of both androgenic hormones and genetic factors. Individuals with this condition appear to be more locally sensitive to androgens, and have higher levels of androgen receptor protein and dihydrotestosterone in the scalp, in comparison to those unaffected.[194] Although dihydrotestosterone is identified as the primary hormone involved in the progress of androgenetic alopecia, it does not possess a unique ability to influence this condition. All anabolic/androgenic steroids stimulate the same cellular receptor, and as a result are capable of providing the necessary androgenic stimulation. Baldness can result from steroid use, even in the absence of steroids that convert to, or are derived from, dihydrotestosterone.

The genetics of androgenetic alopecia are not fully understood. At one time it was believed this condition could be inherited solely from the maternal grandfather. More recent evidence contradicts this notion, however, showing strong support for father-to-son transmission in many cases.[195] A number of genes have been identified as having a potential link to the disorder, including certain variants (polymorphisms) of the androgen receptor gene.[196][197] No single genetic variant alone has yet been able to explain all cases of androgenetic alopecia, however. AGA is now believed to involve several genes (polygenic).[198] The way these genes combine, and the level of androgens in the scalp, may ultimately work together to control the onset and severity of androgenetic alopecia. Estrogen is also known to lengthen the anagen phase,[199] and the pathogenesis of this condition may ultimately involve genes that alter both androgen and estrogen activity.

Treatment for androgenetic alopecia in men usually involves topical minoxidil and oral finasteride, a 5-alpha reductase enzyme inhibitor. Women are typically prescribed anti-androgens and estrogen/progestin drugs. The focus in both cases is on reducing relative androgenic action in the scalp, which may (at least temporarily) stall the condition. With this in mind, many steroid users concerned with hair loss will tailor their drug intake to minimize unnecessary androgenic activity. This usually involves moderate dosing and the careful selection of drugs with high anabolic-to-androgenic ratios, such as oxandrolone, methenolone, or nandrolone. Alternatively, some may choose to use injectable testosterone esters combined with finasteride to reduce scalp DHT conversion. These strategies are met with varying degrees of success.

There has been no study on the role of genetics in baldness linked to steroid abuse. Anecdotally, individuals with existing visible androgenetic alopecia appear to be those most susceptible to the effects of anabolic/androgenic steroids on the scalp. For many of these people, the loss of hair appears significantly accelerated when taking these drugs. On the other hand, this side effect is generally a much less significant issue with individuals that have not noticed thinning beforehand. Many go on to abuse steroids for years without any visible effect at all, making it clear that there is more to this disorder than local androgen levels. It is well understood that androgens play a role in the progression of androgenetic alopecia for those genetically prone. Steroid use can, therefore, coincide with the first noticeable onset of this condition. It is unknown, however, if anabolic/androgenic steroid abuse can cause baldness in an individual that does not carry any genetic susceptibility.

Stunted Growth

Anabolic/androgenic steroids may inhibit linear growth when administered before physical maturity. These hormones actually can have a dichotomous influence on linear height. On one hand, their anabolic effects may increase the retention of calcium in the bones, facilitating linear growth. A number of anabolic steroid programs have been successful in helping children with short stature achieve a faster rate of growth. At the same time, however, anabolic/androgenic steroid use may cause premature closure of the growth plates, which inhibits further linear growth. There have been a number of cases of noticeably stunted growth (short stature) in juvenile athletes that have taken these drugs.[200] The specific outcome of steroid therapy depends on the type and dose of drug administered, the age in which it is administered, the length it is taken, and the responsiveness of the patient.

While androgens, estrogens, and glucocorticoids all inherently participate in bone maturity, estrogen is regarded as the primary inhibitor of linear growth in both men and women.[201] Women are shorter on average than men, and also tend to stop growing at a slightly earlier age, due to the effects of this hormone. Anabolic/androgenic steroids that either convert to estrogen or are inherently estrogenic are, likewise, more likely to inhibit linear growth than other agents. Popular anabolic/androgenic steroids with estrogenic activity include (but are not limited to) boldenone, testosterone, methyltestosterone, methandrostenolone, nandrolone, and oxymetholone. These drugs must be used with additional caution in young patients due to their stronger potential for inducing growth arrest.

Estrogen acts directly on the epiphyseal growth plates to inhibit linear growth. These plates are located at the end of growing bones, and contain a collection of stem-like cells called chondrocytes. These cells proliferate and differentiate to form new bone cells, slowly expanding the length of the bones and the height of the individual. These cells have a finite life span, with programmed senescence (cell death). This will cause the rate of chondrocyte proliferation to slow over time, and eventually stop. The chondrocytes are replaced with blood and bone cells at the point of physical maturity, "fusing" the bones and inhibiting further linear growth. The stimulation of estrogen appears to accelerate bone age advancement by exhausting the proliferative potential of chondrocytes at an earlier time.[202]

Age will also influence a patient's sensitivity to epiphyseal fusion. As young children are far from the point of bone maturity, the inhibitive effects of hormone therapy take longer to manifest in growth cessation. As the juvenile ages, they may become more sensitive to these effects. Studies treating teenage boys (average age 14 years) for tall stature, for example, found that six months of testosterone enanthate (500 mg every two weeks) was sufficient to reduce final height by almost three inches compared to the predicted outcome.[203] This is a moderately supratherapeutic dose, underlining the fact that steroid intake during adolescence can have a very tangible impact on height. This issue may not be as simple as avoiding estrogenic steroids either, as non-estrogenic steroids have also induced skeletal maturation.[204] Individuals remain warned of the potential for growth interruption when anabolic/androgenic steroids are used before physical maturity.

Water and Salt Retention

Anabolic/androgenic steroids may increase the amount of water and sodium stored in the body. This may include increases in both the intracellular and extracellular water compartments. Intracellular fluid refers to water that has been drawn inside the cells. While this does not increase the protein content of the muscles, it does expand the muscle cell, and is often calculated and viewed as a part of total fat free body mass. Extracellular water is stored in the circulatory system, as well as in various body tissues, in the spaces between cells (interstitial). Increases in interstitial fluid can be noticeable and troubling cosmetically. In strong cases this can bring about a very puffy appearance to the body (peripheral or localized edema), with bloating of the hands, arms, body, and face. This may reduce the visibility of muscle features throughout the physique. Excess fluid retention can also be associated with elevated blood pressure,[205] which can increase cardiovascular and renal strain.

Estrogen is a regulator of fluid retention in both men and women.[206] This effect appears to be mediated in part by changes in hypothalamic arginine vasopressin (AVP), the primary hormone involved in controlling water reabsorption in the kidneys.[207] Increased levels of estrogen tend to increase AVP levels, which can promote the increased storage of water. Estrogen also appears to act on the renal tubes in the kidneys in an aldosterone-independent manner to increase the reabsorption of sodium.[208] Sodium is the major electrolyte in the extracellular environment, and helps to regulate the osmotic balance of cells. Higher levels can significantly increase water in the extracellular compartment. Anabolic/androgenic steroids that either convert to estrogen, or possess inherent estrogenic activity, are, likewise, those steroids that are associated with increased extracellular water retention.[209]

Estrogenic anabolic/androgenic steroids are generally favored for mass gaining (bulking) purposes. A steroid user may ignore water retention during this phase of training, occasionally even finding the sheer increases in size to be a welcome benefit. Estrogenic steroids such as testosterone and oxymetholone are also regarded as the strongest mass- and strength-building agents, which may be caused in part by anabolic benefits of elevated estrogenic activity. The excess water stored in the muscles, joints, and connective tissues is also commonly believed to increase an individual's resistance to injury. With the use of many strongly estrogenic anabolic/androgenic steroids, water retention can account for a large portion (35% or more) of the initial body weight gain during steroid treatment. This weight is quickly lost once the steroids are discontinued or estrogenic activity is reduced.

Non-aromatizing steroids such as oxandrolone and stanozolol have also been shown to promote increased water retention, so this effect is not entirely exclusive to aromatizable or estrogenic substances.[210][211] Anabolic steroids with low or no estrogenic action tend to produce modest increases in whole body water and intracellular fluid retention, however, and not in the visible extracellular compartment.[212][213] These steroids are considered to be more cosmetically appealing, and are generally favored by bodybuilders and athletes when looking to improve lean mass and muscle definition. Popular anabolic/androgenic steroids that are associated with low visible water retention include fluoxymesterone, methenolone, nandrolone, oxandrolone, stanozolol, and trenbolone.

Excess water retention may be addressed with the use of ancillary medications such as the anti-estrogen tamoxifen citrate, or an aromatase inhibitor such as anastrozole. By minimizing the activity of estrogens, these drugs can effectively reduce the level of stored water. In most cases where an aromatizable steroid is used, aromatase inhibitors prove to be significantly more effective at achieving this goal. A common practice among bodybuilders during competition is to also use a diuretic, which can shed excess water by directly increasing renal water excretion. This is regarded as the most effective method for rapidly improving muscle definition, but it can also be one of the most acutely risky practices as well. Water retention is not a persistent side effect of steroid use. Excess water is quickly eliminated, and normal water balance returned, once anabolic/androgenic steroid administration is halted.

Physical (Male)

Dysphonia (Vocal Changes)

Although far less common than dysphonia in women, anabolic/androgenic steroids may alter vocal physiology in men. This may include a deepening of the voice. Dysphonia is most common when anabolic/androgenic steroids are administered during adolescence, as the deeper adult voice has not yet been established under the influence of androgens. The administration of anabolic/androgenic steroids before maturity can, likewise, cause a progressive lowering of the vocal pitch, and may trigger pubescent vocal changes in younger patients. Androgens have much less (often minimal) effect on vocal physiology in adulthood. Although a slight lowering of the voice may be noticed with androgen use in some cases, reports of clinically significant changes in the vocal quality of adult men are, likewise, very rare. There has also been an isolated report of stridor (vibrating noise when breathing) and vocal hoarseness in relation to anabolic/androgenic steroid abuse.[214] This instance also involved smoking, however, making the direct influence of steroids more difficult to discern. In general, vocal physiology is well established by adulthood. Aside from very minor reductions in pitch, anabolic/androgenic steroids are not expected to have strong audible effects on the voice.

Gynecomastia

Anabolic/androgenic steroids with significant estrogenic or progestational activity may cause gynecomastia (female breast development in males). This disorder is specifically characterized by the growth of excess glandular tissue in men, due to an imbalance of male and female sex hormones in the breast. Estrogen is the

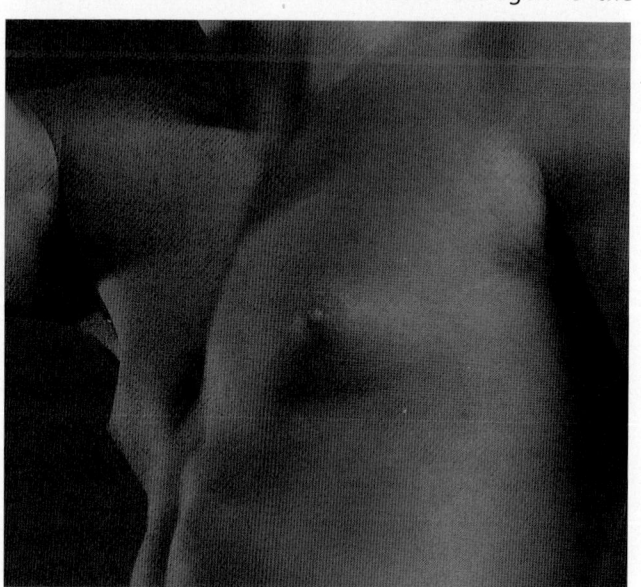

Early gynecomastia.

primary supporter of mammary gland growth, and acts upon receptors in the breast to promote ductal epithelial hyperplasia, ductal elongation/branching, and fibroblast proliferation.[215] Androgens, on the other hand, inhibit glandular tissue growth.[216] High serum androgen levels and low estrogen usually prevent this tissue development in men, but it is possible in both sexes given the right hormonal environment. Gynecomastia is regarded as an unsightly side effect of anabolic/androgenic abuse by most users. In extreme cases the breast may take on a very female looking appearance, which is difficult to hide even with loose clothing.

Gynecomastia tends to develop in a series of progressive stages. The severity of this process will vary depending on the type and dose of drug(s) used, and individual sensitivity to hormones. The first sign is typically pain in the nipple area (gynecodynea). This may quickly coincide with minor swelling around the nipple area (lipomastia). This is sometimes referred to as pseudo-gynecomastia, as it primarily involves fat and not glandular tissue. At this stage, it may be possible to address mild nipple swelling by reducing or eliminating the offending steroidal compounds, and administering an appropriate anti-estrogenic medication for several weeks. If left untreated, however, this may quickly progress to clear gynecomastia, which involves significant fat, fibrous, and glandular tissue growth. The hard tissue growth may be easily felt in the early stages when pinching deeply around the nipple. Noticeable gynecomastia is likely to require corrective cosmetic surgery (male breast reduction).[217]

Although gynecomastia is a very common side effect of steroid abuse, given its clear association with certain drugs or practices, it is also an easily avoidable one. Careful steroid selection and reasonable dosing are usually regarded as the most basic and reliable methods for preventing its onset. Many steroid users also frequently take some form of estrogen maintenance medication, which may effectively counter the effects of elevated estrogenicity. Common options include the anti-estrogen tamoxifen citrate, or an aromatase inhibitor such as anastrozole. The use of a post-cycle hormone recovery program at the conclusion of steroid administration (which usually includes several weeks of anti-estrogen use) is also commonly advised, as gynecomastia is sometimes reported in the post-cycle hormone imbalance phase when steroids are not actually being taken.

It is important to note that progesterone can also augment the stimulatory effect of estrogen on mammary tissue growth.[218] As such, progestational drugs may be able to trigger the onset of gynecomastia in sensitive individuals, even without elevating levels of estrogen. Many anabolic steroids, particularly those derived from nandrolone, are known to exhibit strong progestational activity. While gynecomastia is not a common compliant with these drugs, they are occasionally linked to this side effect in anecdotal reports. The anti-estrogen tamoxifen citrate is usually taken in such instances, as it can offset the effects of estrogen at the receptor, which are still necessary for progestins to impart their growth-promoting effects on the breast.

Physical (Female)

Birth Defects

Anabolic/androgenic steroid exposure to a woman during pregnancy can cause developmental abnormalities in an unborn fetus. Virilization of a female fetus is a particular concern, and may include clitoral hypertrophy or even the growth of ambiguous genitalia (pseudohermaphroditism). Reconstructive surgery will be required to correct these serious developmental abnormalities. Women who are pregnant, or are attempting to become pregnant, should not use or directly handle anabolic/androgenic steroid materials (raw powder, pills, crèmes, patches). Although anabolic/androgenic steroids can reduce sperm count and fertility in men, they are not linked to birth defects when taken by someone fathering a child.

Dysphonia (Vocal Changes)

Anabolic/androgen steroids are commonly linked to a deepening of the voice in females. This is caused by direct androgenic influence on the larynx and muscle tissues involved in vocal physiology, which (in females) are not normally exposed to high androgen levels. Early changes may include a light hoarsening of the voice, with audible shifts in pitch at the high and low end of the vocal spectrum (quiet speaking and voice projection).[219] There is typically a lower general frequency during speech, a reduction of high frequency pitch, and voice instability and cracking. In many cases the changes caused by AAS drugs may resemble those of the pubescent male. If left to progress, these changes may go on to develop into a raspy and recognizable male-characteristic voice.

Deepening of the voice is defined as an androgenic or masculinizing effect. Anabolic/androgenic steroids with higher relative androgenicity such as testosterone, fluoxymesterone, and methandrostenolone, likewise, have a high tendency to produce voice changes when used in females.[220][221][222][223] All anabolic/androgenic steroids are capable of altering the female voice given the right level of stimulation, however. To this point, vocal changes have been reported under therapeutic conditions with even mild anabolic substances such as oxandrolone and nandrolone.[224][225] Care must be taken to monitor the voice during all AAS intake, as changes are often easily generated. Immediately discontinuing anabolic/androgenic steroids may reduce the severity of symptoms, although some changes are likely to persist. Anabolic/androgenic steroid use may, likewise, permanently alter vocal physiology in females.

Enlarged Clitoris (Clitoromegaly)

The male and female reproductive systems differentiate and develop under the influence of estrogen and testosterone. Even as an adult, the female reproductive system remains developmentally responsive to male sex hormones. An elevation of the androgen level in women may stimulate the growth of the clitoris (clitoral hypertrophy). If androgen levels are not abated quickly this may lead to virilization of the external genitalia, characterized by clinically abnormal enlargement of the clitoris (clitoromegaly). With clitoromegaly, the clitoris may begin to resemble a small penis, and may even visibly enlarge during sexual arousal (erection). In more serious cases its association to a male penis can be very striking and clear. Clitoromegaly can be a very embarrassing condition, usually prompting swift intervention when its onset is noticed.

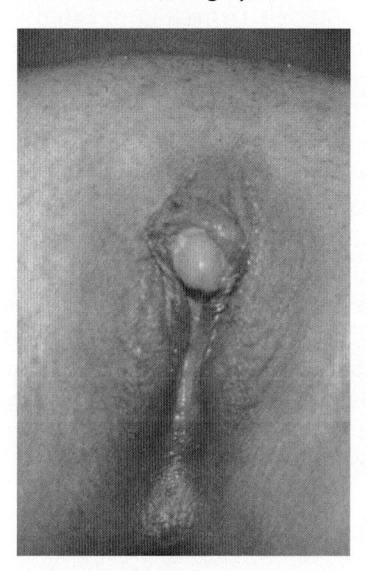

A photograph of distinct clitoromegaly. Here, the clitoris begins to resemble a penis-like structure under androgen influence. If left unabated, this may progress to a more defined phallic abnormality. Source: Copcu et al. Reproductive Health 2004 1:4 doi:10.1186/1742-4755-1-4.

Clitoromegaly is most commonly seen as a congenital disorder, although it may be caused by anabolic/androgenic steroid administration or other pathology in adulthood (acquired clitoromegaly). As a virilizing side effect, clitoromegaly tends to occur in a dose-dependant (androgenicity-dependent) manner. As such, higher doses and more androgenic substances (such as testosterone, trenbolone, and methandrostenolone) are more likely to trigger its onset. Primarily anabolic steroids such nandrolone, stanozolol, and oxandrolone are less androgenic and virilizing, and favored for the treatment of women for this reason. Clitoromegaly caused by steroid use is both avoidable and progressive. Mitigating excess androgenic action early when it is noticed is the most fundamental part of treatment. Reversal of significantly developed tissue, however, will require reconstructive surgery (clitoroplasty).[226] Special care should be taken to preserve the dorsal and ventral neurovascular bundles and normal tissue sensation.[227]

Hair Growth (Hirsutism)

Anabolic/androgenic steroids may cause male-pattern hair growth in females. Medically defined as hirsutism, this condition is characterized by the growth of hair in androgen sensitive areas of the body. With hirsutism, dark coarse hair (terminal hair) may develop on the face, chest, abdomen, and back, areas of the body normally associated with hair growth in men, not women. Treatment for hirsutism typically involves immediate abstinence from anabolic/androgenic steroid intake, and initiation of a strategy to minimize androgen action at the hair follicles. This may include the use of oral estrogens, anti-androgens (spironolactone), or finasteride. Topical ketoconazole, an antifungal agent, has also been used with some success. The response to medical treatments may be slow, and the changes caused by anabolic/androgenic steroid use may persist for a year or longer.[228] Regular hair removal of the affected areas may be necessary. The severity of hirsutism will be related to the androgenicity of the drug(s) taken, the dosage and duration of use, and sensitivity of the individual.

Menstrual Irregularities

Anabolic/androgenic steroids may alter the menstrual cycle in females, resulting in infrequent or absent menses (amenorrhea). Fertility may also be interrupted. Normal menstruation is expected to resume after anabolic/androgenic steroids are discontinued, and the natural hormonal balance is restored. Complete recovery of the female hormonal axis and fertility can take many months in some cases, however, and long-term interruptions of fertility are possible, though unlikely.

Reduced Breast Size

Anabolic/androgenic steroids can inhibit the growth-supporting effects of estrogen on mammary tissues, and may cause a visible reduction in breast size (breast atrophy). Androgen use in females has specifically been shown to cause a reduction in glandular tissue size, and to promote an increase in fibrous connective tissue.[229] These physiological changes are similar to those noted after menopause, when female sex steroids are very low. Reductions in breast size produced by AAS may be very persistent after the discontinuance of drug intake, as there can be substantial local tissue remodeling under excess androgen influence. Women are warned of the potential for substantial physical changes in the breasts with anabolic/androgenic steroid abuse.

Psychological

The effects of anabolic/androgenic steroids on human psychology are complex, controversial, and not fully understood. What is known for certain is that sex steroids influence human psychology. They play a role in an individual's general mood, alertness, aggression, sense of well-being, and many other facets of our psychological state. There are known psychological differences between men and women because of differences in sex steroid levels, and, likewise, altering hormone levels with the administration of exogenous steroids may influence human psychology. The exact strength of this association, however, remains the subject of much research and speculation. In reviewing some of the more substantial data that has been presented thus far, we find a better (though incomplete) understanding of the effects of AAS in several key areas of psychological health.

Aggression

Men tend to be more aggressive than women, a characteristic that has been partly attributed to higher androgen levels.[230] Physiologically, androgens are known to act on the amygdala and hypothalamus, areas of the brain involved in human aggression. They also affect the orbitofrontal cortex, an area involved with impulse control.[231] Steroid abusers commonly report increases in aggression (irritability and bad temper) when taking anabolic/androgenic steroids. In fact, among the illicit steroid-using community, these drugs are often differentiated from one another with regard to their aggression-promoting properties. Many athletes in explosive strength sports even specifically favor highly androgenic drugs such as testosterone, methyltestosterone, and fluoxymesterone due to their perceived greater abilities to support aggression and the competitive drive.[232] While some association between steroid use and aggression is understood, the magnitude of this association remains the subject of much debate.

The psychological effects of escalating dosages of testosterone esters have been examined in a number of placebo-controlled studies. At therapeutic levels, no adverse psychological effects are apparent. If anything, testosterone replacement therapy tends to improve mood and sense of well-being. When used at a contraceptive dosage (200 mg per week), again, no significant psychological effects are seen.[233][234] As the dosage reaches a moderate supratherapeutic range (300 mg per week), psychological side effects such as aggression began to appear in some subjects, but these reports remain mild and infrequent.[235] At a dosage of 500 to 600 mg per week (5 to 6 times the therapeutic level), mild increases in aggression and irritability are frequently reported. Approximately 5% of subjects displayed manic or hypomanic behavior in reaction to this much testosterone, although the vast majority of people still exhibited minor or no psychological change.[236][237]

One extensive placebo-controlled study furthers our understanding of the psychological effects of steroid abuse, often characterized by extreme doses and multi-drug combinations, through its examination of a group of 160 regular users before and during the self-administration of a steroid cycle.[238] A placebo group was also examined, which consisted of people that were unknowingly taking counterfeit medications. Extensive psychological evaluations were taken using System Check List-90 (SCL-90) and the Hostility and Direction of Hostility Questionnaire (HDHQ). Those using placebo steroids did not notice any significant psychological changes. Steroid abuse, however, was associated with higher levels of hostility in all HDHQ measures, with particular increases in acting out, criticism of others, paranoid hostility, guilt, self-criticism, blaming of others, blaming of self, and overall hostility. SCL-90 ratings were also high during steroid abuse for obsessive compulsiveness, interpersonal sensitivity, hostility, phobic anxiety, and paranoid ideation. Hostility measures tended to increase significantly as the level of abuse escalated from light to heavy, although no violent behavior was reported.

Criminality and Violence

Links between anabolic/androgenic steroid abuse and violence have been much more difficult to establish. Most papers suggesting such an association either used correlative data, or discussed individual case studies. These help broaden the scope of research, but are not reliable for proving causality. For example, one study questioned a group of 23 steroid-abusing men, and reported that these men were involved in a significantly greater number of verbal and even physical fights with their girlfriends and wives during the times they were administering AAS drugs.[239] With the known effects of anabolic/androgenic steroids on aggression, this finding is compelling. It may very well be that some men are more susceptible to this type of behavior when abusing AAS than others. A paper like this is not sufficient, however, to substantiate a violent "roid rage". Further research is needed to determine if AAS can even trigger violent behavior in an extremely small minority of users, and if so, what trait(s) makes these individuals susceptible to this reaction when the vast majority of users are not.

Serious criminality has also been difficult to associate with steroid abuse. When discussed, we again tend to see weak correlative data and case studies. For example, one paper in Sweden reports an association between steroid abuse and weapons and fraud crimes.[240] It is uncertain, however, if steroid abuse was actually responsible for this criminality, or just associated with it. It is simply possible these men were more exposed to, or more likely to use, illegal AAS for some unidentified reason. Another paper discussed three individuals with no prior criminal or psychiatric history that were arrested for murder or attempted murder after abusing anabolic/androgenic steroids.[241] While stories like these are interesting (and numerous), with millions of steroid users in the general population they are far from compelling. To date, there is no conclusive medical evidence that anabolic/androgenic steroid abuse can cause violent or serious criminal behavior in a previously mentally stable individual.

Dependency/Addiction

Anabolic/androgenic steroids are considered to be drugs of abuse. Although there is no universally accepted definition for this, abuse is commonly described as the continued use of a substance in spite of adverse consequences. Given the negative health consequences that are associated with supratherapeutic doses of AAS drugs, this classification is a difficult one to dispute. Drugs of abuse are very often also drugs of dependency, which in this context describes an impaired ability to control the use of a substance. There has been a longstanding debate over whether or not anabolic steroids also fit the definition of drugs of dependency. Furthermore, among those that support the notion of an anabolic steroid dependency, there is a split with regard to the nature of this dependency (psychological or physical).

Physical dependency is usually regarded as the most serious form of drug dependency, although both types can be very extreme and troubling depending on the situation. Physical dependency is defined as the need to administer a substance in order for the body to function normally. A physical dependency is usually characterized by drug tolerance, and withdrawal symptoms if the drug is discontinued abruptly. The most well known examples of drugs of physical dependency are opiates such as morphine, hydrocodone, oxycodone, and heroin. Opiates can be very difficult drugs for dependant individuals to quit using, since stopping their use tends to produce extreme withdrawal symptoms including physical pain, sweating, tremors, changes in heart rate and blood pressure, and intense cravings for the drug. The physical symptoms may last for days to weeks after the drug is discontinued, while the psychological symptoms can persist for months longer.

Anabolic/androgenic steroid abuse could be associated with many of the DSM-IV criteria necessary for a diagnosis of both psychological and physical drug dependency. For instance, it is not uncommon for someone to take the drugs in higher doses or for longer periods of time then they had initially planned (criteria #1). Many abusers also have a desire to cut down on their use of these drugs, but concerns over lost muscle size, strength, or performance may prevent this decision (criteria #2). Individuals often continue to abuse steroids in spite of negative health consequences (criteria #5). Steroid abuse is also associated with a diminishing level of effect and escalating dosages (criteria #6). Lastly, steroid discontinuance has been associated with withdrawal symptoms (criteria #7), including reduced sex drive, fatigue, depression, insomnia, suicidal thoughts, restlessness, lack of interest, dissatisfaction with body image, headaches, anorexia, and a desire to take more steroids.[242]

According to the *American Psychiatric Association and its Diagnostic and Statistical Manual of Mental Disorders (DSM-IV)*, three or more of the following criteria must be met for a diagnosis of psychoactive drug dependency.

1. Substance is taken in higher doses or for longer periods than intended.

2. Desire or unsuccessful efforts to cut down or control substance use.

3. Excessive time spent obtaining, using, or recovering from the substance.

4. Important activities are given up because of substance abuse.

5. Continued substance use despite negative psychological or physical consequences.

6. Tolerance, or the need for higher amounts of the substance to achieve desired effect.

7. Withdrawal symptoms.

A drug dependency that is isolated to criteria #1 to #5 would be described as psychological. The meeting of criteria #6 or #7 indicates the dependency is also a physical one.

The physical benefits of anabolic/androgenic steroids complicate the matter of drug dependency a great deal. Unlike narcotics, the main motivator behind the use of steroids is their positive effect on muscle and performance. With this in mind, steroid addiction could actually be a misdiagnosis for muscle dysmorphia in many cases. This is a psychological disorder characterized by persistent feelings of physical inadequacy in spite of extreme muscular development. Steroid abuse (often extreme) is highly common in muscle dysmorphics, along with compulsive resistance training.[243] But steroid abuse is regarded as a symptom of this disorder, not a cause. In a similar sense, the physique-, strength-, and performance-improving qualities of anabolic/androgenic steroids could be driving much or all of the abuse. An analogy would be the so-called addiction to chocolate. Some individuals develop tangible psychological issues surrounding the consumption of chocolate, with uncontrolled binging and negative social and health consequences.[244] But we do not regard chocolate itself as a substance that causes dependency.

There is some evidence that the reinforcing qualities of steroid use go beyond an attraction to their physical benefits. Lab animals such as mice and hamsters will repeatedly self-administer testosterone and other anabolic/androgenic steroids for example, an effect that cannot be caused by a perception of physical change.[245] Testosterone is also known to interact with the mesolimbic dopamine system, which is common with other drugs of abuse.[246,247] Studies additionally suggest that anabolic/androgenic steroids influence dopamine transporter density and increase sensitivity of the brain reward system.[248] Steroids are known to influence psychology, and abusers commonly report an increased sense of wellness, vitality, and confidence when taking AAS drugs. Some speculate this is due in part to an inherent psychoactive effect. Further research is needed to determine if anabolic/androgenic steroids are actually mild psychoactive drugs.

Anabolic/androgenic steroids are not drugs of marked intoxication,[249] which makes them very different from other drugs and abuse or dependency. This makes diagnosing a drug dependency difficult. By definition, drug dependency is related to the abuse of a psychoactive substance, and it is unknown if AAS drugs can accurately be classified as psychoactive substances. At the present time, most experts do not regard anabolic/androgenic steroids as drugs of true physical dependency. It is difficult to correlate the post-cycle hormone imbalance with traditional withdrawal symptoms, and tolerance is really a function of metabolic limits on muscle growth, not necessarily a diminishing biological effect. Individuals remain warned, however, that steroid abuse is commonly associated with the signs of psychological dependency. Further research is needed to evaluate the biological and psychological nature of steroid abuse.

Depression/Suicide

Anabolic/androgenic steroids abuse may be associated with bouts of depression. This is most common after the administration of AAS drugs has been discontinued, especially following high doses or long cycles. During the time that steroids are being administered, natural hormone production is diminished because the body recognizes the excess hormone levels. When the steroid drugs are abruptly discontinued, however, the body can enter a state of temporary hypogonadism (low androgen levels). This may be associated with a number of psychological symptoms including depression, insomnia, and loss of interest. This condition is usually referred to as anabolic steroid withdrawal depression, and can persist for weeks or even months as the body slowly resumes normal hormone production.[250]

The most common method of addressing anabolic steroid withdrawal depression in men is preemptively, with the implementation of an aggressive post-cycle hormone recovery program. These programs are typically based on the combined use of HCG (human chorionic gonadotropin) and anti-estrogenic drugs such as tamoxifen and clomiphene. They are used together in a way that can stimulate and sensitize the hypothalamic pituitary testicular axis, allowing natural hormone production to return more quickly. Alternately or concurrently, fluoxetine (or other antidepressant medications) may help alleviate symptoms of depression following steroid withdrawal, especially when this depression is prolonged or severe.[251] These drugs must be used with caution, however, as they also have been linked with increased thoughts of suicide in some patients.[252]

Although less common, depression is sometimes reported during the active administration of anabolic/androgenic steroids. This may be caused by an imbalance of sex steroid levels, particularly with regard to relative androgenicity or estrogenicity. In more cases than not, it will involve a situation where sufficient androgenicity is not present, usually when primarily anabolic drugs are being taken alone. Given the diverse nature in which sex steroids interact with human psychology, however, it is difficult to clearly outline the parameters necessary for this type of depression to develop. Further confusing the issue is the fact that this depression can involve either elevated or suppressed levels of certain sex steroids. The addition of testosterone to an anabolic steroid cycle causing depression may alleviate the problem in many (but not all) instances, as it can provide both supplemental androgenic and estrogenic action.

Suicide has been linked to anabolic/steroid abuse in rare instances.[253] Such reports are usually case studies, involving individuals that were believed to be psychologically stable before abusing AAS, and who committed suicide during or after use of the drugs. It is known that depression is a common complaint during anabolic steroid withdrawal. It is also known that a small percentage of users are especially sensitive to the psychological effects of anabolic/androgenic steroids, and notice dramatic mood swings, manic behavior, and/or severe depression with their use. It is unknown why these individuals have such extreme reactions, while the vast majority of users notice only mild or moderate changes to their psychological state. Further research is needed to identify and understand these individuals. Readers are cautioned that adverse psychological effects, including severe depression and suicidal thoughts, have been associated with steroid abuse in a small minority of users. Beyond this, there is no compelling evidence suggesting that anabolic/androgenic steroid abuse will lead to suicide in otherwise mentally stable users.

Insomnia

Anabolic/androgenic steroid use may be associated with insomnia. This adverse reaction appears to be related to an imbalance of hormone levels, and has been noticed during both excess and insufficient hormonal states. For example, insomnia is a common complaint among men suffering from low androgen levels (hypogonadism).[254] It is also frequently reported by steroid abusers during the post-cycle refractory period, when endogenous androgen levels are also low due to steroid-induced suppression.[255] At the same time, this side effect is also seen during active AAS administration,[256] when androgen levels are very high. The full etiology of steroid-related insomnia is not fully understood, although increased cortisol or diminished estrogen is commonly blamed.[257][258] Given the complex interactions between sex steroids and the human psyche, it is difficult to predict how and when this adverse reaction will appear. While insomnia may be frequently reported among steroid users, this side effect rarely reaches a clinically significant level.

Reproductive (Male)

Infertility

Anabolic/androgenic steroid use may impair fertility. The human body strives to maintain balance in its sex hormone levels (homeostasis). This balance is regulated largely by the hypothalamic-pituitary-testicular axis (HPTA), which is responsible for controlling the production of testosterone and sperm. The administration of anabolic/androgenic steroids provides additional sex steroid(s) to the body, which the hypothalamus can recognize as excess. It responds to this excess by reducing signals that support the production of pituitary gonadotropins luteinizing hormone (LH) and follicle-stimulating hormone (FSH). LH and FSH normally stimulate the release of testosterone by the testes (gonads), and also increase the quantity and quality of sperm. When LH and FSH levels drop, testosterone levels, sperm concentrations, and sperm quality may all be reduced.

When given in supraphysiological levels, anabolic/androgenic steroids commonly induce oligozoospermia. This is a form of reduced fertility characterized by having less than 20 million spermatozoa per ml of ejaculate. The quality of the sperm may also be impaired under the influence of AAS, as noted by an increase in the number of abnormal or hypokinetic (noticing reduced motion) sperm. Fertility is possible during oligozoospermia, however, as viable sperm are still made by the body. The odds of conception are just significantly lower than when sperm concentrations are normal. In many cases azoospermia is reached during AAS administration, which is defined as having no measurable sperm in the ejaculate. Conception is not possible with true steroid-induced azoospermia. Note that in some cases, fertility has been temporarily restored during active anabolic/androgenic steroid abuse with the use of human chorionic gonadotropin (HCG).[259]

Diminished fertility is considered a reversible side effect of anabolic/androgenic steroid abuse. Sperm concentrations usually return to normal within several months of discontinuing drug intake. A substantial post-cycle recovery program based on the use of HCG, tamoxifen, and clomiphene may significantly shorten the refractory period, and is highly recommended among those in the steroid-using community. In a small percentage of cases, particularly following long periods of heavy steroid abuse, recovery of the HPTA can be very protracted, taking up to a year or longer for full recovery.[260][261] Given the undesirable psychological and physical symptoms that can be associated with a prolonged state of low testosterone levels, such a long recovery window is rarely regarded as acceptable. This will usually prompt an individual to seek medical intervention or initiate an aggressive HPTA recovery program.

The ability of anabolic/androgenic steroids to suppress LH, FSH, and fertility has initiated a great deal of research surrounding their use as male contraceptives. Injectable testosterone has been extensively studied by the World Heath Organization, for example, and was determined to be a safe and moderately effective method of male birth control. In studies which administered 200 mg of testosterone enanthate per week to healthy men, azoospermia was achieved in 65% of patients within six months.[262] Most of the remaining patients were oligozoospermic. This diminished fertility was fully reversible, and baseline sperm concentrations returned within seven months on average after drug discontinuance. A state of full azoospermia is the desired endpoint of male contraception, however, and this has not been reliably achieved with AAS drugs alone, even in high doses.[263] Anabolic/androgenic steroids have, likewise, are not approved for use as male contraceptives.

Libido/Sexual Dysfunction

Anabolic/androgenic steroids may alter sexual desire and functioning. The nature of this alteration, however, can vary depending on individual circumstances. Testosterone is the primary male sex steroid, and is responsible for increasing sexual desire and supporting many male reproductive-system functions.[264] Since all anabolic/androgenic steroids influence the same primary receptor as testosterone, abuse of these drugs (characterized by high levels of stimulation) is usually linked to strong increases in sexual desire, as well as copulation and orgasm frequency.[265] The effect of steroid abuse on erectile function is more variable. In many cases, a significant increase in the frequency and duration of erections is noted. In other instances, however, periodic issues with having or maintaining erections are reported, even when steroid levels are high and libido is significantly increased. Sexual issues are also common after steroid discontinuance, when endogenous androgen levels are low.

Studies with dihydrotestosterone and aromatase inhibition demonstrate that estrogen is not necessary for the support of male libido and sexual functioning.[266] Many non-aromatizable steroids are, therefore, capable of sustaining male sexual functioning given the right level of androgenic stimulation. Difficulties remain possible in many instances, however, especially when primarily anabolic compounds such as methenolone, nandrolone, oxandrolone, and stanozolol are used alone. These drugs many not provide sufficient androgenicity to compensate for the suppression of endogenous testosterone.[267] Given the diverse nature in which sex steroids influence human psychology, the existence of other influencing factors during steroid abuse cannot be excluded, including estrogenic activity.[268] The addition or substitution of testosterone during a cycle is usually regarded as the most reliable way to correct issues with male sexual interest and functioning, as it supplements the full spectrum of sex steroid activity.

Priapism

In very rare instances, anabolic/androgenic steroids have been linked to priapism.[269,270,271] This is a condition characterized by the development of an erection that will not return to its flaccid state within four hours. Priapism is a potentially very serious condition, which can require medical or surgical intervention. If left untreated, priapism can lead to permanent penile damage, erectile dysfunction, or even gangrene, which may necessitate removal of the penis. When priapism is linked to steroid use, testosterone is usually responsible. Furthermore, this condition appears to be more frequent in younger patients undergoing treatment for hypogonadism. This may be due in part to a rapid increase in androgenicity, in a male reproductive system that has not yet been exposed to high levels of stimulation. Priapism is very unlikely to develop in adult steroid abusers.

Prostate Cancer

Prostate cancer is dependent on androgens. This disease will not develop if androgens are eliminated from the body at a young age (as with castration),[272] and abatement of androgenic activity in patients with active disease is regarded as a standard path of treatment. A complete picture of the involvement of androgens, however, remains unclear. Studies show there is no association between the testosterone level and likelihood of developing prostate cancer.[273] On the same note, the administration of exogenous testosterone during androgen replacement therapy seems to have no effect on the risk for developing this disease.[274] A review of the available medical literature also does not support an increased risk of prostate cancer in steroid abusers,[275] which typically endure excessive levels of androgenic stimulation. The present model suggests that while testosterone is a necessary component of prostate cancer, it does not appear to be a direct trigger for its onset.[276]

New diagnoses of prostate cancer are sometimes reported during testosterone replacement therapy and steroid abuse.[277,278] Such reports may be the result of a previously undiagnosed condition or unrelated development of this disease, with androgen stimulation assisting the tumor growth rate. Many forms of prostate cancer possess functional androgen receptors, and are highly androgen responsive. As such, they can be stimulated to grow under the influence of testosterone or other anabolic/androgenic steroids. Given this effect, AAS drugs are usually contraindicated in patients with a history of prostate cancer.[279] While steroid administration appears unlikely to cause prostate cancer, individuals remain warned that the use of testosterone or other AAS drugs by someone with previously undiagnosed (latent) malignant prostate cancer could result in the more rapid advancement of this disease.[280]

Prostate Enlargement

Anabolic/androgenic steroids may influence the size of the prostate. Androgens are integral to the development of the prostate in early life, and are essential to maintaining prostate structure and function throughout adulthood. Increases in the androgen level often result in growth stimulation to this gland (prostate hypertrophy). For example, increased prostate volume has been reported in some patients receiving testosterone injections for the treatment of hypogonadism.[281] While extreme prostate hypertrophy is not common under therapeutic conditions, prostate volume does tend to reach a size that is considered normal for a given androgen level. PSA (prostate-specific antigen) levels have also been shown to increase under the influence of exogenous testosterone in some patients,[283] which is a diagnostic marker of prostate health often correlated with prostate volume.[284,285] Additionally, reducing stimulation of the prostate by lowering the androgen level tends to reduce prostate volume.[286]

Anabolic/androgenic steroid abuse may result in significant increases in prostate volume. In more severe cases, this may lead to benign prostate hypertrophy (BPH). BPH is a common condition in older men, characterized by reduced urine flow, difficulty or discomfort urinating, and changes in urinary frequency. Anecdotal reports of BPH among steroid-using bodybuilders are not common, but do occur with enough frequency to warrant concern. Such reports are most often linked to more androgenic drugs such as testosterone and trenbolone, or the excessive dosing of AAS in general. One of the most extreme reports of prostate hypertrophy came from Dr. John Ziegler, the U.S. Olympic physician accredited with introducing Dianabol to sport.[287] Dr. Ziegler noted that during the mid-1950s, many Russian weightlifters were abusing so much testosterone that they needed catheterization to urinate. Dianabol was released soon after, which is structurally a close derivative of testosterone with reduced androgenicity.

Studies of anabolic/androgenic steroid abusers show a preferential stimulation of the inner prostate under the influence of these drugs, in an area where benign prostate hypertrophy is known to originate.[288] In contrast, prostate cancer usually develops in peripheral areas of the gland. Some association between BPH and prostate cancer is known to exist, however, although the exact nature and strength of this association remains uncertain.[289] PSA values are often (although not always) elevated in both disorders, and serve as a marker of potential trouble. It is important for men to monitor prostate health regularly by digital rectal examinations and blood testing for PSA levels. Anabolic/androgenic steroid use is generally immediately discontinued if signs of BPH or elevated PSA values become apparent.

In addition to androgens, estrogens are also known to be involved in prostate growth and functioning.[290] While androgens are generally stimulatory towards prostate growth, however, estrogen exerts both protective and adverse effects.[291] On the beneficial side, stimulation of estrogen receptor (ER-beta subtype) may help protect the prostate from inflammation, cell hyperplasia, and carcinogenesis. Conversely, stimulation of the alpha subtype of the estrogen receptor is linked to abnormal cell proliferation, inflammation, and carcinogenesis. How the aromatization of testosterone and AAS (which will result in stimulation of both receptor subtypes) will effect prostate hypertrophy remains unclear. Prostate growth and elevated PSA values have been noted during steroid administration with both strongly and mildly estrogenic steroids.[292] Furthermore, the administration of anastrozole (an inhibitor of estrogen synthesis) during testosterone administration does not appear to block stimulation of the prostate.[293] Presently, the most successful strategy to minimizing prostate hypertrophy seems to be focused on reducing relative androgenic, not estrogenic, action.

Testicular Atrophy

Anabolic/androgenic steroids may produce atrophy (shrinkage) of the testicles. Testosterone is synthesized and secreted by the Leydig cells in the testes. Its release is regulated by the hypothalamic-pituitary-testicular axis, a system that is very sensitive to sex steroids. When anabolic steroids are administered, the HPTA will recognize the elevated hormone levels, and respond by reducing the synthesis of testosterone. If the testes are not given ample stimulation, over time they will atrophy, a process that can involve both a loss of testicular volume and shape. This atrophy may or may not be obvious to the individual. In some cases, the testes will appear normal even though their functioning is insufficient. In other cases, shrinkage is very apparent. Visible testicular atrophy is one of the most common side effects of steroid abuse, appearing in more than 50% of all anabolic/androgenic steroid abusers.[294,295]

Although testicular atrophy is very common in frequency, it is also regarded as a temporary reversible side effect.[296] The gonads, by their nature, will vary in size under hormonal influence. Atrophy should not produce permanent damage. Note, however, that it can be a somewhat persistent issue. It may take many weeks or months of sufficient LH stimulation after steroid discontinuance for original testicular volume to be restored. Likewise, testicular atrophy is usually the root cause of prolonged post-cycle hypogonadism. In extreme cases, full recovery can take more than 12 months, and may even require medical intervention. A post-cycle recovery program inclusive of HCG (which mimics luteinizing hormone activity) may be used to minimize this recovery phase.[297] This drug is also frequently effective for maintaining testicular mass when used on a periodic basis during steroid administration.[298] HCG must be used with caution, however, as overuse may cause desensitization of the testes to LH,[299] complicating HPTA recovery.

Some of the more potent anabolic/androgenic steroids, including testosterone, nandrolone, trenbolone, and oxymetholone, appear to be more suppressive of testosterone release than many other AAS drugs. This may be explained in part by the additional estrogenic or progestational activity inherent in these steroids, as estrogens and progestins both also provide negative feedback inhibition of testosterone release.[300] [301] It is important to note, however, that all anabolic/androgenic steroids are capable of suppressing testosterone secretion. This includes primarily anabolic compounds such as methenolone and oxandrolone, which are normally regarded as milder in this regard. While these compounds may be less inhibitive of testosterone synthesis under some therapeutic conditions, when taken in the supratherapeutic doses necessary for physique- or performance-enhancement, significant atrophy and suppression are common, and distinctions less pronounced.

Other

Anaphylactoid Reactions

An anaphylactoid reaction is a serious and potentially life threatening allergic response to the administration of a foreign substance. Symptoms of this disorder include itching of the skin and eyes, swelling of the mucous membranes, hives, lowered blood pressure, abdominal pain, vomiting, and dilated blood vessels. The smooth muscles may also be stimulated to contract, thereby restricting breathing. Anaphylactic shock may develop in severe cases, which is marked by unconsciousness, coma, or death. The physical symptoms of this disorder are medicated by the release of histamine, leukotriene C4, prostaglandin D2, and tryptase. An anaphylactoid reaction has many of the same characteristics as anaphylaxis, although is not immune system mediated. Anaphylactoid reactions are highly uncommon with hormonal medications such as anabolic/androgenic steroids. Warnings of this reaction remain standard on many (often) injectable medications, however. Mild skin reactions may be effectively treated with an antihistamine. More serious manifestations may require IV epinephrine and other supportive care. Given the potential for rapid escalation of this condition, immediate medical attention should be sought if an anaphylactoid reaction develops.

Cancer, Brain

Anabolic/androgenic steroids are not associated with brain cancer. Complications relating to a rare and usually fatal form of cancer called primary central nervous system (brain) lymphoma caused the death of famous American football player Lyle Alzado. This type of brain cancer most commonly appears in immune-compromised patients, such as those suffering from Human Immunodeficiency Virus (HIV), or organ transplant recipients taking immunosuppressive drugs to prevent organ rejection.[302] [303] Before his death, Alzado had self-attributed his cancer to 14 years of anabolic/androgenic steroid abuse.[304] While anabolic/androgenic steroids can be mildly immunosuppressive, these drugs are not associated with extreme clinical immunosuppression that could lead to brain lymphoma. Likewise, there is no clinical evidence or understood mechanism that suggests AAS abuse is responsible for Alzado's death. Even though physicians say there is no proof of an association between performance-enhancing drug abuse and Alzado's cancer,[305] this story is frequently recounted in the media to convey the dangers of steroid abuse.

Cancer, Breast

Although extremely rare, male breast cancer has been associated with the administration of testosterone.[306] It is unknown, however, if the hormone therapy was related to the onset of this disease, or if it was just incidental to its progression and discovery. Androgens generally exhibit inhibitory effects on hormone-responsive breast cancers, and have actually been used in their treatment.[307] Estrogens, on the other hand, can support the growth of many breast tumors. It is not uncommon for elevated estrogen levels to result from testosterone therapy, and at least a supportive role is plausible. The exact relationship between isolated cases of breast carcinoma and testosterone administration in men remains unclear. Testosterone is presently contraindicated in patients with breast cancer.

Insulin Resistance

Anabolic/androgenic steroids may alter insulin sensitivity, an important measure of metabolic health. The effect of these drugs may be variable, however. For example, testosterone administration may improve insulin sensitivity in men with hypogonadism.[308] Oxandrolone (20 mg per day) has also been shown to improve insulin sensitivity in older men (60 to 87 years).[309] These beneficial metabolic outcomes were correlated with reductions in visceral adipose tissue (VAT). This is a deep layer of fat that surrounds the abdominal organs, and is associated with insulin resistance.[310] Insulin resistance may also lead to other health issues including hypertension, elevated triglycerides and cholesterol, and increased risk of diabetes and cardiovascular disease. By reducing VAT levels, testosterone and AAS may improve insulin sensitivity, and potentially metabolic health.

Conversely, anabolic/androgenic steroid abuse has been associated with impaired glucose metabolism.[311] In one study, powerlifters that had abused AAS in high doses for up to seven years were shown to have diminished glucose tolerance and increased insulin resistance.[312] In spite of a long history of resistance exercise, these subjects secreted more insulin in response to measured glucose ingestion than even obese sedentary control subjects. Additional studies with methandrostenolone demonstrated significantly increased insulin secretion and potential resistance.[313] A similar outcome is not found in all AAS studies, however. For example, testosterone enanthate in doses as high as 600 mg per week for 20 weeks failed to produce any changes in insulin sensitivity in healthy young men.[314] Nandrolone decanoate (300 mg per week) also did not impair glucose tolerance, and actually improved insulin independent glucose disposal.[315]

The data concerning the effects of anabolic/androgenic steroids on insulin sensitivity is difficult to interpret. It does appear that when these drugs are used initially, reductions in body fat are common, particularly visceral adipose tissue. This may actually improve insulin sensitivity and the overall metabolic state, and reduce certain specific risk factors for diabetes and cardiovascular disease. Beyond this, the effects of AAS on glucose metabolism are not fully understood, and difficult to predict. Studies using supratherapeutic doses of testosterone and nandrolone have failed to produce any negative changes, suggesting that moderate AAS abuse is probably not associated with impairments in insulin sensitivity. At the same time, studies do suggest that there could be concerns with heavy steroid abuse. Further research is needed is assess the impact of steroid abuse on metabolic health.

Nosebleeds

Anabolic/androgenic steroid use may be associated with periodic nosebleeds. According to one study, approximately 20% of illicit steroid users reported this side effect, making it fairly common.[316] Nosebleeds are not a direct result of androgenic action, but are secondary to steroid-induced increases in blood pressure and/or reductions in blood clotting factors. Although they can be scary, most nosebleeds are harmless, and will not require emergency medical attention. When related to steroid use, however, they may reflect other more serious underlying health issues, particularly hypertension. Nosebleeds that occur under AAS influence usually stop reappearing shortly after drug discontinuance, as blood pressure and/or clotting factors return to their normal pre-treated state.

Sleep Apnea

Obstructive sleep apnea (OSA) is a disorder characterized by brief pauses in breathing during sleep, which occur when the soft tissues in the throat close and block the air passages. Sleep apnea may interfere with normal gas exchange, and can significantly reduce the productivity of sleep. It may also elevate the hematocrit, thicken the blood, and increase the risk of other health issues including hypertension and cardiovascular disease.[317] Sleep apnea can sometimes go undiagnosed for years, as an individual may not be aware of the obstructions during sleep. Symptoms of OSA include daytime sleepiness, snoring, nocturnal awakenings, and morning headaches. Obstructive sleep apnea seems to occur most commonly in overweight individuals, and is related to a combination of hormonal, metabolic, and physical factors.[318,319]

Anabolic/androgenic steroids may be associated with the development of obstructive sleep apnea in a small percentage of individuals. The exact relationship between AAS and OSA, however, remains unclear. This adverse reaction seems to appear in some patients receiving testosterone drugs to treat hypogonadism.[320] More detailed studies have shown that high does of testosterone can disrupt sleep and breathing, as well as increase sleep-related hypoxemia, effects that may precipitate obstructive sleep apnea.[321] While OSA has not been clearly documented in steroid abusers, androgens have been shown to alter the structure and function of the oropharynx in ways that can predispose an individual to this disorder.[322] More research is needed to determine if steroid abuse can trigger OSA in an otherwise healthy person. Individuals with a history of obstructive sleep apnea should not use anabolic/androgenic steroids. Physicians are advised to monitor their patients closely for signs of OSA during AAS therapy.

Acute Steroid Safety: Studies with Real-World Dosages

Few medicines have the type of stigma about them that anabolic/androgenic steroids do. If you mention the decision to use these drugs to the average person, you are likely to be lectured about the tremendous physical and psychological risks you are about to undertake; how your hair might fall out, your testicles will disappear, or the steroids will give you cancer. Or maybe you will just lose you mind to uncontrolled fits of psychotic rage, or suffer a life-threatening heart attack. Clearly, the public has been given a very strong message about steroids: stay far away from them, they are deadly drugs. However, those actually taking anabolic steroids usually see things very differently. They believe the dangers are terribly exaggerated in the media, and the risks of serious injury or death from an isolated steroid cycle are exceedingly low. Which position is correct?

The committed steroid user will usually point out the fact that a review of the medical literature over the past 50 years will show that the overall safety profile of these drugs has been quite favorable. Steroid opponents, on the other hand, point out that an illicit user takes a much larger dose of steroids than those used in medical situations, and are in much greater danger than the patients using them. Who is right? Is the isolated steroid cycle really a serious health risk? One thing that has always confounded this debate is the lack of pertinent medical studies. Medical ethics make high-dosed studies with anabolic/androgenic steroids (which may constitute abuse of the medication) very difficult to design and gain approval for. Only a very small number of clinical studies actually provide environments that could be viewed as relevant to those on both sides of the argument.

In this section, we examine three medical studies that appear highly relevant for examining real-word acute anabolic/androgenic steroid safety. They concern not therapeutic doses, but a supratherapeutic level and duration of intake that any illicit steroid user would recognize as sufficient for improving muscle mass, strength, and performance. In fact, the dosages and administration periods used in these studies reflect those taken by some of the more aggressive steroid-using bodybuilders and strength athletes. A fairly comprehensive set of health markers were assessed during these three investigations, including insulin sensitivity, serum cholesterol and triglyceride, prostate specific antigen (PSA) levels, and liver enzymes. Because of the protocols that were used, these studies give us a fairly good basis to evaluate the negative health impact of anabolic/androgenic steroids, at least as it relates to an isolated cycle.

600 mg/wk of Testosterone

The first is a testosterone dose-response study published in the American Journal of Physiology Endocrinology and Metabolism in July of 2001, which looked at the effects of various doses of testosterone enanthate on body composition, muscle size, strength, power, sexual and cognitive functions, and various markers of health.[323] 61 normal men, ages 18-35, participated in this investigation. They were divided into five groups, with each receiving weekly injections of 25, 50, 125, 300, or 600 milligrams for a period of 20 weeks. This treatment period was preceded by a control (no drug) period of 4 weeks, and followed by a recovery period of 16 weeks. Markers of strength and lean body mass gains were the greatest with larger doses of testosterone, with the 600 mg group gaining slightly over 17 pounds of fat-free mass on average over the 20 weeks of steroid therapy. There were no significant changes in prostate-specific antigen (PSA), liver enzymes (liver stress), sexual activity, or cognitive functioning at any dose. The only negative trait noted was a slight HDL (good) cholesterol reduction in all groups except those taking 25 mg. The worst reduction of 9 points was noted in the 600 mg group, which still averaged 34 points after 20 weeks of treatment. All groups, except this one, remained in the normal reference range for males (40-59 points).

600 mg/wk of Nandrolone

Next we look at a study conducted with HIV+ men, which charted the lean-mass-building effects of nandrolone decanoate[324]. 30 people participated in this investigation, with each given the same (high) weekly dose of this drug. Half underwent resistance training so that two groups (trained and untrained) were formed. The dosing schedule was quite formidable, beginning with 200 mg on the first week, 400 mg on the second, and 600 mg for the remaining 10 weeks of peak therapy. Doses were slowly reduced from weeks 13 to 16 to withdraw patients slowly from the drug. Potential negative metabolic changes were looked at closely, including cholesterol and lipid levels (including subfractions of HDL and LDL), triglycerides, insulin sensitivity, and fasting glucose levels. Even with the high dosages used here, no negative changes were noted in total or LDL cholesterol, triglycerides, or insulin sensitivity. In fact, the group also undergoing resistance exercise noticed significant improvements in LDL particle size distribution, lipoprotein(a) levels, and triglyceride values, which all indicate improved cardiovascular disease risk. Carbohydrate metabolism was also significantly improved in this group. The only negative impact noted during this study was a reduction in HDL (good) cholesterol values similar to that noted with the testosterone study, with an 8-10 point reduction noted between both groups.

100 mg/day of Anadrol

Lastly, we find a study looking at the potent oral steroid oxymetholone (Anadrol).[325] This steroid is thought to be one of the most dangerous ones around by bodybuilders, who as a group seem to treat it with both a lot of respect and caution. It is not common to find them exceeding the doses and intake durations of this investigation, making it a very good representation of real-world Anadrol usage. This study involves 31 elderly men, between the ages of 65 and 80. The men were divided into three groups, with each taking 50 mg, 100 mg, or placebo daily for a 12-week period. Changes in lean body mass and strength were measured, as well as common markers of safety including total, LDL and HDL cholesterol levels, serum triglycerides, PSA (prostate-specific antigen), and liver enzymes. Muscle mass and strength gains were again relative to the dosage taken, with the end results being similar to those noted with 20 weeks of testosterone enanthate therapy at 125 mg or 300 mg per week (about 6.4 and 12 lb of lean body mass gained for the 50 mg and 100 mg doses respectively). There were no significant changes in PSA, total or LDL cholesterol values, or fasting triglycerides; however, there was a significant reduction in HDL cholesterol values (reduced 19 and 23 points for the 50 mg and 100 mg groups respectively). Liver enzymes (transaminases AST and ALT) increased only in the 100 mg group, but the changes were not dramatic, and were not accompanied by hepatic enlargement or the development of any serious liver condition.

Adding It All Up

One hundred and twenty-one men participated in these three studies, which involved the use of moderate to high doses of steroids for periods of three to five months. Although it may be shocking to most opponents of anabolic/androgenic steroid use, an unbiased assessment of the metabolic changes and health risks did not reveal any significant short-term dangers. The main negative impact of steroid use in all three cases was a reduction in good (HDL) cholesterol values, which is a legitimate concern when it comes to assessing one's risk for developing cardiovascular disease. It is uncertain, however, if a short-lived increase in this particular risk factor relates to any tangible damage to one's health over the long-term. It is also unknown how much (if any) this may be offset by the other positive metabolic changes that were seen to accompany combined AAS use and exercise.

Logic would seem to suggest that the isolated use of steroids, under parameters similar to those used in these three studies, should entail relatively minimal risks to health. At the very least, it is extremely difficult to argue that an isolated cycle with a moderate drug dose is tantamount to playing Russian roulette with your body, as most media campaigns against the use of these drugs would seem to suggest. But make no mistake. These same study results consistently demonstrated pro-atherogenic changes in blood lipids with the doses necessary for physique or performance enhancement, and underline how it is that long-term anabolic/androgenic steroid abuse can impair cardiovascular health.

The Endocrinology of Muscle Growth

The road to anabolic insight must include a biological understanding of what muscle growth actually entails. Often simplified by the term "protein synthesis", muscle growth is actually a highly complex process involving much more than just building proteins from amino acids. Muscle hypertrophy, the correct scientific term for the way we adult humans build skeletal muscle, actually requires the fusion of new cells (called satellite cells) with existing muscle fibers. Since this discovery of satellite cells in 1961, a great deal of research into the mechanisms of muscle hypertrophy has been undertaken. Scientists have come to understand that unlike normal muscle cells, these satellite cells can be regenerated throughout adult life. Furthermore, they serve not as functional units of their own, but provide some of the necessary components to repair and rebuild damaged muscle cells. These satellite cells are normally dormant, and sit resting in small indentations on the outer surface of the muscle fibers, waiting for something to trigger them into activation.

Injury or trauma will provide the stimulus necessary to *activate* satellite cells. Once activated, they will begin to divide, multiply, and form into myoblasts (myoblasts are essentially donor cells that express myogenic genes). This stage of hypertrophy is often referred to as satellite cell *proliferation*. The myoblasts will then fuse with existing muscle fibers, donating their nuclei. This stage of the process is usually called *differentiation*. Skeletal muscle cells are multinucleated, which means they possess many nuclei. Increasing the number of nuclei allows the cell to regulate more cytoplasm, which allows more actin and myosin, the two dominant contractile proteins in skeletal muscle, to be produced. This increases the overall cell size and protein content of the muscle cell. Incidentally, the number of nuclei in relation to cross-sectional area also helps to determine the fiber type of the cell, namely slow twitch (aerobic) or fast twitch (anaerobic)[326][327]. It is important to note that we are not increasing muscle cell number with muscle hypertrophy. We are only increasing cell size and protein content, even though we are using satellite cells to help accomplish this. It is possible for myoblasts to fuse together and actually form new muscle fibers. This is called muscle hyperplasia, and equates to the legitimate growth of new muscle tissue. This is, however, not the primary mechanism of muscle growth in adult life.

The Anabolic Chain

Now that we know what muscle hypertrophy is really about, let's look at anabolic stimulus and ongoing regulation. The following is a rundown of the chain of hormones and growth factors that mediate muscle growth, from the initiation of damage, to final recovery, repair, and growth. For the sake of organization, I have presented them in what I consider to be three logical phases of action. These are not scientifically accepted definitions. Additionally, we could continue to go deeper and deeper into each of the various compounds, messengers, binding proteins, and receptors involved in this intricate and amazing biological activity. I believe the included text will demonstrate the process of muscle anabolism in a very tangible way, however, without too much unnecessary information. Each of the key areas of this section can be further researched for more detail if you are interested. For one so inclined, the medical references in the endnotes would be an excellent place to start.

Trigger

We all understand that weight training is fundamental to growing muscle tissue. To date, no "sit on your ass and get huge and ripped" pill has been invented. The reason is that a number of changes take place in your local muscle tissues during intense training that are vital to the growth process. Without these early changes, growth is difficult if not impossible to stimulate. So for our purposes, we will start here. Training is the "trigger" in the anabolic process. More specifically, it is the localized cellular damage that weight training produces that will first set us down the road of anabolism. The body will respond by repairing this damage, and in the process will try to adapt by making itself stronger. Muscle growth is always a circular process, with a step back (damage) being necessary to take any steps forward.

Phase I: Initial Response

The Initial Response phase covers those changes in muscle chemistry that begin immediately, during training, which will lay the groundwork for later repair and growth. In many regards, the Initial Response Phase will control the potential magnitude of other signals to follow. In the anabolic process, this phase is categorized by the release of arachidonic acid from muscle cells, and the formation of active messengers including prostaglandins, cytokines, leukotrienes, and prostacyclins. This begins with the breakdown of the outer phospholipid layer of muscle cells, which is initiated by the cellular disruption of damaging exercise.[328] Phospholipases are released in

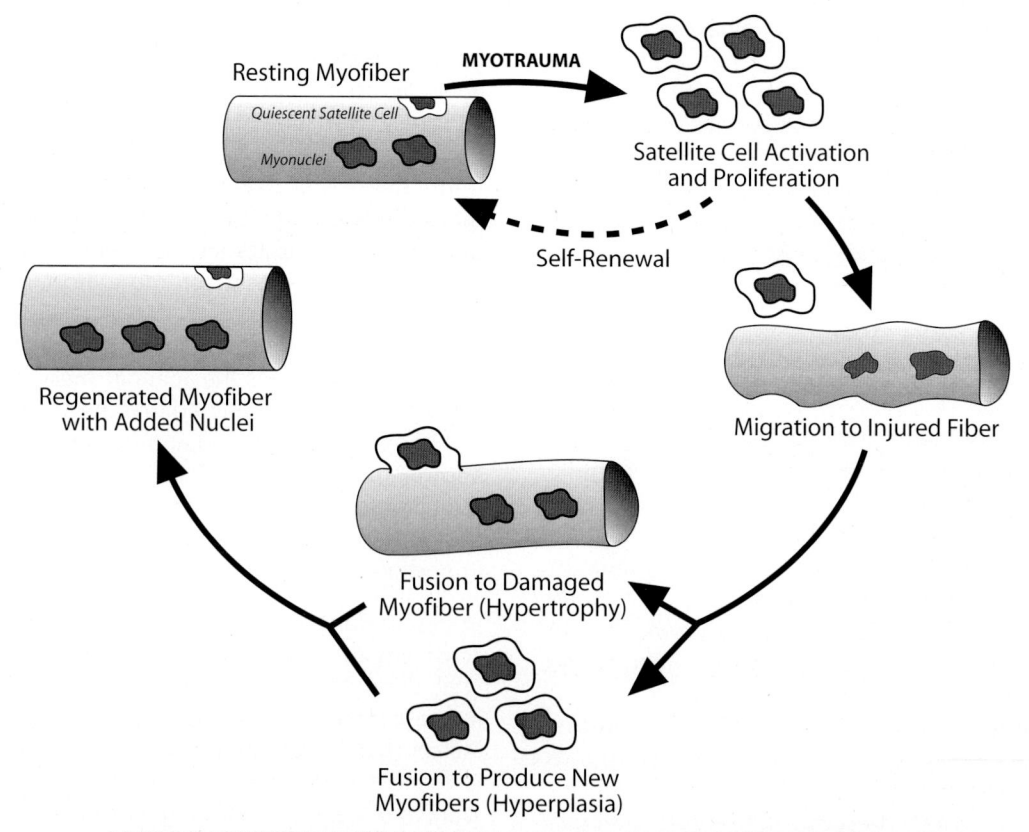

MUSCLE HYPERTROPHY AND THE 4 STAGES OF THE SATELLITE CELL CYCLE

During the *Activation* stage, dormant satellite cells are stimulated to enter the cell cycle. *Proliferation* marks the formation of new myoblasts (active donor cells). These myoblasts will fuse with existing damaged muscle fibers during the *Differentiation* phase. This allows for greater protein synthesis and the expansion of cell size. Quiescence marks the return to a dormant state, where the inactive satellite cells will again rest on the outer layer of the fibers. Myostatin, a known inhibitor of muscle growth, is believed to be a key regulator in this stage.[329][330]

response to this trauma, which causes some of the phospholipids stored in the outer layer of the muscle cells to be released. The eccentric part of the exercise movement is of particular importance here, which is the "negative" part of the lift, where the muscle is stretched under resistance.

The amount of arachidonic acid, which is the central bioactive lipid in the anabolic process, liberated will largely control what occurs during this phase. Arachidonic acid is converted locally and immediately via enzymes to a number of active anabolic end products, the most notable of which (in terms of muscle growth) are prostaglandins, which are produced via interaction with cyclooxygenase enzymes. These prostaglandins (PGE2 and PGF2alpha mainly) will control much of the next phase, identified here as the Localized Tissue Priming phase. Additionally, the prostaglandin PGE2 will work to increase local nitric oxide levels, which is also an active molecule in the anabolic process. It has such actions as

dilating blood vessels (to increase the flow of nutrients and hormones to the muscles) and increasing the production of HGF (hepatocyte growth factor) for satellite cell activation. Arachidonic acid contributes to inflammation and pain signaling as well, and its release plays an integral role in the soreness that follows a productive bout of training.

Training intensity and the relative density of arachidonic acid in the phospholipid layer (arachidonic acid availability is ultimately the rate-limiting step in the formation of anabolic prostaglandins) will dictate how much of this potent lipid can be liberated during exercise. The amount of arachidonic acid stored in skeletal muscle tissue is also in a state of constant flux. A number of factors are involved with its regulation, the most notable of which are dietary intake and daily utilization. Regular resistance training depletes arachidonic acid stores, replacing it with other, more abundant, fatty acids.[331] With less arachidonic acid available, the responsiveness of the prostaglandin system to regular exercise starts to diminish.[332] *Have you ever wondered why you were so sore when you first start training, or after you took a long break? Or why those early workouts tended to be so much more productive than later ones, where you struggle to notice even moderate soreness? Much of this is directly tied to your arachidonic acid stores. The more arachidonic acid you have, the easier it is to liberate during training, and vice versa.* Thankfully, levels can be augmented with dietary intervention (for more information, see the arachidonic acid profile).

Phase II: Localized Tissue Priming

Phase II is characterized by a localized increase in growth factor expression and tissue sensitivity to anabolic hormones. Those who have always wondered why anabolic drugs do not work without training will find a good explanation right here. Simply put, your muscles need to be primed for the actions of these drugs first. One way the body accomplishes this is to increase the density of certain receptors in those specific muscles (fibers really) where it needs to initiate repair. This includes, among others, androgen, IGF-1, MGF, and insulin receptors. Stretch-induced muscle damage and the Phase I response are both principle triggers here. Receptor density regulation is important because it prevents anabolic hormones from stimulating tissue growth in areas of the body that do not require it. Receptor density can, therefore, be as strong a regulating force on the pharmacological activity of anabolic drugs as the serum levels of the drugs themselves.

To put it in perspective, we need to remember that there are two separate components that interact before any message is sent to a muscle cell telling it to increase growth. We have a hormone or growth factor on one hand, such as testosterone, IGF-1, MGF, or insulin, and its corresponding receptor on the other. Injecting exogenous anabolic drugs facilitates greater receptor binding and anabolic signaling by providing more messenger hormones/growth factors (obviously). The more hormones or growth factors you have around the cell, the more binding and activation of receptor sites will take place. We cannot forget, however, that having more receptor sites (instead of more hormones) can also facilitate the process too. More receptors mean the existing hormones or growth factors will find them faster. Faster binding means the anabolic message is sent more quickly, and once completed that the anabolic messenger will be more likely to find another receptor site (to send another message) before it is broken down by enzymes. It is all about how much signal can be sent in a given time period, and both sides of the equation are equally important in determining this.

While on one hand we have an increase in tissue sensitivity to anabolic hormones and growth factors, also vital during the Localized Tissue Priming phase is an increase in the localized expression of certain vital growth factors themselves. This includes IGF-1, MGF, FGF, HGF, TNF, IL-1, and IL-6. These compounds will be released, and will work together on the existing damaged muscle fibers and satellite cells, in a sort of grand symphony of muscle anabolism, with each playing its own vital role in the process. In many cases, the actions of one compound will support the other, either by enhancing its levels, suppressing restricting binding proteins, or supporting its signaling via intertwined mechanisms. A detailed roadmap to all such interactions would go well beyond the scope of this book, and in fact are as of yet not even fully understood to science. A general overview of what is going on with each compound itself, however, is provided

Muscle Damage
Focus on eccentric movement

↓

Phospholipase
Catabolizes outer phospholipid layer

↓

Arachidonic Acid Release
The body's core anabolic lipid

↓

Prostaglandin Formation
And other active end products of arachidonic acid

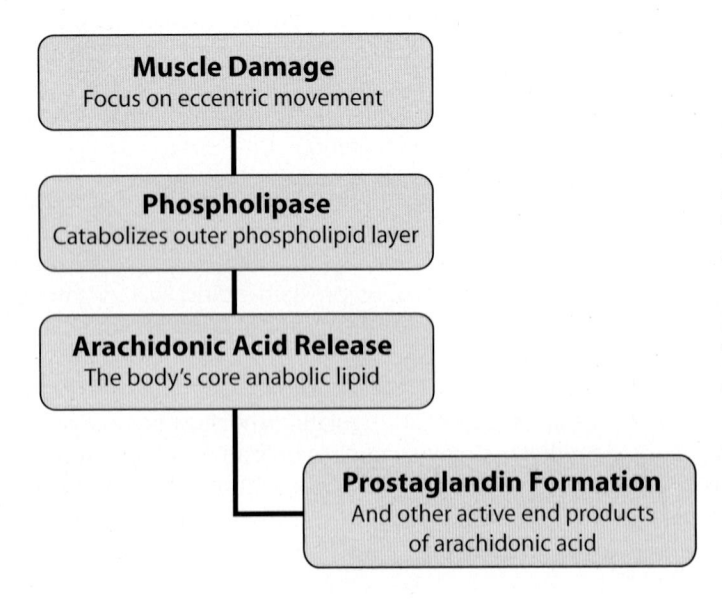

Note: Inhibition of the cyclooxygenase-2 enzyme with anti-inflammatory drugs like ibuprofen, acetaminophen, or aspirin, prevents the formation of active prostaglandins. The anabolic cascade is stalled without sufficient prostaglandin formation (Am J Physiol Endocrinol Metab 282:E551-6), interfering with the normal increase in protein synthesis rates after exercise. It is often advised to use such drugs only when necessary if muscle growth is a key focus.

in our review of Phase III.

Phase III: Repair

Your local muscle tissues are primed during Phases I and II. During Phase III, the hormones and growth factors go to work to finish the job. We categorize this phase as one of ongoing anabolic action, action mediated by the combined effects of many anabolic hormones and growth factors including androgens, insulin, IGF-1, IGF-2, MGF, FGF, HGF, TNF, IL-1, and IL-6. This is the time when repair and hypertrophy are physically taking place in your muscles, and each compound will play an intricate role in the process. We must not forget, however, that everything leading up to this point (the actions in Phase I & II) has still been determining how strong the growth response will be, via modifying receptor densities and hormone/growth factor expression. We will follow the individual actions of the anabolic components very closely here. During the third phase, tissue repair and growth will be finalized with the help of the following hormones and growth factors.

Hepatocyte Growth Factor (HGF): HGF is a heparin-binding growth factor that resides on the outer surface of uninjured cells. Upon injury, it migrates to satellite cells where it triggers their activation and entry into the cell cycle.[333] HGF expression is regulated via nitric oxide release,[334] which is stimulated upon injury to also aid in the flow of nutrients and hormones to the area. PGE2 plays a pivotal role in nitric oxide synthesis and HGF release.[335]

Androgens: Androgens (the hormones that anabolic/androgenic steroids mimic) are strong supporters of protein synthesis rates in skeletal muscle tissue. They are also known to stimulate local IGF-1 expression, so the effects of these hormones extend to the satellite cell cycle (perhaps explaining why they are such strong stimulators of muscle growth). It is also of note that arachidonic acid increases androgen receptor density in skeletal muscle tissue. This helps to further piece together the biochemical links between the Phase I and Phase II response.

Insulin-Like Growth Factor I (IGF-I): IGF-I is an insulin-like hormone with marked anabolic effects. Owing to its name, it also has some insulin-like effects as well. IGF-I increases protein synthesis, and supports the proliferation and differentiation of satellite cells. The prostaglandin PGF2alpha is known to strongly up-regulate local IGF-I receptor expression.[336][337] PGE2 is also believed to play a role in increasing local IGF-1 synthesis.[338]

Insulin-Like Growth Factor II (IGF-II): IGF-II is a second insulin-like growth factor that plays a role in the proliferation of satellite cells. Unlike IGF-I, IGF-II expression does not appear to drastically increase in response to training.[339]

Mechano-Growth Factor (MGF): Mechano-Growth Factor is a recently discovered variant of Insulin-Like Growth Factor I. This growth factor is produced during an alternate splicing sequence of the IGF protein, and plays a strong role in the support of myoblast proliferation. MGF expression, like many of the growth factors discussed here, is strongly up-regulated in muscle tissue in response to stretch stimulus.[340]

Fibroblast Growth Factor (FGF): FGF is actually a family of growth factors, with nine different isoforms (FGF-1 through FGF-9). The full role that FGF plays in muscle hypertrophy in adulthood is not fully understood, however, it is believed to be a strong proliferator of satellite cells, serving to expand their population.[341] FGF's may also play a role in cell differentiation. As with many growth factors, FGF expression up-regulation is proportional to the degree of tissue damage.[342] FGF-2 and FGF-4 seem to be the most prolific representatives of this family in mature muscle tissue.

Insulin: In addition to having some ability to increase protein synthesis and inhibit protein breakdown, insulin is the body's chief nutrient transport hormone. The actions of insulin allow cells to transport glucose and amino acids through the plasma membrane. Insulin receptor expression is strongly up-regulated after traumatic exercise, so as to provide more immediate nutrition to the affected area. This up-regulation has been closely linked to the prostaglandin PGE2.[343][344]

Cytokines (IL-1, IL-6, TNF): Cytokines are a group of immunomodulatory compounds, though in the context of this section we are loosely referring to them as growth factors. The IL cytokines are called interleukins, and TNF is short for Tumor Necrosis Factor. Among other things, cytokines are known to stimulate the migration of lymphocytes, neutrophils, monocytes, and other healing cells to a site of tissue damage, to aid in cell repair. They help in a number of other ways too, such as aiding in the removal of damaged cells and regulating certain inflammatory responses, including the production of some prostaglandins. Prostaglandins are known to play important roles in the expression of all three of the cytokines mentioned here,[345][346] however, they may not be the sole stimulus. Other pathways of arachidonic acid metabolism may also be involved.

Prostaglandins: Although these are the key initial reactionary chemicals, prostaglandins continue to play a role throughout the muscle building process (including Phase III). This includes their support of hormone receptor proliferation, the enhancement of protein synthesis rates, and an intensification of the anabolic signaling of IGF-1 via a shared pathway (PI3K).[347]

Estrogens: Although not specifically highlighted in this outline, estrogens also play a minor role in the anabolic process. This includes helping to increase androgen receptor density in certain tissues (though perhaps not skeletal muscle), stimulating the GH/IGF-1 axis, and enhancing glucose utilization for tissue growth and repair.

Bringing it All Together

So that, in a very loose nutshell, is what is going on inside your body from the time you pick up a weight to the time your muscles are repaired, stronger, and ready for more. If the above seems confusing to you, it should. The fact is, the whole process of muscle growth has been confounding scientists for decades, and undoubtedly will for decades more. We still have a great way to go before being able to explain fully how it is that muscle hypertrophy occurs in humans. But as you can see, we have traveled a great distance as well. During the mid-1960s, scientists were only first learning that we grow muscle with the help of satellite cells. More than forty years later we have identified, and are experimenting with, dozens of growth factors that were unheard of back then. It is a new world today, and despite not having all the answers, we know enough to enhance human performance in many exciting new ways. But please don't mistake the intention of this section. It is not here to give you a functional roadmap of the entire anabolic process, or to guide you in the ultimate polydrug program. It is here simply to open your mind to the true complexity of anabolism. When we start to see muscle growth from its various angles and intricacies, we begin to see our own potential opportunities for successful exploitation. How many of these opportunities you act upon will depend on your own goals and interests. But no matter how much or how little you actually apply this information, I hope you feel better equipped by having it.

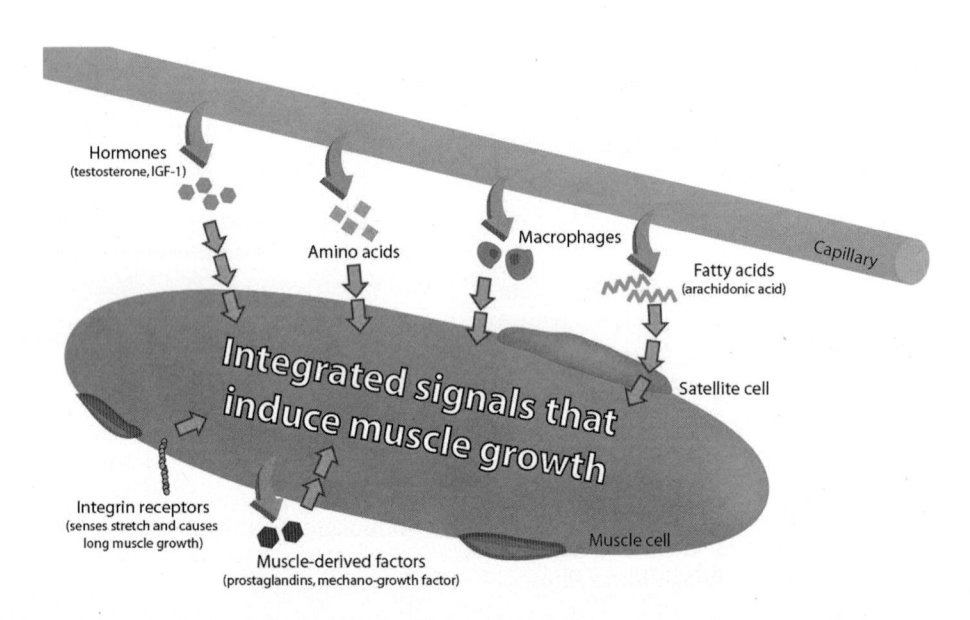

Skeletal muscle growth is a complex process that involves a variety of signaling compounds.

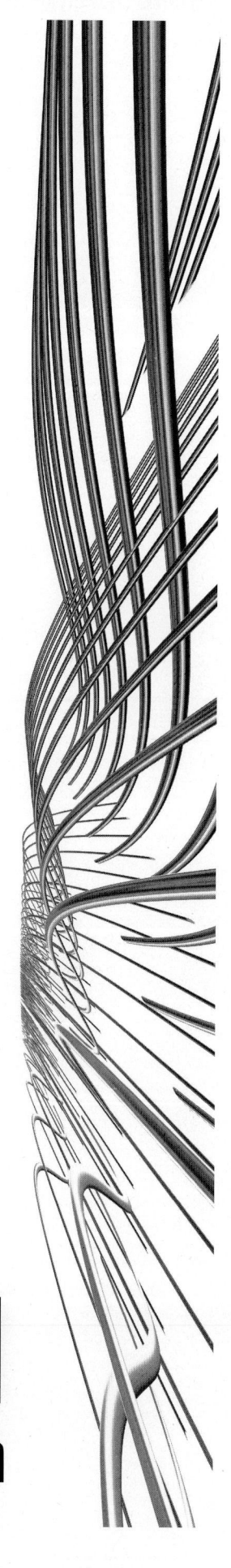

Part II
Practical Application

Steroid Cycles

Anabolic/androgenic steroids are not medically approved to promote excessive muscle mass gains (bodybuilding) or improve athletic performance. Aside from early experimentation on athletes by a handful of sports physicians, an extensive effort to study the physique- and performance-enhancing properties of these drugs, specifically with an eye on developing strategies for using them to maximize benefits and minimize adverse effects, has not been undertaken by the medical community. Because of this, illicit users have been left to develop their own protocols for administering these drugs. The result has been a large variety of different approaches to using these agents, some safer or more effective than others. While it would not be possible to comprehensively evaluate all known approaches, this section will discuss some of the most fundamental and time-proven methods for using AAS.

Steroid Selection

When first considering what steroid(s) to use, one will notice there are many different medications that fall under the category of anabolic/androgenic steroids. This has been the result of many years of development, where specific patients and needs are addressed with drugs that have specific characteristics. For example, some drugs are considered milder (less androgenic), and produce fewer side effects in women and children. Others are more androgenic, which makes them better at supporting sexual functioning in men. Some are injectable medications, and others made for oral administration. There are limits to this diversity, however. All AAS drugs activate the same cellular receptor, and as such share similar protein anabolizing properties. In other words, while different AAS drugs may have some differing properties, if your objective is to gain muscle mass and strength, this could be accomplished with virtually any one of the commercially available agents.

While all AAS drugs may be capable of improving muscle mass, strength, and performance, it would not be correct to say there are no advantages to choosing one agent over another for a particular purpose. Most fundamentally, the quantity and quality of muscle gained may be different from one agent to another. In a general sense, AAS that are also estrogenic tend to be more effective at promoting increases in total muscle size. These steroids also tend to produce visible water (and sometimes fat) retention, however, and are generally favored when raw size is more important than muscle definition. Drugs with low or no significant estrogenicity tend to produce less dramatic size gains in comparison, but the quality is higher, with greater visible muscularity and definition. In reviewing the most popular AAS drugs, we can separate them into these two main categories as follows.

Mass (Bulking):

Methandrostenolone – Oral

Oxymetholone – Oral

Testosterone (cypionate, enanthate) – Injectable

Lean Mass:

Boldenone undecylenate – Injectable

Methenolone enanthate – Injectable

Nandrolone decanoate – Injectable

Oxandrolone – Oral

Stanozolol – Oral

The early stages of AAS use usually involve cycles with a single anabolic/androgenic steroid. Building muscle mass is the most common goal, and usually entails the use of one of the more androgenic substances such as testosterone, methandrostenolone, or oxymetholone. Those looking for lean mass often find favor in such anabolic staples as nandrolone decanoate, oxandrolone, or stanozolol. First time users rarely welcome injecting anabolic/androgenic steroids, and will usually choose an oral compound for the sake of convenience. Methandrostenolone is the most common choice for mass building, and is almost universally regarded as highly effective and only moderately problematic (in terms of estrogenic or androgenic side effects). Stanozolol is the oral anabolic steroid most often preferred for improving lean mass or athletic performance.

The potential for adverse reactions should also be considered when choosing a steroid to use, especially if AAS use is to be regularly repeated. For example, the listed oral medications present greater strain on the cardiovascular system, and are also liver toxic. For these reasons, the injectable medications listed are actually preferred for safety (testosterone most of all). Potential cosmetic side effects may also be taken into account. For example, men with a strong sensitivity to gynecomastia sometimes prefer non-estrogenic drugs such as methenolone, stanozolol, or oxandrolone. Individuals worried about hair loss, on the other hand, may isolate their use to predominantly anabolic drugs, such as nandrolone, methenolone, and oxandrolone. A detailed review of personal goals, health status, and potential side effects of each drug is advised before committing to any AAS regimen.

Dosage

The dosage used is important in determining the level of benefit received. Anabolic/androgenic steroids tend to be most efficient at promoting muscle gains when taken at a moderately supratherapeutic dosage level. Below this (therapeutic), potential anabolic benefits are often counterbalanced, at least to some extent, by the suppression of endogenous testosterone. At very high doses (excessive supratherapeutic), smaller incremental gains are noticed (diminishing returns). In the case of testosterone enanthate or cypionate, for example, a dosage of 100 mg per week is considered therapeutic, and is generally insufficient for noticing strong anabolic benefits. When the dosage is in the 200-600 mg per week range, however, the drug is highly efficient at supporting muscle growth (moderate supratherapeutic). Above this range, a greater level of muscle gain may be noticed, but the amount will be small in comparison to the dosage increase. Below are some commonly recommended dosages for the steroids listed earlier.

- Boldenone undecylenate: 200-400 mg/wk
- Methandrostenolone: 10-30 mg/day
- Methenolone enanthate: 200-400 mg/wk
- Nandrolone decanoate: 200-400 mg/wk
- Oxandrolone: 10-30 mg/day
- Oxymetholone: 50-100 mg/day
- Stanozolol: 10-30 mg/day
- Testosterone (cypionate, enanthate): 200-600 mg/wk

There are additional considerations other than the cost effectiveness of a particular dosage. To begin with, high doses of anabolic/androgenic steroids tend to produce stronger negative cosmetic, psychological, and physical side effects. In light of diminishing returns, the tradeoff between results and adverse reactions becomes less and less favorable. Gains made on lower doses also tend to be better retained after steroid discontinuance than those resulting from excessive intake. It is generally not realistic to expect that rapid double-digit weight gains induced by massive dosing will remain long after a cycle is over. Slower steadier gains are advised. It is also very important to remember that higher doses aren't always what are needed to achieve greater gains. An individual more focused on his or her training and diet will often make better gains on lower dosages of AAS than a less dedicated individual taking higher doses. With this understanding, AAS should only be considered when all other variables of training and diet have been addressed, and always limited to the minimum dosage necessary to achieve the next realistic training/performance goal.

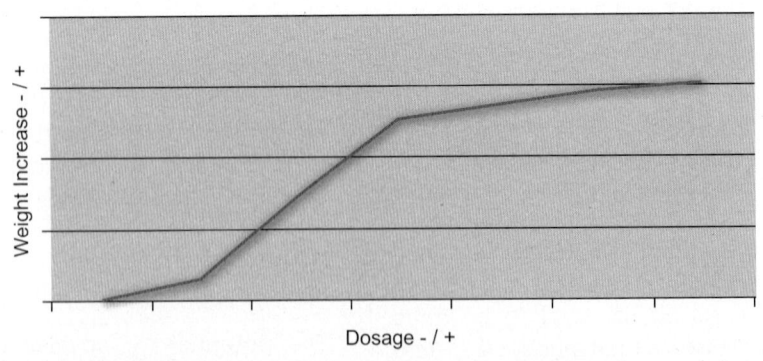

Figure 1. Anabolic/androgenic steroids tend to be most effective in moderately supratherapeutic doses. The anabolic benefits diminish in relation to the amount of drug given at both the high and low ends of the dosage range.

Duration (Cycling)

The administration of anabolic/androgenic steroids at a given dosage will typically produce noticeable increases in muscle size and strength for approximately 6-8 weeks. After this point, the rate of new muscle gain typically slows significantly. A plateau may be reached soon after, where all forward momentum has ceased. To continue making significant progress beyond this point can entail escalating dosages, which is likely to coincide with a greater incidence of adverse reactions and diminishing anabolic returns. Even without dosage escalation, negative health changes are already likely to be apparent, and should be corrected fairly quickly. The practice of extended or continuous steroid administration is discouraged for these reasons. It is generally recommended to use AAS drugs for no longer than 8 weeks at a time (10-12 weeks at the maximum), followed by an equal or longer period of abstinence before another steroid regimen is initiated. This pattern of rotating between "on" and "off" periods is referred to as cycling.

Off-Cycle (Recovery, Bridging, and Tapering)

The period immediately following steroid cession can involve a state of hypogonadism (low androgen levels), and as a result protein catabolism. In an effort to minimize muscle loss, the objective here is usually on restoring natural testosterone production, maintaining an optimal level of muscle stimulation, and remaining dedicated to proper nutrition. A hormonal recovery program is usually initiated, which may involve the use of HCG, tamoxifen, and clomiphene (see PCT: Post Cycle Therapy). A substantial off-cycle period is also advised, involving abstinence from anabolic/androgenic steroids for at least 8-12 weeks. Some AAS abusers have difficulties with complete drug abstinence, and will initiate "bridging" routines between full-dose cycles. This may involve the periodic low-dose administration of an injectable steroid, such as 200 mg of testosterone enanthate or methenolone enanthate every 2-3 weeks. Such practice is discouraged, however, as it can interfere with hormonal recovery, and prevent a return to metabolic homeostasis.

When concluding a cycle, some steroid users also follow a practice of first slowly reducing their dosages (tapering). This tapering may proceed for a 3-4 week period, and will involve an even stepping down of the dose each week until the point of drug discontinuance. It is unknown, however, if such tapering offers any tangible value. This practice has never been evaluated in a clinical setting, and is not widely recommended with steroid medications as it is with some other drugs such as thyroid hormones or antidepressants. Virtually every high-dose AAS administration study can also be found to end at the maximum dosage, with no time allotted to tapering. One flaw in the logic of using a tapering program is that they are ostensibly designed to aid hormone recovery. Recovery is not possible, however, while supraphysiological levels of androgens are present, and such levels are usually found during all weeks of a normal (nonmedical) steroid taper. Individuals remain cautioned that dosage tapering is not a proven way to reduce post-cycle muscle catabolism.

Stacking

As individuals become more experienced with anabolic/androgenic steroid use they may begin experimenting with the use of more than one steroid at a time. This practice is referred to as stacking. Stacking is

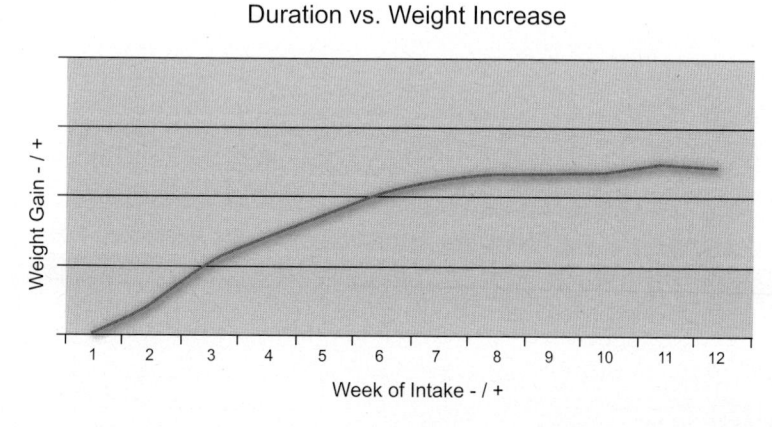

Figure 2. Anabolic/androgenic steroids tend to be most effective at a given dosage for approximately 6-8 weeks. After this point, the rate of new muscle gain will slow, and soon after will usually hit a full plateau.

most common with advanced bodybuilders who find that at a certain level of physical development they begin hitting plateaus that are difficult to break with a previous single-agent approach. In many cases, however, it may simply be the greater cumulative steroid dosage that is necessary for the resumed progress. Stacking usually involves the combination of a more androgenic steroid with one or more primarily anabolic agents. On the anabolic side, common steroids of choice include boldenone, methenolone, nandrolone, oxandrolone, and stanozolol. Testosterone, oxymetholone, or methandrostenolone will serves as the androgenic base of most stacks.

The reasons for stacking androgenic and anabolic steroids together in this manner are two fold. On the one hand, high doses of testosterone, oxymetholone, or methandrostenolone are prone to producing strong androgenic and estrogenic side effects. Stacking first became very popular during the 1960s, a time when effective estrogen maintenance drugs were not widely available. An anabolic-androgen stack allowed the use of a higher total steroid dosage than would be tolerable with a single androgen. Anabolic-androgen pairing also appears to offer efficacy advantages over the use of primarily anabolic agents alone, even when they are taken in higher doses. This conflicts with the original expectations for "anabolic" steroids, which were specifically designed to emphasize muscle-building properties, but is repeatedly noticed by users. The reason the basic androgenic steroids are more anabolically productive is not fully understood, but is believed to involve the interplay of estrogenic hormones, androgenic stimulation in the central nervous system, and potentially other unidentified synergisms necessary for optimal muscle growth.

Today, the availability of drugs that can reduce estrogenic activity makes the continued use of single agent cycles based on a strong androgen like testosterone enanthate or cypionate much more viable than it was decades ago. Side effects like gynecomastia and water retention can now be effectively minimized with anti-estrogens or aromatase inhibitors, even when taking higher doses. Individuals should be aware that stacking is, likewise, not a necessary practice. It is likely to remain commonly applicable in competitive bodybuilding circles, however, or when an individual is sure they have progressed as far as they possibly can with a single-agent approach. Otherwise, for many athletes and recreational bodybuilders, the periodic use of a single steroid will be more than sufficient to maintain optimal levels of muscle mass and performance, and it may never be necessary to deviate from this approach.

Sample Steroid Cycles

The following cycles are presented as examples of common steroid administration protocols. These programs have not been evaluated in a clinical setting for safety and efficacy, and are provided for informational purposes only. These are not recommendations for anabolic/androgenic steroid use. As with any supplemental drug program, it is important to examine your own individual health status, health risks, and performance goals before deciding to engage in any anabolic/androgenic steroid use. For those who have made the decision, it is important to emphasize again that the recommended approach to AAS use is to limit drug intake to the lowest levels necessary to achieve the next rational goal. More aggressive cycles should not be attempted unless one is sure they cannot achieve the results needed on a more moderate program. Note that given the difficulty in predicting androgenic threshold and dosages for female users, the below cycles are examples of programs for men only.

Single Agent Cycles

Dianabol Cycle #1 (Mass)

Products: 100 tablets 5 mg Methandrostenolone

All Weeks: Liver Support: Liver Stabil, Liv-52, or Essentiale Forte (label recommended dosage).

Cholesterol Support: Lipid Stabil (3 caps/day) and Fish Oil (4 g/day).

Estrogen Support: tamoxifen (10-20 mg/day).

Comments: This is a very common first cycle for building muscle mass, and utilizes a single standard bottle of methandrostenolone. This cycle is likely to produce very noticeable muscle growth in a first-time steroid user, often in excess of 8-10lbs of weight gain. This is usually not accompanied by significant visible side effects such as gynecomastia and water retention. Although this is considered a beginner's cycle, methandrostenolone is a c-17 alpha alkylated oral steroid, and presents significant cardiovascular and liver toxicity. The repeated use of such drugs should be limited.

Week	Methandrostenolone
1	10 mg/day
2	10 mg/day
3	15 mg/day
4	15 mg/day
5	20 mg/day

Dianabol Cycle #2 (Mass)

Products: 200 tablets 5 mg Methandrostenolone

All Weeks: Liver Support: Liver Stabil, Liv-52, or Essentiale Forte (label recommended dosage).

Cholesterol Support: Lipid Stabil (3 caps/day) and Fish Oil (4g/day).

Estrogen Support: tamoxifen (20-40 mg/day).

Comments: This is a common follow up to the first Dianabol cycle, utilizing a slightly higher dose and longer duration of intake. The dosages used here are more common for bodybuilding purposes. A slightly greater intensity of adverse reactions is likely.

Week	Methandrostenolone
1	20 mg/day
2	20 mg/day
3	25 mg/day
4	25 mg/day
5	25 mg/day
6	25 mg/day

Testosterone Cycle #1 (Mass)

Products: 10 mL 200 mg/mL Testosterone (enanthate or cypionate)

All Weeks: Cholesterol Support: Lipid Stabil (3 caps/day) and Fish Oil (4 g/day).

Estrogen Support: tamoxifen (20-40 mg/day) or anastrozole (.5 mg/day).

Comments: This mass building cycle is likely to yield similar quantitative results as an early Dianabol cycle, but is favored over the oral for its lower cardiovascular and hepatic strain. The doses used are expected to cause mild shifts in the HDL/LDL cholesterol ratio, but not the substantial changes normally seen with oral anabolic steroids. This sample cycle is likely to present the least amount of health side effects of all listed in this section.

Week	Testosterone
1	200 mg/day
2	200 mg/day
3	300 mg/day
4	300 mg/day
5	300 mg/day
6	350 mg/day
7	350 mg/day

Testosterone Cycle #2 (Mass)

Products: 20 mL 200 mg/mL Testosterone (enanthate or cypionate)

All Weeks: Cholesterol Support: Lipid Stabil (3 caps/day) and Fish Oil (4g/day).

Estrogen Support: tamoxifen (20-40 mg/day) or anastrozole (.5-1mg/day).

Comments: This cycle is a common follow up to the first testosterone only cycle, with a higher dosage and 3 week longer duration of intake. The total testosterone dosage given is double in comparison, and is likely to produce more pronounced estrogenic and androgenic side effects. Cardiovascular strain may be slightly higher than the first cycle, but should remain substantially lower than cycles with oral AAS. Testosterone is arguably the safest, and at the same time one of the most effective, muscle-building steroids available. The exclusive repeated use of a cycle like this would be advised over more adventurous cycling/stacking if possible.

Week	Testosterone
1	200 mg
2	400 mg
3	400 mg
4	400 mg
5	400 mg
6	500 mg
7	500 mg
8	500 mg
9	500 mg
10	200 mg

Sustanon 250 Cycle (Mass)

Products: 15 mL 250 mg/mL Sustanon (testosterone blend)

All Weeks: Cholesterol Support: Lipid Stabil (3 caps/day) and Fish Oil (4g/day).

Estrogen Support: tamoxifen (20-40 mg/day) or anastrozole (.5-1 mg/day).

Comments: This mass building program is similar to the other testosterone cycles, but utilizes Sustanon 250, a form of blended testosterone more widely used in Europe and other regions outside the U.S. The total steroid dosage of this cycle is 3,750 mg, extremely close to the amount used in testosterone cycle #2. A similar level of cardiovascular strain and visible side effects are expected.

Week	Sustanon
1	250 mg
2	250 mg
3	500 mg
4	500 mg
5	500 mg
6	500 mg
7	500 mg
8	500 mg
9	250 mg

Oxymetholone Cycle #1 (Mass)

Products: 50 tablets 50 mg oxymetholone

All Weeks: Liver Support: Liver Stabil, Liv-52, or Essentiale Forte (label recommended dosage).

Cholesterol Support: Lipid Stabil (3 caps/day) and Fish Oil (4g/day).

Estrogen Support: tamoxifen (20-40 mg/day).

Comments: Oxymetholone is commonly regarded as the most potent mass building steroid available. It is also prone to causing both strong estrogenic and androgenic side effects. A steroid novice may gain 15-20 pounds or more on this cycle, although a significant amount of this will be water retention, which will subside soon after drug discontinuance. Oxymetholone is also known for inducing strong cardiovascular and hepatic stress. While this drug may be more convenient to use than an injectable testosterone, it is not regarded as a safe alternative. Repeated use of c-17 alpha alkylated orals like this should be limited.

Week	Oxymetholone
1	50 mg/day
2	50 mg/day
3	50 mg/day
4	75 mg/day
5	75 mg/day
6	75 mg/day

Oxymetholone Cycle #2 (Mass)

Products: 100 tablets 50 mg oxymetholone

All Weeks: Liver Support: Liver Stabil, Liv-52, or Essentiale Forte (label recommended dosage).

Cholesterol Support: Lipid Stabil (3 caps/day) and Fish Oil (4g/day).

Estrogen Support: tamoxifen (20-40 mg/day).

Comments: This is a more popular version of the oxymetholone only cycle. The doses here are more common with experienced steroid users, and more than sufficient to promote strong mass and strength increases. Side effects may be more noticeable than the lower dose cycle, of course, which may necessitate a higher dose of tamoxifen.

Week	Oxymetholone
1	50 mg/day
2	50 mg/day
3	100 mg/day
4	100 mg/day
5	100 mg/day
6	100 mg/day
7	100 mg/day
8	100 mg/day

Stanozolol Cycle #1 (Lean Mass/Cutting)

Products: 200 tablets 2mg Stanozolol

All Weeks: Liver Support: Liver Stabil, Liv-52, or Essentiale Forte (label recommended dosage).

Cholesterol Support: Lipid Stabil (3 caps/day) and Fish Oil (4g/day).

Comments: This is a common first-cycle for an athlete looking for performance improvements or a bodybuilder looking for a lean mass or cutting steroid. This cycle was more common when stanozolol was widely available in 2 mg tablets. Such preparations are now uncommon except in Europe. The dosage used here is low by bodybuilding standards, although similar cycles have been the backbone programs for many athletic competitors, especially during the 1970s and 80's. Significant visible adverse reactions are unlikely at this dosage.

Week	Stanozolol
1	8 mg/day
2	8 mg/day
3	10 mg/day
4	10 mg/day
5	10 mg/day
6	10 mg/day

Stanozolol Cycle #2 (Lean Mass/Cutting)

Products: 200 tablets 5 mg oxymetholone

All Weeks: Liver Support: Liver Stabil, Liv-52, or Essentiale Forte (label recommended dosage).

Cholesterol Support: Lipid Stabil (3 caps/day) and Fish Oil (4g/day).

Comments: This is a stronger version of a cutting/lean mass building cycle utilizing stanozolol. The dosage used here is substantially higher than the first stanozolol cycle, a fact that makes this cycle more properly suited for bodybuilding purposes than Stanozolol Cycle #1. Cardiovascular and hepatic strain will be more notable, and visible side effects more pronounced, than the first cycle. There should be no need to addition an estrogen maintenance drug.

Week	Stanozolol
1	20 mg/day
2	20 mg/day
3	25 mg/day
4	25 mg/day
5	25 mg/day
6	25 mg/day

Stack Cycles

Deca/Dianabol Cycle #1 (Mass)

Products: 10 mL 200 mg/mL nandrolone decanoate

100 tablets 5 mg methandrostenolone

All Weeks: Liver Support: Liver Stabil, Liv-52, or Essentiale Forte (label recommended dosage).

Cholesterol Support: Lipid Stabil (3 caps/day) and Fish Oil (4g/day).

Estrogen Support: tamoxifen (20-40 mg/day).

Comments: This is an extremely old and widely repeated steroid combination, based on the predominantly anabolic steroid nandrolone decanoate. Methandrostenolone serves as the androgenic component of this stack, and is added during week 3, which is a time that side effects of reduced androgenicity (with the exclusive use of nandrolone decanoate) are commonly noticed, such as loss of libido and sexual dysfunction. The doses used in this cycle are not high by most bodybuilding standards, but are sufficient to impart a noticeable increase in muscle size and strength.

Week	Nandrolone	Methandrostenolone
1	200 mg	
2	200 mg	
3	200 mg	10 mg/day
4	200 mg	10 mg/day
5	300 mg	10 mg/day
6	300 mg	15 mg/day
7	300 mg	15 mg/day
8	300 mg	15 mg/day

Deca/Dianabol Cycle #2 (Mass)

Products: 20 mL 200 mg/mL nandrolone decanoate

200 tablets 5 mg methandrostenolone

All Weeks: Liver Support: Liver Stabil, Liv-52, or Essentiale Forte (label recommended dosage).

Cholesterol Support: Lipid Stabil (3 caps/day) and Fish Oil (4g/day).

Estrogen Support: tamoxifen (20-40 mg/day).

Comments: A more popular manifestation of the Deca/Dianabol Cycle, with more commonly accepted dosages for a moderately experienced steroid user. Incidences of side effects are expected to be higher at these dosages, although overall this stack is likely to be less problematic than a combination of testosterone and oxymetholone.

Week	Nandrolone	Methandrostenolone
1	400 mg	
2	400 mg	
3	400 mg	10 mg/day
4	400 mg	10 mg/day
5	400 mg	20 mg/day
6	400 mg	20 mg/day
7	400 mg	20 mg/day
8	400 mg	20 mg/day
9	400 mg	20 mg/day
10	400 mg	20 mg/day

Testosterone/Anadrol Cycle (Mass)

Products: 20 mL 200 mg/mL testosterone (enanthate or cypionate)

100 tablets 50 mg oxymetholone

All Weeks: Liver Support: Liver Stabil, Liv-52, or Essentiale Forte (label recommended dosage).

Cholesterol Support: Lipid Stabil (3 caps/day) and Fish Oil (4g/day).

Estrogen Support: tamoxifen (20-40 mg/day).

Comments: A combination of testosterone and oxymetholone is generally regarded as the most potent 2-drug stack for gaining raw muscle mass. Both drugs will present significant estrogenicity, and will be likely to induce gynecomastia quickly unless an estrogen maintenance drug such as tamoxifen is used. Inexperienced steroid users have been known to gain over 25-30 pounds on a cycle such as this. Water retention will be very high with this stack, however, and a rapid loss of water weight (possibly up to 10 pounds or more) is expected soon after the cycle is discontinued.

Week	Testosterone	Oxymetholone
1	200 mg	
2	400 mg	
3	400 mg	50 mg/day
4	400 mg	50 mg/day
5	400 mg	100 mg/day
6	500 mg	100 mg/day
7	500 mg	100 mg/day
8	500 mg	100 mg/day
9	500 mg	100 mg/day
10	200 mg	100 mg/day

Testosterone/Deca Cycle (Mass)

Products: 10 mL 200 mg/mL nandrolone decanoate

10 mL 200 mg/mL testosterone (enanthate or cypionate)

All Weeks: Cholesterol Support: Lipid Stabil (3 caps/day) and Fish Oil (4g/day).

Estrogen Support: tamoxifen (20-40 mg/day) or anastrozole (.5-1mg/day).

Comments: Testosterone with nandrolone is considered to be one of the most fundamental 2-drug combination stacks. Nandrolone compliments the androgenic base of testosterone by supplementing additional anabolic activity without strong estrogenicity. The resulting stack is almost as productive as a cycle utilizing a higher dose of testosterone alone, but less problematic in terms of estrogenic side effects such as water retention, gynecomastia, and fat buildup. Estrogen conversion is still formidable enough to warrant the use of an estrogen maintenance drug, however, and this stack remains in the realm of mass building instead of lean mass or cutting.

Week	Testosterone	Nandrolone
1	200 mg	200 mg
2	200 mg	200 mg
3	200 mg	200 mg
4	300 mg	300 mg
5	300 mg	300 mg
6	300 mg	300 mg
7	300 mg	300 mg
8	200 mg	200 mg

Andriol/Anavar Cycle (Lean Mass)

Products: 360 capsules Andriol 40 mg

400 tablets oxandrolone 2.5 mg

All Weeks: Liver Support: Liver Stabil, Liv-52, or Essentiale Forte (label recommended dosage).

Cholesterol Support: Lipid Stabil (3 caps/day) and Fish Oil (4g/day).

Comments: This is an effective but mild orals-only lean mass building cycle. Andriol is used as the androgenic base, but in doses that do not greatly exceed normal therapeutic levels. Oxandrolone is non-aromatizable, so significantly elevated estrogenicity is unlikely. Tamoxifen 10-20 mg per day may be used should the testosterone dosage turn out to be problematic. This stack is popular among older men and those not wishing to use injections. The principle drawback with this stack is that it uses a c-17 alpha alkylated oral, and therefore has elevated cardiovascular and liver toxicity. This combination also tends to be very expensive, and is far less cost effective than many stacks based on an injectable testosterone.

Week	Andriol	Oxandrolone
1	240 mg/day	15 mg/day
2	240 mg/day	15 mg/day
3	240 mg/day	15 mg/day
4	240 mg/day	20 mg/day
5	280 mg/day	20 mg/day
6	280 mg/day	20 mg/day
7	280 mg/day	20 mg/day
8	280 mg/day	20 mg/day

Anabolic-Androgenic Bi-Phasic Stack (Lean Mass)

Products: 18 mL methenolone enanthate 100 mg/mL

50 mL boldenone undecylenate 50 mg/mL

20 mL testosterone (enanthate or cypionate) 200 mg/mL

All Weeks: Cholesterol Support: Lipid Stabil (3 caps/day) and Fish Oil (4g/day).

Estrogen Support: tamoxifen (20-40 mg/day) or anastrozole (.5-1mg/day).

Comments: This is a 3-month non-liver-toxic cycle that has 2 distinct phases, mass and lean mass/cutting. The first 6 weeks of training and diet are focused on mass building. Significant estrogenicity will be present in these weeks, and may necessitate the use of tamoxifen or an aromatase inhibitor such as anastrozole to prevent gynecomastia and excessive water retention. Estrogen maintenance drugs may be reduced or possibly eliminated after the start of phase 2, which focuses on increasing the androgen to estrogen ratio and solidifying the muscle mass. A maintenance dosage of testosterone remains during this second phase, in a effort to prevent sexual dysfunction or loss of libido, which often occurs with the use of predominantly anabolic steroids alone.

Week	Testosterone	Boldenone	Methenolone
1	500 mg	200 mg	
2	500 mg	200 mg	
3	600 mg	200 mg	
4	600 mg	200 mg	
5	600 mg	200 mg	
6	600 mg	200 mg	
7	100 mg	200 mg	300 mg
8	100 mg	200 mg	300 mg
9	100 mg	200 mg	300 mg
10	100 mg	200 mg	300 mg
11	100 mg	200 mg	300 mg
12	100 mg	200 mg	300 mg

Testosterone/Anadrol/Trenbolone Cycle (Mass)

Products: 30 mL 200 mg/mL testosterone (enanthate or cypionate)

20 mL 75 mg/mL trenbolone acetate

100 tablets 50 mg oxymetholone

All Weeks: Liver Support: Liver Stabil, Liv-52, or Essentiale Forte (label recommended dosage).

Cholesterol Support: Lipid Stabil (3 caps/day) and Fish Oil (4g/day).

Estrogen Support: tamoxifen (20 mg/day) and anastrozole (.5-1mg/day).

Comments: One of the more extreme mass building cycles in common use among bodybuilders. This stack will impart rapid gains in raw muscle size and strength. This drug combination is highly prone to causing estrogenic and androgenic side effects, including extremely significant levels of water retention. Gynecomastia may also be an issue very early into the cycle. The use of an aromatase inhibitor is likely to be necessary to cut down on the conversion of testosterone to estrogen. Oxymetholone is highly estrogenic but does not aromatize, however, which may necessitate the additional use of tamoxifen. Although often highly problematic with regard to side effects, and therefore rarely recommended to beginners, few steroid combinations can compare to testosterone, oxymetholone, and trenbolone for building rapid muscle mass.

Week	Testosterone	Oxymetholone	Trenbolone
1	300 mg		150 mg
2	600 mg		150 mg
3	600 mg	50 mg	150 mg
4	600 mg	50 mg	150 mg
5	600 mg	100 mg	150 mg
6	600 mg	100 mg	150 mg
7	600 mg	100 mg	150 mg
8	600 mg	100 mg	150 mg
9	600 mg	100 mg	150 mg
10	600 mg	100 mg	150 mg
11	300 mg		

Masteron/Primobolan (Lean Mass/Cutting)

Products: 20 mL 100 mg/mL drostanolone propionate

20 mL 100 mg/mL methenolone enanthate

All Weeks: Cholesterol Support: Lipid Stabil (3 caps/day) and Fish Oil (4g/day)

Comments: This is an effective stack for hardening, cutting, and gaining lean muscle mass. Neither agent is capable of converting to estrogen, so this cycle should significantly elevate the androgen to estrogen ratio. This may assist in the breakdown of fat tissue, enhancing muscle definition. This stack should not present significant liver toxicity, although cholesterol ratios may be significantly altered in light of reduced estrogenic activity.

Week	Drostanolone	Methenolone
1	200 mg	200 mg
2	200 mg	200 mg
3	200 mg	200 mg
4	300 mg	300 mg
5	300 mg	300 mg
6	300 mg	300 mg
7	300 mg	300 mg
8	200 mg	200 mg

Winstrol/Proviron/Trenbolone Cycle (Lean Mass/Cutting)

Products: 250 tablets stanozolol 5 mg

100 tablets mesterolone 25 mg

20 mL trenbolone acetate 75 mg/mL

All Weeks: Liver Support: Liver Stabil, Liv-52, or Essentiale Forte (label recommended dosage).

Cholesterol Support: Lipid Stabil (3 caps/day) and Fish Oil (4g/day).

Comments: Stanozolol and trenbolone are popular steroids during cutting phases of training, and impart strong anabolic and moderate androgenic effects with no significant estrogenicity. This combination helps to impart a strong fat loss/definition-enhancing effect. Two 25 mg tablets of mesterolone have been added per day to supplement additional androgenic activity, which should help maintain normal libido and sexual functioning. Additional anti-estrogenic drugs should not be necessary. Some more aggressive competitive bodybuilders may enhance this cycle by adding rHGH, clenbuterol, and/or thyroid hormones. Higher doses of the individual steroids may also be used, but are expected to impart stronger cardiovascular and hepatic strain, and are generally not advised.

Week	Stanozolol	Mesterolone	Trenbolone
1	20 mg/day	25 mg/day	150 mg
2	20 mg/day	50 mg/day	150 mg
3	20 mg/day	50 mg/day	150 mg
4	20 mg/day	50 mg/day	150 mg
5	25 mg/day	50 mg/day	225 mg
6	25 mg/day	50 mg/day	225 mg
7	25 mg/day	50 mg/day	225 mg
8	25 mg/day	50 mg/day	225 mg

PCT: Post-Cycle Therapy

It is called the "post cycle crash", and is one of the more unwelcome aspects of steroid use. As the saying goes, there is a price to be paid for everything, and in the case of steroids, one of those prices (a temporary one anyway) is your natural hormone production. What happens is quite simple; when you take steroids your body stops making them. Once you stop taking steroids, you can be left with a gap until your body starts making its own again. Here, you can be faced with low levels of androgens and normal levels of corticosteroids. Your body will (should) eventually recognize and fix the imbalance, but it can take weeks or even months. This gap is a bad place to be physiologically, as without normal androgen levels to balance the catabolic effects of corticosteroids, a good deal of your new muscle mass may be lost. To help your body maintain its size, you will want to restore endogenous testosterone production quickly. The methods for doing this seem to be different everywhere you look: "Take HCG, don't take HCG, use an aromatase inhibitor, just take Clomid, forget Clomid and just take Nolvadex." What option is really best? Without an understanding of exactly what is going on in your body, and why certain compounds help to correct the situation, choosing the right Post-Cycle Therapy (PCT) program can be quite confusing. In this section, the roles of anti-estrogens and HCG during this delicate window of time are discussed, while detailing an effective strategy for their use.

The HPTA Axis

The Hypothalamic-Pituitary-Testicular Axis, or HPTA for short, is the thermostat for your body's natural production of testosterone. Too much testosterone, and the furnace will shut off. Not enough, and the heat is turned up (to put it very simply). For the purposes of our discussion, we can look at this regulating process as having three levels. At the top is the hypothalamic region of the brain, which releases the hormone GnRH (Gonadotropin-Releasing Hormone) when it senses a need for more testosterone. GnRH sends a signal to the second level of the axis, the pituitary, which releases Luteinizing Hormone in response. LH for short, this hormone stimulates the testes (level three) to secrete testosterone. The same sex steroids (testosterone, estrogen) that are produced serve to counterbalance things, by providing negative feedback signals (primarily to the hypothalamus and pituitary) to lower the secretion of testosterone. Synthetic steroids send the same negative feedback. This quick background of the testosterone-regulating axis is necessary to furthering our discussion, as we need to first look at the underlying mechanisms involved before we can understand why natural recovery of the HPTA post-cycle is a slow process. Only then can we implement an ancillary drug program to effectively deal with it.

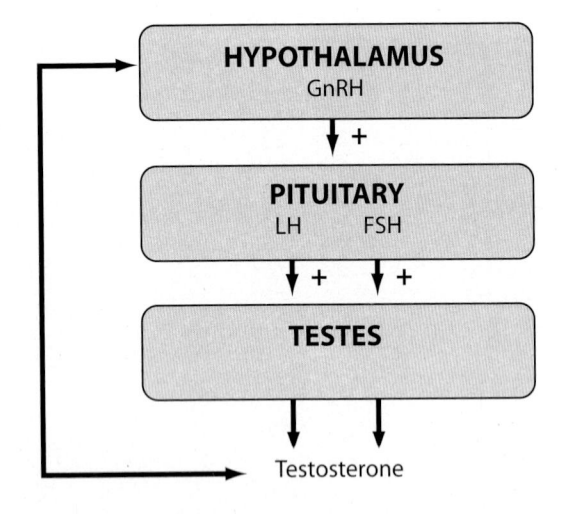

The Hypothalamic-Pituitary-Testicular Axis: The hypothalamus releases Gonadotropin Releasing Hormone (GnRH), which stimulates the pituitary to release luteinizing hormone (LH) and follicle stimulating hormone (FSH). This promotes the release of testosterone from the testes. Testosterone, as well as estrogens and progestins, in turn cause negative feedback inhibition at the hypothalamus (and to some extent the pituitary), lowering the output of gonadotropins and testosterone when too much hormone is present.

Testicular Desensitization

Although steroids suppress testosterone production primarily by lowering the level of gonadotropic hormones, the big roadblock to a restored HPTA after we come off the drugs is surprisingly not LH. This problem was made clearly evident in a study published back in 1975.[348] Here, blood parameters, including testosterone and LH levels, were monitored in male subjects who were given testosterone enanthate injections of 250 mg weekly for 21 weeks. Subjects remained under investigation for an additional 18 weeks after the drug was discontinued. At the start of the study, LH levels became suppressed in direct relation to the rise in testosterone, which was to be expected. Things looked very different, however, once the steroids had been withdrawn (see Figure I). LH levels went on the rise quickly (by the 3rd week), while testosterone barely budged for quite some time. In fact, on average it was more than 10 weeks before any noticeable movement in testosterone production started at all. This lack of correlation makes clear that the problem in getting androgen levels restored is not necessarily the level of LH, but more so testicular atrophy and desensitization to LH. After a period of inactivation, the testes have lost mass (atrophied), making them unable to perform the required workload. The protracted post-cycle window can, likewise, no longer be looked at as one of low testosterone and low LH. Much of it actually involves low testosterone and normal (even high) LH.

The Role of Anti-Estrogens

It is important to understand that anti-estrogens alone are inadequate to restore normal endogenous testosterone production after a cycle. These agents ordinarily increase LH levels by blocking the negative feedback of estrogens. But LH rebounds quickly on its own post-cycle, without help. Plus, there is not an elevated level of estrogen for anti-estrogens to block during this window, as testosterone (now suppressed) is a major substrate used

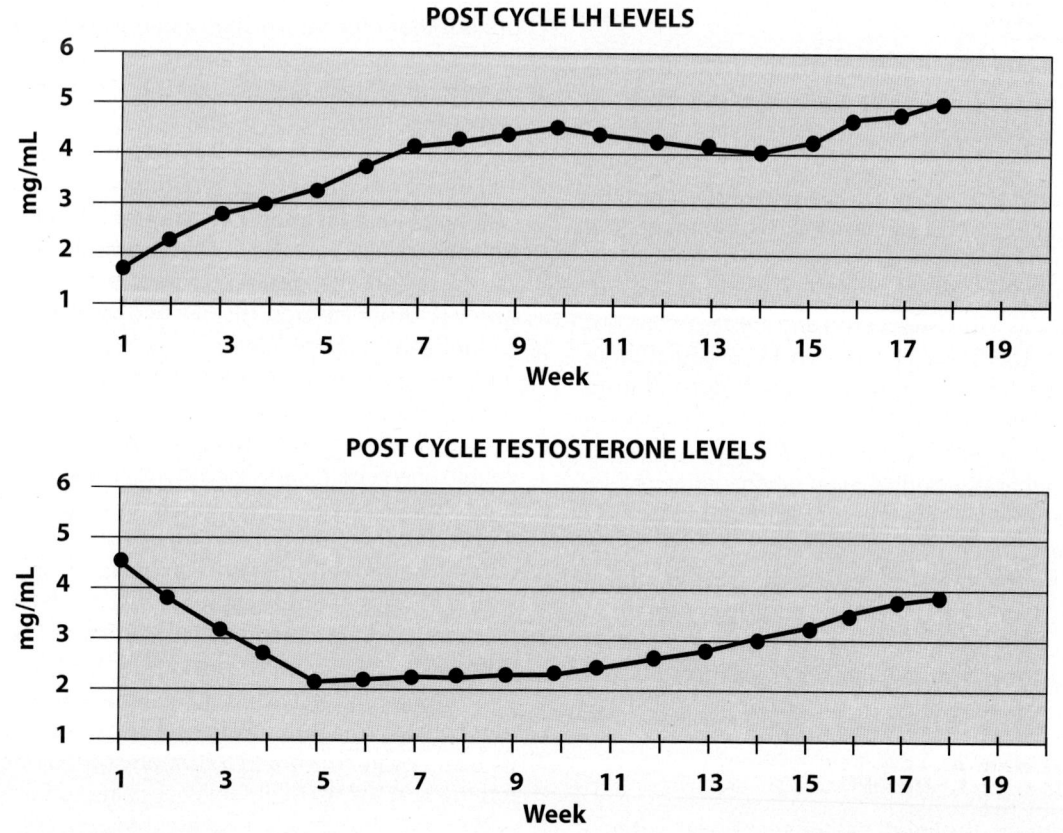

Figure I. LH and Testosterone measurements starting 1 week after the last injection of 250 mg of testosterone enanthate (pretreated measures were 5 mU/mL and 4.5 ng/mL respectively). Note that between weeks 1 and 5, as testosterone levels are declining due to the cessation of exogenous androgen administration, LH levels are already rebounding. From weeks 5 to 10, testosterone levels remain at or very near baseline, despite the substantial increases in LH by this point. No notable rebound in testosterone is noted until after the 10-week mark.

for the synthesis of estrogens in men. Serum estrogen levels are actually lower here, not higher. Any estrogen rebound that occurs post-cycle, likewise, happens with a rebound in testosterone levels, not prior to it (there is an imbalance in the ratio of androgens to estrogens post cycle, but this is another topic altogether). On their own, we are seeing no mechanism in which anti-estrogenic drugs can effectively help here. I can, however, see why this fact would be easy to overlook. The medical literature is filled with references showing anti-estrogenic drugs like Clomid and Nolvadex to increase LH and testosterone levels in men, and in normal situations they indeed perform this function fairly well. Combine this with the fact that just as many studies can be found to show that steroid use lowers LH when suppressing testosterone, and we can see how easy it would be to jump to the conclusion that we need to focus on LH. We would miss the true problem, testicular desensitization, unless we were really looking into the actual recovery rates of the hormones involved. When we do, we immediately see little value in focusing solely on anti-estrogenic drugs.

The Role of HCG

With anti-estrogens alone proving to be ineffective, we are left to focus on a very different level of the HPTA in order to hasten recovery: the testes. For this we will need the injectable drug HCG. If you are not familiar, HCG, or Human Chorionic Gonadotropin, is a prescription fertility agent that mimics the body's natural LH. Although the testes are equally desensitized to this drug as they are to LH (they work through the same receptor), we are administering it as a measured drug and are, therefore, not constrained by the limits of our own LH production. In other words, we can give ourselves a good dose of drug (as much LH as we need, really), shocking the testes with unnaturally high levels of stimulation. We want it to reach a level above what our bodies, even when supported by anti-estrogens, could do on its own. The result should be a more rapid restoration of original testicular mass, which would allow normal levels of testosterone to be output much sooner than without such an ancillary program in place. What we are looking at now is HCG actually being the pivotal post-cycle drug, with anti-estrogens playing more of a supportive role.

The PoWeR PCT Program

The PCT program outlined below represents what I consider to be an ideal and effective post-cycle program. It was developed by the doctors at the Program for Wellness Restoration (PoWeR), who have a formidable history helping patients recover normal hormonal functioning following steroid therapy. One of the key doctors on this program, Dr. Michael Scally, claims to have successfully treated more than 100 cases of hypogonadism/hypogonadotrophic hypogonadism, and is very well known in the field of androgen replacement therapy. PoWeR published this program as part of a recent clinical study, which involved 19 healthy male subjects who were taking suprahysiological (highly suppressive) doses of testosterone cypionate and nandrolone decanoate for 12 weeks. Their HPGA Normalization Protocol focuses on the combined use of HCG, Nolvadex, and Clomid, and is perhaps the only clinically documented post-cycle therapy program to be found in the medical literature (it is amazing how little attention has been paid to hormone normalization in clinical medicine). The most notable variation from a classic PCT stack, such that I have been a longtime supporter of, is the combined use of two anti-estrogens. In this case I cannot say that there is a disadvantage to such use; perhaps it is indeed the better option.

Examining the program closely, we note that the testes are hit hard with HCG at the onset of therapy. Its intake, however, is limited to only 16 days. The doctors undoubtedly recognize that when HCG is taken for too long or at too high a dosage, it can desensitize the LH receptor.[349] This would only further exacerbate the post-cycle problem, not help it. Anti-estrogens are used during and after HCG, with a dosage of 10 mg of Nolvadex and 100 mg of Clomid per day rounding out this compliment of drugs. Clomid is used for a shorter period of time than Nolvadex, likely because of the desensitizing effect it too can have (on the pituitary gland) with continued use. Among other things, these two anti-estrogens will continue to foster LH release as testosterone levels start to go back up, as well as combat any potential estrogenic side effects that may be caused by HCG's up-regulation of testicular aromatase activity.[350] Although in the first couple of weeks the anti-estrogens probably do very little, they should be much more helpful towards the middle and end of the program. During this clinical investigation, normal hormonal function was restored in all subjects within 45 days of drug cessation. This is a definite success, far more favorable than the protracted recovery window noted in studies without post-cycle therapy, such as the 250 mg/week testosterone enanthate investigation highlighted in Figure I. For me, I believe such a detailed recovery program should follow any serious steroid cycle. It is the best way to maintain your gains at their maximum, and that is, after all, what we are after.

HPGA Normalization Protocol (PoWeR)

	Days
Nolvadex	45
Clomid	30
HCG	16

Day After Drug Cessation

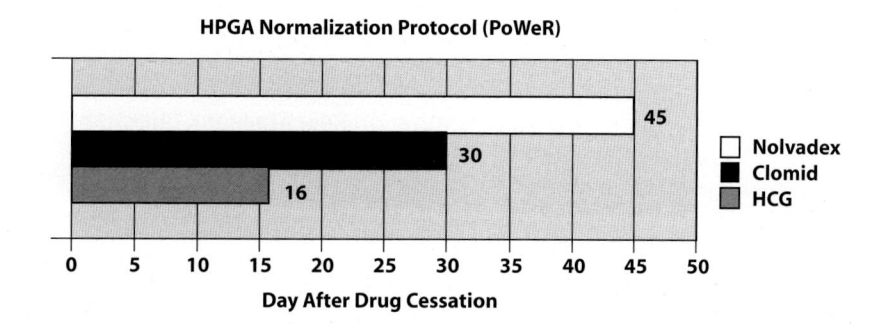

Protocols: Human chorionic gonadotropin (hCG) is taken at 2500IU every other day for 16 days. Clomiphene citrate 50 mg is taken twice per day for 30 days. Tamoxifen citrate is taken 20 mg per day for 45 days.

Injection Protocols

Anabolic/androgenic steroid injections are always given deep in the muscle (intramuscular). Some other performance-enhancing drugs such as human growth hormone and insulin injections are given by injection in the fat layer between the skin and muscle (subcutaneous). The protocols for both injection types are provided. Improper injection technique can result in health complications such as inflammation, bacterial abscess or other infection, scar tissue development, septic shock, or other tissue or nerve injury. Furthermore, the sharing of needles or vials may result in the transmission of blood-borne pathogens including HIV and hepatitis. It is important to closely follow accepted sterility and safety practices for every injection, including the proper disposal of all equipment immediately after use.

General Preparation:

1. Make sure you have all the necessary supplies.

Intramuscular Injection:

(1) 3mL syringe

(1) 22-25g 1-1.5" needle for administering the injection

(1) 21g 1-1.5" needle for drawing solution (if using a multi-dose vial)

(2) Alcohol pads

(1) Dry cotton ball

(1) Plastic bandage

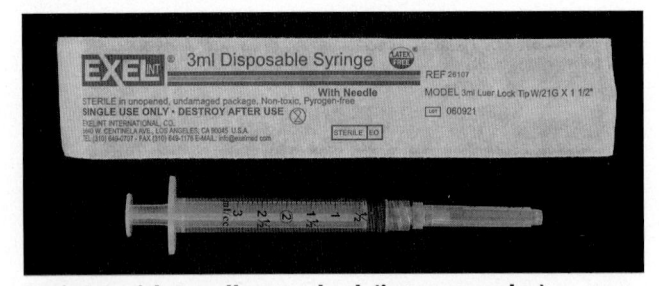

Syringe with needle attached. (intramuscular)

Subcutaneous Injection:

(1) Insulin syringe with needle attached (.5-1mL 27-30g)

(2) Alcohol pads

(1) Dry cotton ball

(1) Plastic bandage

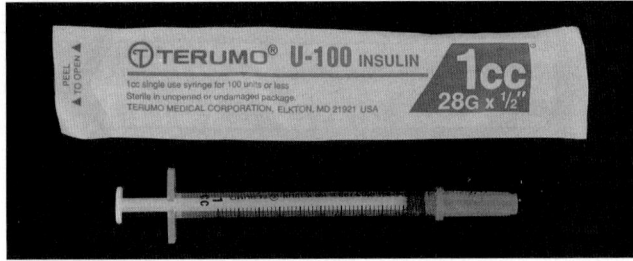

Syringe with needle (insulin)

2. If applicable, keep the administration needle cold by leaving it in the freezer for at least one hour before opening. This will help dull the pinch of penetration.

3. Select a well-lit room with a clean hard surface such as a tabletop or counter to administer the injection.

4. Wash hands thoroughly with soap and warm water.

5. Assure that all injection equipment is sealed and unused. Never reuse needles. Double check the expiration dates on all medications.

6. Clean top of vial thoroughly with an alcohol pad, if applicable. Let air dry for 15 seconds.

Precautions: Do not use injection equipment that is used or has been exposed to air during storage. Never share needles or multi-dose vials. Discard unused portions of the drug at the recommended time.

Drawing Solution into Syringe:

1. Remove syringe from packaging. Attach drawing needle, if applicable.

2. If using a multi-dose vial, fill syringe with air in the amount you are withdrawing. This will help stabilize the pressure and make drawing easier.

3. If using an ampule, break open and place flat on a hard surface. The use of a paper towel to cover the glass top may make breaking easier. Draw solution. Skip below steps and go to Intramuscular or Subcutaneous Injection

Procedure.

4. If using a vial, insert needle through the rubber stopper at a 90-degree angle. Turn the vial upside down with needle attached. Inject air. Slowly withdraw desired amount of solution. You may lightly tap the side of the needle to dislodge air bubbles. Note that small air bubbles are not harmful.

5. Remove needle and syringe from vial, if applicable. Replace cap on the end of needle.

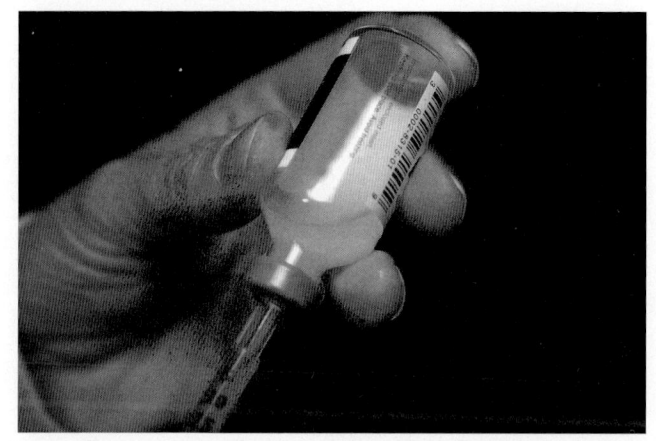

Keep fingers away from needle when drawing.

6. Remove drawing needle and replace with new administration needle, if applicable. This is highly advised with multi-dose vials, as passage through the rubber stopper will have dulled the needle considerably. Remove any air in the tip of the needle, and prepare for injection.

7. Place capped needle back inside wrapper and place on clean surface.

Precautions: Never touch the tip of the exposed syringe, the needle, or the top of the vial stopper after it has been cleaned with alcohol. If you come into contact with these surfaces you should consider the materials contaminated, and should not use them for injection.

Intramuscular Injection Procedure:

Used for all anabolic/androgenic steroid injections.

1. Thoroughly clean the intended site of injection with second alcohol pad. Preferred locations are the upper outer quadrant of the buttocks, or the outer side of the thigh. Let air dry for 15 seconds.

2. Remove needle cap. With free hand, stretch the skin around the site of injection with two fingers. Move the skin over the muscle to the side by 1-1.5" (Z-Track method).

3. In a swift motion, insert the needle into the target muscle at a 90-degree angle with the dominant hand. Make sure the needle is deep within the muscle.

4. Pull back on the plunger (aspirate). If the syringe fills with blood you have hit a blood vessel, and the injection should be aborted.

5. Inject the medication slowly into the muscle.

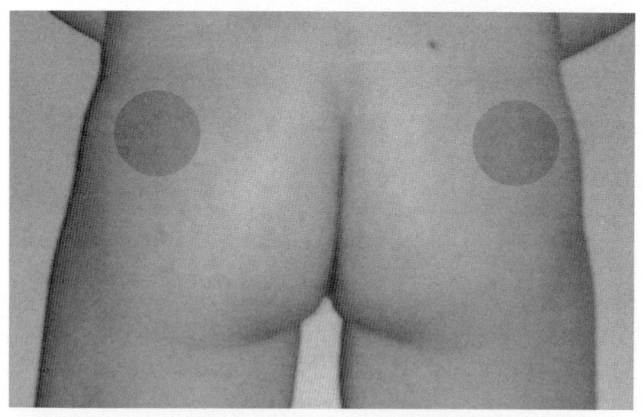

Upper/Outer buttocks is the preferred site for IM injection.

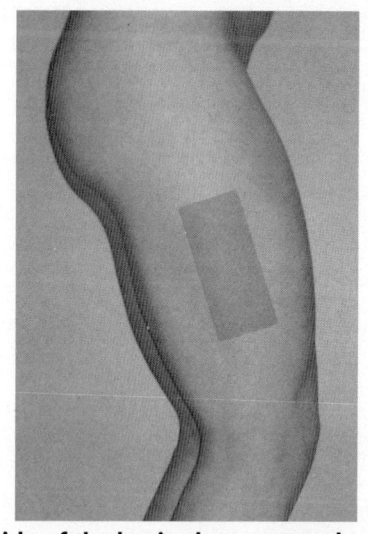

The outer side of the leg is also commonly used.

6. Withdraw the syringe. Release the skin with your other hand. The skin and subcutaneous tissue will rebound, which helps close off the needle shaft and prevent leaking.

7. Dry injection site with dry cotton ball. Cover with plastic bandage if necessary.

Precautions: Never inject into skin that is discolored, broken, or irritated, or if there are lumps, knots, or feelings of pain in the area. Do not inject more than 3mL at one time. Rotate the site of injection so that you do not inject in the same muscle more than once every two weeks.

Subcutaneous Injection Procedure:

1. Thoroughly clean the intended site of injection with second alcohol pad. The preferred location is the lower abdominal region. Let air dry for 15 seconds.

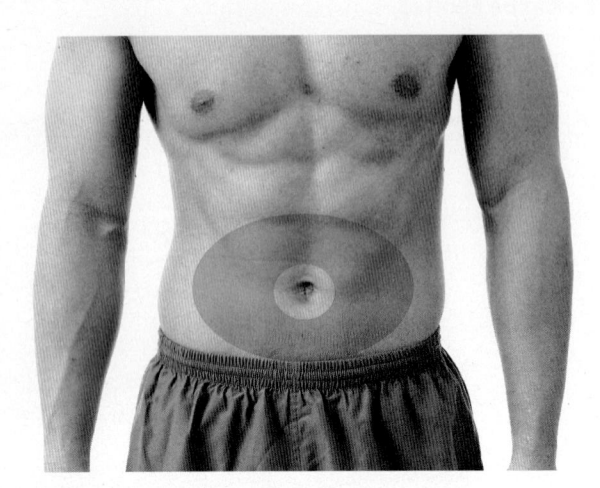

Shaded area denotes site for abdominal subcutaneous injection.

2. Remove needle cap. With free hand, pinch the skin around the site of injection so it is lifted off the muscle.

3. In a swift motion, insert the needle into the target area at a 45-degree angle with dominant hand. Make sure the needle rests within the subcutaneous tissues between the skin and muscle.

4. Inject the medication slowly into the subcutaneous tissue. Do not aspirate.

5. Withdraw the syringe. Release the skin with your other hand.

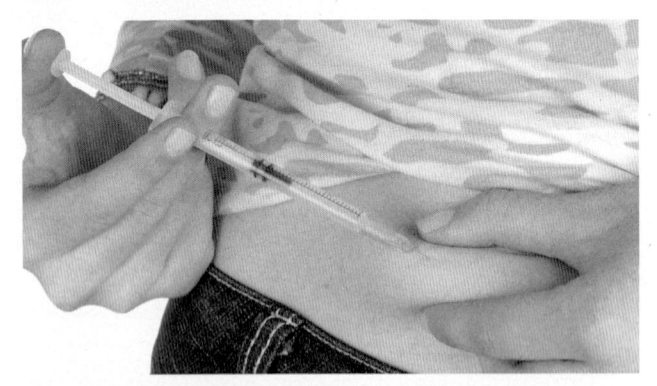

The skin is pinched upwards to facilitate injection into the subcutaneous tissues.

6. Dry injection site with dry cotton ball. Cover with plastic bandage if necessary.

Precautions: Never inject into skin that is discolored, broken, or irritated, or if there are lumps, knots, or feelings of pain in the area. Do not inject more than 1mL at one time. Rotate the site of injection each time so that you are at least 1" away from the last site, and do not return to a previous site until all other available sites have been used. This will help prevent overuse of the same injection area.

Frequently Asked Questions

1) How much weight can someone expect to gain during the first cycle of steroids?

Provided dosing is sufficient, a steroid user can expect to make the most significant progress during their first cycle. Although this will vary from person to person, it is not uncommon for someone to gain 20 pounds of weight or more during a 6-8 week period of AAS use. Some of this may be water retention, although a solid gain of more than 10-15 pounds of muscle mass is possible.

2) Are the gains from steroid use temporary?

Yes, and no. Steroids can help you do two basic things with regard to muscle growth. First, they can allow you to more rapidly reach your genetic limits for muscle growth. Provided you continue to train actively, eat properly, and use an effective PCT program, you should be able to maintain at your genetic limit indefinitely. So in this regard, the early gains do not have to be temporary.

Later, steroids can allow you to push well beyond your genetic limits. It is important to emphasize this, as extreme physical development cannot be maintained long-term without the repeat administration of anabolic substances. The body will always revert back towards its normal metabolic limits once AAS are removed. In this context, some of the gains will not be permanent.

Steroids do permanently alter the physiology of your muscles by adding more cellular nuclei. With higher nuclei content, each muscle cell can manage its volume more efficiently, which allows more rapid expansion. Even after a long period of complete abstinence from training and AAS, the nuclei remain.[351] This may provide a "muscle memory" effect, allowing you to reach your genetic limit (perhaps a slightly extended limit) faster than if you had never used AAS in the past. So in this regard, there are lasting benefits beyond the temporary increase in muscle size itself.

3) Can steroids make me look like a professional bodybuilder?

If you have the underlying genetics to allow for this extreme muscle growth, this may be possible with a lot of hard work and dedication. If you are like the vast majority of people, however, steroids will not be able to make you look like a professional bodybuilder. Genetics are a big factor in determining the ultimate limits to your physique, even in an enhanced state. Many people use steroids and look very big and impressive because of it, but very few users are able to make it to the stage of a professional bodybuilding show.

4) How dangerous is an isolated cycle of steroids?

Anabolic/androgenic steroids are among the safest drugs available, at least in a short-term sense. Fatal overdose is not reasonably possible, and the negative health changes such as alterations in cholesterol, blood pressure, hematocrit, and blood clotting (among other things) are very unlikely to manifest in serious bodily harm or death after an isolated cycle. There are rare deaths from such things as stroke and liver cancer in short-term abusers, but such occurrences are statistically extremely rare in light of the millions of people that use these drugs. If you had to comparatively rate the acute risks of AAS abuse, they would be slightly higher than marijuana, but far less than virtually all other illicit narcotics.

5) How dangerous is long-term steroid use?

The long-term use of steroids for nonmedical reasons can be a significantly unhealthy practice. It has been difficult, however, to quantify the exact risk. The main issue is the fact that AAS abuse can promote heart disease, the number one killer of men. Heart disease is a slow progressive disease, which may build for decades without symptoms. Steroid abuse may accelerate the silent process of plaque deposition in the arteries, and also induce other changes in the cardiovascular system that can increase susceptibility to stroke or heart attack. If death finally occurs, however, it will be difficult for a medical examiner to pinpoint AAS as the cause; too many variables play a role in the etiology of cardiovascular disease. The vast majority of deaths where AAS have contributed go unreported for this reason. The exact mortality rates of long-term steroid abusers have, likewise, been difficult to calculate. According to one population-based study, steroid abusers had a 4.6 times greater risk of early death from all causes including suicide compared to non-users.[352] It is unknown, however, how applicable this number is to the full steroid-using population. It is especially important to closely monitor cardiovascular disease and other health risk factors if long-term steroid use is a practice you will follow.

6) Can steroids be used to enhance an athletic career safely?

The nonmedical use of AAS by definition cannot be defined as a safe practice. However, it can be argued that anabolic/androgenic steroids can be used with high relative safety, even over a period of many years. The guidelines of steroid harm reduction are important to minimizing the negative health effects of these drugs. Provided an individual follows these guidelines and is careful with drug selection, dosages, and durations of intake, follows a diet low in saturated fats, cholesterol, sugar, and refined carbohydrates, actively trains with both resistance and cardiovascular exercise, and uses cholesterol support supplements such as fish oils and Lipid Stabil during all cycles, it may be difficult in many cases to argue high tangible health risks. It takes a great deal of involvement and planning to use AAS in this manner, which is always advised.

7) What are the safest steroids for men?

Testosterone, whatever the form, tends to be the safest steroid for men. When the dose remains within the moderately supratherapeutic range (such as 200-400 mg of an injectable testosterone ester per week), alterations in cardiovascular risks factors are noticed, but not extreme. Some of this has to do with the beneficial cardiovascular effects of estrogen in men. Also considered fairly safe are the common injectable steroids boldenone, nandrolone, and methenolone. Isolating your use to these drugs is recommended over using the full spectrum of oral and injectable steroids.

8) What steroids will not cause hair loss?

For those with a genetic predisposition to hair loss, all anabolic/androgenic steroids are capable of accelerating the process. Slowing the onset of this during AAS use requires a focus on reducing relative androgenicity in the scalp. This can be accomplished with the use of predominantly anabolic drugs such as nandrolone, oxandrolone, or methenolone. Alternately, moderate doses of testosterone can be used with finasteride, a drug that reduces DHT conversion (and androgenic amplification) in the scalp. Still, those genetically prone to hair loss can have problems with any steroid, and are always advised to limit dosing, drug intake durations, and monitor effects on the hairline closely.

9) What are the safest steroids for women?

Women are generally most concerned with the virilizing (masculinizing) effects of anabolic/androgenic steroids. The least virilizing agents are those with the highest relative anabolic to androgenic effect, such as nandrolone, oxandrolone, and methenolone. Care must always be taken, however, as all AAS are based on male sex steroids, and as such can cause masculinizing effects in women.

10) Should I rotate my steroids every few weeks to prevent receptor downregulation?

No, this is not necessary. Anabolic/androgenic steroids all work primarily by attaching to and activating the same receptor. As such, you do not gain anything by switching to a new compound that works via stimulating the same receptor. If tolerance were induced by one AAS compound, it would be extended to all compounds. The plateau effect that is noticed 6-8 weeks into most cycles is poorly understood, but likely related to the new metabolic limits placed on muscle cells under the influence of a certain AAS dosages, not insensitivity to AAS. Classic downregulation does not occur with these drugs, and even if it did, rotating steroids would not prevent it.

11) How likely am I to find real steroids on the black market? Does it matter?

Although exact figures are difficult to calculate, real pharmaceutical anabolic/androgenic steroids are estimated to represent half or less of the products commonly circulated on the black market. In many regions this figure may be below 25%. The majority of products sold presently are counterfeit copies of real AAS, or products made and labeled by underground laboratories. It does matter, because the quality of nonmedical AAS cannot be ensured. These products are generally not advised for use. Given the potential issues with drug safety, it is worthwhile to spend the extra time and money on steroid products you can be assured came from legitimate pharmaceutical channels.

12) What do the anabolic and androgenic reference numbers under the profile for each steroid mean?

These numbers come from early studies measuring the effect of each steroid on certain muscle and sex organ tissues of animals, usually mice. These numbers are useful for assessing the relative anabolic to androgenic balance of each drug in humans. They are not as accurate at assessing the total muscle building potential of each steroid, however, and should not be taken as absolute ratings of potency.

Understanding Blood Tests

The abuse of anabolic/androgenic steroids can have a number of potential negative health consequences, most commonly with regard to cardiovascular and liver health. These issues, however, can almost always be identified in blood work well before physical symptoms become apparent. Cardiovascular disease, for example, is a disease that can take decades to progress. Cholesterol and triglyceride testing can be used to identify and control early risk factors and decisions that would support the disease over time. Liver damage is also generally obvious in liver enzyme tests well before it becomes visibly noticeable to the person. The same holds true for many areas of general health. If you are using steroids, the regular assessment of health with blood work, and the adjustment of therapy when the results call for it, is regarded as the most effective strategy for reducing health risks.

Blood tests with regard to anabolic/androgenic steroids are usually conducted in three separate phases. The first phase looks at your health before steroid use. This is done to asses your current condition and risks before any therapy is initiated, and to set baselines for later comparison. The next is on-cycle testing, which is used to assess the direct impact of the anabolic/androgenic steroid use (what the drugs are actually doing to your body while they are being taken). The latter phase of testing is the follow-up, which is conducted to ensure your original state of good health has been restored once the drugs are no longer in the body. We generally refer to these three phases of testing as Baseline, On-Cycle, and Post-Cycle, respectively.

Baseline (Pre-cycle):

Baseline (pre-cycle) testing is generally very broad. This is done to make sure there are no underlying health conditions that may be worsened by anabolic steroids, and to have a baseline for determining the on-cycle and post-cycle impact. To begin with, a profile of steroid hormones (male users only) is done to identify the current natural state. This can be especially important to know for post-cycle follow up, as the range of what is considered normal for testosterone on a standard blood test can be quite broad. If you started on the high end of normal, for example, you might want to make sure you are not stuck on the low end of normal following your cycles. A full liver panel is usually conducted as well, especially if hepatotoxic oral or injectable steroids are planned. Since cardiovascular disease is one of the most tangible risks with long-term steroid use, lipid profiling is always important, and is usually conducted here and during all other phases of testing. Additionally, other general markers of health are generally examined here including blood, kidney, electrolytes, minerals, glucose, and prostate.

Checklist (minimum):

Hormone (Steroid)

Lipids (Standard Full Set)

Full Liver Panel

Blood

Kidney

Electrolytes, Minerals, and Glucose

Prostate

On-Cycle:

On-cycle testing is usually conducted 3 to 4 weeks after steroid therapy began. The individual will generally look at those indicators of health most directly affected by steroid use. A full lipid examination is conducted, and is often regarded as the single most important set of health tests that can be initiated. It is here that the cardiovascular impact of the steroids will begin to become apparent. One should give special consideration to what these results may mean for their health decades down the road if this type of steroid cycle is to be repeated many times over many years. If hepatotoxic drugs are being used, a full liver panel will be examined. It is also recommended to examine other general health markers here such as blood, kidney, electrolytes, minerals, and glucose.

Checklist (Minimum):

Lipids (Standard Full Set)

Liver Panel, if taking hepatotoxic steroid(s)

Blood

Kidney

Electrolytes, Minerals, and Glucose

Post-Cycle

During the post-cycle testing phase it is common to once again look first at the male steroid hormones. The hope here is to obtain values that closely mirror your pre-treatment levels. Note that there will always be some variation based on the time of the day, and even in the day-to-day results. An exact match is probably not feasible. It is also considered a good idea to look at pituitary LH and FSH, because if testosterone levels come back low it will give you and your physician a better understanding of the cause. High LH/FSH and low testosterone (primary hypogonadism) may simply indicate that your testicles have not yet fully restored their mass. Alternately, low LH/FSH can indicate secondary hypogonadism, which is often cause to initiate corrective therapy with an endocrinologist. A run of other general markers of health are also usually conducted here including lipids, liver, blood, kidney, electrolytes, minerals, glucose, and prostate.

Checklist (Minimum):

Hormone (Steroid, LH/FSH)

Lipids (Standard Full Set)

Liver Panel, if taking hepatotoxic steroid(s)

Blood

Electrolytes, Minerals, and Glucose

Prostate

Blood Tests by Category

Hormone

Steroid (male)

Test Name	Reference Range	
Testosterone, Total	241-827	ng/dL
Testosterone, Free	8.7-25.1	pg/mL
Estradiol	10-53	pg/mL

LH/FSH Panel (male)

Test Name	Reference Range	
LH	2.5-9.8	IU/L
FSH	1.2-5.0	IU/L

Thyroid

Test Name	Reference Range	
TSH	.35-5.5	uIU/mL
Thyroxine (T4)	4.5-12.0	ug/dL
T3 Uptake	24-39	%
Free thyroxine index	1.2-4.9	

Steroid: This set of testing should look at both total and free testosterone. The former measure is most commonly used by physicians to identify the androgen level and determine if there is a need for therapy. The latter measure actually represents the fraction of bioavailable (immediately active) testosterone in the body, and is consequently regarded as more important for assessing the present state of androgenicity. Estradiol is the principle active form of estrogen in the body, and has roles both in potential side effects (gynecomastia, water/fat retention) and hormone balance. This is the estrogen marker most often recommended during hormone profiling.

LH/FSH Panel: Luteinizing hormone (LH) and follicle stimulating hormone (FSH) are responsible for stimulating testosterone production and spermatogenesis in the testes. These measures are most relevant when evaluating the cause and potential treatment options for hypogonadism, not the short-term health impact of anabolic-steroid use. The short-term suppression of LH/FSH is expected with anabolic/androgenic steroid administration.

Thyroid: It is regarded as important to get a baseline measure of thyroid activity, usually once per year. Follow up tests during and after steroid use may be an expense some view as unnecessary. Anabolic/androgenic steroid use is unlikely to permanently affect thyroid function, but may slightly elevate thyroid levels during therapy. A misdiagnosis of hyperthyroidism (overactive thyroid) is sometimes made in light of these elevated numbers. The effect of anabolic/androgenic steroid use on thyroid levels should be taken into account before treatment for hyperthyroid is ordered.

Lipids (Cardiovascular)

Anabolic/androgenic steroids can have strong adverse effects on lipids. The abuse of anabolic/androgenic steroids (particularly long-term abuse) can, likewise, increase the risk for developing cardiovascular disease as assessed by these variables. Mitigating these risks with the careful examination of the lipid profile is regarded as one of the most fundamental of all steroid-related blood tests. While far from comprehensive with regard to assessing total heart disease risk, a full panel examining the variables below (and comparing them to your baseline values) can provide a good snapshot of the cardiovascular impact of anabolic/androgenic steroid use. It is important to measure your blood lipids only after 12 hours of fasting, as food intake can skew the outcome of some measures (particularly triglycerides).

Standard Full Set

Test Name	Reference Range	
Triglycerides	0-149	mg/dL
Cholesterol, Total	100-199	mg/dL
HDL Cholesterol	>40	mg/dL
VLDL Cholesterol	5-40	mg/dL
LDL Cholesterol	<100	mg/dL
LDL/HDL Ratio	<3.6	

LDL/HDL Ratio Risk Assessment	men	women
1/2 Average Risk	1.0	1.5
Average Risk	3.6	3.2
2X Average Risk	6.3	5.0
3X Average Risk	8.0	6.1

Additional Testing

Test Name	Reference Range	
C-reactive Protein	<5	mg/dL
Homocysteine (0-30 years)	4.6-8.1	umol/L
Men (30-59)	6.3-11.2	umol/L
Women (30-59)	4.5-7.9	umol/L
>59 years	5.8-11.9	umol/L

Apo Ratio Testing

Apolipoproteins	men	women
apoB/apoA-I Ratio	<.9	<.8

Apo Ratio Risk Assessment	men	women
Low Risk	<.7	<.6
Average Risk	.7-.9	.6-.8
High Risk	>.9	>.8

Standard Full Set: This is a standard full lipid panel examination. Ideally, all values should be kept within the normal ranges at all times during steroid therapy. Note that the LDL/HDL ratio is regarded as the most important measure of the serum lipid tests, as it reflects the ongoing balance between plaque deposition (LDL) and removal (HDL) in the arteries. The LDL/HDL ratio is used to more closely assess heart disease risk in individuals that have elevated LDL or total cholesterol levels.

Additional Testing: C-reactive protein and homocysteine are two additional markers that are important to examining cardiovascular health. C-reactive protein is a key indicator of inflammation in the body, and homocysteine is involved in blood clotting and LDL cholesterol oxidation. It is also advisable to include these two variables in your cardiovascular testing schedule.

Apo Ratio: Apolipoprotein ratio testing is also recommended. Although not commonly used in general medical practice, apolipoprotein testing is increasingly regarded as a more accurate predictor of cardiovascular disease risk than cholesterol testing. Apolipoprotein B (apoB) is found in all LDL particles, and is responsible for attaching these lipoproteins to the artery walls. Apolipoprotein A-I (apoA-I) is found mainly in HDL particles, and is responsible for initiating beneficial reverse cholesterol transport. ApoA-I enables the HDL particles to pull cholesterol from the artery walls and transport them back to the liver. The ratio of apoB to apoA-I, therefore, appears to reflect a much truer measure of the balance of potentially atherogenic and antiatherogenic particles in the blood. A ratio above .9 is generally regarded as indicative of increased cardiovascular disease risk. Lower ratios reflect reduced cardiovascular disease risk assessments.

Liver Function

Test Name	Reference Range	
Albumin	3.5-5.5	g/dL
Globulin	1.5-4.5	g/dL
Total Protein	6.0-8.5	g/dL
Bilirubin	0.1-1.2	mg/dL
GGT (Gamma GT)	<50	IU/L
ALP (Alkaline Phosphatase)	25-150	IU/L
AST (SGOT)	0-40	IU/L
ALT (SGPT)	0-55	IU/L

A full liver panel is important to assessing hepatic strain. The two markers of liver stress most commonly elevated in abusers of anabolic/androgenic steroids are the enzymes alanine aminotransferase (ALT) and aspartate aminotransferase (AST). ALT and AST are necessary to amino acid metabolism in the liver, and will leak into the bloodstream as the liver becomes inflamed or damaged. These two enzymes are generally regarded as important indicators of early steroid-induced liver toxicity. There have been cases in which substantial liver damage has occurred without substantial elevations in ALT and AST, however, so a more detailed examination of liver enzyme values is always advised.

Alkaline phosphatase (ALP) and gamma-glutamyltranspeptidase (GGT) are known as cholestatic liver enzymes, which mean they diminish or stop the flow of bile (a greenish fluid that aids digestion and is produced in the liver). ALP and GGT are important markers of liver health during steroid use, and should be included in regular blood testing. Elevations in ALP and GGT can indicate bile duct obstruction (intrahepatic cholestasis), which refers to a condition where the liver can no longer properly transport and metabolize bile. Intrahepatic cholestasis is a potentially very serious manifestation of steroid-induced liver toxicity, so elevations in ALP and GGT should not be disregarded.

Mild elevations in ALT and AST may be caused by muscle damage (exercise) and not steroid-induced liver toxicity. A comparison to baseline levels will be important in determining the cause. If the only factor that has changed is the addition of a hepatotoxic anabolic steroid (training is otherwise steady), the drug is likely to blame. It is important to remember that ALP and GGT are not always elevated with early liver strain. Therefore, the elevation of any hepatic markers above the reference range (even if only ALT and AST) can indicate liver toxicity, and should be cause to discontinue the offending steroids and reassess risk.

Muscle Enzyme

Test Name
Creatine Kinase

Reference Range
38-174   u/L

The creatine kinase (CK) enzyme is used as a marker of muscle breakdown, kidney damage, and heart damage. High levels usually indicate heart attack or other organ trauma. This enzyme can also become elevated with exercise that breaks down muscle tissue, especially intense endurance or resistance training. Elevated CK levels caused by high intensity training are often mistaken for organ damage. It is important to further examine other markers of kidney and heart heath before such a determination is made. Note that creatine kinase levels may also be useful in determining if liver strain or heavy training is the cause of mild elevations in liver enzymes ALT and AST. Slight increases in ALT and AST caused by muscle damage will usually coincide with elevated CK and normal ALP and GGT levels.

Blood

Test Name	Reference Range	
WBC	4-11	K/MCL
RBC	81-103	FL
Platelet Count	130-400	K/MCL
Hemoglobin	13-17	g/dL
Hematocrit	40.7-50.3 (men)	%
	36.1-44.3 (women)	%

A full blood count is one of the most commonly run blood tests, and can give you a good snapshot of overall health in many regards. A full blood cell test will give you a measure of white cell count (responsible for fighting infection), platelet count (vital to blood clotting and healing), and red blood cell count (responsible for carrying oxygen). Red and white cell counts will be further subdivided into various individual measurements, often referred to as a differential cell count. Hemoglobin is the specific carrier of gases in red cells, and hematocrit is a measure of the percentage of red blood cells in the total blood volume. Due to their effects on erythropoiesis, anabolic steroids tend to increase red blood cell count, hematocrit, and hemoglobin concentrations. While this may increase oxygen-carrying (aerobic) capacity, as the concentration of red blood cells increases so does the thickness of the blood. Elevated hematocrit can increase the risk of heart attack or stroke.

Kidney

Test Name	Reference Range	
Uric acid	3.0-7.0	mg/dL
Creatinine	.5-1.5	mg/dL
BUN	5-26	mg/dL
BUN/creatinine ratio	8-27	

This panel of tests looks at three primary waste products filtered and excreted through the kidneys, urea, uric acid, and creatinine. Problems here can indicate serious underlying problems with kidney function. Note that Blood Urea Nitrogen (BUN) is often elevated with excess protein consumption, and is used by many physicians as an indicator that too much protein is being consumed for optimal metabolism. The high consumption of meat or creatine supplementation can also elevate creatinine levels, diminishing the value of blood creatinine testing as a marker of kidney health. Electrolyte, mineral, and fasting glucose testing is important to further assessing kidney health, and is advised in addition to the above kidney markers. A quick urine screen for pH, specific gravity, and the presence of sugar, blood, and ketones is also available at most physicians' offices, and is generally advised alongside blood work when possible.

Electrolytes, Minerals, and Glucose

Test Name	Reference Range	
Sodium	136-146	mEq/L
Potassium	3.6-5.2	mEq/L
Chloride	98-109	mEq/L
Bicarbonate (carbon dioxide)	21-30	mEq/L
Phosphorous	2.5-4.5	mg/dL
Calcium	8.5-10.5	mg/dL
Iron	35-185	mcg/dL
Glucose (fasting)	70-110	mg/dL

Electrolyte levels are examined to help detect problems with the fluid and electrolyte balance. Abnormal values may reflect something as small as sodium or potassium deficiency, or a more serious condition such as kidney disease. A variety of other health issues may also become apparent by looking at both electrolyte and mineral levels, giving them somewhat broad prognostic value. Fasting glucose is also examined to determine if the individual may be hypoglycemic (low blood sugar) or hyperglycemic (high blood sugar). Problems with fasting glucose may reflect potentially serious health conditions including metabolic syndrome, diabetes, pancreatic disease, liver disease, kidney failure, or acute stress.

Prostate

Test Name	**Reference Range**
PSA, serum	0.0-4.0 ng/mL

Prostate-specific antigen (PSA) is a protein produced by cells in the prostate gland. Its levels can become elevated in cases of benign prostate hypertrophy or prostate cancer. While it remains unknown if elevating the level of androgens in the body with anabolic/androgenic steroids can increase the risk of prostate cancer, it is known that this disease can be progressed by elevated hormone (androgen and estrogen) levels. The PSA test is regarded as an important diagnostic tool for screening individual prostate cancer risk. If PSA levels are elevated, most will advise against using anabolic/androgenic steroids.

Individual Heath Markers Defined

Alanine Aminotransferase (ALT): An enzyme produced primarily in the liver but also in other tissues. ALT is involved in amino acid and protein metabolism. Used as a primary marker of hepatic strain. Also called Serum Glutamic Pyruvic Transaminase (SGPT).

Albumin: The main protein that circulates in the blood. Produced in the liver and has antioxidant properties. Transports certain hormones, vitamins, and minerals, and plays a role in water balance. Used as an indicator of liver health. Higher levels are optimal.

Alkaline Phosphatase (ALP): A family of cholestatic enzymes produced mainly in the liver, but also in the intestines, kidneys, and bone. Used as a marker of hepatic strain, often relating to disease of the bile ducts.

Apolipoprotein A-I (apoA-I): A constituent of HDL (good) cholesterol, apoA-I is responsible for initiating beneficial reverse cholesterol transport. This process pulls cholesterol particles from the artery walls and transport them back to the liver. Higher levels are optimal.

Apolipoprotein B (apoB): A constituent of LDL (bad) cholesterol, apoB is responsible for attaching these lipoproteins to artery walls. ApoB is a promoter of fatty plaque deposits in the arteries. Lower levels are optimal.

Aspartate Aminotransferase (AST): An enzyme produced primarily in the liver but also in muscle tissue. AST is involved in amino acid and protein metabolism. Used as a marker of hepatic strain, although it is considered less specific than ALT testing. Also called Serum Glutamic-Oxalocetic Transaminase (SGOT).

Basophils: A type of white blood cell. Action not fully understood, but cells are known to carry histamine, heparin, and serotonin. Levels are elevated with allergic reaction and parasitic infection.

Bicarbonate: A measure of carbon dioxide content in the blood, and a common marker of the acid-base balance.

Bilirubin: A waste product made from the breakdown of red blood cells. Excreted into the bile. Regarded as an important indicator of liver health. Elevated levels in the blood indicate liver toxicity.

Blood Urea Nitrogen (BUN): A waste product from the breakdown of proteins, filtered and excreted through the kidneys. Elevated levels may indicate a number of problems including excessive protein intake, kidney damage, dehydration, heart failure, or reduced production of digestive enzymes. Low levels may be indicative of many things including malnutrition or liver damage.

BUN/Creatinine Ratio: The ratio of Blood Urea Nitrogen to Creatinine, used as a marker of kidney and liver health.

C-reactive Protein (CRP): A key marker of inflammation in the body. Elevated levels may indicate increased risk of cardiovascular disease or stroke.

Carbon Dioxide (CO2): Byproduct of respiration, and a common marker of the acid-base balance. See also Bicarbonate.

Calcium: Electrolyte involved in a myriad of body functions including bone metabolism, protein utilization, muscle and nervous system functioning, cardiovascular functioning, blood clotting, and nutrient transport.

Chloride: Electrolyte involved in the regulation of water balance. Elevated levels may indicate a number of things including anemia, dehydration, excess salt consumption, and hyperthyroid. Low levels may indicate heart or kidney failure, severe vomiting, or a number of other health conditions.

Cholesterol, Total: A measure of all fractions of cholesterol in the blood (LDL, VLDL, and HDL). High total cholesterol is regarded as a risk factor for cardiovascular disease.

Cholesterol, HDL: A measure of the beneficial high-density lipoprotein (HDL) fraction of cholesterol, which helps remove plaque deposits from arteries. High levels are optimal. Low levels may be found in cardiovascular disease.

Cholesterol, LDL: A measure of the low-density lipoprotein (LDL) fraction of cholesterol. This is the primary atherogenic particle, meaning it tends to promote the formation of plaque deposits in the arteries. Low levels are optimal.

Cholesterol, VLDL: A measure of the very low-density lipoprotein (LDL) fraction of cholesterol. VLDL contains the highest amount of triglycerides. Considered an atherogenic ("bad") cholesterol particle. Lower levels are optimal.

Cholesterol, LDL/HDL Ratio: A measure of the primary atherogenic particle (LDL) in relation to the primary antiatherogenic particle (HDL). This ratio is generally considered the most important cholesterol test value for assessing cardiovascular disease risk. A low ratio is desirable.

Creatine Kinase: An enzyme found largely in the heart and muscle, and responsible for converting creatine to phosphocreatine. Elevated levels may be linked to a number of things including heart attack, kidney failure, or severe muscle damage.

Creatinine: A waste product of muscle metabolism. Low levels may indicate kidney disease, malnutrition, or liver disease. High levels may indicate a number of things including reduced kidney function or muscle degeneration. Creatine supplementation may also elevate creatinine levels.

Eosinophils: A type of white blood cell. Similar to basophils, eosinophils are used by the body to protect against allergy and parasites. Levels are elevated with infection, and are low with good health.

Estradiol: The principle active form of estrogen. High levels can be associated with water retention, fat buildup, and gynecomastia (men). Also plays a role in prostate hypertrophy. Low levels of estradiol may be associated with increased heart disease risk.

Follicle Stimulating Hormone (FSH): A pituitary hormone involved in reproduction. In men, FSH is mainly responsible for supporting spermatogenesis. In women it supports ovulation.

Gamma-Glutamyl Transpeptidase (GGT): A cholestatic enzyme produced in the bile ducts. GGT is involved in glutathione metabolism and the transport of amino acids and peptides. Used as a marker of hepatic strain.

Globulin: A blood protein similar to albumin. Globulin is responsible for transporting certain hormones, lipids, metals, and antibodies. Levels may be elevated in many conditions including chronic infections, liver disease, arthritis, cancer, or lupus. Lower levels may be found with a number of conditions including suppressed immune system, malnutrition, malabsorption, and liver or kidney disease.

Glucose (fasting): Glucose is the product of carbohydrate metabolism and the primary source of energy for most cells in the body. Fasting glucose levels are elevated in a number of conditions including diabetes, liver disease, metabolic syndrome, pancreatitis, dieting, and stress. Low fasted glucose levels may indicate liver disease, overproduction of insulin, hypothyroidism, or other diseases.

Hematocrit: A measure of the percentage of red cells in the blood. Low levels indicate an anemic condition. High levels may indicate a number of things including dehydration, increased red cell breakdown in the spleen, cardiovascular disease, or respiratory disease. Anabolic steroids may also increase hematocrit.

Hemoglobin: A constituent of red blood cells, and the main carrier of oxygen and carbon dioxide in the blood. Levels may be suppressed with a number of conditions including malnutrition, malabsorption, and anemia. High levels may indicate many things including dehydration, cardiovascular disease, or respiratory disease. Anabolic steroids may also increase hemoglobin levels.

Homocysteine: A compound formed from the metabolism of the amino acid methionine. Involved in blood clotting and LDL cholesterol oxidation. Elevated levels of homocysteine indicate an increased risk of cardiovascular disease and stroke.

Iron: Mineral necessary for many functions including the formation of hemoglobin and certain proteins, and the transport of oxygen. Elevated levels may be caused by many conditions including certain forms of anemia, liver damage, hepatitis, iron poisoning, or vitamin B6 or B12 deficiency. Low levels can indicate a number of things including gastrointestinal blood loss, heavy menstrual bleeding, iron malabsorption, or dietary iron deficiency.

Lactic Acid Dehydrogenase (LDH): An intracellular enzyme found in many tissues including the kidney, heart, skeletal muscle, brain, liver, and lungs. Used as a marker of tissue damage. High levels are found in many conditions including heart attack, anemia, low blood pressure, stroke, liver disease, muscle injury, muscular dystrophy, and pancreatitis.

Luteinizing Hormone (LH): A pituitary hormone responsible for the stimulation of testosterone production in the testes (men). LH primarily supports ovulation in women.

Lymphocytes: A type of white blood cell. Primary role is to fight viral infection. Levels are elevated with active infection. Low levels are associated with suppressed immune system or active bacterial infection (noted by elevated neutrophils).

Mean Corpuscular Volume (MCV): A measure of the size of red blood cells, determined by measuring the volume of a single red blood cell. Useful in determining the cause of anemia. Elevated levels may reflect a number of things including a deficiency of vitamin B6 or folic acid. Low levels may reflect iron deficiency, or other causes.

Mean Corpuscular Hemoglobin (MCH): A measure of the average weight of the hemoglobin in red blood cells. Useful in determining the cause of anemia.

Mean Corpuscular Hemoglobin Concentration (MCHC): A measure of the average concentration of hemoglobin in red blood cells. Useful in evaluating the cause of, and therapy for, anemia. Low levels may indicate blood loss, B6 or iron deficiency, or other causes.

Monocytes: A type of white blood cell. Primary role is to fight severe infection not sufficiently countered by lymphocytes and neutrophils. Levels can be elevated with a number of things including chronic infection and certain cancers. Low levels indicate good health.

Neutrophils: A type of white blood cell, also known as granulocytes. The primary white cell used by the body to fight bacterial infection. Levels are elevated with infection. May be suppressed with compromised immune system or bone marrow.

Phosphorous: An abundant electrolyte involved in a number of body functions including the utilization of carbohydrates, fats, and proteins for cellular maintenance, repair, and growth, the production ATP for the storage of cellular energy, the transport of calcium, the maintenance of osmotic pressure, and the maintenance of heartbeat regularity.

Platelet Count: A measure of the concentration of platelets (also known as thrombocytes) in the blood. Platelets are involved in blood clotting, and protect against excessive bleeding. Elevated levels may be linked with a number of things including dehydration. Low levels are found in suppressed immune system functioning, drug reactions, or deficiencies of vitamin B12 or folic acid, or may have other causes.

Potassium: A key electrolyte necessary for nerve and muscle function, and the transport of nutrients and waste products in and out of cells. Along with sodium it helps maintain the acid-base balance and osmotic pressure. High levels may be caused by a number of things including kidney failure, metabolic or respiratory acidosis, and red blood cell destruction.

Prolactin: A reproductive hormone involved specifically in lactation. Prolactin is sometimes (but not commonly) elevated in steroid abusers, and may be linked to estrogen excess or hormone imbalance. Elevated prolactin may also indicate other issues with the pituitary.

Prostate-specific antigen (PSA): A protein found in prostate cells. Used as a screening for prostate cancer risk. Elevated levels reflect an increased risk of developing prostate cancer. Low levels are desirable, although do not assure against prostate cancer.

Red Blood Cell Count: A measure of the total concentration of red blood cells, responsible for transporting oxygen and carbon dioxide in the body. High red cell counts are seen with a number of conditions including heart disease, dehydration, or pulmonary fibrosis. Low levels may be linked to many things including anemia, bone marrow failure, red blood cell destruction, bleeding, leukemia, and malnutrition.

Red Cell Distribution Width (RDW): A measure of the variation in size between red blood cells. Useful in evaluating the cause of, and therapy for, anemia. Increased values may indicate a number of things including vitamin B12, folic acid, or iron deficiency.

Sodium: An abundant electrolyte necessary for many functions including the maintenance of osmotic pressure, acid-base balance, and nerve impulse activity. Disturbances in the sodium level may be caused by minor things including excessive sweating, vomiting, diarrhea, water intake, or very serious conditions including heart, kidney, or liver disease.

T3 Uptake: This test measures the level of unsaturated thyroxine binding globulin (a carrier of thyroid hormones) in the blood. Increased levels may indicate a number of things including hyperthyroidism (overactive thyroid), liver disease, cancer, and decreased lung function. Low levels may be indicative of hypothyroidism (under active thyroid), excess estrogen levels, pregnancy, or other causes.

Testosterone, Total: The measure of both unbound (active) and bound (inactive) portions of testosterone in the blood.

Testosterone, Free: The measure of free (unbound) testosterone in the blood. This represents the total amount of testosterone immediately available to tissues.

Thyroid-Stimulating Hormone (TSH): A pituitary hormone responsible for stimulating the release of thyroid hormones.

Thyroxine (T4): The more abundant of the two major thyroid hormones (T3 and T4). T4 serves mainly as a reservoir for the more active thyroid hormone (T3), which helps to stabilize and regulate thyroid supply. This is a key marker of the state of thyroid health (low, normal, or overactive).

Thyroxine, Free Index: This measure is a calculation of the amount of unbound (free) T4 in the blood. This is a key marker of the state of thyroid activity (low, normal, or overactive).

Total Protein: A measure of the total serum protein concentration, mainly albumin and globulin. Serum proteins are important to the function and supply of enzymes, hormones, nutrients, and antibodies, and also play a role in maintaining the water and pH balance. Low levels may indicate a number of things including malnutrition, liver disease, malabsorption, diarrhea, or severe burn injury. Elevated levels may indicate infection, liver damage, or other disease.

Triglycerides: The main storage form of fatty acids in the body. May be metabolized and used for energy. Elevated triglyceride levels may contribute to hardening of the arteries (atherosclerosis), and increase the risk of heart disease or stroke. Low levels are optimal.

Urea: (see Blood Urea Nitrogen)

Uric Acid: The waste product of purine metabolism, which is filtered and excreted through the kidneys. Elevated levels may indicate a number of things including gout, infection, kidney damage, and excessive protein intake. Low levels may indicate kidney damage, malnutrition, liver damage, or other causes.

White Blood Cell Count: A measure of the total concentration of white blood cells (also known as leukocytes), responsible for fighting infection and protecting the body from pathogens. A differential measure of white blood cells is usually also taken including neutrophils, eosinophils, basophils, lymphocytes, and monocytes. Levels may be elevated with certain infections or allergic conditions.

Harm Reduction / Safer Use Guidelines

Harm reduction is a concept among healthcare workers that seeks to reduce the negative health consequences of drug abuse. The principles of harm reduction call for an acceptance of the fact that, good or bad, illicit drugs exist in today's society. Instead of ignoring drug users, harm reduction practitioners actively work with them to promote safer use strategies and decrease the health damage of drug abuse. The effort of harm reduction is always helping, not judging, the individual. Although previously focused exclusively on narcotic drugs of abuse, harm reduction principles can (and should) also be developed for steroid users, a group that rarely has the benefit of full physician oversight in its drug programs. In an effort to further this goal, ANABOLICS has outlined the following principles of steroid harm reduction. If followed, these principles should measurably reduce the negative health impact of steroid use, making it a safer (although not completely safe) practice.

Twelve Principles of Anabolic Steroid Harm Reduction

1. Avoid Counterfeit and Underground Steroids. Anabolic steroids produced by illicit manufacturers are often of low quality, and may present additional health risks to the user beyond what are presented by the steroids themselves. Even if they contain actual steroids in properly labeled doses, underground drugs may contain toxic heavy metals, use dirty raw materials, or even carry bacterial, viral, and other forms of contamination. Pharmaceutical drug purity is assured to the public only by an extremely costly, tedious, and methodical process of quality assurance and government oversight. There is little financial and even logistical incentive for most underground drug makers to produce their drugs at such high levels of purity. Counterfeit and underground drugs are not considered equal substitutes for real pharmaceutical products, and should be avoided.

2. Avoid Toxic Oral Steroids. Aside from Andriol, Primobolan, and Proviron, every oral steroid discussed in this reference book is a c-17 alpha alkylated compound and should be avoided whenever possible. While there may be a number of clinical reasons to prescribe such a drug, when used in the higher doses necessary for muscle growth these agents tend to have significant negative impacts on certain health markers. Their most notable effect is to increase the ratio of LDL (bad) to HDL (good) cholesterol in the body, which favors increased plaque deposition in the arteries. Over time this may increase the risk of heart disease. C-17 alpha alkylated steroids are also the drugs exclusively associated with strong liver stress and (rarely) liver cancer. If injection can be tolerated, and moderate physique or performance improvement is the goal, all of the same results can be achieved without oral steroids. Note that injectable forms of otherwise oral steroids (such as stanozolol and methandrostenolone) should also be avoided, as they provide a similar level of hepatic and cardiovascular strain regardless of the differing route of administration.

3. Think of Testosterone First. Of all the anabolic/androgenic steroids produced, testosterone esters like cypionate, enanthate, and Sustanon tend to have the lowest negative impact on health when taken in muscle building and performance-enhancing doses. Testosterone drugs provide a hormone identical to that already produced in the body, presenting the same spectrum of physical and physiological effects. In addition to being one of the most efficient muscle-builders available, testosterone generally has a positive (not negative) effect on libido, supports a positive mood, and supplements necessary estrogen so that cholesterol levels are less negatively shifted. The exclusive use of testosterone drugs for body or performance enhancement is advised if possible.

4. Limit Yourself to the "Safest" Drugs. If the exclusive use of an injectable testosterone is not feasible, limiting use to the safest group of steroids is advised. Of the injectable class, the following drugs have the lowest cardiovascular strain and are recommended: Deca-Durabolin (nandrolone decanoate), Durabolin (nandrolone phenylpropionate), Equipoise (boldenone undecylenate), and Primobolan Depot (methenolone enanthate). If an oral steroid is desired, only Andriol, Primobolan, or Proviron should be used. These drugs are not c-17 alpha alkylated, and can all provide additional steroid activity without the same level of cardiovascular and hepatic strain seen with other common oral steroids including Anadrol (oxymetholone), Anavar (oxandrolone), Dianabol (methandrostenolone), and Winstrol (stanozolol).

5. Use Health Support Supplements. Anabolic/androgenic steroid users can help lower the negative health impact of steroid use with the consumption of natural health support supplements. To begin with, the negative cardiovascular effects of these drugs can be offset (at least to some degree) with cholesterol supplements. Fish oil is recommended as a base, which should be stacked with a number of other clinically studied cholesterol support ingredients including green tea, garlic powder, resveratrol, phytosterols, niacin, and policosinol. The blended product Lipid Stabil (Molecular Nutrition) includes these ingredients and is recommended. Cholesterol support supplements should be taken at all times during anabolic steroid therapy. Next, those taking oral steroids should be reducing liver strain with a liver support supplement. Recommended products include Liver Stabil (Molecular Nutrition), Liv-52 (Himalaya Drug Company), and Essentiale Forte (Aventis). One of these products should be taken at all times during therapy with hepatotoxic agents

6. Always Cycle Steroids. A steroid cycle usually consists of 6 to 12 weeks of drug use followed by an equal period of time or more abstaining from all anabolic/androgenic steroids. This practice is advised for a number of reasons. For one, as you supplement male steroid hormones your body will reduce the production of its own testosterone. Cycling helps reduce the risk of developing long-term fertility and hormonal issues, which are sometimes caused by the uninterrupted use of steroids for many months or years. Cycling also lets your general markers of health (such as cholesterol levels, hematocrit, and blood pressure) return to their normal state periodically, reducing the impact temporary changes may have over time. Those individuals who use anabolic/androgenic steroids for long periods of time without interruption run a greater risk that these negative changes in health markers will result in long-term health issues.

7. Use Reasonable Dosages. High doses of steroids are not necessary to achieve significant muscle growth, especially if moderate physique or performance enhancement is desired. A dosage limit of 400 mg per week on injectables is advised. In the case of testosterone cypionate, 400 mg per week equates to at least 4 to 5 times the level of hormone naturally produced in a healthy male body. This level of use will produce dramatic muscle gain if combined with proper training and diet. In fact, during the 1970s and 80s the dosage range of 200-400 mg per week was considered "standard" for the bodybuilding use of testosterone, nandrolone, boldenone, or methenolone. There is actually little real need for extreme doses of 750-1,000 mg or more of steroid per week, or to supplement an injectable base with additional orals. High doses may produce a faster rate of gain, but are generally not cost effective for the extra muscle they provide. Additionally, high doses of steroids greatly increase cardiovascular strain and the incidence of other side effects.

8. Avoid Aromatase Inhibitors. Aromatase-inhibiting drugs counter estrogenic side effects by preventing the production of estrogen in the body. While an effective practice, they also deprive the body of a hormone that is important to cardiovascular health. In particular, estrogen supports the production of good (HDL) cholesterol, which means that aromatase inhibitors may inadvertently increase the cardiovascular strain of a steroid cycle. If estrogenic side effects are apparent and a reduction or elimination of the offending steroid(s) is not considered an option, the SERM (Selective Estrogen Receptor Modulator) drug Nolvadex could be used instead. This drug offers partial estrogenic action in the liver, which may allow it to counter estrogenic side effects without the same negative shift in cholesterol.

9. Get Regular Blood Tests. Comprehensive blood testing including an examination of hormones, cholesterol, blood cell concentrations, and enzymes is the most useful tool for assessing the negative health impact of steroid use. Changes in cholesterol, for example, can help quantify for the user what effect a particular drug regimen is having on their cardiovascular health. The individual then has the opportunity to better assess long-term risk if this cycle is to be repeated. At a minimum, blood testing should be conducted before a cycle is initiated, 3 to 4 weeks into a cycle, and a couple of months after a cycle. This allows for 1) a baseline for later comparison; 2) a snapshot of the on-cycle health impact; and 3) an opportunity to assess if natural homeostasis has been restored post-cycle.

10. Use Proper Injection Procedures. Careful attention to correct injection procedures can help eliminate some of the complications associated with nonmedical steroid use. Steroids are given via deep intramuscular injections. The most common site of application is the upper outer quadrant of the gluteus muscle, although the drugs are also commonly injected to the upper outer thigh and shoulder. Site injections (in smaller muscle groups like the biceps, triceps, or calf muscles) for cosmetic purposes are discouraged, as they are technically more difficult to navigate and more prone to complications. Comfortable injection volumes should also be used, generally no more than 3 mL per application. Each injection site should be rotated so that the same muscle is not injected more than once every two weeks. A general focus should be made on cleanliness, including the use of alcohol pads on the vials and skin before injection, and the proper disposal of all needles and empty vials/ampules after use.

11. Watch Your Diet. Anabolic/androgenic steroids can allow an individual significantly more latitude with their diet than normal. The caloric demand typically increases due to the effects of these drugs on muscle mass and metabolism, allowing more calories to be consumed each day without adding fat mass. It is important not to let this latitude affect your health in a negative way. Remember, the use of steroids at physique- and performance-enhancing doses is expected to cause an unfavorable shift in cholesterol levels and other cardiovascular health markers, favoring a higher risk of cardiovascular disease. Simultaneously feeding your body greater amounts of saturated fats, cholesterol, and simple carbohydrates can make the impact of these drugs even worse. Diets low in saturated fats, cholesterol, and simple sugars are recommended, and are known to reduce cardiovascular disease risk. Note, however, that diet alone is not effective at countering the negative cardiovascular effects of steroid use, but dietary restrictions can reduce these risks.

12. Always Consider Reward AND Risk. It can be easy to ignore the potential health impact of steroid use when the positive benefits are so rapid and the negative consequences so remote. At the end of the day, however, it is very important to remember that the use of steroids in doses sufficient to support short term muscle gain are virtually always going to have some negative impact on your body. Your cholesterol will shift in an unfavorable direction, your blood pressure may go up a little bit, and you may ever so slightly thicken the ventricles in your heart. Your hormones are out of balance when you take steroids, which will invariably cause other things to go out of balance. Steroid use is rarely dangerous over a short term period. These hormonal drugs are acutely very safe. As use continues over the years, however, these short-term periods accumulate, and total on-cycle time may become very long. Always remember to consider the risks as well as the rewards of each cycle. Choosing your drug program carefully and keeping the negative effects of steroid use in check over the short term is the best way to reduce long term risks.

Counterfeit Steroids

As the name implies, counterfeit steroids are copies of real anabolic/androgenic steroid products, which are made from illicit producers. These drugs are intended for sale on the black market, ultimately to consumers who believe they are buying a legitimate pharmaceutical item from the labeled company. There are many important issues to consider with the potential use of counterfeit steroids. For one, these products are made by criminal operations. The contents of such products, by the very nature of these operations, cannot be verified. In many cases, the counterfeiters will never even use any active steroid at all, and will simply sell an expensive and essentially worthless bottle of inert carriers, fillers, and binders. In other cases, they will substitute lower doses or cheaper steroids to make their profit margins higher.

Even if a counterfeit does contain the active steroid in question, it may not be a clean and safe product. Today, we take for granted the fact that our drug products are made with sterile and pure ingredients. We also give little thought to aseptic processing techniques, which manufacture our drug products free of contamination by harmful bacteria, viruses, or microorganisms. This is especially important with injectable medications, since many of the human body's normal defenses against infection are bypassed when a drug is introduced directly into the body. The theoretical risks of injecting a contaminated drug product are innumerable, and range from simple injection-site infection, to life threatening allergic reactions or illness. These risks are in addition to other serious contamination risks that could be present in any drug product, injected or otherwise. Counterfeiters very rarely produce their steroids with such sophisticated and expensive materials and techniques.

As anyone that studies the illicit anabolic steroid trade knows, high demand and huge profits offer strong incentive for the manufacture of counterfeit drugs. Over the years, this segment of the illegal business has grown exponentially. What was once a problem largely isolated to the United States can now be found in literally every corner of the globe. Counterfeiting is a phenomenon not isolated to anabolic steroids, of course, and is commonly seen when the significant sales of anything valuable are diverted from legitimate to underground sources. Given the nature of drug products, however, the counterfeit steroid phenomenon is an especially important health concern for drug-using bodybuilders. As the number of these products grows, so too does the number of reports of low or no product efficacy, or worse, health consequences including abscess, infection, anaphylaxis, and toxicity caused by heavy metal contamination.

Prevalence Study

By all estimates, counterfeit steroids are very common in all corners of the global steroid black market. Given the illicit nature in which counterfeit steroid products are traded, however, it is difficult to determine the exact prevalence of these drugs. Analysis reports of law enforcement seizures offer an occasional snapshot of the quality of steroid sales in a particular region. One such study was conducted at the Center for Preventative Doping Research in Cologne, Germany, and involved 70 different anabolic steroids and ancillary drug products. All of the samples analyzed were obtained during police raids of three illegal dealers of anabolic steroids. It is important to emphasize that while the amount seized is a fairly large sample for this type of analysis, 70 drug products taken from three dealers is not sufficient to prove any specific market trend, overall counterfeit prevalence, or brand legitimacy.

Overall, more than one-third (34%) of the 50 anabolic steroids tested did not have ingredients that matched their labels, and were clearly made from illicit manufacturers. Of the failing products, nine were identified as copies of known pharmaceutical brands, and would be considered classic counterfeits. These made up 18% of the drug products in inventory by the arrested dealers. The remaining eight (16%) that failed were underground steroid products, which are discussed separately in this book. There were six additional products on the list that passed testing that were made by underground manufacturers (British Dragon, SB Labs, and International Pharmaceuticals). In total, legitimate drug companies did not manufacture 46% of the steroid products that were being sold by these dealers in Germany. The results are probably a good reflection of what is happening on the European market in general. Given the tighter legal controls on steroids in the United States, counterfeit and underground products are expected to make up an even higher percentage of products illegally sold in this market.

Visual Inspection

The researchers in Cologne Germany also made an important observation. Aside from known underground products from labs such as British Dragon, SB Labs, and

International Pharmaceuticals, they noted it was not possible to ascertain what product was real and what was a counterfeit upon visual inspection. While this group may not have had the experience or reference materials necessary to make an up-close product examination, and no product photos were provided in the report to reference, it does underline a problem that the steroid using community has been noticing for a long time, namely counterfeit manufacturing operations are becoming increasingly sophisticated. Now more than ever it can be difficult for someone shopping on the black market to determine product legitimacy before making a purchase and actually consuming the product(s).

The "Best" Products

Of the confiscated German products, those that were manufactured in Western Europe seemed to offer greater assurance of legitimacy than those of other regions. Thailand also remains a common source country for legitimate products not commonly manufactured in Western Europe including oxymetholone and methandrostenolone. This is in great contradiction to the United States, where regional products (U.S. and Canada) are those most likely to be the subject of counterfeiting. Also, the study showed that the less costly testosterone products were most likely to be legitimate, even if they originated outside of Europe. It appears that, at least by way of these three dealers, a good deal of legitimate Karachi Sustanon and Egyptian testosterone enanthate are being imported into Germany. It is of note that the one failure of CID enanthate was due to the inclusion of some testosterone cypionate in addition to the labeled enanthate. It is unknown if this was an error that occurred at the manufacturing plant, or the product was the subject of counterfeiting.

The "Worst" Products

Perhaps due to high recognition and demand, all of the Normal Hellas nandrolone decanoate products tested during this analysis run were determined to be counterfeit. These products were confiscated from each of the three dealers independently. In all cases, these steroid products contained testosterone instead of nandrolone decanoate. This is a common substitution with deviant nandrolone products, as low doses of testosterone can provide a similar level of anabolic effect as nandrolone for some users, with a similar low incidence of side effects. Testosterone is also much less expensive to manufacture in comparison to nandrolone decanoate. The hope is that many users will not be able to identify testosterone as the content. Norma Hellas Deca, therefore, remains a product of extremely high risk on the European and international markets. Great care should be taken to examine any product closely for the required security features shown in this book.

Other Bodybuilding "Ancillary" Drugs

A total of 20 non-steroid drugs were also tested. All products that would be defined as common ancillary drugs including tamoxifen citrate (Nolvadex), clomiphene citrate (Clomid), thyroid hormone, caffeine, and yohimbine hcl turned out to be legitimate. This underlines the lower risk in these ancillary drug items, no doubt due to the lower financial incentive for counterfeiters to duplicate these cheap and easy to access pharmaceuticals. The only non-steroid drugs where there was some substitution noted were in the male sexual performance category, which constitute drugs such as Viagra and Cialis. In most of the individual cases the drugs did test out as labeled. When they did fail testing, however, it was usually for the substitution of active ingredients of the same drug family. Male sexual performance products are known to be an active area of counterfeiting, so care should be taken when purchasing these products from illicit channels as well.

Steroid Analysis Results

Anadrol (oxymetholone):

1. Oxytone 50 mg (SB Labs, Thailand)
Result: PASS

2. Oxytone 50 mg (SB Labs, Thailand)
Result: PASS

3. Oxytone 50 mg (SB Labs, Thailand)
Result: PASS

Deca (nandrolone decanoate):

1. Norma Hellas (100 mg/mL)
Result: FAIL (testosterone)

2. Norma Hellas (100 mg/mL)
Result: FAIL (testosterone)

3. Norma Hellas (100 mg/mL)
Result: FAIL (testosterone)

4. Norma Hellas (100 mg/mL)
Result: FAIL (testosterone)

5. Decabol 250 (British Dragon, Underground)
Result: FAIL (testosterone)

Dianabol (methandrostenolone):

1. Anabol 5 mg (British Dispensary, Thailand)
Result: FAIL (methyltestosterone)

2. Anabol 5 mg (British Dispensary, Thailand)
Result: PASS

3. Anabol 5 mg (British Dispensary, Thailand)
Result: PASS

4. Danabol DS 10 mg (March, Thailand)
Result: PASS

5. Danabol DS 10 mg (March, Thailand)
Result: PASS

6. Naposim 5 mg (Terapia, Romania)
Result: FAIL (methyltestosterone)

Equipoise (boldenone undecylenate):

1. Boldabol 200 (British Dragon, Underground)
Result: PASS

Halotestin (fluoxymesterone):

1. Fluoxymesterone (IP, Underground)
Result: PASS

Primobolan (methenolone enanthate):

1. Primobol 100 (British Dragon, Underground)
Result: FAIL (nandrolone, testosterone)

Proviron (mesterolone):

1. Proviron 25 mg
Result: PASS

Sustanon 250 (testosterone mix):

1. Sustanon 250 (Karachi, Pakistan)
Result: PASS

2. Sustanon 250 (Nile, Egypt)
Result: FAIL (different testosterones)

3. Sustanon 250 (Nile, Egypt)
Result: FAIL (different testosterones)

4. Sustanon 250 (Karachi, Pakistan)
Result: PASS

5. Sustanon 250 (Karachi, Pakistan)
Result: PASS

6. Sustanon 250 (Karachi, Pakistan)
Result: PASS

7. Sustanon 250 (Karachi, Pakistan)
Result: PASS

8. Sustanon 250 (Karachi, Pakistan)
Result: PASS

9. Sustanon 250 (Karachi, Pakistan)
Result: PASS

Testosterone Cypionate:

1. Testex Prolongatum 125 (Q Pharma, Spain)
Result: PASS

2. Testabol 200 (British Dragon, Underground)
Result: FAIL (different testosterones)

Testosterone Enanthate:

1. Testofort 250 mg/mL (Pliva, Pakistan)
Result: PASS

2. Testosterone Depot 250 (Eifelfango, Germany)
Result: PASS

3. Testosterone Depot 250 (Eifelfango, Germany)
Result: PASS

4. Testoviron Depot 250 (Medipharm, Pakistan)
Result: PASS

5. Testoviron Depot 250 (Medipharm, Pakistan)
Result: PASS

6. Cidoteston 250 (CID, Egypt)
Result: FAIL (includes T. cypionate)

7. Cidoteston 250 (CID, Egypt)
Result: PASS

Testosterone Propionate:

1. Testovis 100 mg/mL (SIT, Italy)
Result: PASS

2. Testovis 100 mg/mL (SIT, Italy)
Result: PASS

3. Testovis 100 mg/mL (SIT, Italy)
Result: PASS

4. Testovis 100 mg/mL (SIT, Italy)
Result: PASS

5. Testovis 100 mg/mL (SIT, Italy)
Result: PASS

6. Testabol (British Dragon, Underground)
Result: FAIL (different testosterones)

Trenbolone (various esters):

1. Trenabol 75 (British Dragon, Underground)
Result: FAIL (boldenone, testosterone)

2. Trenabol 100 (British Dragon, Underground)
Result: FAIL (boldenone, testosterone)

3. Tri-Trenabol 150 (British Dragon, Underground)
Result: FAIL (trenbolone, testosterone)

4. Trenabol 200 (British Dragon, Underground)
Result: FAIL (trenbolone, testosterone)

Winstrol (stanozolol):

1. Winstrol Depot 50 mg/mL (Zambon, Spain)
Result: PASS

2. Winstrol Depot 50 mg/mL (Zambon, Spain)
Result: PASS

3. Winstrol Depot 50 mg/mL (Zambon, Spain)
Result: PASS

4. Stanabol 50 (British Dragon, Underground)
Result: PASS

Counterfeit Steroid Identification

This section deals with the most general attributes to look for when attempting to spot counterfeit anabolic steroids. It is important to stress the fact that underground manufacturers are much more advanced today than they were 15 years ago. As the analysis study of black market confiscations in Germany mentions, it is becoming increasingly difficult to identify counterfeit steroids with a general visual inspection. The fakes of today tend to be much better looking, and harder to recognize, than they used to be. The methods mentioned in this section are, therefore, often inadequate for counterfeit identification. Do not be confident if your product passes all points of inspection. It is more important to closely examine each product next to a photograph of a known legitimate version, as well as to determine if the product came through reliable legitimate channels.

Point #1: Matching Labels

Fifteen years ago, many fakes were put together just like the testosterone suspension shown below. The counterfeiter used the same label for both the box and vial to save time and money. In general, be suspicious of any box that carries a sticker instead of print. A legitimate drug company is not going to use a sticker to label a blank cardboard box. There are only a very small number of exceptions to this rule, and they tend to be products of Eastern or South East Asian origin.

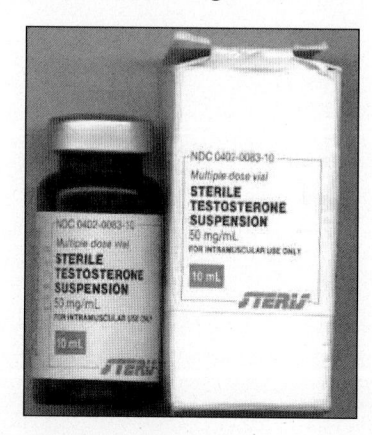

Point #2: Unusual Ampules

When underground manufacturers first began to duplicate ampules, many were quite unusual in appearance. Some leaked, contained air bubbles in the glass, or were uneven. Some were so crooked, that they would fall over if you tried to stand them on a desk. One would want to make sure all ampules are consistent in size and shape, do not leak, and look professional in appearance. Oil levels should be relatively even when they are lined up, and the solution clean (free of particulate) when drawn into a syringe. It should also be sized proportionately to the volume it contains. The pictured ampule of Loniton (left) is very odd, as it can hold about 4 or 5 mL, but is a 1 mL Sustanon clone. Also, some low level counterfeiters will use ampule blanks that can be sealed at home with a flame. These ampules (right photo) look unusual next to the pharmaceutical ampules commonly used.

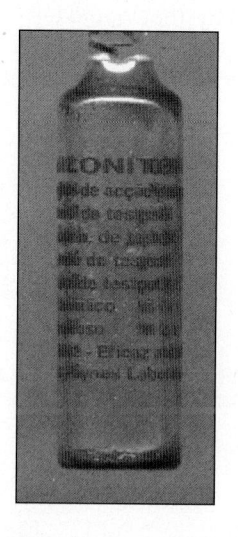

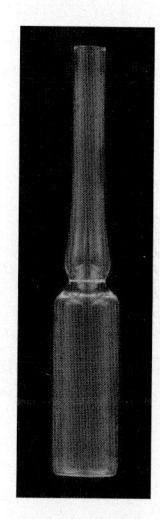

Point #3: Pill Bottles

Bottles of loose pills are among the easiest products to counterfeit. In its most basic form, this requires an ability to scan a legitimate bottle label, and reproduce it on a similar looking pill bottle. Legitimate pill bottles are very rare on the black market in general. This is because this form of packaging is actually very limited in use. Drug companies in the United States do make bottles, but tight controls on prescription AAS make diversion to the black market very unlikely. Pill bottles are also common in some South American and Asian markets. Aside from this, however, most foreign drug markets regard pill bottles as unsanitary. Most manufacturers package their tablets and capsules in foil or foil/plastic push-through strips. All pill bottles should be suspect unless they can be individually verified.

Point #4: Lot Number/Date Code Printing

One will want to examine the lot number and expiration date on the box/vial to determine if it was stamped or printed separately from the rest of the writing. Legitimate drug manufacturers print their boxes and labels in bulk, and apply the lot number and expiration date at the time of packaging. Counterfeiters sometimes include this information with the rest of the printing on the box, as it avoids the need for an extra piece of equipment and an extra step in the manufacturing process. It is best to see some form of stamp or indentation that would tell you for certain the information was added to your product at a later time. Computer printing, which can be difficlt to

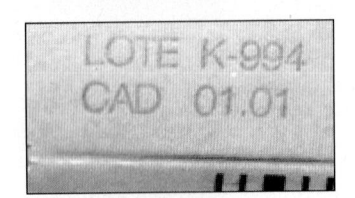

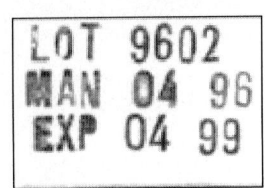

Machine stamping on Real Spanish Primobolan and generic Clomid from Greece.

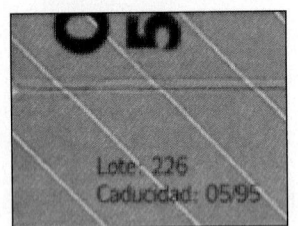

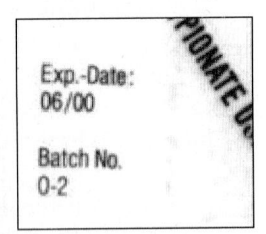

Many counterfeits look like this.

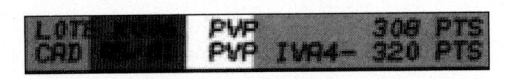

Computer labeling is commonly used on legitimate boxes as well.

dicern from regular printing, is also commonly used on real drugs, however. The two pictured counterfeits clearly have batch and date information that was printed with the rest of the box. Legitimate drug manufacturers will never use this method of coding their items. It is simply too cost ineffective and inflexible. The presence of such printing is regarded as a reliable indication that a particular drug product is counterfeit.

Point #5: (Non-Glossy Surfaces)

Take a minute to look at the area where the dates and lot codes are applied on your box and/or label. This is a particularly important thing to look at if your box is made out of glossy cardboard (it will have a shine to it). Many legitimate pharmaceutical companies will leave a small area on their boxes/labels that does not have a glossy surface. This area may be used for the printing of the lot number and expiration date, which can help prevent smearing of these vital numbers. Although certainly not done in enough frequency to consider this a rule to live by, finding a small non-glossy area on a steroid product for date stamping does show there is extra intricacy to it. Counterfeit drug makers will sometimes overlook small features like this.

Passing Inspection

Remember, anabolic/androgenic steroid counterfeiting is now a highly lucrative business. Counterfeit operations with all forms of sophisticated modern manufacturing equipment have been identified. This includes counterfeiters with an ability to accurately copy foil/plastic tablet strips, single-dose ampules, security features such as holograms and watermarks, pharmacy stickers, date and lot number encoding, and even additional technical details such as Braille lettering and foil inlays. A majority of counterfeit steroids will actually pass the above visual inspection points. They are provided to help weed out some of the more obvious counterfeit products.

Country Specifics

In most countries, a pharmaceutical company is required to meet a specific set of regulations pertaining to the physical packaging of a pharmaceutical product. In some cases these regulations can be used to help evaluate the legitimacy of black market steroids, as all counterfeiters may not have the resources or forethought to implement the required features. Here, we discuss a number of attributes to examine, which should hold true for all of the drugs produced in the specified country.

United States:

First, it is very important to stress the fact that steroids are a controlled substance in the United States. Current controls are very effective at keeping American products off of the black market. It is much easier for the illicit dealers to import or manufacture their own products than it is to get any volume of legitimate American pharmaceuticals to distribute. Be leery of American items you encounter on the black market, as they are in all probability counterfeits. The best rule is to avoid all American items unless you can personally trace them back to a pharmacy.

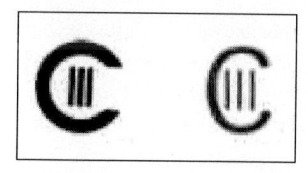

The FDA provides us with a couple of strict requirements, which many counterfeiters overlook. The most predominant is that all legitimate American drugs cannot carry a label that will easily be removed from the vial/bottle. It must be so saturated with glue that you can only remove it in small pieces. This is done to protect the public from the possibility of drug mislabeling. With many U.S. counterfeits, the label can be peeled off the bottle quickly, in one or a few large pieces.

You should also moisten your thumb and rub the expiration date on the box and label. Quite often the ink on the counterfeit will smear and rub off easily. The stamping on a real U.S. pharmaceutical may streak slightly, but should remain intact and legible. Again, this is a requirement to protect consumers.

Additionally, being a Schedule III controlled substance, all commercially available human and veterinary anabolic/androgenic steroids are required to bear the tag "CIII" (see sample picture). The only exceptions would be cattle implant pellets, which are technically not controlled substances, or drugs from compounding pharmacies, which do not have to adhere to the same production guidelines. A small number of lazy counterfeiters continue to duplicate steroids that were manufactured before 1991, when this tag was not present.

The FDA requires that all tablets and capsules are identifiable through unique markings in case they are removed from the packaging. The manufacturer name, or an abbreviation, is usually found on each pill, along with a specific code for the product. Some steroid users have found the Poison Control Center to be a very useful resource in verifying these markings. The Poison Control Center has a full database of pill identification markings at their disposal, and should be able to tell you the drug and dosage based on them. The offices are usually very responsive if you explain it is not an emergency call. If your pill is not found in their database, it should be considered a fake product.

Italy:

All drugs produced in Italy will bear the pictured drug identification sticker. The sticker itself is white, with red and black print. The sticker rests on a laminated surface, so that it can be peeled off and affixed to paperwork. You should never purchase an Italian drug if this sticker is not present. Drugs from Italy will also use abbreviations like Prep, Scad, and Del for the counterpart of lot #, manufacture, and expiration dates. English writing here would indicate counterfeiting.

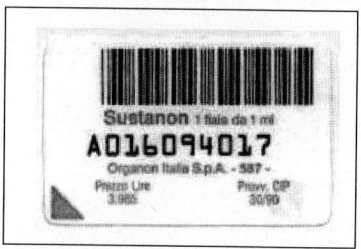

Greece:

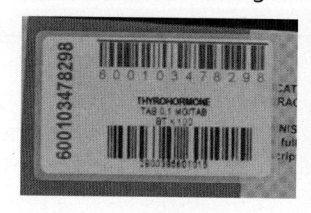

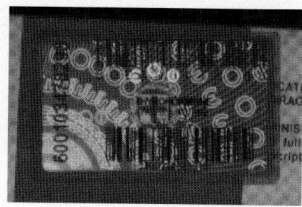

Greece also has a drug ID sticker that must be present on all drugs available for sale. The sticker itself rests on a laminated surface, so that it can be peeled off of the box and affixed to paperwork when a prescription is filled. Most importantly, the sticker will show a hidden mark when placed under UV light. Some counterfeiters have copied these stickers with excellent accuracy, right down to the laminated surface. Copies of the sticker bearing a hidden UV watermark, however, have not been located. Do not purchase any Greek drug without the proper sticker attached.

Spain:

Spanish drugs do not bear a sticker, but instead have an area located on the box that contains a bar code and some drug information. This area will sometimes have indentations in the cardboard, so as to be removable if you tear the surface. At other times, the barcode is simply printed on the box. Spanish drugs also use the abbreviations Lote and Cad for lot number and expiration, respectively. date. Many drug boxes also carry Braille lettering.

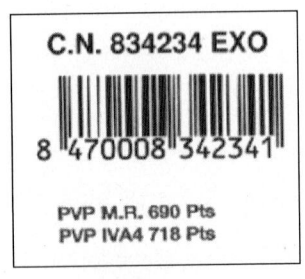

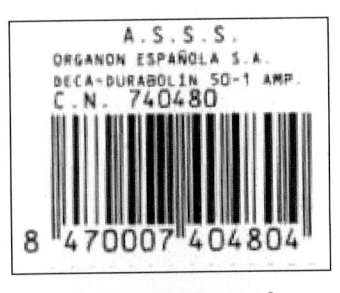

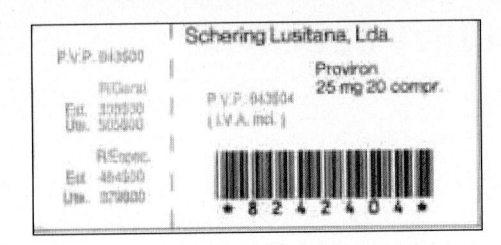

Old one without

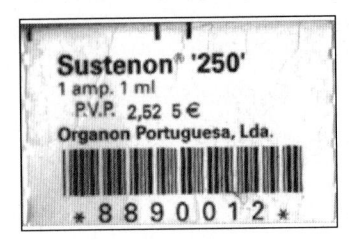

New area with price in Euros

Printed Only

Removable Barcode

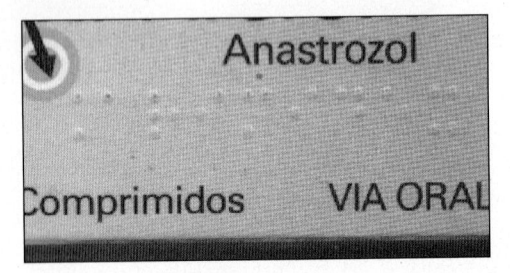

Braille Lettering

France:

Drugs from France will bear a rectangular sticker somewhere on the surface of the box. The text and format is often slightly different item to item. Also, packaging always contains an area with a green and red box. In the sample below, it is in the lower left side of the box.

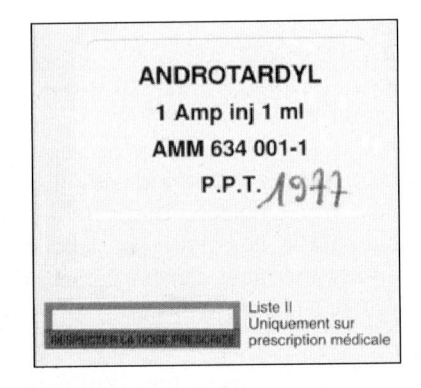

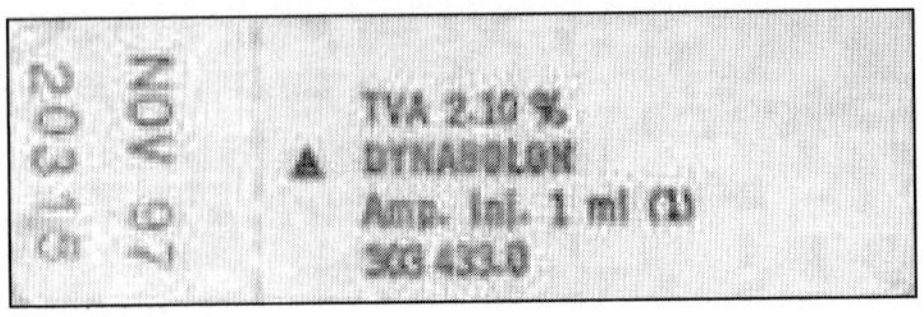

Portugal:

Drug boxes from Portugal contain a rectangular area which displays the bar code and pricing information. This is sometimes found as a sticker, but most commonly it is printed, not stamped, onto the surface. In many cases, the area is indented, so that it can be removed from the box. Drugs from Portugal will also use the abbreviations Lote: and Val. Ate: for lot number and expiration date stampings.

Underground Steroids

An underground steroid is an anabolic/androgenic steroid product that was made by an illegal (underground) laboratory. These drugs are specifically manufactured for sale to athletes and bodybuilders on the black market, and are not available through legitimate channels such as pharmacies and drug distributors. These companies are unlicensed, unregulated, and operate in a completely clandestine manner. At one time the term underground steroid was considered synonymous with counterfeit steroid, but today many people view these two categories as separate. The main point of distinction between an underground steroid and a counterfeit steroid is that the latter is a copy of a legitimate pharmaceutical product, which was made in an effort to deceive the consumer. Underground steroid manufacturers, on the other hand, use distinct brand names that are not to be confused with registered drug companies. They often try to build recognition in the marketplace for their products, and commonly use real steroid ingredients in substantial dosages.

Tighter government enforcement of steroid laws and legitimate distribution channels has fueled an explosion of underground steroid manufacturing operations over the past decade. The business model is now fairly common, and may account for more than 50% of all anabolic/androgenic steroids illegally sold in the United States. The manufacturing process typically involves the sourcing of raw steroid materials from countries where strict regulations concerning the manufacture and sale of drug ingredients are not in place. These ingredients are then smuggled into an area of high regulation such as the United States or Europe, where they are made into individual drug units (vials, ampules, pill bottles, or blister cards) with the use of small-scale packaging machines. In some cases these operations are so large they hire offshore drug manufacturing facilities to assemble their products. Such operations are small in number though, and account for a small portion of the total number of underground laboratories.

Drug Purity

Drug manufacturing safety is a central focus in Western medicine. Pharmaceuticals are intended to treat ill patients, not cause additional harm by being improperly dosed or containing bacteria, heavy metal, or other forms of contamination. Products made for human consumption are only made after government approval by government-licensed companies. These companies are highly regulated and routinely inspected. Their products must only contain materials that come from other licensed suppliers, which also adhere to strict pharmaceutical-grade purity standards (such as USP/BP). These companies must also assemble their products in meticulously scrutinized "clean room" facilities designed to prevent any contamination from air and personnel. Each material or piece of equipment that comes into contact with the drug product must be sterile, and the entire process must result in a preparation that contains exactly and only what the label intends. In short, there is essentially zero margin for error when it comes to pharmaceutical manufacturing.

The above description is in stark contract to the underground steroid manufacturing business. By their very nature, these companies are not under government license or oversight. A majority of underground steroid products will, likewise, not be assembled in a sterile environment, or with the use of expensive pharmaceutical grade materials and equipment. Instead, most are manufactured in a dwelling home or small clandestine business with the use of "food grade" raw materials and manually operated vial/bottle filling and sealing tools. The opportunities for contamination in this type of process are great. By Western medical standards, most underground steroids are, of course, not fit for human consumption. Even so, many consumers still buy these products. They may find attraction to cheaper prices, higher doses, greater selection, or easier availability. Perhaps more simply, they may not be aware of the risks involved. No analysis of product purity specific to underground steroids has previously been published to help consumers weigh these risks.

ANABOLICS Underground Market Analysis

In an effort to help consumers assess the quality and potential health risks of underground steroid products, ANABOLICS undertook a detailed joint drug analysis project in April 2007. This project examined the quality of steroids made from underground facilities, and exceeded the normal scope of testing by examining a number of other variables often overlooked in dosage testing. A total of 14 underground steroid samples were selected for laboratory testing, which included products from Amplio Labs, British Dragon, Diamond Pharma, Generic Anabolics, Generic Pharma, Lizard Laboratories, Medical Inc., Microbiological Labs, Nordic Supplements, Shark Laboratories, SWE Supplements, and Troy Labs. Included in this list were drugs that were made from small underground manufacturers, mid-level operations, and even producers large enough to have their items assembled under contract by drug manufacturing facilities. All 14 samples were analyzed at a registered and licensed facility in the United States.

There were four specific areas of testing for the 2007 market analysis project. The first test was to look for the presence of toxic heavy metals such as lead, tin, mercury, and arsenic. These metals all pose specific threats to health if they accumulate in the body. Those metals considered inert, such as iron and aluminum, were not included. Next, we commissioned the standard steroid quantification testing to see how these products were dosed, then checked for unknown steroidal contaminants. Pharmaceutical grade steroids are highly pure. Unprocessed intermediary chemicals or other contaminants should not appear upon analysis. The presence of unknown steroidal substances would signify that lower quality materials (not made to pharmaceutical standards) were used. Finally, we examined the oil for other substances, such as the flavoring agent 2,4-decadienal. This material is common to food products, and its presence would demonstrate that food-grade oil (not pure pharmaceutical-grade oil for injection) was used during product manufacture.

The specific results for each of the four testing sets are presented in the tables below. Overall, the products examined in this study reflected poorly on the quality of the underground steroid market. To begin with, more than 20% of the products (1 in 5) contained heavy metal contamination. While pre-market testing would have caught this, if such products were ever found on pharmacy shelves in the United States it would trigger an immediate nationwide recall. Next, an examination of basic drug dosing showed many deviations. Approximately 35% of the products were actually significantly overdosed. While this was likely done in an effort to produce a stronger user response and loyal customer base, this is an unacceptable tactic which raises many potential safety issues. In the third set of tests, more than 60% of the samples were shown to contain some type of unidentified steroidal compound. This does not necessarily mean the products were dangerous, as this may simply consist of inert steroid precursors/intermediary compounds. It does, however, show that impure steroid materials were used during the manufacturing process. Lastly, testing for 2,4-decadienal confirmed that at least 14% of the steroids tested used food grade oil, perhaps the type purchased in a grocery store.

Drug Analysis Results

Test #1: Heavy Metals Contamination

Sample	Contamination	Result
1. methandrostenolone	None Detected (<0.002)	PASS
2. testosterone enanthate	None Detected (<0.002)	PASS
3. testosterone enanthate	None Detected (<0.002)	PASS
4. testosterone propionate	None Detected (<0.002)	PASS
5. boldenone undecylenate	Metals Found (>0.002)	FAIL
6. testosterone cypionate	None Detected (<0.002)	PASS
7. boldenone undecylenate	Metals Found (<0.002)	FAIL
8. trenbolone hexahydro.	None Detected (<0.002)	PASS
9. testosterone cypionate	None Detected (<0.002)	PASS
10. methenolone enanthate	Metals Found (>0.002)	FAIL
11. testosterone cypionate	None Detected (<0.002)	PASS

12. nandrolone decanoate	None Detected (<0.002)		PASS
13. methenolone enanthate	None Detected (<0.002)		PASS
14. trenbolone enanthate	None Detected (<0.002)		PASS

Failure Rate: 21%

Test #2: Dosage vs. Label Claim (mg/mL)

Sample	Labeled Dose	Actual Dose	% of Claim	Pass/Fail
1. methandrostenolone	25 mg	115 mg	459%	FAIL
2. testosterone enanthate	250 mg	440 mg	176%	FAIL
3. testosterone enanthate	250 mg	408 mg	163%	FAIL
4. testosterone propionate	75 mg	127 mg	169%	FAIL
5. boldenone undecylenate	200 mg	240 mg	120%	PASS
6. testosterone cypionate	200 mg	204 mg	102%	PASS
7. boldenone undecylenate	200 mg	178 mg	89%	PASS
8. trenbolone hexahydro.	76 mg	190 mg	249%	FAIL
9. testosterone cypionate	200 mg	177 mg	88%	PASS
10. methenolone enanthate	100 mg	54 mg	54%	FAIL
11. testosterone cypionate	250 mg	171 mg	69%	FAIL
12. nandrolone decanoate	250 mg	228 mg	91%	PASS
13. methenolone enanthate	100 mg	78 mg	78%	FAIL
14. trenbolone enanthate	100 mg	0 mg	0%	FAIL

Failure Rate: 64% (+/- >20% of Label Claim)

Test #3: Steroidal Materials Purity

Sample	Contamination	Result
1. methandrostenolone	None Detected	PASS
2. testosterone enanthate	None Detected	PASS
3. testosterone enanthate	Unknown Peak Detected	FAIL
4. testosterone propionate	None Detected	PASS
5. boldenone undecylenate	None Detected	PASS
6. testosterone cypionate	Unknown Peak Detected	FAIL

Sample		Result
7. boldenone undecylenate	None Detected	PASS
8. trenbolone hexahydro.	Unknown Peak Detected	FAIL
9. testosterone cypionate	Unknown Peak Detected	FAIL
10. methenolone enanthate	Unknown Peak Detected	FAIL
11. testosterone cypionate	None Detected	PASS
12. nandrolone decanoate	Unknown Peak Detected	FAIL
13. methenolone enanthate	Unknown Peak Detected	FAIL
14. trenbolone enanthate	Unknown Peak Detected	FAIL

Failure Rate: 57%

Test #4: Oil Purity

Sample	Contamination	Result
1. methandrostenolone	2,4-Decadienal Detected	FAIL
2. testosterone enanthate	None Detected	PASS
3. testosterone enanthate	None Detected	PASS
4. testosterone propionate	None Detected	PASS
5. boldenone undecylenate	None Detected	PASS
6. testosterone cypionate	None Detected	PASS
7. boldenone undecylenate	None Detected	PASS
8. trenbolone hexahydro.	None Detected	PASS
9. testosterone cypionate	None Detected	PASS
10. methenolone enanthate	None Detected	PASS
11. testosterone cypionate	None Detected	PASS
12. nandrolone decanoate	None Detected	PASS
13. methenolone enanthate	2,4-Decadienal Detected	FAIL
14. trenbolone enanthate	None Detected	PASS

Failure Rate: 14%

Conclusions

The scope of testing for this project was fairly limited, and fell well short of the detailed analysis required to validate a real prescription drug product. Still, the standards were rigid enough for a strong majority of the underground steroid products to fail testing. These drugs did not achieve a passing result due to a number of important purity concerns. The reasons being that 1) they contained toxic heavy metals; 2) they were significantly under- or over-dosed; 3) they contained impure (not pharmaceutical grade) raw steroid materials; and/or 4) they were made with food-grade (not pharmaceutical grade) oil. It is important to remember is that this analysis project only covered 14 products, which is a very small number relative to the total number of underground steroid manufacturing operations and products in existence. It is possible that a different set of 14 samples would yield a considerably different set of results. Still, the very high failure rate seen during this investigation appears to underline several important purity concerns with underground steroid products.

Legitimate pharmaceutical products are manufactured under strict conditions for a reason. It is very difficult to maintain an acceptable level of purity without them. Even if pure USP/BP grade materials are being used, it can be very easy for a microscopic biological pathogen or other contaminant to enter a solution unless every single potential source of contamination is addressed. Underground manufacturers have little financial incentive (or often logistical possibility) to make their drugs according to these strict purity standards. Instead, a lower quality ("food grade") level of manufacturing may dominate the underground market. There are likely few exceptions, involving only the largest and most reputable underground operations. While the number of anecdotal reports of injury from underground steroid products appears to be relatively low overall, and admittedly a substantial dose of alcohol in solution will kill most biological contaminants, consumers must be aware that there remains a high likelihood of impurity with underground drugs. By the very nature of these products purity cannot be assured, and results like those of the ANABOLICS Underground Market Analysis only further highlight this. In general, underground steroids should not be considered equal substitutes for licensed pharmaceuticals.

Designer Steroids

There is a fatal flaw in the steroid detection methods used by the various sports agencies. That is, in order to test someone for anabolic steroids, you need to know exactly what you are looking for. You can't just look for "steroids" in the urine, but are forced to test for each specific compound individually. To make things even more complicated, you need to know more than just what these steroids look like chemically before they are administered. You need to know what they are going to look like by the time they appear in the urine, because the original steroids themselves will largely be metabolized into other compounds. For example, nandrolone use is most easily detected by looking for its major metabolites 19-norandrosterone and 19-noretiocholanolone,[353] not nandrolone itself. With this in mind, you need to investigate each potential steroid of "misuse" very closely, and each plan of detection is going to be difficult, and time-consuming, to develop. The past couple of decades have seen a lot of progress in identifying the metabolites unique to most commercially available synthetic steroids. As a result, they are almost all detectable in a urine sample now. In reality, this may still only be a drop in the bucket.

You see, several hundred, if not a thousand or more, different steroids were synthesized and investigated in various laboratories around the world during the heyday of steroid research. In most cases, their anabolic and androgenic potencies were measured, with the same methods that have been used on all of the popular steroids we know today. Only a minute fraction of these research compounds ultimately became commercially available drug products, leaving many potentially excellent steroids by the wayside. This is to be expected in any area of drug research though, as there would be no way for hundreds of similar drugs to exist in the same market. But the early research is still out there, and remains a very valuable source of information for the clever chemists of today.

Some of these old research steroids of the '50s and '60s still exist today, due to the diligence of underground chemists and researchers. We refer to these drugs collectively as "Designer Steroids", and they are here only for the purpose of defeating a drug screen. A true designer steroid is structurally unique next to the known anabolic/androgenic steroids, sharing no common metabolites, so as to be undetectable to even the most thorough steroid test. The thought of tracking down metabolites for all possible steroids compounds, to eliminate the designer steroids issue, seems like an impossible task to say the least. Even if somehow this old research were to be exhausted, and metabolites identified for all known steroids, there are still nearly limitless other ways to alter testosterone, nandrolone, or dihydrotestosterone to make unique new steroids. The designer steroid phenomena could obviously present an overwhelming problem to the sports organizations given present drug testing methods. The athletes can easily stay one or two steps ahead, and nobody on the sidelines is the wiser.

At this point in time, the fact that designer steroids exist is no secret to the sports agencies. It became painfully obvious to the IOC (International Olympic Committee) in March of 2002, when the UCLA Olympic Analytical Lab detected norbolethone, a potent c-17 alpha alkylated nandrolone derivative investigated back in the 1960s, in the urine samples from a female athlete[354](see Drug Profiles: Norbolethone). It turned out to be Tammy Thomas, a 32-year-old cyclist from Colorado Springs. This was the second time she failed a drug test actually, which resulted in a lifetime ban from competition. One of the samples in question was actually flagged previously, with a group of others, because it had extremely low endogenous steroid concentrations (suggesting suppression from exogenous steroid administration). Don Catlin, who runs the UCLA Olympic Analytical Laboratory, would connect it to the designer steroid norbolethone much later. The fact that only one of these samples retroactively tested positive suggests that other designer steroids were being used by competitors in addition to norbolethone.

Catlin was able to obtain a sample of pure norbolethone from the drug company Wyeth, and must have been greatly aided by the fact that metabolites of this steroid had been identified in earlier studies.[355] The procedure for norbolethone detection has now been made available to all testing agencies, and unfortunately it is now unsafe for competition. Its value as a designer steroid has likewise vanished overnight. Perhaps it was a bad idea to use a steroid that actual made it all the way to the point of clinical trials in the U.S., as there is quite a bit of information to be found on it (not having the urinary metabolites study would have made things a lot harder on Catlin). Honestly, I can think of a number of more effective and safer compounds to use than this hideously progestational one (ooh, the water bloat). I don't think the chemist was really thinking this one through very thoroughly, and next time may want to get some help from someone that really knows these agents.

The norbolethone story quietly fell from the public conscience not long after it broke. The number of athletes that ultimately tested positive for the drug was minimal, so it really never evolved into the big scandal that was initially expected. The USADA thrives on negative media attention to steroids, because it leads to more government funding, so no doubt this lack of public outrage was a disappointment. I would suspect many involved were hoping for the global story on par with what happened when Ben Johnson was stripped of his gold medal during the 1988 summer Olympics. This would be of little matter by January 2004, however, because a much bigger doping scandal was about to hit. It involved the use of the designer steroid tetrahydrogestrinone (see Drug Profiles: THG), and this time would snare some of the biggest figures in amateur and professional sports. Not just Olympic competitors, but professional football and baseball players were being listed as potential violators. Many household names were being thrown around, including Jason Giambi, Barry Bonds, and Gary Scheffield. Over 20 athletes ultimately tested positive for THG, or were specifically named for using it in the evidence. The investigation continues today, so this number may rise. Don Catlin was once again the scientist who helped identify this compound in the first place, as well as a method of its detection in urine. This time around, however, he had a lot more help then he did with norbolethone. THG was actually handed over to the IOC testing laboratory in a syringe, by an anonymous coach who did not approve of its use. With the help of an inside informant, USADA got their Ben Johnson story, and then some. THG was at the center of the biggest organized doping scandal in the history of competitive sports, and would come to spark a more vigorous government fight against steroid use than we had yet seen. The steroid-using community is only now beginning to feel the backlash.

I include these stories not because they illustrate victories for the IOC. Quite the contrary, I believe they underline the major failings in current steroid testing methods. These two incidents logically do not represent the only two designer steroids ever used in competitive sports. For one, we surely cannot expect a 100% success rate for the IOC when we know that THG use went completely unnoticed for months, if not years. Nobody knew anything about this steroid until a sample was handed over to the testing facility, which is the same facility that had unwittingly been passing urine samples containing the same steroid just days before. Were it not for the inside source, THG would probably still be in use today. The norbolethone and THG stories spit in the face of those on the sidelines, who insist that drug testing ensures their favorite athlete is drug free. The fact is, many other potent designer steroids are probably out there, either in the books, or in the gym bags, of many of the world's top competitors. It may take years for the next designer compound to be identified by the IOC labs, and perhaps only a matter of weeks for a new one to be synthesized once it is. It is a game the drug testers simply cannot win given the tools they have available to them now. We may see repeats of these scandals in the future, but such events will only exemplify the proficiency of those working against drug testing. They show the public the unshakable will of the athletes who are going to use these agents, not the testing agencies that police them.

Anabolic Steroids and the Law

United States law prohibits the possession of anabolic steroids without a legal medical prescription, imparting severe penalties (including fine and/or imprisonment) for those that choose to violate these laws. Under influence of U.S. government officials, World Anti-Doping Agency (WADA) members, and public criticism following numerous doping scandals, a growing number of countries are following the U.S. by adopting their own laws against the possession of anabolic steroids and other sports doping drugs. In many cases similar severe criminal penalties have been enacted. The following section discusses in more detail various national laws that concern the personal use of anabolic steroids and other related drugs.

United States

Anabolic steroids have been classified as controlled substances in the United States since 1991, with passage of the Anabolic Steroid Control Act of 1990 (Pub. L. No. 101-647, Sec. 1902, 104 Stat. 4851, 1990). This law makes it a criminal offense to sell, distribute, manufacture, or possess anabolic steroids without proper legal authorization. The outlined penalties for possession without a legal prescription include a maximum of 1 year of imprisonment and/or a minimum fine of $1,000. This may be increased to 2 years of imprisonment and/or a $2,500 minimum fine for individuals with a prior drug conviction. Note that this law was amended in 2005 following passage of the Anabolic Steroid Control Act of 2004. The new law added 26 new steroid compounds to the list of controlled substances, and also removed the legal requirement that a compound be proven anabolic in humans before it can be added. This "promotes muscle growth" clause was the key roadblock to removing many of the "legal steroids" of the late 1990s and early 2000s.

State vs. Federal

Criminal laws against the possession of anabolic steroids exist at both the federal and state level in the U.S. Depending on the circumstance, an individual may be charged with a steroid related crime by either the federal government or the state government where the crime took place. Unless the crossing of state lines was involved, most criminal prosecutions for steroid-related crimes take place at the state level in accordance with state laws. Most often the state laws mirror federal statutes very closely,

---

The main body (drug listings) of the Anabolic Steroid Control Act has been included for your review below.

`(A) The term `anabolic steroid' means any drug or hormonal substance, chemically and pharmacologically related to testosterone (other than estrogens, progestins, corticosteroids, and dehydroepiandrosterone), and includes--

`(i) androstanediol--

`(I) 3b,17b-dihydroxy-5a-androstane; and

`(II) 3a,17b-dihydroxy-5a-androstane;

`(ii) androstanedione (5a-androstan-3,17-dione);

`(iii) androstenediol--

`(I) 1-androstenediol (3b,17b-dihydroxy-5a-androst-1-ene);

`(II) 1-androstenediol (3a,17b-dihydroxy-5a-androst-1-ene);

`(III) 4-androstenediol (3b,17b-dihydroxy-androst-4-ene); and

`(IV) 5-androstenediol (3b,17b-dihydroxy-androst-5-ene);

`(iv) androstenedione--

`(I) 1-androstenedione ([5a]-androst-1-en-3,17-dione);

`(II) 4-androstenedione (androst-4-en-3,17-dione); and

`(III) 5-androstenedione (androst-5-en-3,17-dione);

`(v) bolasterone (7a,17a-dimethyl-17b-hydroxyandrost-4-en-3-one);

`(vi) boldenone (17b-hydroxyandrost-1,4,-diene-3-one);

`(vii) calusterone (7b,17a-dimethyl-17b-hydroxyandrost-4-en-3-one);

`(viii) clostebol (4-chloro-17b-hydroxyandrost-4-en-3-one);

`(ix) dehydrochloromethyltestosterone (4-chloro-17b-hydroxy-17a-methyl-androst-1,4-dien-3-one);

`(x) *1-dihydrotestosterone (a.k.a. `1-testosterone') (17b-hydroxy-5a-androst-1-en-3-one);

`(xi) 4-dihydrotestosterone (17b-hydroxy-androstan-3-one);

`(xii) drostanolone (17b-hydroxy-2a-methyl-5a-androstan-3-one);

`(xiii) ethylestrenol (17a-ethyl-17b-hydroxyestr-4-ene);

`(xiv) fluoxymesterone (9-fluoro-17a-methyl-11b,17b-dihydroxyandrost-4-en-3-one);

`(xv) formebolone (2-formyl-17a-methyl-11a,17b-dihydroxyandrost-1,4-dien-3-one);

`(xvi) furazabol (17a-methyl-17b-hydroxyandrostano[2,3-c]-furazan);

`(xvii) 13a-ethyl-17a-hydroxygon-4-en-3-one;

`(xviii) 4-hydroxytestosterone (4,17b-dihydroxy-androst-4-en-3-one);

`(xix) 4-hydroxy-19-nortestosterone (4,17b-dihydroxy-estr-4-en-3-one);

`(xx) mestanolone (17a-methyl-17b-hydroxy-5a-androstan-3-one);

`(xxi) mesterolone (1a-methyl-17b-hydroxy-[5a]-androstan-3-one);

`(xxii) methandienone (17a-methyl-17b-hydroxyandrost-1,4-dien-3-one);

`(xxiii) methandriol (17a-methyl-3b,17b-dihydroxyandrost-5-ene);

`(xxiv) methenolone (1-methyl-17b-hydroxy-5a-androst-1-en-3-one);

`(xxv) methyltestosterone (17a-methyl-17b-hydroxyandrost-4-en-3-one);

`(xxvi) mibolerone (7a,17a-dimethyl-17b-hydroxyestr-4-en-3-one);

`(xxvii) 17a-methyl-*1-dihydrotestosterone (17b-hydroxy-17a-methyl-5a-androst-1-en-3-one) (a.k.a. `17-a-methyl-1-testosterone');

`(xxviii) nandrolone (17b-hydroxyestr-4-en-3-one);

`(xxix) norandrostenediol--

`(I) 19-nor-4-androstenediol (3b, 17b-dihydroxyestr-4-ene);

`(II) 19-nor-4-androstenediol (3a, 17b-dihydroxyestr-4-ene);

`(III) 19-nor-5-androstenediol (3b, 17b-dihydroxyestr-5-ene); and

`(IV) 19-nor-5-androstenediol (3a, 17b-dihydroxyestr-5-ene);

`(xxx) norandrostenedione--

`(I) 19-nor-4-androstenedione (estr-4-en-3,17-dione); and

`(II) 19-nor-5-androstenedione (estr-5-en-3,17-dione;

`(xxxi) norbolethone (13b,17a-diethyl-17b-hydroxygon-4-en-3-one);

`(xxxii) norclostebol (4-chloro-17b-hydroxyestr-4-en-3-one);

`(xxxiii) norethandrolone (17a-ethyl-17b-hydroxyestr-4-en-3-one);

`(xxxiv) oxandrolone (17a-methyl-17b-hydroxy-2-oxa-[5a]-androstan-3-one);

`(xxxv) oxymesterone (17a-methyl-4,17b-dihydroxyandrost-4-en-3-one);

`(xxxvi) oxymetholone (17a-methyl-2-hydroxymethylene-17b-hydroxy-[5a]-androstan-3-one);

`(xxxvii) stanozolol (17a-methyl-17b-hydroxy-[5a]-androst-2-eno[3,2-c]-pyrazole);

`(xxxviii) stenbolone (17b-hydroxy-2-methyl-[5a]-androst-1-en-3-one);

`(xxxix) testolactone (13-hydroxy-3-oxo-13,17-secoandrosta-1,4-dien-17-oic acid lactone);

> '(xl) testosterone (17b-hydroxyandrost-4-en-3-one);
>
> '(xli) tetrahydrogestrinone (13b,17a-diethyl-17b-hydroxygon-4,9,11-trien-3-one);
>
> '(xlii) trenbolone (17b-hydroxyestr-4,9,11-trien-3-one); and
>
> '(xliii) any salt, ester, or ether of a drug or substance described in this paragraph.';

although this is not always the case. There can also be a great deal of variability in how punishments are determined between one state and another. If you are not obtaining medications legally through a physician's prescription, it is advisable to study the steroid laws closely, particularly those of your individual state. The book "Legal Muscle: Anabolics in America" by lawyer Rick Collins [teamlegalmuscle.com] is an excellent review of the legal situation concerning steroids in the U.S., including a detailed breakdown of all state steroid laws.

Austria

The possession of anabolic steroids is not a criminal act according to Austrian law. In 2008, Austrian government officials announced intent to place criminal penalties on steroid possession.

Australia

It is a criminal act to import, supply, use, or possess anabolic steroids in Australia without a prescription from a medical practitioner, dentist, or veterinarian (Poisons and Drugs Act Amendment of 1994). The outlined penalties for possession without a legal prescription include a maximum of 6 months of imprisonment and/or a fine of $5,000.

Canada

Anabolic steroids are included in the Canadian Controlled Drugs and Substances Act as Schedule IV substances. It is illegal to sell, manufacture, or import anabolic steroids into Canada without proper legal authorization. Possession of anabolic steroids for personal use is not a criminal act.

Czech Republic

In 2008 it became a criminal act to manufacture, import, export, store, or distribute anabolic steroids in the Czech Republic. The potential penalties include a maximum of 3 years in prison. It is not a crime to possess steroids for personal use.

Denmark

In Denmark it is a crime to manufacture, import, export, market, dispense, distribute, or possess doping substances including anabolic steroids, human growth hormone, and erythropoietin without proper medical or scientific reason (The Act on Prohibition of Certain Doping Substances No. 232 of 21 April 1999). The potential penalties for possession include a maximum of 2 years in prison.

France

In 2008 it became a criminal offense to manufacture, transport, acquire, or possess doping substances including anabolic steroids, human growth hormone, and erythropoietin in France. The potential penalties for possession include a maximum of 5 years imprisonment and/or a 75,000 Euro fine.

Greece

The possession of anabolic steroids is not a criminal act according to Greek law. In 2008, government officials announced intent to place criminal penalties on steroid possession in Greece.

Sweden

In Sweden it is a crime to import, manufacture, transport, sell, possess, or use doping substances such as anabolic steroids and growth hormone without proper legal authorization (The Swedish Act prohibiting certain doping substances (1991,1969). The potential penalties include a maximum of 2 years in prison. Possession for personal use is usually regarded as a petty offense and given a maximum penalty of 6 months imprisonment.

United Kingdom

The importation, possession, and use of anabolic steroids are not criminal acts according to UK law. There has been a great deal of pressure in recent years from the U.S. and World Anti-Doping Agency to place criminal penalties on the possession of anabolic steroids without a prescription.

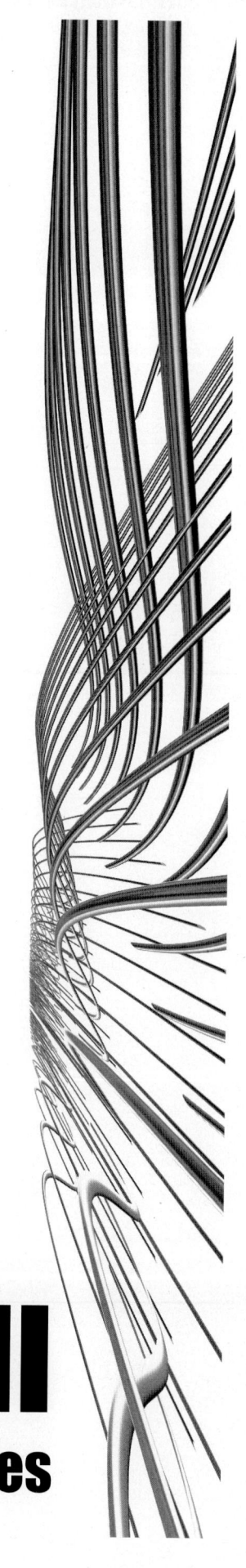

Part III
Drug Profiles

ANABOLIC/ANDROGENIC STEROIDS Drug Profiles

1-Testosterone (dihydroboldenone)

Androgenic	100
Anabolic	200
Standard[356]	Testosterone propionate
Chemical Names	17beta-hydroxyandrost-1-en-3-one
	5alpha-androst-1-en-3-one,17beta-ol
Estrogenic Activity	low
Progestational Activity	no data available

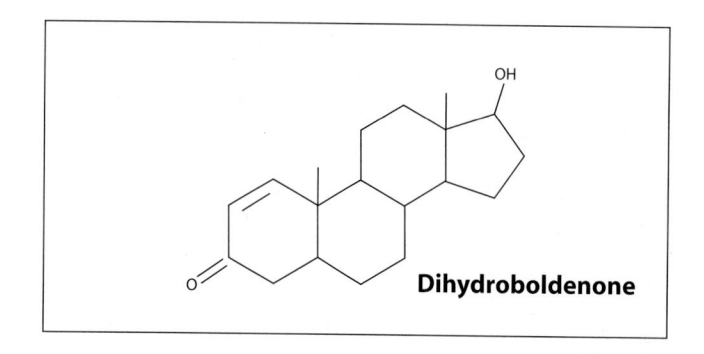

Dihydroboldenone

Description:

1-Testosterone is an anabolic steroid that is derived from dihydrotestosterone. More specifically, it is a dihydro (5-alpha reduced) form of the anabolic steroid boldenone. It is also structurally very similar to Primobolan (methenolone), except that 1-testosterone lacks the additional 1-methyl group used to increase steroid oral bioavailability. The activity of this steroid is that of a strong anabolic agent, with moderate androgenic properties. The standard rat assays show it to be approximately twice as anabolic as testosterone propionate, while it retains a similar level of androgenicity. This gives it an anabolic ratio of about 2, which means it is twice as anabolic as it is androgenic. 1-testosterone is one of the most potent naturally occurring steroids to be isolated, and is valued by bodybuilders for its ability to promote significant muscle tissue gains without water bloat or strong side effects.

History:

Although synthesized some years earlier, the first detailed mention of 1-testosterone in the Western medical literature seems to come in 1962.[357] It was favorably studied (on a limited basis), but never developed as a prescription drug product, likely for a simple lack of financial viability (there are literally thousands of testosterone analogs that have been developed over the years, but certainly no incentive to try and develop all of them into medicines). It was once placed into development as an ether derivative (1-methoxycyclohexyloxy) called mesabolone, but even this was very short lived. 1-testosterone had essentially been lost in the steroid research books for decades, and was all but forgotten. Things changed very quickly in 2002, however, when the drug was released to the U.S. market as a nutritional supplement. Although technically questionable in a legal sense, the popularity of the new hormone was rapid and extreme, and countless OTC 1-testosterone products soon followed.

1-Testosterone is not intrinsically a very orally active hormone. Therefore, it is a little difficult to create a product of high potency with this method of administration. It is very much like taking a powerful hormone such as testosterone, and trying to stuff it in a capsule. The liver is too efficient at breaking steroids down for this to be effective. When 1-testosterone was available as a supplement in the U.S., oil-solubilized softgels using 1-testosterone tetrahydropyranyl ether, hexyldecanoate ester, and undecanoate ester were the most effective products (ANABOLICS author William Llewellyn introduced the first such product). These products resembled Andriol, which dissolves an ester-modified form of testosterone (undecanoate) in oil to help deliver the steroid to the body via the lymphatic system (bypassing the destructive first-pass through the liver).

Some companies were also formulating this steroid in transdermal gels during this time, which is another effective method of getting this hormone into your body. These products were designed in a similar fashion as Androgel, and likely delivered about 10% of the applied dose to the body systemically. Lastly, there were a few products that were made as injectables (1-testosterone cypionate), which reportedly worked very well. This would be the preferred method of using 1-testosterone, although no legitimate prescription drug preparation like this has ever existed (these were essentially injectable drug products created by unregulated supplement companies). While many consumers used them with great success, there was simply no government oversight assuring such products were made to pharmaceutical specifications.

1-Testosterone was sold on the sports supplement market in the U.S. for approximately three years. It was finally classified as a Class III controlled substance in January 2005, as part of an expanded Anabolic Steroid Control Act that was passed by Congress that sought to eliminate OTC steroids. These products were most often described by their manufacturers as prohormones or prosteroids, although were in reality often just unscheduled (unknown to lawmakers) steroids. Given that no legitimate pharmaceutical preparation has ever contained 1-testosterorone, the passing of this law effectively marked the commercial end of this anabolic steroid. At the present time, no 1-testosterone preparations are known to exist, and the agent is once again unavailable to athletes.

How Supplied:

No prescription drug product containing 1-testosterone currently exists. It was sold as an OTC supplement in the U.S. between 2002 and 2005, produced in various oral, transdermal, and injectable forms.

Structural Characteristics:

1-Testosterone is a derivative of dihydrotestosterone. It contains one additional double bond between carbons 1 and 2 (1-ene), which helps to stabilize the 3-keto group and increase the steroid's anabolic properties.

Note that the name 1-testosterone is actually a misnomer, and is not a formal identification for this drug. The term 1-testosterone is more appropriately applied to the steroid boldenone, which consists of a testosterone molecule modified with a 1-ene group. Given the widespread association of 1-testosterone with this steroid, however, it has been identified as such in this reference book.

Side Effects (Estrogenic):

1-Testosterone does metabolize to estrogen in the body, even though there is no evidence that the body can insert a double bond at carbon-4.[358][359] The exact nature of this transformation is unknown. Given experiences with the hormone, 1-testoserone is considered to be only a mild estrogenic steroid. Estrogen-linked side effects are generally not seen when administering this steroid, including gynecomastia, fat deposition, and visibly increased water retention. Gains made with 1-testosterone tend to be quality muscle mass, not the smooth bulk that often accompanies steroids highly open to aromatization. 1-Testosterone is, therefore, a steroid most favored during cutting phases of training, when water and fat retention are major concerns, and sheer mass not the central objective.

Side Effects (Androgenic):

Although classified as an anabolic steroid, androgenic side effects are still possible with this substance. This may include bouts of oily skin, acne, and body/facial hair growth. Anabolic/androgenic steroids may also aggravate male pattern hair loss. Women are warned of the potential virilizing effects of anabolic/androgenic steroids. These may include a deepening of the voice, menstrual irregularities, changes in skin texture, facial hair growth, and clitoral enlargement. Due to its lower relative androgenicity, women often find this preparation an acceptable choice provided low doses are used. Although 1-testosterone is primarily anabolic in nature, strong androgenic side effects are possible with higher doses, and should be carefully monitored. Note that the 5-alpha reductase enzyme does not metabolize 1-testosterone, so its relative androgenicity is not affected by finasteride or dutasteride.

Side Effects (Hepatotoxicity):

1-Testosterone is not known to be a hepatotoxic steroid; liver toxicity is unlikely within normal parameters of use. Note that studies have shown that 1-testosterone significantly increases liver weight (unlike testosterone), suggesting that risk of liver toxicity cannot be completely excluded with high doses or prolonged administration.[360]

Side Effects (Cardiovascular):

Anabolic/androgenic steroids can have deleterious effects on serum cholesterol. This includes a tendency to reduce HDL (good) cholesterol values and increase LDL (bad) cholesterol values, which may shift the HDL to LDL balance in a direction that favors greater risk of arteriosclerosis. The relative impact of an anabolic/androgenic steroid on serum lipids is dependant on the dose, route of administration (oral vs. injectable), type of steroid (aromatizable or non-aromatizable), and level of resistance to hepatic metabolism. 1-Testosterone should have a stronger negative effect on the hepatic management of cholesterol than testosterone or nandrolone due to its weakly aromatized nature, but a weaker impact than most c-17 alpha alkylated steroids. Due to the route of delivery, oral 1-testosterone will have a slightly stronger negative effect on lipids compared to injections. Anabolic/androgenic steroids may also adversely affect blood pressure and triglycerides, reduce endothelial relaxation, and support left ventricular hypertrophy, all potentially increasing the risk of cardiovascular disease and myocardial infarction.

To help reduce cardiovascular strain it is advised to maintain an active cardiovascular exercise program and minimize the intake of saturated fats, cholesterol, and simple carbohydrates at all times during active AAS administration. Supplementing with fish oils (4 grams per day) and a natural cholesterol/antioxidant formula such as Lipid Stabil or a product with comparable ingredients is also recommended.

Side Effects (Testosterone Suppression):

All anabolic/androgenic steroids when taken in doses sufficient to promote muscle gain are expected to suppress endogenous testosterone production. Without the intervention of testosterone-stimulating substances, testosterone levels should return to normal within 1-4 months of drug secession. Note that prolonged hypogonadotrophic hypogonadism can develop secondary to steroid abuse, necessitating medical intervention.

The above side effects are not inclusive. For more detailed discussion of potential side effects, see the Steroid Side Effects section of this book.

Administration (General):

Note that 1-testosterone is slightly an intrinsically irritating substance. This makes injection with the base hormone, even transdermal delivery at times, uncomfortable, producing skin/tissue irritation and redness. Some users even tend to notice a burning sensation when urinating while taking any 1-testosterone product. Although poorly understood, this side effect has never been reported to be dangerous, and is generally looked at as an inconvenience among users.

Administration (Men):

1-Testosterone was never approved for use in humans. Prescribing guidelines are unavailable. For physique- or performance-enhancing purposes, a daily dosage is usually in the range of 100-250 mg with oil-solubilized softgels, or 75-100 mg daily when applied as a transdermal. Injectable dosages would fall in the range of 100-200 mg per week (as 1-testosterone cypionate). The drug is typically taken in cycles of 6-12 weeks. Users of 1-testosterone generally report lean gains in muscle mass, which are often accompanied by body fat reductions and an increased appearance of hardness to the physique.

Administration (Women):

1-Testosterone was never approved for use in humans. Prescribing guidelines are unavailable. For physique- or performance-enhancing purposes, doses of 25 mg daily or less (oil solubilized softgels or transdermal) are usually used. The drug is typically taken in cycles of 4-6 weeks. Given that most preparations contained high concentrations of drug, 1-testosterone was not widely used by females.

Availability:

1-Testosterone is not produced as a prescription drug product. Only residual stock of OTC product is likely to circulate, and should be in very low volume at this time.

20 AET-1 (testosterone buciclate)

Androgenic	100
Anabolic	100
Standard	Standard
Chemical Names	4-androsten-3-one-17beta-ol
	17beta-hydroxy-androst-4-en-3-one
Estrogenic Activity	moderate
Progestational Activity	low

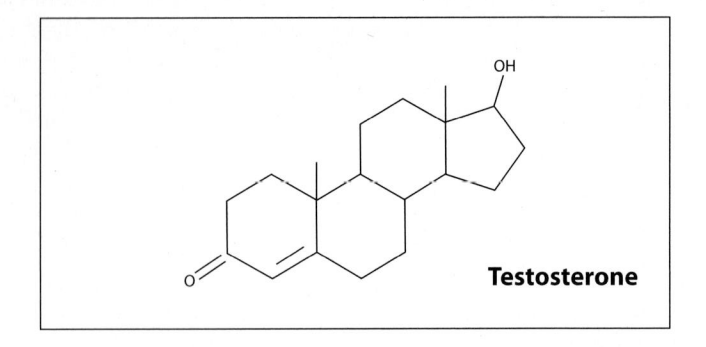

Testosterone

Description:

Testosterone buciclate is a more recently developed injectable testosterone preparation, which utilizes the extremely long, highly oil-soluble, and very slow-acting buciclate ester (also commonly referred to as "20 Aet-1"). At 20 carbon atoms in length, the buciclate ester is the largest ester used to make an injectable steroid preparation. It is about seven times longer than propionate, three times longer than enanthate, and double the length of decanoate. Being that the carbon content of the ester correlates closely to the duration of release, testosterone buciclate is also the longest acting injectable testosterone medication yet to be tested in humans. It appears to be even longer acting than Nebido® (testosterone undecanoate), although both drugs are promising a similar 12-week window of therapeutic effect.

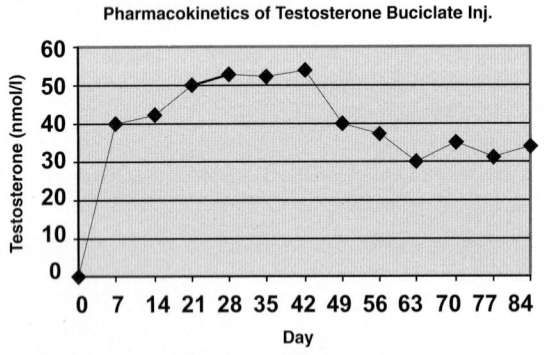

Figure 1. Pharmacokinetics of 600 mg testosterone buciclate injection. Source: Testosterone buciclate (20 Aet-1) in hypogonadal men: pharmacokinetics and pharmacodynamics of the new long-acting androgen ester. Behre HM, Nieschlag E. J Clin Endocrinol Metab. 1992 Nov;75(5):1204-10.

When administered to patients suffering from primary hypogonadism as part of initial clinical studies, a single 600 mg injection of testosterone buciclate was able to maintain therapeutically effective concentrations of testosterone for approximately 12 weeks.[361] No significant peaks were noted in testosterone levels in either group, which are normally observed with esters like enanthate and cypionate. There were no significant side effects, or unfavorable changes in urine flow, PSA (prostate specific antigen) values, or prostate volume. Testosterone buciclate seems to hold a good deal of promise as a slow-acting injectable androgen, with the potential to replace other common esters used for hormone replacement therapy.

History:

Testosterone buciclate was first described in 1986.[362] It was developed as part of a steroid synthesis program that was initiated by the World Health Organization. The focus of this program was to develop longer-acting esters of testosterone, which improved on the disadvantages of existing esters such as enanthate and cypionate, which tended to produce short supraphysiological surges in androgen levels, followed by steadily declining and uneven androgen levels until the next point of administration. Phase-I clinical studies were completed in 1992 (described above), and supported the potential adoption of this agent for the treatment of andropause. Studies conducted three years later suggest the drug may also be useful for male contraception.[363] Testosterone buciclate has already seen a considerable amount of study at this point, but, unlike its similarly slow-acting cousin Nebido®, has yet to be adopted as a prescription drug for widespread use.

How Supplied:

Testosterone buciclate is not currently available as a commercial drug product.

Structural Characteristics:

Testosterone buciclate is a modified form of testosterone, where a carboxylic acid ester (trans-4-n-butylcyclohexyl-carboxylate) has been attached to the 17-beta hydroxyl group. Esterified forms of testosterone are less polar than free testosterone, and are absorbed more slowly from the area of injection. Once in the bloodstream, the ester is removed to yield free (active) testosterone. Esterified forms of testosterone are designed to prolong the window of therapeutic effect following administration, allowing for a less frequent injection schedule compared to injections of free (unesterified) steroid. Testosterone buciclate is designed to maintain physiological levels of testosterone for approximately 12 weeks after injection.

Side Effects (Estrogenic):

Testosterone is readily aromatized in the body to estradiol (estrogen). The aromatase (estrogen synthetase) enzyme is responsible for this metabolism of testosterone. Elevated estrogen levels can cause side effects such as increased water retention, body fat gain, and gynecomastia. Testosterone is considered a moderately estrogenic steroid. An anti-estrogen such as clomiphene citrate or tamoxifen citrate may be necessary to prevent estrogenic side effects. One may alternately use an aromatase inhibitor like Arimidex® (anastrozole), which more efficiently controls estrogen by preventing its synthesis. Aromatase inhibitors can be quite expensive in comparison to anti-estrogens, however, and may also have negative effects on blood lipids.

Estrogenic side effects will occur in a dose-dependant manner, with higher doses (above normal therapeutic levels) of testosterone more likely to require the concurrent use of an anti-estrogen or aromatase inhibitor. Since water retention and loss of muscle definition are common with higher doses of testosterone, this drug is usually considered a poor choice for dieting or cutting phases of training. Its moderate estrogenicity makes it more ideal for bulking phases, where the added water retention will support raw strength and muscle size, and help foster a stronger anabolic environment.

Side Effects (Androgenic):

Testosterone is the primary male androgen, responsible for maintaining secondary male sexual characteristics. Elevated levels of testosterone are likely to produce androgenic side effects including oily skin, acne, and body/facial hair growth. Men with a genetic predisposition for hair loss (androgenetic alopecia) may notice accelerated male pattern balding. Those concerned about hair loss may find a more comfortable option in nandrolone decanoate, which is a comparably less androgenic steroid. Women are warned of the potential virilizing effects of anabolic/androgenic steroids, especially with a strong androgen such as testosterone. These may include deepening of the voice, menstrual irregularities, changes in skin texture, facial hair growth, and clitoral enlargement.

In androgen-responsive target tissues such as the skin, scalp, and prostate, the high relative androgenicity of testosterone is dependant on its reduction to dihydrotestosterone (DHT). The 5-alpha reductase enzyme is responsible for this metabolism of testosterone. The concurrent use of a 5-alpha reductase inhibitor such as finasteride or dutasteride will interfere with site-specific potentiation of testosterone action, lowering the tendency of testosterone drugs to produce androgenic side effects. It is important to remember that both anabolic and androgenic effects are mediated via the cytosolic androgen receptor. Complete separation of testosterone's anabolic and androgenic properties is not possible, even with total 5-alpha reductase inhibition.

Side Effects (Hepatotoxicity):

Testosterone does not have hepatotoxic effects; liver toxicity is unlikely. One study examined the potential for hepatotoxicity with high doses of testosterone by administering 400 mg of the hormone per day (2,800 mg per week) to a group of male subjects. The steroid was taken orally so that higher peak concentrations would be reached in hepatic tissues compared to intramuscular injections. The hormone was given daily for 20 days, and produced no significant changes in liver enzyme values including serum albumin, bilirubin, alanine-amino-transferase, and alkaline phosphatases.[364]

Side Effects (Cardiovascular):

Anabolic/androgenic steroids can have deleterious effects on serum cholesterol. This includes a tendency to reduce HDL (good) cholesterol values and increase LDL (bad) cholesterol values, which may shift the HDL to LDL balance in a direction that favors greater risk of arteriosclerosis. The relative impact of an anabolic/androgenic steroid on serum lipids is dependant on the dose, route of administration (oral vs. injectable), type of steroid (aromatizable or non-aromatizable), and level of resistance to hepatic metabolism. Anabolic/androgenic steroids may also adversely effect blood pressure and triglycerides, reduce endothelial relaxation, and support left ventricular hypertrophy, all potentially increasing the risk of cardiovascular disease and myocardial infarction.

Testosterone tends to have a much less dramatic impact on cardiovascular risk factors than synthetic steroids. This is due in part to its openness to metabolism by the liver, which allows it to have less effect on the hepatic management of cholesterol. The aromatization of testosterone to estradiol also helps to mitigate the negative effects of androgens on serum lipids. In one study, 280 mg per week of testosterone ester (enanthate) had a slight but not statistically significant effect on HDL cholesterol after 12 weeks, but when taken with an aromatase inhibitor a strong (25%) decrease was seen.[365] Studies using 300 mg of testosterone ester (enanthate) per week for twenty weeks without an aromatase inhibitor demonstrated only a 13% decrease in HDL cholesterol, while at 600 mg the reduction reached 21%.[366] The negative impact of aromatase inhibition should be taken into consideration before such drug is added to testosterone therapy.

Due to the positive influence of estrogen on serum lipids, tamoxifen citrate or clomiphene citrate are preferred to aromatase inhibitors for those concerned with cardiovascular health, as they offer a partial estrogenic effect in the liver. This allows them to potentially improve lipid profiles and offset some of the negative effects of androgens. With doses of 600 mg or less per week, the impact on lipid profile tends to be noticeable but not dramatic, making an anti-estrogen (for cardioprotective purposes) perhaps unnecessary. Doses of 600 mg or less per week have also failed to produce statistically significant changes in LDL/VLDL cholesterol, triglycerides, apolipoprotein B/C-III, C-reactive protein, and insulin sensitivity, all indicating a relatively weak impact on cardiovascular risk factors.[367] When used in moderate doses, injectable testosterone esters are usually considered to be the safest of all anabolic/androgenic steroids.

To help reduce cardiovascular strain it is advised to maintain an active cardiovascular exercise program and minimize the intake of saturated fats, cholesterol, and simple carbohydrates at all times during active AAS administration. Supplementing with fish oils (4 grams per day) and a natural cholesterol/antioxidant formula such as Lipid Stabil or a product with comparable ingredients is also recommended.

Side Effects (Testosterone Suppression):

All anabolic/androgenic steroids when taken in doses sufficient to promote muscle gain are expected to suppress endogenous testosterone production. Testosterone is the primary male androgen, and offers strong negative feedback on endogenous testosterone production. Testosterone-based drugs will, likewise, have a strong effect on the hypothalamic regulation of natural steroid hormones. Without the intervention of testosterone stimulating substances, testosterone levels should return to normal within 1-4 months after the drug has fully cleared the body. Note that prolonged hypogonadotrophic hypogonadism can develop secondary to steroid abuse, necessitating medical intervention.

The above side effects are not inclusive. For more detailed discussion of potential side effects, see the Steroid Side Effects section of this book.

Administration (Men):

To treat androgen insufficiency, clinical protocols support the use of 600 mg every twelve weeks. For bodybuilding purposes, supraphysiological (rather than physiological) hormone levels would require injecting the drug on a more regular basis. The most effective use of this compound in a bodybuilding sense would probably entail the injection of two or more doses of 600 mg in the first two weeks of a cycle. After this point another full dose might be given every 7-15 days, depending on the desired potency or other steroids used. The drug could be discontinued 6-9 weeks before the cycle is going to be concluded, and may cause androgen levels to remain elevated 12 weeks or more after the last dose is given. Post-cycle therapy should be planned accordingly. Testosterone is ultimately very versatile, and can be combined with many other anabolic/androgenic steroids depending on the desired effect.

In the context of bodybuilding, testosterone buciclate will be an effective drug, but it is probably not going to win any awards. For one, a cycle based on this compound would be somewhat slower to start than normal, as it will take time and numerous injections for peak blood levels of testosterone to be reached. For the same reason, testosterone buciclate will end up offering its greatest value in cycles lasting more than 4 or 5 months, where its slow-acting nature may be beneficial by allowing a less frequent injection schedule and greater user comfort. In short cycles, this same trait will just be a hindrance, delaying the achievement of supraphysiological testosterone levels (compared to faster testosterone esters) and a strong anabolic effect.

Administration (Women):

Testosterone buciclate has not been studied in women. This drug is not recommended for women for physique- or performance-enhancing purposes due to its strong androgenic nature, tendency to produce virilizing side effects, and very slow- acting characteristics (making blood levels difficult to control).

Availability:

As testosterone buciclate is still really a research drug in Europe, it is not readily available on the black market at this time. It will not be seen in volume until it is adopted for prescription use in a steroid source country, or the various underground labs decide to take an interest in it. Until then, it remains a drug of academic interest only.

Agovirin Depot (testosterone isobutyrate)

Androgenic	100
Anabolic	100
Standard	Standard
Chemical Names	4-androsten-3-one-17beta-ol
	17beta-hydroxy-androst-4-en-3-one
Estrogenic Activity	moderate
Progestational Activity	low

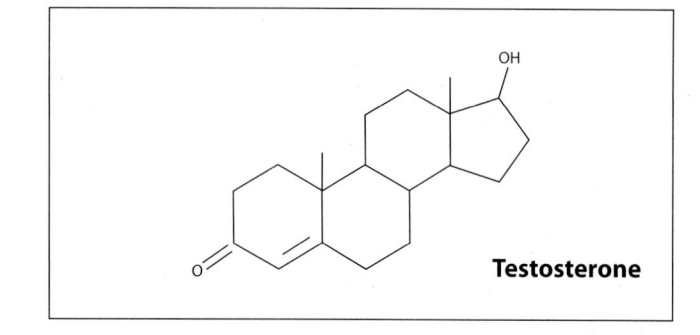

Description:

Testosterone isobutyrate is an injectable steroid preparation that contains the isobutyrate ester of testosterone in a water base. Among bodybuilders, testosterone isobutyrate is often considered analogous to testosterone suspension (no ester). Although both are usually found as water-based suspensions, the pharmacokinetics of the two products are admittedly very different. While testosterone (free) suspension is very fast-acting, requiring injections to be given every few days, testosterone isobutyrate is much slower to release, and is usually administered once every two weeks in a clinical setting. As an injectable testosterone, testosterone isobutyrate is favored for its ability to promote rapid gains in muscle mass and strength.

History:

Injectable testosterone isobutyrate microcrystal suspension was first described in 1952.[368] This agent was developed in an effort to create an injectable (depot) form of testosterone that would be slower acting that regular (free) testosterone suspension or testosterone propionate, the most widely prescribed forms of testosterone at the time. This is accomplished by providing a microcrystalline depot with very low water solubility, delaying the release of free steroid into the bloodstream. Although effective for this purpose, testosterone isobutyrate was developed at a time when many new esters of testosterone were being introduced to the market. By the mid-1950's, testosterone enanthate would emerge as the dominant slow-acting injectable testosterone, and the isobutyrate ester would ultimately see little commercial success.

The only modern steroid product to use testosterone isobutyrate is Agovirin Depot, developed by Biotika in Czechoslovakia. It is primarily prescribed to treat males with insufficient androgen levels and adolescents with delayed puberty, although it is indicated for a variety of other purposes including the treatment of Klinefelter syndrome (a disease where an extra chromosome results in an imbalance of androgenicity and estrogenicity), aplastic anemia, Cushing's syndrome (as an anabolic agent to preserve lean tissue), postmenopausal osteoporosis, advanced breast cancer, mastodynia (breast pain), and cachexia (wasting of the body due to severe illness). Agovirin Depot is still produced by Biotika (currently in the Slovak Republic), and remains a popular export to European black markets.

How Supplied:

Testosterone isobutyrate suspension is available on the human drug market in the Slovak Republic as Agovirin Depot (Biotika). It contains 25 mg/ml of steroid mixed in a water-based solution; packaged in a 2 mL ampule (5 ampules per box). Testosterone isobutyrate has low water solubility; the steroid will noticeably separate from the water-based solution when an ampule is left to sit. A quick shake will temporarily place the drug back into suspension, so that the withdrawn dosage should always be consistent.

Structural Characteristics:

Testosterone isobutyrate is a modified form of testosterone, where a carboxylic acid ester (2-methyl propionic acid) has been attached to the 17-beta hydroxyl group. Esterified forms of testosterone are less polar than free testosterone, and are absorbed more slowly from the area of injection. Once in the bloodstream, the ester is removed to yield free (active) testosterone. Esterified forms of testosterone are designed to prolong the window of therapeutic effect following administration, allowing for a less frequent injection schedule compared to injections of free (unesterified) steroid. Testosterone isobutyrate microcrystalline suspension is designed to provide physiological androgen concentrations for approximately 2 weeks following injection.

Side Effects (Estrogenic):

Testosterone is readily aromatized in the body to estradiol (estrogen). The aromatase (estrogen synthetase) enzyme is responsible for this metabolism of testosterone. Elevated estrogen levels can cause side effects such as increased water retention, body fat gain, and gynecomastia. Testosterone is considered a moderately estrogenic steroid. An anti-estrogen such as clomiphene citrate or tamoxifen citrate may be necessary to prevent estrogenic side effects. One may alternately use an aromatase inhibitor like Arimidex® (anastrozole), which more efficiently controls estrogen by preventing its synthesis. Aromatase inhibitors can be quite expensive in comparison to anti-estrogens, however, and may also have negative effects on blood lipids.

Estrogenic side effects will occur in a dose-dependant manner, with higher doses (above normal therapeutic levels) of testosterone more likely to require the concurrent use of an anti-estrogen or aromatase inhibitor. Since water retention and loss of muscle definition are common with higher doses of testosterone, this drug is usually considered a poor choice for dieting or cutting phases of training. Its moderate estrogenicity makes it more ideal for bulking phases, where the added water retention will support raw strength and muscle size, and help foster a stronger anabolic environment.

Side Effects (Androgenic):

Testosterone is the primary male androgen, responsible for maintaining secondary male sexual characteristics. Elevated levels of testosterone are likely to produce androgenic side effects including oily skin, acne, and body/facial hair growth. Men with a genetic predisposition for hair loss (androgenetic alopecia) may notice accelerated male pattern balding. Those concerned about hair loss may find a more comfortable option in nandrolone decanoate, which is a comparably less androgenic steroid. Women are warned of the potential virilizing effects of anabolic/androgenic steroids, especially with a strong androgen such as testosterone. These may include deepening of the voice, menstrual irregularities, changes in skin texture, facial hair growth, and clitoral enlargement.

In androgen-responsive target tissues such as the skin, scalp, and prostate, the high relative androgenicity of testosterone is dependant on its reduction to dihydrotestosterone (DHT). The 5-alpha reductase enzyme is responsible for this metabolism of testosterone. The concurrent use of a 5-alpha reductase inhibitor such as finasteride or dutasteride will interfere with site-specific potentiation of testosterone action, lowering the tendency of testosterone drugs to produce androgenic side effects. It is important to remember that anabolic and androgenic effects are both mediated via the cytosolic androgen receptor. Complete separation of testosterone's anabolic and androgenic properties is not possible, even with total 5-alpha reductase inhibition.

Side Effects (Hepatotoxicity):

Testosterone does not have hepatotoxic effects; liver toxicity is unlikely. One study examined the potential for hepatotoxicity with high doses of testosterone by administering 400 mg of the hormone per day (2,800 mg per week) to a group of male subjects. The steroid was taken orally so that higher peak concentrations would be reached in hepatic tissues compared to intramuscular injections. The hormone was given daily for 20 days, and produced no significant changes in liver enzyme values including serum albumin, bilirubin, alanine-aminotransferase, and alkaline phosphatases.[369]

Side Effects (Cardiovascular):

Anabolic/androgenic steroids can have deleterious effects on serum cholesterol. This includes a tendency to reduce HDL (good) cholesterol values and increase LDL (bad) cholesterol values, which may shift the HDL to LDL balance in a direction that favors greater risk of arteriosclerosis. The relative impact of an anabolic/androgenic steroid on serum lipids is dependant on the dose, route of administration (oral vs. injectable), type of steroid (aromatizable or non-aromatizable), and level of resistance to hepatic metabolism. Anabolic/androgenic steroids may also adversely effect blood pressure and triglycerides, reduce endothelial relaxation, and support left ventricular hypertrophy, all potentially increasing the risk of cardiovascular disease and myocardial infarction.

Testosterone tends to have a much less dramatic impact on cardiovascular risk factors than synthetic steroids. This is due in part to its openness to metabolism by the liver, which allows it to have less effect on the hepatic management of cholesterol. The aromatization of testosterone to estradiol also helps to mitigate the negative effects of androgens on serum lipids. In one study, 280 mg per week of testosterone ester (enanthate) had a slight but not statistically significant effect on HDL cholesterol after 12 weeks, but when taken with an aromatase inhibitor a strong (25%) decrease was seen.[370] Studies using 300 mg of testosterone ester (enanthate) per week for 20 weeks without an aromatase inhibitor demonstrated only a 13% decrease in HDL cholesterol, while at 600 mg the reduction reached 21%.[371] The negative impact of aromatase inhibition should be taken into consideration before such drug is added to testosterone therapy.

Due to the positive influence of estrogen on serum lipids, tamoxifen citrate or clomiphene citrate are preferred to aromatase inhibitors for those concerned with cardiovascular health, as they offer a partial estrogenic effect in the liver. This allows them to potentially improve lipid profiles and offset some of the negative effects of androgens. With doses of 600 mg or less of testosterone per week, the impact on lipid profile tends to be noticeable but not dramatic, making an anti-estrogen (for cardioprotective purposes) perhaps unnecessary. Doses of 600 mg or less per week have also failed to produce statistically significant changes in LDL/VLDL cholesterol, triglycerides, apolipoprotein B/C-III, C-reactive protein, and insulin sensitivity, all indicating a relatively weak impact on cardiovascular risk factors.[372] When used in moderate doses, injectable testosterone esters are usually considered to be the safest of all anabolic/androgenic steroids.

To help reduce cardiovascular strain it is advised to maintain an active cardiovascular exercise program and minimize the intake of saturated fats, cholesterol, and simple carbohydrates at all times during active AAS administration. Supplementing with fish oils (4 grams per day) and a natural cholesterol/antioxidant formula such as Lipid Stabil or a product with comparable ingredients is also recommended.

Side Effects (Testosterone Suppression):

All anabolic/androgenic steroids when taken in doses sufficient to promote muscle gain are expected to suppress endogenous testosterone production. Testosterone is the primary male androgen, and offers strong negative feedback on endogenous testosterone production. Testosterone-based drugs will, likewise, have a strong effect on the hypothalamic regulation of natural steroid hormones. Without the intervention of testosterone stimulating substances, testosterone levels should return to normal within 1-4 months of drug secession. Note that prolonged hypogonadotrophic hypogonadism can develop secondary to steroid abuse, necessitating medical intervention.

The above side effects are not inclusive. For more detailed discussion of potential side effects, see the Steroid Side Effects section of this book.

Administration (General):

The design of testosterone isobutyrate (as Agovirin Depot) is slightly different than that of most testosterone esters, which are usually made as oily solutions. Agovirin Depot instead contains a microcrystalline aqueous suspension. The crystals form a repository in the muscle following injection, where they slowly dissolve over time. Injections of testosterone isobutyrate may require a large needle (21 gauge), and may result in local irritation, pain, and redness.

Administration (Men):

To treat androgen insufficiency, testosterone isobutyrate suspension is usually administered in a dose of 50-100 mg every 14 days. When used for muscle-building purposes, testosterone isobutyrate suspension is often administered at a dose of 200-400 mg (4-8ml) per week. Although active for longer periods of time, weekly injections would be preferred due to the low dosage and tendency for pain at the site of injection (large injection volumes would not be advised). To reduce injection volume, the weekly dosage may be further subdivided into smaller injections, which are taken every 2nd or 3rd day. Cycles are generally between 6 and 12 weeks in length. This level is sufficient to provide noticeable gains in muscle size and strength. Testosterone drugs are ultimately very versatile, and can be combined with many other anabolic/androgenic steroids depending on the desired effect.

Administration (Women):

Testosterone isobutyrate suspension is not commonly used with women in clinical medicine. When applied, it is usually given in a dose of 25-50 mg every 14 days. Testosterone isobutyrate suspension is not recommended for women for physique- or performance-enhancing purposes due to its strong androgenic nature, tendency to produce virilizing side effects, and slow acting characteristics (making blood levels difficult to control).

Availability:

Agovirin Depot is the dominant form of water-based testosterone on the European black market. Counterfeits do not appear to be a significant problem. This item does not appear on the black market in the United States very often.

Anabol 4-19 (norclostebol acetate)

Androgenic	40
Anabolic	660
Standard	Testosterone

Chemical Names	4-chloro-19-nortestosterone
	4-chloro-estr-4-en-3-one-17beta-ol
Estrogenic Activity	none
Progestational Activity	none

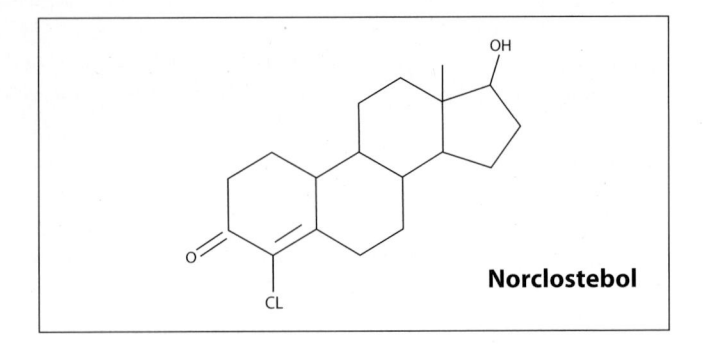

Norclostebol

Description:

Norclostebol acetate is an anabolic steroid that is derived from nandrolone. It is specifically a 4-chloro derivative, further modified with an acetate ester to slightly slow the release of free steroid from the site of injection. An oral form of the same drug was also made, owing to the fact that 4-chloro substitution increases oral bioavailability to some extent. Norclostebol acetate assays out to be very strong compared to testosterone, with approximately 6.6 times the anabolic potency and 40% of the androgenicity. Comparisons to testosterone propionate, perhaps more valid given the use of an ester, put this steroid at about equal in anabolic potency (112%), with only 20-25% of the androgenicity. Although the exact real-world relevance of these figures remains to be seen, when put into use this agent is very likely to behave as a favorable and primarily anabolic drug, with a low tendency to produce side effects.

History:

Norclostebol acetate was first described in 1956.[373.] It was developed into a medicine by Piam, which sold it briefly decades ago under the trade name Anabol 4-19. The 4-19 referred to the unique structural modifications to the steroid, namely that it was a 4-chloro 19-nortestosterone (nandrolone) derivative. Like its cousin Megagrisevit (clostebol acetate), norclostebol acetate was manufactured in both oral and injectable forms. The drug was ultimately less successful than even Megagrisevit (which also was a poor performer internationally), probably because it was developed during a very competitive time in the industry, when many effective agents were vying for pharmacy dollars. Anabol 4-19 was abandoned by the manufacturer many years ago, and has been unavailable for so long that few athletes have any memory of it.

How Supplied:

Norclostebol acetate is no longer available as a commercial agent.

Structural Characteristics:

Norclostebol is a modified form of nandrolone. It differs by the introduction of a hydroxyl group at carbon 4, which inhibits aromatization and reduces relative steroid androgenicity. Norclostebol acetate contains norclostebol modified with the addition of carboxylic acid ester (acetic acid) at the 17-beta hydroxyl group, so that the free steroid is released more slowly from the area of injection.

Side Effects (Estrogenic):

Norclostebol is not aromatized by the body, and is not measurably estrogenic. An anti-estrogen is not necessary when using this steroid, as gynecomastia should not be a concern even among sensitive individuals. Since estrogen is the usual culprit with water retention, norclostebol instead produces a lean, quality look to the physique with no fear of excess subcutaneous fluid retention. This makes it a favorable steroid to use during cutting cycles, when water and fat retention are major concerns.

Side Effects (Androgenic):

Although classified as an anabolic steroid, androgenic side effects are still possible with this substance. This may include bouts of oily skin, acne, and body/facial hair growth. Anabolic/androgenic steroids may also aggravate male pattern hair loss. Women are also warned of the potential virilizing effects of anabolic/androgenic steroids. These may include a deepening of the voice, menstrual irregularities, changes in skin texture, facial hair growth, and clitoral enlargement. Additionally, norclostebol is not extensively metabolized by the 5-alpha reductase enzyme, so its relative androgenicity is not greatly altered by the concurrent use of finasteride or dutasteride. Note that norclostebol is a steroid with relatively low androgenic activity relative to its tissue-building actions, making the threshold for strong androgenic side effects comparably higher than with more androgenic agents such as testosterone, methandrostenolone, or fluoxymesterone.

Side Effects (Hepatotoxicity):

Norclostebol is not a c17-alpha alkylated compound, and not known to have hepatotoxic effects. Liver toxicity is unlikely.

Side Effects (Cardiovascular):

Anabolic/androgenic steroids can have deleterious effects on serum cholesterol. This includes a tendency to reduce HDL (good) cholesterol values and increase LDL (bad) cholesterol values, which may shift the HDL to LDL balance in a direction that favors greater risk of arteriosclerosis. The relative impact of an anabolic/androgenic steroid on serum lipids is dependant on the dose, route of administration (oral vs. injectable), type of steroid (aromatizable or non-aromatizable), and level of resistance to hepatic metabolism. Norclostebol should have a stronger negative effect on the hepatic management of cholesterol than testosterone or nandrolone due to its non-aromatizable nature, but a much weaker impact than c-17 alpha alkylated steroids. Anabolic/androgenic steroids may also adversely effect blood pressure and triglycerides, reduce endothelial relaxation, and support left ventricular hypertrophy, all potentially increasing the risk of cardiovascular disease and myocardial infarction.

To help reduce cardiovascular strain it is advised to maintain an active cardiovascular exercise program and minimize the intake of saturated fats, cholesterol, and simple carbohydrates at all times during active AAS administration. Supplementing with fish oils (4 grams per day) and a natural cholesterol/antioxidant formula such as Lipid Stabil or a product with comparable ingredients is also recommended.

Side Effects (Testosterone Suppression):

All anabolic/androgenic steroids when taken in doses sufficient to promote muscle gain are expected to suppress endogenous testosterone production. Without the intervention of testosterone stimulating substances, testosterone levels should return to normal within 1-4 months of drug secession. Note that prolonged hypogonadotrophic hypogonadism can develop secondary to steroid abuse, necessitating medical intervention.

The above side effects are not inclusive. For more detailed discussion of potential side effects, see the Steroid Side Effects section of this book.

Administration (Men):

Norclostebol acetate has been successfully used in clinical doses as low as 5-20 mg, which increased nitrogen retention for as long as 2 weeks.[374] Effective doses for physique- or performance-enhancing purposes would fall in the range of 100-400 mg per week, taken for 6-12 weeks. Given the fast-acting nature of acetate injectables, the weekly dosage is generally subdivided into injections given at least every third day. An effective oral daily dosage falls in the range of 75-100 mg, although would be less cost-effective and produce stronger negative changes in blood lipids than the injectable. Cycles (oral or injectable) would generally last 6-12 weeks. Use of norclostebol acetate will not effect rapid mass gains, but is likely to produce slow but steady increases in strength and lean muscle tissue, with a concurrent increase in fat loss and muscle definition.

Administration (Women):

Norclostebol acetate has been successfully used in clinical doses as low as 5-20 mg, which increased nitrogen retention for as long as 2 weeks. Effective doses for physique- or performance-enhancing purposes fall in the range of 50-75 mg per week for the injectable, or 25-50 mg daily for the oral, taken for no longer than 6 weeks. Note that virilizing side effects are still possible with use, and should be carefully monitored.

Availability:

Norclostebol acetate is no longer available as a prescription agent at this time, and is unavailable on the black market.

Anabolicum Vister (quinbolone)

Androgenic	20
Anabolic	60
Standard	Methyltestosterone (oral)

Chemical Names	1,4-androstadiene-3-one,17beta-cyclopentenyl
	1-dehydrotestosterone cyclopentenyl
Estrogenic Activity	low
Progestational Activity	no data available (low)

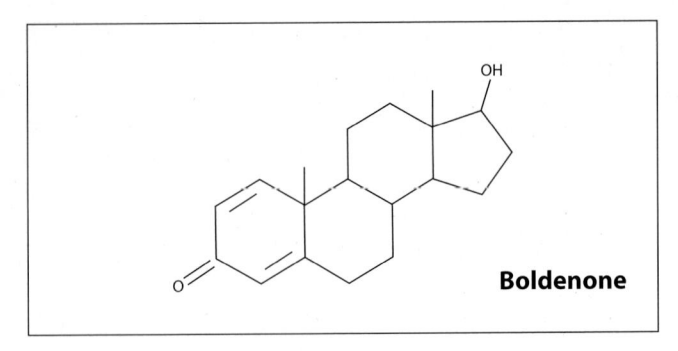

Boldenone

Description:

Quinbolone is a modified form of the anabolic steroid boldenone. This agent is chemically identical to Equipoise®, except in this case the boldenone base has a 17-beta cyclopentenyl (enol) ether attached instead of an undecylenate ester. The ether functions very much like an ester, increasing the fat solubility of the compound. It, however, is used here to increase the oral bioavailability of the hormone, not to prolong its release from an injection site. The design of this steroid is, likewise, very similar to that of Andriol® (testosterone undecanoate), which is also orally administered. With an approximate 7% level of bioavailability, Andriol reminds us that this type of steroid delivery is not very efficient, although with frequent dosing a steady blood hormone level could be achieved. With sufficient dosing the effects of this drug would be qualitatively very similar to those reported with Equipoise®, providing strength and lean mass gains with low to moderate estrogenic and androgenic activity.

History:

Quinbolone was first described in 1962.[375] It was developed during a time when there was growing concern about the hepatotoxicity of oral c-17 alpha alkylated steroids. The focus with this steroid was likely to create a non-toxic clinical alternative to other anabolic agents like methyltestosterone and methandrostenolone, a purpose for which it seemed sufficiently (although not perfectly) suited, at least for some applications. The technology was developed under Alberto Ercoli of Vister Research Laboratories in Casatenovo Italy. Quinbolone was based on Ercoli's early work with ethers and steroid hormones, first published in 1956.[376] He had actually previously worked with enol ethers of a large number of active steroids, including testosterone, nandrolone, dihydrotestosterone, and methyltestosterone. Quinbolone would be the first commercial ether-modified anabolic steroid to be sold.

Parke Davis released quinbolone as a prescription agent during the mid-1960's, sold in Italy under the Anabolicum Vister brand name. This product was manufactured in two distinct forms. The first was an oral soft-gelatin capsule, which carried the steroid dissolved in oil, similar to Andriol. The second was an oral solution, which was administered in measured oral doses similar to those in a bottle of cough syrup. The main clinical uses for Anabolicum Vister seemed to focus on those populations most susceptible to the side effects of anabolic/androgenic steroid therapy, namely women, children, and the elderly. In spite of a seemingly favorable safety record with these groups, quinbolone was withdrawn from the Italian market during the 1970's. Peculiarly, quinbolone was only sold in Italy, and never had much success with bodybuilders outside of this country.

How Supplied:

Quinbolone is no longer commercially available. When produced, it was supplied in the form of 10 mg oral soft gelatin capsules and bottles of oral solution.

Structural Characteristics:

Boldenone is a modified form of testosterone. It differs by the introduction of a double bond between carbons 1 and 2, which reduces its relative estrogenicity and androgenicity. Quinbolone contains boldenone modified with the addition of an enol ether (cyclopentenyl) at the 17-beta hydroxyl group. The ether-modified hormone is more fat soluble than base (free) boldenone, and is dissolved in a carrier intended for oral administration. Significant absorption of oral quinbolone takes place through the lymphatic route, bypassing the first pass through the liver.

Side Effects (Estrogenic):

Boldenone is aromatized in the body to estradiol (estrogen). Elevated estrogen levels can cause side effects such as increased water retention, body fat gain, and gynecomastia. Boldenone is considered a mildly estrogenic steroid. Aromatization studies suggest that its rate of conversion to estradiol is roughly half that of testosterone. The tendency to develop noticeable estrogenic side effects with boldenone should be slightly higher than nandrolone, but much lower than with testosterone. Estrogenic side effects are usually not pronounced unless this drug is taken in moderate doses. An anti-estrogen such as clomiphene citrate or tamoxifen citrate might be used to help mitigate these side effects, should they become present. One may alternately use an aromatase inhibitor like Arimidex® (anastrozole), although it is considerably more expensive, and may negatively affect blood lipids.

Side Effects (Androgenic):

Although classified as an anabolic steroid, androgenic side effects are still common with this substance, especially with higher doses. This may include bouts of oily skin, acne, and body/facial hair growth. Anabolic/androgenic steroids may also aggravate male pattern hair loss. Women are also warned of the potential virilizing effects of anabolic/androgenic steroids. These may include a deepening of the voice, menstrual irregularities, changes in skin texture, facial hair growth, and clitoral enlargement.

Note that while boldenone does reduce to a more potent androgen (dihydroboldenone) via the 5alpha reductase enzyme in androgen-responsive target tissues such as the skin, scalp, and prostate, its affinity to do so in the human body is extremely low.[377] The relative androgenicity of boldenone is, therefore, not significantly affected by finasteride or dutasteride.

Side Effects (Hepatotoxicity):

Quinbolone is not c-17 alpha alkylated, and not known to have hepatotoxic effects. Liver toxicity is unlikely.

Side Effects (Cardiovascular):

Anabolic/androgenic steroids can have deleterious effects on serum cholesterol. This includes a tendency to reduce HDL (good) cholesterol values and increase LDL (bad) cholesterol values, which may shift the HDL to LDL balance in a direction that favors greater risk of arteriosclerosis. The relative impact of an anabolic/androgenic steroid on serum lipids is dependant on the dose, route of administration (oral vs. injectable), type of steroid (aromatizable or non-aromatizable), and level of resistance to hepatic metabolism. Anabolic/androgenic steroids may also adversely affect blood pressure and triglycerides, reduce endothelial relaxation, and support left ventricular hypertrophy, all potentially increasing the risk of cardiovascular disease and myocardial infarction. Boldenone is likely to have a less dramatic impact on cardiovascular risk factors than synthetic oral anabolic steroids. This is due in part to its openness to metabolism by the liver, which allows it to have less effect on the hepatic management of cholesterol. The aromatization of boldenone to estradiol may also help to mitigate the negative effects of androgens on serum lipids.

To help reduce cardiovascular strain it is advised to maintain an active cardiovascular exercise program and minimize the intake of saturated fats, cholesterol, and simple carbohydrates at all times during active AAS administration. Supplementing with fish oils (4 grams per day) and a natural cholesterol/antioxidant formula such as Lipid Stabil or a product with comparable ingredients is also recommended.

Side Effects (Testosterone Suppression):

All anabolic/androgenic steroids when taken in doses sufficient to promote muscle gain are expected to suppress endogenous testosterone production. Without the intervention of testosterone stimulating substances, testosterone levels should return to normal within 1-4 months of drug secession. Note that prolonged hypogonadotrophic hypogonadism can develop secondary to steroid abuse, necessitating medical intervention.

The above side effects are not inclusive. For more detailed discussion of potential side effects, see the Steroid Side Effects section of this book.

Administration (General):

This steroid should always be taken with meals, preferably containing a moderate fat content (20 grams) to maximize lymphatic absorption. Very low bioavailability is likely when taken in the fasted state. The total daily dosage should be divided into a minimum of two applications, taken in the morning and evening, to maintain more consistent elevations of serum boldenone levels.

Administration (Men):

When used for physique- or performance-enhancing purposes, an effective oral daily dosage of quinbolone seemed to fall in the range of 80-120 mg (8-12 capsules) per day, taken for 6-12 weeks. The drug was generally considered too weak for bulking purposes, and was most often combined with other (more potent) anabolic/androgenic steroids in order to achieve desired results. When taken alone, the gains produced with this agent were generally mild due to its low relative oral bioavailability. Higher doses could produce a more profound anabolic response, but were generally not feasible.

Administration (Women):

When used for physique- or performance-enhancing purposes, an effective oral daily dosage of quinbolone was typically in the range of 30-40 mg (3-4 capsules) daily, taken for 4-6 weeks. Women that had been afraid to experiment with Equipoise for fear of its slow rate of metabolic clearance would have found this steroid more favorable.

Availability:

Italy was the only country making this steroid commercially, and now that it is discontinued, quinbolone is no longer available.

Anadrol®-50 (oxymetholone)

Androgenic	45
Anabolic	320
Standard	Methyltestosterone (oral)
Chemical Names	2-hydroxymethylene-17a-methyl- dihydrotestosterone
	4,5-dihydro-2-hydroxymethylene-17-alpha-methyltestosterone
	17alpha-methyl-2-hydroxymethylene-17-hydroxy-5alpha-androstan-3-one
Estrogenic Activity	high
Progestational Activity	not significant

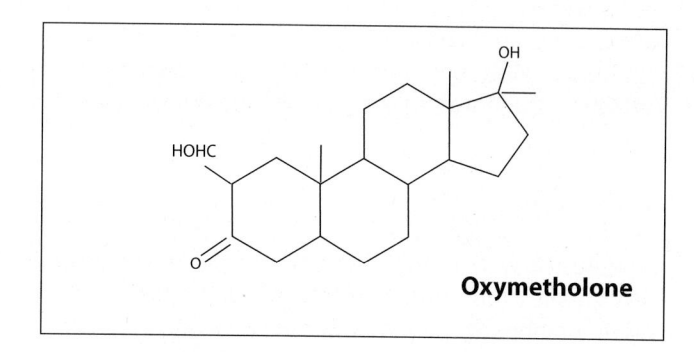

Oxymetholone

Description:

Oxymetholone is a potent oral anabolic steroid derived from dihydrotestosterone. More specifically, it is a close cousin of methyldihydrotestosterone (mestanolone), differing only by the addition of a 2-hydroxymethylene group. This creates a steroid with considerably different activity than mestanolone, however, such that it is very difficult to draw comparisons between the two. For starters, oxymetholone is a very potent anabolic hormone. Dihydrotestosterone and mestanolone are both very weak in this regard, owing to the fact that these molecules are not very stable in the high enzyme (3-alpha hydroxysteroid dehydrogenase) environment of muscle tissue. Oxymetholone remains highly active here instead, as is reported in standard animal assay tests demonstrating a significantly higher anabolic activity than testosterone or methyltestosterone. Such assays suggest the androgenicity of oxymetholone is also very low (1/4th to 1/7th its anabolic activity), although real world results in humans suggest it is decidedly higher than that.

Oxymetholone is considered by many to be the most powerful steroid commercially available. A steroid novice experimenting with this agent is likely to gain 20 to 30 pounds of massive bulk, and it can often be accomplished within 6 weeks of use. This steroid produces a lot of water retention, so a good portion of this gain is going to be water weight. This is often of little consequence to the user, who may be feeling very big and strong while taking oxymetholone. Although the smooth look that results from water retention is often not attractive, it can aid quite a bit to the level of size and strength gained. The muscle is fuller, will contract better, and is provided a level of protection in the form of extra water held into and around connective tissues. This will allow for more elasticity, and will hopefully decrease the chance for injury when lifting heavy. It should be noted, however, that a very rapid gain in mass might also place too much stress on your connective tissues. The tearing of pectoral and biceps tissue is commonly associated with heavy lifting while massing up on steroids, and oxymetholone is a common offender. There can be such a thing as gaining too fast.

History:

Oxymetholone was first described in 1959.[378] The agent was released in the United States as a prescription drug during the early 1960's, sold under the brand names Anadrol-50 (Syntex) and Androyd (Parke Davis & Co.). Syntex developed the agent, and would hold patent rights to it until their expiration many years later. The drug was originally approved for use in conditions where anabolic action was necessary. Indicated uses included geriatric debilitation, chronic underweight states, pre- and postoperative preservation of lean mass, convalescence from infection, gastrointestinal disease, osteoporosis, and general catabolic conditions. The recommended dose for such uses was usually 2.5 mg three times per day. The drug was originally supplied in a 2.5 mg, 5 mg, or 10 mg tablet.

In spite of the many potential therapeutic uses or a strong anabolic activity of this drug, the FDA soon strictly narrowed the indicated uses of oxymetholone. By the mid-1970's, the drug was FDA approved only for the indicated treatment of anemia characterized by deficient red blood cell (RBC) production. Admittedly the stimulation of erythropoiesis is an affect that is characteristic of nearly all anabolic steroids, which as a group tend to increase RBC concentrations. Oxymetholone, however, seemed fairly reliable in this regard; demonstrating an increase in erythropoietin levels as much as 5 fold.[379] This has led to its adoption for this relatively new medical use, as well as the institution of a higher (50 mg) dosage with the updated Anadrol-50 product, necessary for a stronger effect on RBC count. The Parke Davis item would not be brought up to the higher dosage, however, and was discontinued.

Recent years have brought fourth a number of new treatments for anemia, most notably Epogen (recombinant erythropoietin) and related erythropoietic peptides. These drugs directly mimic the body's natural red blood cell producing hormone, and as such provide a much more focused form of therapy, with less of the unrelated side effects one would have to endure with the use of a strong androgen. Although Anadrol was once viewed as an effective drug for this purpose, sales were now dropping. Financial disinterest finally prompted Syntex to halt production of the U.S. Anadrol 50 in 1993, which was around the same time they decided to drop this item in a number of foreign countries. Plenastril from Switzerland and Austria were dropped; following soon was Oxitosona from Spain. During the mid-1990's, many Athletes feared oxymetholone was on the way out for good.

In July 1997, Syntex sold all rights to Anadrol-50 in the U.S., Canada, and Mexico to Unimed Pharmaceuticals. Unimed reintroduced Anadrol-50 to the U.S. market in 1998, this time targeting HIV/AIDS patients. Patients with HIV are commonly anemic, often caused by the disease itself, opportunistic infections, or the antiretroviral drugs used to treat the disease. The anemia in HIV patients is typically categorized by impaired red blood cell production in bone marrow, the FDA approved indication for oxymetholone use. Adding to this, oxymetholone was showing great promise in studies combating HIV associated wasting. Unimed soon initiated Phase II/III trials with Anadrol for HIV wasting syndrome, and continued to research its use for treating such things as chronic obstructive pulmonary disease and lipodystrophy (a disorder characterized by a selective loss of body fat, insulin resistance, diabetes, high triglycerides levels, and a fatty liver).

In April 2006, Solvay Pharmaceuticals (parent company of Unimed) sold the rights to Anadrol-50 to Alaven Pharmaceutical, LLC. Alaven continues to market the drug in the United States, although given the transition it is uncertain what additional uses the company plans to pursue with oxymetholone. At the present time the only FDA approved indication remains that of treating red blood cell deficient anemia. Syntex seems to have removed itself from the oxymetholone market globally, discontinuing product or transferring license to other companies whenever possible. Oxymetholone remains available outside of the United States, although it is mostly still sold in smaller and less tightly regulated markets.

How Supplied:

Oxymetholone is available in select human drug markets. Composition and dosage may vary by country and manufacturer. Most brands contain 50 mg of steroid per tablet.

Structural Characteristics:

Oxymetholone is a modified form of dihydrotestosterone. It differs by 1) the addition of a methyl group at carbon 17-alpha, which helps protect the hormone during oral administration, and 2) the introduction of a 2-hydroxymethylene group, which inhibits its metabolism by the 3-hsd enzyme and greatly enhances the anabolic and relative biological activity of methyldihydrotestosterone.

Side Effects (Estrogenic):

Oxymetholone is a highly estrogenic steroid. Gynecomastia is often a concern during treatment, and may present itself quite early into a cycle (particularly when higher doses are used). At the same time water retention can become a problem, causing a notable loss of muscle definition as both subcutaneous water retention and fat levels build. To avoid strong estrogenic side effects, it may be necessary to use an anti-estrogen such as Nolvadex® or Clomid®.

It is important to note that oxymetholone does not directly convert to estrogen in the body. This steroid is a derivative of dihydrotestosterone, and as such cannot be aromatized. Anti-aromatase compounds such as Cytadren and Arimidex® will, likewise, not effect the relative estrogenicity of this steroid. Some have suggested that the high level of estrogenic activity in oxymetholone is actually due to the drug acting as a progestin, similar to nandrolone. The side effects of both estrogens and progestins can be very similar, which might have made this explanation a plausible one. There was a medical study examining the progestational activity of oxymetholone, however, and it determined that there was no such activity present.[380] With such findings, it seems most plausible that oxymetholone can activate the estrogen receptor, similar to, but more profoundly than, the estrogenic androgen methandriol.

Side Effects (Androgenic):

Although oxymetholone is classified as an anabolic steroid, androgenic side effects are still possible with this substance. These may include bouts of oily skin, acne, and body/facial hair growth. Higher doses are more likely to cause such side effects. Anabolic/androgenic steroids may also aggravate male pattern hair loss. Women are additionally warned of the potential virilizing effects of anabolic/androgenic steroids. These may include a deepening of the voice, menstrual irregularities, changes in skin texture, facial hair growth, and clitoral enlargement. While Anadrol is classified as an anabolic steroid, it does retain a notable androgenic component.

It is interesting to note that oxymetholone does exhibit

some tendency to convert to dihydrotestosterone in the body, although this does not occur via the 5-alpha reductase enzyme. Oxymetholone is already a dihydrotestosterone-based steroid, so no such alteration can take place. Aside from the added c-17 alpha alkylation (discussed below), oxymetholone differs from DHT only by the addition of a 2-hydroxymethylene group. This grouping can be removed metabolically, reducing oxymetholone to the potent androgen 17alpha-methyl dihydrotestosterone (mestanolone).[381] There is little doubt that this biotransformation contributes at least on some level to the androgenic nature of this steroid. Note that since 5-alpha reductase is not involved, the relative androgenicity of oxymetholone is not affected by the concurrent use of finasteride or dutasteride.

Side Effects (Hepatotoxicity):

Oxymetholone is a c17-alpha alkylated compound. This alteration protects the drug from deactivation by the liver, allowing a very high percentage of the drug entry into the bloodstream following oral administration. C17-alpha alkylated anabolic/androgenic steroids can be hepatotoxic. Prolonged or high exposure may result in liver damage. In rare instances life-threatening dysfunction may develop. It is advisable to visit a physician periodically during each cycle to monitor liver function and overall health. Intake of c17-alpha alkylated steroids is commonly limited to 6-8 weeks, in an effort to avoid escalating liver strain.

Oxymetholone has a saturated A-ring, which slightly reduces its relative hepatotoxicity.[382] Still, this agent, particularly at the doses commonly used, can present substantial hepatotoxicity to the user. Studies administering 50 mg or 100 mg daily to 31 elderly men for 12 weeks produced significant increases in liver enzymes (transaminases AST and ALT) only in patients taking 100 mg. A second study administering 50 mg daily to 30 patients for up to and exceeding one year (in some patients) has demonstrated elevations in γ-glutamyltransferase (GGT) in 17% of patients, significant increases in bilirubin in 10%, and serum albumin increases in 20%.[383] One patient developed a liver tumor that could have been peliosis hepatitis, a life-threatening adverse event characterized by blood filled cysts in the liver. A small number of other cases of peliosis hepatitis have been linked to oxymetholone, suggesting the potential for hepatotoxicity should still be carefully considered before use.

The use of a liver detoxification supplement such as Liver Stabil, Liv-52, or Essentiale Forte is advised while taking any hepatotoxic anabolic/androgenic steroids.

Side Effects (Cardiovascular):

Anabolic/androgenic steroids can have deleterious effects on serum cholesterol. This includes a tendency to reduce HDL (good) cholesterol values and increase LDL (bad) cholesterol values, which may shift the HDL to LDL balance in a direction that favors greater risk of arteriosclerosis. The relative impact of an anabolic/androgenic steroid on serum lipids is dependant on the dose, route of administration (oral vs. injectable), type of steroid (aromatizable or non-aromatizable), and level of resistance to hepatic metabolism. Anabolic/androgenic steroids may also adversely affect blood pressure and triglycerides, reduce endothelial relaxation, and support left ventricular hypertrophy, all potentially increasing the risk of cardiovascular disease and myocardial infarction.

Oxymetholone has a strong effect on the hepatic management of cholesterol due to its structural resistance to liver breakdown and route of administration. Studies administering 50 mg or 100 mg daily to a group of elderly men for 12 weeks have demonstrated insignificant increases in LDL cholesterol, accompanied by very significant (dramatic) suppressions of HDL cholesterol (reduced 19 and 23 points in the 50 mg and 100 mg groups, respectively).[384] The use of oxymetholone should be undertaken only after careful consideration in people with high cholesterol or a familial history of heart disease.

To help reduce cardiovascular strain it is advised to maintain an active cardiovascular exercise program and minimize the intake of saturated fats, cholesterol, and simple carbohydrates at all times during active AAS administration. Supplementing with fish oils (4 grams per day) and a natural cholesterol/antioxidant formula such as Lipid Stabil or a product with comparable ingredients is also recommended.

Side Effects (Testosterone Suppression):

All anabolic/androgenic steroids when taken in doses sufficient to promote muscle gain are expected to suppress endogenous testosterone production. Without the intervention of testosterone stimulating substances, testosterone levels should return to normal within 1-4 months of drug secession. Note that prolonged hypogonadotrophic hypogonadism can develop secondary to steroid abuse, necessitating medical intervention.

Note that when discontinuing oxymetholone, the crash can be as equally powerful as the on-cycle results. To begin with, the level of water retention will quickly diminish, dropping the user's body weight dramatically. This should be expected, and not of much concern. What is usually of most concern is restoring endogenous testosterone production with a proper PCT program (see: Post Cycle Therapy in this book). Before going off, some alternately choose to first switch over to a milder injectable like Deca-Durabolin® for several weeks. This is in an effort to "harden up the new mass," and can prove to be an effective practice, at least from a mental standpoint. A drop of weight is likely when making the switch, although the end result is still often viewed as allowing the retention of more (quality) muscle mass. It is sort of stepping down, first off the water retention, and weeks later finally off the hormones. Remember ancillaries though, as testosterone production will not be rebounding during Deca therapy.

The above side effects are not inclusive. For more detailed discussion of potential side effects, see the Steroid Side Effects section of this book.

Administration (General):

Studies have shown that taking an oral anabolic steroid with food may decrease its bioavailability.[385] This is caused by the fat-soluble nature of steroid hormones, which can allow some of the drug to dissolve with undigested dietary fat, reducing its absorption from the gastrointestinal tract. For maximum utilization, this steroid should be taken on an empty stomach.

Administration (Men):

Early prescribing guidelines recommended a dosage of 2.5 mg three times per day to reverse the wasting process and provide solid weight gain. Doses as high as 30 mg were employed in some cases. Current prescribing guidelines recommend a dosage of 1-5 mg per kilogram of bodyweight per day for treating anemia, although do indicate that a dose of 1-2mg per kilogram is typically sufficient. At a dose of 5 mg per kg of weight, a 175-pound person would take a dose of approximately 400 mg per day. The same patient would take approximately 150 mg (3 tablets) per day at the common 2mg/kg dosage. Therapy is usually given for a minimum of three to six months. When used for physique- or performance-enhancing purposes, an effective oral daily dosage would fall in the range of 25-150 mg, taken in cycles lasting no more than 6-8 weeks to minimize hepatotoxicity. This level is sufficient for dramatic increases in muscle mass and strength. Higher doses are rarely administered due to the strong estrogenic nature of the drug, as well as the high potential for hepatotoxicity.

Administration (Women):

Prescribing information for oxymetholone in the U.S. makes no distinction with the dose for females. Oxymetholone is generally not recommended for women for physique- or performance-enhancing purposes due to its very strong nature and tendency to produce virilizing side effects.

Availability:

Oxymetholone remains widely available on the black market. Although there are many counterfeits in circulation, there are also enough legitimate companies making the drug to make some good suggestions when shopping.

Androlic continues to be sold in Thailand, manufactured by the drug firm British Dispensary. It comes in a dark plastic bottle with a silver cap and bright green label. The tablets themselves should be green, with a hexagon shape and company snake emblem stamped in its surface.

Anadrol 50® (U.S.) is rarely found on the black market, due mainly to its high cost at the pharmacy and very tight controls on its distribution. Never purchase this product on the black market unless you can personally trace it to someone receiving it from a doctor. Note that counterfeits have already circulated with such accuracy that they were unknowingly being distributed in the U.S. through legitimate pharmacies. All Anadrol-50 tablets are white, scored, and embossed with 0055 and ALAVEEN.

Iran has become an active source country for steroids as of late, and their generic oxymetholone product from Alhavi is one of their most popular exports. This product carries one hundred 50 mg tablets in a dark amber glass bottle. The bottle itself is sealed with a strip of holographic tape, which carries an embedded image of the company name. The company Iran Hormone also makes a generic, which comes in foil and plastic strips of 10 tablets.

Oxymetholone is still available in Turkey under the Anapolon brand name. These are packaged in a foil & plastic push-through strip of 20 tablets, 1 strip per box. The back reads Anapolon Tablet, Oksimetolon 50 mg in black ink. There are a good number of counterfeits of this brand, so shop carefully. Note that the real tablets are a sort of off white to yellowish color. A very good looking fake is currently circulating that uses pure white tablets. They are easy to spot once you know to look for this. Avoid. Also, some counterfeiters have been making mistakes on the company logo. Be sure the letters Al touch in the logo, to form one graphic. Often the fakers just use two separate letters to form a logo, which make a close, but not perfect, match.

Anemoxic from Jinan Pharmaceuticals in China is a popular export product. It comes in foil and plastic strips holding 20 tablets each. Each box carries a holographic security sticker on the back to deter counterfeiting.

Oxybolone from Greece is in circulation. It should carry a pharmacy sticker that will show a hidden image under black light.

Oxitoland from Landerlan in Paraguay is another popular item on the black market, particularly in South America. Counterfeits have not yet been a significant problem.

Han Seo, Han Bul, Korea United, and Dongindang produce generic Oxymetholone in Korea. The product from Han Seo is most popular. There are numerous fakes of "Korean Anadrol," making them risky purchases.

Anadur® (nandrolone hexyloxyphenylpropionate)

Androgenic	37
Anabolic	125
Standard	Testosterone

Chemical Names	19-nortestosterone hexyloxyphenylpropionate
	17beta-Hydroxyestra-4-en-3-one hexyloxyphenylpropionate
Estrogenic Activity	low
Progestational Activity	moderate

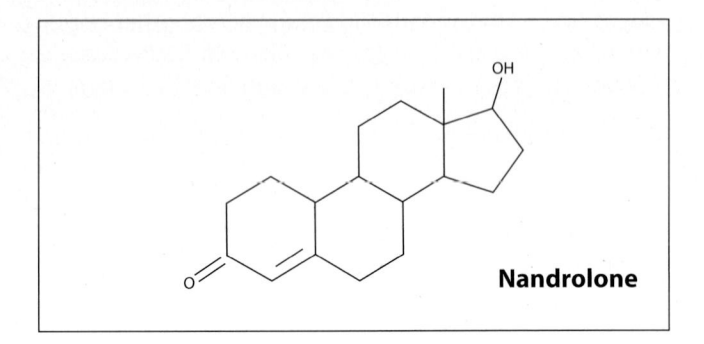

Description:

Nandrolone hexyloxyphenylpropionate is a slow-acting injectable form of the anabolic steroid nandrolone. Hexyloxyphenylpropionate, also called parahexyloxyphenylpropionate, is a fairly unusual nandrolone ester in a structural sense. It is essentially nandrolone phenylpropionate, which has been extended with a tail of one additional oxygen atom and 6 more carbons. It is the largest, and likely the slowest acting, ester of nandrolone to ever be introduced into clinical medicine. It is considerably slower acting than the popular Deca-Durabolin (nandrolone decanoate), and generally would be administered once every three to four weeks in a medical setting. Nandrolone hexyloxyphenylpropionate is no longer manufactured, but when available was favored by athletes and bodybuilders for its ability to promote slow steady gains in lean mass with low estrogenic and androgenic side effects.

History:

Nandrolone hexyloxyphenylpropionate was first described in 1960.[386] It was developed into a medicine shortly after, and was sold mainly under the Anadur brand name in such markets as Austria, Sweden, Switzerland, Belgium, Netherlands, and Germany. Anadur persisted through the early 1990's, and, following some mergers and acquisitions, was sold mainly by Kabi Pharmacia. Kabi would also sell the drug in France, but under the brand name Anador. Indicated uses for the drug included osteoporosis, chronic renal and intestinal disorders, and radiation and chemotherapy induced suppression of red blood cells (anemia). It was also used as a general lean-tissue-building anabolic, with certain diseased states, injury, or convalescence.

Nandrolone hexyloxyphenylpropionate was not widely distributed outside of Europe, and in spite of a long history of relative safety, would not last as a medicinal product. The 1995 merger of Kabi with Upjohn formed the company Pharmacia & Upjohn, and would soon spell the commercial end to Anadur. Pharmacia & Upjohn did continue to market the drug in Austria, but only briefly, and soon refined its offerings to eliminate all forms of nandrolone hexyloxyphenylpropionate in all countries. It is of note that this ester of nandrolone was also sold by Leo in Spain (Anadur), Lundbeck in Denmark (Anadur), Eczacibasi in Turkey (Anadur), and by Xponei in Greece (Anadurin), much under direct license with Kabi. All such preparations have since been discontinued as well, however, and nandrolone hexyloxyphenylpropionate is no longer available as a commercial medicine.

How Supplied:

Nandrolone hexyloxyphenylpropionate is no longer available as a prescription drug product. When supplied, it usually contained 25 mg/mL or 50 mg/mL of steroid dissolved in oil in a 1 mL or 2 mL ampule.

Structural Characteristics:

Nandrolone hexyloxyphenylpropionate is a modified form of nandrolone, where a carboxylic acid ester (parahexyloxyphenylpropionic acid) has been attached to the 17-beta hydroxyl group. Esterified steroids are less polar than free steroids, and are absorbed more slowly from the area of injection. Once in the bloodstream, the ester is removed to yield free (active) nandrolone. Esterified steroids are designed to prolong the window of therapeutic effect following administration, allowing for a less frequent injection schedule compared to injections of free (unesterified) steroid. Nandrolone hexyloxyphenylpropionate is designed to provide a slow release of nandrolone for up to four weeks following injection.

Side Effects (Estrogenic):

Nandrolone has a low tendency for estrogen conversion, estimated to be only about 20% of that seen with testosterone.[387] This is because while the liver can convert nandrolone to estradiol, in other more active sites of steroid aromatization such as adipose tissue nandrolone is far less open to this process.[388] Consequently, estrogen related side effects are a much lower concern with this drug than with testosterone. Elevated estrogen levels may still be noticed with higher dosing, however, and may cause side effects such as increased water retention, body fat gain, and gynecomastia. An anti-estrogen such as clomiphene citrate or tamoxifen citrate may be necessary to prevent estrogenic side effects if they occur. One may alternately use an aromatase inhibitor like Arimidex® (anastrozole), which more efficiently controls estrogen by preventing its synthesis. Aromatase inhibitors can be quite expensive in comparison to anti-estrogens, however, and may also have negative effects on blood lipids.

It is of note that nandrolone has some activity as a progestin in the body.[389] Although progesterone is a c-19 steroid, removal of this group as in 19-norprogesterone creates a hormone with greater binding affinity for its corresponding receptor. Sharing this trait, many 19-nor anabolic steroids are shown to have some affinity for the progesterone receptor as well.[390] The side effects associated with progesterone are similar to those of estrogen, including negative feedback inhibition of testosterone production and enhanced rate of fat storage. Progestins also augment the stimulatory effect of estrogens on mammary tissue growth. There appears to be a strong synergy between these two hormones here, such that gynecomastia might even occur with the help of progestins, without excessive estrogen levels. The use of an anti-estrogen, which inhibits the estrogenic component of this disorder, is often sufficient to mitigate gynecomastia caused by nandrolone.

Side Effects (Androgenic):

Although classified as an anabolic steroid, androgenic side effects are still possible with this substance, especially with higher doses. This may include bouts of oily skin, acne, and body/facial hair growth. Anabolic/androgenic steroids may also aggravate male pattern hair loss. Women are warned of the potential virilizing effects of anabolic/androgenic steroids. These may include a deepening of the voice, menstrual irregularities, changes in skin texture, facial hair growth, and clitoral enlargement. Nandrolone is a steroid with relatively low androgenic activity relative to its tissue-building actions, making the threshold for strong androgenic side effects comparably higher than with more androgenic agents such as testosterone, methandrostenolone, or fluoxymesterone. It is also important to point out that due to its mild androgenic nature and ability to suppress endogenous testosterone, nandrolone is prone to interfering with libido in males when used without another androgen.

Note that in androgen-responsive target tissues such as the skin, scalp, and prostate, the relative androgenicity of nandrolone is reduced by its reduction to dihydronandrolone (DHN).[391] [392] The 5-alpha reductase enzyme is responsible for this metabolism of nandrolone. The concurrent use of a 5-alpha reductase inhibitor such as finasteride or dutasteride will interfere with site-specific reduction of nandrolone action, considerably increasing the tendency of nandrolone to produce androgenic side effects. Reductase inhibitors should be avoided with nandrolone if low androgenicity is desired.

Side Effects (Hepatotoxicity):

Nandrolone is not c-17 alpha alkylated, and not known to have hepatotoxic effects. Liver toxicity is unlikely.

Side Effects (Cardiovascular):

Anabolic/androgenic steroids can have deleterious effects on serum cholesterol. This includes a tendency to reduce HDL (good) cholesterol values and increase LDL (bad) cholesterol values, which may shift the HDL to LDL balance in a direction that favors greater risk of arteriosclerosis. The relative impact of an anabolic/androgenic steroid on serum lipids is dependant on the dose, route of administration (oral vs. injectable), type of steroid (aromatizable or non-aromatizable), and level of resistance to hepatic metabolism. Studies administering 600 mg of nandrolone decanoate per week for 10 weeks demonstrated a 26% reduction in HDL cholesterol levels.[393] This suppression is slightly greater than that reported with an equal dose of testosterone enanthate, and is in agreement with earlier studies showing a slightly stronger negative impact on HDL/LDL ratio with nandrolone decanoate as compared to testosterone cypionate.[394] Nandrolone injectables, however, should still have a significantly weaker impact on serum lipids than c-17 alpha alkylated agents. Anabolic/androgenic steroids may also adversely affect blood pressure and triglycerides, reduce endothelial relaxation, and support left ventricular hypertrophy, all potentially increasing the risk of cardiovascular disease and myocardial infarction.

To help reduce cardiovascular strain it is advised to maintain an active cardiovascular exercise program and minimize the intake of saturated fats, cholesterol, and simple carbohydrates at all times during active AAS administration. Supplementing with fish oils (4 grams per day) and a natural cholesterol/antioxidant formula such as Lipid Stabil or a product with comparable ingredients is

also recommended.

Side Effects (Testosterone Suppression):

All anabolic/androgenic steroids when taken in doses sufficient to promote muscle gain are expected to suppress endogenous testosterone production. For sake of comparison, studies administering 100 mg per week of nandrolone decanoate for 6 weeks have demonstrated an approximate 57% reduction in serum testosterone levels during therapy. At a dosage of 300 mg per week, this reduction reached 70%.[395] It is believed that the progestational activity of nandrolone notably contributes to the suppression of testosterone synthesis during therapy, which can be marked in spite of a low tendency for estrogen conversion.[396] Without the intervention of testosterone stimulating substances, testosterone levels should return to normal within 2-6 months of drug secession. Note that prolonged hypogonadotrophic hypogonadism can develop secondary to steroid abuse, necessitating medical intervention.

The above side effects are not inclusive. For more detailed discussion of potential side effects, see the Steroid Side Effects section of this book.

Administration (Men):

When used for physique- or performance-enhancing purposes, a dose of 200-400 mg given every week to 10 days was most common, taken in cycles eight to twelve weeks in length. This level is sufficient for most users to notice measurable gains in lean muscle mass and strength, which should be accompanied by a low level of estrogenic and androgenic activity.

Administration (Women):

When used for physique- or performance-enhancing purposes, a dosage of 50 mg per week, or 100 mg every 10-14 days, was most common. Although only slightly androgenic, women are occasionally confronted with virilization symptoms when taking this compound. Should virilizing side effects become a concern, the drug should be discontinued immediately to help prevent their permanent appearance. After a sufficient period of withdrawal, the shorter acting nandrolone Durabolin® might be considered a safer (more controllable) option. This drug stays active for only several days, greatly reducing the withdrawal time if indicated.

Availability:

Nandrolone hexyloxyphenylpropionate is no longer available as a commercial drug product. Avoid all products labeled to contain this steroid.

Anatrofin (stenbolone acetate)

Androgenic	115-130
Anabolic	300
Standard	Testosterone
Chemical Names	2-methyl-5a-androst-1-en-17b-ol-3-one
Estrogenic Activity	none
Progestational Activity	no data available

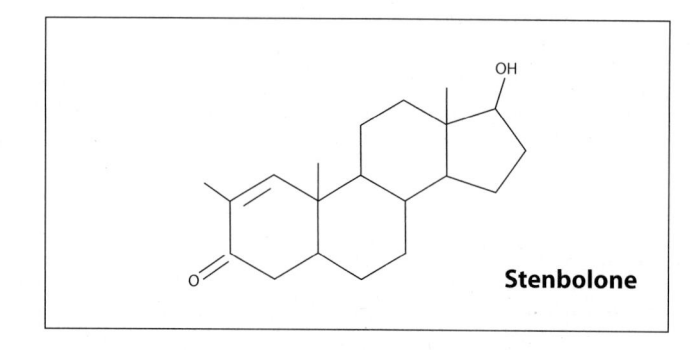

Description:

Stenbolone acetate is an injectable anabolic steroid derived from dihydrotestosterone. Stenbolone was actually developed on a 1-testosterone backbone, differing only by the addition of a 2-methyl group. The resulting steroid remains very similar to its non-methylated base, with only modest differences in anabolic and androgenic potency. On the tissue-building side, stenbolone is probably a little weaker on a milligram for milligram basis than 1-testosterone, although it is difficult to make direct comparisons. As an androgen, stenbolone is also probably slightly weaker than 1-testosterone, when you are talking milligram for milligram dose, although the anabolic/androgenic ratio (the more relevant measure) remains very similar. When compared to testosterone, standard assays suggest that stenbolone has roughly three times greater anabolic effect, and somewhere between 15% and 30% more androgenic activity.

History:

Schering AG in Germany introduced stenbolone acetate in 1961. Approximately two years later, Syntex would introduce the drug to the United Kingdom, and soon after Mexico, under the brand name Anatrofin. Farmacologico Latino also sold this drug in Spain, under the generic name Stenbolone.[397] It was reportedly applied (most commonly) as an injectable alternative to Anadrol in cases of Anemia, although little information about the clinical use of this agent survives today. The distribution of stenbolone acetate did not expand from its original markets, and ultimately enjoyed a relatively short lifespan as a pharmaceutical product. The last commercial preparation containing this ingredient was reportedly withdrawn from market (voluntarily) in the early 1980s. Its demise was likely financially driven, as Anatrofin disappeared at a time when many pharmaceutical manufacturers were dropping their lesser-used anabolic/androgenic steroids.

European bodybuilders were disappointed when Anatrofin was removed from the global market a couple of decades ago. Its loss was a hard felt one, very much like the old Primobolan acetate injectables. Old timers often claimed that the likes of this steroid were never replaced with the other popular non-aromatizable anabolics. Whether or not this is based on realistic experience or simple nostalgia remains to be seen. It is difficult today to say how different this agent ultimately is from methenolone or 1-testosterone, close chemical and pharmacological relatives which we have much more modern experience with. Until such time as this agent goes into wide-scale production again, which seems unlikely (at least as a prescription product), the true nature of stenbolone will remain elusive to the modern bodybuilding community. This steroid does, however, remain as an interesting chapter in the history of anabolic steroids.

How Supplied:

Stenbolone acetate is no longer available as a prescription drug product. When manufactured, it contained 25 mg, 50 mg, or 100 mg of steroid per milliliter of oil, packaged in 1 ml glass ampules.

Structural Characteristics:

Stenbolone is a derivative of dihydrotestosterone. It contains one additional double bond between carbons 1 and 2, and one additional methyl group at carbon 2, which helps to stabilize the 3-keto group and increase the steroid's anabolic properties. Anatrofin makes use of stenbolone with a carboxylic acid ester (acetic acid) attached to the 17-beta hydroxyl group. Esterified steroids are less polar than free steroids, and are absorbed more slowly from the area of injection. Once in the bloodstream, the ester is removed to yield free (active) stenbolone. Esterified steroids are designed to prolong the window of therapeutic effect following administration, allowing for a less frequent injection schedule compared to injections of free (unesterified) steroid.

Side Effects (Estrogenic):

Stenbolone is not aromatized by the body, and is not measurably estrogenic. An anti-estrogen is not necessary when using this steroid, as gynecomastia should not be a concern even among sensitive individuals. Since estrogen is the usual culprit with water retention, this steroid instead produces a lean, quality look to the physique with no fear of excess subcutaneous fluid retention. This makes it a favorable steroid to use during cutting cycles, when water and fat retention are major concerns.

Side Effects (Androgenic):

Although classified as an anabolic steroid, androgenic side effects are still possible with this substance, particularly with higher than normal therapeutic doses. This may include bouts of oily skin, acne, and body/facial hair growth. Anabolic/androgenic steroids may also aggravate male pattern hair loss. Women are warned of the potential virilizing effects of anabolic/androgenic steroids. These may include a deepening of the voice, menstrual irregularities, changes in skin texture, facial hair growth, and clitoral enlargement. Stenbolone is a steroid with relatively low androgenic activity relative to its tissue-building actions, making the threshold for strong androgenic side effects comparably higher than with more androgenic agents such as testosterone, methandrostenolone, or fluoxymesterone. Note that stenbolone is unaffected by the 5-alpha reductase enzyme, so its relative androgenicity is not affected by the concurrent use of finasteride or dutasteride.

Side Effects (Hepatotoxicity):

Stenbolone is not a c17-alpha alkylated compound, and not known to have hepatotoxic effects. Liver toxicity is unlikely.

Side Effects (Cardiovascular):

Anabolic/androgenic steroids can have deleterious effects on serum cholesterol. This includes a tendency to reduce HDL (good) cholesterol values and increase LDL (bad) cholesterol values, which may shift the HDL to LDL balance in a direction that favors greater risk of arteriosclerosis. The relative impact of an anabolic/androgenic steroid on serum lipids is dependant on the dose, route of administration (oral vs. injectable), type of steroid (aromatizable or non-aromatizable), and level of resistance to hepatic metabolism. Stenbolone should have a stronger negative effect on the hepatic management of cholesterol than testosterone or nandrolone due to its non-aromatizable nature, but a much weaker impact than c-17 alpha alkylated steroids. Anabolic/androgenic steroids may also adversely affect blood pressure and triglycerides, reduce endothelial relaxation, and support left ventricular hypertrophy, all potentially increasing the risk of cardiovascular disease and myocardial infarction.

To help reduce cardiovascular strain it is advised to maintain an active cardiovascular exercise program and minimize the intake of saturated fats, cholesterol, and simple carbohydrates at all times during active AAS administration. Supplementing with fish oils (4 grams per day) and a natural cholesterol/antioxidant formula such as Lipid Stabil or a product with comparable ingredients is also recommended.

Side Effects (Testosterone Suppression):

All anabolic/androgenic steroids when taken in doses sufficient to promote muscle gain are expected to suppress endogenous testosterone production. Without the intervention of testosterone-stimulating substances, testosterone levels should return to normal within 1-4 months of drug secession. Note that prolonged hypogonadotrophic hypogonadism can develop secondary to steroid abuse, necessitating medical intervention.

The above side effects are not inclusive. For more detailed discussion of potential side effects, see the Steroid Side Effects section of this book.

Administration (Men):

The usual dosage among male athletes is in the range of 200-300 mg per week, taken for 8 to 12 weeks. This level of use is sufficient to notice moderate increases in strength and lean mass. Note that due to the short-acting nature of acetate esters, the weekly dosage is typically divided into three separate applications.

Administration (Women):

Female athletes would likely notice excellent gains and minimal virilizing activities on a dosage of 25-100 mg per week, taken in cycles no longer than 4 to 6 weeks. Note that due to the short acting nature of acetate esters, the weekly dosage is typically divided into two or three separate applications.

Availability:

Stenbolone acetate is no longer manufactured as a prescription drug product, and is unavailable on the black market.

Anavar (oxandrolone)

Androgenic	24
Anabolic	322-630
Standard	Methyltestosterone (oral)
Chemical Names	17b-hydroxy-17a-methyl-2-oxa-5a-androstane-3-one
Estrogenic Activity	none
Progestational Activity	none

Oxandrolone

Description:

Oxandrolone is an oral anabolic steroid derived from dihydrotestosterone. It was designed to have a very strong separation of anabolic and androgenic effect, and no significant estrogenic or progestational activity. Oxandrolone is noted for being quite mild as far as oral steroids are concerned, well tailored for the promotion of strength and quality muscle tissue gains without significant side effects. Milligram for milligram it displays as much as six times the anabolic activity of testosterone in assays, with significantly less androgenicity.[398] This drug is a favorite of dieting bodybuilders and competitive athletes in speed/anaerobic performance sports, where its tendency for pure tissue gain (without fat or water retention) fits well with the desired goals.

History:

Oxandrolone was first described in 1962.[399] It was developed into a medicine several years later by pharmaceutical giant G.D. Searle & Co. (now Pfizer), which sold it in the United States and the Netherlands under the Anavar trade name. Searle also sold/licensed the drug under different trade names including Lonavar (Argentina, Australia), Lipidex (Brazil), Antitriol (Spain), Anatrophill (France), and Protivar. Oxandrolone was designed to be an extremely mild oral anabolic, one that could even be used safely by women and children. In this regard Searle seems to have succeeded, as Anavar has shown a high degree of therapeutic success and tolerability in men, women, and children alike. During its early years, Anavar had been offered for a number of therapeutic applications, including the promotion of lean tissue growth during catabolic illness, the promotion of lean tissue growth following surgery, trauma, infection, or prolonged corticosteroid administration, or the support of bone density in patients with osteoporosis.

By the 1980's, the FDA had slightly refined the approved applications of oxandrolone to include the promotion of weight gain following surgery, chronic infection, trauma, or weight loss without definite pathophysiologic reason. In spite of its ongoing track record of safety, Searle decided to voluntarily discontinue the sale of Anavar on July 1, 1989. Lagging sales and growing public concern about the athletic use of anabolic steroids appeared to be at the root of this decision. With the Anavar brand off the market, oxandrolone had completely vanished from U.S. pharmacies. Soon after, oxandrolone products in international markets (often sold by or under license from Searle) began to disappear as well, as the leading global manufacturer of the drug continued its withdrawal from the anabolic steroid business. For several years during the early 1990's, it looked as if Anavar might be on its way out of commerce for good.

It would be approximately six years before oxandrolone tablets would be back on the U.S. market. The product returned to pharmacy shelves in December 1995, this time under the Oxandrin name by Bio-Technology General Corp. (BTG). BTG would continue selling it for the FDA approved uses involving lean mass preservation, but had also been granted orphan-drug status for the treatment of AIDS wasting, alcoholic hepatitis, Turner's syndrome in girls, and constitutional delay of growth and puberty in boys. Orphan drug status gave BTG a 7-year monopoly on the drug for these new uses, allowing them to protect a very high selling price. Many patients were outraged to learn that the drug would cost them (at wholesale price) between $3.75 and $30 per day, which was many times more costly than Anavar had been just several years back. The release of a 10 mg tablet from BTG several years later did little to reduce the relative cost of the drug.

Oxandrin® continues to be sold in the U.S., but is now under the Savient label (formerly known as BTG). It is currently approved by the FDA for "adjunctive therapy to promote weight gain after weight loss following extensive surgery, chronic infections, or severe trauma and in some patients who without definite pathophysiologic reasons fail to gain or to maintain normal weight, to offset the protein catabolism associated with prolonged administration of corticosteroids, and for the relief of the bone pain frequently accompanying osteoporosis." Savient remains heavily invested in Oxandrin, which as of 2005 accounted for 52% of its net sales. Generic versions of the drug are expected to be approved in the U.S. very shortly, however, and promise to reduce the price of oxandrolone therapy. Outside of the U.S., oxandrolone remains available, although not widely.

How Supplied:

Oxandrolone is available in select human drug markets. Composition and dosage may vary by country and manufacturer. The original Anavar brand contained 2.5 mg of steroid per tablet. Oxandrin contains 2.5 mg or 10 mg per tablet. Other modern brands commonly contain 2.5 mg, 5 mg, or 10 mg of steroid per tablet.

Structural Characteristics:

Oxandrolone is a modified form of dihydrotestosterone. It differs by: 1) the addition of a methyl group at carbon 17-alpha to protect the hormone during oral administration and 2) the substitution of carbon-2 in the A-ring with an oxygen atom. Oxandrolone is the only commercially available steroid with such a substitution to its basic ring structure, an alteration that considerably increases the anabolic strength of the steroid (partly by making it resistant to metabolism by 3-hydroxysteroid dehydrogenase in skeletal muscle tissue).

Side Effects (Estrogenic):

Oxandrolone is not aromatized by the body, and is not measurably estrogenic. Oxandrolone also offers no related progestational activity.[400] An anti-estrogen is not necessary when using this steroid, as gynecomastia should not be a concern even among sensitive individuals. Since estrogen is the usual culprit with water retention, oxandrolone instead produces a lean, quality look to the physique with no fear of excess subcutaneous fluid retention. This makes it a favorable steroid to use during cutting cycles, when water and fat retention are major concerns. Oxandrolone is also very popular among athletes in strength/speed sports such as sprinting, swimming, and gymnastics. In such disciplines one usually does not want to carry around excess water weight, and may find the raw muscle-growth brought about by oxandrolone to be quite favorable over the lower quality mass gains of aromatizable agents.

Side Effects (Androgenic):

Although classified as an anabolic steroid, androgenic side effects are still possible with this substance. This may include bouts of oily skin, acne, and body/facial hair growth. Anabolic/androgenic steroids may also aggravate male pattern hair loss. Women are warned of the potential virilizing effects of anabolic/androgenic steroids. These may include a deepening of the voice, menstrual irregularities, changes in skin texture, facial hair growth, and clitoral enlargement. Oxandrolone is a steroid with low androgenic activity relative to its tissue-building actions, making the threshold for strong androgenic side effects comparably higher than with more androgenic agents such as testosterone, methandrostenolone, or fluoxymesterone.

The low androgenic activity of oxandrolone is due in part to it being a derivative of dihydrotestosterone. This creates a less androgenic steroid because the agent lacks the capacity to interact with the 5-alpha reductase enzyme and convert to a more potent "di-hydro" form. This is unlike testosterone, which is several times more active in androgen responsive target tissues such as the scalp, skin, and prostate (where 5-alpha reductase is present in high amounts) due to its conversion to DHT. In essence, oxandrolone has a more balanced level of potency between muscle and androgenic target tissues. This is a similar situation as is noted with Primobolan and Winstrol, which are also derived from dihydrotestosterone and not known to be very androgenic substances.

Side Effects (Hepatotoxicity):

Oxandrolone is a c17-alpha alkylated compound. This alteration protects the drug from deactivation by the liver, allowing a very high percentage of the drug entry into the bloodstream following oral administration. C17-alpha alkylated anabolic/androgenic steroids can be hepatotoxic. Prolonged or high exposure may result in liver damage. In rare instances life-threatening dysfunction may develop. It is advisable to visit a physician periodically during each cycle to monitor liver function and overall health. Intake of c17-alpha alkylated steroids is commonly limited to 6-8 weeks, in an effort to avoid escalating liver strain.

Oxandrolone appears to offer less hepatic stress than other c-17 alpha alkylated steroids. The manufacturer identifies oxandrolone as a steroid that is not extensively metabolized by the liver like other 17-alpha alkylated orals, which may be a factor in its reduced hepatotoxicity. This is evidenced by the fact that more than a third of the compound is still intact when excreted in the urine.[401] Another study comparing the effects of oxandrolone to other alkylated agents including methyltestosterone, norethandrolone, fluoxymesterone, and methandriol demonstrated that oxandrolone causes the lowest sulfobromophthalein (BSP; a marker of liver stress) retention of the agents tested.[402] 20 mg of oxandrolone produced 72% less BSP retention than an equal dosage of fluoxymesterone, which is a considerable difference being that they are both 17-alpha alkylated.

A more recent study looked at escalating doses (20 mg, 40 mg, and 80 mg) of oxandrolone in 262 HIV+ men. The drug was administered for a period of 12 weeks. The group taking 20 mg of oxandrolone per day showed no statistically significant trends of hepatotoxicity in liver enzyme (AST/ALT; aminotransferase and alanine aminotransferase) values. Those men taking 40 mg noticed a mean increase of approximately 30-50% in liver enzyme values, while the group of men taking 80 mg noticed an approximate 50-100% increase. Approximately 10-11% of the patients in the 40 mg group noticed World Health Organization grade III and IV toxicity according to AST and ALT values. This figure jumped to 15% in the 80 mg group. While serious hepatotoxicity cannot be excluded with oxandrolone, these studies do suggest that it is measurably safer than other alkylated agents.

The use of a liver detoxification supplement such as Liver Stabil, Liv-52, or Essentiale Forte is advised while taking any hepatotoxic anabolic/androgenic steroids.

Side Effects (Cardiovascular):

Anabolic/androgenic steroids can have deleterious effects on serum cholesterol. This includes a tendency to reduce HDL (good) cholesterol values and increase LDL (bad) cholesterol values, which may shift the HDL to LDL balance in a direction that favors greater risk of arteriosclerosis. The relative impact of an anabolic/androgenic steroid on serum lipids is dependant on the dose, route of administration (oral vs. injectable), type of steroid (aromatizable or non-aromatizable), and level of resistance to hepatic metabolism. Oxandrolone has a strong effect on the hepatic management of cholesterol due to its structural resistance to liver breakdown, non-aromatizable nature, and route of administration. In the previously cited study in HIV+ males, 20 mg of oxandrolone daily for 12 weeks caused a mean serum HDL reduction of 30%. HDL values were suppressed 33% in the 40 mg group, and 50% in the 80 mg group. This was accompanied by a statistically significant increase in LDL values (approximately 30-33%) in the 40 mg and 80 mg groups, further increasing atherogenic risk. Anabolic/androgenic steroids may also adversely effect blood pressure and triglycerides, reduce endothelial relaxation, and support left ventricular hypertrophy, all potentially increasing the risk of cardiovascular disease and myocardial infarction.

At one time oxandrolone was looked at as a possible drug for those suffering from disorders of high cholesterol or triglycerides. Early studies showed it to be capable of lowering total cholesterol and triglyceride values in certain types of hyperlipidemic patients, which was thought to signify potential for this drug as a lipid-lowering agent.[403] With further investigation it was found, however, that any lowering of total cholesterol values was accompanied by a redistribution in the ratio of good (HDL) to bad (LDL) cholesterol that favored greater atherogenic risk.[404,405] This negates any positive effect this drug might have on triglycerides or total cholesterol, and actually makes it a potential danger in terms of cardiac risk, especially when taken for prolonged periods of time. Today we understand that as a group, anabolic/androgenic steroids tend to produce unfavorable changes in lipid profiles, and are really not useful in disorders of lipid metabolism. As an oral c17 alpha alkylated steroid, oxandrolone is even more risky to use in this regard than an esterified injectable such as a testosterone or nandrolone.

To help reduce cardiovascular strain it is advised to maintain an active cardiovascular exercise program and minimize the intake of saturated fats, cholesterol, and simple carbohydrates at all times during active AAS administration. Supplementing with fish oils (4 grams per day) and a natural cholesterol/antioxidant formula such as Lipid Stabil or a product with comparable ingredients is also recommended.

Side Effects (Testosterone Suppression):

All anabolic/androgenic steroids when taken in doses sufficient to promote muscle gain are expected to suppress endogenous testosterone production. Oxandrolone is no exception. In the above-cited study on HIV+ males, twelve weeks of 20 mg or 40 mg per day caused an approximate 45% reduction in serum testosterone levels. The group taking 80 mg noticed a 66% decrease in testosterone. Similar trends of decrease were noticed in LH production, with the 20 mg and 40 mg doses causing a 25-30% reduction, and the 80 mg group noticing a decline of more than 50%. Additionally, studies on boys with constitutionally delayed puberty have demonstrated significant suppression of endogenous LH and testosterone with as little as 2.5 mg per day.[406] Without the intervention of testosterone stimulating substances, testosterone levels should return to normal within 1-4 months of drug secession. Note that prolonged hypogonadotrophic hypogonadism can develop secondary to steroid abuse, necessitating medical intervention.

The above side effects are not inclusive. For more detailed discussion of potential side effects, see the Steroid Side Effects section of this book.

Administration (General):

Studies have shown that taking an oral anabolic steroid with food may decrease its bioavailability.[407] This is caused by the fat-soluble nature of steroid hormones, which can allow some of the drug to dissolve with undigested dietary fat, reducing its absorption from the gastrointestinal tract. For maximum utilization, this steroid should be taken on an empty stomach.

Administration (Men):

The original prescribing guidelines for Anavar called for a daily dosage of between 2.5 mg and 20 mg per day (5-10 mg being most common). This was usually recommended for a period of two to four weeks, but occasionally it was taken for as long as three months. The dosing guidelines recommended with the current U.S. production form of the drug (Oxandrin, Savient Pharmaceuticals) also call for between 2.5 and 20 mg of drug per day, taken in intermittent cycles of 2 to 4 weeks. The usual dosage for physique- or performance-enhancing purposes is in the range of 15-25 mg per day, taken for 6 to 8 weeks. These protocols are not far removed from those of normal therapeutic situations.

Oxandrolone is often combined with other steroids for a more dramatic result. For example, while bulking one might opt to add in 200-400 mg of a testosterone ester (cypionate, enanthate, or propionate) per week. The result should be a considerable gain in new muscle mass, with a more comfortable level of water and fat retention than if taking a higher dose of testosterone alone. For dieting phases, one might alternately combine oxandrolone with a non-aromatizing steroid such as 150 mg per week of a trenbolone ester or 200-300 mg of Primobolan® (methenolone enanthate). Such stacks are highly favored for increasing definition and muscularity. An in-between (lean mass gain) might be to add in 200-400 mg of a low estrogenic compound like Deca-Durabolin® (nandrolone decanoate) or Equipoise® (boldenone undecylenate).

Administration (Women):

The original prescribing guidelines for Anavar did not offer separate dosing recommendations for women, although it was indicated that women who were pregnant, or may become pregnant, should not use the drug. The current guidelines for Oxandrin also do not make special dosing recommendations for women. Women who fear the masculinizing effects of many steroids would be quite comfortable using this drug, as these properties are very rarely seen with low doses. For physique- or performance-enhancing purposes, a daily dosage of 5-10 mg should illicit considerable growth without the noticeable androgenic side effects of other drugs. This would be taken for no longer than 4-6 weeks. Eager females may wish to add another mild anabolic such as Winstrol®, Primobolan® or Durabolin®. When combined with such anabolics, the user should notice faster, more pronounced muscle-building effects, but it may also increase the likelihood of seeing androgenic side effects (or hepatotoxicity in the case of Winstrol).

Availability:

Oxandrolone has been limited in supply, and scarce on the black market, for many years now. There are a number of legitimate brands still made, however. Below are some of the more popular items on the black market.

Atlantis (Mexico) produces an oxandrolone product called Xtendrol. It carries 2.5 mg of steroid per tablet, and comes in a box of 30 tablets each. This is a legitimate human-use pharmaceutical company, with products sold through real pharmacies in Mexico.

Bonavar from Body Research (Thailand) seems to be in production again. Be sure your product looks like the legitimate item in the product identification section, as counterfeits of the Body Research line are known to exist.

Oxandrolone is sold in the U.S. by Savient Pharmaceuticals under the Oxandrin brand name. It comes in both 2.5 mg and 10 mg tablet strengths. High price at the pharmacy precludes any reasonable entry into the black market. This would be a high-risk item regardless, as real U.S. steroids rarely circulate the black market.

Balkan Pharmaceuticals in Moldova produces an oxandrolone product called Oxandrolon. It comes packaged in foil and plastic strips of 20 tablets each. Counterfeits have not yet been a problem.

Oxandroland frm Landerlan in Paraguay is a common product in recent years, especially throughout South America. It comes in bottles of 100 tablets each.

Xenion Pharma Co. in Myanmar produces an oxandrolone product called Oxanol. It carries 5 mg of steroid per tablet, and comes 60 tabs to a box. The pills themselves are white in color, and are imprinted with the characters "OXA 5.0" on one side and the company logo on the reverse. Twenty tablets are sealed in each foil and plastic strip.

Andractim® (dihydrotestosterone)

Androgenic	30-260
Anabolic	60-220
Standard	Testosterone, T. propionate
Chemical Names	5-alpha-androstan-3-one-17beta-ol 5-alpha-androstanolone
Estrogenic Activity	none
Progestational Activity	none

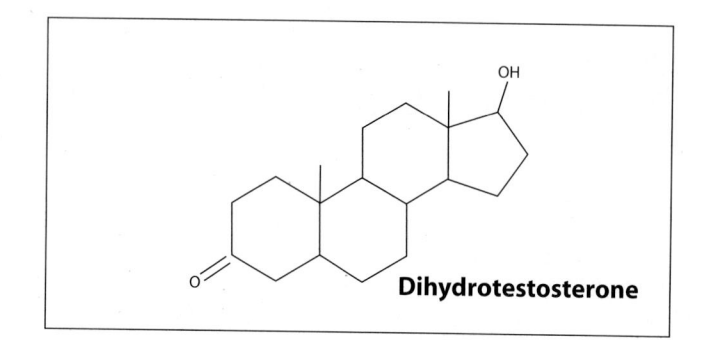

Dihydrotestosterone

Description:

Andractim is a prescription steroid preparation that contains the potent androgenic steroid dihydrotestosterone. This product comes in the form of a transdermal gel, typically containing 2.5% dihydrotestosterone by weight in an 80gram tube. As with Androgel, roughly 10% of the active steroid will make it into circulation with each application. This would equate to 80 doses of 25 mg, with each dose delivering approximately 2.5 mg of steroid to the body. Dihydrotestosterone itself is the most active androgen in the human body, displaying an ability to bind and activate the androgen receptor at least three or four times greater than that of its parent steroid testosterone. This trait, however, is not accompanied by equally powerful anabolic tendencies. In the case of dihydrotestosterone, we have a steroid that is almost purely androgenic, with only minimal muscle-building (anabolic) action.

Dihydrotestosterone is a weak muscle builder because it is extremely open to alteration by the 3-alpha-hydroxysteroid-dehydrogenase enzyme, responsible for breaking down active steroids like DHT into their inactive metabolites. 3a-HSD is present in high quantities in muscle tissue, running interference between the outer cell membrane and the androgen receptors that all steroid hormones are trying to reach. In humans, little DHT ends up actually reaching this receptor. Testosterone is very resistant to this enzyme, however, which allows it to be a much more effective muscle-building agent. 3a-HSD steroid deactivation in muscle tissue causes the same problem with Proviron (1-methyl-dihydrotestosterone). DHT and Proviron both have very effective uses in areas such as fat loss, hardening, increasing CNS activity, and pure strength gains, but they do not perform well as anabolic agents.

History:

Dihydrotestosterone was first synthesized in 1935.[408] This strong androgen was put into consistent medical use during the late 1950's, after a series of experiments demonstrating that it had measurable anabolic effects. Prior to this it was largely believed that DHT was exclusively an androgenic substance, and was of little value clinically. Dihydrotestosterone gels were developed more recently, and have been investigated for a number of medical purposes. At present, these preparations are primarily indicated for the treatment of androgen deficiency, gynecomastia, and insufficient genital growth. Transdermal DHT has been successful as an androgen replacement medication in older men at risk for developing prostate hypertrophy largely because of its non-aromatizable nature,[409][410] as this disorder is fueled partly by estrogens. The latter two indications are considered local applications of the drug, and the DHT gel is applied directly to the tissues requiring treatment.

The primary manufacturer of dihydrotestosterone gel globally is Besins International, based in France. Besins produces the drug under the Andractim name, selling it in France and scarcely in other parts of Europe. Dihydrotestosterone gels are found much less commonly outside of Europe, and presently no such preparation is commercially available in the United States. In 1995, U.S. manufacturer Unimed Pharmaceuticals purchased the rights to Andractim from Besins in the U.S., Mexico, and Canada. The firm announced an interest in the drug for several uses, including androgen replacement in men over age sixty, treating benign prostate hypertrophy, and combating HIV- associated wasting. Its use as an anabolic may be desirable with HIV because it had been determined that many patients lack an ability to properly convert testosterone to DHT, and therefore lack sufficient levels of this important androgen. It appears that Unimed has since sold its interests in the anabolic steroid market, however, leaving the potential reemergence of dihydrotestosterone in the U.S. in question.

How Supplied:

Hydroalcoholic transdermal dihydrotestosterone gels are available in select human drug markets. Composition and dosage may vary by country and manufacturer, but usually contain 2.5% dihydrotestosterone by weight.

Structural Characteristics:

Andractim® is a hydroalcoholic gel containing 2.5% of dihydrotestosterone (free) by weight. It is designed to provide a continuous transdermal delivery of dihydrotestosterone for 24 hours following application to the skin. Approximately 10% of the applied dose is absorbed across the skin during each 24-hour period.

Side Effects (Estrogenic):

Dihydrotestosterone is not aromatized by the body, and is not measurably estrogenic. An anti-estrogen is not necessary when using this steroid, as gynecomastia and water retention should not be concerns even among sensitive individuals. DHT also has inherent anti-estrogenic properties, competing with other substrates for binding to the aromatase enzyme. Percutaneous dihydrotestosterone may be an effective option for the treatment of gynecomastia. Studies have reported a good level of success when treating certain forms of this disorder with Andractim, the drug affecting the ratio of androgenic to estrogenic action in the breast area enough that a notable regression of mammary tissue has been achieved in many cases.[411][412]

Side Effects (Androgenic):

Dihydrotestosterone is the strongest natural male androgen. Higher than normal therapeutic doses are likely to produce androgenic side effects including oily skin, acne, and body/facial hair growth. Men with a genetic predisposition for hair loss (androgenetic alopecia) may notice accelerated male pattern balding. Women are warned of the potential virilizing effects of anabolic/androgenic steroids, especially with a strong androgen such as dihydrotestosterone. These may include deepening of the voice, menstrual irregularities, changes in skin texture, facial hair growth, and clitoral enlargement. Note that the 5-alpha reductase enzyme does not metabolize dihydrotestosterone, so its relative androgenicity is not affected by finasteride or dutasteride.

Side Effects (Hepatotoxicity):

Dihydrotestosterone does not have hepatotoxic effects; liver toxicity is unlikely.

Side Effects (Cardiovascular):

Anabolic/androgenic steroids can have deleterious effects on serum cholesterol. This includes a tendency to reduce HDL (good) cholesterol values and increase LDL (bad) cholesterol values, which may shift the HDL to LDL balance in a direction that favors greater risk of arteriosclerosis. The relative impact of an anabolic/androgenic steroid on serum lipids is dependant on the dose, route of administration (oral vs. injectable), type of steroid (aromatizable or non-aromatizable), and level of resistance to hepatic metabolism. Anabolic/androgenic steroids may also adversely affect blood pressure and triglycerides, reduce endothelial relaxation, and support left ventricular hypertrophy, all potentially increasing the risk of cardiovascular disease and myocardial infarction. Therapeutic doses of dihydrotestosterone used to correct insufficient androgen production in otherwise healthy aging men are unlikely to increase atherogenic risk. Higher doses are likely to increase atherogenic risk, but less dramatically than equivalent doses of synthetic oral anabolic/androgenic steroids.

To help reduce cardiovascular strain it is advised to maintain an active cardiovascular exercise program and minimize the intake of saturated fats, cholesterol, and simple carbohydrates at all times during active AAS administration. Supplementing with fish oils (4 grams per day) and a natural cholesterol/antioxidant formula such as Lipid Stabil or a product with comparable ingredients is also recommended.

Side Effects (Testosterone Suppression):

All anabolic/androgenic steroids when taken in doses sufficient to promote muscle gain are expected to suppress endogenous testosterone production. Without the intervention of testosterone stimulating substances, testosterone levels should return to normal within 1-4 months of drug secession. Note that prolonged hypogonadotrophic hypogonadism can develop secondary to steroid abuse, necessitating medical intervention.

The above side effects are not inclusive. For more detailed discussion of potential side effects, see the Steroid Side Effects section of this book.

Administration (Men):

To treat androgen insufficiency, hydroalcoholic transdermal dihydrotestosterone gels have been used in doses ranging from 16 to 64mg per day (1.6-6.4mg of hormone delivered). For physique- or performance-enhancing purposes, higher doses would be necessary to achieve strong supraphysiological levels of dihydrotestosterone. Logical effective doses begin in the range of 50-100 mg per day, or 5-10 mg of hormone delivered systemically. Dihydrotestosterone is of little value for building muscle, and is most commonly applied for cutting or pure-strength-promoting purposes.

Administration (Women):

Hydroalcoholic transdermal dihydrotestosterone gel is not recommended for women for physique- or performance-enhancing purposes due to its strong androgenic nature and tendency to produce virilizing side effects.

Availability:

Andractim is not widely available, and is rarely seen on the black market. It is sold in several countries, but steroid dealers and consumers just do not pay enough attention to it for it to circulate in any volume. When found, an Andractim product is likely to be legitimate.

Andriol® (testosterone undecanoate)

Androgenic	100
Anabolic	100
Standard	Standard
Chemical Names	4-androsten-3-one-17beta-ol
	17beta-hydroxy-androst-4-en-3-one
Estrogenic Activity	moderate
Progestational Activity	low

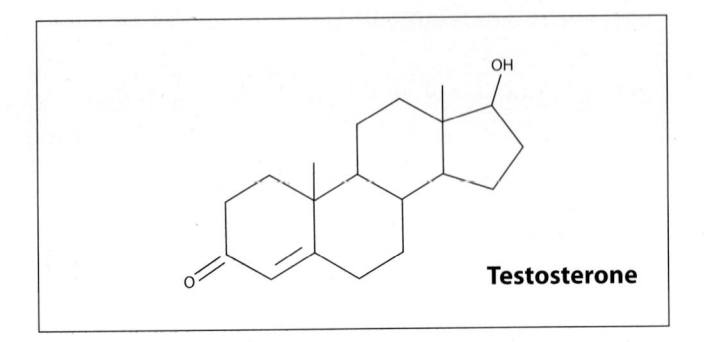

Description:

Andriol® is an oral testosterone preparation that contains 40 mg of testosterone undecanoate (in an oil base) in a soft gelatin capsule. This drug is very different than most oral anabolic steroids, which are usually c-17 alpha alkylated to survive first pass metabolism through the liver. Instead, esterification and suspension in oil allows the testosterone undecanoate in Andriol® to be partially absorbed through the lymphatic system along with dietary fat. This bypasses the destructive first-pass through liver, providing sustained physiological levels of testosterone to the body. The actual oral bioavailability of Andriol is estimated to be approximately 7%. In design, this steroid is essentially a non-toxic and orally active testosterone, intended to provide a unique alternative to testosterone injections and other hepatotoxic oral anabolic/androgenic steroids.

History:

Oral testosterone undecanoate capsules were developed by international drug giant Organon, and first introduced into clinical trials during the early 1980's. The drug was soon approved for use as a prescription agent in a number of countries around the globe, generally under the Andriol brand name, although Organon has also marketed it as Androxon, Panteston, Restandol, Undestor, and Virigen in certain markets. This drug preparation is indicated for testosterone replacement therapy in males with conditions associated with insufficient endogenous androgen production. Although there is a large market for androgen replacement drugs in the United States, the drug is not approved for sale on the U.S. market. It has been approved as a prescription agent in the bordering markets of Mexico and Canada, however.

In 2003, Organon began replacing its Andriol products with Andriol® Testocaps®. The new formulation improves on the storage limitations of the original Andriol preparations, which needed to be kept under refrigeration at the pharmacy. The drug was stored at room temperature once dispensed, as the product needed to be consumed at room temperature. Outside of refrigeration, however, the drug functionally had only a 3-month shelf life. The new Andriol Testocaps are designed to always be stored at room temperature, and have a shelf life of 3 years. The new formulation is considered to be bioequivalent to the older version, and can be substituted in patients without any change in dosage.[413] Given the handling advantages and bioequivalency, it is likely that the new Testocaps will slowly come to replace all of the older Andriol preparations.

In spite of its wide availability, Andriol has never been a popular item among athletes. This is likely due to the high relative cost of the drug, and its low potency compared to other pharmaceutical preparations, particularly injectable testosterone compounds and the more potent synthetic oral anabolic steroids. Still, Andriol remains a product of choice among those athletes not interested in using injectable medications and preferring to avoid the greater risks of hepatotoxicity and lipid alterations inherent in c-17 alpha alkylated orals. Today, decades after its initial release, Organon remains the sole global producer of prescription oral testosterone undecanoate. Andriol itself has maintained a prominent share of the global hormone replacement market since the 1990's.

How Supplied:

Oral testosterone undecanoate preparations are available in various human drug markets. The older formulations supply 40 mg of testosterone undecanoate in oleic acid, contained in small soft gelatin capsules. Andriol Testocaps supplies 40 mg of testosterone undecanoate in castor oil and propylene glycol monolaurate, contained in small soft gelatin capsules. Packaging is commonly as bottles of 30 or 60 capsules, or foil/plastic strips of 10 capsules. Subtracting the ester weight, each 40 mg Andriol capsule contains 25.3mg of (base) testosterone.

Structural Characteristics:

Andriol® contains testosterone that has been modified with the addition of carboxylic acid ester (undecanoic acid) at the 17-beta hydroxyl group. The esterified hormone is more fat soluble than base (free) testosterone, and has been dissolved in oil and encapsulated for oral administration. Significant absorption of oral testosterone undecanoate takes place through the lymphatic route, bypassing the first pass through the liver. Andriol® is designed to provide a peak in testosterone levels several hours after administration, and with repeated dosing maintain physiological concentrations for 24 hours.

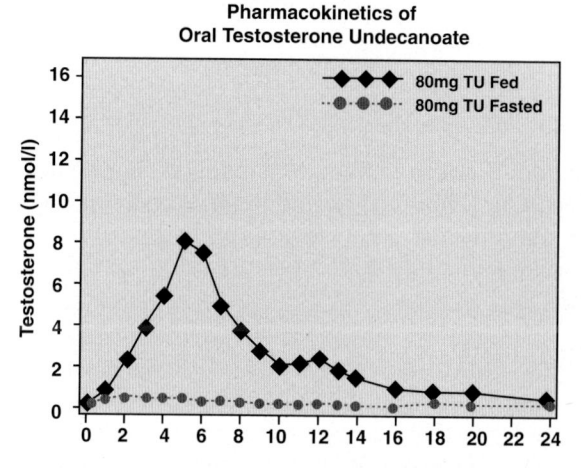

Figure 1. Median response pharmacokinetics after oral administration of 80 mg of testosterone undecanoate in fasted and fed states. Testosterone absorption is impaired when taken without meals. Source: Andriol Testocaps online information, Organon. Citation Bachus et al, 2001. Andriol.com.

Side Effects (Estrogenic):

Testosterone is readily aromatized in the body to estradiol (estrogen). The aromatase (estrogen synthetase) enzyme is responsible for this metabolism of testosterone. Elevated estrogen levels can cause side effects such as increased water retention, body fat gain, and gynecomastia. Testosterone is considered a moderately estrogenic steroid. Exceeding therapeutic doses will increase the likelihood of estrogenic side effects. In such cases, an anti-estrogen such as clomiphene citrate or tamoxifen citrate is commonly applied to prevent estrogenic side effects. One may alternately use an aromatase inhibitor like Arimidex® (anastrozole), which more efficiently controls estrogen by preventing its synthesis. Aromatase inhibitors can be quite expensive in comparison to anti-estrogens, however, and may also have negative effects on blood lipids.

Side Effects (Androgenic):

Testosterone is the primary male androgen, responsible for maintaining secondary male sexual characteristics. Taking oral testosterone undecanoate in doses exceeding normal therapeutic levels is likely to produce androgenic side effects including oily skin, acne, and body/facial hair growth. Men with a genetic predisposition for hair loss (androgenetic alopecia) may notice accelerated male pattern balding. Women are warned of the potential virilizing effects of anabolic/androgenic steroids, especially with a strong androgen such as testosterone. These may include deepening of the voice, menstrual irregularities, changes in skin texture, facial hair growth, and clitoral enlargement.

In androgen-responsive target tissues such as the skin, scalp, and prostate, the high relative androgenicity of testosterone is dependant on its reduction to dihydrotestosterone (DHT). The 5-alpha reductase enzyme is responsible for this metabolism of testosterone. The concurrent use of a 5-alpha reductase inhibitor such as finasteride or dutasteride will interfere with site-specific potentiation of testosterone action, lowering the tendency of testosterone drugs to produce androgenic side effects. It is important to remember that anabolic and androgenic effects are both mediated via the cytosolic androgen receptor. Complete separation of testosterone's anabolic and androgenic properties is not possible, even with total 5-alpha reductase inhibition.

Side Effects (Hepatotoxicity):

Testosterone does not have hepatotoxic effects; liver toxicity is unlikely. One study examined the potential for hepatotoxicity with high doses of oral testosterone by administering 400 mg of the hormone per day (2,800 mg per week) to a group of male subjects. The hormone was given daily for 20 days, and produced no significant changes in liver enzyme values including serum albumin, bilirubin, alanine-amino-transferase, and alkaline phosphatases.[414] No study in which liver enzymes were examined has demonstrated an adverse hepatotoxic effect from Andriol, including an examination of patients on continuous therapy for 10 years.[415]

Side Effects (Cardiovascular):

Anabolic/androgenic steroids can have deleterious effects on serum cholesterol. This includes a tendency to reduce HDL (good) cholesterol values and increase LDL (bad) cholesterol values, which may shift the HDL to LDL balance in a direction that favors greater risk of arteriosclerosis. The relative impact of an anabolic/androgenic steroid on serum lipids is dependant on the dose, route of administration (oral vs. injectable), type of steroid (aromatizable or non-aromatizable), and level of resistance to hepatic metabolism. Anabolic/androgenic steroids may also adversely effect blood pressure and triglycerides, reduce endothelial relaxation, and support left ventricular hypertrophy, all potentially increasing the risk of cardiovascular disease and myocardial infarction. Therapeutic doses of oral testosterone undecanoate used to correct insufficient androgen production in otherwise healthy aging men are unlikely to increase atherogenic risk, and may actually improve lipid profiles and cardiovascular risk factors.[416]

To help reduce cardiovascular strain it is advised to maintain an active cardiovascular exercise program and minimize the intake of saturated fats, cholesterol, and simple carbohydrates at all times during active AAS administration. Supplementing with fish oils (4 grams per day) and a natural cholesterol/antioxidant formula such as Lipid Stabil or a product with comparable ingredients is also recommended.

Side Effects (Testosterone Suppression):

All anabolic/androgenic steroids when taken in doses sufficient to promote muscle gain are expected to suppress endogenous testosterone production. Testosterone is the primary male androgen, and offers strong negative feedback on endogenous testosterone production. Testosterone-based drugs will, likewise, have a strong effect on the hypothalamic regulation of natural steroid hormones. Without the intervention of testosterone-stimulating substances, testosterone levels should return to normal within 1-4 months of drug secession. Note that prolonged hypogonadotrophic hypogonadism can develop secondary to steroid abuse, necessitating medical intervention.

The above side effects are not inclusive. For more detailed discussion of potential side effects, see the Steroid Side Effects section of this book.

Administration (General):

Andriol should always be taken with meals, preferably containing a moderate fat content (20 grams) to maximize lymphatic absorption. Very low bioavailability has been reported when taken in the fasted state. The total daily dosage should be divided into a minimum of two applications, taken in the morning and evening, to maintain more consistent elevations of serum testosterone.

Administration (Men):

For the treatment of low androgen levels, prescribing guidelines for Andriol recommend an initial dosage of 120-160 mg daily for 2-3 weeks. Based on the level of effect, a daily maintenance dosage of 40-120 mg is usually continued at this point. For bodybuilding purposes, higher doses would be required to reach strong supraphysiological levels of testosterone. This would generally call for a minimum dosage of 240-280 mg per day (6-8 capsules), taken in cycles of 6-8 weeks. A more common effective dosage, however, would fall in the range of 400-480 mg (10 to 12 capsules) per day. These doses can be quite costly given the relative price of Andriol preparations, making injectable testosterones much more cost effective and popular. Given the relative low potency of Andriol, when taken by athletes it is most commonly used in combination with other agents. Testosterone drugs are ultimately very versatile, and can be stacked with many other anabolic/androgenic steroids depending on the desired effect.

Administration (Women):

Andriol is not prescribed to women in clinical medicine. This drug is not recommended for women for physique- or performance-enhancing purposes due to its strong androgenic nature and tendency to produce virilizing side effects.

Availability:

Andriol® and Andriol® Testocaps® are both difficult formulations to duplicate, so counterfeits are not a common problem. With legit Andriol® (older) we are looking for a brown/red colored capsule that contains oil inside. It is completely sealed and does not pull apart. The Testocaps® are also soft oval glossy capsules, but these are made out of a transparent orange gelatin mixture. Inside there is a yellow oily liquid. DV3 and ORG are printed on the surface of both types of capsules. Legitimate Organon oral testosterone undecanoate is sold under the brand names Andriol®, Andriol® Testocaps®, Androxon, Panteston, Restandol, Undestor, and Virigen.

Androderm® (testosterone)

Androgenic	100
Anabolic	100
Standard	Standard
Chemical Names	4-androsten-3-one-17beta-ol
Estrogenic Activity	moderate
Progestational Activity	low

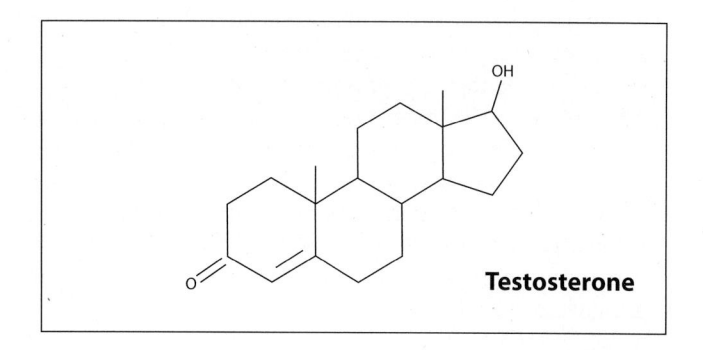

Testosterone

Description:

Androderm® is a testosterone delivery system that utilizes an adhesive "patch" to deliver the hormone transdermally. The testosterone itself is dissolved in an alcoholic gel similar to AndroGel®, except here the gel is contained in a protected external drug reservoir. This design provides approximately double the hormone bioavailability of AndroGel®, and also severely limits the transfer of testosterone to other people during rigorous skin-to-skin contact. The patches come in two strengths, 2.5 mg and 5 mg, indicating the amount of testosterone each is to supply systemically over a 24-hour period (they contain 12.2 and 24.3mg of testosterone respectively). Androderm® was designed to mimic the natural circadian rhythm of testosterone release in healthy young men, higher during the first 12 hours and lower during the next 12 hours of each day. The clinical significance of this, if any, is not known.

History:

Androderm® was developed in the United States by TheraTech (Salt Lake City). It was approved for sale as a prescription agent by the Food and Drug Administration in September 1995, and is indicated for testosterone replacement therapy in men with a deficiency or absence of endogenous testosterone. This includes cases of primary hypogonadism, which may be caused by cryptorchidism, bilateral torsion, orchitis, vanishing testis syndrome, orchiectomy, Klinefelter's syndrome, chemotherapy, or alcohol/heavy metal toxicity. It is also prescribed to treat hypogonadotrophic hypogonadism, including patients with luteinizing hormone or luteinizing hormone-releasing hormone (LHRH) deficiency caused by tumors, injury, or radiation. Primary hypogonadism is usually characterized by low testosterone and high gonadotropin (LH/FSH) levels, while hypogonadotrophic hypogonadism is usually associated with low testosterone and low to normal gonadotropin levels. Watson currently sells this product in the United States under the Androderm® brand name. In Europe, the ATMOS® brand from Astra is most commonly found.

How Supplied:

TheraTech's transdermal testosterone system is available in select human drug markets, where it is commonly sold as Androderm® or ATMOS®. It is produced in two strengths, one containing 12.2mg of testosterone, and one containing 24.3mg of testosterone. These are intended to deliver approximately 2.5 mg and 5 mg of testosterone systemically to the patient over a 24-hour period.

Structural Characteristics:

Androderm® is a transdermal drug delivery system that contains an alcoholic gel of testosterone (free) enclosed in an adhesive patch with a protected drug reservoir. It is designed to provide steady but varying levels of testosterone transdermally during each 24-hour period of application.

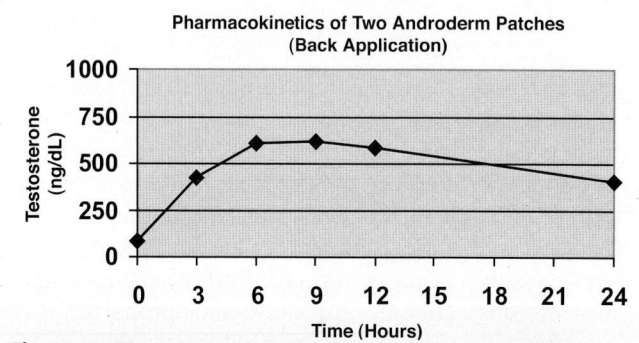

Figure 1. Mean serum testosterone concentrations (ng/dL) measured during single-dose applications of two Androderm 2.5 mg systems applied at night to the back. The figures reflect the greatest response in a study comparing four different sites of application (abdomen, back, thigh and upper arm) in 34 hypogonadal men. Source: Androderm® prescribing information. Watson Pharma, Inc.

Side Effects (Estrogenic):

Testosterone is readily aromatized in the body to estradiol (estrogen). The aromatase (estrogen synthetase) enzyme is responsible for this metabolism of testosterone. Elevated estrogen levels can cause side effects such as increased water retention, body fat gain, and gynecomastia. Testosterone is considered a moderately estrogenic steroid. Exceeding therapeutic doses will increase the likelihood of estrogenic side effects. In such cases, an anti-estrogen such as clomiphene citrate or tamoxifen citrate is commonly applied to prevent estrogenic side effects. One may alternately use an aromatase inhibitor like Arimidex® (anastrozole), which more efficiently controls estrogen by preventing its synthesis. Aromatase inhibitors can be quite expensive in comparison to anti-estrogens, however, and may also have negative effects on blood lipids.

Side Effects (Androgenic):

Testosterone is the primary male androgen, responsible for maintaining secondary male sexual characteristics. Exceeding therapeutic doses is likely to produce androgenic side effects including oily skin, acne, and body/facial hair growth. Men with a genetic predisposition for hair loss (androgenetic alopecia) may notice accelerated male pattern balding. Women are warned of the potential virilizing effects of anabolic/androgenic steroids, especially with a strong androgen such as testosterone. These may include deepening of the voice, menstrual irregularities, changes in skin texture, facial hair growth, and clitoral enlargement.

In androgen-responsive target tissues such as the skin, scalp, and prostate, the high relative androgenicity of testosterone is dependant on its reduction to dihydrotestosterone (DHT). The 5-alpha reductase enzyme is responsible for this metabolism of testosterone. The concurrent use of a 5-alpha reductase inhibitor such as finasteride or dutasteride will interfere with site-specific potentiation of testosterone action, lowering the tendency of testosterone drugs to produce androgenic side effects. It is important to remember that anabolic and androgenic effects are both mediated via the cytosolic androgen receptor. Complete separation of testosterone's anabolic and androgenic properties is not possible, even with total 5-alpha reductase inhibition.

Side Effects (Hepatotoxicity):

Testosterone does not have hepatotoxic effects; liver toxicity is unlikely. One study examined the potential for hepatotoxicity with high doses of testosterone by administering 400 mg of the hormone per day (2,800 mg per week) to a group of male subjects. The steroid was taken orally so that higher peak concentrations would be reached in hepatic tissues compared to intramuscular injections. The hormone was given daily for 20 days, and produced no significant changes in liver enzyme values including serum albumin, bilirubin, alanine-aminotransferase, and alkaline phosphatases.[417]

Side Effects (Cardiovascular):

Anabolic/androgenic steroids can have deleterious effects on serum cholesterol. This includes a tendency to reduce HDL (good) cholesterol values and increase LDL (bad) cholesterol values, which may shift the HDL to LDL balance in a direction that favors greater risk of arteriosclerosis. The relative impact of an anabolic/androgenic steroid on serum lipids is dependant on the dose, route of administration (oral vs. injectable), type of steroid (aromatizable or non-aromatizable), and level of resistance to hepatic metabolism. Anabolic/androgenic steroids may also adversely affect blood pressure and triglycerides, reduce endothelial relaxation, and support left ventricular hypertrophy, all potentially increasing the risk of cardiovascular disease and myocardial infarction. Therapeutic doses of testosterone used to correct insufficient androgen production in otherwise healthy aging men are unlikely to increase atherogenic risk, and may actually reduce the risk of cardiovascular mortality.[418]

To help reduce cardiovascular strain it is advised to maintain an active cardiovascular exercise program and minimize the intake of saturated fats, cholesterol, and simple carbohydrates at all times during active AAS administration. Supplementing with fish oils (4 grams per day) and a natural cholesterol/antioxidant formula such as Lipid Stabil or a product with comparable ingredients is also recommended.

Side Effects (Testosterone Suppression):

All anabolic/androgenic steroids when taken in doses sufficient to promote muscle gain are expected to suppress endogenous testosterone production. Testosterone is the primary male androgen, and offers strong negative feedback on endogenous testosterone production. Testosterone-based drugs will, likewise, have a strong effect on the hypothalamic regulation of natural steroid hormones. Without the intervention of testosterone-stimulating substances, testosterone levels should return to normal within 1-4 months of drug secession. Note that prolonged hypogonadotrophic hypogonadism can develop secondary to steroid abuse, necessitating medical intervention.

The above side effects are not inclusive. For more detailed discussion of potential side effects, see the Steroid Side Effects section of this book.

Administration (General):

Androderm® is applied daily (before bed) to intact, clean, dry skin of the back, upper arms, thighs, and/or abdomen. The site(s) of application should be rotated so that no patch is reapplied to the same area in less than 7 days. Lower bioavailability may be noticed in some areas of the body, such as the chest and calves. Androderm should not be applied to the scrotum. It should also not be applied over a bony area of the body, or any part of the body that could be subject to prolonged pressure during sleep or sitting. Application to these sites has been associated with burn-like blister reactions. Skin irritation causes approximately 1 in 20 patients to discontinue treatment. Irritation may be ameliorated by treatment of the affected area with over-the-counter topical hydrocortisone cream applied after the patch is removed. A small amount of prescription 0.1% triamcinolone acetonide cream may also be applied to the center of each patch before application, which should reduce irritation and not significantly alter the transdermal absorption of testosterone. Many OTC ointments will significantly reduce the penetration of testosterone when applied to the skin before use, and should be avoided.

Administration (Men):

To treat androgen insufficiency, the prescribing guidelines for Androderm® recommend two 2.5 mg patches or one 5 mg patch per day. Morning serum testosterone levels are later measured, at which point the physician may adjust upwards or downwards if necessary. For physique- or performance-enhancing purposes, higher doses would be necessary to achieve supraphysiological levels of testosterone. This would require at least three or four 5 mg or eight 2.5 mg patches per day, delivering approximately 15-20 mg of testosterone. This level is sufficient for most users to notice gains in muscle size and strength, although this is not a very realistic idea in a practical sense. Lower doses may be used, but typically when accompanied by other anabolic/androgenic steroids. Testosterone is ultimately very versatile, and can be combined with many other anabolic/androgenic steroids to tailor the desired effect.

Administration (Women):

Androderm® is not FDA approved for use in women. Testosterone is not recommended for women for physique- or performance-enhancing purposes due to its strong androgenic nature and tendency to produce virilizing side effects.

Availability:

Given their high relative price and low delivery of testosterone, Androderm® and ATMOS® are not commonly traded on the black market. Counterfeits have not yet been reported. These preparations can probably be considered real if located.

AndroGel® (testosterone)

Androgenic	100
Anabolic	100
Standard	Standard
Chemical Names	4-androsten-3-one-17beta-ol
	17beta-hydroxy-androst-4-en-3-one
Estrogenic Activity	moderate
Progestational Activity	low

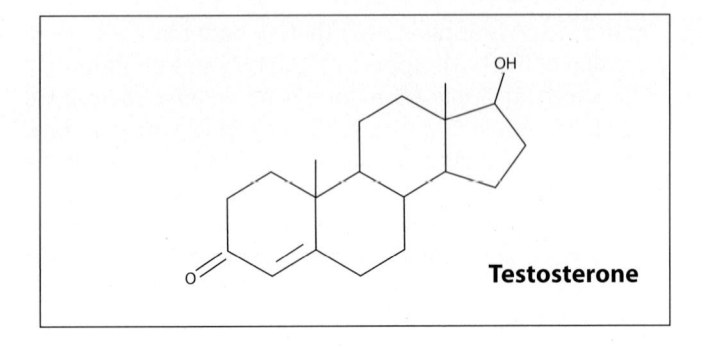

Description:

AndroGel® is a transdermal hydroalcoholic testosterone gel that contains a 1% concentration of testosterone by weight. It was originally released in 2.5 gram and 5-gram sachets, equating to a total per-application testosterone dose of 25 mg and 50 mg respectively. The AndroGel® prescribing information states that the product has a transdermal bioavailability of approximately 10%. This means that each 2.5 or 5 gram dose will deliver approximately 2.5 mg or 5 mg of hormone systemically. With this mode of administration, testosterone levels begin to elevate approximately 30 minutes after the gel is applied to the body, and substantial elevations in serum androgen levels are achieved within 4 hours. Testosterone levels will remain elevated for approximately 24 hours after administration, so that that the drug is applied once per day. Regular dosing will provide a steady hormone balance over each 24-hour period.

History:

AndroGel® was developed in the United States by Unimed Pharmaceuticals, a division of Solvay. It was approved by the FDA for sale as a prescription drug in February of 2000. It is indicated for use in adult males with conditions associated with a deficiency or absence of endogenous testosterone. This includes cases of primary hypogonadism, which may be caused by cryptorchidism, bilateral torsion, orchitis, vanishing testis syndrome, orchiectomy, Klinefelter's syndrome, chemotherapy, or alcohol/heavy metal toxicity. It is also prescribed to treat hypogonadotrophic hypogonadism, including patients with luteinizing hormone or luteinizing hormone-releasing hormone (LHRH) deficiency caused by tumors, injury, or radiation. Primary hypogonadism is usually characterized by low testosterone and high gonadotropin (LH/FSH) levels, while hypogonadotrophic hypogonadism is usually associated with low testosterone and low to normal gonadotropin levels. AndroGel® is said to have a clinical success rate of 87%, perhaps owing to the greater patient comfort and compliance this form of testosterone offers in comparison with hormone injections.

Other transdermal testosterone hydroalcoholic gels have been released in the U.S. and abroad since the introduction of AndroGel®. Testim® by Auxilium Pharmaceuticals is perhaps the most well-known competing brand, sold widely in the U.S. and Europe. This product also comes in the form of a 1% testosterone gel claiming a 10% level of bioavailability. Studies have demonstrated that Testim® delivers as much as 38% more free testosterone for a given dose compared to AndroGel®, however.[419] Testim® is noted to use a thicker and stickier gel compared to AndroGel®, which may explain the greater transfer of hormone. In January 2006, the FDA approved the first generic testosterone gel in the U.S., made by Watson Pharmaceuticals. Testosterone gels are one of the most popular methods of testosterone delivery in clinical medicine at the present time, and are likely to be soon found in every market globally that supports an active hormone replacement therapy industry.

How Supplied:

Hydroalcoholic transdermal testosterone gels are available in many human drug markets. Composition and dosage may vary by country and manufacturer, but usually contain 1% testosterone by weight; packaged in volume tubes or single-dose packets containing 2.5 grams or 5 grams of gel. AndroGel® (U.S.) is also produced in a pump dispenser containing 75 grams of gel, which delivers 60 metered applications of 1.25 grams each.

Structural Characteristics:

AndroGel® is a hydroalcoholic gel containing 1% of testosterone (free) by weight. It is designed to provide a continuous transdermal delivery of testosterone for 24 hours following application to the skin. Approximately 10% of the applied dose is absorbed across the skin during each

24-hour period.

Steady-State Testosterone Concentrations at Day 30 (10g Androgel)

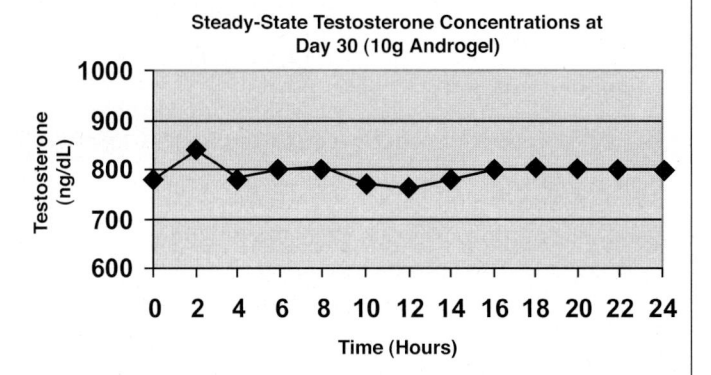

Figure 1. Steady-State Testosterone concentrations in blood, measured 30 days after beginning therapy with Androgel (10g application). Drug was applied to the body once daily.

Side Effects (Estrogenic):

Testosterone is readily aromatized in the body to estradiol (estrogen). The aromatase (estrogen synthetase) enzyme is responsible for this metabolism of testosterone. Elevated estrogen levels can cause side effects such as increased water retention, body fat gain, and gynecomastia. Testosterone is considered a moderately estrogenic steroid. Exceeding therapeutic doses will increase the likelihood of estrogenic side effects. In such cases, an anti-estrogen such as clomiphene citrate or tamoxifen citrate is commonly applied to prevent estrogenic side effects. One may alternately use an aromatase inhibitor like Arimidex® (anastrozole), which more efficiently controls estrogen by preventing its synthesis. Aromatase inhibitors can be quite expensive in comparison to anti-estrogens, however, and may also have negative effects on blood lipids.

Side Effects (Androgenic):

Testosterone is the primary male androgen, responsible for maintaining secondary male sexual characteristics. Exceeding normal therapeutic doses is likely to produce androgenic side effects including oily skin, acne, and body/facial hair growth. Men with a genetic predisposition for hair loss (androgenetic alopecia) may notice accelerated male pattern balding. Women are warned of the potential virilizing effects of anabolic/androgenic steroids, especially with a strong androgen such as testosterone. These may include deepening of the voice, menstrual irregularities, changes in skin texture, facial hair growth, and clitoral enlargement.

In androgen-responsive target tissues such as the skin, scalp, and prostate, the high relative androgenicity of testosterone is dependant on its reduction to dihydrotestosterone (DHT). The 5-alpha reductase enzyme is responsible for this metabolism of testosterone. The concurrent use of a 5-alpha reductase inhibitor such as finasteride or dutasteride will interfere with site-specific potentiation of testosterone action, lowering the tendency of testosterone drugs to produce androgenic side effects. It is important to remember that anabolic and androgenic effects are both mediated via the cytosolic androgen receptor. Complete separation of testosterone's anabolic and androgenic properties is not possible, even with total 5-alpha reductase inhibition.

Side Effects (Hepatotoxicity):

Testosterone does not have hepatotoxic effects; liver toxicity is unlikely. One study examined the potential for hepatotoxicity with high doses of testosterone by administering 400 mg of the hormone per day (2,800 mg per week) to a group of male subjects. The steroid was taken orally so that higher peak concentrations would be reached in hepatic tissues compared to intramuscular injections. The hormone was given daily for 20 days, and produced no significant changes in liver enzyme values including serum albumin, bilirubin, alanine-aminotransferase, and alkaline phosphatases.[420]

Side Effects (Cardiovascular):

Anabolic/androgenic steroids can have deleterious effects on serum cholesterol. This includes a tendency to reduce HDL (good) cholesterol values and increase LDL (bad) cholesterol values, which may shift the HDL to LDL balance in a direction that favors greater risk of arteriosclerosis. The relative impact of an anabolic/androgenic steroid on serum lipids is dependant on the dose, route of administration (oral vs. injectable), type of steroid (aromatizable or non-aromatizable), and level of resistance to hepatic metabolism. Anabolic/androgenic steroids may also adversely effect blood pressure and triglycerides, reduce endothelial relaxation, and support left ventricular hypertrophy, all potentially increasing the risk of cardiovascular disease and myocardial infarction. Therapeutic doses of testosterone used to correct insufficient androgen production in otherwise healthy aging men are unlikely to increase atherogenic risk, and may actually reduce the risk of cardiovascular mortality.[421]

To help reduce cardiovascular strain it is advised to maintain an active cardiovascular exercise program and minimize the intake of saturated fats, cholesterol, and simple carbohydrates at all times during active AAS administration. Supplementing with fish oils (4 grams per

day) and a natural cholesterol/antioxidant formula such as Lipid Stabil or a product with comparable ingredients is also recommended.

Side Effects (Testosterone Suppression):

All anabolic/androgenic steroids when taken in doses sufficient to promote muscle gain are expected to suppress endogenous testosterone production. Testosterone is the primary male androgen, and offers strong negative feedback on endogenous testosterone production. Testosterone-based drugs will, likewise, have a strong effect on the hypothalamic regulation of natural steroid hormones. Without the intervention of testosterone-stimulating substances, testosterone levels should return to normal within 1-4 months of drug secession. Note that prolonged hypogonadotrophic hypogonadism can develop secondary to steroid abuse, necessitating medical intervention.

The above side effects are not inclusive. For more detailed discussion of potential side effects, see the Steroid Side Effects section of this book.

Administration (General):

Testosterone hydroalcoholic gel is applied daily (preferably in the morning) to intact, clean, dry skin of the shoulders, upper arms, and/or abdomen. Patients should be careful about transferring testosterone to their female partner(s). The prescribing information for AndroGel® suggests that patients wash their hands immediately with soap and water after application, and also recommends covering the application site(s) with clothing after the gel has dried. Studies with AndroGel® have demonstrated that female partners of male patients noticed as much as a doubling of serum testosterone levels following 15 minutes of rigorous skin-on-skin contact. This contact was initiated between 2 and 12 hours after drug administration. Testosterone transfer was completely avoided when the male subjects wore a shirt.

Administration (Men):

To treat androgen insufficiency, the prescribing guidelines for AndroGel® recommend initiating therapy with a 5g daily dose (delivering 5 mg of testosterone systemically). Serum testosterone levels are measured after 14 days, at which point the physician may adjust upwards to 7.5g or 10g if necessary. For physique- or performance-enhancing purposes, higher doses would be necessary to achieve supraphysiological levels of testosterone. The most common dose here is 20 grams per day, which delivers approximately 20 mg of testosterone. This level is sufficient for most users to notice significant gains in muscle size and strength. Lower doses are also regularly used by some athletes, but typically when accompanied by other anabolic/androgenic steroids. Testosterone is ultimately very versatile, and can be combined with many other anabolic/androgenic steroids to tailor the desired effect.

Administration (Women):

Hydroalcoholic transdermal testosterone gels are not FDA approved for use in women. Testosterone is not recommended for women for physique- or performance-enhancing purposes due to its strong androgenic nature and tendency to produce virilizing side effects.

Availability:

Given their high relative price and low delivery of testosterone, hydroalcoholic transdermal testosterone gels are not commonly traded on the black market. Counterfeits have not yet been widely reported. The various AndroGel® and Testim® preparations can probably be considered real if located.

Andromar Retard (testosterone cyclohexylpropionate)

Androgenic	100
Anabolic	100
Standard	Standard

Chemical Names	4-androsten-3-one-17beta-ol
	17beta-hydroxy-androst-4-en-3-one
Estrogenic Activity	moderate
Progestational Activity	low

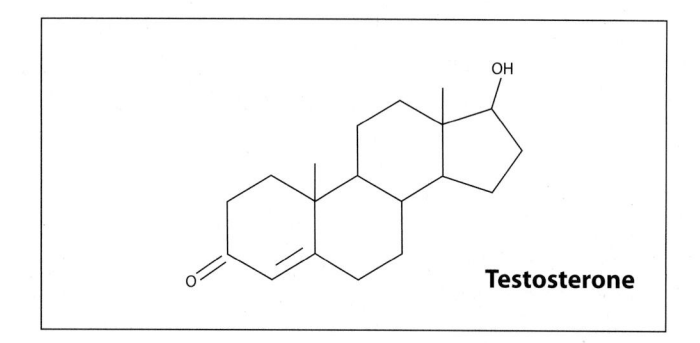

Testosterone

Description:

Testosterone cyclohexylpropionate, or CHP for short, is a slow acting injectable ester of the primary male androgen testosterone. The cyclohexylpropionate ester is very similar in structure to the cypionate (cyclopentylpropionate) ester, different only by the inclusion of a cyclohexane ring (6 carbon atoms) instead of cyclopentane ring (5 carbon atoms). Given the close similarity of these two compounds, one would expect the release duration of testosterone CHP to be very similar to that of testosterone cypionate, perhaps only slightly longer lasting in effect given the greater size/carbon content of the ester. As a testosterone drug, testosterone CHP is capable of imparting rapid gains in muscle size and strength.

History:

Testosterone cyclohexylpropionate was first released commercially during the mid-1970's. It was sold mainly in Europe, under such brand names as Femalon 25, Andromar Retard, and Testosterone Retard Theramex. The Theramex product was the longest lasting of the group, and was sold for approximately 17 years on the French drug market (1974-1991). It contained a steroid concentration of 296mg/mL, 148mg/mL, or 37mg/mL in a 1 mL ampule, which equates to 200 mg, 100 mg, or 25 mg of active testosterone, respectively. The 296mg/mL version was the most popular one located on the black market, for obvious reasons. Today, testosterone cyclohexylpropionate is no longer available. No residual stock of the Theramex product is left in commerce at this time, and all other commercial brands were removed from market years before the Theramex brand.

How Supplied:

Testosterone cyclohexylpropionate is no longer commercially available. When produced, it contained varying amounts of steroid in an oily solution.

Structural Characteristics:

Testosterone cyclohexylpropionate is a modified form of testosterone, where a carboxylic acid ester (cyclohexylpropionic acid) has been attached to the 17-beta hydroxyl group. Esterified forms of testosterone are less polar than free testosterone, and are absorbed more slowly from the area of injection. Once in the bloodstream, the ester is removed to yield free (active) testosterone. Esterified forms of testosterone are designed to prolong the window of therapeutic effect following administration, allowing for a less frequent injection schedule compared to injections of free (unesterified) steroid.

Side Effects (Estrogenic):

Testosterone is readily aromatized in the body to estradiol (estrogen). The aromatase (estrogen synthetase) enzyme is responsible for this metabolism of testosterone. Elevated estrogen levels can cause side effects such as increased water retention, body fat gain, and gynecomastia. Testosterone is considered a moderately estrogenic steroid. An anti-estrogen such as clomiphene citrate or tamoxifen citrate may be necessary to prevent estrogenic side effects. One may alternately use an aromatase inhibitor like Arimidex® (anastrozole), which more efficiently controls estrogen by preventing its synthesis. Aromatase inhibitors can be quite expensive in comparison to anti-estrogens, however, and may also have negative effects on blood lipids.

Estrogenic side effects will occur in a dose-dependant manner, with higher doses (above normal therapeutic levels) of testosterone cypionate more likely to require the concurrent use of an anti-estrogen or aromatase inhibitor. Since water retention and loss of muscle definition are common with higher doses of testosterone, this drug is usually considered a poor choice for dieting or cutting phases of training. Its moderate estrogenicity makes it more ideal for bulking phases, where the added water retention will support raw strength and muscle size, and help foster a stronger anabolic environment.

Side Effects (Androgenic):

Testosterone is the primary male androgen, responsible for maintaining secondary male sexual characteristics. Elevated levels of testosterone are likely to produce androgenic side effects including oily skin, acne, and body/facial hair growth. Men with a genetic predisposition for hair loss (androgenetic alopecia) may notice accelerated male pattern balding. Those concerned about hair loss may find a more comfortable option in nandrolone decanoate, which is a comparably less androgenic steroid. Women are warned of the potential virilizing effects of anabolic/androgenic steroids, especially with a strong androgen such as testosterone. These may include deepening of the voice, menstrual irregularities, changes in skin texture, facial hair growth, and clitoral enlargement.

In androgen-responsive target tissues such as the skin, scalp, and prostate, the high relative androgenicity of testosterone is dependant on its reduction to dihydrotestosterone (DHT). The 5-alpha reductase enzyme is responsible for this metabolism of testosterone. The concurrent use of a 5-alpha reductase inhibitor such as finasteride or dutasteride will interfere with site-specific potentiation of testosterone action, lowering the tendency of testosterone drugs to produce androgenic side effects. It is important to remember that anabolic and androgenic effects are both mediated via the cytosolic androgen receptor. Complete separation of testosterone's anabolic and androgenic properties is not possible, even with total 5-alpha reductase inhibition.

Side Effects (Hepatotoxicity):

Testosterone does not have hepatotoxic effects; liver toxicity is unlikely. One study examined the potential for hepatotoxicity with high doses of testosterone by administering 400 mg of the hormone per day (2,800 mg per week) to a group of male subjects. The steroid was taken orally so that higher peak concentrations would be reached in hepatic tissues compared to intramuscular injections. The hormone was given daily for 20 days, and produced no significant changes in liver enzyme values including serum albumin, bilirubin, alanine-amino-transferase, and alkaline phosphatases.[422]

Side Effects (Cardiovascular):

Anabolic/androgenic steroids can have deleterious effects on serum cholesterol. This includes a tendency to reduce HDL (good) cholesterol values and increase LDL (bad) cholesterol values, which may shift the HDL to LDL balance in a direction that favors greater risk of arteriosclerosis. The relative impact of an anabolic/androgenic steroid on serum lipids is dependant on the dose, route of administration (oral vs. injectable), type of steroid (aromatizable or non-aromatizable), and level of resistance to hepatic metabolism. Anabolic/androgenic steroids may also adversely affect blood pressure and triglycerides, reduce endothelial relaxation, and support left ventricular hypertrophy, all potentially increasing the risk of cardiovascular disease and myocardial infarction.

Testosterone tends to have a much less dramatic impact on cardiovascular risk factors than synthetic steroids. This is due in part to its openness to metabolism by the liver, which allows it to have less effect on the hepatic management of cholesterol. The aromatization of testosterone to estradiol also helps to mitigate the negative effects of androgens on serum lipids. In one study, 280 mg per week of testosterone ester (enanthate) had a slight but not statistically significant effect on HDL cholesterol after 12 weeks, but when taken with an aromatase inhibitor a strong (25%) decrease was seen.[423] Studies using 300 mg of testosterone ester (enanthate) per week for 20 weeks without an aromatase inhibitor demonstrated only a 13% decrease in HDL cholesterol, while at 600 mg the reduction reached 21%.[424] The negative impact of aromatase inhibition should be taken into consideration before such drug is added to testosterone therapy.

Due to the positive influence of estrogen on serum lipids, tamoxifen citrate or clomiphene citrate are preferred to aromatase inhibitors for those concerned with cardiovascular health, as they offer a partial estrogenic effect in the liver. This allows them to potentially improve lipid profiles and offset some of the negative effects of androgens. With doses of 600 mg or less per week, the impact on lipid profile tends to be noticeable but not dramatic, making an anti-estrogen (for cardioprotective purposes) perhaps unnecessary. Doses of 600 mg or less per week have also failed to produce statistically significant changes in LDL/VLDL cholesterol, triglycerides, apolipoprotein B/C-III, C-reactive protein, and insulin sensitivity, all indicating a relatively weak impact on cardiovascular risk factors.[425] When used in moderate doses, injectable testosterone esters are usually considered to be the safest of all anabolic/androgenic steroids.

To help reduce cardiovascular strain it is advised to maintain an active cardiovascular exercise program and minimize the intake of saturated fats, cholesterol, and simple carbohydrates at all times during active AAS administration. Supplementing with fish oils (4 grams per day) and a natural cholesterol/antioxidant formula such as Lipid Stabil or a product with comparable ingredients is

also recommended.

Side Effects (Testosterone Suppression):

All anabolic/androgenic steroids when taken in doses sufficient to promote muscle gain are expected to suppress endogenous testosterone production. Testosterone is the primary male androgen, and offers strong negative feedback on endogenous testosterone production. Testosterone-based drugs will, likewise, have a strong effect on the hypothalamic regulation of natural steroid hormones. Without the intervention of testosterone-stimulating substances, testosterone levels should return to normal within 1-4 months of drug secession. Note that prolonged hypogonadotrophic hypogonadism can develop secondary to steroid abuse, necessitating medical intervention.

The above side effects are not inclusive. For more detailed discussion of potential side effects, see the Steroid Side Effects section of this book.

Administration (Men):

Although active in the body for a longer time, testosterone cyclohexylpropionate was usually injected on a weekly basis for muscle-building purposes. The usual dosage among male athletes is in the range of 300-600 mg per week, taken in cycles 6 to 12 weeks in length. This level is sufficient for most users to notice exceptional gains in muscle size and strength. Testosterone is ultimately very versatile, and can be combined with many other anabolic/androgenic steroids to tailor the desired effect.

Administration (Women):

Testosterone cyclohexylpropionate is not recommended for women for physique- or performance-enhancing purposes due to its strong androgenic nature, tendency to produce virilizing side effects, and slow-acting characteristics (making blood levels difficult to control).

Availability:

Testosterone cyclohexylpropionate is not currently found on the black market; no known legitimate sources for the drug are known to exist.

Andronaq (testosterone suspension)

Androgenic	100
Anabolic	100
Standard	Standard
Chemical Names	4-androsten-3-one-17beta-ol
	17beta-hydroxy-androst-4-en-3-one
Estrogenic Activity	moderate
Progestational Activity	low

Testosterone

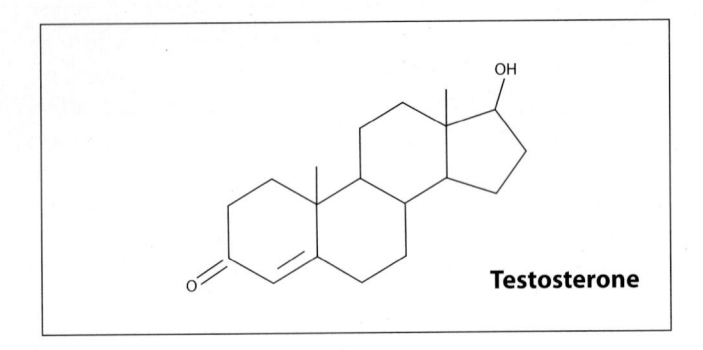

Description:

Testosterone suspension is an injectable preparation containing testosterone (no ester), usually in a water base. Among bodybuilders, "suspension" is known to be an extremely potent mass agent. It is often said to be the most powerful injectable steroid available, producing very rapid gains in muscle mass and strength. This is largely due to the very fast action of the drug. When using a slow-acting oil-based steroid like Sustanon® 250, it can take weeks before a peak testosterone level is reached. With suspension, it is just a matter of hours. This will usually result in the athlete starting to notice size and strength gains by the end of the first week. By the time the athlete is 30 days into a cycle of suspension, the length it will usually take for Sustanon® 250 to really begin working consistently, the mass gains are already (generally) very extreme.

History:

Testosterone suspension is one of the oldest anabolic/androgenic steroids, dating all the way back to the 1930's. Used generically to describe any injectable form of free testosterone, testosterone suspension predates the development of slow-acting (depot) injections of esterified testosterone by several years. Even after the development of esterified derivates, testosterone suspension remained on the U.S. and other select drug markets. For example, testosterone propionate and testosterone enanthate were both commercially available by the 1950's, yet testosterone suspension remained a regularly produced item in the U.S. for decades more. Previous American trade names for the drug have include Sterotate (Ulmer), Andronaq (Central), Aquaspension Testosterone (Pitman-Moore), Injectable Aqueous Testosterone (Arlington-Funk), Virosterone (Endo), and Testosterone Aqueous (National Drug). A full accounting of the former generic manufacturers and brand names for this drug would be too numerous to list.

Testosterone suspension shares a clinical application history similar to that of other testosterone products. Early prescribing guidelines called for its use to ameliorate a loss of sex drive, impotence, and general loss of vitality in aging males with declining hormone levels. Testosterone was/is also used to treat pubertal adolescents with undescended testicles. With women, the drug was commonly prescribed for the treatment of excessive or painful lactation following childbirth, as well as inoperable mammary cancer. By the 1990's, however, the FDA had refined the approved uses for testosterone suspension slightly, which began to focus more tightly on the treatment of male androgen insufficiency. The drug may, however, still be used as a secondary therapy in inoperable breast cancer, although its high tendency to produce virilization makes it an uncommon choice.

Although the number of products containing testosterone suspension steadily dwindled over the years, the drug enjoyed uninterrupted availability on the U.S. prescription drug market all the way up to 1998. That year, the FDA had taken action against Steris Laboratories (a subsidiary of Henry Schein), which at the time was the principal U.S. supplier for testosterone products (manufacturing them for their label and several other brands). The firm was also the last remaining producer of testosterone suspension. The dispute arose over Steris' inventory reports for their Class III drugs. The FDA forced the company to suspend production of all C-III pharmaceuticals until certain "discrepancies" could be addressed. Years later, Steris was able to resume producing testosterone drugs again, but by this time had made the decision not to resume making testosterone suspension. Currently, testosterone suspension is still available in the U.S., but only through private compounding pharmacies, which may produce the drug on special order from a licensed doctor.

How Supplied:

Testosterone suspension is available in select human and veterinary drug markets. Composition and dosage may vary by country and manufacturer, but usually contain 50 mg/ml or 100 mg/ml of steroid mixed in a water-based solution. Testosterone has low water solubility, so the steroid will noticeably separate from a water-based solution when a vial or ampule is left to sit. A quick shake will temporarily place the drug back into suspension, so that the withdrawn dosage should always be consistent.

Structural Characteristics:

Testosterone suspension contains (free) testosterone in a water-based suspension, although oils are sometime also used as carriers. Without esterification, testosterone has a short half-life in the body. Testosterone suspension may require a minimum of 2-3 injections per week to maintain consistent hormone elevations. When calculating dose, especially when moving from one testosterone preparation to another, it is also important to remember that testosterone suspension contains more active testosterone per milligram than its esterified derivatives. For example, when the weight of the ester is taken into account, 100 mg of testosterone enanthate actually only provides 72mg of raw testosterone.

Side Effects (Estrogenic):

Testosterone is readily aromatized in the body to estradiol (estrogen). The aromatase (estrogen synthetase) enzyme is responsible for this metabolism of testosterone. Elevated estrogen levels can cause side effects such as increased water retention, body fat gain, and gynecomastia. Testosterone is considered a moderately estrogenic steroid. An anti-estrogen such as clomiphene citrate or tamoxifen citrate may be necessary to prevent estrogenic side effects. One may alternately use an aromatase inhibitor like Arimidex® (anastrozole), which more efficiently controls estrogen by preventing its synthesis. Aromatase inhibitors can be quite expensive in comparison to anti-estrogens, however, and may also have negative effects on blood lipids.

Estrogenic side effects will occur in a dose-dependant manner, with higher doses (above normal therapeutic levels) of testosterone more likely to require the concurrent use of an anti-estrogen or aromatase inhibitor. Since water retention and loss of muscle definition are common with higher doses of testosterone, this drug is usually considered a poor choice for dieting or cutting phases of training. Its moderate estrogenicity makes it more ideal for bulking phases, where the added water retention will support raw strength and muscle size, and help foster a stronger anabolic environment.

Side Effects (Androgenic):

Testosterone is the primary male androgen, responsible for maintaining secondary male sexual characteristics. Elevated levels of testosterone are likely to produce androgenic side effects including oily skin, acne, and body/facial hair growth. Men with a genetic predisposition for hair loss (androgenetic alopecia) may notice accelerated male pattern balding. Those concerned about hair loss may find a more comfortable option in nandrolone decanoate, which is a comparably less androgenic steroid. Women are warned of the potential virilizing effects of anabolic/androgenic steroids, especially with a strong androgen such as testosterone. These may include deepening of the voice, menstrual irregularities, changes in skin texture, facial hair growth, and clitoral enlargement.

In androgen-responsive target tissues such as the skin, scalp, and prostate, the high relative androgenicity of testosterone is dependant on its reduction to dihydrotestosterone (DHT). The 5-alpha reductase enzyme is responsible for this metabolism of testosterone. The concurrent use of a 5-alpha reductase inhibitor such as finasteride or dutasteride will interfere with site-specific potentiation of testosterone action, lowering the tendency of testosterone drugs to produce androgenic side effects. It is important to remember that anabolic and androgenic effects are both mediated via the cytosolic androgen receptor. Complete separation of testosterone's anabolic and androgenic properties is not possible, even with total 5-alpha reductase inhibition.

Side Effects (Hepatotoxicity):

Testosterone does not have hepatotoxic effects; liver toxicity is unlikely. One study examined the potential for hepatotoxicity with high doses of testosterone by administering 400 mg of the hormone per day (2,800 mg per week) to a group of male subjects. The steroid was taken orally so that higher peak concentrations would be reached in hepatic tissues compared to intramuscular injections. The hormone was given daily for 20 days, and produced no significant changes in liver enzyme values including serum albumin, bilirubin, alanine-amino-transferase, and alkaline phosphatases.[426]

Side Effects (Cardiovascular):

Anabolic/androgenic steroids can have deleterious effects on serum cholesterol. This includes a tendency to reduce HDL (good) cholesterol values and increase LDL (bad) cholesterol values, which may shift the HDL to LDL balance in a direction that favors greater risk of arteriosclerosis. The relative impact of an anabolic/androgenic steroid on serum lipids is dependant on the dose, route of administration (oral vs. injectable), type of steroid (aromatizable or non-aromatizable), and level of resistance to hepatic metabolism. Anabolic/androgenic steroids may also adversely affect blood pressure and triglycerides, reduce endothelial relaxation, and support left ventricular hypertrophy, all potentially increasing the risk of cardiovascular disease and myocardial infarction.

Testosterone tends to have a much less dramatic impact on cardiovascular risk factors than synthetic steroids. This is due in part to its openness to metabolism by the liver, which allows it to have less effect on the hepatic management of cholesterol. The aromatization of testosterone to estradiol also helps to mitigate the negative effects of androgens on serum lipids. In one study, 280 mg per week of testosterone ester (enanthate) had a slight but not statistically significant effect on HDL cholesterol after 12 weeks, but when taken with an aromatase inhibitor a strong (25%) decrease was seen.[427] Studies using 300 mg of testosterone ester (enanthate) per week for 20 weeks without an aromatase inhibitor demonstrated only a 13% decrease in HDL cholesterol, while at 600 mg the reduction reached 21%.[428] The negative impact of aromatase inhibition should be taken into consideration before such drug is added to testosterone therapy.

Due to the positive influence of estrogen on serum lipids, tamoxifen citrate or clomiphene citrate are preferred to aromatase inhibitors for those concerned with cardiovascular health, as they offer a partial estrogenic effect in the liver. This allows them to potentially improve lipid profiles and offset some of the negative effects of androgens. With doses of 600 mg or less of testosterone per week, the impact on lipid profile tends to be noticeable but not dramatic, making an anti-estrogen (for cardioprotective purposes) perhaps unnecessary. Doses of 600 mg or less per week have also failed to produce statistically significant changes in LDL/VLDL cholesterol, triglycerides, apolipoprotein B/C-III, C-reactive protein, and insulin sensitivity, all indicating a relatively weak impact on cardiovascular risk factors.[429] When used in moderate doses, injectable testosterone esters are usually considered to be the safest of all anabolic/androgenic steroids.

To help reduce cardiovascular strain it is advised to maintain an active cardiovascular exercise program and minimize the intake of saturated fats, cholesterol, and simple carbohydrates at all times during active AAS administration. Supplementing with fish oils (4 grams per day) and a natural cholesterol/antioxidant formula such as Lipid Stabil or a product with comparable ingredients is also recommended.

Side Effects (Testosterone Suppression):

All anabolic/androgenic steroids when taken in doses sufficient to promote muscle gain are expected to suppress endogenous testosterone production. Testosterone is the primary male androgen, and offers strong negative feedback on endogenous testosterone production. Testosterone-based drugs will, likewise, have a strong effect on the hypothalamic regulation of natural steroid hormones. Without the intervention of testosterone-stimulating substances, testosterone levels should return to normal within 1-4 months of drug secession. Note that prolonged hypogonadotrophic hypogonadism can develop secondary to steroid abuse, necessitating medical intervention.

The above side effects are not inclusive. For more detailed discussion of potential side effects, see the Steroid Side Effects section of this book.

Administration (General):

Testosterone suspension contains undissolved testosterone particles, which form a short-acting repository in the muscle following injection. Depending on the size of the particles and other agents present, injections of testosterone suspension may result in local irritation, pain, and redness. Veterinary testosterone suspensions may use large particles that require a needle as large as 21 gauge for injection, for example, and can be very uncomfortable to use. Modern testosterone suspension preparations made for human use often contain microcrystalline steroid particles. These crystals are highly refined, and are too small to see with the naked eye. This design provides significantly more patient comfort than less refined products, and is generally well tolerated.

Administration (Men):

To treat androgen insufficiency, the prescribing guidelines for testosterone suspension recommend a dose of 25-50 mg, which is given 2-3 times per week. When used for muscle-building purposes, testosterone suspension is often administered at a dose of 100-200 mg per injection, which is given every 2nd or 3rd day. Athletes looking to achieve an extremely rapid bulk gain will inject as much as 100 mg daily. In most cases this higher dose can be amazing, the user seeming to just inflate with bloated muscle mass in a very short period of time. Back when they were being manufactured, the U.S. 30 mL vials (100 mg/mL) were always the most sought after for this procedure, as each would run the cycle for about a month. Although this drug does require a frequent injection schedule, a well-refined suspension should pass through a needle as fine as 27 gauge (insulin). This allows the user more available injection sites, hitting the smaller muscle groups such as the deltoid, triceps, and calves.

Those looking for only a potent mass agent are often extremely happy with the results provided by testosterone suspension; this product certainly has a strong reputation for performing. But those athletes who want not just quantity but quality are likely to be disappointed, as the muscle mass gain is not going to be a hard, dense one. In fact, the user will often have to contend with excessive fat and water-weight gains when building their physique with this drug, and will often seek the benefit of cutting agents soon afterwards to clean up the look of muscularity. Alternately, one could make use of a smaller dosage of testosterone suspension, which would allow for less estrogen buildup. In such a scenario, one could stack it with any of a variety of other less or non-aromatizable steroids, depending on the desired goals.

Administration (Women):

Testosterone suspension is rarely used with women in clinical medicine. When applied, it is most often used as a secondary treatment for inoperable breast cancer. Doses given for this application may reach 100 mg three times per week, a level well into the threshold likely to cause strong virilizing side effects. Testosterone suspension is not recommended for women for physique- or performance-enhancing purposes due to its strong androgenic nature and tendency to produce virilizing side effects.

Availability:

Testosterone suspension is not abundant on the black market at this time. Few legitimate brands still exist, and of those very small quantities of product are diverted for illicit sale.

Bolfortan (testosterone nicotinate)

Androgenic	100
Anabolic	100
Standard	Standard |//
Chemical Names	4-androsten-3-one-17beta-ol
	17beta-hydroxy-androst-4-en-3-one
Estrogenic Activity	moderate
Progestational Activity	low

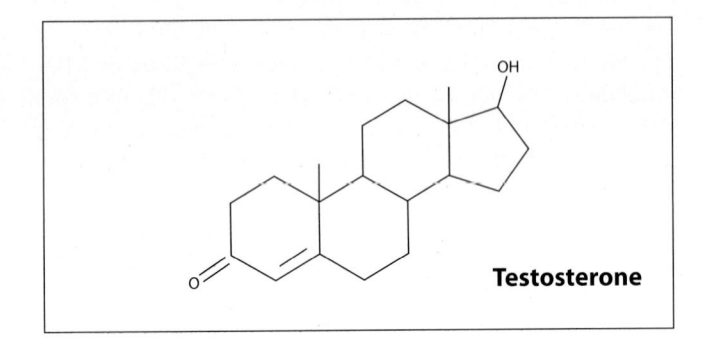

Testosterone

Description:

Testosterone nicotinate is an injectable form of the primary male androgen testosterone. This compound uses an unusual chemical group to extend the biological activity of testosterone, namely nicotinic acid. Nicotinic acid is also known as niacin, a well-known vitamin of the B complex family. Niacin is occasionally used as an ester with other medications to improve the pharmacokinetic profile of a delivered agent, although little is known about its application with an injectable androgenic steroid. As an injectable testosterone, it is certain, however, that testosterone nicotinate is an effective mass- and strength-building drug.

History:

Testosterone nicotinate was originally developed in the U.S. in 1962, but is most known as a commercial drug product by Lannacher Heilmittel GmbH in Austria. It was sold to the Austrian drug market during the 1960's and 70's under the brand name of Bolfortan. No other brands of this drug were known to exist worldwide, making this a very rare form of testosterone. As a result, a great deal of mystique had come to surround this steroid. Many American bodybuilders came to identify Bolfortan as an agent utilized only by certain circles of elite European athletes, and attributed an unusually high level of anabolic potency to this compound. In reality, however, this was simply one of many different injectable esters of testosterone, with similar relatively anabolic potency as other testosterone drugs. Testosterone nicotinate ultimately had a short life on the Austrian drug market, and was all but a myth by the time the early steroid-era of 1980's and 90's was in full swing.

How Supplied:

Testosterone nicotinate is no longer commercially available. When produced, it was supplied in the form of a 1 mL ampule containing 50 mg/ml of steroid in a water-based suspension.

Structural Characteristics:

Testosterone nicotinate is a modified form of testosterone, where a carboxylic acid ester (3-pyridinecarboxylic acid) has been attached to the 17-beta hydroxyl group. Esterified forms of testosterone are less polar than free testosterone, and are absorbed more slowly from the area of injection. Once in the bloodstream, the ester is removed to yield free (active) testosterone. Esterified forms of testosterone are designed to prolong the window of therapeutic effect following administration, allowing for a less frequent injection schedule compared to injections of free (unesterified) steroid.

Side Effects (Estrogenic):

Testosterone is readily aromatized in the body to estradiol (estrogen). The aromatase (estrogen synthetase) enzyme is responsible for this metabolism of testosterone. Elevated estrogen levels can cause side effects such as increased water retention, body fat gain, and gynecomastia. Testosterone is considered a moderately estrogenic steroid. An anti-estrogen such as clomiphene citrate or tamoxifen citrate may be necessary to prevent estrogenic side effects. One may alternately use an aromatase inhibitor like Arimidex® (anastrozole), which more efficiently controls estrogen by preventing its synthesis. Aromatase inhibitors can be quite expensive in comparison to anti-estrogens, however, and may also have negative effects on blood lipids.

Estrogenic side effects will occur in a dose-dependant manner, with higher doses (above normal therapeutic levels) of testosterone more likely to require the concurrent use of an anti-estrogen or aromatase inhibitor. Since water retention and loss of muscle definition are common with higher doses of testosterone, this drug is usually considered a poor choice for dieting or cutting phases of training. Its moderate estrogenicity makes it more ideal for bulking phases, where the added water retention will support raw strength and muscle size, and help foster a stronger anabolic environment.

Side Effects (Androgenic):

Testosterone is the primary male androgen, responsible for maintaining secondary male sexual characteristics. Elevated levels of testosterone are likely to produce androgenic side effects including oily skin, acne, and body/facial hair growth. Men with a genetic predisposition for hair loss (androgenetic alopecia) may notice accelerated male pattern balding. Those concerned about hair loss may find a more comfortable option in nandrolone decanoate, which is a comparably less androgenic steroid. Women are warned of the potential virilizing effects of anabolic/androgenic steroids, especially with a strong androgen such as testosterone. These may include deepening of the voice, menstrual irregularities, changes in skin texture, facial hair growth, and clitoral enlargement.

In androgen-responsive target tissues such as the skin, scalp, and prostate, the high relative androgenicity of testosterone is dependant on its reduction to dihydrotestosterone (DHT). The 5-alpha reductase enzyme is responsible for this metabolism of testosterone. The concurrent use of a 5-alpha reductase inhibitor such as finasteride or dutasteride will interfere with site-specific potentiation of testosterone action, lowering the tendency of testosterone drugs to produce androgenic side effects. It is important to remember that anabolic and androgenic effects are both mediated via the cytosolic androgen receptor. Complete separation of testosterone's anabolic and androgenic properties is not possible, even with total 5-alpha reductase inhibition.

Side Effects (Hepatotoxicity):

Testosterone does not have hepatotoxic effects; liver toxicity is unlikely. One study examined the potential for hepatotoxicity with high doses of testosterone by administering 400 mg of the hormone per day (2,800 mg per week) to a group of male subjects. The steroid was taken orally so that higher peak concentrations would be reached in hepatic tissues compared to intramuscular injections. The hormone was given daily for 20 days, and produced no significant changes in liver enzyme values including serum albumin, bilirubin, alanine-amino-transferase, and alkaline phosphatases.[430]

Side Effects (Cardiovascular):

Anabolic/androgenic steroids can have deleterious effects on serum cholesterol. This includes a tendency to reduce HDL (good) cholesterol values and increase LDL (bad) cholesterol values, which may shift the HDL to LDL balance in a direction that favors greater risk of arteriosclerosis. The relative impact of an anabolic/androgenic steroid on serum lipids is dependant on the dose, route of administration (oral vs. injectable), type of steroid (aromatizable or non-aromatizable), and level of resistance to hepatic metabolism. Anabolic/androgenic steroids may also adversely affect blood pressure and triglycerides, reduce endothelial relaxation, and support left ventricular hypertrophy, all potentially increasing the risk of cardiovascular disease and myocardial infarction.

Testosterone tends to have a much less dramatic impact on cardiovascular risk factors than synthetic steroids. This is due in part to its openness to metabolism by the liver, which allows it to have less effect on the hepatic management of cholesterol. The aromatization of testosterone to estradiol also helps to mitigate the negative effects of androgens on serum lipids. In one study, 280 mg per week of testosterone ester (enanthate) had a slight but not statistically significant effect on HDL cholesterol after 12 weeks, but when taken with an aromatase inhibitor a strong (25%) decrease was seen.[431] Studies using 300 mg of testosterone ester (enanthate) per week for 20 weeks without an aromatase inhibitor demonstrated only a 13% decrease in HDL cholesterol, while at 600 mg the reduction reached 21%.[432] The negative impact of aromatase inhibition should be taken into consideration before such drug is added to testosterone therapy.

Due to the positive influence of estrogen on serum lipids, tamoxifen citrate or clomiphene citrate are preferred to aromatase inhibitors for those concerned with cardiovascular health, as they offer a partial estrogenic effect in the liver. This allows them to potentially improve lipid profiles and offset some of the negative effects of androgens. With doses of 600 mg or less of testosterone per week, the impact on lipid profile tends to be noticeable but not dramatic, making an anti-estrogen (for cardioprotective purposes) perhaps unnecessary. Doses of 600 mg or less per week have also failed to produce statistically significant changes in LDL/VLDL cholesterol, triglycerides, apolipoprotein B/C-III, C-reactive protein, and insulin sensitivity, all indicating a relatively weak impact on cardiovascular risk factors.[433] When used in moderate doses, injectable testosterone esters are usually considered to be the safest of all anabolic/androgenic steroids.

To help reduce cardiovascular strain it is advised to maintain an active cardiovascular exercise program and minimize the intake of saturated fats, cholesterol, and simple carbohydrates at all times during active AAS administration. Supplementing with fish oils (4 grams per

day) and a natural cholesterol/antioxidant formula such as Lipid Stabil or a product with comparable ingredients is also recommended.

Side Effects (Testosterone Suppression):

All anabolic/androgenic steroids when taken in doses sufficient to promote muscle gain are expected to suppress endogenous testosterone production. Testosterone is the primary male androgen, and offers strong negative feedback on endogenous testosterone production. Testosterone-based drugs will, likewise, have a strong effect on the hypothalamic regulation of natural steroid hormones. Without the intervention of testosterone-stimulating substances, testosterone levels should return to normal within 1-4 months of drug secession. Note that prolonged hypogonadotrophic hypogonadism can develop secondary to steroid abuse, necessitating medical intervention.

The above side effects are not inclusive. For more detailed discussion of potential side effects, see the Steroid Side Effects section of this book.

Administration (General):

Bolfortan was known to use a large particle size, requiring injections with a very large (20-gauge) needle. The design of this steroid is such that steroid crystals form a repository in the muscle following injection, where they would slowly dissolve over time. Injections could result in local irritation, pain, and redness. Although this was an effective method of delivering testosterone, patient comfort was likely not ideal with this formulation.

Administration (Men):

As an injectable testosterone, a weekly cumulative dosage of 200-400 mg would be sufficient to promote muscle mass and strength gains. This could be broken up into 2-3 separate injections per week. Higher doses than 400 mg per week would be more difficult given the relatively low dose of this steroid at its time of availability (50 mg/ml).

Administration (Women):

In modern clinical medicine, testosterone compounds are rarely used with women. Testosterone nicotinate is not recommended for women for physique- or performance-enhancing purposes due to its strong androgenic nature and tendency to produce virilizing side effects.

Availability:

Testosterone nicotinate is no longer commercially available. The raw material is available from certain manufacturers, and may turn up in black market (underground) preparations.

Cheque Drops® (mibolerone)

Androgenic	1,800
Anabolic	4,100
Standard	Methyltestosterone (oral)

Chemical Names	7,17-dimethyl-19-norandrost-4-en-3-one-17b-ol
	17beta-Hydroxy-7alpha,17-dimethylestr-4-en-3-one
Estrogenic Activity	high
Progestational Activity	high

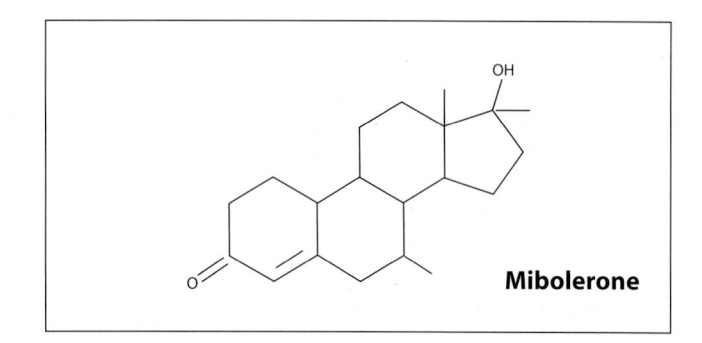

Description:

Mibolerone is an oral anabolic steroid, structurally derived from nandrolone. This agent is specifically 7,17-dimethylated nandrolone, significantly more potent as an anabolic and androgenic agent than its non-methylated parent. Over the years, mibolerone has earned a reputation among bodybuilders as being one of the strongest steroids ever made. This is correct in a technical sense, as it is one of only a select few commercial steroid products effective in microgram, not milligram, amounts. During standard animal assays, mibolerone was determined to have 41 times the anabolic activity of methyltestosterone when given orally. In contrast, it had only 18 times the androgenic activity. Although both properties are strongly pronounced with this agent, it retains a primarily anabolic character (in a relative sense). Estrogenic and progestational properties are also very pronounced with this drug, however. Among athletes it is most commonly applied during bulking phases of training, or to stimulate aggression before a workout or competition.

History:

Mibolerone was first described in 1963.[434] It was developed into a veterinary medicine during the 1960's by Upjohn, which sold the drug under the brand name Cheque Drops. The preparation contained 100 mcg/ml of steroid in a 55 mL bottle, for a total steroid content of 5.5 milligrams (illustrating the high relative potency of mibolerone). Pharmacia & Upjohn later also sold a preparation called Cheque Medicated Dog Food, of obvious composition. The drug was administered orally, and had been used to interrupt the estrous cycle of female dogs, preventing them from going into heat. It is approved for use in an animal for no longer than 24 months. Use of the drug is considered carefully by most veterinarians, mainly because longer-term administration can produce side effects such as clitoral enlargement, aggression, urinary difficulties, and liver damage.

Among athletes, mibolerone has always been seen with a high level of mystique, perhaps partly due to its limited availability. Those actually familiar with the Upjohn (then Pharmacia & Upjohn) product were likely disappointed during the early 2000's, when the Cheque products were officially discontinued by the manufacturer. The company, now Pfizer Animal Health, presently lists no mibolerone-containing products on its inventory, despite retaining the rights to market the drug. Mibolerone is still available in the U.S., but only in generic form from a private compounding pharmacy, obtained under special order by a licensed veterinarian. The removal of the Pharmacia & Upjohn products from the U.S. market marked the commercial end of mibolerone. No prescription preparation, human or veterinary, is currently known to contain mibolerone worldwide.

How Supplied:

Mibolerone is no longer available as a prescription drug product. When produced it most commonly came in the form of an oral solution based in propylene glycol, carrying 100mcg of steroid per milliliter in a 55 mL bottle.

Structural Characteristics:

Mibolerone is a modified form of nandrolone. It differs by 1) the addition of a methyl group at carbon 17-alpha to protect the hormone during oral administration and 2) the introduction of a methyl group at carbon 7 (alpha), which inhibits 5-alpha reduction and increases relative androgenicity. 7,17-dimethylated steroids also tend to be very resistant to metabolism and serum-binding proteins, greatly enhancing their relative biological activity.

Side Effects (Estrogenic):

Mibolerone is aromatized by the body, and is considered a highly estrogenic steroid due to its conversion to 7,17-dimethylestradiol (an estrogen with high biological activity). Gynecomastia may be a concern during treatment, especially when higher than normal therapeutic doses are used. At the same time water retention can become a problem, causing a notable loss of muscle definition as both subcutaneous water retention and fat levels build. To avoid strong estrogenic side effects, it may be necessary to use an anti-estrogen such as Nolvadex®. One may alternately use an aromatase inhibitor like Arimidex® (anastrozole), which is a more effective remedy for estrogen control. Aromatase inhibitors, however, can be quite expensive in comparison to standard estrogen maintenance therapies, and may also have negative effects on blood lipids.

It is of note that mibolerone also displays strong activity as a progestin in the body. The side effects associated with progesterone are similar to those of estrogen, including negative feedback inhibition of testosterone production and enhanced rate of fat storage. Progestins also augment the stimulatory effect of estrogens on mammary tissue growth. There appears to be a strong synergy between these two hormones here, such that gynecomastia might even occur with the help of progestins without excessive estrogen levels being present. The use of an anti-estrogen, which inhibits the estrogenic component of this disorder, is often sufficient to mitigate gynecomastia caused by mibolerone.

Side Effects (Androgenic):

Although classified as an anabolic steroid, androgenic side effects are still common with this substance. This may include bouts of oily skin, acne, and body/facial hair growth. Anabolic/androgenic steroids may also aggravate male pattern hair loss. Individuals sensitive to the androgenic effects of this steroid may find a milder anabolic such as Deca-Durabolin® to be more comfortable. Women are additionally warned of the potential virilizing effects of anabolic/androgenic steroids. These may include a deepening of the voice, menstrual irregularities, changes in skin texture, facial hair growth, and clitoral enlargement. Note that 7-methylation inhibits steroid 5-alpha reduction.[435] The relative androgenicity of mibolerone is not affected by the concurrent use of finasteride or dutasteride.

Side Effects (Hepatotoxicity):

Mibolerone is a c17-alpha alkylated compound. This alteration protects the drug from deactivation by the liver, allowing a very high percentage of the drug entry into the bloodstream following oral administration. C17-alpha alkylated anabolic/androgenic steroids can be hepatotoxic. Prolonged or high exposure may result in liver damage. In rare instances life-threatening dysfunction may develop. It is advisable to visit a physician periodically during each cycle to monitor liver function and overall health. Intake of c17-alpha alkylated steroids is commonly limited to 6-8 weeks, in an effort to avoid escalating liver strain. Severe liver complications are rare given the periodic nature in which most people use oral anabolic/androgenic steroids, although cannot be excluded with this steroid, especially with high doses and/or prolonged administration periods. Note that U.S. prescribing information for Cheque Drops mentions only one human study being conducted on mibolerone, and that the study was terminated early due to high hepatotoxicity.

The use of a liver detoxification supplement such as Liver Stabil, Liv-52, or Essentiale Forte is advised while taking any hepatotoxic anabolic/androgenic steroids.

Side Effects (Cardiovascular):

Anabolic/androgenic steroids can have deleterious effects on serum cholesterol. This includes a tendency to reduce HDL (good) cholesterol values and increase LDL (bad) cholesterol values, which may shift the HDL to LDL balance in a direction that favors greater risk of arteriosclerosis. The relative impact of an anabolic/androgenic steroid on serum lipids is dependant on the dose, route of administration (oral vs. injectable), type of steroid (aromatizable or non-aromatizable), and level of resistance to hepatic metabolism. Mibolerone has a strong effect on the hepatic management of cholesterol due to its structural resistance to liver breakdown and route of administration. Anabolic/androgenic steroids may also adversely affect blood pressure and triglycerides, reduce endothelial relaxation, and support left ventricular hypertrophy, all potentially increasing the risk of cardiovascular disease and myocardial infarction.

To help reduce cardiovascular strain it is advised to maintain an active cardiovascular exercise program and minimize the intake of saturated fats, cholesterol, and simple carbohydrates at all times during active AAS administration. Supplementing with fish oils (4 grams per day) and a natural cholesterol/antioxidant formula such as Lipid Stabil or a product with comparable ingredients is also recommended.

Side Effects (Testosterone Suppression):

All anabolic/androgenic steroids when taken in doses sufficient to promote muscle gain are expected to suppress endogenous testosterone production. Without the intervention of testosterone-stimulating substances, testosterone levels should return to normal within 1-4 months of drug secession. Note that prolonged hypogonadotrophic hypogonadism can develop secondary to steroid abuse, necessitating medical intervention.

The above side effects are not inclusive. For more detailed discussion of potential side effects, see the Steroid Side Effects section of this book.

Administration (General):

Studies have shown that taking an oral anabolic steroid with food may decrease its bioavailability.[436] This is caused by the fat-soluble nature of steroid hormones, which can allow some of the drug to dissolve with undigested dietary fat, reducing its absorption from the gastrointestinal tract. For maximum utilization, this steroid should be taken on an empty stomach.

Administration (Men):

Mibolerone was never approved for use in humans. Prescribing guidelines are unavailable. In the athletic arena, the drug is used intermittently due to its high level of hepatotoxicity, with cycles usually lasting no more than 6 weeks followed by 6-8 weeks off. A daily dosage of 200 to 500mcg is most common for bodybuilding purposes. This level is typically sufficient for gains in strength and muscle mass (bulk). The high progestational and estrogenic activity of mibolerone makes it of little value in speed and endurance sports, causing an unwanted retention of water weight.

Administration (Women):

Mibolerone was never approved for use in humans. Prescribing guidelines are unavailable. Mibolerone is generally not recommended for women for physique- or performance-enhancing purposes due to its very strong nature and tendency to produce virilizing side effects.

Availability:

As mentioned above, Pharmacia & Upjohn no longer makes this product. It is still being sold as a compounded veterinary medicine in the United States, however. No commercial preparations are known worldwide. While real Cheque Drops are gone, mibolerone has seen a small rebirth on the underground drug market.

Danocrine® (danazol)

Androgenic	37
Anabolic	125
Standard	Testosterone

Chemical Names	17alpha-Pregna-2,4-dien-20-yno[2,3-d]isoxazol-17-ol
Estrogenic Activity	none
Progestational Activity	none

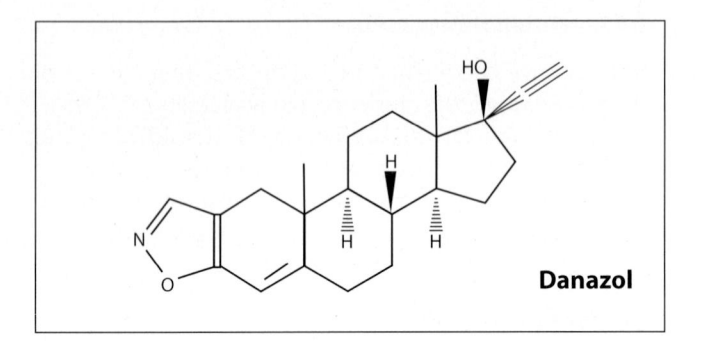

Description:

Danazol is a synthetic androgen derived from ethisterone (ethinyltestosterone), which is a synthetic oral progestin. Although steroidal in structure, danazol is technically classified as an anti-gonadotropin agent. This means that its main function is to suppress LH and FSH, which may also suppress the body's release of sex hormones like testosterone and estrogen. Danazol is used clinically to treat certain hormone-related disorders, not to build muscle. It appears to have little if any anabolic effect, and at best slight androgenic activity. It is also described as being non-estrogenic and non-progestational. This drug is not widely used by athletes, offering little tangible benefits in spite of its structural similarity to other steroids.

History:

Danazol first appeared on the U.S. prescription drug market in the mid-1970's. It was initially indicated for the treatment of endometriosis amenable to hormonal management, and only in those patients who failed to respond, or could not take, other drugs. Danazol works by inhibiting the output of LH and FSH, which in turn may cause normal and ectopic endometrial tissue to become inactive, producing atrophy and regression. More modern applications for the drug include endometriosis, fibrocystic breast disease, and hereditary angioedema. Due to that fact that its main activity is that of an anti-gonadotropic agent, and not as an anabolic steroid, it was deemed there would be little chance for abuse with this drug. It was likewise never registered as a controlled substance in the United States.

Athletes rarely use danazol, mainly because it has little to nothing to offer. Some steroid reference materials have recommended its use to combat the feminization caused by other aromatizable steroids. It is assumed that its androgenic activity will be enough to counter this, however, it excludes the fact that this drug remains a fairly weak androgen. The fact remains that anti-estrogens are fundamentally more appropriate for such situations. In their absence, one could find a number of more effective options before trying danazol. Today, most athletes pay absolutely no attention to this drug, so it is rarely encountered. Many newer medications have taken a good deal of the market share away from danazol in recent years as well, although there are also many situations in which this drug is still appropriate to prescribe. It remains available in the U.S. and many markets abroad.

How Supplied:

Danazol is available in a variety of human drug markets. Composition and dosage may vary by country and manufacturer, but typically come in capsules containing 50 mg, 100 mg, or 200 mg of drug each.

Side Effects (Estrogenic):

Danazol is described as having no appreciable estrogenic activity. Therapy with this drug may cause side effects relating to low serum estrogen, including hot flashes, flushing, sweating, nervousness, emotional variability, and vaginal itching and dryness.

Side Effects (Androgenic):

Danazol is a weak androgen, and may produce side effects, particularly in women more susceptible to the androgenic effects of steroids. These include oily skin, acne, deepening of the voice, menstrual irregularities, changes in skin texture, facial hair growth, and in rare cases clitoral enlargement.

Side Effects (Hepatotoxicity):

Danazol is a c17-alpha alkylated compound. This alteration protects the drug from deactivation by the liver, allowing a very high percentage of the drug entry into the bloodstream following oral administration. C17-alpha alkylated steroids can be hepatotoxic. Prolonged or high exposure may result in liver damage. In rare instances life-threatening dysfunction may develop. It is advisable to visit a physician periodically during use to monitor liver function and overall health.

The use of a liver detoxification supplement such as Liver Stabil, Liv-52, or Essentiale Forte is advised while taking any hepatotoxic anabolic/androgenic steroids.

Side Effects (Testosterone Suppression):

Danazol is a strong antigonadotropin, and will suppress serum testosterone levels in men (and to a lesser extent women). Testicular atrophy may be a side effect of therapy.

The above side effects are not inclusive. For more detailed discussion of potential side effects, see the Steroid Side Effects section of this book.

Administration (Men):

Danazol is used clinically in doses of 200 mg two to three times per day to treat hereditary angioedema. A lower long-term maintenance dose is later established. Danazol is generally not recommended for physique- or performance-enhancing purposes due to its weak anabolic and androgenic nature and strong tendency to suppress gonadotropin levels.

Administration (Women):

Danazol is used clinically in doses ranging from 100 mg to 800 mg per day depending on the disorder and individual treatment required. Therapy is often continued for 6-9 months. Danazol is generally not recommended for physique- or performance-enhancing purposes due to its weak anabolic and androgenic nature and strong tendency to suppress gonadotropin levels.

Availability:

Danazol is not widely sold on the black market, due to limited demand.

Deca-Durabolin® (nandrolone decanoate)

Androgenic	37
Anabolic	125
Standard	Testosterone
Chemical Names	19-norandrost-4-en-3-one-17beta-ol
	17beta-hydroxy-estr-4-en-3-one
Estrogenic Activity	low
Progestational Activity	moderate

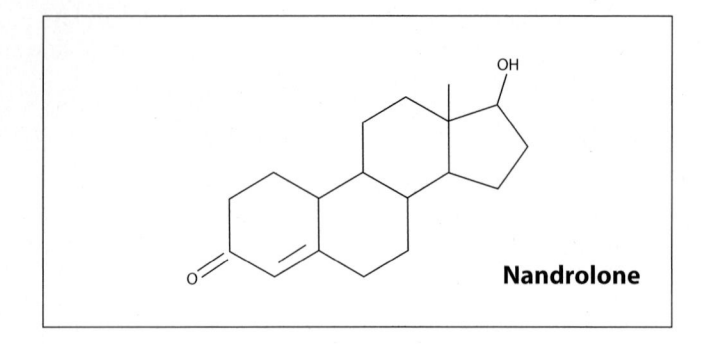

Nandrolone

Description:

Nandrolone decanoate is an injectable form of the anabolic steroid nandrolone. The decanoate ester provides a slow release of nandrolone from the site of injection, lasting for up to three weeks. Nandrolone is very similar to testosterone in structure, although it lacks a carbon atom at the 19th position (hence its other name, 19-nortestosterone). Like testosterone, nandrolone exhibits relatively strong anabolic properties. Unlike testosterone, however, its tissue-building activity is accompanied by weak androgenic properties. Much of this has to do with the reduction of nandrolone to a weaker steroid, dihydronandrolone, in the same androgen-responsive target tissues that potentate the action of testosterone (by converting it to DHT). The mild properties of nandrolone decanoate have made it one of the most popular injectable steroids worldwide, highly favored by athletes for its ability to promote significant strength and lean muscle mass gains without strong androgenic or estrogenic side effects.

History:

Nandrolone decanoate was first described in 1960,[437] and became a prescription medication in 1962. It was developed by the international pharmaceuticals giant Organon, and sold under the brand name Deca-Durabolin. The name Deca-Durabolin denotes that the product contains a variant of Organon's previously popular nandrolone injectable Durabolin (nandrolone phenylpropionate) using an ester of 10 carbon atoms. Organon expanded the market for nandrolone decanoate very rapidly following its release. Probably owing to a combination of its favorable properties and the large market presence of Organon, Deca-Durabolin soon became one of the most widely distributed anabolic steroids in the world.

When first introduced to the United States, nandrolone decanoate (like Durabolin) was prescribed for a variety of ailments. Listed indications included pre- and postoperative use for building lean mass, osteoporosis, advanced breast cancer, weight loss due to convalescence or disease, geriatric states (general weakness and frailty), burns, severe trauma, ulcers, adjunct therapy with certain forms of anemia, and selective cases of growth and development retardation in children. The drug was initially sold in a dosage of only 50 mg/ml, owing to the very low recommended doses (usually 50-100 mg every 3-4 weeks). The drug was soon updated to include a 100 mg/ml version, reflecting the need for higher doses in some situations, particularly those with refractory anemia and advanced breast cancer. Later, a 200 mg/ml product was released by Organon as well.

Although the drug had been applied favorably for a great many medical uses for approximately a decade, by the mid-1970's the indicated uses for nandrolone decanoate were being refined, both in the U.S. and abroad. FDA approved prescribing information from 1975 lists nandrolone decanoate as "probably effective" as adjunct therapy in senile and postmenopausal osteoporosis, as well as for treating pituitary-deficient dwarfism until growth hormone is more available. It was also deemed "possibly effective" in aiding the retention of lean mass, controlling advanced breast cancer, and as adjunctive therapy for certain types of anemia. More time was given to investigate the potential "less than effective" uses of the drug.

Modern (approved) medical applications for the drug are even more refined than they were in the mid-1970's. In the United States, the drug is now only FDA approved for treating anemia, although it is often also used "off label" to preserve lean mass in HIV positive patients and others suffering from wasting diseases. Outside of the U.S., Organon seems to support the use of this drug mainly with patients suffering from severe anemia, osteoporosis, and advanced breast cancer. The Organon Deca-Durabolin brand of nandrolone decanoate remains widely available today. In addition, nandrolone decanoate is produced as a generic drug in many countries, and is also manufactured under numerous other distinctive brand names, both for human and veterinary use.

How Supplied:

Nandrolone decanoate is widely available in human and veterinary drug markets. Composition and dosage may vary by country and manufacturer, but usually contain 25 mg/ml, 50 mg/ml, 100 mg/ml, or 200 mg/ml of steroid dissolved in oil.

Structural Characteristics:

Nandrolone decanoate is a modified form of nandrolone, where a carboxylic acid ester (decanoic acid) has been attached to the 17-beta hydroxyl group. Esterified steroids are less polar than free steroids, and are absorbed more slowly from the area of injection. Once in the bloodstream, the ester is removed to yield free (active) nandrolone. Esterified steroids are designed to prolong the window of therapeutic effect following administration, allowing for a less frequent injection schedule compared to injections of free (unesterified) steroid. Nandrolone decanoate provides a sharp spike in nandrolone release 24-48 hours following deep intramuscular injection, which steadily declines to near baseline levels approximately two weeks later. The mean depot-release half-life of nandrolone decanoate is 8 days.

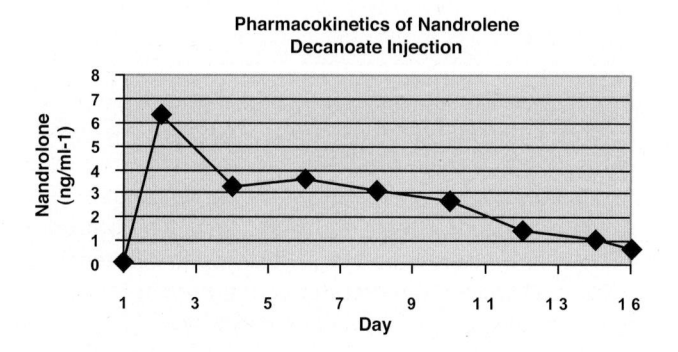

Figure 1. Pharmacokinetics of 200 mg Nandrolone Decanoate injection. Source: Pharmacokinetic parameters of nandrolone (19-nortestosterone) after intramuscular administration of nandrolone decanoate (Deca-Durabolin®) to healthy volunteers. Wijnand H, Bosch A, Donker C. Acta Endocrinol 1985 supp 271 19-30.

Side Effects (Estrogenic):

Nandrolone has a low tendency for estrogen conversion, estimated to be only about 20% of that seen with testosterone.[438] This is because while the liver can convert nandrolone to estradiol, in other more active sites of steroid aromatization such as adipose tissue nandrolone is far less open to this process.[439] Consequently, estrogen-related side effects are a much lower concern with this drug than with testosterone. Elevated estrogen levels may still be noticed with higher dosing, however, and may cause side effects such as increased water retention, body fat gain, and gynecomastia. An anti-estrogen such as clomiphene citrate or tamoxifen citrate may be necessary to prevent estrogenic side effects if they occur. One may alternately use an aromatase inhibitor like Arimidex® (anastrozole), which more efficiently controls estrogen by preventing its synthesis. Aromatase inhibitors can be quite expensive in comparison to anti-estrogens, however, and may also have negative effects on blood lipids.

It is of note that nandrolone has some activity as a progestin in the body.[440] Although progesterone is a c-19 steroid, removal of this group as in 19-norprogesterone creates a hormone with greater binding affinity for its corresponding receptor. Sharing this trait, many 19-nor anabolic steroids are shown to have some affinity for the progesterone receptor as well.[441] The side effects associated with progesterone are similar to those of estrogen, including negative feedback inhibition of testosterone production and enhanced rate of fat storage. Progestins also augment the stimulatory effect of estrogens on mammary tissue growth. There appears to be a strong synergy between these two hormones here, such that gynecomastia might even occur with the help of progestins, without excessive estrogen levels. The use of an anti-estrogen, which inhibits the estrogenic component of this disorder, is often sufficient to mitigate gynecomastia caused by nandrolone.

Side Effects (Androgenic):

Although classified as an anabolic steroid, androgenic side effects are still possible with this substance, especially with higher doses. This may include bouts of oily skin, acne, and body/facial hair growth. Anabolic/androgenic steroids may also aggravate male pattern hair loss. Women are warned of the potential virilizing effects of anabolic/androgenic steroids. These may include a deepening of the voice, menstrual irregularities, changes in skin texture, facial hair growth, and clitoral enlargement. Nandrolone is a steroid with relatively low androgenic activity relative to its tissue-building actions, making the threshold for strong androgenic side effects comparably higher than with more androgenic agents such as testosterone, methandrostenolone, or fluoxymesterone. It is also important to point out that due to its mild androgenic nature and ability to suppress endogenous testosterone, nandrolone is prone to interfering with libido in males when used without another androgen.

Note that in androgen-responsive target tissues such as the skin, scalp, and prostate, the relative androgenicity of nandrolone is reduced by its reduction to dihydronandrolone (DHN).[442][443] The 5-alpha reductase enzyme is responsible for this metabolism of nandrolone. The concurrent use of a 5-alpha reductase inhibitor such as finasteride or dutasteride will interfere with site-specific reduction of nandrolone action, considerably increasing the tendency of nandrolone to produce androgenic side effects. Reductase inhibitors should be avoided with nandrolone if low androgenicity is desired.

Side Effects (Hepatotoxicity):

Nandrolone is not c-17 alpha alkylated, and not known to have hepatotoxic effects in healthy subjects. Liver toxicity is unlikely.

Side Effects (Cardiovascular):

Anabolic/androgenic steroids can have deleterious effects on serum cholesterol. This includes a tendency to reduce HDL (good) cholesterol values and increase LDL (bad) cholesterol values, which may shift the HDL to LDL balance in a direction that favors greater risk of arteriosclerosis. The relative impact of an anabolic/androgenic steroid on serum lipids is dependant on the dose, route of administration (oral vs. injectable), type of steroid (aromatizable or non-aromatizable), and level of resistance to hepatic metabolism. Studies administering 600 mg of nandrolone decanoate per week for 10 weeks demonstrated a 26% reduction in HDL cholesterol levels.[444] This suppression is slightly greater than that reported with an equal dose of testosterone enanthate, and is in agreement with earlier studies showing a slightly stronger negative impact on HDL/LDL ratio with nandrolone decanoate as compared to testosterone cypionate.[445] Nandrolone decanoate should still have a significantly weaker impact on serum lipids than c-17 alpha alkylated agents. Anabolic/androgenic steroids may also adversely affect blood pressure and triglycerides, reduce endothelial relaxation, and support left ventricular hypertrophy, all potentially increasing the risk of cardiovascular disease and myocardial infarction.

To help reduce cardiovascular strain it is advised to maintain an active cardiovascular exercise program and minimize the intake of saturated fats, cholesterol, and simple carbohydrates at all times during active AAS administration. Supplementing with fish oils (4 grams per day) and a natural cholesterol/antioxidant formula such as Lipid Stabil or a product with comparable ingredients is also recommended.

Side Effects (Testosterone Suppression):

All anabolic/androgenic steroids when taken in doses sufficient to promote muscle gain are expected to suppress endogenous testosterone production. Studies administering 100 mg per week of nandrolone decanoate for 6 weeks have demonstrated an approximate 57% reduction in serum testosterone levels during therapy. At a dosage of 300 mg per week, this reduction reached 70%.[446] It is believed that the progestational activity of nandrolone notably contributes to the suppression of testosterone synthesis during therapy, which can be marked in spite of a low tendency for estrogen conversion.[447] Without the intervention of testosterone-stimulating substances, testosterone levels should return to normal within 2-6 months of drug secession. Note that prolonged hypogonadotrophic hypogonadism can develop secondary to steroid abuse, necessitating medical intervention.

The above side effects are not inclusive. For more detailed discussion of potential side effects, see the Steroid Side Effects section of this book.

Administration (Men):

For general anabolic effects, early prescribing guidelines recommend a dosage of 50-100 mg every 3-4 weeks for 12 weeks. To treat renal anemia, the prescribing guidelines for nandrolone decanoate recommend a dosage of 100-200 mg per week. The usual dosage for physique- or performance-enhancing purposes is the range of 200-600 mg per week, taken in cycles 8 to 12 weeks in length. This level is sufficient for most users to notice measurable gains in lean muscle mass and strength. It is often stated that nandrolone decanoate will exhibit its optimal effect (best gain/side effect ratio) at 2mg per pound of bodyweight/weekly, although individual differences in response will likely dictate varying ideal doses for different users. Deca is not known as a very "fast" builder. The muscle-building effect of this drug is quite noticeable, but not dramatic. In general, one can expect to gain muscle weight at about half the rate of that with an equal amount of testosterone.

Nandrolone decanoate is often combined with other steroids for an enhanced effect. A combination of 200-400 mg/week of nandrolone decanoate and 10-20 mg daily of Winstrol®, for example, is noted to greatly enhance the look of muscularity and definition when dieting/cutting. A strong non-aromatizing androgen like Halotestin® or trenbolone could also be used, again providing an enhanced level of hardness and density to the muscles. Being a moderately strong muscle builder, nandrolone can also be incorporated into bulk cycles with acceptable results. The classic "Deca and D-bol" stack (usually 200-400 mg of nandrolone decanoate per week and 15-25 mg of Dianabol per day) has been a bodybuilding basic for decades, and always seems to provide excellent muscle growth. A stronger androgen such as Anadrol 50® or testosterone could also be substituted, producing greater results, but with more water retention.

Administration (Women):

For general anabolic effects, early prescribing guidelines recommend a dosage of 50-100 mg every 3-4 weeks for 12 weeks. To treat renal anemia, the prescribing guidelines for nandrolone decanoate recommend a dosage of 50-100 mg per week. When used for physique- or performance-enhancing purposes, a dosage of 50 mg per week is most common, taken for 4-6 weeks. Although only slightly androgenic, women are occasionally confronted with virilization symptoms when taking this compound. Studies have demonstrated high tolerability (minor but statistically insignificant incidence of virilizing side effects) with a dose of 100 mg every other week for 12 weeks,[448] while long-term studies (+12 months of use) have demonstrated virilizing side effects on a dose as low as 50 mg every 2-3 weeks.[449] Should virilizing side effects become a concern, nandrolone decanoate should be discontinued immediately to help prevent their permanent appearance. After a sufficient period of withdrawal, the shorter-acting nandrolone Durabolin® might be considered a safer option. This drug stays active for only several days, greatly reducing the withdrawal time if indicated.

Availability:

Deca-Durabolin is one of the most widely duplicated steroids in the world, with fakes taking on many different forms. Legitimate drugs are also widely sold. Below are some of the more popular items currently found on the U.S. black market.

Organon no longer sells Deca-Durabolin in the United States. Watson Labs and Schein Pharmaceuticals also discontinued their generics as well. This drug is presently unavailable in the U.S.

Balkan Pharmaceuticals in Moldova produces a nandrolone decanoate product called Nandrolona D. It comes packaged in 1 mL ampules. Counterfeits have not yet been a problem.

Decaland frm Landerlan in Paraguay is a common product in recent years, especially throughout South America. It comes in 10 mL multi-dose vials.

Norma Hellas Deca (100 mg/mL nandrolone decanoate in 2 mL vials) from Greece is a good product, but also widely counterfeited. One should only purchase this steroid when packaged in a box with paperwork. The firm has recently started using a patented photochromic label to deter counterfeiting, which carries a metallic/holographic watermark of the Norma Hellas logo. This is a very difficult feature to duplicate, and should provide very strong assurance of a legitimate purchase.

Greek Deca-Durabolin from Organon is another widely counterfeited product. It is one of only a handful of European nandrolone injectables to be found in multi-dosed vials, making it an easy target for counterfeiters that lack the capacity to produce glass ampules. Make sure you purchase this product only when it comes in a box with the proper Greek drug ID sticker. As with all Greek drugs, the sticker should show a hidden mark under UV light.

Greek Extraboline may be in circulation, and is generally regarded as a high quality item on par with Organon Deca-Durabolin. This also makes it a common target of counterfeiting. As with all Greek drugs, only buy this when properly boxed so you can place the peel-off pharmacy sticker under UV lighting to look for the hidden watermark. All Extraboline in circulation will also carry a holographic image directly on the vial label. Finding this feature should assure a legitimate purchase.

PB Labs in India is still producing Deca-Pronabol 200. This comes in the form of a 1 mL ampule containing 200 mg of steroid. This item is scarce on the black market these days, probably because India is not a very hot source country, and other cheaper forms of Deca are more easily found.

The Indian export firm Alpha-Pharma also makes a nandrolone decanoate product. It comes in 2mL multi-dose vials containing 200mg each.

Delatestryl® (testosterone enanthate)

Androgenic	100
Anabolic	100
Standard	Standard

Chemical Names	4-androsten-3-one-17beta-ol
	17beta-hydroxy-androst-4-en-3-one
Estrogenic Activity	moderate
Progestational Activity	low

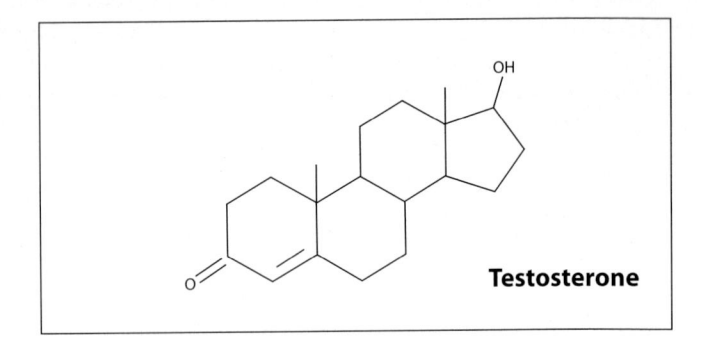

Testosterone

Description:

Testosterone enanthate is a slow-acting injectable form of the androgen testosterone. Following deep intramuscular injection, the drug is designed to provide a sustained release of testosterone into the bloodstream for approximately 2 to 3 weeks. In order to maintain normal physiological levels of testosterone during androgen replacement therapies, injections of testosterone enanthate are usually required at least every two weeks, although more meticulous physicians will administer the drug weekly. As with all testosterone injectables, testosterone enanthate is highly favored by athletes for its ability to promote strong increases in muscle mass and strength.

History:

Testosterone enanthate first appeared on Western drug markets during the early 1950's. It was the first slow-acting oil-based injectable ester of testosterone to be widely adopted in Western medicine, and effectively replaced testosterone propionate and testosterone suspension for most therapeutic uses. The first brand of this drug to be sold in the U.S. was Delatestryl® by Squibb. Over the years the Delatestryl® brand has changed hands several times, most notably to Mead Johnson, BTG, Savient, and in December 2005, Indevus. The most prominent brand of testosterone enanthate outside of the United States is Testoviron®, a drug that has seen uninterrupted production by the same manufacturer (Schering AG, Germany) for more than 50 years. Globally, the Testoviron® brand from Schering is the single most widely used injectable testosterone preparation.

Testosterone enanthate is most often used clinically to replace normal levels of testosterone in adult males suffering diminished androgen levels. This may manifest itself with a loss of libido, lean muscle mass, and normal energy and vigor. Testosterone enanthate is also used to treat undescended testicles and delayed puberty in adolescent males, and occasionally as a secondary medication during inoperable breast cancer in women. This form of testosterone has also been studied with great success as a male birth control option.[450] Weekly injections of 200 mg were shown to efficiently lower sperm production for most men within three months of treatment, a state of suppression that remained until after the drug was discontinued. With the current stigma surrounding anabolic/androgenic steroids, however, it is unlikely that such therapy will become adopted in Western medical practice. Today, in spite of the growing number of alternative therapies, testosterone enanthate remains the most widely prescribed form of testosterone in the world.

How Supplied:

Testosterone enanthate is widely available in human and veterinary drug markets. Composition and dosage may vary by country and manufacturer, but usually contain 50 mg/ml, 100 mg/ml, 200 mg/ml, or 250 mg/ml of steroid dissolved in oil.

Structural Characteristics:

Testosterone enanthate is a modified form of testosterone, where a carboxylic acid ester (enanthoic acid) has been attached to the 17-beta hydroxyl group. Esterified forms of testosterone are less polar than free testosterone, and are absorbed more slowly from the area of injection. Once in the bloodstream, the ester is removed to yield free (active) testosterone. Esterified forms of testosterone are designed to prolong the window of therapeutic effect following administration, allowing for a less frequent injection schedule compared to injections of free (unesterified) steroid. The half-life of testosterone enanthate is approximately eight days after injection.

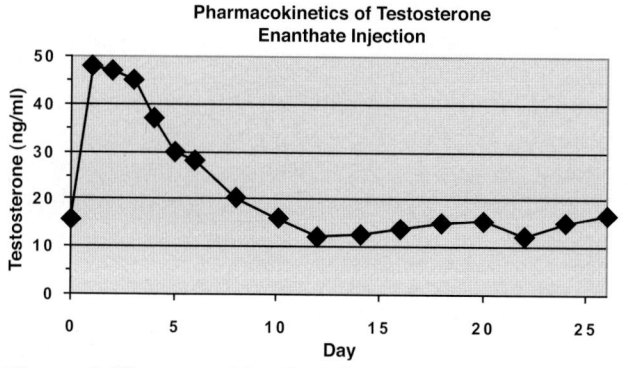

Figure 1. Pharmacokinetics of 194mg testosterone enanthate injection. Source: Comparison of testosterone, dihydrotestosterone, luteinizing hormone, and follicle-stimulating hormone in serum after injection of testosterone enanthate or testosterone cypionate. Schulte-Beerbuhl M, Nieschlag E. Fertility and Sterility 33 (1980):201-3.

Side Effects (Estrogenic):

Testosterone is readily aromatized in the body to estradiol (estrogen). The aromatase (estrogen synthetase) enzyme is responsible for this metabolism of testosterone. Elevated estrogen levels can cause side effects such as increased water retention, body fat gain, and gynecomastia. Testosterone is considered a moderately estrogenic steroid. An anti-estrogen such as clomiphene citrate or tamoxifen citrate may be necessary to prevent estrogenic side effects. One may alternately use an aromatase inhibitor like Arimidex® (anastrozole), which more efficiently controls estrogen by preventing its synthesis. Aromatase inhibitors can be quite expensive in comparison to anti-estrogens, however, and may also have negative effects on blood lipids.

Estrogenic side effects will occur in a dose-dependant manner, with higher doses (above normal therapeutic levels) of testosterone more likely to require the concurrent use of an anti-estrogen or aromatase inhibitor. Since water retention and loss of muscle definition are common with higher doses of testosterone, this drug is usually considered a poor choice for dieting or cutting phases of training. Its moderate estrogenicity makes it more ideal for bulking phases, where the added water retention will support raw strength and muscle size, and help foster a stronger anabolic environment.

Side Effects (Androgenic):

Testosterone is the primary male androgen, responsible for maintaining secondary male sexual characteristics. Elevated levels of testosterone are likely to produce androgenic side effects including oily skin, acne, and body/facial hair growth. Men with a genetic predisposition for hair loss (androgenetic alopecia) may notice accelerated male pattern balding. Those concerned about hair loss may find a more comfortable option in nandrolone decanoate, which is a comparably less androgenic steroid. Women are warned of the potential virilizing effects of anabolic/androgenic steroids, especially with a strong androgen such as testosterone. These may include deepening of the voice, menstrual irregularities, changes in skin texture, facial hair growth, and clitoral enlargement.

In androgen-responsive target tissues such as the skin, scalp, and prostate, the high relative androgenicity of testosterone is dependant on its reduction to dihydrotestosterone (DHT). The 5-alpha reductase enzyme is responsible for this metabolism of testosterone. The concurrent use of a 5-alpha reductase inhibitor such as finasteride or dutasteride will interfere with site-specific potentiation of testosterone action, lowering the tendency of testosterone drugs to produce androgenic side effects. It is important to remember that anabolic and androgenic effects are both mediated via the cytosolic androgen receptor. Complete separation of testosterone's anabolic and androgenic properties is not possible, even with total 5-alpha reductase inhibition.

Side Effects (Hepatotoxicity):

Testosterone does not have hepatotoxic effects; liver toxicity is unlikely. One study examined the potential for hepatotoxicity with high doses of testosterone by administering 400 mg of the hormone per day (2,800 mg per week) to a group of male subjects. The steroid was taken orally so that higher peak concentrations would be reached in hepatic tissues compared to intramuscular injections. The hormone was given daily for 20 days, and produced no significant changes in liver enzyme values including serum albumin, bilirubin, alanine-amino-transferase, and alkaline phosphatases.[451]

Side Effects (Cardiovascular):

Anabolic/androgenic steroids can have deleterious effects on serum cholesterol. This includes a tendency to reduce HDL (good) cholesterol values and increase LDL (bad) cholesterol values, which may shift the HDL to LDL balance in a direction that favors greater risk of arteriosclerosis. The relative impact of an anabolic/androgenic steroid on serum lipids is dependant on the dose, route of administration (oral vs. injectable), type of steroid (aromatizable or non-aromatizable), and level of resistance to hepatic metabolism. Anabolic/androgenic steroids may also adversely effect blood pressure and triglycerides, reduce endothelial relaxation, and support left ventricular hypertrophy, all potentially increasing the risk of cardiovascular disease and myocardial infarction.

Testosterone tends to have a much less dramatic impact on cardiovascular risk factors than synthetic steroids. This is due in part to its openness to metabolism by the liver, which allows it to have less effect on the hepatic management of cholesterol. The aromatization of testosterone to estradiol also helps to mitigate the negative effects of androgens on serum lipids. In one study, 280 mg per week of testosterone ester (enanthate) had a slight but not statistically significant effect on HDL cholesterol after 12 weeks, but when taken with an aromatase inhibitor a strong (25%) decrease was seen.[452] Studies using 300 mg of testosterone ester (enanthate) per week for 20 weeks without an aromatase inhibitor demonstrated only a 13% decrease in HDL cholesterol, while at 600 mg the reduction reached 21%.[453] The negative impact of aromatase inhibition should be taken into consideration before such drug is added to testosterone therapy.

Due to the positive influence of estrogen on serum lipids, tamoxifen citrate or clomiphene citrate are preferred to aromatase inhibitors for those concerned with cardiovascular health, as they offer a partial estrogenic effect in the liver. This allows them to potentially improve lipid profiles and offset some of the negative effects of androgens. With doses of 600 mg or less per week, the impact on lipid profile tends to be noticeable but not dramatic, making an anti-estrogen (for cardioprotective purposes) perhaps unnecessary. Doses of 600 mg or less per week have also failed to produce statistically significant changes in LDL/VLDL cholesterol, triglycerides, apolipoprotein B/C-III, C-reactive protein, and insulin sensitivity, all indicating a relatively weak impact on cardiovascular risk factors.[454] When used in moderate doses, injectable testosterone esters are usually considered to be the safest of all anabolic/androgenic steroids.

To help reduce cardiovascular strain it is advised to maintain an active cardiovascular exercise program and minimize the intake of saturated fats, cholesterol, and simple carbohydrates at all times during active AAS administration. Supplementing with fish oils (4 grams per day) and a natural cholesterol/antioxidant formula such as Lipid Stabil or a product with comparable ingredients is also recommended.

Side Effects (Testosterone Suppression):

All anabolic/androgenic steroids when taken in doses sufficient to promote muscle gain are expected to suppress endogenous testosterone production. Testosterone is the primary male androgen, and offers strong negative feedback on endogenous testosterone production. Testosterone-based drugs will, likewise, have a strong effect on the hypothalamic regulation of natural steroid hormones. Without the intervention of testosterone-stimulating substances, testosterone levels should return to normal within 1-4 months of drug secession. Note that prolonged hypogonadotrophic hypogonadism can develop secondary to steroid abuse, necessitating medical intervention.

As with all anabolic/androgenic steroids, it is unlikely that one will retain every pound of new bodyweight after a cycle is concluded. This is especially true when withdrawing from a strong (aromatizing) androgen like testosterone, as much of the new weight gain is likely to be in the form of water retention; quickly eliminated after drug discontinuance. An imbalance of anabolic and catabolic hormones during the post-cycle recovery period may further create an environment that is unfavorable for the retention of muscle tissue. Proper ancillary drug therapy is usually recommended to help restore hormonal balance more quickly, ultimately helping the user retain more muscle tissue.

The above side effects are not inclusive. For more detailed discussion of potential side effects, see the Steroid Side Effects section of this book.

Administration (Men):

To treat androgen insufficiency, the prescribing guidelines for testosterone enanthate call for a dosage of 50-400 mg every 2 to 4 weeks. Although active in the body for a longer time, testosterone enanthate is usually injected on a weekly basis for muscle-building purposes. The usual dosage for physique- or performance-enhancing purposes is in the range of 200-600 mg per week, taken in cycles 6 to 12 weeks in length. This level is sufficient for most users to notice exceptional gains in muscle size and strength.

Testosterone is usually incorporated into bulking phases of training, when added water retention will be of little consequence, the user more concerned with raw mass than definition. Some do incorporate the drug into cutting cycles as well, but typically in lower doses (100-200 mg per week) and/or when accompanied by an aromatase inhibitor to keep estrogen levels under control. Testosterone enanthate is a very effective anabolic drug, and is often used alone with great benefit. Some, however, find a need to stack it with other anabolic/androgenic steroids for a stronger effect, in which case an additional 200-400 mg per week of boldenone undecylenate, methenolone enanthate, or nandrolone decanoate should provide substantial results with no significant hepatotoxicity. Testosterone is ultimately very versatile, and can be combined with many other anabolic/androgenic steroids to tailor the desired effect.

Administration (Women):

Testosterone enanthate is rarely used with women in clinical medicine. When applied, it is most often used as a secondary medication during inoperable breast cancer, when other therapies have failed to produce a desirable effect and suppression of ovarian function is necessary. Testosterone enanthate is not recommended for women for physique- or performance-enhancing purposes due to its strong androgenic nature, tendency to produce virilizing side effects, and slow-acting characteristics (making blood levels difficult to control).

Availability:

Worldwide, enanthate is the most abundantly produced ester of testosterone, and consequently is also the one most commonly found on the black market. It would be impossible to describe every product that you may come across when shopping in detail here, but some advice concerning products most popular right now is provided below.

Delatestryl is the most well-known brand of enanthate in the U.S. at this time. It comes in both 1 mL pre-loaded syringes and 5 mL multi-dose vials, the latter being the only form really found on the black market (and rarely at that, due to strict controls). Note that the vials are short, and carry a label with metallic backing you can see through the glass. Looking for this will help assure you are getting the real thing, if somehow you luck out and come across a vial. Delatestryl from Canada is made to similar specifications (see the included photos).

Watson and Paddock both make generic versions in the U.S. They are packaged in 5 mL and 10 mL multi-dose vials. Be leery of either product if you are offered it from a steroid dealer, however, given the very low tendency for U.S. drugs to be diverted to the black market. Most will be counterfeit.

Norma Hellas (Greece), makers of Norma Hellas Nandrolone, recently added a generic 250 mg/mL testosterone enanthate injectable to their product offerings. It comes in a single dark amber 1 mL glass ampule, and is packaged 1 ampule per box. Be sure to look at the Greek Pharmacy sticker under UV light to assure you have a legitimate product.

Schering's Testoviron® is one of the most popular individual brands worldwide. It comes in 1 mL ampules only, and the various preparations usually look very similar to each other. They are made of clear glass, and most often have a green ring and blue dot on the tip. Most are wrapped in a white paper label.

CID makes a product in Egypt called Cidoteston. It carries the standard 250 mg dosage per 1 mL ampule. Note that newer versions have silkscreen printing directly on the glass, which replaced early batches of Cidoteston with paper labels.

The French product Testosterone Heptylate Theramex also circulates on the black market. Note that heptylate is not a unique ester of testosterone as described by other writers. It is simply another word for enanthate. Make sure to buy this item only when in the proper box, sitting (in pairs) in a foil-lined plastic tray. You are much more likely to get a fake product if buying loose ampules.

Androtardyl is also produced in France, and occasionally circulates on the black market. Again, be sure to look for the proper box before buying.

Testo-Enant is another brand in Europe, this one being made by Geymonat in Italy. These ampules contain 250 mg of steroid, either in 1 mL or 2 mL of oil. Currently fakes are not a problem; however, this steroid is not found on the black market in high volumes.

Galenika makes Testosteron Depo in Serbia. These 1 mL ampules contain 250 mg/mL of steroid, and are extremely cheap at the retail level in their country of origin.

Jelfa in Poland is still making Testosteronum Prolongatum, a 100 mg/mL enanthate product. Each box contains five 1 mL ampules, which are themselves made of clear glass and carry a paper label. Fakes of this product do not appear to be an issue at this time.

Testoviron Depot from German Remedies in India has changed its packaging recently. The new product comes packaged in blister packs, instead of the old boxes with a tray for 10 ampules.

The Indian export firm Alpha-Pharma also makes a testosterone enanthate, called Testobolin. It comes in 1 mL glass ampules.

Testofort Inj from Albert Davis Pakistan is commonly seen on the black market. It contains 250 mg/ml of steroid in 1 mL ampules. Three ampules come packaged to each cardboard box.

Geofman Pharmaceuticals also makes a generic in Pakistan. The product contains 250 mg of steroid in each 1 mL ampule. Like Testofort, three ampules are contained in each box. Note that the lot number and expiration date are electronically printed on the bottom inside flap of the box, in addition to the proper placement on the outside.

Aburaihan makes a generic enanthate in Iran, which is

becoming increasingly popular on the black market. Note that many fakes are already circulating of this product as well. The current popular fakes have a noticeable mistake on the placement of the company logo (see pictures).

Balkan Pharmaceuticals in Moldova makes a testosterone enanthate product called Testosterona E. It comes in 1 mL ampules. Counterfeits are not known to be a problem.

Depo®-Testosterone (testosterone cypionate)

Androgenic	100
Anabolic	100
Standard	Standard
Chemical Names	4-androsten-3-one-17beta-ol
	17beta-hydroxy-androst-4-en-3-one
Estrogenic Activity	moderate
Progestational Activity	low

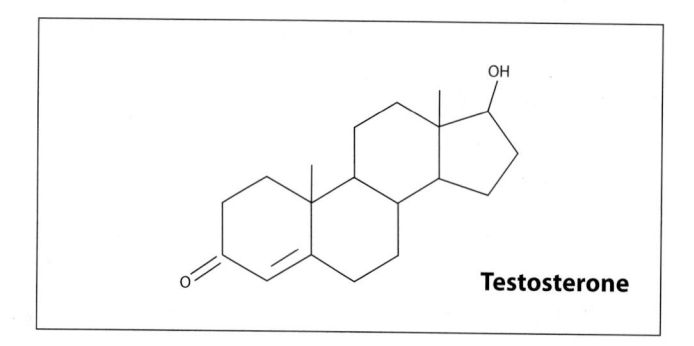

Description:

Testosterone cypionate is a slow-acting injectable ester of the primary male androgen testosterone. Testosterone is also the principle anabolic hormone in men, and is the basis of comparison by which all other anabolic/androgenic steroids are judged. As with all testosterone injectables, testosterone cypionate is highly favored by athletes for its ability to promote strong increases in muscle mass and strength. It is interesting to note that while a large number of other steroidal compounds have been made available since testosterone injectables, they are still considered to be the dominant bulking agents among bodybuilders. There is little argument that these are among the most powerful mass drugs available, testosterone cypionate included.

History:

Testosterone cypionate first appeared on the U.S. drug market during the mid-1950's under the brand name of Depo-Testosterone cyclopentylpropionate (soon abridged to simply Depo-Testosterone). It was developed by the pharmaceutical giant Upjohn, and is still sold to this day by the same company under the same trade name (although now they are called Pharmacia & Upjohn). This is a drug with limited global availability, and has historically been (largely) identified as an American item. It is not surprising that American athletes have long favored this form of testosterone over testosterone enanthate, the dominant slow-acting ester of testosterone on the global market. This preference, however, is likely rooted in history and availability, not actual therapeutic advantages.

Testosterone cypionate and testosterone enanthate provide extremely comparable patterns of testosterone release. Not only are physical advantages not possible in one over the other, but actual differences in pharmacokinetic patterns are hard to notice (these two drugs are for all intents and purposes functionally interchangeable). The only key difference between the two seems to be in the area of patient comfort. Cypionic acid is less irritating at the site of injection than enanthoic acid (enanthate) for a small percentage of patients. This makes testosterone cypionate a more favorable choice for those with recurring issues of injection-site pain with testosterone enanthate. This difference likely had something to do with the early development of this testosterone ester as a commercial drug product.

The main use of testosterone cypionate in clinical medicine has historically been the treatment of low androgen levels in males, although many other applications have existed for this drug as well. During the 1960's, for example, the drug's prescribing recommendations called for such uses as supporting bone structure maturity, treating menorrhagia (heavy menstrual bleeding) and excessive lactation in females, and increasing muscle mass and combating osteoporosis in the elderly. It was also being recommended for increasing male fertility, whereby induced testosterone/spermatogenesis suppression (caused by administering 200 mg of testosterone cypionate per week for 6 to 10 weeks) was potentially followed by a period of rebound spermatogenesis (due to temporarily higher than normal gonadotropin levels).

By the 1970's, the FDA had been granted much stronger control over the prescription drug market, and the broad uses in which testosterone cypionate was first indicated were now being refined. For example, "testosterone rebound therapy" as a way to increase male fertility was proving to be unreliable, especially in the face of newer more effective medications, and was soon eliminated from prescribing guidelines. So too was the recommendation for its use to treat things like excessive menstrual bleeding and lactation. In general, testosterone therapy was being pulled back to focus mainly on male androgen deficiency, and less on other applications, especially when involving populations more susceptible to androgenic side effects, such as women and the elderly.

Today, testosterone cypionate remains readily available on the U.S. prescription drug market, where it is FDA-approved for hormone replacement therapy in men with conditions associated with a deficiency of endogenous testosterone, and as a secondary treatment for inoperable metastatic breast cancer in women (although it is not widely used for this purpose anymore). Testosterone cypionate is currently available outside of the United States, but not widely. Known international sources for the drug include Canada, Australia, Spain, Brazil, and South Africa (see: Drug Availability Tables for more detailed information).

How Supplied:

Testosterone cypionate is available in select human and veterinary drug markets. Composition and dosage may vary by country and manufacturer, but usually contain 50 mg/ml, 100 mg/ml, 125 mg/ml, or 200 mg/ml of steroid dissolved in oil.

Structural Characteristics:

Testosterone cypionate is a modified form of testosterone, where a carboxylic acid ester (cyclopentylpropionic acid) has been attached to the 17-beta hydroxyl group. Esterified forms of testosterone are less polar than free testosterone, and are absorbed more slowly from the area of injection. Once in the bloodstream, the ester is removed to yield free (active) testosterone. Esterified forms of testosterone are designed to prolong the window of therapeutic effect following administration, allowing for a less frequent injection schedule compared to injections of free (unesterified) steroid. The half-life of testosterone cypionate is approximately 8 days after injection.

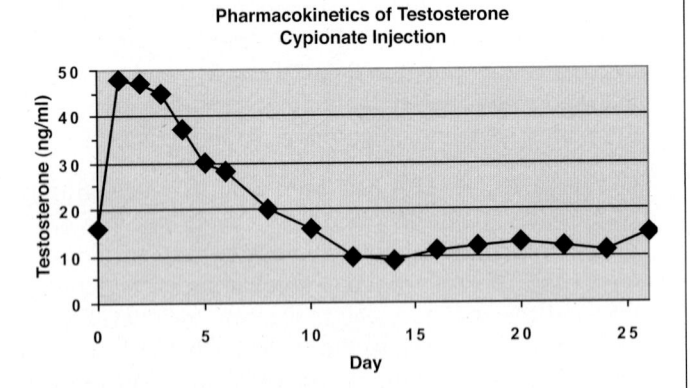

Figure 1. Pharmacokinetics of 200 mg testosterone cypionate injection. Source: Comparison of testosterone, dihydrotestosterone, luteinizing hormone, and follicle-stimulating hormone in serum after injection of testosterone enanthate or testosterone cypionate. Schulte-Beerbuhl M, Nieschlag E. Fertility and Sterility 33 (1980):201-3.

Side Effects (Estrogenic):

Testosterone is readily aromatized in the body to estradiol (estrogen). The aromatase (estrogen synthetase) enzyme is responsible for this metabolism of testosterone. Elevated estrogen levels can cause side effects such as increased water retention, body fat gain, and gynecomastia. Testosterone is considered a moderately estrogenic steroid. An anti-estrogen such as clomiphene citrate or tamoxifen citrate may be necessary to prevent estrogenic side effects. One may alternately use an aromatase inhibitor like Arimidex® (anastrozole), which more efficiently controls estrogen by preventing its synthesis. Aromatase inhibitors can be quite expensive in comparison to anti-estrogens, however, and may also have negative effects on blood lipids.

Estrogenic side effects will occur in a dose-dependant manner, with higher doses (above normal therapeutic levels) of testosterone cypionate more likely to require the concurrent use of an anti-estrogen or aromatase inhibitor. Since water retention and loss of muscle definition are common with higher doses of testosterone cypionate, this drug is usually considered a poor choice for dieting or cutting phases of training. Its moderate estrogenicity makes it more ideal for bulking phases, where the added water retention will support raw strength and muscle size, and help foster a stronger anabolic environment.

Side Effects (Androgenic):

Testosterone is the primary male androgen, responsible for maintaining secondary male sexual characteristics. Elevated levels of testosterone are likely to produce androgenic side effects including oily skin, acne, and body/facial hair growth. Men with a genetic predisposition for hair loss (androgenetic alopecia) may notice accelerated male pattern balding. Those concerned about hair loss may find a more comfortable option in nandrolone decanoate, which is a comparably less androgenic steroid. Women are warned of the potential virilizing effects of anabolic/androgenic steroids, especially with a strong androgen such as testosterone. These may include deepening of the voice, menstrual irregularities, changes in skin texture, facial hair growth, and clitoral enlargement.

In androgen-responsive target tissues such as the skin, scalp, and prostate, the high relative androgenicity of testosterone is dependant on its reduction to dihydrotestosterone (DHT). The 5-alpha reductase enzyme is responsible for this metabolism of testosterone. The concurrent use of a 5-alpha reductase inhibitor such as finasteride or dutasteride will interfere with site-specific potentiation of testosterone action, lowering the tendency of testosterone drugs to produce androgenic side effects. It is important to remember that anabolic and androgenic effects are both mediated via the cytosolic androgen receptor. Complete separation of testosterone's anabolic and androgenic properties is not possible, even with total 5-alpha reductase inhibition.

Side Effects (Hepatotoxicity):

Testosterone does not have hepatotoxic effects; liver toxicity is unlikely. One study examined the potential for hepatotoxicity with high doses of testosterone by administering 400 mg of the hormone per day (2,800 mg per week) to a group of male subjects. The steroid was taken orally so that higher peak concentrations would be reached in hepatic tissues compared to intramuscular injections. The hormone was given daily for 20 days, and produced no significant changes in liver enzyme values including serum albumin, bilirubin, alanine-aminotransferase, and alkaline phosphatases.[455]

Side Effects (Cardiovascular):

Anabolic/androgenic steroids can have deleterious effects on serum cholesterol. This includes a tendency to reduce HDL (good) cholesterol values and increase LDL (bad) cholesterol values, which may shift the HDL to LDL balance in a direction that favors greater risk of arteriosclerosis. The relative impact of an anabolic/androgenic steroid on serum lipids is dependant on the dose, route of administration (oral vs. injectable), type of steroid (aromatizable or non-aromatizable), and level of resistance to hepatic metabolism. Anabolic/androgenic steroids may also adversely affect blood pressure and triglycerides, reduce endothelial relaxation, and support left ventricular hypertrophy, all potentially increasing the risk of cardiovascular disease and myocardial infarction.

Testosterone tends to have a much less dramatic impact on cardiovascular risk factors than synthetic steroids. This is due in part to its openness to metabolism by the liver, which allows it to have less effect on the hepatic management of cholesterol. The aromatization of testosterone to estradiol also helps to mitigate the negative effects of androgens on serum lipids. In one study, 280 mg per week of testosterone ester (enanthate) had a slight but not statistically significant effect on HDL cholesterol after 12 weeks, but when taken with an aromatase inhibitor a strong (25%) decrease was seen.[456] Studies using 300 mg of testosterone ester (enanthate) per week for 20 weeks without an aromatase inhibitor demonstrated only a 13% decrease in HDL cholesterol, while at 600 mg the reduction reached 21%.[457] The negative impact of aromatase inhibition should be taken into consideration before such drug is added to testosterone therapy.

Due to the positive influence of estrogen on serum lipids, tamoxifen citrate or clomiphene citrate are preferred to aromatase inhibitors for those concerned with cardiovascular health, as they offer a partial estrogenic effect in the liver. This allows them to potentially improve lipid profiles and offset some of the negative effects of androgens. With doses of 600 mg or less per week, the impact on lipid profile tends to be noticeable but not dramatic, making an anti-estrogen (for cardioprotective purposes) perhaps unnecessary. Doses of 600 mg or less per week have also failed to produce statistically significant changes in LDL/VLDL cholesterol, triglycerides, apolipoprotein B/C-III, C-reactive protein, and insulin sensitivity, all indicating a relatively weak impact on cardiovascular risk factors.[458] When used in moderate doses, injectable testosterone esters are usually considered to be the safest of all anabolic/androgenic steroids.

To help reduce cardiovascular strain it is advised to maintain an active cardiovascular exercise program and minimize the intake of saturated fats, cholesterol, and simple carbohydrates at all times during active AAS administration. Supplementing with fish oils (4 grams per day) and a natural cholesterol/antioxidant formula such as Lipid Stabil or a product with comparable ingredients is also recommended.

Side Effects (Testosterone Suppression):

All anabolic/androgenic steroids when taken in doses sufficient to promote muscle gain are expected to suppress endogenous testosterone production. Testosterone is the primary male androgen, and offers strong negative feedback on endogenous testosterone production. Testosterone-based drugs will, likewise, have a strong effect on the hypothalamic regulation of natural steroid hormones. Without the intervention of testosterone-stimulating substances, testosterone levels should return to normal within 1-4 months of drug secession. Note that prolonged hypogonadotrophic hypogonadism can develop secondary to steroid abuse, necessitating medical intervention.

As with all anabolic/androgenic steroids, it is unlikely that one will retain every pound of new bodyweight after a cycle is concluded. This is especially true when withdrawing from a strong (aromatizing) androgen like testosterone cypionate, as much of the new weight gain is likely to be in the form of water retention, quickly eliminated after drug discontinuance. An imbalance of anabolic and catabolic hormones during the post-cycle recovery period may further create an environment that is unfavorable for the retention of muscle tissue. Proper ancillary drug therapy is usually recommended to help restore hormonal balance more quickly, ultimately helping the user retain more muscle tissue.

Another way to lessen the post-cycle "crash" is to first replace testosterone cypionate with a milder anabolic such as nandrolone decanoate or methenolone enanthate. The new steroid would be administered alone for one to two more months, at a dosage of 200-400 mg per week. In this "stepping down" procedure the user is attempting to eliminate the watery bulk of a testosterone-based drug while simultaneously preserving the solid muscularity underneath. This practice can prove to be effective, even if mainly for psychological reasons (some may view it as simply dividing the crash into water and hormonal stages). Testosterone-stimulating drugs are still typically used at the conclusion of therapy, as endogenous testosterone production will not rebound during the administration of nandrolone decanoate or methenolone enanthate.

The above side effects are not inclusive. For more detailed discussion of potential side effects, see the Steroid Side Effects section of this book.

Administration (Men):

To treat androgen insufficiency, the prescribing guidelines for testosterone cypionate call for a dosage of 50-400 mg every two to four weeks. Although active in the body for a longer time, testosterone cypionate is usually injected on a weekly basis for physique- or performance-enhancing purposes. The usual dosage is in the range of 200-600 mg per week, taken in cycles 6 to 12 weeks in length. This level is sufficient for most users to notice exceptional gains in muscle size and strength.

Testosterone is usually incorporated into bulking phases of training, when added water retention will be of little consequence, the user more concerned with raw mass than definition. Some do incorporate the drug into cutting cycles as well, but typically in lower doses (100-200 mg per week) and/or when accompanied by an aromatase inhibitor to keep estrogen levels under control. Testosterone cypionate is a very effective anabolic drug, and is often used alone with great benefit. Some, however, find a need to stack it with other anabolic/androgenic steroids for a stronger effect, in which case an additional 200-400 mg per week of boldenone undecylenate, methenolone enanthate, or nandrolone decanoate should provide substantial results with no significant hepatotoxicity. Testosterone is ultimately very versatile, and can be combined with many other anabolic/androgenic steroids to tailor the desired effect.

While large doses are generally not advised, some bodybuilders have been known to use excessively high dosages of this drug (1,000 mg per week or more). This was much more common before the 1990's, when cypionate vials were usually very cheap and easy to find. A "more is better" attitude is easy to justify when paying only $20 for a 10cc vial (today the typical price for a single injection). At dosages of 800-1000 mg per week or more, water retention will likely account for more of the additional weight gain than new muscle tissue. The practice of "megadosing" is inefficient (not to mention potentially dangerous), especially when we take into account the typical high cost of steroids today.

Administration (Women):

Testosterone cypionate is rarely used with women in clinical medicine. When applied, it is most often used as a secondary medication during inoperable breast cancer, when other therapies have failed to produce a desirable effect and suppression of ovarian function is necessary. Testosterone cypionate is not recommended for women for physique- or performance-enhancing purposes due to its strong androgenic nature, tendency to produce virilizing side effects, and slow-acting characteristics (making blood levels difficult to control).

Availability:

Testosterone cypionate can be found in fair volume on the black market, although it appears less commonly than testosterone enanthate. Below are some of the more popular items.

Depo-Testosterone from Pharmacia (formerly Upjohn) is the most popular brand of cypionate in the U.S. This is a high-profile target of counterfeiters. Be careful to examine the packaging closely, and to compare it to the photos in the picture library. Note that all legitimate boxes will carry a "Jh" symbol hidden on one of the top inside flaps. It will appear when placed under UV light.

Watson Labs, Sicor, and Sandoz make generic testosterone cypionate products in the U.S. They come packaged in multiple-dose vials. As with all U.S. drugs, it is not advisable to buy these products blindly off the black market. U.S. drugs are rarely diverted for black market sale, and most found there are fakes. Look at these drugs only if you can track them back to a pharmacy or legitimate prescription.

There are several pharmacies custom-compounding testosterone cypionate for doctors that specialize in androgen replacement therapy, but these products rarely circulate on the black market. Some photos were included in the picture library for your reference.

Body Research in Thailand distributes Cypionax, a drug made by T.P. Drug Laboratories. This is one of only a few registered testosterone products in Thailand.

Testex Prolongatum is still available from Spain. This

steroid is produced by Laboratorios Q Pharma. It is packaged in 2 mL dark glass ampules with grey silkscreen lettering. It comes in two doses, containing a total of 100 mg or 250 mg of steroid. Testex has always been a high-risk item on the black market, so be careful when shopping.

Deposteron is still made by Novaquimica in Brazil, and makes its way to the U.S. from time to time. Note that they are now using dark amber glass for the ampules instead of clear. Due to the fact that plain ampules are very easy to duplicate, it would be best to trust this product only when it is packaged in the appropriate box.

Balkan Pharmaceuticals in Moldova makes a testosterone cypionate product called Testosterona C. It comes in 1 mL ampules. Counterfeits are not known to be a problem.

Found in Chile is a high-dose cypionate product called ciclo-6. The product is manufactured by the firm Drag Pharma, and contains 300 mg/ml of steroid in a 2 mL ampule (600 mg of cypionate in total).

Miro Depo from Korea is still found in the U.S. from time to time, but not abundantly. Note that this product uses multi-dose vials, which sit in a foil-topped plastic tray. Obtaining this item with the full packaging is the best way to guarantee authenticity, although fakes of this item have not been a problem so far.

Deposterona (testosterone blend)

Androgenic	100
Anabolic	100
Standard	Standard
Chemical Names	4-androsten-3-one-17beta-ol
	17beta-hydroxy-androst-4-en-3-one
Estrogenic Activity	moderate
Progestational Activity	low

Testosterone

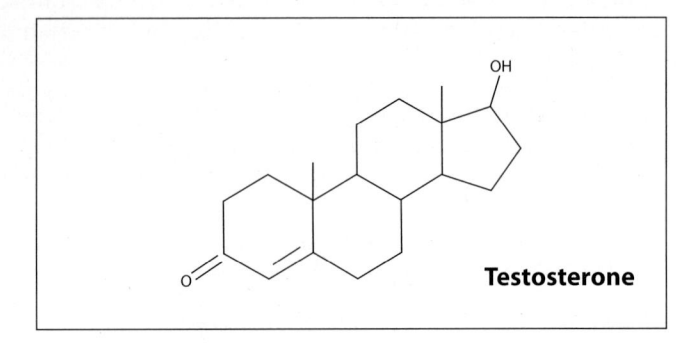

Description:

Deposterona is an injectable veterinary steroid preparation that contains a blend of three different testosterone esters. Each milliliter contains 12mg of testosterone acetate, 12mg of testosterone valerate, and 36mg of testosterone undecanoate, for a total steroid concentration of 60 mg/mL. This is currently the only commercial steroid product available that contains testosterone valerate, which is a short to medium acting ester with a half-life approximately double that of testosterone propionate.[459] With its blend of slow- and fast-acting esters, Deposterona is essentially a low-dosed alternative to Sustanon, although given the use of testosterone undecanoate it will be longer acting with more unbalanced pharmacokinetics.

History:

Deposterona was developed by Syntex Animal Health Company several decades ago, and has been sold on the Mexican veterinary drug market since. It is used primarily to treat impotence, weakness, fatigue, and hypogonadism in male breeding animals (cows, pigs, canines, and sheep), and also as a general protein-sparing anabolic. Deposterona is now sold under the Fort Dodge Animal Health label, which acquired Syntex Animal Health in the mid-1990's.

How Supplied:

Deposterona is available on the Mexican veterinary drug market. It contains 12mg of testosterone acetate, 12mg of testosterone valerate, and 36mg of testosterone undecanoate per milliliter of oil; packaged in a 10 mL multi-dose vial. Twelve vials are packed in each box.

Structural Characteristics:

Deposterona contains a mixture of three testosterone compounds, which where modified with the addition of carboxylic acid esters (acetic, valeric, and undecanoic acids) at the 17-beta hydroxyl group. Esterified forms of testosterone are less polar than free testosterone, and are absorbed more slowly from the area of injection. Once in the bloodstream, the ester is removed to yield free (active) testosterone. Esterified forms of testosterone are designed to prolong the window of therapeutic effect following administration, allowing for a less frequent injection schedule compared to injections of free (unesterified) steroid.

Side Effects (Estrogenic):

Testosterone is readily aromatized in the body to estradiol (estrogen). The aromatase (estrogen synthetase) enzyme is responsible for this metabolism of testosterone. Elevated estrogen levels can cause side effects such as increased water retention, body fat gain, and gynecomastia. Testosterone is considered a moderately estrogenic steroid. An anti-estrogen such as clomiphene citrate or tamoxifen citrate may be necessary to prevent estrogenic side effects. One may alternately use an aromatase inhibitor like Arimidex® (anastrozole), which more efficiently controls estrogen by preventing its synthesis. Aromatase inhibitors can be quite expensive in comparison to anti-estrogens, however, and may also have negative effects on blood lipids.

Estrogenic side effects will occur in a dose-dependant manner, with higher doses (above normal therapeutic levels) of testosterone more likely to require the concurrent use of an anti-estrogen or aromatase inhibitor. Since water retention and loss of muscle definition are common with higher doses of testosterone, this drug is usually considered a poor choice for dieting or cutting phases of training. Its moderate estrogenicity makes it more ideal for bulking phases, where the added water retention will support raw strength and muscle size, and help foster a stronger anabolic environment.

Side Effects (Androgenic):

Testosterone is the primary male androgen, responsible for

maintaining secondary male sexual characteristics. Elevated levels of testosterone are likely to produce androgenic side effects including oily skin, acne, and body/facial hair growth. Men with a genetic predisposition for hair loss (androgenetic alopecia) may notice accelerated male pattern balding. Those concerned about hair loss may find a more comfortable option in nandrolone decanoate, which is a comparably less androgenic steroid. Women are warned of the potential virilizing effects of anabolic/androgenic steroids, especially with a strong androgen such as testosterone. These may include deepening of the voice, menstrual irregularities, changes in skin texture, facial hair growth, and clitoral enlargement.

In androgen-responsive target tissues such as the skin, scalp, and prostate, the high relative androgenicity of testosterone is dependant on its reduction to dihydrotestosterone (DHT). The 5-alpha reductase enzyme is responsible for this metabolism of testosterone. The concurrent use of a 5-alpha reductase inhibitor such as finasteride or dutasteride will interfere with site-specific potentiation of testosterone action, lowering the tendency of testosterone drugs to produce androgenic side effects. It is important to remember that anabolic and androgenic effects are both mediated via the cytosolic androgen receptor. Complete separation of testosterone's anabolic and androgenic properties is not possible, even with total 5-alpha reductase inhibition.

Side Effects (Hepatotoxicity):

Testosterone does not have hepatotoxic effects; liver toxicity is unlikely. One study examined the potential for hepatotoxicity with high doses of testosterone by administering 400 mg of the hormone per day (2,800 mg per week) to a group of male subjects. The steroid was taken orally so that higher peak concentrations would be reached in hepatic tissues compared to intramuscular injections. The hormone was given daily for 20 days, and produced no significant changes in liver enzyme values including serum albumin, bilirubin, alanine-amino-transferase, and alkaline phosphatases.[460]

Side Effects (Cardiovascular):

Anabolic/androgenic steroids can have deleterious effects on serum cholesterol. This includes a tendency to reduce HDL (good) cholesterol values and increase LDL (bad) cholesterol values, which may shift the HDL to LDL balance in a direction that favors greater risk of arteriosclerosis. The relative impact of an anabolic/androgenic steroid on serum lipids is dependant on the dose, route of administration (oral vs. injectable), type of steroid (aromatizable or non-aromatizable), and level of resistance to hepatic metabolism. Anabolic/androgenic steroids may also adversely affect blood pressure and triglycerides, reduce endothelial relaxation, and support left ventricular hypertrophy, all potentially increasing the risk of cardiovascular disease and myocardial infarction.

Testosterone tends to have a much less dramatic impact on cardiovascular risk factors than synthetic steroids. This is due in part to its openness to metabolism by the liver, which allows it to have less effect on the hepatic management of cholesterol. The aromatization of testosterone to estradiol also helps to mitigate the negative effects of androgens on serum lipids. In one study, 280 mg per week of testosterone ester (enanthate) had a slight but not statistically significant effect on HDL cholesterol after 12 weeks, but when taken with an aromatase inhibitor a strong (25%) decrease was seen.[461] Studies using 300 mg of testosterone ester (enanthate) per week for 20 weeks without an aromatase inhibitor demonstrated only a 13% decrease in HDL cholesterol, while at 600 mg the reduction reached 21%.[462] The negative impact of aromatase inhibition should be taken into consideration before such drug is added to testosterone therapy.

Due to the positive influence of estrogen on serum lipids, tamoxifen citrate or clomiphene citrate are preferred to aromatase inhibitors for those concerned with cardiovascular health, as they offer a partial estrogenic effect in the liver. This allows them to potentially improve lipid profiles and offset some of the negative effects of androgens. With doses of 600 mg or less per week, the impact on lipid profile tends to be noticeable but not dramatic, making an anti-estrogen (for cardioprotective purposes) perhaps unnecessary. Doses of 600 mg or less per week have also failed to produce statistically significant changes in LDL/VLDL cholesterol, triglycerides, apolipoprotein B/C-III, C-reactive protein, and insulin sensitivity, all indicating a relatively weak impact on cardiovascular risk factors.[463] When used in moderate doses, injectable testosterone esters are usually considered to be the safest of all anabolic/androgenic steroids.

To help reduce cardiovascular strain it is advised to maintain an active cardiovascular exercise program and minimize the intake of saturated fats, cholesterol, and simple carbohydrates at all times during active AAS administration. Supplementing with fish oils (4 grams per day) and a natural cholesterol/antioxidant formula such as Lipid Stabil or a product with comparable ingredients is also recommended.

Side Effects (Testosterone Suppression):

All anabolic/androgenic steroids when taken in doses

sufficient to promote muscle gain are expected to suppress endogenous testosterone production. Testosterone is the primary male androgen, and offers strong negative feedback on endogenous testosterone production. Testosterone-based drugs will, likewise, have a strong effect on the hypothalamic regulation of natural steroid hormones. Without the intervention of testosterone-stimulating substances, testosterone levels should return to normal within 1-4 months of drug secession. Note that prolonged hypogonadotrophic hypogonadism can develop secondary to steroid abuse, necessitating medical intervention.

The above side effects are not inclusive. For more detailed discussion of potential side effects, see the Steroid Side Effects section of this book.

Administration (Men):

For bodybuilding purposes, Deposterona is usually injected on at least a weekly basis, in a dosage of 120-360 mg (2-6 ml). Dividing the weekly dosage into two or more smaller applications can reduce injection volume. Cycles are generally between 6 and 12 weeks in length. This level is sufficient to provide noticeable gains in muscle size and strength. Testosterone drugs are ultimately very versatile, and can be combined with many other anabolic/androgenic steroids depending on the desired effect.

Administration (Women):

Deposterona is not recommended for women for performance-enhancing purposes due to its strong androgenic nature, tendency to produce virilizing side effects, and slow-acting characteristics (making blood levels difficult to control).

Availability:

Because it contains such a low concentration of steroid, Deposterona is not in high demand among athletes. As such, this product is not readily smuggled into the U.S. This does, however, also make Deposterona a product of low interest to counterfeiters.

Dianabol® (methandrostenolone, methandienone)

Androgenic	40-60
Anabolic	90-210
Standard	Methyltestosterone (oral)
Chemical Names	17a-methyl-17b-hydroxy-1,4-androstadien-3-one 1-Dehydro- 17a-methyltestosterone
Estrogenic Activity	moderate
Progestational Activity	not significant

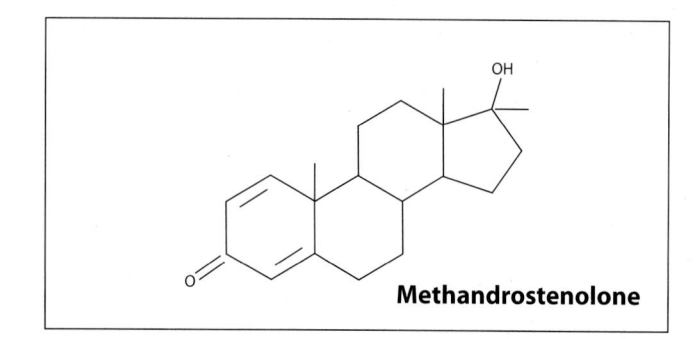

Methandrostenolone

Description:

Dianabol is the most recognized trade name for the drug methandrostenolone, also referred to as methandienone in many countries. Methandrostenolone is a derivative of testosterone, modified so that the hormone's androgenic (masculinizing) properties are reduced and its anabolic (tissue building) properties preserved. Having a lower level of relative androgenicity than testosterone, methandrostenolone is classified as an "anabolic" steroid, although quite a distinct androgenic side is still present. This drug was designed, and is principally sold, as an oral medication, although it can also be found in a number of injectable veterinary solutions. Dianabol is today, and has historically been, the most commonly used oral anabolic/androgenic steroid for physique and performance-enhancing purposes.

History:

Methandrostenolone was first described in 1955.[464] It was released to the U.S. prescription drug market in 1958, under the brand name Dianabol by Ciba Pharmaceuticals. Ciba developed methandrostenolone into a medicine with the help of Dr. John Ziegler, who was the team physician for a number of U.S. Olympic teams, including weightlifting. Ziegler makes note in Bob Goldman's Death in the Locker Room that he was first exposed to steroids at the 1956 World Games, seeing that the Russians were heavily abusing testosterone on their strength athletes. According to Ziegler, the hormone was having noticeable side effects, and one athlete had such profound prostate enlargement that he was forced to urinate with the aid of a catheter. While working with Ciba, the company tested a steroid (synthesized earlier) that had reduced androgenicity compared to testosterone, but with retained tissue-building (anabolic) properties. This had been accomplished by altering the basic chemical structure of testosterone in a way that altered its metabolism and disposition in the body. With the help of Dr. Ziegler, Ciba brought to market one of the most effective oral "anabolic" steroid medicines ever known, methandrostenolone. The success of the drug was rapid and far-reaching.

Dr. Ziegler's athletes were quickly making great advancements in their competitive careers with the help of the drug. According to reports, Ziegler too seemed to be very impressed, at least for a while.[465] But by the early 1960's, it was starting to look like Dianabol had sparked a great wave of steroid abuse in competitive sports. Dr. Ziegler's early recommendations, which depending on the source called for as little as 5 mg per day or as much as 15 mg per day, were being largely ignored, as athletes developed their own more aggressive (and potentially dangerous) dosing strategies. Dr. Ziegler soon became disgusted with the misuse of the drug, and would eventually become a voice of opposition to sports doping. By 1967, approximately 10 years after first introducing Dianabol to his athletes, he had categorically condemned the use of anabolic steroids in sports.[466]

As early as 1965, Dianabol was already starting to fall under scrutiny of the U.S. Food and Drug Administration. That year the FDA requested Ciba clarify Dianabol's medical uses, which were then stated to include helping patients in debilitated states and those with weakened bones. In 1970, the FDA accepted that Dianabol was "Probably Effective" in treating post-menopausal osteoporosis and pituitary-deficient dwarfism. These changes were reflected in the drug's prescribing recommendations during the 1970's, and Ciba was allowed to continue selling and studying the agent. Ciba eventually lost patent protection, however, and companies like Parr, Barr, Bolar, and Rugby were soon cutting deeply into their market with their own generic version of the drug.

By the early-80's the FDA had withdrawn its "Probably Effective" position on the pituitary-deficient dwarfism, and continued to press Ciba for more data. Sufficient clarification never came, and in 1983 Ciba officially withdrew Dianabol from the U.S. market.[467] Perhaps financial disinterest had a hand in their abandoned push to keep the drug approved. The FDA pulled all generic forms of methandrostenolone from the U.S. market in 1985, a time when most Western nations were also eliminating the drug, finding its existence to be justified mainly by sports doping. Methandrostenolone is still produced today, but typically in nations with loose prescription drug regulations, and by companies that still prefer to cater to an underground athletic market.

How Supplied:

Methandrostenolone is widely available in both human and veterinary drug markets. Composition and dosage may vary by country and manufacturer. Methandrostenolone was designed as an oral anabolic steroid containing 2.5 mg or 5 mg of steroid per tablet (Dianabol). Modern brands usually contain 5 mg or 10 mg per tablet. Methandrostenolone can also be found in injectable veterinary preparations. These are typically oil-based solutions that carry 25 mg/ml of steroid.

Structural Characteristics:

Methandrostenolone is a modified form of testosterone. It differs by: 1) the addition of a methyl group at carbon 17-alpha to protect the hormone during oral administration and 2) the introduction of a double bond between carbons 1 and 2, which reduces its relative androgenicity. The resulting steroid also has a much weaker relative binding affinity for the androgen receptor than testosterone, but at the same time displays a much longer half-life and lower affinity for serum-binding proteins in comparison. These features (among others) allow methandrostenolone to be a very potent anabolic steroid in spite of a weaker affinity for receptor binding. Recent studies have additionally confirmed that its primary mode of action involves interaction with the cellular androgen receptor.[468]

Side Effects (Estrogenic):

Methandrostenolone is aromatized by the body, and is a moderately estrogenic steroid.[469] Gynecomastia is often a concern during treatment, and may present itself quite early into a cycle (particularly when higher doses are used). At the same time water retention can become a problem, causing a notable loss of muscle definition as both subcutaneous water retention and fat levels build. Sensitive individuals may therefore want to keep the estrogen under control with the addition of an anti-estrogen such as Nolvadex® and/or Proviron®. One may alternately use an aromatase inhibitor like Arimidex® (anastrozole), which is a more effective remedy for estrogen control. Aromatase inhibitors, however, can be quite expensive in comparison to standard estrogen maintenance therapies, and may also have negative effects on blood lipids.

It is interesting to note that methandrostenolone is structurally identical to boldenone, except that it contains the added c17-alpha-methyl group. This fact makes clear the impact of altering a steroid in such a way, as these two compounds appear to act very differently in the body. A key dissimilarity seems to lie in the tendency for estrogenic side effects. Equipoise® (boldenone undecylenate) is known to be quite mild in this regard, and users commonly take this drug without the need to add an anti-estrogen. Methandrostenolone is much more estrogenic, often necessitating anti-estrogen use. But this difference is not caused by methandrostenolone being more easily aromatized. In fact, the 17-alpha methyl group and c1-2 double bond both slow the process of aromatization considerably. The issue actually is caused by methandrostenolone converting to 17alpha-methylestradiol, a more biologically active form of estrogen than estradiol.

Side Effects (Androgenic):

Although classified as an anabolic steroid, androgenic side effects are still common with this substance. This may include bouts of oily skin, acne, and body/facial hair growth. Anabolic/androgenic steroids may also aggravate male pattern hair loss. Individuals sensitive to the androgenic effects of methandrostenolone may find a milder anabolic such as Deca-Durabolin® to be more comfortable. Women are additionally warned of the potential virilizing effects of anabolic/androgenic steroids. These may include a deepening of the voice, menstrual irregularities, changes in skin texture, facial hair growth, and clitoral enlargement.

While methandrostenolone does convert to a more potent steroid via interaction with the 5-alpha reductase enzyme (the same enzyme responsible for converting testosterone to dihydrotestosterone), it has an extremely low affinity to do so.[470] The androgenic metabolite 5-alpha dihydromethandrostenolone is produced only in trace amounts, so the relative androgenicity of methandrostenolone is not significantly affected by finasteride or dutasteride.

Side Effects (Hepatotoxicity):

Methandrostenolone is a c17-alpha alkylated compound. This alteration protects the drug from deactivation by the liver, allowing a very high percentage of the drug entry into the bloodstream following oral administration. C17-alpha alkylated anabolic/androgenic steroids can be hepatotoxic. Prolonged or high exposure may result in liver damage. In rare instances life-threatening dysfunction may develop. It is advisable to visit a physician periodically during each cycle to monitor liver function and overall health. Intake of c17-alpha alkylated steroids is commonly limited to 6-8 weeks, in an effort to avoid escalating liver strain.

Studies have shown that several weeks of methandrostenolone administration offers minimal hepatic stress so long as it is given at a dosage of 10 mg per day or below. At a dose of 15 mg per day, a majority of patients will begin to demonstrate disturbed liver function as measured by clinically elevated bromosulphalein retention (a marker of hepatic stress).[471] Even at 2.5 and 5 mg per day, elevations in BSP retention have been reported in patients. Severe liver complications are rare given the periodic nature in which most people use oral anabolic/androgenic steroids, although cannot be excluded with methandrostenolone, especially with high doses and/or prolonged administration periods.

The use of a liver detoxification supplement such as Liver Stabil, Liv-52, or Essentiale Forte is advised while taking any hepatotoxic anabolic/androgenic steroids.

Side Effects (Cardiovascular):

Anabolic/androgenic steroids can have deleterious effects on serum cholesterol. This includes a tendency to reduce HDL (good) cholesterol values and increase LDL (bad) cholesterol values, which may shift the HDL to LDL balance in a direction that favors greater risk of arteriosclerosis. The relative impact of an anabolic/androgenic steroid on serum lipids is dependant on the dose, route of administration (oral vs. injectable), type of steroid (aromatizable or non-aromatizable), and level of resistance to hepatic metabolism. Methandrostenolone has a strong effect on the hepatic management of cholesterol due to its structural resistance to liver breakdown and route of administration. Anabolic/androgenic steroids may also adversely affect blood pressure and triglycerides, reduce endothelial relaxation, and support left ventricular hypertrophy, all potentially increasing the risk of cardiovascular disease and myocardial infarction.

To help reduce cardiovascular strain it is advised to maintain an active cardiovascular exercise program and minimize the intake of saturated fats, cholesterol, and simple carbohydrates at all times during active AAS administration. Supplementing with fish oils (4 grams per day) and a natural cholesterol/antioxidant formula such as Lipid Stabil or a product with comparable ingredients is also recommended.

Side Effects (Testosterone Suppression):

All anabolic/androgenic steroids when taken in doses sufficient to promote muscle gain are expected to suppress endogenous testosterone production. Methandrostenolone is no exception, and is noted for its strong influence on the hypothalamic-pituitary-testicular axis. Clinical studies giving 15 mg per day to resistance-training males for 8 weeks caused the mean plasma testosterone level to fall by 69%.[472] Without the intervention of testosterone-stimulating substances, testosterone levels should return to normal within 1-4 months of drug secession. Note that prolonged hypogonadotrophic hypogonadism can develop secondary to steroid abuse, necessitating medical intervention.

The above side effects are not inclusive. For more detailed discussion of potential side effects, see the Steroid Side Effects section of this book.

Administration (General):

Studies have shown that taking an oral anabolic steroid with food may decrease its bioavailability.[473] This is caused by the fat-soluble nature of steroid hormones, which can allow some of the drug to dissolve with undigested dietary fat, reducing its absorption from the gastrointestinal tract. For maximum utilization, this steroid should be taken on an empty stomach.

Administration (Men):

The original prescribing guidelines for Dianabol called for a daily dosage of 5 mg. This was to be administered on an intermittent basis, with the drug taken for no more than 6 consecutive weeks. Thereafter, a break of 2 to 4 weeks was advised before therapy was resumed. For physique- or performance-enhancing purposes, the drug is also used intermittently, with cycles usually lasting between 6 and 8 weeks in length followed by 6-8 weeks off. Although a low dose of 5 mg daily may be effective for improving performance, athletes typically take much higher amounts. A daily dosage of three to six 5 mg tablets (15-30 mg) is most common, and typically produces very dramatic results. Some venture even higher in dosage, but this practice usually leads to a more profound incidence of side effects, and is generally discouraged.

Dianabol stacks well with a variety of other steroids. It is noted to mix particularly well with the mild anabolic Deca-Durabolin®, for example. Together one can expect exceptional muscle and strength gains, with side effects not much worse than one would expect from Dianabol alone. For sheer mass, a long-acting testosterone ester like enanthate or cypionate can be used. With the high estrogenic/androgenic properties of this androgen, however, side effects should be more pronounced. Gains would be pronounced as well, which usually makes such an endeavor worthwhile to the user. As discussed earlier, ancillary drugs can be added to reduce the side effects associated with this kind of cycle.

The half-life of Dianabol is only about 3 to 5 hours. A single daily dosage schedule will produce a varying blood level, with ups and downs throughout the day. The user, likewise, has a choice, to either split up the tablets during the day or to take them all at one time. The usual recommendation has been to divide them and try to regulate the concentration in your blood. This, however, will produce a lower peak blood level than if the tablets were taken all at once, so there may be a trade-off with this option. Both options work fine, but anecdotal evidence seems to support single daily doses as being better for overall results. With such a schedule, it seems logical that taking the pills earlier in the day would be optimal. This would allow a considerable number of daytime hours for an androgen-rich metabolism to heighten the uptake of nutrients, especially the critical hours following training.

Administration (Women):

Being moderately androgenic, Dianabol is really only a popular steroid with men. When used by women, strong virilization symptoms are possible. Some do experiment with it, however, and often find low doses (2.5-5 mg) of this steroid quite effective for new muscle growth. Studies have demonstrated that a majority of women will notice acne, which is indicative of androgenicity, at a dosage of only 10 mg per day. Children are likely to notice virilizing effects with as little as 2.5 mg per day.

Availability:

Legitimate pharmaceutical forms of methandrostenolone are scare. Western medicine has completely done away with this steroid, where it is thought to hold no real therapeutic value. Its potential existence is viewed as supporting doping/performance-enhancement only. Therefore, you are not going to come across legitimate Dianabol from the U.S., Canada, or Western Europe. This drug is made exclusively in areas such as Asia, South America (limited), and Eastern Europe. Ignore anything labeled as Italian or Spanish, etc. They will not be legitimate. In regards to some of the most popular legitimate brands on the black market, here is what to look for.

British Dispensary Anabol tablets from Thailand are still very popular. Due to rampant counterfeiting, the manufacturer has instituted three security guards. One is a hologram sticker, which is affixed to each 1,000-count tub of tablets. Second, the tablets themselves are imprinted with the company's snake emblem. Lastly, the 1,000-count tub bears the company logo formed into the plastic top. Note that Anabol is in such high demand that some advanced counterfeiters have been duplicating British Dispensary's holograms, custom tablet dyes, and logo-impressed plastic bottles. They look good, but all fakes thus far have minor deviations from the original. Be sure to compare your product's features to the real Anabol photos very closely. Note that the product carries a computer printed lot number and expiration date, similar to Anabol 10.

British Dispensary also manufactures a 10 mg version of Anabol called Anabol 10. This product carries the same security features as the regular Anabol product, but in a smaller yellow and white package. The tablets themselves are identical in shape to the 5 mg version, and also carry the company logo stamped into them. The only difference is their color, which is yellow instead of pink.

Generic "Russian D-Bol" (METAHAPOCTEHOROH) is still being produced in Russia by Akrikhin (the name looks like Akpnxnh in Cyrillic). The current box is purple in color, and carries 10 strips of 10 tablets each. This has always been a highly regarded form of Dianabol. As such, it has also been a regularly counterfeited one. Most of the fakes have been poor copies of the original, often coming as bottles of loose tablets instead of proper foil and plastic push-through strips. That is not to say locating the current production version in tablet strips assures a safe purchase, however, so take care to compare your product to the original photos closely. Note that the manufacturer has started making a version of this product for the Ukrainian market. This product can be identified by the company name, which appears as Akpixih on the packaging. Some have mistakenly identified these as fakes, believing this to be a typographical error.

Naposim from Rumania is still available. It comes in a white box, containing 10 triangle stamped pills to each foil and plastic strip. Note that the foil strip on real Naposim has date and lot number stampings on both ends. Some fakes in the past have overlooked this, placing them only on one end. Additionally, there is a little nipple in the center of each pill bubble on the real Naposim strip. Fakes of this product have been located in the past with smooth pill bubbles. Also, be sure the triangle on your tablets is sharp and even. One recent fake has been seen with stampings that look more like Star Trek emblems than triangles. Also, note that some strips are found with the generic name metandienona instead of metandienonum. This is simply how the company labels the product for export.

Danabol DS from Body Research/March Pharmaceutical

Company in Thailand are also available. The tablets are made in the form of distinct small blue heart shapes. Body Research products are often counterfeited, so take care when shopping.

Methandon and Melic from Thailand are both legit items, and come packed in containers of 1,000 tablets each. Both of these products are relatively rare on the black market these days, although it is believed that both are still in production. Their lack of abundance may simply be due to the far greater popularity and recognition of Anabol, which continues to dominate the Thai Dianabol market in spite of growing competition. Both products have pink 5-sided tablets like Anabol, and are very similar in appearance without the bottles. The Methandon product (which used to use plain white tablets) is the most distinct, as it carries the letters "ES" etched into them.

Anabolex 3mg tabs from the Dominican Republic are still a safe buy. Note that each pill contains an added 1.5 mg of Periactin, used as an appetite stimulant. It's an antihistamine and may cause drowsiness. Make sure your product is packaged in the modern-style blue pouches, not the older plain white ones. These are long off the market at this point.

Metanabol from Poland is another legit brand, but be sure to purchase these only in strips of 20 tabs, as shown in the picture library.

Balkan Pharmaceuticals in Moldova makes a methandrostenolone product called Danabol. It comes in foil and plastic strips of 20 tablets each. Both 10 mg and 50 mgversions are produced. Counterfeits are not known to be a problem.

Jinan Pharmaceuticals makes a 10 mg version in China for export called Anahexia. It comes in foil and plastic strips of 20 tablets each.

Dimethyltrienolone

Androgenic	>10,000
Anabolic	>10,000
Standard	Methyltestosterone (oral)
Chemical Names	
Estrogenic Activity	none
Progestational Activity	high

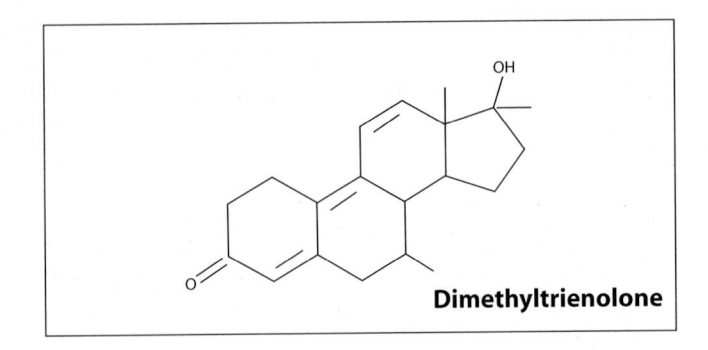

Description:

Dimethyltrienolone is a potent oral steroid derived from nandrolone. It is a close cousin of methyltrienolone, differing only by an additional 7-alpha methyl group. This is a modification that only appears a couple of times in commercial steroid medicine, but when it does it seems to have a powerful effect. Its main function is to reduce binding to serum proteins, increasing the percentage of free (active) steroid in the blood and overall steroid potency. We see this with bolasterone, a powerful dimethylated derivative of testosterone that displays nearly six times greater anabolic potency than methyltestosterone. 7-Methylation also appears on Cheque Drops (mibolerone), a 7,17-dimethylated nandrolone with about 41 times the oral anabolic potency of methyltestosterone. Dimethyltrienolone is in the same class as a dimethylated form of trenbolone. It is an extremely potent oral anabolic and androgenic steroid, perhaps far more than any other agent developed before or after. This agent is not widely used by athletes, however, given that it was never produced commercially.

History:

Dimethyltrienolone was first described in 1967.[474] This agent is one of a great many potent anabolic steroids that has been developed but never introduced into a commercial drug market. As such, it is a research compound only, and there is no human data on it to report. There are, of course, a great many compounds that fit this description that are not included in this reference. What makes this particular steroid stand out from the others is its sheer potency. More to the point, dimethyltrienolone is perhaps the most potent anabolic steroid that has ever been developed and assayed for effect. This agent is very similar in structure to Metribolone (methyltrienolone), which was determined to be not only extremely potent, but also the most hepatotoxic steroid ever developed at the time of its testing. That steroid is certainly an agent of extreme proportions, and dimethyltrienolone is only going to be a more potent (and potentially more toxic) derivative.

When this steroid was assayed for anabolic and androgenic effect back in 1967, the results were indeterminate. They were indeterminate because the values were so high they could not be accurately calculated given the parameters of the study. The study itself was very typical. As would be expected of an oral steroid, methyltestosterone was used as the standard of comparison. The animals (rats) were dosed and later sacrificed. Ventral prostate and seminal vesicles were weighed to measure androgenic effect, and levator ani was used for anabolic potency (the same three values that were the standard of analysis for steroids in the 1960's and '70's). In regards to all three measures, dimethyltrienolone was shown to be more than 100 times stronger in effect than methyltestosterone. The numbers, when reported in percentages, simply read "> 10,000" (greater than 10,000%) on all 3 tests. I was unable to find further oral assays on this steroid, making the exact potency (by these experiments or others) unknown.

How Supplied:

Dimethyltrienolone is not available as a commercial agent.

Structural Characteristics:

Dimethyltrienolone is a modified form of nandrolone. It differs by: 1) the addition of a methyl group at carbon 17-alpha to protect the hormone during oral administration, 2) the introduction of double bonds at carbons 9 and 11, which increases its binding affinity and slows its metabolism, and 3) the introduction of a methyl group at carbon 7 (alpha), which inhibits steroid attachment to serum-binding proteins like SHBG (Sex Hormone Binding Globulin) and greatly enhances relative biological activity.

Side Effects (Estrogenic):

Dimethyltrienolone is not aromatized by the body, and is not believed to be measurably estrogenic. It is of note, however, that dimethyltrienolone likely displays significant binding affinity for the progesterone receptor. The side effects associated with progesterone are similar to those of estrogen, including negative feedback inhibition of testosterone production and enhanced rate of fat storage. Progestins also augment the stimulatory effect of estrogens on mammary tissue growth. There appears to be a strong synergy between these two hormones here, such that gynecomastia might even occur with the help of progestins, without excessive estrogen levels. The use of an anti-estrogen, which inhibits the estrogenic component of this disorder, is often sufficient to mitigate gynecomastia caused by progestational anabolic/androgenic steroids.

Side Effects (Androgenic):

Although classified as an anabolic steroid, androgenic side effects are still likely with this substance. This may include bouts of oily skin, acne, and body/facial hair growth. Anabolic/androgenic steroids may also aggravate male pattern hair loss. Women are also warned of the potential virilizing effects of anabolic/androgenic steroids. These may include a deepening of the voice, menstrual irregularities, changes in skin texture, facial hair growth, and clitoral enlargement. Additionally, the 5-alpha reductase enzyme does not metabolize dimethyltrienolone, so its relative androgenicity is not affected by finasteride or dutasteride.

Side Effects (Hepatotoxicity):

Dimethyltrienolone is a c17-alpha alkylated compound. This alteration protects the drug from deactivation by the liver, allowing a very high percentage of the drug entry into the bloodstream following oral administration. C17-alpha alkylated anabolic/androgenic steroids can be hepatotoxic. Prolonged or high exposure may result in liver damage. In rare instances life-threatening dysfunction may develop. It is advisable to visit a physician periodically during each cycle to monitor liver function and overall health. Intake of c17-alpha alkylated steroids is commonly limited to 6-8 weeks, in an effort to avoid escalating liver strain. Note that dimethyltrienolone is an exceedingly potent oral steroid, with a very high level of resistance to hepatic metabolism. This makes dimethyltrienolone exceedingly liver toxic.

The use of a liver detoxification supplement such as Liver Stabil, Liv-52, or Essentiale Forte is advised while taking any hepatotoxic anabolic/androgenic steroids.

Side Effects (Cardiovascular):

Anabolic/androgenic steroids can have deleterious effects on serum cholesterol. This includes a tendency to reduce HDL (good) cholesterol values and increase LDL (bad) cholesterol values, which may shift the HDL to LDL balance in a direction that favors greater risk of arteriosclerosis. The relative impact of an anabolic/androgenic steroid on serum lipids is dependant on the dose, route of administration (oral vs. injectable), type of steroid (aromatizable or non-aromatizable), and level of resistance to hepatic metabolism. Although not extensively studied in humans, the high relative potency and non-aromatizable nature of dimethyltrienolone suggests that this agent is extremely prone to negatively altering lipid values and increasing atherogenic risk. Anabolic/androgenic steroids may also adversely affect blood pressure and triglycerides, reduce endothelial relaxation, and support left ventricular hypertrophy, all potentially increasing the risk of cardiovascular disease and myocardial infarction.

To help reduce cardiovascular strain it is advised to maintain an active cardiovascular exercise program and minimize the intake of saturated fats, cholesterol, and simple carbohydrates at all times during active AAS administration. Supplementing with fish oils (4 grams per day) and a natural cholesterol/antioxidant formula such as Lipid Stabil or a product with comparable ingredients is also recommended.

Side Effects (Testosterone Suppression):

All anabolic/androgenic steroids when taken in doses sufficient to promote muscle gain are expected to suppress endogenous testosterone production. Without the intervention of testosterone-stimulating substances, testosterone levels should return to normal within 1-4 months of drug secession. Note that prolonged hypogonadotrophic hypogonadism can develop secondary to steroid abuse, necessitating medical intervention.

The above side effects are not inclusive. For more detailed discussion of potential side effects, see the Steroid Side Effects section of this book.

Administration (General):

Studies have shown that taking an oral anabolic steroid with food may decrease its bioavailability.[475] This is caused by the fat-soluble nature of steroid hormones, which can allow some of the drug to dissolve with undigested dietary fat, reducing its absorption from the gastrointestinal tract. For maximum utilization, dimethyltrienolone should be taken on an empty stomach.

Administration (Men):

Dimethyltrienolone was never approved for use in humans. Prescribing guidelines are unavailable. This agent is generally not recommended for physique- or performance-enhancing purposes due to its high level of hepatotoxicity. Those absolutely insisting on its use need to take its level of liver toxicity very seriously. At the very least, routine blood tests should be conducted to ensure the agent is not imparting damage. Drug duration is also usually very limited, typically to 4 weeks of use or less. The relative potency of dimethyltrienolone is extremely high, requiring doses as little as .25 (1/4) milligram per day for a pronounced anabolic effect (.25 to 1mg likely being the chosen range). It needs to be emphasized again that there are many other steroids out there worth using before this one, which are not going to be as dangerous. No compound, no matter how potent, is magic, and dimethyltrienolone is one of those steroids that should probably just be left alone.

Administration (Women):

Dimethyltrienolone was never approved for use in humans. Prescribing guidelines are unavailable. This agent is not recommended for women for physique- or performance-enhancing purposes due to its extremely strong toxicity and tendency to produce virilizing side effects.

Availability:

Dimethyltrienolone is not produced as a prescription steroid product in any part of the world. This agent is available as a black market designer compound, however. Those contemplating the use of underground forms of dimethyltrienolone should consider that such agents are being released for human use without any government approval or consideration to its safety.

Dinandrol (nandrolone blend)

Androgenic	37
Anabolic	125
Standard	Testosterone
Chemical Names	19-norandrost-4-en-3-one-17beta-ol
	17beta-hydroxy-estr-4-en-3-one
Estrogenic Activity	low
Progestational Activity	moderate

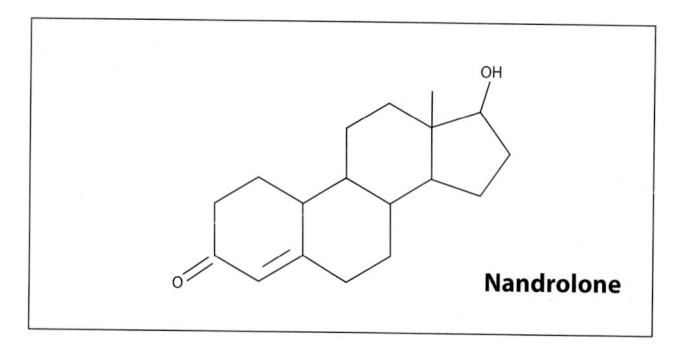

Nandrolone

Description:

Dinandrol is an injectable anabolic steroid preparation that contains a mixture of nandrolone phenylpropionate and nandrolone decanoate. The two steroids are present in a concentration of 40 mg/mL and 60 mg/mL, respectively. With a blend of fast- and slow-acting esters, this product was outwardly designed as a nandrolone equivalent of Sustanon or Testoviron. Given that nandrolone decanoate already provides its peak steroid release approximately 24-48 hours post injection, however, as with Sustanon and Testoviron, a more even and sustained release of hormone is not actually achieved. Instead, Dinandrol can be looked at as a form of Deca-Durabolin that has a sharper short-term spike of nandrolone following each injection, perhaps making it best to inject twice weekly as opposed to once. As with all nandrolone injectables, this preparation is favored by athletes and bodybuilders for its ability to promote moderate to strong gains in lean muscle mass, with minimal estrogenic or androgenic side effects.

History:

Dinandrol is a product of Xelox Pharma Co. in the Philippines. Xelox is a licensed drug company, although most of its steroid products are developed for export sales only. The packaging for Dinandrol lists the indicated uses for the drug as being aplastic anemia, anemia caused by cytotoxic drugs, or anemia caused by chronic renal failure. Owing to the fact that Deca-Durabolin is also approved for use in anemic patients in many markets, this drug could be viewed as a cheaper and often acceptable (although not ideal) therapeutic alternative. Still, it is estimated that the majority of steroid product that is traded on the international market is diverted to off-label use by athletes and bodybuilders, usually in Europe and the United States, so it is uncertain how widely this drug is dispensed to legitimate patients. Dinandrol is occasionally smuggled into the United States, though remains more widely distributed on less tightly controlled European markets.

How Supplied:

Dinandrol is manufactured by Xelox Pharma in the Philippines. It contains 100 mg/mL of steroid in oil in a 2 mL vial.

Structural Characteristics:

Dinandrol contains a mixture of two nandrolone compounds, which where modified with the addition of carboxylic acid esters (propionic phenyl ester and decanoic acids) at the 17-beta hydroxyl group. Esterified steroids are less polar than free steroids, and are absorbed more slowly from the area of injection. Once in the bloodstream, the ester is removed to yield free (active) nandrolone. Esterified steroids are designed to prolong the window of therapeutic effect following administration, allowing for a less frequent injection schedule compared to injections of free (unesterified) steroid.

Side Effects (Estrogenic):

Nandrolone has a low tendency for estrogen conversion, estimated to be only about 20% of that seen with testosterone.[476] This is because while the liver can convert nandrolone to estradiol, in other more active sites of steroid aromatization such as adipose tissue nandrolone is far less open to this process.[477] Consequently, estrogen related side effects are a much lower concern with this drug than with testosterone. Elevated-estrogen levels may still be noticed with higher dosing, however, and may cause side effects such as increased water retention, body fat gain, and gynecomastia. An anti-estrogen such as clomiphene citrate or tamoxifen citrate may be necessary to prevent estrogenic side effects if they occur. One may alternately use an aromatase inhibitor like Arimidex® (anastrozole), which more efficiently controls estrogen by preventing its synthesis. Aromatase inhibitors can be quite expensive in comparison to anti-estrogens, however, and may also have negative effects on blood lipids.

It is of note that nandrolone has some activity as a progestin in the body.[478] Although progesterone is a c-19 steroid, removal of this group as in 19-norprogesterone creates a hormone with greater binding affinity for its corresponding receptor. Sharing this trait, many 19-nor anabolic steroids are shown to have some affinity for the progesterone receptor as well.[479] The side effects associated with progesterone are similar to those of estrogen, including negative feedback inhibition of testosterone production and enhanced rate of fat storage. Progestins also augment the stimulatory effect of estrogens on mammary tissue growth. There appears to be a strong synergy between these two hormones here, such that gynecomastia might even occur with the help of progestins, without excessive estrogen levels. The use of an anti-estrogen, which inhibits the estrogenic component of this disorder, is often sufficient to mitigate gynecomastia caused by nandrolone.

Side Effects (Androgenic):

Although classified as an anabolic steroid, androgenic side effects are still possible with this substance, especially with higher doses. This may include bouts of oily skin, acne, and body/facial hair growth. Anabolic/androgenic steroids may also aggravate male pattern hair loss. Women are warned of the potential virilizing effects of anabolic/androgenic steroids. These may include a deepening of the voice, menstrual irregularities, changes in skin texture, facial hair growth, and clitoral enlargement. Nandrolone is a steroid with relatively low androgenic activity relative to its tissue-building actions, making the threshold for strong androgenic side effects comparably higher than with more androgenic agents such as testosterone, methandrostenolone, or fluoxymesterone. It is also important to point out that due to its mild androgenic nature and ability to suppress endogenous testosterone, nandrolone is prone to interfering with libido in males when used without another androgen.

Note that in androgen-responsive target tissues such as the skin, scalp, and prostate, the relative androgenicity of nandrolone is reduced by its reduction to dihydronandrolone (DHN).[480] [481] The 5-alpha reductase enzyme is responsible for this metabolism of nandrolone. The concurrent use of a 5-alpha reductase inhibitor such as finasteride or dutasteride will interfere with site-specific reduction of nandrolone action, considerably increasing the tendency of nandrolone to produce androgenic side effects. Reductase inhibitors should be avoided with nandrolone if low androgenicity is desired.

Side Effects (Hepatotoxicity):

Nandrolone is not c-17 alpha alkylated, and not known to have hepatotoxic effects. Liver toxicity is unlikely.

Side Effects (Cardiovascular):

Anabolic/androgenic steroids can have deleterious effects on serum cholesterol. This includes a tendency to reduce HDL (good) cholesterol values and increase LDL (bad) cholesterol values, which may shift the HDL to LDL balance in a direction that favors greater risk of arteriosclerosis. The relative impact of an anabolic/androgenic steroid on serum lipids is dependant on the dose, route of administration (oral vs. injectable), type of steroid (aromatizable or non-aromatizable), and level of resistance to hepatic metabolism. Studies administering 600 mg of nandrolone decanoate per week for 10 weeks demonstrated a 26% reduction in HDL cholesterol levels.[482] This suppression is slightly greater than that reported with an equal dose of testosterone enanthate, and is in agreement with earlier studies showing a slightly stronger negative impact on HDL/LDL ratio with nandrolone decanoate as compared to testosterone cypionate.[483] Nandrolone injectables, however, should still have a significantly weaker impact on serum lipids than c-17 alpha alkylated agents. Anabolic/androgenic steroids may also adversely affect blood pressure and triglycerides, reduce endothelial relaxation, and support left ventricular hypertrophy, all potentially increasing the risk of cardiovascular disease and myocardial infarction.

To help reduce cardiovascular strain it is advised to maintain an active cardiovascular exercise program and minimize the intake of saturated fats, cholesterol, and simple carbohydrates at all times during active AAS administration. Supplementing with fish oils (4 grams per day) and a natural cholesterol/antioxidant formula such as Lipid Stabil or a product with comparable ingredients is also recommended.

Side Effects (Testosterone Suppression):

All anabolic/androgenic steroids when taken in doses sufficient to promote muscle gain are expected to suppress endogenous testosterone production. Studies administering 100 mg per week of nandrolone decanoate for 6 weeks have demonstrated an approximate 57% reduction in serum testosterone levels during therapy. At a dosage of 300 mg per week, this reduction reached 70%.[484] It is believed that the progestational activity of nandrolone notably contributes to the suppression of testosterone synthesis during therapy, which can be marked in spite of a low tendency for estrogen conversion.[485] Without the intervention of testosterone-stimulating substances, testosterone levels should return to normal within 2-6 months of drug secession. Note that prolonged hypogonadotrophic hypogonadism can develop secondary to steroid abuse, necessitating medical intervention.

The above side effects are not inclusive. For more detailed discussion of potential side effects, see the Steroid Side Effects section of this book.

Administration (Men):

To treat aplastic anemia, prescribing guidelines recommend a dosage of 50-200 mg per week. A 200 mg per week dose is recommended for anemia due to renal failure or cytotoxic therapy. When used for physique- or performance-enhancing purposes, a dose of 200-600 mg per week is most common, taken in cycles 8 to 12 weeks in length. This level is sufficient for most users to notice measurable gains in lean muscle mass and strength, which should be accompanied by a low level of estrogenic and androgenic activity. Due to the fast-acting nature of nandrolone phenylpropionate, the total weekly dosage is often divided into two separate applications, spaced several days apart. Note that as a nandrolone injectable, Dinandrol seems to fit well for both bulking and cutting purposes, and can reasonably replace Deca-Durabolin in most cycles.

Administration (Women):

To treat aplastic anemia, prescribing guidelines recommend a dosage of 50-200 mg per week. A 100 mg per week dose is recommended for anemia due to renal failure, and 200 mg per week for anemia caused by cytotoxic therapy. When used for physique- or performance-enhancing purposes, a dosage of 50 mg per week is most common, which is taken for 4 to 6 weeks. Although only slightly androgenic, women are occasionally confronted with virilization symptoms when taking this compound, even when taking recommended therapeutic doses. Should virilizing side effects become a concern, the drug should be discontinued immediately to help prevent their permanent appearance. After a sufficient period of withdrawal, the shorter acting nandrolone Durabolin® might be considered a safer (more controllable) option. This drug stays active for only several days, greatly reducing the withdrawal time if indicated.

Availability:

Dinandrol is commonly found on the black market. Its packaging is unique, and would seemingly be difficult and costly to duplicate. To begin with, the product carries a sticker bearing the company logo, which, once removed to open the box, reads VOID. You also open the box to find the vials sitting in a clear-plastic tray that bears the firm's name (Xelox). It is not printed on the tray but molded directly into the plastic, which would obviously be some task for an underground manufacturer to duplicate. Counterfeits of Dinandrol are currently not known to be a problem.

Drive® (boldenone/methylandrostenediol blend)

Androgenic	
Anabolic	
Standard	

Chemical Names	
Estrogenic Activity	
Progestational Activity	

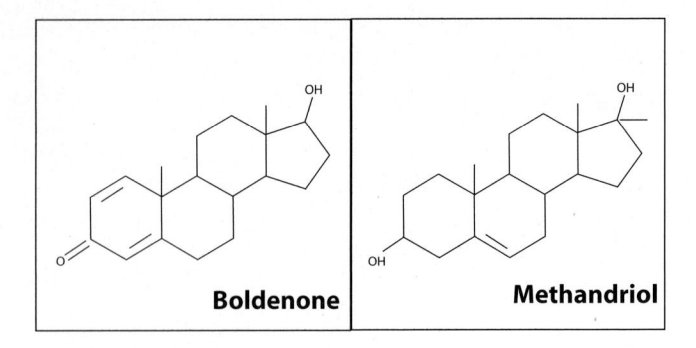

Description:

Drive is an Australian injectable veterinary steroid preparation that contains a blend of methandriol dipropionate and boldenone undecylenate. The two steroids are present in a dose of 25 mg/mL and 30 mg/mL respectively, for a total steroid concentration of 55 mg/mL. Boldenone undecylenate is a highly common steroid most notably identified with the preparation Equipoise®. Methandriol dipropionate, however, is very rarely seen on the U.S. black market. Its character is that of a moderately strong anabolic steroid, which is accompanied by a notable androgenic component. When combined with boldenone, the result is a moderately androgenic/anabolic blend inclined to produce notable muscle mass and strength gains, usually without excessive water retention.

History:

Drive is a product of RWR Veterinary Products (formerly a subsidiary of Nature Vet), sold only on the Australian veterinary drug market. It is designed for use in horses, typically as a general anabolic or health tonic drug for when an animal is weak from vigorous performance. It is supposed to aid the growth of muscle tissue, help avoid dehydration, and improve the digestion of dietary proteins. The dosage used for an adult 1,100lb horse is 5 mL (110 mg) every two weeks. Australia is a country with a robust veterinary drug market, known to carry a variety of unusual steroids and odd multi-component steroid blends. Drive is perhaps the most well-known of these products. Being that it is neither the most concentrated preparation nor the most effective, however, much of its popularity is likely due to its well-coined trade name and early sales history. Drive remains on the Australina market today, although tight controls and its relatively low per-milliliter steroid concentration make diversion for athletic use much less common than it was many years ago.

How Supplied:

Drive is available on the Australian veterinary drug market. It contains 55 mg/mL of steroid in oil in a 10 mL vial.

Structural Characteristics:

For a more comprehensive discussion of the individual steroids boldenone undecylenate and methandriol dipropionate, refer to their respective profiles.

Side Effects (Estrogenic):

Methylandrostendiol is not directly aromatized by the body, although one of its known metabolites is methyltestosterone, which can aromatize. Methyandrostenediol is also believed to have some inherent estrogenic activity.[486] Combined with boldenone, which also aromatizes, Drive is considered a moderately estrogenic steroid. Gynecomastia is possible during treatment, but generally only when higher doses are used. Water and fat retention can also become issues, again depending on dose. Sensitive individuals may need to add an anti-estrogen such as Nolvadex® to minimize related side effects.

Side Effects (Androgenic):

Although classified as an anabolic steroid preparation, androgenic side effects are still common with this substance. This may include bouts of oily skin, acne, and body/facial hair growth. Anabolic/androgenic steroids may also aggravate male pattern hair loss. Women are warned of the potential virilizing effects of anabolic/androgenic steroids. These may include a deepening of the voice, menstrual irregularities, changes in skin texture, facial hair growth, and clitoral enlargement.

Side Effects (Hepatotoxicity):

Methylandrostenediol is a c17-alpha alkylated compound. This alteration protects the drug from deactivation by the liver, allowing a very high percentage of the drug entry into the bloodstream following oral administration. C17-alpha alkylated anabolic/androgenic steroids can be hepatotoxic. Prolonged or high exposure may result in liver damage. In rare instances life-threatening dysfunction may develop. It is advisable to visit a physician periodically during each cycle to monitor liver function and overall health. Intake of c17-alpha alkylated steroids is commonly limited to 6-8 weeks, in an effort to avoid escalating liver strain. Injectable forms of the drug may present slightly less strain on the liver by avoiding the first pass metabolism of oral dosing, although may still present substantial hepatotoxicity.

Side Effects (Cardiovascular):

Anabolic/androgenic steroids can have deleterious effects on serum cholesterol. This includes a tendency to reduce HDL (good) cholesterol values and increase LDL (bad) cholesterol values, which may shift the HDL to LDL balance in a direction that favors greater risk of arteriosclerosis. The relative impact of an anabolic/androgenic steroid on serum lipids is dependant on the dose, route of administration (oral vs. injectable), type of steroid (aromatizable or non-aromatizable), and level of resistance to hepatic metabolism. Methylandrostenediol has a strong effect on the hepatic management of cholesterol due to its structural resistance to liver breakdown and (with the oral) route of administration. Anabolic/androgenic steroids may also adversely affect blood pressure and triglycerides, reduce endothelial relaxation, and support left ventricular hypertrophy, all potentially increasing the risk of cardiovascular disease and myocardial infarction.

To help reduce cardiovascular strain it is advised to maintain an active cardiovascular exercise program and minimize the intake of saturated fats, cholesterol, and simple carbohydrates at all times during active AAS administration. Supplementing with fish oils (4 grams per day) and a natural cholesterol/antioxidant formula such as Lipid Stabil or a product with comparable ingredients is also recommended.

Side Effects (Testosterone Suppression):

All anabolic/androgenic steroids when taken in doses sufficient to promote muscle gain are expected to suppress endogenous testosterone production. Without the intervention of testosterone-stimulating substances, testosterone levels should return to normal within 1-4 months of drug secession. Note that prolonged hypogonadotrophic hypogonadism can develop secondary to steroid abuse, necessitating medical intervention.

The above side effects are not inclusive. For more detailed discussion of potential side effects, see the Steroid Side Effects section of this book.

Administration (Men):

Drive has not been approved for use in humans. Prescribing guidelines are unavailable. Typical dosing schedule for physique- or performance-enhancing purposes would be in the range of 220 mg (4mL) to 440 mg (8mL) per week, a level that should provide quality lean mass gain without strong bloating or body fat retention. Due to the high injection volume and fast-acting nature of methandriol dipropionate, the total weekly dosage is commonly divided into 2-3 smaller applications.

Administration (Women):

Drive has not been approved for use in humans. Prescribing guidelines are unavailable. Drugs containing methylandrostenediol are generally not recommended for women for physique- or performance-enhancing purposes due to its androgenic nature and tendency to produce virilizing side effects.

Availability:

Drive is rarely smuggled into the U.S. in noticeable quantity, but can be found on occasion. Its packaging is quite simple and easy to duplicate; most product bearing this name on the black market is actually counterfeit.

Durabolin® (nandrolone phenylpropionate)

Androgenic	37
Anabolic	125
Standard	Testosterone
Chemical Names	19-norandrost-4-en-3-one-17beta-ol
	17beta-hydroxy-estr-4-en-3-one
Estrogenic Activity	low
Progestational Activity	moderate

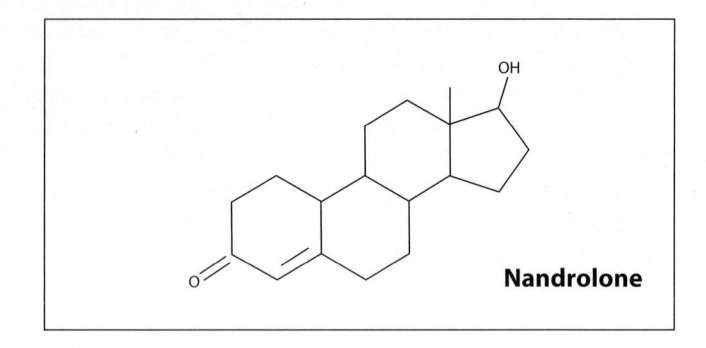

Nandrolone

Description:

Nandrolone phenylpropionate is an injectable form of the anabolic steroid nandrolone. The properties of this drug are strikingly similar to those of Deca-Durabolin®, which uses the slower acting drug nandrolone decanoate. The primary difference between these two preparations is the speed in which nandrolone is released into the blood. While nandrolone decanoate provides a release of nandrolone from the area of injection lasting approximately 3 weeks, nandrolone phenylpropionate is active for only about a week. In clinical situations, Deca-Durabolin can thus be injected once every 2 or 3 weeks, while Durabolin® is usually administered every several days to once weekly. Otherwise, the two drugs are virtually interchangeable. Like Deca-Durabolin, Durabolin is valued by athletes and bodybuilders for its abilities to promote strength and lean muscle mass gains without significant estrogenic or androgenic side effects.

History:

Nandrolone phenylpropionate was first described in 1957.[487] It became a prescription medication shortly after, sold by the international pharmaceuticals giant Organon under the brand name Durabolin. When first introduced to the United States, indicated uses of nandrolone phenylpropionate included pre- and postoperative lean mass retention, osteoporosis, advanced breast cancer, weight loss due to convalescence or disease, geriatric states (general weakness and frailty), burns, severe trauma, ulcers, adjunct therapy with certain forms of anemia, and selective cases of growth and development retardation in children. During the 1970's, the FDA began revising the indicated uses of this drug, however, and they were soon significantly narrowed. Moving forward, the drug was mainly being indicated for the treatment of advanced metastatic breast cancer, and as adjunct therapy for the treatment of senile and post-menopausal osteoporosis.

Durabolin was a key focus of Organon's marketing efforts only for well less than a decade following its release. Once Deca-Durabolin was introduced during the 1960's, this shorter-acting counterpart, although still available, started to take a back seat. Durabolin was not completely abandoned by Organon, however, partly due to the fact that it was given a slightly different set of therapeutic uses in certain countries, and therefore continued to hold onto a niche market. As the size of the anabolic steroid market continued to grow throughout the 1970's and '80's, it was nandrolone decanoate that was attracting the most attention of other drug manufacturers. Numerous drug companies had produced their own versions of nandrolone phenylpropionate over the years, however, and the drug remains fairly available today. Organon continues to sell its original brand of Durabolin as well, but only in select markets, most notably Portugal, India, Malaysia, Indonesia, Netherlands, Finland, and Taiwan.

How Supplied:

Nandrolone phenylpropionate is available in select human drug markets. Composition and dosage may vary by country and manufacturer, but usually contain 25 mg/mL or 50 mg/mL of steroid dissolved in oil.

Structural Characteristics:

Nandrolone phenylpropionate is a modified form of nandrolone, where a carboxylic acid ester (propionic phenyl ester) has been attached to the 17-beta hydroxyl group. Esterified steroids are less polar than free steroids, and are absorbed more slowly from the area of injection. Once in the bloodstream, the ester is removed to yield free (active) nandrolone. Esterified steroids are designed to prolong the window of therapeutic effect following administration, allowing for a less frequent injection schedule compared to injections of free (unesterified) steroid. Nandrolone phenylpropionate provides a sharp spike in nandrolone release 24-48 hours following deep intramuscular injection, and declines to near baseline levels within a week.

Side Effects (Estrogenic):

Nandrolone has a low tendency for estrogen conversion, estimated to be only about 20% of that seen with testosterone.[488] This is because while the liver can convert nandrolone to estradiol, in other more active sites of steroid aromatization such as adipose tissue nandrolone is far less open to this process.[489] Consequently, estrogen-related side effects are a much lower concern with this drug than with testosterone. Elevated estrogen levels may still be noticed with higher dosing, however, and may cause side effects such as increased water retention, body fat gain, and gynecomastia. An anti-estrogen such as clomiphene citrate or tamoxifen citrate may be necessary to prevent estrogenic side effects if they occur. One may alternately use an aromatase inhibitor like Arimidex® (anastrozole), which more efficiently controls estrogen by preventing its synthesis. Aromatase inhibitors can be quite expensive in comparison to anti-estrogens, however, and may also have negative effects on blood lipids.

It is of note that nandrolone has some activity as a progestin in the body.[490] Although progesterone is a c-19 steroid, removal of this group as in 19-norprogesterone creates a hormone with greater binding affinity for its corresponding receptor. Sharing this trait, many 19-nor anabolic steroids are shown to have some affinity for the progesterone receptor as well.[491] The side effects associated with progesterone are similar to those of estrogen, including negative feedback inhibition of testosterone production and enhanced rate of fat storage. Progestins also augment the stimulatory effect of estrogens on mammary tissue growth. There appears to be a strong synergy between these two hormones here, such that gynecomastia might even occur with the help of progestins, without excessive estrogen levels. The use of an anti-estrogen, which inhibits the estrogenic component of this disorder, is often sufficient to mitigate gynecomastia caused by nandrolone.

Side Effects (Androgenic):

Although classified as an anabolic steroid, androgenic side effects are still possible with this substance, especially with higher doses. This may include bouts of oily skin, acne, and body/facial hair growth. Anabolic/androgenic steroids may also aggravate male pattern hair loss. Women are warned of the potential virilizing effects of anabolic/androgenic steroids. These may include a deepening of the voice, menstrual irregularities, changes in skin texture, facial hair growth, and clitoral enlargement. Nandrolone is a steroid with relatively low androgenic activity relative to its tissue-building actions, making the threshold for strong androgenic side effects comparably higher than with more androgenic agents such as testosterone, methandrostenolone, or fluoxymesterone. It is also important to point out that due to its mild androgenic nature and ability to suppress endogenous testosterone, nandrolone is prone to interfering with libido in males when used without another androgen.

Note that in androgen-responsive target tissues such as the skin, scalp, and prostate, the relative androgenicity of nandrolone is reduced by its reduction to dihydronandrolone (DHN).[492][493] The 5-alpha reductase enzyme is responsible for this metabolism of nandrolone. The concurrent use of a 5-alpha reductase inhibitor such as finasteride or dutasteride will interfere with site-specific reduction of nandrolone action, considerably increasing the tendency of nandrolone to produce androgenic side effects. Reductase inhibitors should be avoided with nandrolone if low androgenicity is desired.

Side Effects (Hepatotoxicity):

Nandrolone is not c-17 alpha alkylated, and not known to have hepatotoxic effects. Liver toxicity is unlikely.

Side Effects (Cardiovascular):

Anabolic/androgenic steroids can have deleterious effects on serum cholesterol. This includes a tendency to reduce HDL (good) cholesterol values and increase LDL (bad) cholesterol values, which may shift the HDL to LDL balance in a direction that favors greater risk of arteriosclerosis. The relative impact of an anabolic/androgenic steroid on serum lipids is dependant on the dose, route of administration (oral vs. injectable), type of steroid (aromatizable or non-aromatizable), and level of resistance to hepatic metabolism. Studies administering 600 mg of nandrolone decanoate per week for 10 weeks demonstrated a 26% reduction in HDL cholesterol levels.[494] This suppression is slightly greater than that reported with an equal dose of testosterone enanthate, and is in agreement with earlier studies showing a slightly stronger negative impact on HDL/LDL ratio with nandrolone decanoate as compared to testosterone cypionate.[495] Nandrolone should still have a significantly weaker impact on serum lipids than c-17 alpha alkylated agents. Anabolic/androgenic steroids may also adversely effect blood pressure and triglycerides, reduce endothelial relaxation, and support left ventricular hypertrophy, all potentially increasing the risk of cardiovascular disease and myocardial infarction.

To help reduce cardiovascular strain it is advised to maintain an active cardiovascular exercise program and minimize the intake of saturated fats, cholesterol, and simple carbohydrates at all times during active AAS administration. Supplementing with fish oils (4 grams per

day) and a natural cholesterol/antioxidant formula such as Lipid Stabil or a product with comparable ingredients is also recommended.

Side Effects (Testosterone Suppression):

All anabolic/androgenic steroids when taken in doses sufficient to promote muscle gain are expected to suppress endogenous testosterone production. Studies administering 100 mg injection of nandrolone phenylpropionate demonstrated a rapid suppression of serum testosterone following a single injection. Testosterone levels declined to approximately 30% of initial level by day 3 after drug administration, and stayed suppressed for approximately 13 days. Regular use is expected to significantly lengthen the endogenous hormone recovery window. It is believed that the progestational activity of nandrolone notably contributes to the suppression of testosterone synthesis during therapy, which can be marked in spite of a low tendency for estrogen conversion.[496] Without the intervention of testosterone-stimulating substances, testosterone levels should return to normal within 2-6 months of drug secession. Note that prolonged hypogonadotrophic hypogonadism can develop secondary to steroid abuse, necessitating medical intervention.

The above side effects are not inclusive. For more detailed discussion of potential side effects, see the Steroid Side Effects section of this book.

Administration (Men):

For general anabolic effects, early prescribing guidelines recommend a dosage of 25-50 mg per week for 12 weeks. The usual dosage for physique- or performance-enhancing purposes is in the range of 200-400 mg per week, taken in cycles 8 to 12 weeks in length. This level is sufficient for most users to notice measurable gains in lean muscle mass and strength. Note that due to the fast-acting nature of the phenylpropionate ester, the weekly dosage is usually subdivided into 2 separate applications spaced evenly apart.

Administration (Women):

For general anabolic effects, early prescribing guidelines recommend a dosage of 25-50 mg per week for 12 weeks. When used for physique- or performance-enhancing purposes, a dosage of 50 mg per week (given in a single weekly injection) is most common, taken for cycle lasting 4 to 6 weeks. Higher doses or longer durations of use are discouraged due to potential for androgenic side effects. Although only slightly androgenic, women are occasionally confronted with virilization symptoms when taking this compound. Should virilizing side effects become a concern, nandrolone phenylpropionate should be discontinued immediately to help prevent a permanent appearance.

Availability:

Although produced in a fair number of countries, Durabolin® in not commonly found due to the high selling price and low strength of the Organon preparations. A single 50 mg ampule could cost as much as $15 when sold on the black market, which is usually the same price for 200 mg. Often the only strength available is the 25 mg version, which can be even less cost effective. The Organon preparations are not subject to high levels of counterfeiting, and can usually be trusted when located.

Superanabolon from Spofa in the Czech Republic is also still in manufacture. It contains only 25 mg of steroid per 1 mL ampule, which makes it in relatively low demand among athletes. Still, it is a reputable product, with no major problems of fakes.

Iran Hormone (Iran) makes a 25 mg/mL generic nandrolone phenylpropionate in 1 mL ampules. Counterfeits are not known to be a problem.

Dynabol® (nandrolone cypionate)

Androgenic	37
Anabolic	125
Standard	Testosterone
Chemical Names	19-norandrost-4-en-3-one-17beta-ol
	17beta-hydroxy-estr-4-en-3-one
Estrogenic Activity	low
Progestational Activity	moderate

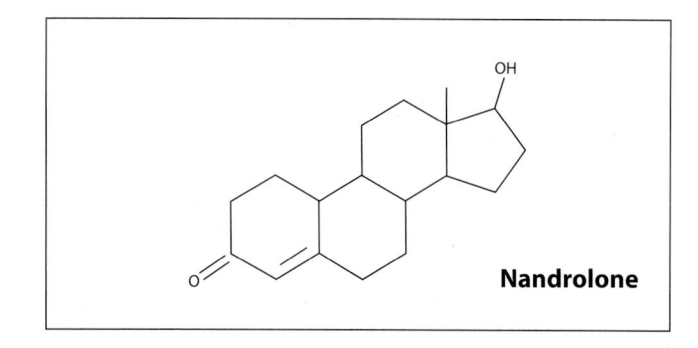

Nandrolone

Description:

Nandrolone cypionate is an injectable form of the anabolic steroid nandrolone. This ester provides a pattern of hormone release virtually identical to that of testosterone cypionate, with peak levels of drug being noted approximately 24-48 hours after administration, and a substantial hormone release sustained for about weeks. In this case the active hormone is nandrolone, which is a moderately strong anabolic steroid that carries mild estrogenic and androgenic properties. This product is essentially identical in overall effect to Deca-Durabolin® (nandrolone decanoate), producing measurable gains in strength and lean muscle mass, which tend to be accompanied by a low level of side effects. The one point of difference is that nandrolone cypionate may appear to be a faster-acting compound to some users. Otherwise, there is no discernable difference between the two compounds, and nandrolone cypionate could replace nandrolone decanoate in virtually all cycles.

History:

Nandrolone cypionate was first developed during the 1960's. It was sold for a brief time as a human-use pharmaceutical, under such brand names as Anabo, Depo-Nortestonate, Nortestrionate, and Sterocrinolo. Such preparations did not last, however, and in recent years the drug has been available only as a product of veterinary medicine. The most notable appearance has come from Jurox in Australia, which marketed a 50 mg/mL version of the drug called Dynabol 50. Jurox also included nandrolone cypionate as part of an anabolic steroid blend called Nandrabolin. Both products, however, were discontinued in 2001, when Jurox scaled back its steroid line. This was likely done in response to media criticisms of heavy Australian veterinary exports to Mexico, which largely fuel the American black market.

The discontinued Jurox products were quickly transferred to SYD Group in Australia, assuring they would not be completely eliminated from commerce. They were subsequently reintroduced to market in 2002, under the names Anabolic DN and Anabolic NA, respectively. The new names made loose reference to the former Jurox trademarks, likely in an effort to retain some of the original market for the products. SYD Group had also introduced a high-dose version of Anabolic DN directly to the Mexican veterinary drug market, but the product has since been withdrawn. This time the product was discontinued following U.S. DEA charges against the firm, alleging that they were conspiring to illegally export Mexican steroids to the U.S. Today, the Anabolic DN and Anabolic NA products remain available on the Australian veterinary drug market, although tight controls limit diversion for off-label use.

How Supplied:

Nandrolone cypionate is available on the Australian veterinary drug markets. It is supplied as 50 mg/mL of steroid dissolved in oil, in a 10 mL vial.

Structural Characteristics:

Nandrolone cypionate is a modified form of nandrolone, where a carboxylic acid ester (cyclopentylpropionic acid) has been attached to the 17-beta hydroxyl group. Esterified steroids are less polar than free steroids, and are absorbed more slowly from the area of injection. Once in the bloodstream, the ester is removed to yield free (active) nandrolone. Esterified steroids are designed to prolong the window of therapeutic effect following administration, allowing for a less-frequent injection schedule compared to injections of free (unesterified) steroid. Nandrolone cypionate provides a sharp spike in nandrolone release 24-48 hours following deep intramuscular injection, and sustains a substantial release of hormone for approximately 2 weeks.

Side Effects (Estrogenic):

Nandrolone has a low tendency for estrogen conversion,

estimated to be only about 20% of that seen with testosterone.[497] This is because while the liver can convert nandrolone to estradiol, in other more active sites of steroid aromatization such as adipose tissue nandrolone is far less open to this process.[498] Consequently, estrogen-related side effects are a much lower concern with this drug than with testosterone. Elevated estrogen levels may still be noticed with higher dosing, however, and may cause side effects such as increased water retention, body fat gain, and gynecomastia. An anti-estrogen such as clomiphene citrate or tamoxifen citrate may be necessary to prevent estrogenic side effects if they occur. One may alternately use an aromatase inhibitor like Arimidex® (anastrozole), which more efficiently controls estrogen by preventing its synthesis. Aromatase inhibitors can be quite expensive in comparison to anti-estrogens, however, and may also have negative effects on blood lipids.

It is of note that nandrolone has some activity as a progestin in the body.[499] Although progesterone is a c-19 steroid, removal of this group as in 19-norprogesterone creates a hormone with greater binding affinity for its corresponding receptor. Sharing this trait, many 19-nor anabolic steroids are shown to have some affinity for the progesterone receptor as well.[500] The side effects associated with progesterone are similar to those of estrogen, including negative feedback inhibition of testosterone production and enhanced rate of fat storage. Progestins also augment the stimulatory effect of estrogens on mammary tissue growth. There appears to be a strong synergy between these two hormones here, such that gynecomastia might even occur with the help of progestins, without excessive estrogen levels. The use of an anti-estrogen, which inhibits the estrogenic component of this disorder, is often sufficient to mitigate gynecomastia caused by nandrolone.

Side Effects (Androgenic):

Although classified as an anabolic steroid, androgenic side effects are still possible with this substance, especially with higher doses. This may include bouts of oily skin, acne, and body/facial hair growth. Anabolic/androgenic steroids may also aggravate male pattern hair loss. Women are warned of the potential virilizing effects of anabolic/androgenic steroids. These may include a deepening of the voice, menstrual irregularities, changes in skin texture, facial hair growth, and clitoral enlargement. Nandrolone is a steroid with relatively low androgenic activity relative to its tissue-building actions, making the threshold for strong androgenic side effects comparably higher than with more androgenic agents such as testosterone, methandrostenolone, or fluoxymesterone. It is also important to point out that due to its mild androgenic nature and ability to suppress endogenous testosterone, nandrolone is prone to interfering with libido in males when used without another androgen.

Note that in androgen-responsive target tissues such as the skin, scalp, and prostate, the relative androgenicity of nandrolone is reduced by its reduction to dihydronandrolone (DHN).[501] [502] The 5-alpha reductase enzyme is responsible for this metabolism of nandrolone. The concurrent use of a 5-alpha reductase inhibitor such as finasteride or dutasteride will interfere with site-specific reduction of nandrolone action, considerably increasing the tendency of nandrolone to produce androgenic side effects. Reductase inhibitors should be avoided with nandrolone if low androgenicity is desired.

Side Effects (Hepatotoxicity):

Nandrolone is not c-17 alpha alkylated, and not known to have hepatotoxic effects. Liver toxicity is unlikely.

Side Effects (Cardiovascular):

Anabolic/androgenic steroids can have deleterious effects on serum cholesterol. This includes a tendency to reduce HDL (good) cholesterol values and increase LDL (bad) cholesterol values, which may shift the HDL to LDL balance in a direction that favors greater risk of arteriosclerosis. The relative impact of an anabolic/androgenic steroid on serum lipids is dependant on the dose, route of administration (oral vs. injectable), type of steroid (aromatizable or non-aromatizable), and level of resistance to hepatic metabolism. Studies administering 600 mg of nandrolone decanoate per week for 10 weeks demonstrated a 26% reduction in HDL cholesterol levels.[503] This suppression is slightly greater than that reported with an equal dose of testosterone enanthate, and is in agreement with earlier studies showing a slightly stronger negative impact on HDL/LDL ratio with nandrolone decanoate as compared to testosterone cypionate.[504] Nandrolone injectables, however, should still have a significantly weaker impact on serum lipids than c-17 alpha alkylated agents. Anabolic/androgenic steroids may also adversely affect blood pressure and triglycerides, reduce endothelial relaxation, and support left ventricular hypertrophy, all potentially increasing the risk of cardiovascular disease and myocardial infarction.

To help reduce cardiovascular strain it is advised to maintain an active cardiovascular exercise program and minimize the intake of saturated fats, cholesterol, and simple carbohydrates at all times during active AAS administration. Supplementing with fish oils (4 grams per day) and a natural cholesterol/antioxidant formula such as

Lipid Stabil or a product with comparable ingredients is also recommended.

Side Effects (Testosterone Suppression):

All anabolic/androgenic steroids when taken in doses sufficient to promote muscle gain are expected to suppress endogenous testosterone production. For sake of comparison, studies administering 100 mg per week of nandrolone decanoate for 6 weeks have demonstrated an approximate 57% reduction in serum testosterone levels during therapy. At a dosage of 300 mg per week, this reduction reached 70%.[505] It is believed that the progestational activity of nandrolone notably contributes to the suppression of testosterone synthesis during therapy, which can be marked in spite of a low tendency for estrogen conversion.[506] Without the intervention of testosterone-stimulating substances, testosterone levels should return to normal within 2-6 months of drug secession. Note that prolonged hypogonadotrophic hypogonadism can develop secondary to steroid abuse, necessitating medical intervention.

The above side effects are not inclusive. For more detailed discussion of potential side effects, see the Steroid Side Effects section of this book.

Administration (Men):

When used for physique- or performance-enhancing purposes, a dose of 200-400 mg per week is most common, taken in cycles 8 to 12 weeks in length. This level is sufficient for most users to notice measurable gains in lean muscle mass and strength, which should be accompanied by a low level of estrogenic and androgenic activity. Although higher doses (450-600 mg) may produce a stronger anabolic effect, given the relatively low concentration in which this drug is found (50 mg/mL), doses above 400 mg are not commonly applied. Instead, the drug is often stacked with another agent, usually an androgen such as an injectable testosterone, which also helps offset the very low level of androgenicity of nandrolone. An oral steroid with pronounced androgenicity, such as methandrostenolone or oxymetholone, is sometimes used as well, but will also present some hepatotoxicity and have a stronger effect on serum lipids (negatively).

Administration (Women):

When used for physique- or performance-enhancing purposes, a dosage of 50 mg per week is most common. Although only slightly androgenic, women are occasionally confronted with virilization symptoms when taking this compound. Should virilizing side effects become a concern, nandrolone cypionate should be discontinued immediately to help prevent their permanent appearance. After a sufficient period of withdrawal, the shorter-acting nandrolone Durabolin® might be considered a safer (more controllable) option. This drug stays active for only several days, greatly reducing the withdrawal time if indicated.

Availability:

The only remaining pure nandrolone cypionate product is Anabolic DN from Australia, produced only in a 50 mg/mL concentration. It comes in the form of a 10 mL vial, which is contained in an orange tube.

Dynabolon® (nandrolone undecanoate)

Androgenic	37
Anabolic	125
Standard	Testosterone

Chemical Names	19-norandrost-4-en-3-one-17beta-ol
	17beta-hydroxy-estr-4-en-3-one
Estrogenic Activity	low
Progestational Activity	moderate

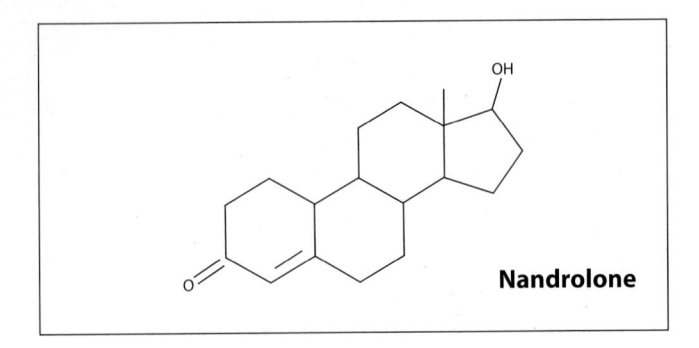

Description:

Nandrolone undecanoate is an injectable form of the anabolic steroid nandrolone. The ester applied here is one carbon atom longer than decanoate, and consequently forms a very slightly longer-lasting drug deposit at the site of injection. With proper attention paid to carrier, concentration, volume, and pharmacokinetics, it would likely even be possible to formulate this steroid into a very long-acting drug preparation, one similar to testosterone undecanoate (Nebido) in appearance. Even without a further protracted therapeutic window, nandrolone undecanoate can be comfortably injected once every 1 to 2 weeks, which reflects its slow-acting nature. Although no longer available, this agent was once highly favored by athletes and bodybuilders for its ability to promote slow steady gains in lean mass with minimal estrogenic or androgenic side effects.

History:

Nandrolone undecanoate was developed during the 1960's, and was subsequently sold as Dynabolon in Italy (Chrinos) and France (Theramex), and as Psychobolan in Germany (Theramex). The Italian product was moved to the new Farmasister label years later, but retained the original Dynabolon trade name. Dynabolon was generally indicated for use in patients suffering from malnutrition, catabolic states, or recovering from major surgery. It was also used to combat osteoporosis, including the treatment of androgen-sensitive populations such as women and the elderly. Nandrolone undecanoate seems to have exhibited a fair safety record, yet in spite of this, the three known commercial preparations did not last on their respective prescription drug markets. Psychobolan from Germany and Dynabolon from Farmasister in Italy were discontinued many years ago, and Dynabolon from France finally followed before the close of the 1990's. Presently, no legitimate pharmaceutical preparation containing nandrolone undecanoate is known to exist.

How Supplied:

Nandrolone undecanoate is no longer available as a prescription drug product. When manufactured, it was supplied at a concentration of 80.5 mg/mL dissolved in oil and sealed in a 1 mL ampule. Each ampule provided the equivalent of 50 mg of nandrolone base.

Structural Characteristics:

Nandrolone undecanoate is a modified form of nandrolone, where a carboxylic acid ester (undecanoic acid) has been attached to the 17-beta hydroxyl group. Esterified steroids are less polar than free steroids, and are absorbed more slowly from the area of injection. Once in the bloodstream, the ester is removed to yield free (active) nandrolone. Esterified steroids are designed to prolong the window of therapeutic effect following administration, allowing for a less-frequent injection schedule compared to injections of free (unesterified) steroid. Nandrolone undecanoate is designed to provide a slow release of nandrolone for up to 3 to 4 weeks following injection.

Side Effects (Estrogenic):

Nandrolone has a low tendency for estrogen conversion, estimated to be only about 20% of that seen with testosterone.[507] This is because while the liver can convert nandrolone to estradiol, in other more active sites of steroid aromatization such as adipose tissue nandrolone is far less open to this process.[508] Consequently, estrogen-related side effects are a much lower concern with this drug than with testosterone. Elevated estrogen levels may still be noticed with higher dosing, however, and may cause side effects such as increased water retention, body fat gain, and gynecomastia. An anti-estrogen such as clomiphene citrate or tamoxifen citrate may be necessary to prevent estrogenic side effects if they occur. One may alternately use an aromatase inhibitor like Arimidex® (anastrozole), which more efficiently controls estrogen by preventing its synthesis. Aromatase inhibitors can be quite expensive in comparison to anti-estrogens, however, and may also have negative effects on blood lipids.

It is of note that nandrolone has some activity as a progestin in the body.[509] Although progesterone is a c-19 steroid, removal of this group as in 19-norprogesterone creates a hormone with greater binding affinity for its corresponding receptor. Sharing this trait, many 19-nor anabolic steroids are shown to have some affinity for the progesterone receptor as well.[510] The side effects associated with progesterone are similar to those of estrogen, including negative feedback inhibition of testosterone production and enhanced rate of fat storage. Progestins also augment the stimulatory effect of estrogens on mammary tissue growth. There appears to be a strong synergy between these two hormones here, such that gynecomastia might even occur with the help of progestins, without excessive estrogen levels. The use of an anti-estrogen, which inhibits the estrogenic component of this disorder, is often sufficient to mitigate gynecomastia caused by nandrolone.

Side Effects (Androgenic):

Although classified as an anabolic steroid, androgenic side effects are still possible with this substance, especially with higher doses. This may include bouts of oily skin, acne, and body/facial hair growth. Anabolic/androgenic steroids may also aggravate male pattern hair loss. Women are warned of the potential virilizing effects of anabolic/androgenic steroids. These may include a deepening of the voice, menstrual irregularities, changes in skin texture, facial hair growth, and clitoral enlargement. Nandrolone is a steroid with relatively low androgenic activity relative to its tissue-building actions, making the threshold for strong androgenic side effects comparably higher than with more androgenic agents such as testosterone, methandrostenolone, or fluoxymesterone. It is also important to point out that due to its mild androgenic nature and ability to suppress endogenous testosterone, nandrolone is prone to interfering with libido in males when used without another androgen.

Note that in androgen-responsive target tissues such as the skin, scalp, and prostate, the relative androgenicity of nandrolone is reduced by its reduction to dihydronandrolone (DHN).[511] [512] The 5-alpha reductase enzyme is responsible for this metabolism of nandrolone. The concurrent use of a 5-alpha reductase inhibitor such as finasteride or dutasteride will interfere with site-specific reduction of nandrolone action, considerably increasing the tendency of nandrolone to produce androgenic side effects. Reductase inhibitors should be avoided with nandrolone if low androgenicity is desired.

Side Effects (Hepatotoxicity):

Nandrolone is not c-17 alpha alkylated, and not known to have hepatotoxic effects. Liver toxicity is unlikely.

Side Effects (Cardiovascular):

Anabolic/androgenic steroids can have deleterious effects on serum cholesterol. This includes a tendency to reduce HDL (good) cholesterol values and increase LDL (bad) cholesterol values, which may shift the HDL to LDL balance in a direction that favors greater risk of arteriosclerosis. The relative impact of an anabolic/androgenic steroid on serum lipids is dependant on the dose, route of administration (oral vs. injectable), type of steroid (aromatizable or non-aromatizable), and level of resistance to hepatic metabolism. Studies administering 600 mg of nandrolone decanoate per week for 10 weeks demonstrated a 26% reduction in HDL cholesterol levels.[513] This suppression is slightly greater than that reported with an equal dose of testosterone enanthate, and is in agreement with earlier studies showing a slightly stronger negative impact on HDL/LDL ratio with nandrolone decanoate as compared to testosterone cypionate.[514] Nandrolone injectables, however, should still have a significantly weaker impact on serum lipids than c-17 alpha alkylated agents. Anabolic/androgenic steroids may also adversely affect blood pressure and triglycerides, reduce endothelial relaxation, and support left ventricular hypertrophy, all potentially increasing the risk of cardiovascular disease and myocardial infarction.

To help reduce cardiovascular strain it is advised to maintain an active cardiovascular exercise program and minimize the intake of saturated fats, cholesterol, and simple carbohydrates at all times during active AAS administration. Supplementing with fish oils (4 grams per day) and a natural cholesterol/antioxidant formula such as Lipid Stabil or a product with comparable ingredients is also recommended.

Side Effects (Testosterone Suppression):

All anabolic/androgenic steroids when taken in doses sufficient to promote muscle gain are expected to suppress endogenous testosterone production. For sake of comparison, studies administering 100 mg per week of nandrolone decanoate for 6 weeks have demonstrated an approximate 57% reduction in serum testosterone levels during therapy. At a dosage of 300 mg per week, this reduction reached 70%.[515] It is believed that the progestational activity of nandrolone notably contributes to the suppression of testosterone synthesis during therapy, which can be marked in spite of a low tendency for estrogen conversion.[516] Without the intervention of testosterone-stimulating substances, testosterone levels should return to normal within 2-6 months of drug secession. Note that prolonged hypogonadotrophic hypogonadism can develop secondary to steroid abuse, necessitating medical intervention.

The above side effects are not inclusive. For more detailed discussion of potential side effects, see the Steroid Side Effects section of this book.

Administration (Men):

Nandrolone undecanoate was used clinically at a dose of 1 ampule every 1 to 2 weeks. A total of 3 to 6 ampules were used for a given 6-week period of therapy. When used for physique- or performance-enhancing purposes, a dose of 3 to 4 ampules (241.5 to 322mg) per week is most common, taken in cycles 8 to 12 weeks in length. This level is sufficient for most users to notice measurable gains in lean muscle mass and strength, which should be accompanied by a low level of estrogenic and androgenic activity. Higher doses (400-600 mg per week) will impart a stronger anabolic effect, but can be difficult given the relatively low concentration this steroid was manufactured in. Instead, many opted to combine this agent with other anabolic/androgenic steroids for a stronger effect. Given its properties, it seems to fit well for both bulking and cutting purposes, and can reasonably replace Deca-Durabolin in such cycles.

Administration (Women):

Nandrolone undecanoate was used clinically at a dose of 1 ampule every 1 to 2 weeks. A total of 3 to 6 ampules were used for a given 6-week period of therapy. When used for physique- or performance-enhancing purposes, a dosage of 1 ampule (80.5 mg) every 10 days was most common, which is taken for 4 to 6 weeks. Although only slightly androgenic, women are occasionally confronted with virilization symptoms when taking this compound. Should virilizing side effects become a concern, the drug should be discontinued immediately to help prevent their permanent appearance. After a sufficient period of withdrawal, the shorter acting nandrolone Durabolin® might be considered a safer (more controllable) option. This drug stays active for only several days, greatly reducing the withdrawal time if indicated.

Availability:

Nandrolone undecanoate is no longer available as a prescription drug product. Some underground preparations are known to exist, but are of unverified quality.

Emdabol (thiomesterone)

Androgenic	61
Anabolic	456
Standard	Methyltestosterone (oral)
Chemical Names	1,7-bis(acetylthio)-17b-hydroxy-17-methylandrost-4-en-3-one
Estrogenic Activity	none
Progestational Activity	none

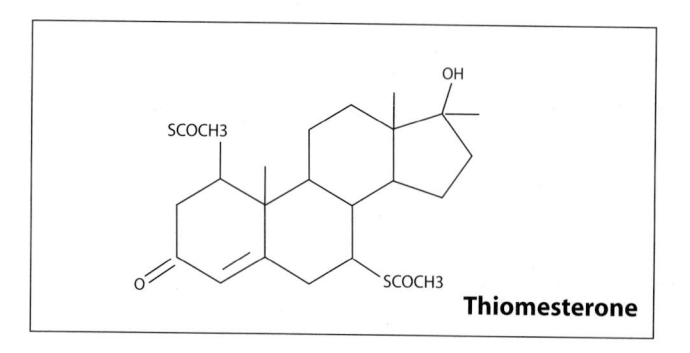

Thiomesterone

Description:

Thiomesterone is an oral anabolic steroid that is derived from testosterone. It is a close chemical cousin of methyltestosterone, although in spite of this association the agent is far more anabolic than it is androgenic in nature. More specifically, standard laboratory assays show that its anabolic potency exceeds its androgenic by a factor of 7.5. Milligram for milligram it is also about 4.5 times more anabolic than methyltestosterone, while having only about 60% of its androgenic component. Although these values may vary somewhat with humans, in regards to potency and anabolic/androgenic separation, thiomesterone is still very much in the same class as the popular anabolics stanozolol and oxandrolone. This drug, though scarcely used by athletes, especially in modern years, was highly valued for its ability to promote lean gains in muscle size and strength without water retention or significant side effects.

History:

Thiomesterone was first described in 1964.[517] It was developed by E. Merck AG, and presented as a medicine at the 16th German Therapy Congress and Pharmaceutical Exhibition.[518] Merck had given the agent the trivial name thiomesterone (tiomesterone), and would sell it in Germany under the trademark name Emdabol. This steroid was designed for oral administration, and was indicated for all consumptive illnesses and for cachectic states. Essentially, it was applied as a general anabolic substance when weight gain (lean body mass) was necessary due to severe illness or debilitation. Merck described the drug to the public for the first time in 1964, stating, "Its anabolic activity is twice that of methyltestosterone. It has an extremely favorable anabolic/androgenic index and is said to exhibit no gestagenic or mineralocorticoid side-effects."

Following the release of the drug in Germany, thiomesterone would be produced by AB Drago in Sweden, sold as Protabol. Merck would also sell it for a brief time in Spain as Vitabonifen Forte, which was a vitamin preparation that included thiomesterone and other ingredients. Vitabonifen Forte was used to treat a loss of strength with aging, lean body mass wasting, and osteoporosis. This preparation also included bromelains, which are concentrated proteolytic enzymes from the pineapple plant used to help aid the digestion of proteins from whole foods. Outside of Europe, the drug was even more scarcely produced. The only preparation of note was Emdabolin, made by Chugai Labs in Tokyo, Japan. All such thiomesterone preparations have since been removed from commerce, however, and the drug is no longer available to athletes as a commercial product.

Thiomesterone was always more whisper than substance in athletic circles. While available, it saw extremely limited use even by European athletes, due to its very limited supply. It has, likewise, gone practically unseen in the United States. Thirty years ago, American bodybuilders were treated only to rumors of thiomesterone, and how this rare and highly coveted steroid was the holy grail of anabolic steroids. Nobody could obtain a cycle to vary its effect, however, which only further fed the myth. Little was known about the compound in the West at the time; even its chemical structure was elusive. Dan Duchaine mentions in his Underground Steroid Handbook II only, "This is the elusive thiomesterone, always written up in the research as the most promising, most potent anabolic with no androgenic side effects. Let me know if you ever find any." Few other books even discussed it at all.

Although there has been little real-world feedback on this steroid over the years to make reference of, there is enough known about its pharmacological properties to paint a more complete picture than we had before. As detailed above, its anabolic and androgenic properties were assayed, and were shown to be quite favorable. Studies published in 1966 also showed that thiomesterone was more effective than equal doses of methyltestosterone, methandrostenolone, or methenolone acetate for blocking the catabolic actions of corticosteroid treatment on bone mass.[519] Still, its effects are consistent with that of other potent anabolic agents, and nothing unusual has been found of note. While thiomesterone may indeed be an effective drug with a low inclination for side effects, it is certainly not the "pure" anabolic agent it was rumored to be thirty years ago. Simply stated, it is a steroid that retains very favorable properties if one is looking for a primarily tissue-building (as opposed to masculinizing) steroid, and would behave in a very similar manner to Anavar (oxandrolone) for most users.

How Supplied:

Thiomesterone is no longer available as a prescription agent. When manufactured, it came in the form of an oral tablet.

Structural Characteristics:

Thiomesterone is a modified form of testosterone. It differs by 1) the addition of a methyl group at carbon 17-alpha, which helps protect the hormone during oral administration, and 2) the addition of two thioacetyl groups, one at carbon 1 and the other at carbon 7, which inhibit aromatization and 5-alpha reduction and shift the anabolic to androgenic ratio in favor of the former. Thiomesterone has significantly enhanced anabolic potency relative to methyltestosterone, with reduced androgenicity.

Side Effects (Estrogenic):

Thiomesterone is not aromatized by the body, and is not measurably estrogenic. An anti-estrogen is not necessary when using this steroid, as gynecomastia should not be a concern even among sensitive individuals. Since estrogen is the usual culprit with water retention, clostebol instead produces a lean, quality look to the physique with no fear of excess subcutaneous fluid retention. This makes it a favorable steroid to use during cutting cycles, when water and fat retention are major concerns.

Side Effects (Androgenic):

Although classified as an anabolic steroid, androgenic side effects are still possible with this substance. This may include bouts of oily skin, acne, and body/facial hair growth. Anabolic/androgenic steroids may also aggravate male pattern hair loss. Women are also warned of the potential virilizing effects of anabolic/androgenic steroids. These may include a deepening of the voice, menstrual irregularities, changes in skin texture, facial hair growth, and clitoral enlargement. Additionally, the 5-alpha reductase enzyme does not metabolize thiomesterone, so its relative androgenicity is not affected by finasteride or dutasteride. Note that thiomesterone is a steroid with very low androgenic activity relative to its tissue-building actions, making the threshold for strong androgenic side effects comparably higher than with more androgenic agents such as testosterone, methandrostenolone, or fluoxymesterone.

Side Effects (Hepatotoxicity):

Thiomesterone is a c17-alpha alkylated compound. This alteration protects the drug from deactivation by the liver, allowing a very high percentage of the drug entry into the bloodstream following oral administration. C17-alpha alkylated anabolic/androgenic steroids can be hepatotoxic. Prolonged or high exposure may result in liver damage. In rare instances life-threatening dysfunction may develop. It is advisable to visit a physician periodically during each cycle to monitor liver function and overall health. Intake of c17-alpha alkylated steroids is commonly limited to 6-8 weeks, in an effort to avoid escalating liver strain.

The use of a liver detoxification supplement such as Liver Stabil, Liv-52, or Essentiale Forte is advised while taking any hepatotoxic anabolic/androgenic steroids.

Side Effects (Cardiovascular):

Anabolic/androgenic steroids can have deleterious effects on serum cholesterol. This includes a tendency to reduce HDL (good) cholesterol values and increase LDL (bad) cholesterol values, which may shift the HDL to LDL balance in a direction that favors greater risk of arteriosclerosis. The relative impact of an anabolic/androgenic steroid on serum lipids is dependant on the dose, route of administration (oral vs. injectable), type of steroid (aromatizable or non-aromatizable), and level of resistance to hepatic metabolism. Although not extensively studied in humans, the high relative potency and non-aromatizable nature of thiomesterone suggests that this agent is extremely prone to negatively altering lipid values and increasing atherogenic risk. Anabolic/androgenic steroids may also adversely affect blood pressure and triglycerides, reduce endothelial relaxation, and support left ventricular hypertrophy, all potentially increasing the risk of cardiovascular disease and myocardial infarction.

To help reduce cardiovascular strain it is advised to maintain an active cardiovascular exercise program and minimize the intake of saturated fats, cholesterol, and simple carbohydrates at all times during active AAS administration. Supplementing with fish oils (4 grams per day) and a natural cholesterol/antioxidant formula such as Lipid Stabil or a product with comparable ingredients is also recommended.

Side Effects (Testosterone Suppression):

All anabolic/androgenic steroids when taken in doses sufficient to promote muscle gain are expected to suppress endogenous testosterone production. Without the intervention of testosterone-stimulating substances, testosterone levels should return to normal within 1-4 months of drug secession. Note that prolonged hypogonadotrophic hypogonadism can develop secondary to steroid abuse, necessitating medical intervention.

The above side effects are not inclusive. For more detailed discussion of potential side effects, see the Steroid Side Effects section of this book.

Administration (General):

Studies have shown that taking an oral anabolic steroid with food may decrease its bioavailability.[520] This is caused by the fat-soluble nature of steroid hormones, which can allow some of the drug to dissolve with undigested dietary fat, reducing its absorption from the gastrointestinal tract. For maximum utilization, this steroid should be taken on an empty stomach.

Administration (Men):

Effective doses for physique- or performance-enhancing purposes fall in the range of 15-25 mg per day, taken for no more than 6-8 weeks to minimize hepatic stress. Here, one is likely to see measurable lean tissue gains, modest strength increases, greater muscle definition, and heightened vascularity. Thiomesterone is a very versatile steroid in general, and should stack well with other mild injectable anabolics like Primobolan or Deca-Durabolin for cutting cycles, or stronger androgens/aromatizable steroids like testosterone or boldenone for bulking phases. The fact that estrogen levels will be kept low makes this agent very favorable when it comes to tightening up or contest preparations. Its low androgenic and estrogenic components, however, may put many of this drug's more sensitive users at risk for incurring a loss of libido and even lethargic side effects. This is often corrected by the addition of some other aromatizable or more androgenic compound (testosterone would be the preferred remedy).

Administration (Women):

Effective doses for physique- or performance-enhancing purposes fall in the range of 5 mg per day or less, taken for no longer than 4-6 weeks to minimize the chance for virilizing side effects. Note that while thiomesterone is highly anabolic relative to its androgenic properties, side effects are still possible, and should be carefully monitored.

Availability:

Thiomesterone is no longer available as a prescription agent at this time, and is unavailable on the black market.

Equilon 100 (boldenone blend)

Androgenic	50
Anabolic	100
Standard	Testosterone
Chemical Names	1,4-androstadiene-3-one,17beta-ol / 1-dehydrotestosterone
Estrogenic Activity	low
Progestational Activity	no data available (low)

Boldenone

Description:

Equilon is an injectable steroid containing a blend of four boldenone esters. Specifically, each milliliter contains 10 mg of boldenone acetate, 30 mg of boldenone propionate, 40 mg of boldenone cypionate, and 20 mg of boldenone undecylenate. The total steroid concentration of the product is 100 mg/mL. As a boldenone product, Equilon provides a strong anabolic effect with only moderate androgenic and estrogenic activity. The main difference between Equilon and the more popular boldenone injectable Equipoise lies in the pharmacokinetics of the preparations. Serum levels of boldenone are likely to peak more quickly with Equilon due to the inclusion of short chain esters, even if only slightly. The time to peak release with Equipoise shouldn't be more than several days, however, and it is highly likely that its release pattern would actually be more even over time compared to Equilon. Still, this item could essentially be considered a close counterpart of Equipoise, and for all intents and purposes could replace Equipoise milligram for milligram in most applications.

History:

Equilon is a product of WDV Pharma Co., Ltd, a veterinary steroid manufacturer based in Yangon, Myanmar. This is the same company that makes a seven-ester blend of testosterone called Equitest, which has garnered some attention in the athletic community due to its unusual nature. As with Equitest, the target species of this product is horses and cattle, though it is widely diverted for human use. It is indicated for the treatment of animals suffering from debilitating conditions, which may be aided by the lean-tissue preserving and anti-catabolic effects of anabolic steroids. The recommended dose is 1-3ml given to the animal every 10 days, as needed.

Equilon is the first multi-component boldenone product to be commercially developed, and in this regard it too stands out as a unique product. The design of this preparation is supposed to be such that boldenone levels spike very quickly due to the acetate and propionate, the two "fast-acting" esters, but are sustained in a more even pattern due to their combination with "slow-acting" esters cypionate and undecylenate. In reality, however, such slow/fast blends tend to be more a product of marketing than science, as even the supposed slow-acting esters like cypionate and undecylenate produce their peak hormone release within a few days of injection at most. Regardless, products like this tend to have strong market value, so Equilon is likely to sit well with bodybuilders who have liked Equipoise in the past.

How Supplied:

Equilon is manufactured in Myanmar only. The product is supplied in a multi-dose glass vial (6ml), which contains an oily solution; each milliliter contains 10 mg of boldenone acetate, 30 mg of boldenone propionate, 40 mg of boldenone cypionate, and 20 mg of boldenone undecylenate.

Structural Characteristics:

Boldenone is a modified form of testosterone. It differs by the introduction of a double bond between carbons 1 and 2, which reduces its relative estrogenicity and androgenicity. Equilon contains boldenone modified with the addition of carboxylic acid esters (acetic, propionic, cyclopentylpropionic, and undecylenoic acids) at the 17-beta hydroxyl group. Esterified steroids are less polar than free steroids, and are absorbed more slowly from the area of injection. Once in the bloodstream, the ester is removed to yield free (active) boldenone. Esterified steroids are designed to prolong the window of therapeutic effect following administration, allowing for a less frequent injection schedule compared to injections of free (unesterified) steroid. Equilon is designed to provide a peak release of boldenone approximately 24-48 hours after injection, and sustain hormone release for approximately 21-28 days.

Side Effects (Estrogenic):

Boldenone is aromatized in the body to estradiol (estrogen). Elevated estrogen levels can cause side effects such as increased water retention, body fat gain, and gynecomastia. Boldenone is considered a mildly estrogenic steroid. Aromatization studies suggest that its rate of conversion to estradiol is roughly half that of testosterone.[521] The tendency to develop noticeable estrogenic side effects with boldenone should be slightly higher than nandrolone, but much lower than with testosterone. Estrogenic side effects are usually not pronounced unless this drug is taken in doses above 200-400 mg per week. An anti-estrogen such as clomiphene citrate or tamoxifen citrate might be used to help mitigate these side effects, should they become present. One may alternately use an aromatase inhibitor like Arimidex® (anastrozole), although it is considerably more expensive, and may negatively effect blood lipids.

Side Effects (Androgenic):

Although classified as an anabolic steroid, androgenic side effects are still common with this substance, especially with higher doses. This may include bouts of oily skin, acne, and body/facial hair growth. Anabolic/androgenic steroids may also aggravate male pattern hair loss. Women are also warned of the potential virilizing effects of anabolic/androgenic steroids. These may include a deepening of the voice, menstrual irregularities, changes in skin texture, facial hair growth, and clitoral enlargement.

Note that while boldenone does reduce to a more potent androgen (dihydroboldenone) via the 5-alpha reductase enzyme in androgen-responsive target tissues such as the skin, scalp, and prostate, its affinity to do so in the human body is extremely low.[522] The relative androgenicity of boldenone is, therefore, not significantly affected by finasteride or dutasteride.

Side Effects (Hepatotoxicity):

Boldenone is not c-17 alpha alkylated, and not known to have hepatotoxic effects. Liver toxicity is unlikely.

Side Effects (Cardiovascular):

Anabolic/androgenic steroids can have deleterious effects on serum cholesterol. This includes a tendency to reduce HDL (good) cholesterol values and increase LDL (bad) cholesterol values, which may shift the HDL to LDL balance in a direction that favors greater risk of arteriosclerosis. The relative impact of an anabolic/androgenic steroid on serum lipids is dependant on the dose, route of administration (oral vs. injectable), type of steroid (aromatizable or non-aromatizable), and level of resistance to hepatic metabolism. Anabolic/androgenic steroids may also adversely affect blood pressure and triglycerides, reduce endothelial relaxation, and support left ventricular hypertrophy, all potentially increasing the risk of cardiovascular disease and myocardial infarction. Boldenone is likely to have a less dramatic impact on cardiovascular risk factors than synthetic oral anabolic steroids. This is due in part to its openness to metabolism by the liver, which allows it to have less effect on the hepatic management of cholesterol. The aromatization of boldenone to estradiol may also help to mitigate the negative effects of androgens on serum lipids.

To help reduce cardiovascular strain it is advised to maintain an active cardiovascular exercise program and minimize the intake of saturated fats, cholesterol, and simple carbohydrates at all times during active AAS administration. Supplementing with fish oils (4 grams per day) and a natural cholesterol/antioxidant formula such as Lipid Stabil or a product with comparable ingredients is also recommended.

Side Effects (Testosterone Suppression):

All anabolic/androgenic steroids when taken in doses sufficient to promote muscle gain are expected to suppress endogenous testosterone production. Without the intervention of testosterone-stimulating substances, testosterone levels should return to normal within 1-4 months of drug secession. Note that prolonged hypogonadotrophic hypogonadism can develop secondary to steroid abuse, necessitating medical intervention.

The above side effects are not inclusive. For more detailed discussion of potential side effects, see the Steroid Side Effects section of this book.

Administration (Men):

Although it stays active for a much longer time, Equilon is typically injected at least weekly for physique- or performance-enhancing purposes. It is most commonly used at a dosage of 200-400 mg (2-4ml) per week for 6-12 weeks. This level is sufficient to notice significant increases in strength and lean mass.

Administration (Women):

When used for physique- or performance-enhancing purposes, women take much lower doses of boldenone than men. This would suggest typically 50-75 mg of Equilon per week. Women should take caution with the slow-acting characteristics of this preparation, which make blood levels difficult to control and slow to decline should virilization symptoms become present.

Availability:

Equilon is not widely distributed on the black market, mainly because it is only produced by one company and is not well known among the athletic community. It still can be located on occasion, however. Counterfeits are not known to be a significant problem.

Equipoise® (boldenone undecylenate)

Androgenic	50
Anabolic	100
Standard	Testosterone
Chemical Names	1,4-androstadiene-3-one,17beta-ol 1-dehydrotestosterone
Estrogenic Activity	low
Progestational Activity	no data available (low)

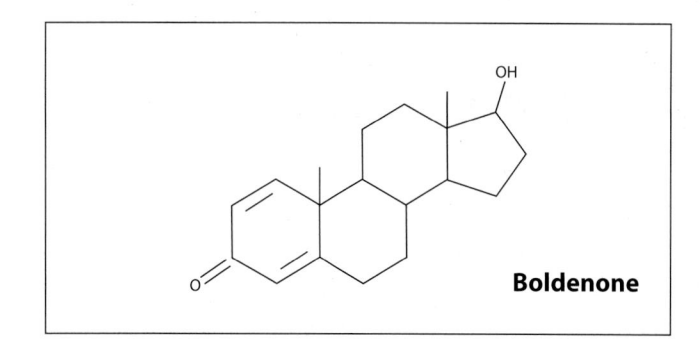

Description:

Boldenone undecylenate is an injectable veterinary steroid that exhibits strong anabolic and moderately androgenic properties. The undecylenate ester extends the activity of the drug greatly (the undecylenate ester is only one carbon atom longer than decanoate), so that injections need to be repeated only once every 3 or 4 weeks. The well-balanced anabolic and androgenic properties of this drug are greatly appreciated by athletes, who generally consider it to be a stronger, slightly more androgenic, alternative to Deca-Durabolin®. It is generally cheaper, and could replace Deca in most cycles without greatly changing the end result. Boldenone undecylenate is also commonly known as a drug capable of increasing red blood cell production, although there should be no confusion that this is an effect characteristic of nearly all anabolic/androgenic steroids.

History:

Ciba reportedly patented boldenone as a synthetic anabolic steroid in 1949. During the 1950's and '60's, the firm developed several experimental esters of the drug, and would later release a long-acting form of the agent (briefly) in the form of boldenone undecylenate. It would be sold under the brand name Parenabol, which likely referred to its characteristics as a parenteral (injectable) anabolic agent. Parenabol saw some clinical use during the late '60's and early '70's, mainly as a lean-tissue-preserving anabolic agent in cases of wasting, and for the retention of bone mass with osteoporosis. Boldenone undecylenate was a short-lived preparation on human medical markets, however, and would be discontinued globally before the end of the 1970's. Squibb would ultimately be most famous for introducing this agent in the veterinary market, and would sell it under its now most famous trade name, Equipoise.

In the veterinary market, boldenone undecylenate is most commonly applied to horses, although in many regions it is indicated for use in other animals as well. It generally exhibits a pronounced effect on lean bodyweight, appetite, and general disposition of the animal. The Equipoise brand was sold under the Squibb label until 1985, when Solvay acquired Squibb's U.S. animal health business. Equipoise would be sold under the Solvay label for the next several years, until Wyeth finally acquired the animal health division of Solvay in 1995. The division was formed into Fort Dodge Animal Health, which continues to market Equipoise in the U.S. and certain markets abroad today. Many other generic and brand name forms of boldenone undecylenate exist in numerous international drug markets, owing to the fact that any patents on boldenone undecylenate have long since expired.

How Supplied:

Boldenone undecylenate is widely available in veterinary drug markets. Composition and dosage may vary by country and manufacturer; the majority of products are supplied as multi-dose glass vials containing an oily solution; usually carrying 25 mg/ml or 50 mg/ml of steroid.

Structural Characteristics:

Boldenone is a modified form of testosterone. It differs by the introduction of a double bond between carbons 1 and 2, which reduces its relative estrogenicity and androgenicity. Equipoise® contains boldenone modified with the addition of carboxylic acid ester (undecylenoic acid) at the 17-beta hydroxyl group. Esterified steroids are less polar than free steroids, and are absorbed more slowly from the area of injection. Once in the bloodstream, the ester is removed to yield free (active) boldenone. Esterified steroids are designed to prolong the window of therapeutic effect following administration, allowing for a less frequent injection schedule compared to injections of free (unesterified) steroid. Boldenone undecylenate is designed to provide a peak release of boldenone within a few days after injection, and sustain hormone release for approximately 21-28 days.

It is interesting to note that structurally boldenone and methandrostenolone (Dianabol) are almost identical. In the case of boldenone (as applied here), the compound uses a 17-beta ester (undecylenate) to facilitate administration, while methandrostenolone accomplishes this with the use of a 17-alpha alkyl group. Aside from this, the molecules are the same. Of course they act quite differently in the body, which goes to show that the 17-methylation affects more than just the oral efficacy of an anabolic/androgenic steroid.

Side Effects (Estrogenic):

Boldenone is aromatized in the body to estradiol (estrogen). Elevated estrogen levels can cause side effects such as increased water retention, body fat gain, and gynecomastia. Boldenone is considered a mildly estrogenic steroid. Aromatization studies suggest that its rate of conversion to estradiol is roughly half that of testosterone.[523] The tendency to develop noticeable estrogenic side effects with boldenone should be slightly higher than nandrolone, but much lower than with testosterone. Estrogenic side effects are usually not pronounced unless this drug is taken in doses above 200-400 mg per week. An anti-estrogen such as clomiphene citrate or tamoxifen citrate might be used to help mitigate these side effects, should they become present. One may alternately use an aromatase inhibitor like Arimidex® (anastrozole), although it is considerably more expensive, and may negatively affect blood lipids.

Side Effects (Androgenic):

Although classified as an anabolic steroid, androgenic side effects are still common with this substance, especially with higher doses. This may include bouts of oily skin, acne, and body/facial hair growth. Anabolic/androgenic steroids may also aggravate male pattern hair loss. Women are also warned of the potential virilizing effects of anabolic/androgenic steroids. These may include a deepening of the voice, menstrual irregularities, changes in skin texture, facial hair growth, and clitoral enlargement.

Note that while boldenone does reduce to a more potent androgen (dihydroboldenone) via the 5-alpha reductase enzyme in androgen-responsive target tissues such as the skin, scalp, and prostate, its affinity to do so in the human body is extremely low.[524] The relative androgenicity of boldenone is, therefore, not significantly affected by finasteride or dutasteride.

Side Effects (Hepatotoxicity):

Boldenone is not c-17 alpha alkylated, and not known to have hepatotoxic effects. Liver toxicity is unlikely.

Side Effects (Cardiovascular):

Anabolic/androgenic steroids can have deleterious effects on serum cholesterol. This includes a tendency to reduce HDL (good) cholesterol values and increase LDL (bad) cholesterol values, which may shift the HDL to LDL balance in a direction that favors greater risk of arteriosclerosis. The relative impact of an anabolic/androgenic steroid on serum lipids is dependant on the dose, route of administration (oral vs. injectable), type of steroid (aromatizable or non-aromatizable), and level of resistance to hepatic metabolism. Anabolic/androgenic steroids may also adversely affect blood pressure and triglycerides, reduce endothelial relaxation, and support left ventricular hypertrophy, all potentially increasing the risk of cardiovascular disease and myocardial infarction. Boldenone is likely to have a less dramatic impact on cardiovascular risk factors than synthetic oral anabolic steroids. This is due in part to its openness to metabolism by the liver, which allows it to have less effect on the hepatic management of cholesterol. The aromatization of boldenone to estradiol may also help to mitigate the negative effects of androgens on serum lipids.

To help reduce cardiovascular strain it is advised to maintain an active cardiovascular exercise program and minimize the intake of saturated fats, cholesterol, and simple carbohydrates at all times during active AAS administration. Supplementing with fish oils (4 grams per day) and a natural cholesterol/antioxidant formula such as Lipid Stabil or a product with comparable ingredients is also recommended.

Side Effects (Testosterone Suppression):

All anabolic/androgenic steroids when taken in doses sufficient to promote muscle gain are expected to suppress endogenous testosterone production. Without the intervention of testosterone-stimulating substances, testosterone levels should return to normal within 1-4 months of drug secession. Note that prolonged hypogonadotrophic hypogonadism can develop secondary to steroid abuse, necessitating medical intervention.

The above side effects are not inclusive. For more detailed discussion of potential side effects, see the Steroid Side Effects section of this book.

Administration (Men):

Although it stays active for a much longer time, boldenone undecylenate is injected at least weekly for physique- or performance-enhancing purposes. It is most commonly used at a dosage of 200-400 mg (4-8ml, 50 mg version) per week. The dosage schedule can be further divided to reduce the volume of each injection if necessary, perhaps administering the drug two to three times per week. One should also take caution to rotate injection sites regularly, so as to avoid irritation or infection.

Not a rapid mass builder, boldenone undecylenate instead provides a slow but steady gain of strength and quality muscle mass. The positive effects of this drug become most apparent when it is used for longer cycles, usually lasting 8 weeks or more in duration. The muscle gained should also not be the smooth bulk associated with testosterone, but more defined and solid. Since water bloat is not contributing greatly to the diameter of the muscle, more of the visible size gained on a cycle of boldenone undecylenate should be retained after the drug has been discontinued.

Boldenone undecylenate is a very versatile drug, and can be combined with a number of other agents depending on the desired result. For mass, it is commonly stacked with an injectable testosterone such as enanthate or cypionate. This should produce strong gains in muscle size and strength, without the same intensity of side effects of using testosterone (at a higher dose) alone. During a cutting phase, muscle hardness and density can be greatly improved when combining boldenone undecylenate with a non-aromatizable steroid such as trenbolone acetate or methenolone enanthate. Oral c-17 alpha alkylated agents such as fluoxymesterone or stanozolol may also be used, but will present some level of hepatotoxicity. For some, even the low buildup of estrogen associated with this compound is enough to relegate its use to bulking cycles only.

Administration (Women):

When used for physique- or performance-enhancing purposes, women take much lower doses of boldenone undecylenate than men, typically 50-75 mg per week. Women should take caution with the slow-acting characteristics of this preparation, which make blood levels difficult to control and slow to decline should virilization symptoms become present.

Availability:

Boldenone undecylenate is widely traded on the black market. Counterfeits are also common. Below are some of the more popular legitimate brands in circulation.

Equipoise® is produced in the United States by the Fort Dodge Company. The Fort Dodge products are sold readily in Mexico, and afterwards smuggled back into the U.S. Legitimate vials are made of clear glass, and carry a label with a shiny metallic surface on the under side. Fakes are very abundant of this item, however, so be careful while shopping.

Ganabol, which is produced in a number of South American countries, is still a popular brand in the United States as well. It is seen in two strengths (25 mg/mL and 50 mg/mL) and in five sizes (10, 50, 100, 250, and 500 mL). There have been numerous fakes of this product in the past, so be careful when shopping.

The Legacy brand name product from Tecnoquimicas in Argentina seems to be reaching the U.S. as of late, at least in small volume. This product carries 50 mg/mL of steroid in a 50 mL vial. At this time the Legacy product is very low on the radar, and probably can be trusted when located.

The brands Boldenona and Boldegan from Gen-Far are also popular in South America, and occasionally smuggled into the United States. These are low-dose (50 mg/mL) preparations. Like Ganabol, they come in a variety of vial sizes. Counterfeits do not appear to be a big issue at this time, making these products fairly trustworthy items when located on the black market.

Equitest 200 (Testosterone blend)

Androgenic	100
Anabolic	100
Standard	Standard
Chemical Names	4-androsten-3-one-17beta-ol
	17beta-hydroxy-androst-4-en-3-one
Estrogenic Activity	moderate
Progestational Activity	low

Testosterone

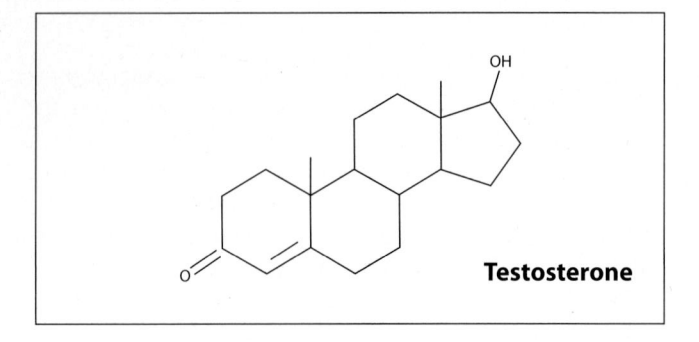

Description:

Equitest 200 is an injectable steroid preparation that contains seven different esters of testosterone. Specifically, each milliliter of oil contains 10 mg of testosterone acetate, 30 mg of testosterone propionate, 20 mg of testosterone phenylpropionate, 20 mg of testosterone caproate, 40 mg of testosterone heptanoate (enanthate), 20 mg of testosterone cyclopentylpropionate (cypionate), and 60 mg of testosterone Decanoate. This blended ester formulation is supposed to result in a rapid increase in testosterone level, followed by a sustained hormone elevation for approximately 3 weeks. The design of this steroid is very similar to Sustanon®, although it contains a slightly different and more extensive blend of testosterones. As a testosterone product, Equitest is capable of producing rapid gains in size and strength.

Upon close analysis, Equitest offers no real advantages over Sustanon. Its seven esters all have very similar pharmacokinetic properties to the four esters found in Sustanon, and will display a great deal of similarity in regards to the pattern of testosterone release. Furthermore, blended-ester preparations like these are pharmacologically inferior to testosterone cypionate or enanthate to begin with, as they provide a stronger supraphysiological spike of testosterone the first days of therapy, and an overall greater imbalance between the beginning and later days of each application window. The seven esters are good for marketing, however, as many buyers will identify this product as containing seven different steroids in one.

History:

Equitest 200 was developed by WDV Pharma, which is a veterinary drug manufacturer based in Myanmar. This company has been operating since the early 1990's, and offers a full line of veterinary drug products (only a few are anabolic steroids). The small size and remoteness of this company in relation to the most active steroid markets would normally have allowed it to stay very low on the radar. However, a couple of their products are unusual enough to catch the attention of dealers and importers looking for marketable items to sell. This includes the seven-testosterone blend of Equitest, as well as their 4-component boldenone injectable called Equilon 100. Equitest 200 remains available today, but is not widely distributed on the global market.

How Supplied:

Equitest 200 is produced as a veterinary drug product in Myanmar. It contains 200 mg of testosterone ester per milliliter; packaged in 6ml vials.

Structural Characteristics:

Equitest 200 contains a mixture of seven testosterone compounds, which where modified with the addition of carboxylic acid esters (acetic, propionic, propionic phenyl ester, caproic, enanthoic, cyclopentylpropionic, and decanoic acids) at the 17-beta hydroxyl group. Esterified forms of testosterone are less polar than free testosterone, and are absorbed more slowly from the area of injection. Once in the bloodstream, the ester is removed to yield free (active) testosterone. Esterified forms of testosterone are designed to prolong the window of therapeutic effect following administration, allowing for a less frequent injection schedule compared to injections of free (unesterified) steroid. Equitest 200 is designed to provide a rapid peak in testosterone levels (24-48 hours after injection), and maintain elevated concentrations for approximately 21 days.

Side Effects (Estrogenic):

Testosterone is readily aromatized in the body to estradiol (estrogen). The aromatase (estrogen synthetase) enzyme is responsible for this metabolism of testosterone. Elevated estrogen levels can cause side effects such as increased water retention, body fat gain, and gynecomastia.

Testosterone is considered a moderately estrogenic steroid. An anti-estrogen such as clomiphene citrate or tamoxifen citrate may be necessary to prevent estrogenic side effects. One may alternately use an aromatase inhibitor like Arimidex® (anastrozole), which more efficiently controls estrogen by preventing its synthesis. Aromatase inhibitors can be quite expensive in comparison to anti-estrogens, however, and may also have negative effects on blood lipids.

Estrogenic side effects will occur in a dose-dependant manner, with higher doses (above normal therapeutic levels) of testosterone more likely to require the concurrent use of an anti-estrogen or aromatase inhibitor. Since water retention and loss of muscle definition are common with higher doses of testosterone, this drug is usually considered a poor choice for dieting or cutting phases of training. Its moderate estrogenicity makes it more ideal for bulking phases, where the added water retention will support raw strength and muscle size, and help foster a stronger anabolic environment.

Side Effects (Androgenic):

Testosterone is the primary male androgen, responsible for maintaining secondary male sexual characteristics. Elevated levels of testosterone are likely to produce androgenic side effects including oily skin, acne, and body/facial hair growth. Men with a genetic predisposition for hair loss (androgenetic alopecia) may notice accelerated male pattern balding. Those concerned about hair loss may find a more comfortable option in nandrolone decanoate, which is a comparably less androgenic steroid. Women are warned of the potential virilizing effects of anabolic/androgenic steroids, especially with a strong androgen such as testosterone. These may include deepening of the voice, menstrual irregularities, changes in skin texture, facial hair growth, and clitoral enlargement.

In androgen-responsive target tissues such as the skin, scalp, and prostate, the high relative androgenicity of testosterone is dependant on its reduction to dihydrotestosterone (DHT). The 5-alpha reductase enzyme is responsible for this metabolism of testosterone. The concurrent use of a 5-alpha reductase inhibitor such as finasteride or dutasteride will interfere with site-specific potentiation of testosterone action, lowering the tendency of testosterone drugs to produce androgenic side effects. It is important to remember that anabolic and androgenic effects are both mediated via the cytosolic androgen receptor. Complete separation of testosterone's anabolic and androgenic properties is not possible, even with total 5-alpha reductase inhibition.

Side Effects (Hepatotoxicity):

Testosterone does not have hepatotoxic effects; liver toxicity is unlikely. One study examined the potential for hepatotoxicity with high doses of testosterone by administering 400 mg of the hormone per day (2,800 mg per week) to a group of male subjects. The steroid was taken orally so that higher peak concentrations would be reached in hepatic tissues compared to intramuscular injections. The hormone was given daily for 20 days, and produced no significant changes in liver enzyme values including serum albumin, bilirubin, alanine-aminotransferase, and alkaline phosphatases.[525]

Side Effects (Cardiovascular):

Anabolic/androgenic steroids can have deleterious effects on serum cholesterol. This includes a tendency to reduce HDL (good) cholesterol values and increase LDL (bad) cholesterol values, which may shift the HDL to LDL balance in a direction that favors greater risk of arteriosclerosis. The relative impact of an anabolic/androgenic steroid on serum lipids is dependant on the dose, route of administration (oral vs. injectable), type of steroid (aromatizable or non-aromatizable), and level of resistance to hepatic metabolism. Anabolic/androgenic steroids may also adversely affect blood pressure and triglycerides, reduce endothelial relaxation, and support left ventricular hypertrophy, all potentially increasing the risk of cardiovascular disease and myocardial infarction.

Testosterone tends to have a much less dramatic impact on cardiovascular risk factors than synthetic steroids. This is due in part to its openness to metabolism by the liver, which allows it to have less effect on the hepatic management of cholesterol. The aromatization of testosterone to estradiol also helps to mitigate the negative effects of androgens on serum lipids. In one study, 280 mg per week of testosterone ester (enanthate) had a slight but not statistically significant effect on HDL cholesterol after 12 weeks, but when taken with an aromatase inhibitor a strong (25%) decrease was seen.[526] Studies using 300 mg of testosterone ester (enanthate) per week for 20 weeks without an aromatase inhibitor demonstrated only a 13% decrease in HDL cholesterol, while at 600 mg the reduction reached 21%.[527] The negative impact of aromatase inhibition should be taken into consideration before such drug is added to testosterone therapy.

Due to the positive influence of estrogen on serum lipids, tamoxifen citrate or clomiphene citrate are preferred to aromatase inhibitors for those concerned with cardiovascular health, as they offer a partial estrogenic effect in the liver. This allows them to potentially improve lipid profiles and offset some of the negative effects of androgens. With doses of 600 mg or less per week, the impact on lipid profile tends to be noticeable but not dramatic, making an anti-estrogen (for cardioprotective purposes) perhaps unnecessary. Doses of 600 mg or less per week have also failed to produce statistically significant changes in LDL/VLDL cholesterol, triglycerides, apolipoprotein B/C-III, C-reactive protein, and insulin sensitivity, all indicating a relatively weak impact on cardiovascular risk factors.[528] When used in moderate doses, injectable testosterone esters are usually considered to be the safest of all anabolic/androgenic steroids.

To help reduce cardiovascular strain it is advised to maintain an active cardiovascular exercise program and minimize the intake of saturated fats, cholesterol, and simple carbohydrates at all times during active AAS administration. Supplementing with fish oils (4 grams per day) and a natural cholesterol/antioxidant formula such as Lipid Stabil or a product with comparable ingredients is also recommended.

Side Effects (Testosterone Suppression):

All anabolic/androgenic steroids when taken in doses sufficient to promote muscle gain are expected to suppress endogenous testosterone production. Testosterone is the primary male androgen, and offers strong negative feedback on endogenous testosterone production. Testosterone-based drugs will, likewise, have a strong effect on the hypothalamic regulation of natural steroid hormones. Without the intervention of testosterone-stimulating substances, testosterone levels should return to normal within 1-4 months of drug secession. Note that prolonged hypogonadotrophic hypogonadism can develop secondary to steroid abuse, necessitating medical intervention.

The above side effects are not inclusive. For more detailed discussion of potential side effects, see the Steroid Side Effects section of this book.

Administration (Men):

For bodybuilding purposes, this drug is usually injected on a weekly basis, at a dosage of 200-600 mg. Cycles are generally between 6 and 12 weeks in length. This level is sufficient to provide excellent gains in muscle size and strength. Testosterone drugs are ultimately very versatile, and can be combined with many other anabolic/androgenic steroids depending on the desired effect.

Administration (Women):

Equitest 200 is not recommended for women for physique- or performance-enhancing purposes due to its strong androgenic nature, tendency to produce virilizing side effects, and slow-acting characteristics (making blood levels difficult to control).

Availability:

Equitest 200 is circulated on the black market, but not in high volume. Counterfeits are not yet known to be a significant problem.

Ermalone (mestanolone)

Androgenic	78-254
Anabolic	107
Standard	Testosterone
Chemical Name	17a-methyl-4,5a-dihydrotestosterone
Estrogenic Activity	none
Progestational Activity	none

Description:

Mestanolone is an oral analog of dihydrotestosterone. This steroid is a 17-alpha methylated form of this potent endogenous androgen, being essentially (in structure) to DHT what methyltestosterone is to testosterone. Overall, mestanolone has an activity profile not very dissimilar from the hormone it is derived from. For starters, like DHT, mestanolone is primarily androgenic in nature, displaying a low level of anabolic activity. Both DHT and mestanolone are also devoid of estrogenic activity, which eliminates the chance for estrogenic side effects like water retention, fat deposition, and gynecomastia. In fact, both should be measurably anti-estrogenic in effect, inhibiting the aromatase enzyme in a competitive and dose-dependant manner. Among athletes, this drug is valued for its ability to promote pure strength gains and improved aggression and focus, with minimal gains in total bodyweight.

History:

Dihydrotestosterone was first synthesized in 1935.[529] Mestanolone, trivial name for the 17-alpha alkylated form of dihydrotestosterone, was produced shortly after. To spite such an old history as an investigatory agent, however, this steroid has been scarcely used in clinical medicine. The only noteworthy preparation to appear during the last forty years has been Ermalone, which was manufactured for a short period of time by Roussel Pharmaceuticals in Germany. It has since been discontinued, however. Many things probably led to the general abandonment of this steroid in the pharmaceutical industry, including an increased number of alternative agents, a lack of financial viability, and a reassessment of its tissue-building and hepatotoxic properties.

Most of the studies on mestanolone took place during the 1950's and '60's. This was a period when a great deal of drug development was taking place. Many new compounds were being introduced, and many old ones were being reassessed for potential value. Although mestanolone had been synthesized long before, the drug was seeing revitalized interest by researchers due to more recent assays showing that the agent could provide both strong androgenic and anabolic effects. For a short period of time it was believed that mestanolone would be a palatable tissue-building agent. Not long after, however, the general consensus about this agent came to be that it was an androgen, not really a strong anabolic, and that its risk profile (hepatotoxicity, lipid alterations) probably did not warrant its use over other commercial androgen preparations.

Although it had a weak history as a prescription medicine, mestanolone was one of the oldest and most-valued secrets of the East German doping machine, the infamous state-sponsored doping program of the 1970s and '80s that developed advanced systematic techniques designed to assist drug-tested athletes avoid detection. This program allowed East German athletes to evade countless urine tests and become a dominant force in Olympic sports throughout much of the Cold War era. Mestanolone was valued not for its potency as a muscle builder, but for its abilities as a pure and powerful androgen. Its effects were largely focused on the central nervous system and neuromuscular interaction. Athletes would routinely comment that while the drug would not make them huge, it was very capable of improving speed, strength, aggression, endurance, and resistance to stress. Drug tested or not, mestanolone remains intrinsically valuable today as a fast-acting oral androgen capable of providing tangible benefits to many users.

How Supplied:

Mestanolone is no longer available as a prescription agent. When manufactured, it came in the form of an oral tablet.

Structural Characteristics:

Mestanolone is a modified form of dihydrotestosterone. It differs by the addition of a methyl group at carbon 17-

alpha, which helps protect the hormone during oral administration.

Side Effects (Estrogenic):

Mestanolone is not aromatized by the body, and is not measurably estrogenic. An anti-estrogen is not necessary when using this steroid, as gynecomastia should not be a concern even among sensitive individuals. Note that due to its structural similarity to dihydrotestosterone, mestanolone likely also has inherent anti-estrogenic properties, competing with aromatizable substrates for binding to the aromatase enzyme.

Side Effects (Androgenic):

Mestanolone is an androgen. Higher than normal therapeutic doses are likely to produce androgenic side effects including oily skin, acne, and body/facial hair growth. Men with a genetic predisposition for hair loss (androgenetic alopecia) may notice accelerated male pattern balding. Women are warned of the potential virilizing effects of anabolic/androgenic steroids, especially with such a strong androgen. These may include deepening of the voice, menstrual irregularities, changes in skin texture, facial hair growth, and clitoral enlargement. Note that mestanolone is unaffected by the 5-alpha reductase enzyme, so its relative androgenicity is not affected by the concurrent use of finasteride or dutasteride.

Side Effects (Hepatotoxicity):

Mestanolone is a c17-alpha alkylated compound. This alteration protects the drug from deactivation by the liver, allowing a very high percentage of the drug entry into the bloodstream following oral administration. C17-alpha alkylated anabolic/androgenic steroids can be hepatotoxic. Prolonged or high exposure may result in liver damage. In rare instances life-threatening dysfunction may develop. It is advisable to visit a physician periodically during each cycle to monitor liver function and overall health. Intake of c17-alpha alkylated steroids is commonly limited to 6-8 weeks, in an effort to avoid escalating liver strain.

The use of a liver detoxification supplement such as Liver Stabil, Liv-52, or Essentiale Forte is advised while taking any hepatotoxic anabolic/androgenic steroids.

Side Effects (Cardiovascular):

Anabolic/androgenic steroids can have deleterious effects on serum cholesterol. This includes a tendency to reduce HDL (good) cholesterol values and increase LDL (bad) cholesterol values, which may shift the HDL to LDL balance in a direction that favors greater risk of arteriosclerosis. The relative impact of an anabolic/androgenic steroid on serum lipids is dependant on the dose, route of administration (oral vs. injectable), type of steroid (aromatizable or non-aromatizable), and level of resistance to hepatic metabolism. Mestanolone has a strong effect on the hepatic management of cholesterol due to its non-aromatizable nature, structural resistance to liver breakdown, and route of administration. Anabolic/androgenic steroids may also adversely affect blood pressure and triglycerides, reduce endothelial relaxation, and support left ventricular hypertrophy, all potentially increasing the risk of cardiovascular disease and myocardial infarction.

To help reduce cardiovascular strain it is advised to maintain an active cardiovascular exercise program and minimize the intake of saturated fats, cholesterol, and simple carbohydrates at all times during active AAS administration. Supplementing with fish oils (4 grams per day) and a natural cholesterol/antioxidant formula such as Lipid Stabil or a product with comparable ingredients is also recommended.

Side Effects (Testosterone Suppression):

All anabolic/androgenic steroids when taken in doses sufficient to promote muscle gain are expected to suppress endogenous testosterone production. Without the intervention of testosterone-stimulating substances, testosterone levels should return to normal within 1-4 months of drug secession. Note that prolonged hypogonadotrophic hypogonadism can develop secondary to steroid abuse, necessitating medical intervention.

The above side effects are not inclusive. For more detailed discussion of potential side effects, see the Steroid Side Effects section of this book.

Administration (Men):

Effective doses for physique- or performance-enhancing purposes fall in the range of 10-20 mg per day, taken for no more than 6-8 weeks to minimize hepatic stress. At this level mestanolone should impart considerable strength gains, and may also aid in the speed performance of competitive athletes. Provided diet is adequate, this androgen should also promote fat loss, and will increase muscular definition by reducing the level of water retention.

Administration (Women):

Mestanolone is not recommended for women for physique- or performance-enhancing purposes due to its strong androgenic nature and tendency to produce virilizing side effects.

Availability:

Mestanolone is no longer in commercial production. Several underground laboratories have released products containing the agent, however, making it available on the black market.

Esiclene® (formebolone, formyldienolone)

Androgenic	no data available
Anabolic	no data available
Standard	
Chemical Names	11alpha,17beta-Dihydroxy-17-methyl-3-oxoandrosta-1,4-dien-2-carboxaldehyde Formyldienolone
Estrogenic Activity	none
Progestational Activity	no data available (low)

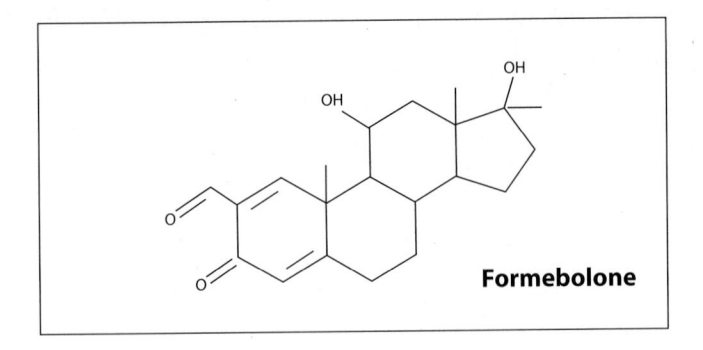

Formebolone

Description:

Formebolone is an anabolic steroid derived from testosterone. More specifically, it is a close cousin of Dianabol, although this steroid has been extensively modified in comparison. Among other traits, formebolone is unable to convert to estrogen, and exhibits even less relative androgenicity in comparison. The drug is generally viewed as a very weak anabolic by athletes, and is not commonly used for building muscle. It is, however, very effective in one very novel way. When given by injection, the drug formebolone irritates the muscle tissue at the site of administration. The body will respond to this with a localized inflammation, which will cause an increase in the overall diameter of the treated muscle. This irritation can be uncomfortable, however, so each ampule of LPB Esiclene contains 20 mg of added lidocaine (a local painkiller) to make the injection less painful. While this does compensate somewhat, Esiclene is still relatively uncomfortable to use. The procedure is usually endured for the results, which can be dramatic in a very short period of time.

History:

Formebolone was first extensively studied in Italy during the early 1970's.[530][531][532] It was developed as a steroid with increased anabolic activity and reduced androgenicity compared to testosterone, with a focus on the tissue-building functions of the hormone and reducing its unwanted side effects. It was produced as both an oral and injectable medication, and was distributed in Europe. The most notable manufacturer was LPB in Italy, which sold the drug under the Esiclene brand name. It was also sold in Portugal as Esiclene (Biofarma), and in Spain as Hubernol (Hubber). Formebolone was used clinically as an anabolic agent, often to treat populations susceptible to the androgenic effects of steroids including women, the elderly, and children. In 1985, the drug was even tried as a growth-promoting agent in children with short stature, and produced significant increases in bone mass and linear height.[533] It was proving to be a favorable and mild anabolic agent, with minimal side effects when used in clinical doses.

In spite of its favorable efficacy and patient safety record, formebolone was ultimately not very successful as a commercial steroid product. Its availability would soon be in question. Of the listed brands, Hubernol from Spain would be the first product to be voluntarily withdrawn from the marketplace by its manufacturer. Esiclene by Biofarma soon followed. Towards the end of the 1990's, the last remaining preparations worldwide to contain formebolone were the Esiclene products from LPB in Italy. Their producer too would soon discontinue these offerings, and by 2004, most residual stock of Esiclene had completely dried up. For the first time since its release decades earlier, the drug had officially gone out of commerce. Formebolone remains unavailable to bodybuilders today as a prescription preparation.

How Supplied:

Formebolonee is not available as a prescription drug product. When manufactured, it was commonly found in the form of 5 mg tablets and a 2mg/ml injectable solution.

Structural Characteristics:

Formebolone is a modified form of testosterone. It differs by 1) the addition of a methyl group at carbon 17-alpha, which helps protect the hormone during oral administration, 2) the introduction of a double bond between carbons 1 and 2 (1-ene), which shifts the anabolic to androgenic ratio in favor of the former, 3) the attachment of hydroxylgroup at carbon 11, which inhibits steroid aromatization (the modification at C-2 also accomplishes this), and 4) the attachment of a formyl group at carbon 2, which further reduces the androgenic to anabolic ratio and overall potency of the steroid.

Side Effects (Estrogenic):

Formebolone is not aromatized by the body, and is not

measurably estrogenic. An anti-estrogen is not necessary when using this steroid, as gynecomastia should not be a concern even among sensitive individuals. Since estrogen is the usual culprit with water retention, this steroid instead produces a lean, quality look to the physique with no fear of excess subcutaneous fluid retention. This makes it a favorable steroid to use during cutting cycles, when water and fat retention are major concerns.

Side Effects (Androgenic):

Although formebolone is classified as an anabolic steroid, androgenic side effects are still possible with this substance. These may include bouts of oily skin, acne, and body/facial hair growth. Doses higher than normally prescribed are more likely to cause such side effects. Anabolic/androgenic steroids may also aggravate male pattern hair loss. Women are additionally warned of the potential virilizing effects of anabolic/androgenic steroids. These may include a deepening of the voice, menstrual irregularities, changes in skin texture, facial hair growth, and clitoral enlargement. Formebolone is unaffected by the 5-alpha reductase enzyme, so its relative androgenicity is not affected by the concurrent use of finasteride or dutasteride. Note that formebolone is a steroid with relatively low androgenic activity relative to its tissue-building actions, making the threshold for strong androgenic side effects comparably higher than with more androgenic agents such as testosterone, methandrostenolone, or fluoxymesterone.

Side Effects (Hepatotoxicity):

Formebolone is a c17-alpha alkylated compound. This alteration protects the drug from deactivation by the liver, allowing a very high percentage of the drug entry into the bloodstream following oral administration. C17-alpha alkylated anabolic/androgenic steroids can be hepatotoxic. Prolonged or high exposure may result in liver damage. In rare instances life-threatening dysfunction may develop. It is advisable to visit a physician periodically during each cycle to monitor liver function and overall health. Intake of c17-alpha alkylated steroids is commonly limited to 6-8 weeks, in an effort to avoid escalating liver strain.

The use of a liver detoxification supplement such as Liver Stabil, Liv-52, or Essentiale Forte is advised while taking any hepatotoxic anabolic/androgenic steroids.

Side Effects (Cardiovascular):

Anabolic/androgenic steroids can have deleterious effects on serum cholesterol. This includes a tendency to reduce HDL (good) cholesterol values and increase LDL (bad) cholesterol values, which may shift the HDL to LDL balance in a direction that favors greater risk of arteriosclerosis. The relative impact of an anabolic/androgenic steroid on serum lipids is dependant on the dose, route of administration (oral vs. injectable), type of steroid (aromatizable or non-aromatizable), and level of resistance to hepatic metabolism. Formebolone has a strong effect on the hepatic management of cholesterol due to its non-aromatizable nature, structural resistance to liver breakdown, and route of administration (the oral should have a slightly stronger negative impact here compared to the injectable). Anabolic/androgenic steroids may also adversely affect blood pressure and triglycerides, reduce endothelial relaxation, and support left ventricular hypertrophy, all potentially increasing the risk of cardiovascular disease and myocardial infarction.

To help reduce cardiovascular strain it is advised to maintain an active cardiovascular exercise program and minimize the intake of saturated fats, cholesterol, and simple carbohydrates at all times during active AAS administration. Supplementing with fish oils (4 grams per day) and a natural cholesterol/antioxidant formula such as Lipid Stabil or a product with comparable ingredients is also recommended.

Side Effects (Testosterone Suppression):

All anabolic/androgenic steroids when taken in doses sufficient to promote muscle gain are expected to suppress endogenous testosterone production. Without the intervention of testosterone-stimulating substances, testosterone levels should return to normal within 1-4 months of drug secession. Note that prolonged hypogonadotrophic hypogonadism can develop secondary to steroid abuse, necessitating medical intervention.

The above side effects are not inclusive. For more detailed discussion of potential side effects, see the Steroid Side Effects section of this book.

Administration (General):

Studies have shown that taking an oral anabolic steroid with food may decrease its bioavailability.[534] This is caused by the fat-soluble nature of steroid hormones, which can allow some of the drug to dissolve with undigested dietary fat, reducing its absorption from the gastrointestinal tract. For maximum utilization, oral forms of this steroid should be taken on an empty stomach.

Administration (Men):

A common clinical dose of formebolone is estimated to be 5 mg per day; actual prescribing guidelines are unavailable. In the athletic arena, an effective oral daily dosage falls in the range of 15-40 mg, taken in cycles lasting no more than 6-8 weeks to minimize hepatotoxicity. This level is sufficient for noticeable increases in lean tissue mass, strength, and hardness, with little "bulking" effect to be seen. When the injectable form of formebolone is used for site enhancement, it is important to note that the swelling produced by this drug is only temporary. It will usually take only a week after the last injection was given for the swelling to subside. For this reason, injectable Esiclene is really only used during the last week or two before a competition. It is also usually injected on a daily basis into each lagging muscle site. Those trying to stretch out the dosage schedule may opt to inject every other day, but generally no longer of an interval is used. When stretched too many days apart, the accumulated swelling will likely not reach a desirable point.

In order to keep this procedure more comfortable, the full dosage is not to be given from the onset of the regimen. Instead, the user will generally begin with half of an ampule, or 1 mL (2mg) per muscle. After a number of days the dosage is increased to 2 mL, or a full ampule for each individual injection site. After continuing at this dosage for a week or two, one can possibly see an increase of 1 or 1.5 inches in their arm and calf measurements. This is clearly a tremendous improvement for only two weeks' use. In addition, those who have used this steroid often report the drug produces an increase in overall muscle hardness. This is an added benefit when preparing for a contest, as a large, hard, and defined muscle body is the obvious goal. Over the years, a large number of male and female competitors have relied heavily on this drug for their exceptional show physiques. Esiclene injections have no doubt been the difference between winning and losing for many competitors.

It is also very important to stress that injectable Esiclene does not work well as a site-enhancement agent for every muscle group. Bodybuilders experimenting with this compound have generally found that it is most effective with the smaller muscle groups such as the biceps, deltoid, and calf. The resultant swelling will equate to a very favorable size increase in these small muscles, looking much larger and fuller, but natural. When trying to inject Esiclene into larger muscles like the chest, back, and legs, however, one can run into trouble. The result in this case can be a very uneven look, producing lumps in the muscle body instead of a total overall size increase. For this reason, the large muscle groups are usually off limits unless the user is very experienced with the practice and his or her personal results with it.

Administration (Women):

A common clinical dose of formebolone is estimated to be 5 mg per day; actual prescribing guidelines are unavailable. In the athletic arena, an effective oral daily dosage falls in the range of 5-10 mg, taken in cycles lasting no more than 4-6 weeks. Virilizing effects are unlikely at this level of use, although cannot be excluded.

Availability:

All forms of Esiclene have been discontinued, and are no longer available on the black market.

Estandron (testosterone/estrogen blend)

Androgenic	
Anabolic	
Standard	
Chemical Names	
Estrogenic Activity	
Progestational Activity	

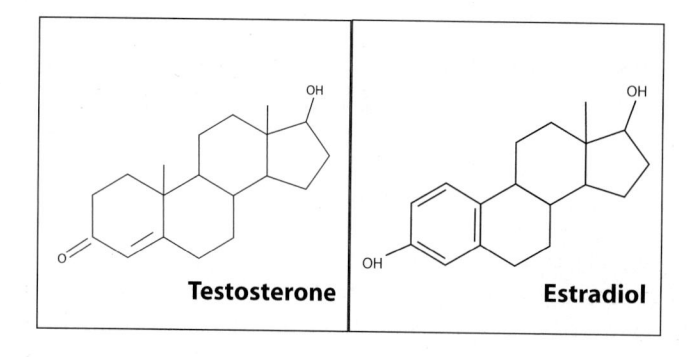

Description:

Estandron is a combination testosterone and estrogen product made for injection. This particular product is made by Organon, although many variants of such a testosterone plus estrogen formulations can be found. At first glance the constituents of Estandron look very familiar to Sustanon 100. It begins with a small dose of testosterone propionate (20 mg), followed by equal amounts of testosterone phenylpropionate and testosterone isocaproate (40 mg of each). The result is a 100 mg/mL mix of testosterone that is ester-for-ester and milligram-for-milligram equivalent to this lower-dosed version of Sustanon. The only differences are the addition of 1mg of estradiol benzoate and 4mg of estradiol phenylpropionate, which have been included to provide estrogen to the patient as well (this product is intended for clinical use with women). While this preparation does carry a formidable dose of testosterone, it is not widely used by athletes and bodybuilders, particularly men, due to its high level of estrogenicity.

History:

Estandron is but one of many combination testosterone/estrogen products developed over the years. These products have historically been used with women in clinical medicine when the anabolic/androgenic effects of testosterone are desired in addition to the therapeutic benefits of estrogens. This includes the treatment of osteoporosis, menopause, breast cancer, and the suppression of lactation. Such applications are not as popular today as they were in the past, however, given that many other medications are available that are better suited for the needs of patients. The one key exception is the recent reemergence of low doses of testosterone with estrogen replacement therapy for menopause, which is proving to have numerous benefits with women when it comes to the support of lean tissue mass, bone density, energy, and sexual vigor. Estandron is often used specifically for the loss of libido and energy with menopause, although it contains far too much testosterone to be widely used for this purpose.

Estandron is not widely used outside of clinical medicine. Some female bodybuilders interested in testosterone do experiment with this drug, believing the added estrogen makes it a drug for women. While true in a clinical sense, when used at the higher doses needed for bodybuilding purposes, testosterone is generally not recommended for women. The very rare male athlete will attempt its use, and may find that the estrogen helps with lipid values. Most will not go near the drug though, given that the estrogenicity of testosterone is usually more than enough to deal with during a cycle. Estandron is still fairly available for those interested, although Organon seems to be supporting the drug much less these days. It has already been discontinued in some European markets, including Italy and Austria. The most notable countries it is still being sold in include the Netherlands (Estandron Prolongatum), Chile (Estandron Prolongado), Brazil (Estandron P), Egypt (Estandron), and Turkey (Estandron Prolongatum).

How Supplied:

Estandron is available in select human drug markets. All products are supplied in 1 mL glass ampules or pre-loaded syringes containing an oily solution; sold by or under license from Organon.

Structural Characteristics:

Estandron contains a mixture of three testosterone compounds, which where modified with the addition of carboxylic acid esters (propionic, propionic phenyl ester, and isocaproic acids) at the 17-beta hydroxyl group. The preparation also contains two esterified forms of estrogen: estradiol benzoate and estradiol phenylpropionate. Esterified steroids are less polar than free steroids, and are absorbed more slowly from the area of injection. Once in the bloodstream, the ester is removed to yield free (active) hormone. Estandron is designed to provide a rapid peak in testosterone and estrogen levels (24-48 hours after injection), and maintain physiological concentrations for approximately 21-28 days.

Side Effects (Estrogenic):

Testosterone is readily aromatized in the body to estradiol (estrogen). Additionally, this preparation contains two forms of active estrogen. Elevated estrogen levels can cause side effects such as increased water retention, body fat gain, and gynecomastia. This steroid preparation is considered to be highly estrogenic. An anti-estrogen such as clomiphene citrate or tamoxifen citrate may be necessary to prevent estrogenic side effects. One may alternately use an aromatase inhibitor like Arimidex® (anastrozole), although it will not have an effect on the additional estrogens present in the preparation. Since water retention and loss of muscle definition are common with highly estrogenic steroid products, this drug is usually considered a poor choice for dieting or cutting phases of training. It would only be appropriate during bulking phases, where the added water retention will support raw strength and muscle size, and help foster a stronger anabolic environment.

Side Effects (Androgenic):

Testosterone is the primary male androgen, responsible for maintaining secondary male sexual characteristics. Elevated levels of testosterone are likely to produce androgenic side effects including oily skin, acne, and body/facial hair growth. Men with a genetic predisposition for hair loss (androgenetic alopecia) may notice accelerated male pattern balding. Those concerned about hair loss may find a more comfortable option in nandrolone decanoate, which is a comparably less androgenic steroid. Women are warned of the potential virilizing effects of anabolic/androgenic steroids, especially with a strong androgen such as testosterone. These may include deepening of the voice, menstrual irregularities, changes in skin texture, facial hair growth, and clitoral enlargement.

Side Effects (Hepatotoxicity):

Testosterone and estrogen do not have hepatotoxic effects; liver toxicity is unlikely.

Side Effects (Cardiovascular):

Anabolic/androgenic steroids can have deleterious effects on serum cholesterol. This includes a tendency to reduce HDL (good) cholesterol values and increase LDL (bad) cholesterol values, which may shift the HDL to LDL balance in a direction that favors greater risk of arteriosclerosis. The relative impact of an anabolic/androgenic steroid on serum lipids is dependant on the dose, route of administration (oral vs. injectable), type of steroid (aromatizable or non-aromatizable), and level of resistance to hepatic metabolism. Testosterone tends to have a much less dramatic impact on cardiovascular risk factors than synthetic steroids. This is due in part to its openness to metabolism by the liver, which allows it to have less effect on the hepatic management of cholesterol. The aromatization of testosterone to estradiol also helps to mitigate the negative effects of androgens on serum lipids. The added estrogens in this product may further help to offset some of the androgenic effect on lipid values, and the preparation may, therefore, have a weaker impact on cholesterol than a comparably dosed straight testosterone product. Anabolic/androgenic steroids may also adversely affect blood pressure and triglycerides, reduce endothelial relaxation, and support left ventricular hypertrophy, all potentially increasing the risk of cardiovascular disease and myocardial infarction.

To help reduce cardiovascular strain it is advised to maintain an active cardiovascular exercise program and minimize the intake of saturated fats, cholesterol, and simple carbohydrates at all times during active AAS administration. Supplementing with fish oils (4 grams per day) and a natural cholesterol/antioxidant formula such as Lipid Stabil or a product with comparable ingredients is also recommended.

Side Effects (Testosterone Suppression):

All anabolic/androgenic steroids when taken in doses sufficient to promote muscle gain are expected to suppress endogenous testosterone production. Testosterone is the primary male androgen, and offers strong negative feedback on endogenous testosterone production. The added estrogens will also provide negative-feedback suppression. This preparation should have a strong effect on the hypothalamic regulation of natural steroid hormones. Without the intervention of testosterone stimulating substances, testosterone levels should return to normal within 1-4 months of drug secession. Note that prolonged hypogonadotrophic hypogonadism can develop secondary to steroid abuse, necessitating medical intervention.

The above side effects are not inclusive. For more detailed discussion of potential side effects, see the Steroid Side Effects section of this book.

Administration (General):

Testosterone propionate is often regarded as a painful injection. This is due to the very short carbon chain of the propionic acid ester, which can be irritating to tissues at the site of injection. Many sensitive individuals choose to stay away from this steroid completely, their bodies reacting with a pronounced soreness and low-grade fever that may last for a few days after each injection.

Administration (Men):

Estandron is not approved for use in men. Prescribing guidelines are unavailable. When used for physique- or performance-enhancing purposes (very rarely), this steroid preparation is usually included in a stack with other compounds, in an effort to offset some of the negative effects of testosterone on lipid values. Here, it is administered at a dosage of 1 ampule per week, and usually taken for no longer than 6-12 weeks. This level will provide a replacement level dose of testosterone to help support muscle growth during a bulking phase, and should also provide a sufficient level of estrogen to affect lipids positive (compared to testosterone alone). Higher doses are likely to exacerbate estrogen-related side effects, and are generally not advised. This product is not widely used by male athletes and bodybuilders due to the estrogen content.

Administration (Women):

Estandron is used with women to treat a loss of libido and energy with menopause, when estrogens alone were insufficient to elicit a desired response. The recommended dose is 1 ampule every 4 weeks. This interval may be extended if the level is deemed to provide too much androgenic stimulation. Estandron is not generally recommended for women for physique- or performance-enhancing purposes due to its strong androgenic nature, tendency to produce virilizing side effects, and slow acting characteristics (making blood levels difficult to control). For those that choose to administer the drug, it is recommended to stay within normal prescribing guidelines, as increasing the dose above the recommended level is very likely to induce significant virilizing side effects.

Availability:

Given the extremely poor demand for mixed testosterone and estrogen preparations in general on the black market, Estandron is scarcely seen in circulation. It does occasionally appear, and when it does it is usually trusted, as it is highly unlikely this drug will be counterfeited. There is very little financial motive to do so (and in all probability it would be a losing investment for anyone that tried). If you do come across one of the various Organon preparations, and have a need for it, you can probably make your purchase with confidence that you are getting what you paid for.

Fherbolico (nandrolone cyclohexylpropionate)

Androgenic	37
Anabolic	125
Standard	Testosterone

Chemical Names	19-norandrost-4-en-3-one-17beta-ol
	17beta-hydroxy-estr-4-en-3-one
Estrogenic Activity	low
Progestational Activity	moderate

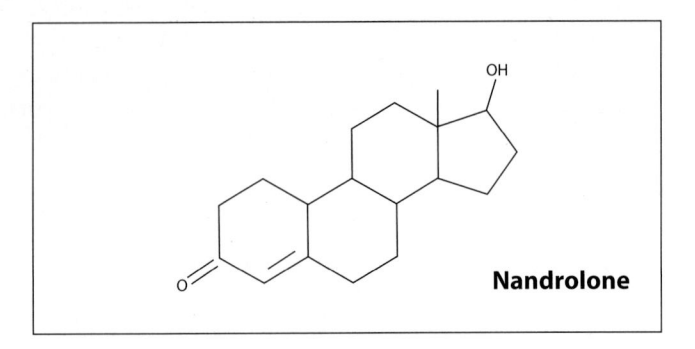

Nandrolone

Description:

Nandrolone cyclohexylpropionate is an injectable form of the anabolic steroid nandrolone. The cyclohexylpropionate ester used here is very similar in structure to cypionate (cyclopentylpropionate). It differs only by the use of a 6-carbon-atom cyclohexane ring, instead of cypionate's 5-carbon-atom cyclopentane ring. This agent is slightly longer acting than nandrolone cypionate, and could be comfortably injected on a bi-weekly basis in a clinical setting. As a nandrolone injectable, this drug is highly similar in appearance to Deca-Durabolin (nandrolone decanoate), exhibiting relatively strong anabolic properties and a low level of relative androgenicity and estrogenicity. Nandrolone cyclohexylpropionate is favored by athletes and bodybuilders for its ability to promote significant strength and lean muscle mass gains without excessive side effects.

History:

Nandrolone cyclohexylpropionate was first described in 1962. It was developed into a medicine shortly thereafter, although its adoption by pharmaceutical companies was not as rapid and widespread as the phenylpropionate and decanoate esters of nandrolone. The most notable brand name of reference for nandrolone cyclohexylpropionate was Fherbolico, which was manufactured by Fher in Spain, It has also been sold under such brand names as Anabolicum "Sanabo", Androl, Megabolin, and Proteron-Depot. The drug was used principally as an anabolic to aid in the gain of lean bodyweight, as well as to combat osteoporosis. Given its mild androgenic nature, it was often applied to androgen-sensitive patients, including women and the elderly.

Most of the early preparations containing nandrolone cyclohexylpropionate have been removed from the market over the years. Given the high relative safety of nandrolone preparations, such decisions were probably voluntary ones by the manufacturers, likely based on financial considerations. By the 1980's and 1990's, nandrolone decanoate, and to a lesser extent nandrolone phenylpropionate, dominated the global nandrolone market, and there was not a great deal of money being made with the lesser-known esters. Some isolated preparations containing nandrolone cyclohexylpropionate are still being manufactured, however, so the drug remains available in commerce. More recent products known to still use this steroid are Sanabolicum by the Nile Company in Egypt, Sanabolicum-Vet by Werfft-Chemie in Austria, and Genadrag by Drag Pharma in Chile, the latter being the most commonly located form of the drug in recent years.

How Supplied:

Nandrolone cyclohexylpropionate is available in select human and veterinary drug markets. Composition and dosage may vary by country and manufacturer, but usually contain 25 mg/mL or 50 mg/mL of steroid dissolved in oil.

Structural Characteristics:

Nandrolone cyclohexylpropionate is a modified form of nandrolone, where a carboxylic acid ester (cyclohexylpropionic acid) has been attached to the 17-beta hydroxyl group. Esterified steroids are less polar than free steroids, and are absorbed more slowly from the area of injection. Once in the bloodstream, the ester is removed to yield free (active) nandrolone. Esterified steroids are designed to prolong the window of therapeutic effect following administration, allowing for a less frequent injection schedule compared to injections of free (unesterified) steroid. Nandrolone cyclohexylpropionate provides a sharp spike in nandrolone release 24-48 hours following deep intramuscular injection, which steadily declines to near baseline levels approximately 2 weeks later.

Side Effects (Estrogenic):

Nandrolone has a low tendency for estrogen conversion,

estimated to be only about 20% of that seen with testosterone.[535] This is because while the liver can convert nandrolone to estradiol, in other more active sites of steroid aromatization such as adipose tissue nandrolone is far less open to this process.[536] Consequently, estrogen-related side effects are a much lower concern with this drug than with testosterone. Elevated estrogen levels may still be noticed with higher dosing, however, and may cause side effects such as increased water retention, body fat gain, and gynecomastia. An anti-estrogen such as clomiphene citrate or tamoxifen citrate may be necessary to prevent estrogenic side effects if they occur. One may alternately use an aromatase inhibitor like Arimidex® (anastrozole), which more efficiently controls estrogen by preventing its synthesis. Aromatase inhibitors can be quite expensive in comparison to anti-estrogens, however, and may also have negative effects on blood lipids.

It is of note that nandrolone has some activity as a progestin in the body.[537] Although progesterone is a c-19 steroid, removal of this group as in 19-norprogesterone creates a hormone with greater binding affinity for its corresponding receptor. Sharing this trait, many 19-nor anabolic steroids are shown to have some affinity for the progesterone receptor as well.[538] The side effects associated with progesterone are similar to those of estrogen, including negative feedback inhibition of testosterone production and enhanced rate of fat storage. Progestins also augment the stimulatory effect of estrogens on mammary tissue growth. There appears to be a strong synergy between these two hormones here, such that gynecomastia might even occur with the help of progestins, without excessive estrogen levels. The use of an anti-estrogen, which inhibits the estrogenic component of this disorder, is often sufficient to mitigate gynecomastia caused by nandrolone.

Side Effects (Androgenic):

Although classified as an anabolic steroid, androgenic side effects are still possible with this substance, especially with higher doses. This may include bouts of oily skin, acne, and body/facial hair growth. Anabolic/androgenic steroids may also aggravate male pattern hair loss. Women are warned of the potential virilizing effects of anabolic/androgenic steroids. These may include a deepening of the voice, menstrual irregularities, changes in skin texture, facial hair growth, and clitoral enlargement. Nandrolone is a steroid with relatively low androgenic activity relative to its tissue-building actions, making the threshold for strong androgenic side effects comparably higher than with more androgenic agents such as testosterone, methandrostenolone, or fluoxymesterone. It is also important to point out that due to its mild androgenic nature and ability to suppress endogenous testosterone, nandrolone is prone to interfering with libido in males when used without another androgen.

Note that in androgen-responsive target tissues such as the skin, scalp, and prostate, the relative androgenicity of nandrolone is reduced by its reduction to dihydronandrolone (DHN).[539][540] The 5-alpha reductase enzyme is responsible for this metabolism of nandrolone. The concurrent use of a 5-alpha reductase inhibitor such as finasteride or dutasteride will interfere with site-specific reduction of nandrolone action, considerably increasing the tendency of nandrolone to produce androgenic side effects. Reductase inhibitors should be avoided with nandrolone if low androgenicity is desired.

Side Effects (Hepatotoxicity):

Nandrolone is not c-17 alpha alkylated, and not known to have hepatotoxic effects. Liver toxicity is unlikely. Note that one case of intrahepatic cholestasis has been documented in a patient receiving long-term nandrolone cyclohexylpropionate.[541]

Side Effects (Cardiovascular):

Anabolic/androgenic steroids can have deleterious effects on serum cholesterol. This includes a tendency to reduce HDL (good) cholesterol values and increase LDL (bad) cholesterol values, which may shift the HDL to LDL balance in a direction that favors greater risk of arteriosclerosis. The relative impact of an anabolic/androgenic steroid on serum lipids is dependant on the dose, route of administration (oral vs. injectable), type of steroid (aromatizable or non-aromatizable), and level of resistance to hepatic metabolism. Studies administering 600 mg of nandrolone decanoate per week for 10 weeks demonstrated a 26% reduction in HDL cholesterol levels.[542] This suppression is slightly greater than that reported with an equal dose of testosterone enanthate, and is in agreement with earlier studies showing a slightly stronger negative impact on HDL/LDL ratio with nandrolone decanoate as compared to testosterone cypionate.[543] Nandrolone injectables, however, should still have a significantly weaker impact on serum lipids than c-17 alpha alkylated agents. Anabolic/androgenic steroids may also adversely affect blood pressure and triglycerides, reduce endothelial relaxation, and support left ventricular hypertrophy, all potentially increasing the risk of cardiovascular disease and myocardial infarction.

To help reduce cardiovascular strain it is advised to maintain an active cardiovascular exercise program and minimize the intake of saturated fats, cholesterol, and simple carbohydrates at all times during active AAS administration. Supplementing with fish oils (4 grams per day) and a natural cholesterol/antioxidant formula such as Lipid Stabil or a product with comparable ingredients is also recommended.

Side Effects (Testosterone Suppression):

All anabolic/androgenic steroids when taken in doses sufficient to promote muscle gain are expected to suppress endogenous testosterone production. For sake of comparison, studies administering 100 mg per week of nandrolone decanoate for 6 weeks have demonstrated an approximate 57% reduction in serum testosterone levels during therapy. At a dosage of 300 mg per week, this reduction reached 70%.[544] It is believed that the progestational activity of nandrolone notably contributes to the suppression of testosterone synthesis during therapy, which can be marked in spite of a low tendency for estrogen conversion.[545] Without the intervention of testosterone-stimulating substances, testosterone levels should return to normal within 2-6 months of drug secession. Note that prolonged hypogonadotrophic hypogonadism can develop secondary to steroid abuse, necessitating medical intervention.

The above side effects are not inclusive. For more detailed discussion of potential side effects, see the Steroid Side Effects section of this book.

Administration (Men):

When used for physique- or performance-enhancing purposes, a dose of 200-400 mg per week is most common, taken in cycles 8 to 12 weeks in length. This level is sufficient for most users to notice measurable gains in lean muscle mass and strength, which should be accompanied by a low level of estrogenic and androgenic activity. Although higher doses (450-600 mg) may produce a stronger anabolic effect, given the relatively low concentration this drug is found in (25 mg/mL and 50 mg/mL), doses above 400 mg are not commonly applied. Instead, the drug is often stacked with another agent, usually an androgen such as an injectable testosterone, which also helps offset the very low level of androgenicity of nandrolone. An oral steroid with pronounced androgenicity, such as methandrostenolone or oxymetholone, is sometimes used as well, but will also present some hepatotoxicity and have a stronger effect on serum lipids (negatively).

Administration (Women):

When used for physique- or performance-enhancing purposes, a dosage of 50 mg per week is most common. Although only slightly androgenic, women are occasionally confronted with virilization symptoms when taking this compound. Should virilizing side effects become a concern, nandrolone cyclohexylpropionate should be discontinued immediately to help prevent their permanent appearance. After a sufficient period of withdrawal, the shorter-acting nandrolone Durabolin® might be considered a safer (more controllable) option. This drug stays active for only several days, greatly reducing the withdrawal time if indicated.

Availability:

Nandrolone cyclohexylpropionate is not commonly in circulation, but can be found on occasion. There are at most a few low-dose products in manufacture worldwide to choose from, which have the added benefit of being very low on the radar for importers, dealers, and buyers alike. Counterfeiters presently have just as little interest in this steroid as consumers, so should you find one of the available products, the odds it will be fake are probably much lower than with most steroids. At this time you probably have the best chance of finding the Genadrag brand, which is produced by Drag Pharma in Santiago Chile. Genadrag comes packaged in a bright orange and white box, and bears a relatively simple-looking orange and white or blue and white sticker on a dark amber 10 mL vial.

Finajet (trenbolone acetate)

Androgenic	500
Anabolic	500
Standard	Nandrolone acetate
Chemical Name	17beta-Hydroxyestra-4,9,11-trien-3-one
Estrogenic Activity	none
Progestational Activity	moderate

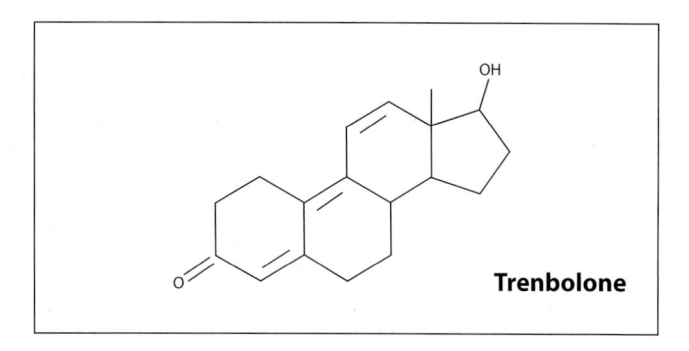

Trenbolone

Description:

Trenbolone acetate is an injectable (generally) anabolic steroid derived from nandrolone. Its activity is quite removed from its structural parent, however, such that direct comparisons between the two are difficult. Trenbolone is a non-estrogenic steroid, and is considerably more anabolic and androgenic than nandrolone on a milligram for milligram basis. In appearance, it is much more commonly compared to a stronger androgen such as drostanolone, than it is to nandrolone. It is also estimated to display about three times more androgenic potency than testosterone, making it one of the strongest injectable anabolic steroids ever commercially manufactured. Among athletes, this steroid is highly valued for its ability to increase muscle hardness, definition, and raw strength, without unwanted water retention and fat mass gains. It is considered a drug of choice for contest bodybuilders, yet remains very popular with recreational users simply looking to refine their physiques.

History:

Trenbolone acetate was first closely studied in 1967, described during a series of experiments into synthetic anabolic steroids by Roussel-UCLAF.[546] By the early 1970's, trenbolone acetate was being sold in England by Hoechst as Finajet, and in France as Finaject by Roussel. Roussel AG in Germany was parent to both companies. Trenbolone acetate is a drug of veterinary medicine, although a longer-acting ester of trenbolone (see: Parabolan) was once sold for human consumption as well. Trenbolone acetate is used, almost exclusively, to increase the rate of weight gain and improve feed efficiency of cattle shortly before slaughter. Essentially, the drug is utilized to increase product profitability, as measured in total pounds of salable meat. It is generally used right up to the point of slaughter, with no withholding period. Meat products sold in many areas of the world will often contain small amounts of residual trenbolone metabolites as a result of this practice.

Trenbolone acetate first became popular among U.S. bodybuilders during the 1980's, a time when the drug was being smuggled in from Europe in high volume. It was identified (rightly so) as a powerful anabolic and androgenic agent, and quickly became a drug of choice among American competitive bodybuilders. Although extremely hot for a brief period of time, the supply of trenbolone acetate ended abruptly in 1987, as Hoechst-Roussel decided to voluntarily discontinue sale of all injectable forms of this medication. Although unconfirmed, the growing public concern about sports doping likely had much to do with this decision, as the discontinuation of "controversial" steroids was very common during the late 1980's and early 1990's. This event marked the end of legitimate medicines containing trenbolone acetate for injection.

Around the same time as we were seeing the demise of Finajet and Finaject, Hoechst-Roussell was introducing trenbolone acetate to the U.S. market as Finaplix cattle implant pellets. This came subsequent to the FDA's approval for such products in 1987. The pellets were designed for subcutaneous implantation into the ear of the cattle with a handheld implant gun, and are far too large to be implanted in humans without minor surgery. Remarkably, trenbolone acetate pellets are exempt from U.S. controlled substance laws. This is presumably to make it easy and affordable for livestock owners to have access to the growth-promoting agent. If a veterinarian were needed every time these products were to be used, they might be too troublesome or cost prohibitive to consider. Admittedly, since these products come in the form of pellets, they are not in a form suitable for human consumption either, making their exemption seem a little more reasonable than at first glance.

Human administration of Finaplix pellets can be difficult to accomplish, but it is still widely done. Most commonly, two to four implant pellets are ground up and mixed with a 50/50 water and DMSO solution, which is applied to the skin daily. This home-brew transdermal mix is effective, but also tends to carry a strong odor of garlic (an effect of the DMSO). Others simply grind up a few pellets with the back of a spoon and inhale (snort) them. Here, the drug enters the blood stream through the mucous membrane, a poor but still useful means of delivery for steroid hormones. Those who have tried this often claim it is not as irritating as they had imagined it would be. Alternately, some athletes opt to simply consume the drug orally. Although not an ideal mode of delivery, trenbolone displays a moderate level of oral bioavailability, and can be used in this manner given adequate dosing.

More adventurous individuals have made it a practice to mix their own injections with Finaplix. The pellets are ground into a fine powder (usually anywhere from 2 to 6 pellets), and then are added to sterile water, propylene glycol, or an oil-based injectable steroid or veterinary vitamin. This is usually repeated twice weekly, although some do manage to undertake this practice more frequently. Since this is not being done in a controlled sterile environment, however, one is obviously risking infection (or worse) by doing this. Starting in the late 1990's, some stores began selling kits that contain all the necessary ingredients to separate the binders from the active steroid and brew a relatively pure injectable. These kits have grown in popularity over the years, and are usually reviewed favorably, although are not considered a substitute for sterile pharmaceutical medications.

Finaplix® is presently available in the U.S. and some markets abroad, although it is now being sold by Intervet instead of Hoechst-Roussel Agri-vet. This product comes in two forms, Finaplix-H and Finaplix-S, which denotes if the product was intended for a Heifer or a Steer respectively. The total dosages of both products are different, with the "H" version containing 100 20 mg trenbolone acetate pellets (2,000 mg) and the "S" version only 70 (1,400 mg). Ivy Animal Health (U.S.) has introduced two competing products of equivalent makeup as well, sold as Component-TH and Component-TS. There are also the Revalor and Synovex+ brands that contain trenbolone acetate with an added (usually unwanted) dose of estrogen. Additionally, although no other legitimate medicines containing trenbolone acetate exist, the drug is produced (for injection and oral use) by a number of export and underground steroid manufacturers.

How Supplied:

Trenbolone acetate is available in select veterinary drug markets. It generally comes in the form of implant pellets containing 20 mg of trenbolone acetate each. Injectable preparations containing 30 mg/ml of steroid in oil were formerly sold.

Structural Characteristics:

Trenbolone is a modified form of nandrolone. It differs by the introduction of double bonds at carbons 9 and 11, which inhibit aromatization (9-ene), increase androgen-binding affinity,[547] and slow its metabolism. The resulting steroid is significantly more potent as both an anabolic and an androgen than its nandrolone base. Trenbolone acetate contains trenbolone modified with the addition of carboxylic acid ester (acetic acid) at the 17-beta hydroxyl group, so that the free steroid is released more slowly from the area of injection.

Side Effects (Estrogenic):

Trenbolone is not aromatized by the body, and is not measurably estrogenic. It is of note, however, that this steroid displays significant binding affinity for the progesterone receptor (slightly stronger than progesterone itself).[548,549] The side effects associated with progesterone are similar to those of estrogen, including negative feedback inhibition of testosterone production and enhanced rate of fat storage. Progestins also augment the stimulatory effect of estrogens on mammary tissue growth. There appears to be a strong synergy between these two hormones here, such that gynecomastia might even occur with the help of progestins, without excessive estrogen levels. The use of an anti-estrogen, which inhibits the estrogenic component of this disorder, is often sufficient to mitigate gynecomastia caused by progestational anabolic/androgenic steroids. Note that progestational side effects are more common when trenbolone is being taken with other aromatizable steroids.

Side Effects (Androgenic):

Although classified as an anabolic steroid, trenbolone is sufficiently androgenic. Androgenic side effects are still common with this substance, and may include bouts of oily skin, acne, and body/facial hair growth. Anabolic/androgenic steroids may also aggravate male pattern hair loss. Women are also warned of the potential virilizing effects of anabolic/androgenic steroids. These may include a deepening of the voice, menstrual irregularities, changes in skin texture, facial hair growth, and clitoral enlargement. Additionally, the 5-alpha reductase enzyme does not metabolize trenbolone,[550] so its relative androgenicity is not affected by finasteride or dutasteride.

Side Effects (Hepatotoxicity):

Trenbolone is not c-17 alpha alkylated, and is generally not considered a hepatotoxic steroid; liver toxicity is unlikely. This steroid does have a strong level of resistance to hepatic breakdown, however, and severe liver toxicity has been noted in bodybuilders abusing trenbolone.[551] Although unlikely, hepatotoxicity cannot be completely excluded, especially with high doses.

Side Effects (Cardiovascular):

Anabolic/androgenic steroids can have deleterious effects on serum cholesterol. This includes a tendency to reduce HDL (good) cholesterol values and increase LDL (bad) cholesterol values, which may shift the HDL to LDL balance in a direction that favors greater risk of arteriosclerosis. The relative impact of an anabolic/androgenic steroid on serum lipids is dependant on the dose, route of administration (oral vs. injectable), type of steroid (aromatizable or non-aromatizable), and level of resistance to hepatic metabolism. Due to its non-aromatizable nature and strong resistance to metabolism, trenbolone has a moderate to strong (negative) impact on lipid values and atherogenic risk. Anabolic/androgenic steroids may also adversely affect blood pressure and triglycerides, reduce endothelial relaxation, and support left ventricular hypertrophy, all potentially increasing the risk of cardiovascular disease and myocardial infarction.

To help reduce cardiovascular strain it is advised to maintain an active cardiovascular exercise program and minimize the intake of saturated fats, cholesterol, and simple carbohydrates at all times during active AAS administration. Supplementing with fish oils (4 grams per day) and a natural cholesterol/antioxidant formula such as Lipid Stabil or a product with comparable ingredients is also recommended.

Side Effects (Testosterone Suppression):

All anabolic/androgenic steroids when taken in doses sufficient to promote muscle gain are expected to suppress endogenous testosterone production. Without the intervention of testosterone-stimulating substances, testosterone levels should return to normal within 1-4 months of drug secession. Note that prolonged hypogonadotrophic hypogonadism can develop secondary to steroid abuse, necessitating medical intervention. In experimental studies, trenbolone was determined to be approximately three times stronger at suppressing gonadotropins than testosterone on a milligram for milligram basis.

The above side effects are not inclusive. For more detailed discussion of potential side effects, see the Steroid Side Effects section of this book.

Administration (Men):

Trenbolone acetate was never approved for use in humans. Prescribing guidelines are unavailable. An effective dosage for physique- or performance-enhancing purposes generally falls in the range of 100-300 mg per week, taken for 6 to 8 weeks. Due to the short-acting nature of acetate esters, the total week's dosage is subdivided into 2-3 smaller applications. Effective oral doses tend to fall in the range of 100-200 mg per day, taken for no longer than 6-8 weeks to minimize any potential hepatic strain. This level is sufficient to notice strong increases in strength and lean tissue mass, with a low level of unwanted side effects. Lack of estrogenic activity has made trenbolone very appealing for competitive athletes looking to shed fat, while at the same time trying to avoid water retention. Here, trenbolone may provide the high androgen content needed in order to elicit a very hard, defined physique.

While it is a noteworthy hardening agent, this is not the only benefit of trenbolone acetate. It is also a strong anabolic, with muscle-building properties often compared to testosterone and Dianabol, but without the same level of water retention. This may be a little generous of a description, as its lack of estrogenic activity does seem to hurt this agent in its abilities to promote muscle mass gains. While trenbolone is often recommended as a great addition to a mass cycle, it is rarely reported to be a very powerful agent when used alone. Results are most often reported as moderate lean tissue growth accompanied by exceptional hardening and fat loss. Although perhaps it is not quite as potent as the more estrogenic bulking agents if sheer mass is the goal, trenbolone is still a better builder milligram for milligram than nandrolone, and likely the most anabolic of all the non-estrogenic commercial steroids.

For stacking, trenbolone is a very versatile steroid, and seems to work exceptionally well with other agents for both bulking and cutting purposes. For cutting, bodybuilders often stack it with a mild anabolic like Winstrol® or Primobolan®. Without extra water beneath your skin, the mix will elicit a very solid, well-defined hardness to the physique. For lean mass gains, Deca-Durabolin® or Equipoise® are popular additions. Here again, trenbolone will greatly enhance and solidify the new muscle growth. When looking purely for mass, trenbolone pairs well with testosterone, Anadrol 50®, or Dianabol. The result is typically the rapid and substantial gain of somewhat solid muscle mass. In the Underground Steroid Hanbook II, Dan Duchaine describes the mix of trenbolone, testosterone, and Anadrol as the "Most Effective" stack for men, and states, "I've not encountered any other stack that will put weight and strength on like this one." This particular drug combination has subsequently become quite popular.

Administration (Women):

Trenbolone acetate was never approved for use in humans. Prescribing guidelines are unavailable. This agent is not recommended for women for physique- or performance-enhancing purposes due to strong androgenic nature and tendency to produce virilizing side effects.

Availability:

Finaplix® and competing trenbolone acetate pellets are available through many veterinary and black market suppliers. These pellets are difficult to administer, however they are also not commonly subject to counterfeiting. This is the only legitimate form of trenbolone acetate in the U.S.

Moving on from Finaplix pellets, legitimate pharmaceutical preparations using trenbolone acetate are scarce.

Trenol 50 is manufactured in Myanmar by WDV Pharmaceuticals. This 50 mg/ml 6ml multi-dose vial provides a decent amount of steroid, although it does not make its way to the U.S. very often. WDV products seem most popular in areas of Eastern Europe, and to a lesser extent Western Europe.

Most other forms are from underground manufacturers, and therefore are of unverifiable quality.

Genabol (norbolethone)

Androgenic	17
Anabolic	350
Standard	Testosterone propionate

Chemical Names 13-ethyl-17-hydroxy-18,19-dinor-17a-pregn-4-en-3-one
13,17-alpha-diethyl-17-hydroxygon-4-en-3-one

Estrogenic Activity	moderate
Progestational Activity	moderate

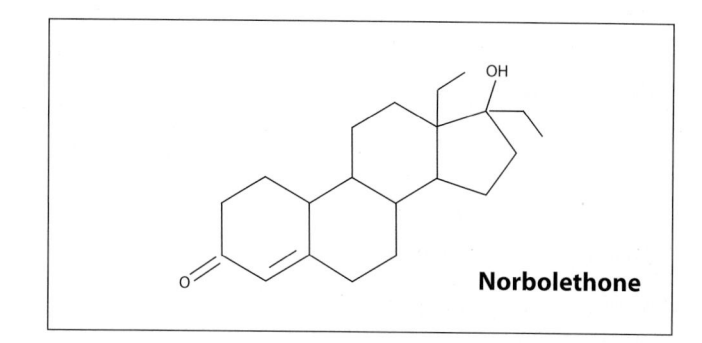

Norbolethone

Description:

Norbolethone is an orally active derivative of nandrolone. Structurally, this steroid differs from normethandrolone (Orgasteron) only by the substitution of the 13-methyl group with an ethyl. As is common for a member of the nandrolone family, norbolethone is more anabolic than androgenic in nature. Early animal studies place the anabolic index of this agent at 20 as compared to oral methyltestosterone (the standard of comparison for oral anabolic/androgenic steroids), meaning that it has 20 times higher anabolic than androgenic activity. Although this figure may not translate perfectly to real-world human use, we can still expect a favorable balance of anabolic to androgenic effect. Comparisons to other commercially available agents would probably place norbolethone in a similar category to norethandrolone, both being effective anabolic derivatives of nandrolone, but with some additional estrogenic and progestational activity that makes them somewhat dissimilar to more purely anabolic agents such as Winstrol, Primobolan, and Anavar. Norbolethone is most appropriately considered a bodybuilding drug, and is less ideally suited for the needs of competitive athletes.

History:

Norbolethone was first described in 1963.[552] The drug was developed by Wyeth (Genabol, 2.5 mg), and put into human clinical trials between 1964 and 1972. It was investigated as a potential medicine to treat low body weight and children with short stature.[553][554][555][556] Effective doses used in the studies were as low as 1.25 mg per day in children, but generally included a common adult dose of 2.5 mg to 10 mg per day. A detailed series of investigations into the metabolic effects of norbolethone (using 2.5 mg to 10 mg per day for up to 6 weeks) in adult and elderly men and women recovering from surgery or illness in 1968 determined that optimal protein retention was achieved at 7.5 mg per day (10 mg per day was shown to offer no advantage in this study).[557] Although the drug was deemed highly anabolic with minimal androgenic properties, and effective doses had been determined, norbolethone was ultimately never released as a commercial prescription agent. As such, after the clinical trials were published, little mention was made of this drug for approximately thirty years.

Norbolethone was thrown into headlines in mid-2002, when it was announced that Dr. Don Catlin of the UCLA Analytical Laboratories had discovered that athletes were using this drug to beat the drug screens being conducted at his facility. Because norbolethone was never sold as a commercial steroid, the athletic bodies were not looking for it during earlier tests. A private chemist (later identified as Patrick Arnold) realized this, and manufactured it for the specific purpose of beating the drug screen. Catlin was clued into its use after identifying several "negative" samples that had signs of endogenous steroid suppression (potentially indicating steroid use). The norbolethone doping scandal that resulted was the first modern appearance of the "designer steroid" phenomenon. These are non-commercial steroids that do not show up on a drug screen by virtue of their anonymity. For as long as they are not known to drug-testing facilities, they will not be detected. Drugs like norbolethone are highly valued commodities among competitive athletes.

Once Catlin identified norbolethone, he promptly devised and released a method for the detection of its metabolites in the urine.[558] Several world-class athletes were ultimately suspended for using this drug during competition, including U.S. Olympic cyclist Tammy Thomas. With this press release, norbolethone immediately lost any value it formerly had as an undetectable designer steroid. It has been "discovered," so to speak, and is now actively screened for during any serious steroid urinalysis test. There is little doubt that most of the athletes that were using this compound have long since abandoned it and moved on to better things. Charlie Francis, the man who coached Ben Johnson when he tested positive for steroids at the 1988 Summer Games, would later comment that norbolethone was being widely used at the 2000 Sydney Games, two years before the IOC caught wind of its existence.[559]

How Supplied:

Norbolethone is not available as a prescription drug product. When produced as an experimental drug by Wyeth it was found in the form of a 2.5 mg tablet.

Structural Characteristics:

Norbolethone is a modified form of nandrolone. It differs by 1) the addition of an ethyl group at carbon 17-alpha to protect the hormone during oral administration and 2) the introduction of an ethyl group at carbon 13-alpha, which seems to intensify steroid anabolic activity.

Side Effects (Estrogenic):

Norbolethone has not been extensively studied in humans. Based on its structure, it is expected that norbolethone is aromatized. It should convert to a synthetic estrogen with a high level of biological activity (13,17alpha-diethyl-estradiol). This should be a moderately estrogenic steroid. Gynecomastia may be a concern during treatment, particularly with higher doses. At the same time water retention can become a problem, causing a notable loss of muscle definition as both subcutaneous water retention and fat levels build. Sensitive individuals may want to keep the estrogen under control with the addition of an anti-estrogen such as Nolvadex®. One may alternately use an aromatase inhibitor like Arimidex® (anastrozole), which is a more effective remedy for estrogen control. Aromatase inhibitors, however, can be quite expensive in comparison to standard estrogen maintenance therapies, and may also have negative effects on blood lipids.

Based on its structure, it is expected that norbolethone has some activity as a progestin in the body. The side effects associated with progesterone are similar to those of estrogen, including negative feedback inhibition of testosterone production and enhanced rate of fat storage. Progestins also augment the stimulatory effect of estrogens on mammary tissue growth. There appears to be a strong synergy between these two hormones here, such that gynecomastia might even occur with the help of progestins without excessive estrogen levels being present. The use of an anti-estrogen, which inhibits the estrogenic component of this disorder, is often sufficient to mitigate gynecomastia caused by progestational anabolic steroids.

Side Effects (Androgenic):

Although classified as an anabolic steroid, androgenic side effects are still possible with this substance. This may include bouts of oily skin, acne, and body/facial hair growth. Anabolic/androgenic steroids may also aggravate male pattern hair loss. Women are additionally warned of the potential virilizing effects of anabolic/androgenic steroids. These may include a deepening of the voice, menstrual irregularities, changes in skin texture, facial hair growth, and clitoral enlargement. Note that in androgen-responsive target tissues such as the skin, scalp, and prostate, structure suggests that the relative androgenicity of norbolethone is reduced by its reduction to dihydo-norbolethone. The concurrent use of a 5-alpha reductase inhibitor such as finasteride or dutasteride may interfere with site-specific reduction of norbolethone action, increasing the tendency of the drug to produce androgenic side effects. Reductase inhibitors should be avoided with this steroid if maintaining low relative androgenicity is desired.

Side Effects (Hepatotoxicity):

Norbolethone is a c17-alpha alkylated compound. This alteration protects the drug from deactivation by the liver, allowing a very high percentage of the drug entry into the bloodstream following oral administration. C17-alpha alkylated anabolic/androgenic steroids can be hepatotoxic. Prolonged or high exposure may result in liver damage. In rare instances life-threatening dysfunction may develop. It is advisable to visit a physician periodically during each cycle to monitor liver function and overall health. Intake of c17-alpha alkylated steroids is commonly limited to 6-8 weeks, in an effort to avoid escalating liver strain. Severe liver complications are rare given the periodic nature in which most people use oral anabolic/androgenic steroids, although cannot be excluded with this steroid, especially with high doses and/or prolonged administration periods. Studies examining the sulfobromophthalein (BSP) retention effects of norbolethone and sixteen other anabolic/androgenic steroids in animals determined the drug to be among the most active.[560] Increased BSP retention is a common marker of hepatic stress. Later studies in humans determined that the drug was well tolerated in doses of 10 mg per day or less for up to 6 weeks of continuous use.

The use of a liver detoxification supplement such as Liver Stabil, Liv-52, or Essentiale Forte is advised while taking any hepatotoxic anabolic/androgenic steroids.

Side Effects (Cardiovascular):

Anabolic/androgenic steroids can have deleterious effects

on serum cholesterol. This includes a tendency to reduce HDL (good) cholesterol values and increase LDL (bad) cholesterol values, which may shift the HDL to LDL balance in a direction that favors greater risk of arteriosclerosis. The relative impact of an anabolic/androgenic steroid on serum lipids is dependant on the dose, route of administration (oral vs. injectable), type of steroid (aromatizable or non-aromatizable), and level of resistance to hepatic metabolism. Norbolethone has a strong effect on the hepatic management of cholesterol due to its structural resistance to liver breakdown and route of administration. Anabolic/androgenic steroids may also adversely affect blood pressure and triglycerides, reduce endothelial relaxation, and support left ventricular hypertrophy, all potentially increasing the risk of cardiovascular disease and myocardial infarction.

To help reduce cardiovascular strain it is advised to maintain an active cardiovascular exercise program and minimize the intake of saturated fats, cholesterol, and simple carbohydrates at all times during active AAS administration. Supplementing with fish oils (4 grams per day) and a natural cholesterol/antioxidant formula such as Lipid Stabil or a product with comparable ingredients is also recommended.

Side Effects (Testosterone Suppression):

All anabolic/androgenic steroids when taken in doses sufficient to promote muscle gain are expected to suppress endogenous testosterone production. Without the intervention of testosterone-stimulating substances, testosterone levels should return to normal within 1-4 months of drug secession. Note that prolonged hypogonadotrophic hypogonadism can develop secondary to steroid abuse, necessitating medical intervention.

The above side effects are not inclusive. For more detailed discussion of potential side effects, see the Steroid Side Effects section of this book.

Administration (General):

Studies have shown that taking an oral anabolic steroid with food may decrease its bioavailability.[561] This is caused by the fat-soluble nature of steroid hormones, which can allow some of the drug to dissolve with undigested dietary fat, reducing its absorption from the gastrointestinal tract. For maximum utilization, this steroid should be taken on an empty stomach.

Administration (Men):

Norbolethone was never approved for use in humans. Prescribing guidelines are unavailable. Human studies determined an optimal clinical dose to be 7.5 mg per day. When used for physique- or performance-enhancing purposes, a dosage of 10-15 mg per day would be applied, taken for 6-8 weeks. The results at these doses should be measurable improvements in strength and muscle size, which may be accompanied by increased water retention, fat gain, and a loss of definition.

Administration (Women):

Norbolethone was never approved for use in humans. Prescribing guidelines are unavailable. Human studies determined an optimal clinical dose to be 7.5 mg per day. When used for physique- or performance-enhancing purposes, a dosage of 5 mg per day would likely be applied, taken for 4-6 weeks. Although primarily anabolic in nature, women are still warned of the potential for virilizing activities, especially with higher doses.

Availability:

Norbolethone is currently unavailable on the black market.

Halodrol (chlorodehydromethylandrostenediol)

Androgenic	no data available
Anabolic	no data available
Standard	Methyltestosterone (oral)
Chemical Name	4-chloro-17a-methylandrosta-1,4-dien-3,17-diol
Estrogenic Activity	none
Progestational Activity	no data available (low)

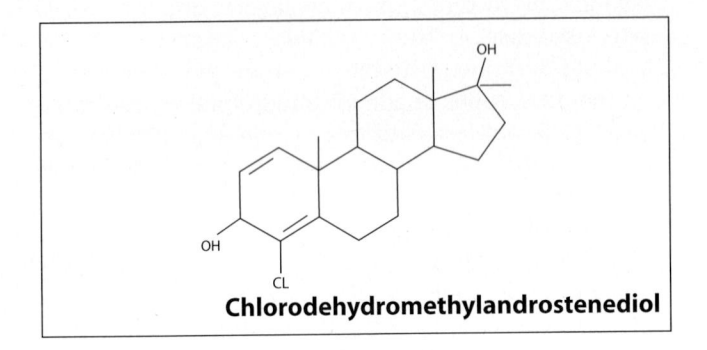

Description:

Chlorodehydromethylandrostenediol (CDMA) is an oral anabolic steroid derived from testosterone. It is extremely close in structure to chlorodehydromethyltestosterone (Oral Turinabol), differing only by the substitution of the basic steroid 3-keto group with a 3-hydroxyl. It is essentially a "diol" form of Oral Turinabol, and with this understanding is often described as a "prohormone" or "prosteroid" to this well-known and highly valued anabolic steroid. While some conversion to active chlorodehydromethyltestosterone is assumed, based on its structure it is likely that this conversion is far from complete, and that much of the anabolic and androgenic activity received with use is intrinsic to CDMA. This steroid is non-aromatizable, and exhibits a greater tendency for anabolic as compared to androgenic effect.

History:

Chlorodehydromethylandrostenediol was first described in 2005, when it was introduced to the U.S. supplement market as a "prosteroid" by Gaspari Nutrition. The agent was considered a "grey market" product, containing a drug that was not technically illegal due to it not being specifically listed in previous controlled substance laws. The designation of nutritional supplement, however, was viewed as highly controversial. In November 2005, Halodrol was the subject of a scathing article in the Washington Post for its unrestricted and likely illegal OTC sale.[562] Don Catlin of the UCLA Olympic Analytical Laboratory analyzed the product for the Post, and described Halodrol as containing, "a steroid that closely resembles Oral-Turinabol, the principal steroid used to fuel East Germany's secret, systematic sports doping program." Catlin also claimed that the product contained desoxymethytestosterone (Madol), something the manufacturer has denied.

Although no specific action was taken on the part of the FDA concerning chlorodehydromethylandrostenediol, the manufacturer voluntarily discontinued its sale in mid-2006, likely fearing government sanctions if it continued to manufacture the agent indefinitely. During its brief period of time, Halodrol was an extremely well-selling item, and by some estimates was the single best selling hormonal product ever sold over the counter in the U.S., with total sales estimated to be in the tens of millions of dollars. Today, the original Halodrol-50 product from Gaspari is no longer manufactured, and few companies will market the active drug for fear of FDA scrutiny. In September 2006, Gaspari introduced a replacement formula for Halodrol called Halodrol Liquigels, which includes arachidonic acid (profiled in this book), an aromatase inhibitor, and several other ingredients to impart an anabolic effect.

How Supplied:

Chlorodehydromethylandrostenediol is not available as a prescription drug product. When manufactured as a supplement, it contained 50 mg of steroid per tablet.

Structural Characteristics:

Chlorodehydromethylandrostenediol is a modified form of testosterone. It differs by 1) the addition of a methyl group at carbon 17-alpha, which helps protect the hormone during oral administration, 2) the introduction of a double bond between carbons 1 and 2 (1-ene), which shifts the anabolic to androgenic ratio in favor of the former, 3) the attachment of a chloro group at carbon 4, which inhibits steroid aromatization and reduces relative androgenicity, and 4) the substitution of 3-keto with 3-hydroxyl, which reduces relative steroid activity.

Side Effects (Estrogenic):

Chlorodehydromethylandrostenediol is not aromatized by the body, and is not measurably estrogenic. An anti-estrogen is not necessary when using this steroid, as gynecomastia should not be a concern even among sensitive individuals. Since estrogen is the usual culprit with water retention, this steroid instead produces a lean, quality look to the physique with no fear of excess subcutaneous fluid retention. This makes it a favorable steroid to use during cutting cycles, when water and fat retention are major concerns.

Side Effects (Androgenic):

Although chlorodehydromethylandrostenediol is classified as an anabolic steroid, androgenic side effects are still possible with this substance. These may include bouts of oily skin, acne, and body/facial hair growth. Higher doses are more likely to cause such side effects. For those with a genetic predisposition, anabolic/androgenic steroids may also aggravate male pattern hair loss. Women are additionally warned of the potential virilizing effects of anabolic/androgenic steroids. These may include a deepening of the voice, menstrual irregularities, changes in skin texture, body and facial hair growth, and clitoral enlargement. Note that chlorodehydromethylandrostenediol is not extensively metabolized by the 5-alpha reductase enzyme, so its relative androgenicity is not greatly altered by the concurrent use of finasteride or dutasteride.

Side Effects (Hepatotoxicity):

Chlorodehydromethylandrostenediol is a c17-alpha alkylated compound. This alteration protects the drug from deactivation by the liver, allowing a very high percentage of the drug entry into the bloodstream following oral administration. C17-alpha alkylated anabolic/androgenic steroids can be hepatotoxic. Prolonged or high exposure may result in liver damage. In rare instances life-threatening dysfunction may develop. It is advisable to visit a physician periodically during each cycle to monitor liver function and overall health. Intake of c17-alpha alkylated steroids is commonly limited to 6-8 weeks, in an effort to avoid escalating liver strain.

The use of a liver detoxification supplement such as Liver Stabil, Liv-52, or Essentiale Forte is advised while taking any hepatotoxic anabolic/androgenic steroids.

Side Effects (Cardiovascular):

Anabolic/androgenic steroids can have deleterious effects on serum cholesterol. This includes a tendency to reduce HDL (good) cholesterol values and increase LDL (bad) cholesterol values, which may shift the HDL to LDL balance in a direction that favors greater risk of arteriosclerosis. The relative impact of an anabolic/androgenic steroid on serum lipids is dependant on the dose, route of administration (oral vs. injectable), type of steroid (aromatizable or non-aromatizable), and level of resistance to hepatic metabolism. Chlorodehydromethylandrostenediol has a strong effect on the hepatic management of cholesterol due to its non-aromatizable nature, structural resistance to liver breakdown, and route of administration. Anabolic/androgenic steroids may also adversely affect blood pressure and triglycerides, reduce endothelial relaxation, and support left ventricular hypertrophy, all potentially increasing the risk of cardiovascular disease and myocardial infarction.

To help reduce cardiovascular strain it is advised to maintain an active cardiovascular exercise program and minimize the intake of saturated fats, cholesterol, and simple carbohydrates at all times during active AAS administration. Supplementing with fish oils (4 grams per day) and a natural cholesterol/antioxidant formula such as Lipid Stabil or a product with comparable ingredients is also recommended.

Side Effects (Testosterone Suppression):

All anabolic/androgenic steroids when taken in doses sufficient to promote muscle gain are expected to suppress endogenous testosterone production. Without the intervention of testosterone-stimulating substances, testosterone levels should return to normal within 1-4 months of drug secession. Note that prolonged hypogonadotrophic hypogonadism can develop secondary to steroid abuse, necessitating medical intervention.

The above side effects are not inclusive. For more detailed discussion of potential side effects, see the Steroid Side Effects section of this book.

Administration (General):

Studies have shown that taking an oral anabolic steroid with food may decrease its bioavailability.[563] This is caused by the fat-soluble nature of steroid hormones, which can allow some of the drug to dissolve with undigested dietary fat, reducing its absorption from the gastrointestinal tract. For maximum utilization, this steroid should be taken on an empty stomach.

Administration (Men):

Chlorodehydromethylandrostenediol was never approved for use in humans. Prescribing guidelines are unavailable. When used for physique- or performance-enhancing purposes, an effective oral daily dosage falls in the range of 50-100 mg, taken in cycles lasting no more than 6-8 weeks to minimize hepatotoxicity. This level is sufficient for noticeable increases in lean muscle mass and strength. Higher doses will impart a stronger effect, but are also more likely to present significant hepatotoxicity.

Administration (Women):

Chlorodehydromethylandrostenediol was never

approved for use in humans. Prescribing guidelines are unavailable. Chlorodehydromethylandrostenediol is generally not recommended for women for physique- or performance-enhancing purposes due to its high per-tablet dosage and the possibility of virilizing side effects. Low doses (12.5 mg per day or less) are unlikely to produce virilizing side effects, provided it was used for brief periods of 4-6 weeks. Note that as with all anabolic/androgenic steroids, the chance for virilization cannot be completely excluded.

Availability:

Halodrol-50 is no longer available, although old lots may circulate on the black market. Several other generics or spin-off brands may also still be in circulation.

Halotestin® (fluoxymesterone)

Androgenic	850
Anabolic	1,900
Standard	Methyltestosterone (oral)
Chemical Names	9a-fluoro-11b,17b-dihydroxy-17a-methyl-4-androsten-3-one
	9a-fluoro-11b-hydroxy-17a-methyltestosterone
Estrogenic Activity	none
Progestational Activity	no data available (low)

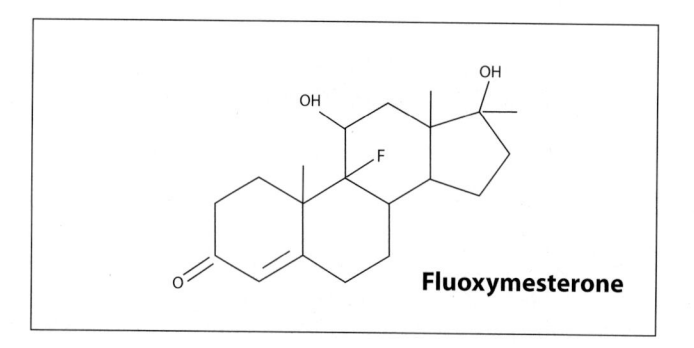

Description:

Fluoxymesterone is an oral anabolic steroid derived from testosterone. More specifically, it is a methyltestosterone derivative, differing by the addition of 11-beta-hydroxy and 9-alpha-fluoro groups. The result is a potent orally active non-aromatizable steroid that exhibits extremely strong androgenic properties. Fluoxymesterone is considerably more androgenic than testosterone, while at the same time the anabolic effects of this agent are considered to be moderate in comparison. This makes fluoxymesterone a great strength drug, but not the most ideal agent for gaining muscle mass. The predominant effects seen when taking fluoxymesterone are increased strength, increased muscle density, and increased definition, with only modest size increases.

History:

Fluoxymesterone was first described in 1956.[564] It was assayed that same year, and shown to possess approximately 20 times the anabolic potency of methyltestosterone[565] (its relative anabolic effect in humans would not be quite as strong in comparison). It was introduced to the U.S. prescription drug market shortly after under the brand name Halotestin (Upjohn), and soon after that as Ultandren (Ciba). The drug was initially described as halogenated derivative of testosterone, possessing up to 5 times greater anabolic and androgenic potency than methyltestosterone. Early prescribing guidelines recommended its use in both sexes for the promotion of lean tissue repair and growth following such conditions as burns, delayed healing of fractures, chronic malnutrition, debilitating diseases, convalescence, paraplegia, and catabolism induced by long-term administration of cortisone. It was also used in males to treat insufficient androgen levels, and in women to treat abnormal bleeding in the uterus and advanced breast cancer.

By the mid-1970's, the FDA had been granted much more control over the U.S. drug market. One of the first major changes with steroid medicine came when the FDA required strong substantiation for each potential use of a drug. The prescribing guidelines for fluoxymesterone were soon refined to state that the drug was "effective" for treating various forms of androgen deficiency in males, and reducing the severity of postpartum breast pain and treating androgen-responsive inoperable breast cancer in females. It was also listed as "probably effective" in treating postmenopausal osteoporosis. Current prescribing guidelines for fluoxymesterone list only the uses of treating androgen deficiency in males and breast cancer in females.

In recent years, fluoxymesterone has become viewed more and more as a controversial medication in the eyes of most clinicians. Its hepatotoxicity and potential negative impact of lipids and cardiovascular risk factors are often cited as reasons for avoiding the use of this agent in otherwise healthy males for treating androgen insufficiency. Today, testosterone preparations (injections, gels, patches, implants, etc.) are preferred for this purpose, and they supplement the same androgens missing from the body (testosterone, DHT), not more toxic synthetic derivatives. Fluoxymesterone remains for sale in the U.S. under the brand name Halotestin, sold by Pharmacia (formerly Upjohn). Declining financial interest had caused most generics to be withdrawn from the U.S. market years ago. Fluoxymesterone remains available in only limited supply outside of the United States.

How Supplied:

Fluoxymesterone is available in select human drug markets. Composition and dosage may vary by country and manufacturer, although generally contain 2mg, 2.5 mg, 5 mg, or 10 mg per tablet.

Structural Characteristics:

Fluoxymesterone is a modified form of testosterone. It differs by 1) the addition of a methyl group at carbon 17-

alpha, which helps protect the hormone during oral administration, 2) the introduction of a fluoro group at carbon 9 (alpha) and 3) the attachment of a hydroxyl group at carbon 11 (beta), which inhibits steroid aromatization. The latter two modifications also greatly enhance the androgenic and relative biological activity of the steroid over 17-alpha methyltestosterone.

Side Effects (Estrogenic):

Fluoxymesterone is not aromatized by the body, and is not measurably estrogenic. An anti-estrogen is not necessary when using this steroid, as gynecomastia should not be a concern even among sensitive individuals. Since estrogen is the usual culprit with water retention, this steroid instead produces a lean, quality look to the physique with no fear of excess subcutaneous fluid retention. This makes it a favorable steroid to use during cutting cycles, when water and fat retention are major concerns.

Side Effects (Androgenic):

Fluoxymesterone is classified as an androgen. Androgenic side effects are common with this substance, and may include bouts of oily skin, acne, and body/facial hair growth. Anabolic/androgenic steroids may also aggravate male pattern hair loss. Those genetically prone to male pattern hair loss may wish to opt for a milder, less androgenic, anabolic steroid. As a potent androgen, this steroid may also increase aggressiveness. Women are additionally warned of the potential virilizing effects of anabolic/androgenic steroids. These may include a deepening of the voice, menstrual irregularities, changes in skin texture, facial hair growth, and clitoral enlargement.

Fluoxymesterone appears to be a good substrate for the 5-alpha reductase enzyme. This is evidenced by the fact that a large number of its metabolites are found to be 5-alpha reduced androgens,[566] which coupled with its outward androgenic nature, suggests that this steroid is converting to a much more active steroid in androgen responsive target tissues such as the skin, scalp and prostate. It may be possible to reduce the relative androgenicity of fluoxymesterone by the concurrent use of finasteride or dutasteride.

It is also of note that fluoxymesterone has been shown to possess usual androgenic properties. In human studies published back in 1961, the steroid displayed a much stronger tendency to promote phallic enlargement compared to other androgenic effects such as hair growth, libido, and changes in vocal pitch.[567] Fluoxymesterone was offering a somewhat different androgenic profile compared to testosterone, and as such demonstrated that it was possible, at some level, to actually tailor drug effect within the broad category of androgenic action. Fluoxymesterone remains considered an androgen, but studies like the above suggest that it may not offer a complete biological equivalent to testosterone where androgenicity is concerned.

Side Effects (Hepatotoxicity):

Fluoxymesterone is a c17-alpha alkylated compound. This alteration protects the drug from deactivation by the liver, allowing a very high percentage of the drug entry into the bloodstream following oral administration. C17-alpha alkylated anabolic/androgenic steroids can be hepatotoxic. Prolonged or high exposure may result in liver damage. In rare instances life-threatening dysfunction may develop. It is advisable to visit a physician periodically during each cycle to monitor liver function and overall health. Intake of c17-alpha alkylated steroids is commonly limited to 6-8 weeks, in an effort to avoid escalating liver strain. Studies administering 20 mg of fluoxymesterone to a group of nine male subjects for two weeks resulted in most patients (6/9) noticing abnormal sulfobromophthalein (BSP) retention,[568] a marker of liver stress.

The use of a liver detoxification supplement such as Liver Stabil, Liv-52, or Essentiale Forte is advised while taking any hepatotoxic anabolic/androgenic steroids.

Side Effects (Cardiovascular):

Anabolic/androgenic steroids can have deleterious effects on serum cholesterol. This includes a tendency to reduce HDL (good) cholesterol values and increase LDL (bad) cholesterol values, which may shift the HDL to LDL balance in a direction that favors greater risk of arteriosclerosis. The relative impact of an anabolic/androgenic steroid on serum lipids is dependant on the dose, route of administration (oral vs. injectable), type of steroid (aromatizable or non-aromatizable), and level of resistance to hepatic metabolism. Fluoxymesterone has a strong effect on the hepatic management of cholesterol due to its structural resistance to liver breakdown and route of administration. Anabolic/androgenic steroids may also adversely affect blood pressure and triglycerides, reduce endothelial relaxation, and support left ventricular hypertrophy, all potentially increasing the risk of cardiovascular disease and myocardial infarction.

To help reduce cardiovascular strain it is advised to maintain an active cardiovascular exercise program and minimize the intake of saturated fats, cholesterol, and simple carbohydrates at all times during active AAS administration. Supplementing with fish oils (4 grams per

day) and a natural cholesterol/antioxidant formula such as Lipid Stabil or a product with comparable ingredients is also recommended.

Side Effects (Testosterone Suppression):

All anabolic/androgenic steroids when taken in doses sufficient to promote muscle gain are expected to suppress endogenous testosterone production. Without the intervention of testosterone-stimulating substances, testosterone levels should return to normal within 1-4 months of drug secession. Note that prolonged hypogonadotrophic hypogonadism can develop secondary to steroid abuse, necessitating medical intervention.

Studies administering 10 mg, 20 mg, or 30 mg of fluoxymesterone to nine healthy male subjects for up to 12 weeks have demonstrated the strong suppression of endogenous testosterone levels, with inconsistent effects on gonadotropin levels. Although not fully understood, fluoxymesterone is proposed to have a direct suppressive effect on testicular steroidogenesis that is not mediated by the suppression gonadotropins.[569]

The above side effects are not inclusive. For more detailed discussion of potential side effects, see the Steroid Side Effects section of this book.

Administration (General):

Studies have shown that taking an oral anabolic steroid with food may decrease its bioavailability.[570] This is caused by the fat-soluble nature of steroid hormones, which can allow some of the drug to dissolve with undigested dietary fat, reducing its absorption from the gastrointestinal tract. For maximum utilization, this steroid should be taken on an empty stomach.

Administration (Men):

To treat androgen insufficiency, early prescribing guidelines for fluoxymesterone called for a dose of 2-10 mg per day. Modern prescribing guidelines call for a daily dosage of 5-20 mg. Therapy is usually initiated at the full 20 mg dosage, which is later adjusted downward to meet the individual needs of the patient. The drug would be continued long-term unless laboratory tests (lipids, liver enzymes, etc.) or side effects contraindicate its continued use. For physique- or performance-enhancing purposes, an effective oral daily dosage would fall in the range of 10-40 mg, taken in cycles lasting no more than 6-8 weeks to minimize hepatotoxicity. This level is sufficient for measurable increases in muscle strength, which may be accompanied by modest increases in lean muscle mass.

Fluoxymesterone is commonly used by athletes in weight-restricted sports like wrestling, powerlifting, and boxing, due to the fact that strength gained from the drug is usually not accompanied by great increases in bodyweight. When properly used, it can allow a competitor to stay within a specified weight range, yet drastically improve his performance. Fluoxymesterone is also commonly used for bodybuilding contest preparation. When the competitor has an acceptably low body fat percentage, the strong androgen level (in absence of excess estrogen) can elicit an extremely hard and defined ("ripped") look to the muscles. The shift in androgen/estrogen ratio additionally seems to bring about a state in which the body may be more inclined to burn off excess fat and prevent new fat storage. The "hardening" effect of fluoxymesterone would, therefore, be somewhat similar to that seen with trenbolone, although it will be without the same level of mass gain.

In cutting phases, a milder anabolic such as Deca-Durabolin® or Equipoise® is commonly stacked with fluoxymesterone, as they provide good anabolic effect without excessive estrogen buildup. Here, fluoxymesterone provides a well-needed androgenic component, helping to promote a more solid and defined gain in muscle mass, with less interference with energy and libido, than might be obtained with a primarily anabolic agent alone. Perhaps Primobolan®-Depot would be an even better choice, as with such a combination there is no buildup of estrogen, and likewise even less worry of water and fat retention. For mass, one might alternately use an injectable testosterone. A mix of 400 mg per week of testosterone enanthate and 20-30 mg daily of fluoxymesterone, for example, often provides exceptional increases in strength and lean muscle mass. A more significant level of androgenic side effects usually accompanies such a combination, however, as both compounds exhibit strong androgenic activity in the body.

Administration (Women):

Fluoxymesterone is most often used as a secondary medication during inoperable androgen-sensitive breast cancer, when other therapies have failed to produce a desirable effect. The dosage used for this application is 10-40 mg per day. Virilizing effects are common at doses of only 10-15 mg per day in these patients. Fluoxymesterone is not recommended for women for physique- or performance-enhancing purposes due to its strong androgenic nature and tendency to produce virilizing side effects.

Availability:

Since fluoxymesterone is only used for a few specific purposes, it is not in high demand among athletes. Likewise it is not a very popular item on the black market.

Investing in the manufacture of a counterfeit version would probably not pay off well, no doubt the reason we haven't seen much yet. Most forms of fluoxymesterone found in circulation will, therefore, be legitimate, though the occasional counterfeits are located. Currently, the most popular item found on the black market is the Stenox brand from Mexico, which is sold in boxes of 20 tablets. Although the dosage of these tablets is only 2.5 mg, the low price usually asked for this preparation more than compensates.

Havoc (methepitiostane)

Androgenic	91
Anabolic	1100
Standard	Methyltestosterone (oral)

Chemical Name	2alpha,3alpha-epithio-17alpha-methyl-5alpha-androstan-17beta-ol
Estrogenic Activity	none
Progestational Activity	none

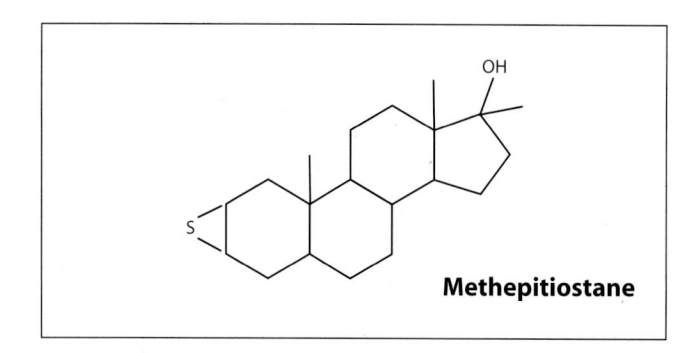

Methepitiostane

Description:

Methepitiostane is an oral anabolic steroid derived from dihydrotestosterone. This agent is a c17-alpha alkylated analog of epitiostane (see Thioderon), and like this drug also displays a favorable balance between anabolic and androgenic effect. In this case, however, the separation is considerably more pronounced, with the drug exhibiting an anabolic effect that is roughly 12 times more pronounced than its androgenic effect. That is according to the standard animal assays, which often vary somewhat to experiences in humans. This drug was never clinical tested in humans, so what is known of it is based on a small number of animal experiments, and structural and anecdotal observations. What can be stated with certainty if that methepitiostane is a primarily anabolic steroid with a pronounced level of activity, and is effective for the promotion of lean mass and strength gains. It likely also imparts some anti-estrogenic effect, further strengthening the association between this agent and dieting, cutting, and lean muscle mass phases of training as opposed to bulking.

History:

Methepitiostane was first described in 1966, during investigations into a series of A-ring modified androstane derivatives.[571] That same year it was assayed for anabolic and androgenic potency via the standard rat assays, and demonstrated both pronounced anabolic properties and very weak relative androgenicity.[572] The assay results were probably most similar to desoxymethyltestosterone (Madol), although methepitiostane is about half as androgenic. Although the results of the early testing were very favorable, this agent never progressed to the point of being a commercial steroid product or even tested on human subjects. Like a great many steroids, it was examined but not actualized as a prescription product. For forty years, the agent would be lost to the public, existing as an item of research interest only.

Methepitiostane would emerge from research obscurity at the end of 2006, when a new company called Recomp Performance Nutrition introduced it to the U.S. market under the trade name Havoc. It would be sold openly as a dietary supplement. This channel of sales does not reflect a weak potency or "non-steroid" classification, however, as methepitiostane is very much a potent drug. It is being sold as such due to the fact that the U.S. dietary supplement market is not tightly regulated, and the drug was never classified (specifically according to the law) as an anabolic steroid. While regulations do exist that would prevent the sale of an unapproved new drug as a food supplement, they do not carry the same weight as the anabolic steroid laws, and have historically not been aggressively enforced. Methepitiostane remains on sale as of December 2006, although the manufacturer has stated that they plan to discontinue the product very shortly.

How Supplied:

Methepitiostane was never approved as a prescription drug preparation. It is being sold in the U.S. supplement market under the trade name Havoc, and is supplied in the form of capsules containing 10 mg of steroid.

Structural Characteristics:

Methepitiostane is a modified form of dihydrotestosterone. It differs by 1) the addition of a 17-alpha methyl group, which helps protect the steroid from metabolism during oral administration, and 2) the replacement of 3-keto with 2,3alpha-epithio, which increases anabolic strength while reducing relative androgenicity.

Side Effects (Estrogenic):

Methepitiostane is not aromatized by the body, and is not measurably estrogenic. Furthermore, its non-methylated analog mepitiostane (Thioderon) is used clinically for its inherent antiestrogenic effect. Some level of antiestrogenic effect is also assumed with methepitiostane. An anti-estrogen is, likewise, not necessary when using this steroid, as gynecomastia should not be a concern even among sensitive individuals. Since estrogen is the usual culprit with water retention, this steroid instead produces a lean, quality look to the physique with no fear of excess subcutaneous fluid retention. This makes it a favorable steroid to use during cutting cycles, when water and fat retention are major concerns. Note that some users may notice lethargy with this steroid, which may be due, in part, to its low androgenic or estrogenic component. Stacking it with an aromatizable androgen like testosterone should alleviate this problem.

Side Effects (Androgenic):

Although classified as an anabolic steroid, androgenic side effects are still possible with this substance, especially with higher doses. This may include bouts of oily skin, acne, and body/facial hair growth. Anabolic/androgenic steroids may also aggravate male pattern hair loss. Women are warned of the potential virilizing effects of anabolic/androgenic steroids. These may include a deepening of the voice, menstrual irregularities, changes in skin texture, facial hair growth, and clitoral enlargement. Methepitiostane is a steroid with very low androgenic activity relative to its tissue-building actions, making the threshold for strong androgenic side effects comparably higher than with more androgenic agents such as testosterone, methandrostenolone, or fluoxymesterone. Note that methepitiostane is unaffected by the 5-alpha reductase enzyme, so its relative androgenicity is not affected by the concurrent use of finasteride or dutasteride.

Side Effects (Hepatotoxicity):

Methepitiostane is a c17-alpha alkylated compound. This alteration protects the drug from deactivation by the liver, allowing a very high percentage of the drug entry into the bloodstream following oral administration. C17-alpha alkylated anabolic/androgenic steroids can be hepatotoxic. Prolonged or high exposure may result in liver damage. In rare instances life-threatening dysfunction may develop. It is advisable to visit a physician periodically during each cycle to monitor liver function and overall health. Intake of c17-alpha alkylated steroids is commonly limited to 6-8 weeks, in an effort to avoid escalating liver strain.

The use of a liver detoxification supplement such as Liver Stabil, Liv-52, or Essentiale Forte is advised while taking any hepatotoxic anabolic/androgenic steroids.

Side Effects (Cardiovascular):

Anabolic/androgenic steroids can have deleterious effects on serum cholesterol. This includes a tendency to reduce HDL (good) cholesterol values and increase LDL (bad) cholesterol values, which may shift the HDL to LDL balance in a direction that favors greater risk of arteriosclerosis. The relative impact of an anabolic/androgenic steroid on serum lipids is dependant on the dose, route of administration (oral vs. injectable), type of steroid (aromatizable or non-aromatizable), and level of resistance to hepatic metabolism. Methepitiostane has a strong effect on the hepatic management of cholesterol due to its structural resistance to liver breakdown, non-aromatizable nature, and route of administration. Anabolic/androgenic steroids may also adversely affect blood pressure and triglycerides, reduce endothelial relaxation, and support left ventricular hypertrophy, all potentially increasing the risk of cardiovascular disease and myocardial infarction.

To help reduce cardiovascular strain it is advised to maintain an active cardiovascular exercise program and minimize the intake of saturated fats, cholesterol, and simple carbohydrates at all times during active AAS administration. Supplementing with fish oils (4 grams per day) and a natural cholesterol/antioxidant formula such as Lipid Stabil or a product with comparable ingredients is also recommended.

Side Effects (Testosterone Suppression):

All anabolic/androgenic steroids when taken in doses sufficient to promote muscle gain are expected to suppress endogenous testosterone production. Without the intervention of testosterone stimulating substances, testosterone levels should return to normal within 1-4 months of drug secession. Note that prolonged hypogonadotrophic hypogonadism can develop secondary to steroid abuse, necessitating medical intervention.

The above side effects are not inclusive. For more detailed discussion of potential side effects, see the Steroid Side Effects section of this book.

Administration (Men):

Methepitiostane was never approved for use in humans. Prescribing guidelines are unavailable. An effective dosage for physique- or performance-enhancing purposes falls in the range of 10-20 mg daily. This is usually taken for no longer than 6-8 weeks, in an effort to avoid significant liver strain. At this level the drug should impart a measurable but moderate lean-mass-building effect, which, depending on dietary and metabolic factors, may be accompanied by measurable fat loss and an increase in definition. Doses of 30 mg per day are also commonly used, however given the high relative potency of the steroid may present significant hepatotoxicity. When administered, higher doses are usually taken for durations lasting no longer than 4-6 weeks.

Administration (Women):

Methepitiostane was never approved for use in humans. Prescribing guidelines are unavailable. An effective dosage for physique- or performance-enhancing purposes would be around 5 mg per day. This would be taken for no longer than 4-6 weeks, in an effort to avoid significant liver strain or virilizing side effects. Given that complete separation of anabolic and androgenic effect has not been achieved with any steroid, this agent is still capable of producing virilizing activity given the right dose or individual sensitivity.

Availability:

Methepitiostane is currently only produced in U.S. as a sports nutrition product, sold as Havoc and under numerous other brand names.

Hydroxytest (hydroxytestosterone)

Androgenic	25
Anabolic	65
Standard	Testosterone
Chemical Names	4-hydroxy-androsten-3-one-17beta-ol
	4,17-dihydroxyandrost-4-en-3-one
Estrogenic Activity	none
Progestational Activity	no data available (low)

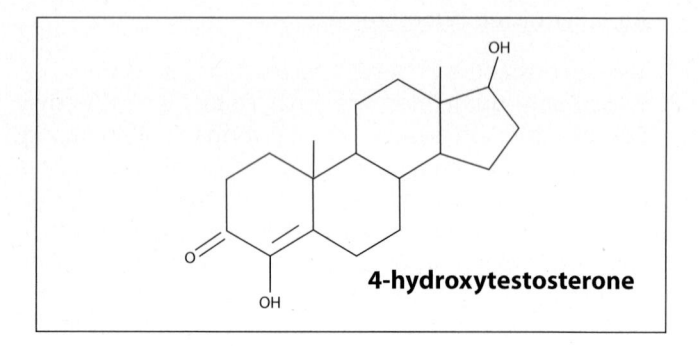

4-hydroxytestosterone

Description:

Hydroxytestosterone is an anabolic steroid that, as its name would indicate, is a close structural relative of testosterone. More specifically, it is testosterone with an added 4-hydroxl group, an alteration that drastically alters the activity of this steroid. In action it is only moderately anabolic and androgenic, with both traits significantly reduced in potency compared to testosterone. When looking at its activity profile, hydroxytestosterone is classified as an anabolic steroid, with a much lower level of relative androgenicity compared to the primary male androgen. This steroid is additionally non-estrogenic (anti-estrogenic actually), and as such tends to promote lean mass and strength gains, whereas testosterone is primarily thought of as a bulking agent. Ultimately, this steroid bears little resemblance to the androgen that it is so closely related to on a molecular level, and is often applied in very different circumstances by athletes.

History:

Hydroxytestosterone was originally developed by the pharmaceutical manufacturing giant G.D. & Searle. Methods for its synthesis were first patented in 1956.[573] Studies on its pharmacology were published soon after, and have determined that (when given by injection as an acetate) this steroid had approximately 65% of the anabolic potency of testosterone propionate, with only 25% of the androgenicity.[574] [575] This makes hydroxytestosterone a fairly favorable anabolic drug, displaying a much lower tendency to produce androgenic side effects than to increase protein synthesis. In spite of this, however, the drug never did make it to the shelf as a commercial prescription steroid product. It simply lay lost in the research books for decades, the manufacturer and patent holder probably finding little financial incentive to market it next to the many other anabolic agents available.

Hydroxytestosterone emerged from its research obscurity in 2004, when it was sold very briefly in the United States as an OTC nutritional supplement. This had to do simply with the fact that the steroid was naturally occurring, and (not being developed into a medicine) had not been identified by lawmakers at the time the first Anabolic Steroid Control Act went into effect. It was not specifically included, and thus exempt. As with all naturally occurring non-methylated steroid hormones, however, hydroxytestosterone is not intrinsically very orally active, and pharmaceutical delivery (injection) was not viable as a supplement. Hydroxytestosterone will work, but you must get the steroid into your body first. This necessitated the development of commercial ester-modified softgels (similar to Andriol in design), as well as transdermal formulas (similar to Androgel). Some consumers also made their own injections out of raw hydroxytestosterone powder. While the latter option may be preferred in a bioavailability sense, such practices were generally not recommended, as they were not inclined to produce a sterile pharmaceutical-quality medicine.

This steroid was generally a very effective one, and when sold as a supplement, seemed to be well-tolerated by consumers. There were no reports of acute side effects beyond those produced by the normal androgenic properties of the drug. Still, this agent would be very short-lived on the consumer market. By late 2004, Congress had passed an amendment to the original Anabolic Steroid Control Act that would add a number of OTC compounds to the Federal list of controlled drugs, hydroxytestosterone included. The amended law went into effect in early 2005. All supplement products containing this anabolic steroid were subsequently removed from market. Residual stock was generally pulled from commerce at the same time as well. Presently, hydroxytestosterone is again unavailable to athletes. Its future development into a commercial medicine seems highly unlikely.

How Supplied:

Hydroxytestosterone is not available as a commercial

agent. When produced as a supplement it was found in various oral and transdermal doses.

Structural Characteristics:

Hydroxytestosterone is a modified form of testosterone. It differs by the introduction of a hydroxyl group at carbon 4, which inhibits aromatization and reduces relative steroid androgenicity.

Side Effects (Estrogenic):

Hydroxytestosterone is not aromatized by the body, and is not measurably estrogenic. Estrogenic side effects such as increased water retention, fat gain, and gynecomastia are not likely with use. Note that hydroxytestosterone also has strong aromatase-inhibiting activities. This steroid differs from the suicide aromatase inhibitor formestane (4-hydroxyandrostenedione) only in that it is the active form of the steroid (17-beta hydroxysteroid) instead of the inactive dione (17-ketosteroid), and in the body is a precursor to formestane. Both formestane and hydroxytestosterone directly inhibit the aromatase enzyme, although the former (possessing a 3-keto group) is a more appropriate fit for the enzyme, and is therefore comparably more effective.[576] Regardless of its lower potency, hydroxytestosterone will still effectively lower serum estrogen, reducing the estrogenic side effects caused by the aromatization of other steroid compounds. This agent may, therefore, be looked at as a dual-purpose anabolic/aromatase-inhibiting drug.

Side Effects (Androgenic):

Although classified as an anabolic steroid, androgenic side effects are still possible with this substance. This may include bouts of oily skin, acne, and body/facial hair growth. Anabolic/androgenic steroids may also aggravate male pattern hair loss. Women are also warned of the potential virilizing effects of anabolic/androgenic steroids. These may include a deepening of the voice, menstrual irregularities, changes in skin texture, facial hair growth, and clitoral enlargement. Note that hydroxytestosterone is not extensively metabolized by the 5-alpha reductase enzyme, so its relative androgenicity is not greatly altered by the concurrent use of finasteride or dutasteride.

Side Effects (Hepatotoxicity):

Hydroxytestosterone is not a c17-alpha alkylated compound, and not known to have hepatotoxic effects. Liver toxicity is unlikely.

Side Effects (Cardiovascular):

Anabolic/androgenic steroids can have deleterious effects on serum cholesterol. This includes a tendency to reduce HDL (good) cholesterol values and increase LDL (bad) cholesterol values, which may shift the HDL to LDL balance in a direction that favors greater risk of arteriosclerosis. The relative impact of an anabolic/androgenic steroid on serum lipids is dependant on the dose, route of administration (oral vs. injectable), type of steroid (aromatizable or non-aromatizable), and level of resistance to hepatic metabolism. Hydroxytestosterone should have a stronger negative effect on the hepatic management of cholesterol than testosterone or nandrolone due to its non-aromatizable nature, but a much weaker impact than c-17 alpha alkylated steroids. Anabolic/androgenic steroids may also adversely affect blood pressure and triglycerides, reduce endothelial relaxation, and support left ventricular hypertrophy, all potentially increasing the risk of cardiovascular disease and myocardial infarction.

To help reduce cardiovascular strain it is advised to maintain an active cardiovascular exercise program and minimize the intake of saturated fats, cholesterol, and simple carbohydrates at all times during active AAS administration. Supplementing with fish oils (4 grams per day) and a natural cholesterol/antioxidant formula such as Lipid Stabil or a product with comparable ingredients is also recommended.

Side Effects (Testosterone Suppression):

All anabolic/androgenic steroids when taken in doses sufficient to promote muscle gain are expected to suppress endogenous testosterone production. Without the intervention of testosterone-stimulating substances, testosterone levels should return to normal within 1-4 months of drug secession. Note that prolonged hypogonadotrophic hypogonadism can develop secondary to steroid abuse, necessitating medical intervention.

The above side effects are not inclusive. For more detailed discussion of potential side effects, see the Steroid Side Effects section of this book.

Administration (Men):

Hydroxytestosterone was never produced as a prescription medication. Prescribing guidelines are unavailable. Effective doses for physique- or performance-enhancing purposes are in the range of 200-400 mg per week by injection, or 100-300 mg daily if taking an oil-solubilized oral product or transdermal. Maximum aromatase inhibition is likely reached by 250 mg per week when given by injection, or 100-200 mg per day when taking oral softgels. Users often keep the doses limited to this range if estrogen minimization is the main focus. Hydroxytestosterone and formestane may not be quite as potent as the selective third generation non-steroidal aromatase inhibitors Arimidex or Femara, but they do seem to do a much better job here than the "standard issue" estrogen receptor antagonists Nolvadex and Clomid (especially when it comes to shedding water and producing the tight "high androgen" look). As with all effective aromatase inhibitors, its estrogen-lowering action is likely to be accompanied by a negative lowering of HDL (good) cholesterol levels. For this reason hydroxytestosterone should never be used for long periods of time, and regular doctor's checkups are recommended during use.

Administration (Women):

Hydroxytestosterone was never produced as a prescription medication. Prescribing guidelines are unavailable. Hydroxytestosterone is not recommended for women for physique- or performance-enhancing purposes due to its strong anti-estrogenic nature and tendency to produce virilizing side effects

Availability:

Hydroxytestosterone is not available as a prescription agent at this time.

Laurabolin® (nandrolone laurate)

Androgenic	37
Anabolic	125
Standard	Testosterone
Chemical Names	19-norandrost-4-en-3-one-17beta-ol 17beta-hydroxy-estr-4-en-3-one
Estrogenic Activity	low
Progestational Activity	moderate

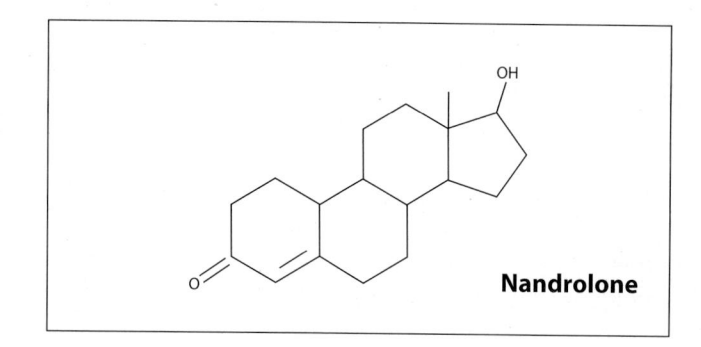

Nandrolone

Description:

Nandrolone laurate is an injectable form of the anabolic steroid nandrolone. The laurate ester applied here is two carbon atoms longer than decanoate, and consequently this agent forms a slightly longer-lasting drug deposit around the area of injection than Deca-Durabolin. Given its strong delayed-release properties, it is possible to administer nandrolone laurate once every three to four weeks in a medical setting. As a nandrolone injectable, this drug provides a moderately strong anabolic effect, which is accompanied by a low level of estrogenic and androgenic properties. Although not widely used, nandrolone laurate is favored by athletes and bodybuilders for its ability to promote slow steady gains in lean mass with minimal side effects.

History:

Nandrolone laurate was developed during the 1960's, a time when many new nandrolone esters were being synthesized and investigated. This long-acting ester of nandrolone is usually identified as a veterinary drug, but was actually prescribed to humans before it was adopted for animal use. The only brand name of reference is Clinibolin, which was sold for a brief time on the German drug market around the end of the 1960's. Nandrolone laurate was ultimately short-lived as a human medication, however, and from this point on would be used exclusively in veterinary preparations. There is nothing particular that makes the drug poorly suited for human use, and its discontinuance probably had much more to do with the dominance of Organon's Deca-Durabolin, which made nandrolone laurate fairly superfluous as a prescription drug, than any faults of the drug itself.

As a veterinary drug, nandrolone laurate is most commonly identified with the Laurabolin brand name. Laurabolin is manufactured by Intervet, and is found in a variety of countries including Mexico, Chile, The Netherlands, Australia, and Colombia. It is used with cats, dogs, horses, pigs and cattle, typically to offset malnutrition caused by viral or parasitic illness, to treat anemia, counter the catabolic effects of corticosteroids, and to improve the overall physical condition of highly active or elderly animals. The Laurabolin brand has also been sold at one time by Werfft-Chemie in Austria and Vemie in Germany, however these products have since been discontinued. In addition to the Laurabolin brand name, the drug had also been marketed in the past under the trade names Fortadex (Hydro, Germany), Fortabol (Parfam, Mexico), and Lauradrol 250 (Loeffler, Mexico). Today, only the Intervet products are known to exist.

How Supplied:

Nandrolone laurate is available in select veterinary drug markets. Composition and dosage may vary by country and manufacturer, but usually contain 20 mg/mL or 50 mg/mL of steroid dissolved in oil.

Structural Characteristics:

Nandrolone laurate is a modified form of nandrolone, where a carboxylic acid ester (lauric acid) has been attached to the 17-beta hydroxyl group. Esterified steroids are less polar than free steroids, and are absorbed more slowly from the area of injection. Once in the bloodstream, the ester is removed to yield free (active) nandrolone. Esterified steroids are designed to prolong the window of therapeutic effect following administration, allowing for a less frequent injection schedule compared to injections of free (unesterified) steroid. Nandrolone laurate is designed to provide a slow release of nandrolone for up to 3 to 4 weeks following injection.

Side Effects (Estrogenic):

Nandrolone has a low tendency for estrogen conversion, estimated to be only about 20% of that seen with testosterone.[577] This is because while the liver can convert nandrolone to estradiol, in other more active sites of steroid aromatization such as adipose tissue nandrolone is far less open to this process.[578] Consequently, estrogen-related side effects are a much lower concern with this drug than with testosterone. Elevated estrogen levels may still be noticed with higher dosing, however, and may cause side effects such as increased water retention, body fat gain, and gynecomastia. An anti-estrogen such as clomiphene citrate or tamoxifen citrate may be necessary to prevent estrogenic side effects if they occur. One may alternately use an aromatase inhibitor like Arimidex® (anastrozole), which more efficiently controls estrogen by preventing its synthesis. Aromatase inhibitors can be quite expensive in comparison to anti-estrogens, however, and may also have negative effects on blood lipids.

It is of note that nandrolone has some activity as a progestin in the body.[579] Although progesterone is a c-19 steroid, removal of this group as in 19-norprogesterone creates a hormone with greater binding affinity for its corresponding receptor. Sharing this trait, many 19-nor anabolic steroids are shown to have some affinity for the progesterone receptor as well.[580] The side effects associated with progesterone are similar to those of estrogen, including negative feedback inhibition of testosterone production and enhanced rate of fat storage. Progestins also augment the stimulatory effect of estrogens on mammary tissue growth. There appears to be a strong synergy between these two hormones here, such that gynecomastia might even occur with the help of progestins, without excessive estrogen levels. The use of an anti-estrogen, which inhibits the estrogenic component of this disorder, is often sufficient to mitigate gynecomastia caused by nandrolone.

Side Effects (Androgenic):

Although classified as an anabolic steroid, androgenic side effects are still possible with this substance, especially with higher doses. This may include bouts of oily skin, acne, and body/facial hair growth. Anabolic/androgenic steroids may also aggravate male pattern hair loss. Women are warned of the potential virilizing effects of anabolic/androgenic steroids. These may include a deepening of the voice, menstrual irregularities, changes in skin texture, facial hair growth, and clitoral enlargement. Nandrolone is a steroid with relatively low androgenic activity relative to its tissue-building actions, making the threshold for strong androgenic side effects comparably higher than with more androgenic agents such as testosterone, methandrostenolone, or fluoxymesterone. It is also important to point out that due to its mild androgenic nature and ability to suppress endogenous testosterone, nandrolone is prone to interfering with libido in males when used without another androgen.

Note that in androgen-responsive target tissues such as the skin, scalp, and prostate, the relative androgenicity of nandrolone is reduced by its reduction to dihydronandrolone (DHN).[581] [582] The 5-alpha reductase enzyme is responsible for this metabolism of nandrolone. The concurrent use of a 5-alpha reductase inhibitor such as finasteride or dutasteride will interfere with site-specific reduction of nandrolone action, considerably increasing the tendency of nandrolone to produce androgenic side effects. Reductase inhibitors should be avoided with nandrolone if low androgenicity is desired.

Side Effects (Hepatotoxicity):

Nandrolone is not c-17 alpha alkylated, and not known to have hepatotoxic effects. Liver toxicity is unlikely.

Side Effects (Cardiovascular):

Anabolic/androgenic steroids can have deleterious effects on serum cholesterol. This includes a tendency to reduce HDL (good) cholesterol values and increase LDL (bad) cholesterol values, which may shift the HDL to LDL balance in a direction that favors greater risk of arteriosclerosis. The relative impact of an anabolic/androgenic steroid on serum lipids is dependant on the dose, route of administration (oral vs. injectable), type of steroid (aromatizable or non-aromatizable), and level of resistance to hepatic metabolism. Studies administering 600 mg of nandrolone decanoate per week for 10 weeks demonstrated a 26% reduction in HDL cholesterol levels.[583] This suppression is slightly greater than that reported with an equal dose of testosterone enanthate, and is in agreement with earlier studies showing a slightly stronger negative impact on HDL/LDL ratio with nandrolone decanoate as compared to testosterone cypionate.[584] Nandrolone injectables, however, should still have a significantly weaker impact on serum lipids than c-17 alpha alkylated agents. Anabolic/androgenic steroids may also adversely affect blood pressure and triglycerides, reduce endothelial relaxation, and support left ventricular hypertrophy, all potentially increasing the risk of cardiovascular disease and myocardial infarction.

To help reduce cardiovascular strain it is advised to maintain an active cardiovascular exercise program and minimize the intake of saturated fats, cholesterol, and simple carbohydrates at all times during active AAS administration. Supplementing with fish oils (4 grams per day) and a natural cholesterol/antioxidant formula such as Lipid Stabil or a product with comparable ingredients is also recommended.

Side Effects (Testosterone Suppression):

All anabolic/androgenic steroids when taken in doses sufficient to promote muscle gain are expected to suppress endogenous testosterone production. For sake of comparison, studies administering 100 mg per week of nandrolone decanoate for 6 weeks have demonstrated an approximate 57% reduction in serum testosterone levels during therapy. At a dosage of 300 mg per week, this reduction reached 70%.[585] It is believed that the progestational activity of nandrolone notably contributes to the suppression of testosterone synthesis during therapy, which can be marked in spite of a low tendency for estrogen conversion.[586] Without the intervention of testosterone-stimulating substances, testosterone levels should return to normal within 2-6 months of drug secession. Note that prolonged hypogonadotrophic hypogonadism can develop secondary to steroid abuse, necessitating medical intervention.

The above side effects are not inclusive. For more detailed discussion of potential side effects, see the Steroid Side Effects section of this book.

Administration (Men):

Nandrolone laurate is not approved for use in humans. Prescribing guidelines are unavailable. When used for physique- or performance- enhancing purposes, a dose of 200-400 mg given every 7-10 days is most common, taken in cycles 8 to 12 weeks in length. This level is sufficient for most users to notice measurable gains in lean muscle mass and strength, which should be accompanied by a low level of estrogenic and androgenic activity. Higher doses (450-600 mg every 7-10 days) will impart a stronger anabolic effect, but can be difficult given the relatively low concentration this steroid is usually found in. Instead, many opt to combine this agent with other anabolic/androgenic steroids. Given its properties, it seems to fit well for both bulking and cutting purposes, and can reasonably replace Deca-Durabolin in cycles.

Administration (Women):

Nandrolone laurate is not approved for use in humans. Prescribing guidelines are unavailable. When used for physique- or performance- enhancing purposes, a dosage of 100 mg every 10-14 days is most common, taken for 4 to 6 weeks. Although only slightly androgenic, women are occasionally confronted with virilization symptoms when taking this compound. Should virilizing side effects become a concern, the drug should be discontinued immediately to help prevent their permanent appearance. After a sufficient period of withdrawal, the shorter-acting nandrolone Durabolin® might be considered a safer (more controllable) option. This drug stays active for only several days, greatly reducing the withdrawal time if indicated.

Availability:

The Intervet brand name Laurabolin product from Mexico is still circulating, although counterfeits are also made.

In the past, Fortabol was found on very rare occasion in the U.S. This product includes 20 mg nandrolone laurate with an added amount of Vitamin A. Since the dosage was so low, this brand was really only beneficial to women. This brand is now out of commerce.

Although even less common than other brands, Intervet sells Laurabolin in several European and South American countries. These are of similar mixed reliability to Mexican Laurabolin.

Libriol (nandrolone/methandriol blend)

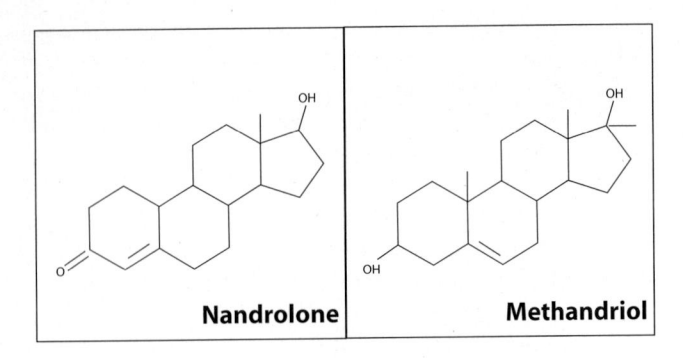

Androgenic

Anabolic

Standard

Chemical Names

Estrogenic Activity

Progestational Activity

Description:

Libriol is an Australian injectable veterinary steroid preparation that contains a blend of methandriol dipropionate and nandrolone phenylpropionate. The two steroids are present in a dose of 45 mg/mL and 30 mg/mL respectively. This adds up to a total steroid concentration of 75 mg/mL. As a blend of methandriol and nandrolone, Libriol can be categorized as a moderately strong anabolic steroid with mild androgenic properties. It is also mildly estrogenic, owing to its methandriol content. This preparation can essentially be viewed as a fast-acting version of Ranvet's Tribolin. Although not widely available, this product is an effective muscle-building drug, which generally produces lean gains as opposed to strong mass increases.

History:

Libriol is a product of RWR Veterinary Products (formerly a subsidiary of Nature Vet), sold only on the Australian veterinary drug market. It is used exclusively for horses, generally racehorses that need rehabilitation or improvements in general health and performance. The drug combination is prescribed to increase lean muscularity of the animal, help maintain proper fluid levels and avoid dehydration, and to improve the digestion and assimilation of proteins from feed. For a horse weighing approximately 1,100 pounds (500kg), a dosage of 5 mL (350 mg) is generally administered once every 2 weeks. As a "pre-stacked" steroid preparation, this steroid has piqued a great deal of interest among bodybuilders historically, and at one time would fetch a fairly high price on the black market due to the uniqueness of its formulation.

Libriol has been on the Australian market for many years, and remains available today in spite of the growing publicity paid to sports doping and the declining interest of legitimate companies to market these drugs. It is of note that RWR discontinued use of the long-standing Libriol trade name in 2005, however, registering a new trade name for the product, RWR 4 Fillies. The same nandrolone/methandriol formulation thus remains available on the Australian market, for those veterinarians that have come to rely on Libriol as an effective anabolic/tonic aid. Due to tight government controls, it is unlikely that much volume of the new RWR 4 Fillies product will be diverted for athletic use. Given the low per-milliliter steroid concentration and diverse competition of today's market, this product is additionally much less desirable than it used to be.

How Supplied:

Libriol is available on the Australian veterinary drug market, sold presently under the trade name RWR 4 Fillies. It contains 75 mg/mL of steroid in oil in a 10 mL vial.

Structural Characteristics:

For a more comprehensive discussion of the individual steroids nandrolone phenylpropionate and methandriol dipropionate, refer to their respective profiles.

Side Effects (Estrogenic):

Methylandrostendiol is not directly aromatized by the body, although one of its known metabolites is methyltestosterone, which can aromatize. Methylandrostenediol is also believed to have some inherent estrogenic activity.[587] Combined with nandrolone, which also weakly aromatizes, Libriol is considered a weakly to moderately estrogenic steroid. Gynecomastia is possible during treatment, but generally only when higher doses are used. Water and fat retention can also become issues, again depending on dose. Sensitive individuals may need to addition an anti-estrogen such as Nolvadex® to minimize related side effects.

Side Effects (Androgenic):

Although classified as an anabolic steroid preparation,

androgenic side effects are still common with this substance. This may include bouts of oily skin, acne, and body/facial hair growth. Anabolic/androgenic steroids may also aggravate male pattern hair loss. Women are warned of the potential virilizing effects of anabolic/androgenic steroids. These may include a deepening of the voice, menstrual irregularities, changes in skin texture, facial hair growth, and clitoral enlargement.

Side Effects (Hepatotoxicity):

Methylandrostenediol is a c17-alpha alkylated compound. This alteration protects the drug from deactivation by the liver, allowing a very high percentage of the drug entry into the bloodstream following oral administration. C17-alpha alkylated anabolic/androgenic steroids can be hepatotoxic. Prolonged or high exposure may result in liver damage. In rare instances life-threatening dysfunction may develop. It is advisable to visit a physician periodically during each cycle to monitor liver function and overall health. Intake of c17-alpha alkylated steroids is commonly limited to 6-8 weeks, in an effort to avoid escalating liver strain. Injectable forms of the drug may present slightly less strain on the liver by avoiding the first-pass metabolism of oral dosing, although may still present substantial hepatotoxicity.

The use of a liver detoxification supplement such as Liver Stabil, Liv-52, or Essentiale Forte is advised while taking any hepatotoxic anabolic/androgenic steroids.

Side Effects (Cardiovascular):

Anabolic/androgenic steroids can have deleterious effects on serum cholesterol. This includes a tendency to reduce HDL (good) cholesterol values and increase LDL (bad) cholesterol values, which may shift the HDL to LDL balance in a direction that favors greater risk of arteriosclerosis. The relative impact of an anabolic/androgenic steroid on serum lipids is dependant on the dose, route of administration (oral vs. injectable), type of steroid (aromatizable or non-aromatizable), and level of resistance to hepatic metabolism. Methylandrostenediol has a strong effect on the hepatic management of cholesterol due to its structural resistance to liver breakdown and (with the oral) route of administration. Anabolic/androgenic steroids may also adversely affect blood pressure and triglycerides, reduce endothelial relaxation, and support left ventricular hypertrophy, all potentially increasing the risk of cardiovascular disease and myocardial infarction.

To help reduce cardiovascular strain it is advised to maintain an active cardiovascular exercise program and minimize the intake of saturated fats, cholesterol, and simple carbohydrates at all times during active AAS administration. Supplementing with fish oils (4 grams per day) and a natural cholesterol/antioxidant formula such as Lipid Stabil or a product with comparable ingredients is also recommended.

Side Effects (Testosterone Suppression):

All anabolic/androgenic steroids when taken in doses sufficient to promote muscle gain are expected to suppress endogenous testosterone production. Without the intervention of testosterone-stimulating substances, testosterone levels should return to normal within 1-4 months of drug secession. Note that prolonged hypogonadotrophic hypogonadism can develop secondary to steroid abuse, necessitating medical intervention.

The above side effects are not inclusive. For more detailed discussion of potential side effects, see the Steroid Side Effects section of this book.

Administration (Men):

Libriol has not been approved for use in humans. Prescribing guidelines are unavailable. Typical dosing schedule for physique- or performance-enhancing purposes would be in the range of 225 mg (3cc's) to 450 mg (6cc's) per week, a level that should provide quality lean mass gain without bloating or significant body fat retention. Due to the fast-acting nature of the esters used, the total weekly dosage is commonly divided into 2-3 smaller applications.

Administration (Women):

Libriol has not been approved for use in humans. Prescribing guidelines are unavailable. Drugs containing methylandrostenediol are generally not recommended for women for physique- or performance-enhancing purposes due to its androgenic nature and tendency to produce virilizing side effects.

Availability:

Libriol (RWR 4 Fillies) is not widely available on the black market due to strict controls over steroid distribution channels in Australia. The manufacturer also claims to be very diligent in trying to limit diversion of the product. As such, most products sold on the black market labeled as Libriol/RWR 4 Fillies are actually counterfeits.

Madol (desoxymethyltestosterone)

Androgenic	187
Anabolic	1,200
Standard	Methyltestosterone (oral)
Chemical Names	17a-methyl-17b-hydroxy-5a-androst-2-ene
Estrogenic Activity	none
Progestational Activity	no data available

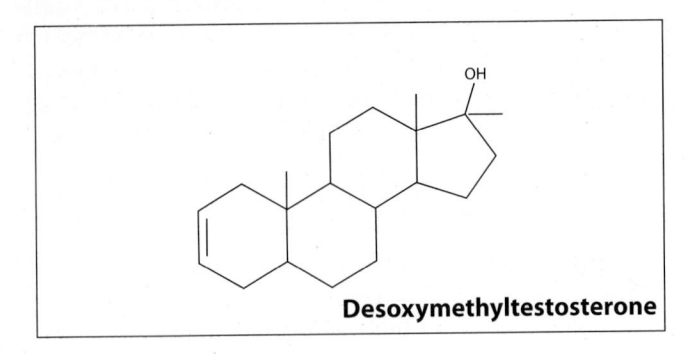

Description:

Madol (desoxymethyltestosterone; also known as DMT) is a potent synthetic oral anabolic steroid. Desoxymethyltestosterone is thought of as a cousin to methyltestosterone, although the association between the two steroids is very loose. The unique thing about desoxymethyltestosterone is that it is structurally a 2-ene compound, lacking the 3-keto group present on most commercial anabolic steroids. This lack of a 3-keto group, however, does not mean desoxymethyltestosterone is a weak compound. Quite the contrary, it is an exceedingly potent oral steroid. According to the standard rat assays, desoxymethyltestosterone exceeds methyltestosterone in oral potency by a factor of 12.[588] At the same time, its androgenicity is recorded to be only 87% higher, giving desoxymethyltestosterone an extremely favorable anabolic to androgenic ratio (measured to be nearly 6.5:1). The resulting steroid is considerably different than methyltestosterone, a drug which is both significantly weaker mg for mg than desoxymethyltestosterone, and possesses a much more formidable androgenic component.

History:

Desoxymethyltestosterone was first described in 1963.[589] This agent was never made available as a commercial prescription drug product, and saw only limited investigation in animals during the mid-1960's before disappearing into research obscurity. This agent remained hidden in the library bookshelves for decades, until reemerging in 2005 as a new "designer steroid" of interest to international sports doping officials. This was due to the confiscation of a sample of DMT at the Canadian border in December of 2003, where it was found in the possession of Canadian sprinter Derek Dueck during a routine vehicle inspection. The DMT sample remained nameless in a Customs warehouse for over a year, until officials from the World Anti-Doping Agency (WADA) finally had it tested and identified. Desoxymethyltestosterone is only the third never commercially marketed anabolic steroid found to be in use by athletes, following norbolethone and THG.

Although at one point DMT could have been considered an effective and "invisible" designer steroid for use while competing in drug-tested sports, this is no longer the case. The UCLA Olympic Laboratory was successful in its quest to outline methods for detecting desoxymethyltestosterone in the urine, and these methods have been made available to all Olympic drug-testing labs. They have also been published, and as such are available to any other agency that wants to take an interest in its detection as well. Any sport that has its athletes' urine samples analyzed at an accredited laboratory will likely be checking for DMT at this point. Still, it is an oral steroid, and likely most metabolites are cleared from the body within a few weeks of stopping its use (not unlike most oral steroids). This agent is likely still around in some competitive circles, taunting testing officials with its relatively rapid rate of clearance.

Desoxymethyltestosterone was never sold as a commercial prescription anabolic steroid; however, it did appear on the sports nutrition market in 2005 under the brand name ErgoMax LMG (Lean Mass Generator), and subsequently other brand names. This drug is in sort of a grey area legally. It is not yet listed on any State or Federal law as an anabolic steroid, and is not subject to criminal possession laws. But at the same time, it is clearly synthetic, and therefore not legal to sell as a dietary supplement. The FDA had acknowledged the presence of DMT in the supplement market in late 2005, and claimed they were investigating the issue and planning to take action. This resulted in the voluntary withdrawal of desoxymethyltestosterone-containing products from the U.S. marketplace. Today, desoxymethyltestosterone is scarcely available, with residual stock and a very small number of clone products being traded overseas.

It should be noted that manufacture of this steroid is not extremely easy. The first hints of this came from the World Anti-Doping Agency, who reported that the confiscated sample of DMT was shown to be very impure upon analysis. It was principally comprised of four different steroidal components: DMT, its unmethylated analog, and isomers of these two steroids bearing a 3-ene structure instead of 2-ene. DMT is likely the only highly effective anabolic steroid in the group, making it obvious the blend is an issue of manufacturing contamination and not functionality. The same issue appeared again when Don Catlin and his staff at the UCLA Olympic Analytical Laboratory began working on methods for detecting DMT in urine. The procedure required they obtain samples of DMT to work with, which was accomplished by chemically modifying the available starting material 5-alpha-androst-2-ene-17-one. Even the laboratory material they had to work with was shown to be a mixture of both 2-ene and 3-ene isomers (in approximately a 4:1 ratio) upon analysis, an unexpected but now consistent result. Although marketed as such, the existence of pure DMT products has not been independently confirmed. The same purity issues may apply to other (perhaps all) DMT-containing products.

How Supplied:

Desoxymethyltestosterone is not available as a prescription drug product.

Structural Characteristics:

Desoxymethyltestosterone is a modified form of dihydrotestosterone. It differs by 1) the addition of a methyl group at carbon 17-alpha, which helps protect the hormone during oral administration, 2) the introduction of a double bond between carbons 2 and 3 (2-ene) and 3) the removal of the 3-keto group (des-oxy). The latter two modifications greatly enhance the anabolic and relative biological activity of the steroid, partly by preventing the reduction of DMT to inactive 3-hydroxysteroid metabolites.

Side Effects (Estrogenic):

Desoxymethyltestosterone is not aromatized by the body, and is not known to be measurably estrogenic. An anti-estrogen should not be necessary when using this steroid. Since estrogen is the usual culprit with water retention, this steroid instead tends to produces a lean, quality look to the physique for most users. This makes it a favorable steroid to use during cutting cycles, when water and fat retention are major concerns. Note that some sensitive individuals do report estrogen-like side effects from this steroid, which suggests that it may have some low level of estrogen or progesterone receptor binding.

Side Effects (Androgenic):

Although desoxymethyltestosterone is classified as an anabolic steroid, androgenic side effects are still possible with this substance. These may include bouts of oily skin, acne, and body/facial hair growth. Higher doses are more likely to cause such side effects. Anabolic/androgenic steroids may also aggravate male pattern hair loss. Women are additionally warned of the potential virilizing effects of anabolic/androgenic steroids. These may include a deepening of the voice, menstrual irregularities, changes in skin texture, facial hair growth, and clitoral enlargement. Desoxymethyltestosterone is unaffected by the 5-alpha reductase enzyme, so its relative androgenicity is not affected by the concurrent use of finasteride or dutasteride.

Side Effects (Hepatotoxicity):

Desoxymethyltestosterone is a c17-alpha alkylated compound. This alteration protects the drug from deactivation by the liver, allowing a very high percentage of the drug entry into the bloodstream following oral administration. C17-alpha alkylated anabolic/androgenic steroids can be hepatotoxic. Prolonged or high exposure may result in liver damage. In rare instances life-threatening dysfunction may develop. It is advisable to visit a physician periodically during each cycle to monitor liver function and overall health. Intake of c17-alpha alkylated steroids is commonly limited to 6-8 weeks, in an effort to avoid escalating liver strain.

The use of a liver detoxification supplement such as Liver Stabil, Liv-52, or Essentiale Forte is advised while taking any hepatotoxic anabolic/androgenic steroids.

Side Effects (Cardiovascular):

Anabolic/androgenic steroids can have deleterious effects on serum cholesterol. This includes a tendency to reduce HDL (good) cholesterol values and increase LDL (bad) cholesterol values, which may shift the HDL to LDL balance in a direction that favors greater risk of arteriosclerosis. The relative impact of an anabolic/androgenic steroid on serum lipids is dependant on the dose, route of administration (oral vs. injectable), type of steroid (aromatizable or non-aromatizable), and level of resistance to hepatic metabolism. Desoxymethyltestosterone has a strong effect on the hepatic management of cholesterol due to its non-aromatizable nature, structural resistance to liver breakdown, and route of administration. Anabolic/androgenic steroids may also adversely affect blood pressure and triglycerides, reduce endothelial relaxation, and support left ventricular hypertrophy, all potentially increasing the risk of cardiovascular disease and myocardial infarction.

To help reduce cardiovascular strain it is advised to maintain an active cardiovascular exercise program and minimize the intake of saturated fats, cholesterol, and simple carbohydrates at all times during active AAS administration. Supplementing with fish oils (4 grams per day) and a natural cholesterol/antioxidant formula such as Lipid Stabil or a product with comparable ingredients is also recommended.

Side Effects (Testosterone Suppression):

All anabolic/androgenic steroids when taken in doses sufficient to promote muscle gain are expected to suppress endogenous testosterone production. Without the intervention of testosterone-stimulating substances, testosterone levels should return to normal within 1-4 months of drug secession. Note that prolonged hypogonadotrophic hypogonadism can develop secondary to steroid abuse, necessitating medical intervention.

The above side effects are not inclusive. For more detailed discussion of potential side effects, see the Steroid Side Effects section of this book.

Administration (General):

Studies have shown that taking an oral anabolic steroid with food may decrease its bioavailability.[590] This is caused by the fat-soluble nature of steroid hormones, which can allow some of the drug to dissolve with undigested dietary fat, reducing its absorption from the gastrointestinal tract. For maximum utilization, this steroid should be taken on an empty stomach.

Administration (Men):

Desoxymethyltestosterone was never approved for use in humans; actual prescribing guidelines are unavailable. In the athletic arena, an effective oral daily dosage would fall in the range of 5-15 mg, taken in cycles lasting no more than 6-8 weeks to minimize hepatotoxicity. This level is sufficient for measurable increases in lean muscle mass and strength. Note that a dosage of 5-15 mg per day could relate to as much as 10-30 mg when using an impure "supplement" product containing a mixture of DMT and its isomers. Desoxymethyltestosterone is considered a very versatile steroid, and while it is most ideally used during cutting phases of training, is potent enough to stack with other agents for bulking purposes as well.

Administration (Women):

Desoxymethyltestosterone was never approved for use in humans; actual prescribing guidelines are unavailable. In the athletic arena, an effective oral daily dosage would fall in the range of 1-2mg, taken in cycles lasting no more than 4-6 weeks to minimize the impact of DMT's hepatotoxicity and virilizing activities.

Availability:

Desoxymethyltestosterone is only available in underground or black market preparations. A number of such products may be located at this time; however, all are lacking any verifiable quality controls (as is the nature of illicitly manufactured and traded products). Numerous such products have been found to be of acceptable quality by consumers, however.

William Llewellyn's ANABOLICS, 9th ed.

Masteron® *(drostanolone propionate)*

Androgenic	25-40
Anabolic	62-130
Standard	Testosterone

Chemical Names	2alpha-methyl-androstan-3-one-17beta-ol
	2alpha-methyl-dihydrotestosterone
Estrogenic Activity	none
Progestational Activity	no data available (low)

Drostanolone

Description:

Drostanolone propionate is an injectable anabolic steroid derived from dihydrotestosterone (DHT). Here, the DHT backbone has been modified with a 2-methyl group to increase its anabolic properties, making this agent significantly more effective at promoting the growth of muscle tissue than its non-methylated parent. Drostanolone propionate is described in product literature as a "steroid with powerful anabolic and anti-estrogenic properties," and indeed does seem to share some of both properties. Admittedly, however, its anabolic properties are more properly described as moderate, especially when placed in the context of other agents. The drug is most often used by dieting bodybuilders and athletes in speed sports, where it is highly favored for its ability to produce solid increases in lean muscle mass and strength, which are usually accompanied by reductions in body fat level and minimal side effects.

History:

Drostanolone propionate was first described in 1959.[591] Syntex developed the agent alongside such other well-known steroids as Anadrol and methyldrostanolone (Superdrol), also first described in the same paper. Drostanolone propionate would be introduced as a prescription drug product approximately a decade later. Lilly had an agreement with Syntex to split certain research and development costs in exchange for the rights to market the results of that research. Lilly would, therefore, sell drostanolone propionate in the U.S. under the Drolban brand name, while Syntex would sell/license it in other markets. Products included Masteron in Belgium (Sarva-Syntex) and Portugal (Cilag), Masteril in the U.K. and Bulgaria, and Metormon in Spain. Drostanolone propionate was also found in such popular preparations as Permastril (Cassenne, France), Mastisol (Shionogi, Japan), and Masterid (Grunenthal, Germany Democratic Republic).

The U.S. Food and Drug Administration approved drostanolone propionate for the treatment of advanced inoperable breast cancer in postmenopausal women. This remained the principle clinical indication for the agent in all international markets as well. The prescribing literature reminds doctors and female patients that there is considerably less virilization with drostanolone propionate as compared to equal doses of testosterone propionate, suggesting this was a much more comfortable alternative to testosterone injections for the given audience. Still, the given dosage level (300 mg per week) was relatively high, and the literature also reminds us that mild virilization symptoms still commonly occur, such as deepening of the voice, acne, facial hair growth, and enlargement of the clitoris. It also reports that marked virilization sometimes follows long-term therapy.

While highly popular among athletes during the 1970's and '80's, drostanolone propionate ultimately enjoyed limited success as a prescription agent. Manufacturers began voluntarily discontinuing sale of the agent in various markets before long, likely due to the advent of more effective therapies for breast cancer, as well as the slow decline in steroid prescriptions for this phase of treatment. One of the first preparations to go was the U.S. Drolban, which was removed from market during the late 1980's. Permastril and Metormon were soon dropped as well. The last remaining Western preparation containing drostanolone propionate was Masteron from Belgium, which disappeared by the late 1990's. Drostanolone propionate remains listed on the U.S. Pharmacopias, suggesting there is presently no legal roadblock to its sale, although its reemergence as a prescription drug product seems highly unlikely.

How Supplied:

Drostanolone propionate is no longer available as a prescription drug preparation. When produced, it was supplied in the form of 1 mL and 2 mL ampules and 10 mL vials containing 50 mg/ml or 100 mg/ml of steroid in oil.

Structural Characteristics:

Drostanolone (also known as dromostanolone) is a modified form of dihydrotestosterone. It differs by the introduction of a methyl group at carbon-2 (alpha), which considerably increases the anabolic strength of the steroid by heightening its resistance to metabolism by the 3-hydroxysteroid dehydrogenase enzyme in skeletal muscle tissue. Drostanolone propionate is a modified form of drostanolone, where a carboxylic acid ester (propionic acid) has been attached to the 17-beta hydroxyl group. Esterified steroids are less polar than free steroids, and are absorbed more slowly from the area of injection. Once in the bloodstream, the ester is removed to yield free (active) drostanolone. Esterified steroids are designed to prolong the window of therapeutic effect following administration, allowing for a less frequent injection schedule compared to injections of free (unesterified) steroid. The half-life of drostanolone propionate is approximately two days after injection.

Side Effects (Estrogenic):

Drostanolone is not aromatized by the body, and is not measurably estrogenic. An anti-estrogen is not necessary when using this steroid, as gynecomastia should not be a concern even among sensitive individuals. Since estrogen is the usual culprit with water retention, drostanolone instead produces a lean, quality look to the physique with no fear of excess subcutaneous fluid retention. This makes it a favorable steroid to use during cutting cycles, when water and fat retention are major concerns. As a non-aromatizable DHT derivative, drostanolone may impart an anti-estrogenic effect, the drug competing with other (aromatizable) substrates for binding to the aromatase enzyme.

Side Effects (Androgenic):

Although classified as an anabolic steroid, androgenic side effects are still possible with this substance, especially with higher than normal therapeutic doses. This may include bouts of oily skin, acne, and body/facial hair growth. Anabolic/androgenic steroids may also aggravate male pattern hair loss. Women are warned of the potential virilizing effects of anabolic/androgenic steroids. These may include a deepening of the voice, menstrual irregularities, changes in skin texture, facial hair growth, and clitoral enlargement. Drostanolone is a steroid with relatively low androgenic activity relative to its tissue-building actions, making the threshold for strong androgenic side effects comparably higher than with more androgenic agents such as testosterone, methandrostenolone, or fluoxymesterone. Note that drostanolone is unaffected by the 5-alpha reductase enzyme, so its relative androgenicity is not affected by the concurrent use of finasteride or dutasteride.

Side Effects (Hepatotoxicity):

Drostanolone is not c17-alpha alkylated, and not known to have hepatotoxic properties. Liver toxicity is unlikely.

Side Effects (Cardiovascular):

Anabolic/androgenic steroids can have deleterious effects on serum cholesterol. This includes a tendency to reduce HDL (good) cholesterol values and increase LDL (bad) cholesterol values, which may shift the HDL to LDL balance in a direction that favors greater risk of arteriosclerosis. The relative impact of an anabolic/androgenic steroid on serum lipids is dependant on the dose, route of administration (oral vs. injectable), type of steroid (aromatizable or non-aromatizable), and level of resistance to hepatic metabolism. Drostanolone should have a stronger negative effect on the hepatic management of cholesterol than testosterone or nandrolone due to its non-aromatizable nature, but a weaker impact than c-17 alpha alkylated steroids. Anabolic/androgenic steroids may also adversely affect blood pressure and triglycerides, reduce endothelial relaxation, and support left ventricular hypertrophy, all potentially increasing the risk of cardiovascular disease and myocardial infarction.

To help reduce cardiovascular strain it is advised to maintain an active cardiovascular exercise program and minimize the intake of saturated fats, cholesterol, and simple carbohydrates at all times during active AAS administration. Supplementing with fish oils (4 grams per day) and a natural cholesterol/antioxidant formula such as Lipid Stabil or a product with comparable ingredients is also recommended.

Side Effects (Testosterone Suppression):

All anabolic/androgenic steroids when taken in doses sufficient to promote muscle gain are expected to suppress endogenous testosterone production. Without the intervention of testosterone-stimulating substances, testosterone levels should return to normal within 1-4 months of drug secession. Note that prolonged hypogonadotrophic hypogonadism can develop secondary to steroid abuse, necessitating medical intervention.

The above side effects are not inclusive. For more detailed discussion of potential side effects, see the Steroid Side Effects section of this book.

Administration (Men):

Drostanolone propionate was not FDA approved for use in men. Prescribing guidelines are unavailable. For physique- or performance-enhancing purposes, this drug is usually injected three times per week. The total weekly dosage is typically 200-400 mg, which is taken for 6-12 weeks. This level of use is sufficient to provide measurable gains in lean muscle mass and strength.

Drostanolone propionate is often combined with other steroids for an enhanced effect. Common stacks include an injectable anabolic such as Deca-Durabolin® (nandrolone decanoate) or Equipoise® (boldenone undecylenate), which can provide notably enhanced muscle gains without excessive water retention. For mass gains, it is often combined with an injectable testosterone. The result here can be solid muscle gain, with a lower level of water retention and other estrogenic side effects than if these steroids were used alone (usually in higher doses). Masteron, however, is most commonly applied during cutting phases of training. Here it is often combined with other non-aromatizable steroids such as Winstrol®, Primobolan®, Parabolan, or Anavar, which can greatly aid muscle retention and fat loss, during a period which can be very catabolic without steroids.

Administration (Women):

The prescribing guidelines for Drolban recommended a dose of 100 mg given three times per week. Therapy is given for a minimum of 8 to 12 weeks before an evaluation of its efficacy is made. If successful, the drug may be continued for as long as satisfactory results are obtained. Note that virilization symptoms were common at the recommended dosage. When used for physique- or performance-enhancing purposes, a dosage of 50 mg per week is most common, taken for 4 to 6 weeks. Virilization symptoms are rare in doses of 100 mg per week or below. Note that due to the short-acting nature of the propionate ester, the total weekly dosage is usually subdivided into smaller injections given once every second or third day.

Availability:

The original Syntex Masteron is now unavailable on the black market. It was discontinued in Europe years ago. No old lots should still be circulating, meaning that there is no legitimate source for brand name product Masteron anywhere.

Other legitimate pharmaceutical brands are almost nonexistent. There is a version of drostanolone sold in Myanmar by the Xelox Company called Dromostan. It contains base drostanolone only, not drostanolone propionate. Although unconfirmed by lab testing, this is a legit company, hopefully making a legit product. If so, it would be only the second real drostanolone currently sold worldwide. Due to the lack of an ester, injections would best be given every 2 days with this product, just short of the 3-4 typically used with Masteron.

In addition to the above, there are numerous underground labs producing drostanolone propionate at this time. Again, make sure you understand the inherent risks of buying underground products before making such a purchase. These risks can involve more than just the loss of money, as underground products are not often produced in a proper sterile (pharmaceutical level) environment.

Megagrisevit-Mono® (clostebol acetate)

Androgenic	25
Anabolic	46
Standard	Testosterone
Chemical Names	4-chloro-testosterone
	4-chloro-androsten-3-one-17beta-ol
Estrogenic Activity	none
Progestational Activity	no data available (low)

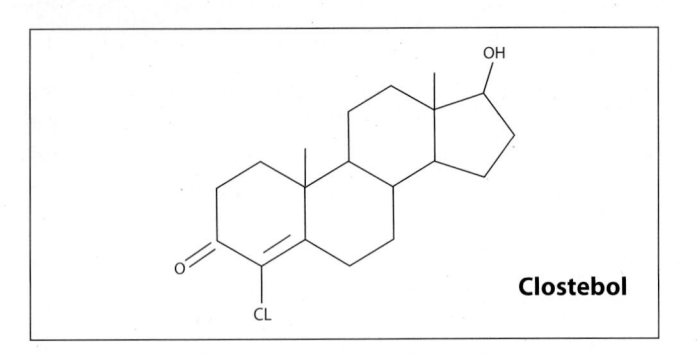

Description:

Clostebol acetate is an anabolic steroid that is derived from testosterone. Clostebol is 4-chloro-testosterone, a modification that makes this steroid a low strength anabolic compound with minimal androgenic potency. This analog of testosterone is also not 17-alpha alkylated and does not aromatize, so there is little worry of water retention, gynecomastia, or liver toxicity during use. The hydrogen substitution at the 4 position does not greatly enhance the oral efficacy of this drug, however, so the injectable is much more potent on a milligram for milligram basis, and generally preferred. Although a derivative of the potent androgen testosterone, clostebol is certainly far removed from its parent steroid in action, and generally favored by athletes for its mildness, not raw power.

History:

Clostebol acetate was first described in 1956.[592] It was developed into a medicine in Europe, where it was sold as Steranabol (Farmitalia, Germany) and Turinabol (Jenapharm, GDR). This anabolic steroid had generally been indicated for the treatment of osteoporosis, although it has reportedly been used with success for a wide variety of ailments including anorexia and liver disease. Both oral and injectable forms of the drug were produced, although the injectable was more popularly used. Clostebol acetate was commonly used with women and the elderly in European medicine, making clear the relative mildness of this anabolic. The side effects of anabolic/androgenic steroids can be much more pronounced in these populations, so typically very weak androgens are shown to be the most tolerable here.

Although quite favorable in effect and patient comfort, clostebol acetate was never a widely successful anabolic, and saw only limited use in a small number of markets. As such, its future would be a tenuous one. The Turinabol product from Jenapharm would disappear by the reunification of Germany, and the Steranabol brand would soon be replaced with lower dosed vitamin fortified versions of the drug sold by Farmitalia under the new Megagrisevit brand name. Pharmacia would acquire Farmitalia in 1993, although for a short point thereafter Megagrisevit was still being manufactured under the Pharmacia label. This did not last long, however, and Pharmacia eventually tightened up its line and removed this steroid from its offerings. Clostebol acetate had also appeared for some time in Japan, sold as Macrobin by the firm Teikoku, but this product too has since been discontinued.

Although the more functional injectable preparations of this steroid are off the market, clostebol acetate is still manufactured in a number of dermal preparations. The most recognizable such product has been Alfa-Trofodermin from Italy, although it has also been sold in such products as Neobol (Mexico), Trofodermin (Chile, Brazil), and Novaderm (Brazil). Dermal preparations of clostebol acetate are generally used to treat ulcers and wounds, and often include some neomycin to help accelerate healing. The doses of steroid used in these products is generally very small, however, and, combined with poor systemic delivery, are not of much use to athletes. In addition, this steroid has even been included in certain ophthalmologic solutions, which are even less practical to use for performance-enhancing purposes, and of less interest. Given that Megagrisevit was the last remaining effective oral or injectable steroid product to contain clostebol acetate, this drug is now essentially a defunct item as far as the athletic use of steroids are concerned.

How Supplied:

Clostebol acetate is no longer available as a commercial oral or injectable agent. When produced (Steranabol) it contained 20 mg/ml of steroid in a 2 mL glass ampule or 15 mg per tablet.

Structural Characteristics:

Clostebol is a modified form of testosterone. It differs by the introduction of a hydroxyl group at carbon 4, which inhibits aromatization and reduces relative steroid androgenicity. Clostebol acetate contains clostebol modified with the addition of carboxylic acid ester (acetic acid) at the 17-beta hydroxyl group, so that the free steroid is released more slowly from the area of injection.

Side Effects (Estrogenic):

Clostebol is not aromatized by the body, and is not measurably estrogenic. An anti-estrogen is not necessary when using this steroid, as gynecomastia should not be a concern even among sensitive individuals. Since estrogen is the usual culprit with water retention, clostebol instead produces a lean, quality look to the physique with no fear of excess subcutaneous fluid retention. This makes it a favorable steroid to use during cutting cycles, when water and fat retention are major concerns.

Side Effects (Androgenic):

Although classified as an anabolic steroid, androgenic side effects are still possible with this substance. This may include bouts of oily skin, acne, and body/facial hair growth. Anabolic/androgenic steroids may also aggravate male pattern hair loss. Women are also warned of the potential virilizing effects of anabolic/androgenic steroids. These may include a deepening of the voice, menstrual irregularities, changes in skin texture, facial hair growth, and clitoral enlargement. Additionally, clostebol is not extensively metabolized by the 5-alpha reductase enzyme, so its relative androgenicity is not greatly altered by the concurrent use of finasteride or dutasteride. Note that clostebol is a steroid with low androgenic activity relative to its tissue-building actions, making the threshold for strong androgenic side effects comparably higher than with more androgenic agents such as testosterone, methandrostenolone, or fluoxymesterone.

Side Effects (Hepatotoxicity):

Clostebol is not a c17-alpha alkylated compound, and not known to have hepatotoxic effects. Liver toxicity is unlikely.

Side Effects (Cardiovascular):

Anabolic/androgenic steroids can have deleterious effects on serum cholesterol. This includes a tendency to reduce HDL (good) cholesterol values and increase LDL (bad) cholesterol values, which may shift the HDL to LDL balance in a direction that favors greater risk of arteriosclerosis. The relative impact of an anabolic/androgenic steroid on serum lipids is dependant on the dose, route of administration (oral vs. injectable), type of steroid (aromatizable or non-aromatizable), and level of resistance to hepatic metabolism. Clostebol should have a stronger negative effect on the hepatic management of cholesterol than testosterone or nandrolone due to its non-aromatizable nature, but a much weaker impact than c-17 alpha alkylated steroids. Anabolic/androgenic steroids may also adversely affect blood pressure and triglycerides, reduce endothelial relaxation, and support left ventricular hypertrophy, all potentially increasing the risk of cardiovascular disease and myocardial infarction.

To help reduce cardiovascular strain it is advised to maintain an active cardiovascular exercise program and minimize the intake of saturated fats, cholesterol, and simple carbohydrates at all times during active AAS administration. Supplementing with fish oils (4 grams per day) and a natural cholesterol/antioxidant formula such as Lipid Stabil or a product with comparable ingredients is also recommended.

Side Effects (Testosterone Suppression):

All anabolic/androgenic steroids when taken in doses sufficient to promote muscle gain are expected to suppress endogenous testosterone production. Without the intervention of testosterone-stimulating substances, testosterone levels should return to normal within 1-4 months of drug secession. Note that prolonged hypogonadotrophic hypogonadism can develop secondary to steroid abuse, necessitating medical intervention.

The above side effects are not inclusive. For more detailed discussion of potential side effects, see the Steroid Side Effects section of this book.

Administration (Men):

Clostebol acetate is generally used in clinical doses of 30 mg per week by injection or 15 mg 2-3 times per day orally. The drug is administered for 3 consecutive weeks, followed by a break for 3 weeks. It is resumed at this point if indicated. Effective doses for physique- or performance-enhancing purposes fall in the range of 100-300 mg per week, taken for 6-12 weeks. Given the fast-acting nature of acetate injectables, the weekly dosage is generally subdivided into injections given at least every third day. With the low dosage of previous commercial clostebol acetate products, daily injectable were most common. Given the lower bioavailability and higher price, oral forms of the drug were not commonly used by athletes. When administered, a daily dosage of 60-90 mg appeared to be the most common.

The anabolic effect of this drug is fairly weak, so clostebol acetate is most often utilized in combination with other steroids for a stronger effect. The general application is to use it for contest preparations with other non-aromatizing anabolics such as Winstrol® or oxandrolone. Here, a daily dose of 20 mg may be added in with an average dose (20-30 mg per day) of the oral anabolic, which together should provide the user a nice muscle building effect without any water retention. The effect of clostebol would be somewhat similar to that seen with the old Primobolan® acetate ampules, although Megagrisevit is somewhat weaker in effect. Some also opt to use this compound in addition with strong non-aromatizing androgens such as trenbolone, Halotestin®, or Proviron®. The result in such cases can be an even more pronounced effect of muscle definition, although this will be accompanied by a much stronger set of side effects.

Administration (Women):

Clostebol acetate is generally used in clinical doses 30 mg per week by injection or 15 mg 2-3 times per day orally. The drug is administered for 3 consecutive weeks, followed by a break for 3 weeks. The drug is resumed at this point if indicated. Effective doses for physique- or performance-enhancing purposes fall in the range of 50-75 mg per week for the injectable, or 30-60 mg daily for the oral, taken for no longer than 6 weeks.

Availability:

Clostebol acetate is no longer available as a prescription agent at this time, and is unavailable on the black market.

MENT (methylnortestosterone acetate)

Androgenic	650
Anabolic	2,300
Standard	Testosterone propionate
Chemical Names	19-norandrost-4-en-3-one-17beta-ol
	17beta-hydroxy-estr-4-en-3-one
Estrogenic Activity	low
Progestational Activity	moderate

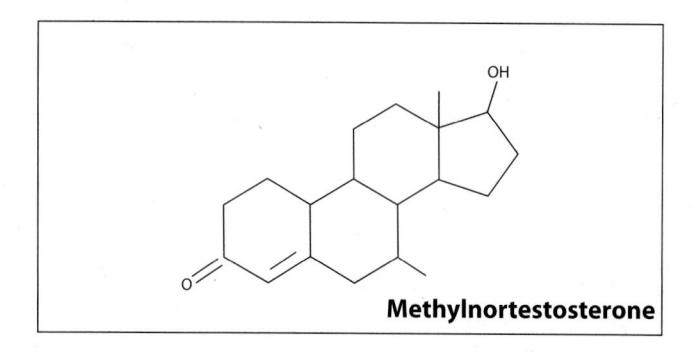

Methylnortestosterone

Description:

MENT, short for methylnortestosterone (acetate), is a synthetic anabolic steroid derived from nandrolone. This agent is also called trestolone acetate, although not as commonly. The trivial name methylnortestosterone is vague, and can also be applied to other steroids. In this case the "methyl" in the name, which is commonly associated with C-17 alpha alkylated androgens like methyltestosterone, methandrostenolone, or oxymetholone, is referring to a modification at C-7. This gives MENT a considerably different appearance than 17-methylnoretestosterone (Orgasteron). Of most obvious significance is its method of use. Although perhaps possessing a moderate level of oral bioavailability, this nandrolone derivative was not designed for oral administration. It is much more effective when administered to the body directly, by injection, implant, or transdermal gel. In character, MENT is a strongly anabolic steroid, which is accompanied by moderate androgenic and estrogenic properties.

General steroid potency is usually increased with 7-methylation, a trait well illustrated with MENT. When methylation increases steroid potency it is usually due to one or a couple of things, most notably increased resistance to hepatic metabolism (breakdown) or reduced affinity for constrictive binding proteins. In the case of MENT, we see a steroid with relatively fast metabolic breakdown, but no binding to SHBG (Sex Hormone-Binding Globulin).[593] Therefore, reduced binding to serum proteins seems to be partly responsible for making MENT a more potent steroid. When assayed in 1963, scientists reported an anabolic effect that was between 3.5 and 23 times greater than testosterone, while being only 3-6 times more androgenic.[594][595] When investigated in primates in 1998, it was shown to have 10 times more anabolic potency than testosterone, with only 2 times the stimulatory action on the prostate.[596] Its relative androgen receptor binding affinity was investigated a year later, and provided further explanation for the strong anabolic effect of this steroid. Here, MENT was shown to bind the androgen receptor more strongly than testosterone, nandrolone, or dihydrotestosterone.[597]

History:

MENT (methylnortestosterone acetate) was first described in 1963.[598] The early 1960's were part of the heyday of anabolic steroid development, with new compounds being introduced into the journals almost every week. Like a great many of the effective steroids studied during this era, however, MENT didn't make its way to becoming a commercial drug product. For about four decades it sat gathering dust on the bookshelves, next to many other effective but anonymous compounds. Historically, lack of early financial support has been a death sentence for anabolic steroids. If a company isn't there in the beginning to spend the millions necessary to develop it into an actual prescription product, it isn't going to go anywhere later on. The money simply wasn't there for MENT in the 1960s, and it died. For a long time this agent remained a "nothing" in the world of steroids.

But things changed for MENT around the turn of the century, in a very dramatic fashion. On October 30, 2000, international drug giant Schering AG made a public announcement that it had entered into a partnership to research, develop, and market methylnortestosterone acetate for both male contraceptive and hormone replacement use. This followed several years of sporadic but positive studies on this agent. The ball was set in motion, and this old steroid, which scientists had ignored for over thirty years, was suddenly amidst a hotbed of new research and speculation, the likes of which it had never seen before. In their press release, Schering AG makes promise of a new androgen that offers the anabolic and endocrine benefits of an injectable testosterone, but with less prostate growth, and more patient comfort. In other words, Schering is saying that MENT looks to be an easier to administer and equally useful steroid as testosterone, without the same issues concerning androgenicity.

The principle attraction Schering has to MENT is probably not necessarily its potency, but its ability to duplicate the positive effects of testosterone on muscle mass and male sexual function while minimizing stimulatory action on the prostate. Prostate cancer and benign prostate enlargement are very common problems among males in the U.S., and both diseases are fueled at least partly by androgens. This has led to a great deal of caution when it comes to androgen replacement therapy in older men. Although the medical data is still inconclusive in this regard, many physicians fear that the androgenicity of testosterone may lead to ill effects. After all, increases in PSA values with testosterone use in older men are well documented.[599] Perhaps MENT is being introduced to alleviate this concern. Noticing the lower relative androgenicity of MENT, researchers concluded over a decade ago that it might be a far better option for hormone replacement therapy. To quote the researchers from the NY Center for Biomedical Research exactly, "We conclude that the use of MENT instead of T for androgen replacement therapy could have health-promoting effects by reducing the occurrence of prostate disease."[600] This is quite a statement, especially when we remember it concerns the use of a synthetic anabolic steroid.

Looking a little more closely at some of the recent studies conducted on MENT, we see a general trend of success and relative safety. Perhaps the most noteworthy to examine is the multinational clinical study that was conducted between 2002 and 2003.[601] It involved the use of MENT implants as long-term contraceptives in males. In this experiment, thirty-six men were enrolled in three separate clinics residing in Germany, Chile, and the Dominical Republic (12 men at each). The study protocols itself called for the use of the implants for 6, 9, or 12 months, and required periodic examinations to measure their effects and potential risks. Three different dosages were used, which consisted of administering one, two, or four implants at the onset of the investigation. Each implant is designed to deliver about 400mcg of steroid per day, which equates to daily doses of .4mg, .8mg, or 1.6mg of steroid. The release rate is slowly reduced as the implant loses surface area, however, reaching approximately 200mcg per day by the one-year mark.

The results of the clinical trial were very promising. Four MENT implants (1.6mg/day) suppressed spermatogenesis with similar effectiveness as testosterone implants, testosterone enanthate injections, and testosterone undecanoate injections (all of which have been investigated successfully as contraceptives). MENT was able to produce azoospermia in 82% of treated subjects, a figure that was actually higher than reported with 200 mg of testosterone enanthate per week (which produced azoospermia in 65-66% of normal male subjects by 6 months). As far as negative side effects, they were few. Two subjects noted increases in blood pressure that went outside the normal range, and one was forced to discontinue the study because of it (though no ill effect was noted). Otherwise, there was generally just a very small rise in systolic pressure (+4.8), and no significant changes in lipids (including cholesterol and triglycerides) or PSA values. Furthermore, prostate volume was slightly reduced (not increased) in all groups. Liver enzymes were increased slightly, but stayed within the normal range in all subjects. The mean time to the recovery of normal sperm production after discontinuance was 3 months, similar to that reported in a 1990 World Heath Organization study with 200 mg weekly of testosterone enanthate. Overall, MENT performed admirably, with a very notable (acceptable) level of effect, and minimal side effects. And what is more, the drug may be effective when being implanted as infrequently as once per year.

Another study of interest examined the ability of MENT implants to restore sexual behavior and function in hypogonadal (low testosterone) men.[602] This, of course, is one of the principle objectives of androgen replacement therapy. This investigation took place in two clinics, one based in Ireland and the other Hong Kong. Twenty men participated in total, 10 at each location. The study was a double crossover investigation comparing the effects of testosterone enanthate (200 mg every 3 weeks) to that of two MENT implants (delivering .8mg of drug per day). This means that each of the twenty men had an opportunity to try both drugs, which were taken on two separate occasions between washout periods. Only minor differences in response were noted between MENT and conventional androgen replacement therapy, and both drugs were effective in restoring sexual behavior and erection frequency. MENT, at a dosage of 2 implants delivering approximately .8mg of drug per day, proved to be an effective option for androgen replacement therapy.

If Schering does market this drug as an implant, it will be impractical to use for bodybuilding purposes. At best it will need to be broken down and made into an injectable somehow. The clinical study discussed above used implants containing about 140 mg of steroid each. Given the same in a production drug, more than one implant will be needed for a workable cycle. There is some investigation into its use as an oral,[603] which does seem feasible (although not ideal from a cost effectiveness standpoint). The key to this steroid's success with bodybuilders will really be the development of a commercial injectable. This will likely follow the release of Schering's product; perhaps even precede it. The raw powder is already available from suppliers overseas, so it should not take long for some veterinary or underground manufacturer to perceive value in this new agent. An acetate version will probably be closely followed by a slower-acting MENT ester, perhaps even something basic like MENT cypionate or MENT enanthate.

How Supplied:

MENT is not yet available as a prescription drug product.

Structural Characteristics:

MENT is a modified form of nandrolone. It differs by the addition of a methyl group at carbon 7-alpha to increase steroid potency and relative androgenicity. MENT generally refers to methylnortestosterone acetate, modified with the addition of carboxylic acid ester (acetic acid) at the 17-beta hydroxyl group to help extend the activity of the steroid during injection or implantation.

Side Effects (Estrogenic):

MENT is aromatized by the body, and converts to a synthetic estrogen with a high level of biological activity (7alpha-methyl-estradiol).[604] As a result, it is a moderately estrogenic steroid. Gynecomastia is possible during treatment, particularly when higher doses are used. At the same time water retention can become a problem, causing a notable loss of muscle definition as both subcutaneous water retention and fat levels build. Sensitive individuals may want to keep the estrogen under control with the addition of an anti-estrogen such as Nolvadex®. One may alternately use an aromatase inhibitor like Arimidex® (anastrozole), which is a more effective remedy for estrogen control. Aromatase inhibitors, however, can be quite expensive in comparison to standard estrogen maintenance therapies, and may also have negative effects on blood lipids. Note that there is no mention of gynecomastia in any of the human clinical studies that have been conducted on this agent. Estrogenicity does not appear to be much of a problem when used at appropriate therapeutic dosages.

Note that studies have also shown MENT to strongly bind the progesterone receptor, as well as to produce progestational effects on uterine weight in immature rabbits.[605] Further examination, however, confuses this determination. The effects of MENT on uterine weight were not blocked by concurrent use of an anti-progestin (mifepristone) or anti-estrogen, suggesting that neither progestational nor estrogenic activity was responsible for this effect. Given the use of only this one limited model, the known binding of MENT to the progesterone receptor, and the tendency for nandrolone-derived drugs to offer at least some progestational activity, moderate activity will be assumed until it can be discounted.

The side effects associated with progesterone are similar to those of estrogen, including negative feedback inhibition of testosterone production and enhanced rate of fat storage. Progestins also augment the stimulatory effect of estrogens on mammary tissue growth. There appears to be a strong synergy between these two hormones here, such that gynecomastia might even occur with the help of progestins without excessive estrogen levels being present. The use of an anti-estrogen, which inhibits the estrogenic component of this disorder, may be sufficient to mitigate gynecomastia caused by progestational anabolic/androgenic steroids.

Side Effects (Androgenic):

Although classified as an anabolic steroid, androgenic side effects are still possible with this substance. This may include bouts of oily skin, acne, and body/facial hair growth. Anabolic/androgenic steroids may also aggravate male pattern hair loss. Individuals sensitive to the androgenic effects of this steroid may find a milder anabolic such as Deca-Durabolin® to be more comfortable. Women are additionally warned of the potential virilizing effects of anabolic/androgenic steroids. These may include a deepening of the voice, menstrual irregularities, changes in skin texture, facial hair growth, and clitoral enlargement.

Note that one well-understood function of 7-methylation is to block steroid 5-alpha reduction. As such, this derivative of nandrolone cannot be converted to a "dihydro" metabolite.[606] With nandrolone and most of its analogs, this reduction means a less androgenic steroid. Dihydronandrolone is weaker than nandrolone, so relative binding is reduced in target tissues with high reductase concentrations. Not being able to convert to a weaker steroid here, MENT is going to display more relative androgenicity than nandrolone. Reductase inhibitors, likewise, will not affect the relative androgenicity of MENT. Greater androgenicity was deemed a desirable trait during development, as it allows MENT to more effectively support male sex characteristics and libido compared to the weakly androgenic nandrolone.

Side Effects (Hepatotoxicity):

MENT is not a c17-alpha alkylated compound, and not known to have hepatotoxic effects. Liver toxicity is unlikely.

Side Effects (Cardiovascular):

Anabolic/androgenic steroids can have deleterious effects on serum cholesterol. This includes a tendency to reduce HDL (good) cholesterol values and increase LDL (bad) cholesterol values, which may shift the HDL to LDL balance in a direction that favors greater risk of arteriosclerosis. The relative impact of an anabolic/androgenic steroid on serum lipids is dependant on the dose, route of administration (oral vs. injectable), type of steroid (aromatizable or non-aromatizable), and level of resistance to hepatic metabolism. MENT is likely to have a moderate effect on the hepatic management of cholesterol due to its aromatizable nature and route of administration. Anabolic/androgenic steroids may also adversely affect blood pressure and triglycerides, reduce endothelial relaxation, and support left ventricular hypertrophy, all potentially increasing the risk of cardiovascular disease and myocardial infarction.

To help reduce cardiovascular strain it is advised to maintain an active cardiovascular exercise program and minimize the intake of saturated fats, cholesterol, and simple carbohydrates at all times during active AAS administration. Supplementing with fish oils (4 grams per day) and a natural cholesterol/antioxidant formula such as Lipid Stabil or a product with comparable ingredients is also recommended.

Side Effects (Testosterone Suppression):

All anabolic/androgenic steroids when taken in doses sufficient to promote muscle gain are expected to suppress endogenous testosterone production. Without the intervention of testosterone-stimulating substances, testosterone levels should return to normal within 1-4 months of drug secession. Note that prolonged hypogonadotrophic hypogonadism can develop secondary to steroid abuse, necessitating medical intervention.

The above side effects are not inclusive. For more detailed discussion of potential side effects, see the Steroid Side Effects section of this book.

Administration (Men):

MENT has not yet been developed into a commercial drug product. Prescribing guidelines are unavailable. MENT is a relatively potent steroid, so an effective dose for bodybuilders is going to be small. As a drug 10 times more anabolic than testosterone by some studies, and 20 times more effective at suppressing spermatogenesis than testosterone enanthate in others, we should commonly see daily doses under 10 mg (maybe 3-6mg most commonly). If prepared as an oil-based injectable (with acetate ester), this would mean shots of roughly 10-20 mg every two to three days. Compare this to trenbolone, which is usually given in doses of 75-100 mg per shot under the same schedule (and this is a particularly potent steroid). Some might find good effect at 10 mg daily or above, although high doses will likely amplify potential side effects, and are not recommended.

MENT should stack well with a variety of different steroids, possibly for both cutting and bulking phases of training depending on individual sensitivity to its estrogenic and progestational properties. For simplicity, this might mean using it with drugs like testosterone cypionate or enanthate (200-400 mg per week), Dianabol (20-35 mg per day), or Anadrol (50-100 mg per day) when looking for sheer size, milder anabolics like nandrolone decanoate or boldenone undecylenate (200-400 mg per week) for lean mass, or non-aromatizable drugs like Primobolan (200-400 mg per week), Winstrol (20-35 mg per day), or Anavar (15-20 mg per day) while cutting. Remember that c-17 alpha alkylated substances impart some hepatotoxictiy, and may greatly amplify the negative effects of steroid therapy on serum lipids.

Administration (Women):

MENT has not yet been developed into a commercial drug product. Prescribing guidelines are unavailable. Given its high level of potency, effective doses in women would likely be measured in microgram amounts. The drug would also generally be taken in cycles lasting 4 weeks or less. Note that virilizing side effects are still possible with primarily anabolic substances, and need to be carefully monitored.

Availability:

No legitimate medical preparation containing MENT is yet available. Black market preparations are likely to surface, but as is the nature of such preparations will lack verifiable purity and legitimacy.

Metandren (methyltestosterone)

Androgenic	94-130
Anabolic	115-150
Standard	Testosterone

Chemical Names	17b-hydroxy-17a-methyl-4-androsten-3-one
	17alpha-methylandrost-4-en-3-one-17b-ol
Estrogenic Activity	high
Progestational Activity	not significant

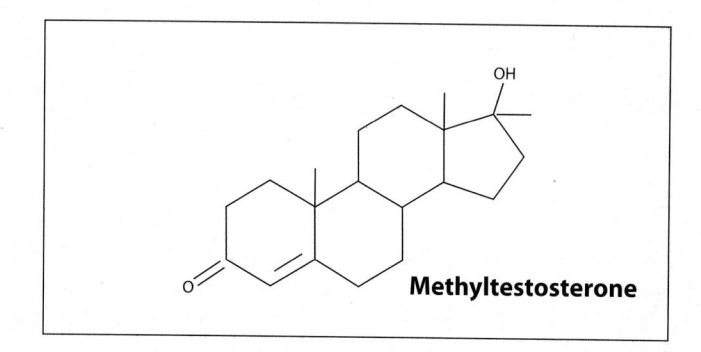

Description:

Methyltestosterone is an orally available form of the primary male androgen testosterone. Looking at the structure of this steroid, we see it is basically just testosterone with an added methyl group at the c-17 alpha position (a c-17 alpha alkylated substance), which allows for oral administration. The resultant compound "methylated-testosterone" was among the first functional oral steroids to be produced. This field of research has consequently improved greatly over the years, and today methyltestosterone is quite crude in comparison to many of the other orals that were subsequently developed. The action of this steroid is moderately anabolic and androgenic, with high estrogenic activity due to its aromatization to 17-alpha methyl estradiol. This generally makes methyltestosterone too troublesome (in terms of estrogenic side effects) to use for muscle-building purposes.

History:

Methyltestosterone was first described in 1935,[607] and was one of the first oral androgens to be used in clinical medicine (it follows Proviron, the first oral androgen, by one year). Its main clinical use at the time of development was as an oral medication to replace testosterone (and its anabolic and/or androgenic activity) in males when endogenous levels were insufficient (Andropause), although the drug was adopted for a number of other uses over the years as well. These include the treatment of cryptorchidism (undescended testicles), breast cancer in postmenopausal women, excessive lactation and breast pain after pregnancy in mothers not nursing, osteoporosis, and, more recently, female menopause (supporting the overall energy and sexual interest of the patient).

In addition to standard tablets and capsules, methyltestosterone has also been commercially prepared in sublingual or buccal tablets. Metandren Linguets from Ciba Pharmaceutical Company were perhaps the most recognized, and were popularly sold from the 1950's to 1990's. These tablets were placed under the tongue or between the gum and cheek and left to dissolve, delivering the drug to circulation via the mucous membranes, bypassing the liver. Sublingual or buccal intake approximately doubles the bioavailability of methyltestosterone, and also provides peak levels of drug rapidly (approximately 1 hour after dosing instead of 2 hours). Although Ciba's Metandren Linguets are no longer commercially available, numerous other sublingual/buccal methyltestosterone tablets are still in production today.

Methyltestosterone remains a controversial steroid. Although it has a long history, and arguably a justifiable safety record, it is no longer widely used, and is even being withdrawn from many drug markets. The German Endocrine Society made an official statement that methyltestosterone was obsolete in 1981, and the drug would be removed from German pharmacies some seven years later. Most European nations followed suit. The drug remains available in the United States, although most clinicians generally find it to be a poor choice and don't prescribe it. Its potential hepatotoxicity is usually cited as a reason, especially when long-term androgen therapy is contemplated. The one exception seems to be the growing interest in using oral methyltestosterone in low doses to treat female menopause. Early success with Estratest (Solvay) seems to indicate future expansion for this application. Although many markets no longer produce this drug, especially as a single-ingredient product, methyltestosterone remains widely produced in many others.

How Supplied:

Methyltestosterone is widely available in human drug markets. Composition and dosage may vary by country and manufacturer.

Structural Characteristics:

Methyltestosterone is a modified form of testosterone. It differs by the addition of a methyl group at carbon 17-alpha, which helps protect the hormone during oral administration. As is typical with c17-alpha alkylation, the resulting steroid has lower anabolic activity than its parent testosterone.

Side Effects (Estrogenic):

Methyltestosterone is aromatized by the body, and is highly estrogenic due to its conversion to 17-alpha methylestradiol, a synthetic estrogen with high biological activity. 17-alpha methylation actually slows the rate of aromatization, although the potent nature of 17-methylestradiol more than compensates for this. Gynecomastia is often a concern during treatment, and may present itself quite early into a cycle (particularly when higher doses are used). At the same time water retention can become a problem, causing a notable loss of muscle definition as both subcutaneous water retention and fat levels build. To avoid strong estrogenic side effects, it may be necessary to use an anti-estrogen such as Nolvadex®. One may alternately use an aromatase inhibitor like Arimidex® (anastrozole), which is a more effective remedy for estrogen control. Aromatase inhibitors, however, can be quite expensive in comparison to standard estrogen maintenance therapies, and may also have negative effects on blood lipids.

Side Effects (Androgenic):

Methyltestosterone is classified as an androgen. Androgenic side effects are common with this substance, and may include bouts of oily skin, acne, and body/facial hair growth. Higher doses are more likely to cause such side effects. Anabolic/androgenic steroids may also aggravate male pattern hair loss. Those genetically prone to male pattern hair loss may wish to opt for a milder, less androgenic, anabolic steroid. As a potent androgen, this steroid may also increase aggressiveness. Women are additionally warned of the potential virilizing effects of anabolic/androgenic steroids. These may include a deepening of the voice, menstrual irregularities, changes in skin texture, facial hair growth, and clitoral enlargement. Like testosterone, methyltestosterone converts to a more potent steroid via interaction with the 5-alpha reductase enzyme, in this case 17-alpha-methyldihydrotestosterone. The relative androgenicity of methyltestosterone may be reduced, although not completely eliminated, by the concurrent use of finasteride or dutasteride.

Side Effects (Hepatotoxicity):

Methyltestosterone is a c17-alpha alkylated compound. This alteration protects the drug from deactivation by the liver, allowing a very high percentage of the drug entry into the bloodstream following oral administration. C17-alpha alkylated anabolic/androgenic steroids can be hepatotoxic. Prolonged or high exposure may result in liver damage. In rare instances life-threatening dysfunction may develop. It is advisable to visit a physician periodically during each cycle to monitor liver function and overall health. Intake of c17-alpha alkylated steroids is commonly limited to 6-8 weeks, in an effort to avoid escalating liver strain.

Methyltestosterone was the first oral steroid linked to hepatic damage. This may be, in part, related to the early widespread use of the compound, as the drug generally displays acceptable safety when used in clinically prescribed dosages (serious liver toxicity cannot be completely excluded, however, even at clinical doses). When taken at a dose of 30 mg daily for 5 weeks, hepatotoxicity, as measured by bromosulphalein (BSP) retention, was low in one study.[608] In a separate investigation, a majority of patients noticed significant BSP retention after only 2 weeks of therapy with 67mg daily.[609] Severe liver complications are rare given the periodic nature in which most people use oral anabolic/androgenic steroids, although cannot be excluded with methyltestosterone, especially with high doses and/or prolonged administration periods.

The use of a liver detoxification supplement such as Liver Stabil, Liv-52, or Essentiale Forte is advised while taking any hepatotoxic anabolic/androgenic steroids.

Side Effects (Cardiovascular):

Anabolic/androgenic steroids can have deleterious effects on serum cholesterol. This includes a tendency to reduce HDL (good) cholesterol values and increase LDL (bad) cholesterol values, which may shift the HDL to LDL balance in a direction that favors greater risk of arteriosclerosis. The relative impact of an anabolic/androgenic steroid on serum lipids is dependant on the dose, route of administration (oral vs. injectable), type of steroid (aromatizable or non-aromatizable), and level of resistance to hepatic metabolism.

Methyltestosterone has a strong effect on the hepatic management of cholesterol due to its structural resistance to liver breakdown and route of administration. Studies have demonstrated an approximate 35% decrease in HDL cholesterol and a 30% increase in LDL cholesterol with 40 mg per day.[610] These changes occurred within 2-4 weeks of the initiation of therapy, and persisted for 2 weeks after discontinuation of the drug. Anabolic/androgenic steroids may also adversely affect blood pressure and triglycerides, reduce endothelial relaxation, and support left ventricular hypertrophy, all potentially increasing the risk of cardiovascular disease and myocardial infarction.

To help reduce cardiovascular strain it is advised to maintain an active cardiovascular exercise program and minimize the intake of saturated fats, cholesterol, and simple carbohydrates at all times during active AAS administration. Supplementing with fish oils (4 grams per day) and a natural cholesterol/antioxidant formula such as Lipid Stabil or a product with comparable ingredients is also recommended.

Side Effects (Testosterone Suppression):

All anabolic/androgenic steroids when taken in doses sufficient to promote muscle gain are expected to suppress endogenous testosterone production. Without the intervention of testosterone-stimulating substances, testosterone levels should return to normal within 1-4 months of drug secession. Note that prolonged hypogonadotrophic hypogonadism can develop secondary to steroid abuse, necessitating medical intervention.

The above side effects are not inclusive. For more detailed discussion of potential side effects, see the Steroid Side Effects section of this book.

Administration (General):

Studies have shown that taking an oral anabolic steroid with food may decrease its bioavailability.[611] This is caused by the fat-soluble nature of steroid hormones, which can allow some of the drug to dissolve with undigested dietary fat, reducing its absorption from the gastrointestinal tract. For maximum utilization, this steroid should be taken on an empty stomach.

Administration (Men):

To treat androgen insufficiency, prescribing guidelines call for a daily dosage of 10-40 mg. The dose is reduced by 50% when administered in sublingual or buccal form. The drug would be used for extended periods so long as the patent's laboratory results (hepatotoxicity, serum lipids, etc.) do not necessitate its discontinuance. When used for physique- or performance-enhancing purposes, a daily dosage of 10-50 mg is most commonly used, taken in cycles lasting no more than 6-8 weeks in length. Methyltestosterone is most commonly used not as an anabolic, but to stimulate aggression in the user. Powerlifters, bodybuilders, and competitive athletes often attempt to harness this effect, looking for extra intensity in a training session or competition. Aside from this, methyltestosterone offers little except side effects. It is quite toxic, elevating liver enzymes and causing acne, gynecomastia, aggression, and water retention quite easily. Were one to tolerate these side effects, methyltestosterone will offer only poor quality (bulky) gains. One should also be prepared for a substantial loss of size and bodyweight at the conclusion of each cycle with methyltestosterone, due to the high level of water excretion once the drug is discontinued (during administration water retention will account for a considerable percentage of the total weight gain).

Administration (Women):

Methyltestosterone is not widely used with women in clinical medicine. When applied, it is most often used as a secondary medication during inoperable breast cancer, when other therapies have failed to produce a desirable effect. The dosage used for this application can be as high as 200 mg per day. Low doses of methyltestosterone have been used in recent years to treat the symptoms of menopause. An example is the product Estratest, which contains esterified estrogens and 2.5 mg of methyltestosterone. A dosage of 1 tablet per day may improve energy, libido, and overall wellness of the patient, as well as combat osteoporosis (while estrogen replacement may halt calcium loss in the bones, testosterone tends to increase calcium stores). Methyltestosterone is generally not recommended for women for physique- or performance-enhancing purposes due to its strong androgenic nature and tendency to produce virilizing side effects.

Availability:

Methyltestosterone is produced by a good number of pharmaceutical manufacturers. It is, likewise, found in a variety of countries, usually selling for an extremely low price (especially in bulk). Methyltestosterone is, therefore, a popular ingredient in many counterfeit (oral) preparations. An inexperienced buyer can easily mistake the effect of this drug for whatever is written on the label, unaware of the cheap steroid actually being administered.

Although there are a number of legit preparations that might be found on the black market, the only common form of methyltestosterone these days are the Teston tablets from Greece. Counterfeits do not appear to be a significant problem.

Methandriol (methylandrostenediol)

Androgenic	30-60
Anabolic	20-60
Standard	Testosterone propionate
Chemical Name	17-alpha-methylandrost-5-ene-3,17-beta-diol
Estrogenic Activity	low to moderate
Progestational Activity	no data available (low)

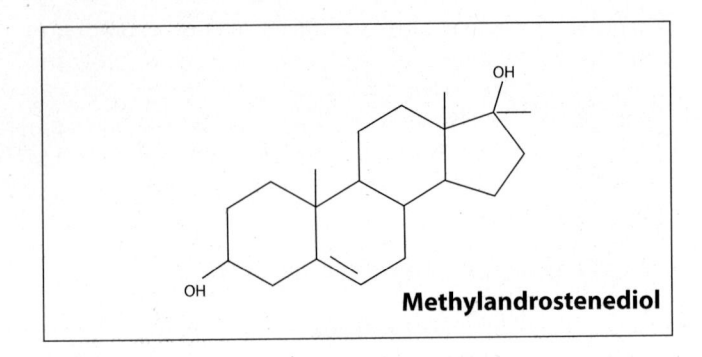

Description:

Methylandrostenediol (methandriol for short) is an anabolic steroid derived from dihydrotestosterone. The drug itself is manufactured in two very distinct forms. The first is unesterified (straight) methylandrostenediol, which is used when making an oral medication with this steroid (although an injectable once existed in the U.S.). It is also found as esterified methylandrostenediol dipropionate, which is prepared as an injectable. The added propionate esters in the injectable form extend the activity of the drug for several days. Basically, methandriol drugs are altered c-17 alkylated forms of 5-androstenediol. Methandriol is classified as a weak anabolic with weak androgenic properties. It also seems to display some level of estrogenic activity, making this steroid less ideal for dieting. The drug is generally considered too mild, and is not widely popular among bodybuilders and athletes. Sometimes, however, it is used in place of other anabolic/androgenic agents in bulking stacks when available.

History:

Methylandrostenediol was first described in 1935,[612] making this a very old agent as far as synthetic anabolic steroids are concerned. Methylandrostendiol was developed into a medicine by Organon, which sold it in the United States under the Stenediol brand name in both oral (methylandrostenediol) and injectable (methylandrostendiol dipropionate) forms. Many other generics and other brands of methylandrostenediol soon followed, and the drug was a popular anabolic agent in the United States during the 1950's. Methylandrostenediol was essentially the first steroid perceived to have a notable separation of anabolic (higher) and androgenic (lower) effect, a persistent goal of pharmaceutical developers. Early product literature described it as, "a steroid which has considerable of the male hormone's tissue-building action without to the same extent causing virilization."[613] It was indicated for use as a, "tissue-builder in cases of retarded growth or failure to gain weight accompanied by protein wastage, negative nitrogen balance, or failure to build body proteins."

Early assessments of methylandrostenediol being primarily anabolic in nature did not hold up well with later extensive use in humans. It was eventually determined that in doses sufficient to promote weight gain, its anabolic properties were accompanied by significant androgenic activity. Ultimately, this drug would be viewed as one of balanced anabolic and androgenic action, not as a highly anabolic agent as originally thought. Organon would go on to develop more effective anabolic agents, such as their 19-nor series of drugs including Durabolin, Deca-Durabolin, and Maxibolin, and eventually discontinued the Stenediol products. The other U.S. brand and generic forms of the drug would follow as well, although methylandrostenediol would persist in the U.S. scene for some time. Currently, no domestic source of the drug exists, although it is still found in certain international markets. It seems most prominent in Australia at the present time, where it remains included in a number of veterinary anabolic steroid products.

How Supplied:

Methylandrostendiol is available in select human and veterinary drug markets. Composition and dosage may vary by country and manufacturer.

Structural Characteristics:

Methylandrostendiol is a modified form of dihydrotestosterone. It differs by: 1) the addition of a methyl group at carbon 17-alpha to protect the hormone during oral administration and 2) the introduction of a double bond between carbons 5 and 6, which seems to increase the anabolic strength of the steroid (partly by making it resistant to metabolism by 3-hydroxysteroid dehydrogenase in skeletal muscle tissue). Methylandrostenediol dipropionate contains methylandrostenediol modified with the addition of 2 carboxylic acid esters (propionic acid) at the 3-beta and 17-beta hydroxyl groups, which delay the release of free methylandrostenediol from the site of injection (depot).

Side Effects (Estrogenic):

Methylandrostendiol is not directly aromatized by the body, although one of its known metabolites is methyltestosterone, which can aromatize. Methlyandrostenediol is also believed to have some inherent estrogenic activity. It is, likewise, considered a weakly to moderately estrogenic steroid. Gynecomastia is possible during treatment, but generally only when higher doses are used. Water and fat retention can also become issues, again depending on dose. Sensitive individuals may need to addition an anti-estrogen such as Nolvadex® to minimize related side effects.

Side Effects (Androgenic):

Although often classified as an anabolic steroid, methylandrostenediol is sufficiently androgenic. Androgenic side effects are common with this substance. This may include bouts of oily skin, acne, and body/facial hair growth. Anabolic/androgenic steroids may also aggravate male pattern hair loss. Women are warned of the potential virilizing effects of anabolic/androgenic steroids. These may include a deepening of the voice, menstrual irregularities, changes in skin texture, facial hair growth, and clitoral enlargement. Note that methylandrostenediol is not affected by 5-alpha reductase, so the relative androgenicity of this steroid is not affected by the concurrent use of finasteride or dutasteride.

Side Effects (Hepatotoxicity):

Methylandrostenediol is a c17-alpha alkylated compound. This alteration protects the drug from deactivation by the liver, allowing a very high percentage of the drug entry into the bloodstream following oral administration. C17-alpha alkylated anabolic/androgenic steroids can be hepatotoxic. Prolonged or high exposure may result in liver damage. In rare instances life-threatening dysfunction may develop. It is advisable to visit a physician periodically during each cycle to monitor liver function and overall health. Intake of c17-alpha alkylated steroids is commonly limited to 6-8 weeks, in an effort to avoid escalating liver strain. Injectable forms of the drug may present slightly less strain on the liver by avoiding the first pass metabolism of oral dosing, although may still present substantial hepatotoxicity.

The use of a liver detoxification supplement such as Liver Stabil, Liv-52, or Essentiale Forte is advised while taking any hepatotoxic anabolic/androgenic steroids.

Side Effects (Cardiovascular):

Anabolic/androgenic steroids can have deleterious effects on serum cholesterol. This includes a tendency to reduce HDL (good) cholesterol values and increase LDL (bad) cholesterol values, which may shift the HDL to LDL balance in a direction that favors greater risk of arteriosclerosis. The relative impact of an anabolic/androgenic steroid on serum lipids is dependant on the dose, route of administration (oral vs. injectable), type of steroid (aromatizable or non-aromatizable), and level of resistance to hepatic metabolism. Methylandrostenediol has a strong effect on the hepatic management of cholesterol due to its structural resistance to liver breakdown and (with the oral) route of administration. Anabolic/androgenic steroids may also adversely affect blood pressure and triglycerides, reduce endothelial relaxation, and support left ventricular hypertrophy, all potentially increasing the risk of cardiovascular disease and myocardial infarction.

To help reduce cardiovascular strain it is advised to maintain an active cardiovascular exercise program and minimize the intake of saturated fats, cholesterol, and simple carbohydrates at all times during active AAS administration. Supplementing with fish oils (4 grams per day) and a natural cholesterol/antioxidant formula such as Lipid Stabil or a product with comparable ingredients is also recommended.

Side Effects (Testosterone Suppression):

All anabolic/androgenic steroids when taken in doses sufficient to promote muscle gain are expected to suppress endogenous testosterone production. Without the intervention of testosterone-stimulating substances, testosterone levels should return to normal within 1-4 months of drug secession. Note that prolonged hypogonadotrophic hypogonadism can develop secondary to steroid abuse, necessitating medical intervention.

The above side effects are not inclusive. For more detailed discussion of potential side effects, see the Steroid Side Effects section of this book.

Administration (General):

Studies have shown that taking an oral anabolic steroid with food may decrease its bioavailability. This is caused by the fat-soluble nature of steroid hormones, which can allow some of the drug to dissolve with undigested dietary fat, reducing its absorption from the gastrointestinal tract. For maximum utilization, oral forms of this steroid should be taken on an empty stomach.

Administration (Men):

Early prescribing guidelines for Stenediol recommend a dosage of 25 mg given 2 to 5 times per week by oral, buccal, or intramuscular route. For physique- or performance-enhancing purposes, a typical dosage is in the range of 25-50 mg daily for the oral form, and 200-400 mg per week with the injectable. In order to keep blood levels more even with the injectable, it is generally administered once every three to four days. Cycles generally last for no more than 6 to 8 weeks, in an effort to minimize hepatotoxicity and strain on the liver and cholesterol values. This level of use is sufficient for moderate gains in muscle size and strength, which may be accompanied by a low level of water retention.

While it may be possible to use methylandrostenediol alone for muscle-building purposes, it is most often combined with other anabolics for a stronger effect. Combined with Deca-Durabolin® or Equipoise®, for example, measurable gains of hard muscle mass, without an extreme level of water retention, may be noticed. This is the general composition of most Australian vet blends that include methylandrostenediol. When looking for a more pronounced gain in mass, a stronger androgen such as testosterone may be added. The resulting growth can be quite exceptional, but the user will also have to deal with a much stronger set of estrogenic side effects. The drug sometimes also combines well with non-aromatizing anabolics such as Winstrol®, Primobolan®, or oxandrolone. The result here should be a more pronounced effect on muscle hardness, with a moderate gain of solid lean tissue.

Administration (Women):

Early prescribing guidelines for Stenediol recommend a dosage of 25 mg given 2 to 5 times per week by oral, buccal, or intramuscular route. Methylandrostenediol is generally not recommended for women for physique- or performance-enhancing purposes due to its androgenic nature and tendency to produce virilizing side effects.

Availability:

Methylandrostenediol is not commonly found on the black market. The only place it is produced in abundance is Australia, where a number of veterinary preparations still include methandriol in their blends. These occasionally do reach the U.S., often selling for a high price.

Methosarb (calusterone)

Androgenic	20
Anabolic	no data available
Standard	Testosterone

Chemical Names 17beta-Hydroxy-7beta,17-dimethylandrost-4-en-3-one
7b,17a-dimethyltestosterone

Estrogenic Activity	no data available
Progestational Activity	no data available

Calusterone

Description:

Calusterone is an oral androgen structurally related to methyltestosterone. It differs only by the addition of a methyl group at C-7 beta, which studies have shown eliminates or considerably reduces steroid (anabolic/androgenic) activity. The drug was developed as a less-toxic alternative to other androgens used for breast cancer, such as testosterone propionate and fluoxymesterone, which tend to induce strong virilizing side effects in women. What was produced was a steroid with minimal anabolic effect and low to moderate androgenic activity, far removed from its 7-alpha isomer cousin (bolasterone) in overall appearance. Although technically an androgen with some inherent value as such, calusterone has never been popular with athletes, and likely has very little to offer when compared with numerous other commercial anabolic agents.

History:

Calusterone was first described in 1959.[614] It was FDA approved for sale in the U.S. as a prescription drug product in 1973.[615] It was developed into a medicine by The Upjohn Company, and sold under the Methosarb brand name. It was reportedly also sold in other (limited) drug markets as Riedemil. Calusterone was indicated for the treatment of advanced inoperable or metastatic breast cancer in postmenopausal women or those that have had their ovarian function terminated as a course of therapy. According to early product literature, the drug was effective in approximately 25% of patients receiving it, provided that they met a series of criteria for therapy first. The drug was also investigated successfully in men with breast cancer,[616] a rare but not unseen occurrence. Aside from its actions relating to breast cancer in women, calusterone was not FDA approved for use in any other forms of treatment, as an anabolic agent or otherwise.

When calusterone was first introduced, it was described as an improved synthetic androgen for breast cancer treatment, with increased therapeutic potential and reduced toxicity compared to testosterone.[617] It was believed that the molecule had been modified in such as way as to eliminate many of its undesirable traits. Ultimately, these notions were poorly supported by medical investigations, and the drug seemed to perform with a comparable level of efficacy, and similar side effects, to other forms of androgen therapy. Calusterone was voluntarily removed from the U.S. drug market by the 1980's, and was officially removed from the FDA's list of therapeutic substances in 2001 at the request of Pharmacia & Upjohn. The drug remains unavailable today worldwide.

How Supplied:

Calusterone is no longer available as a prescription drug product. When manufactured, it came in the form of a 50 mg tablet.

Structural Characteristics:

Calusterone is a modified form of testosterone. It differs by 1) the addition of a methyl group at carbon 17-alpha, which helps protect the hormone during oral administration, and 2) the introduction of a methyl group at carbon 7 (beta), which significantly reduces its relative biological activity.

Side Effects (Estrogenic):

Calusterone is not described as a steroid with significant estrogenic activity. Studies have demonstrated that this agent actually reduces the binding capacity of estrogen to its corresponding receptor.[618] It may, likewise, offer some level of anti-estrogenic effect.

Side Effects (Androgenic):

Calusterone is classified as an androgen. Androgenic side effects are common with this substance, and may include bouts of oily skin, acne, and body/facial hair growth. Anabolic/androgenic steroids may also aggravate male pattern hair loss. Those genetically prone to male pattern hair loss may wish to opt for a milder, less androgenic, anabolic steroid. Women are additionally warned of the potential virilizing effects of anabolic/androgenic steroids. These may include a deepening of the voice, menstrual irregularities, changes in skin texture, facial hair growth, and clitoral enlargement.

Side Effects (Hepatotoxicity):

Calusterone is a c17-alpha alkylated compound. This alteration protects the drug from deactivation by the liver, allowing a very high percentage of the drug entry into the bloodstream following oral administration. C17-alpha alkylated anabolic/androgenic steroids can be hepatotoxic. Prolonged or high exposure may result in liver damage. In rare instances life-threatening dysfunction may develop. It is advisable to visit a physician periodically during each cycle to monitor liver function and overall health. Intake of c17-alpha alkylated steroids is commonly limited to 6-8 weeks, in an effort to avoid escalating liver strain. Studies administering 200 mg per day for at least 3 months have demonstrated increased sulfobromophthalein (BSP) retention, a marker of hepatic stress, in approximately one third of patients.[619]

The use of a liver detoxification supplement such as Liver Stabil, Liv-52, or Essentiale Forte is advised while taking any hepatotoxic anabolic/androgenic steroids.

Side Effects (Cardiovascular):

Anabolic/androgenic steroids can have deleterious effects on serum cholesterol. This includes a tendency to reduce HDL (good) cholesterol values and increase LDL (bad) cholesterol values, which may shift the HDL to LDL balance in a direction that favors greater risk of arteriosclerosis. The relative impact of an anabolic/androgenic steroid on serum lipids is dependant on the dose, route of administration (oral vs. injectable), type of steroid (aromatizable or non-aromatizable), and level of resistance to hepatic metabolism. Calusterone is expected to have a strong effect on the hepatic management of cholesterol due to its structural resistance to liver breakdown and route of administration. Anabolic/androgenic steroids may also adversely affect blood pressure and triglycerides, reduce endothelial relaxation, and support left ventricular hypertrophy, all potentially increasing the risk of cardiovascular disease and myocardial infarction.

To help reduce cardiovascular strain it is advised to maintain an active cardiovascular exercise program and minimize the intake of saturated fats, cholesterol, and simple carbohydrates at all times during active AAS administration. Supplementing with fish oils (4 grams per day) and a natural cholesterol/antioxidant formula such as Lipid Stabil or a product with comparable ingredients is also recommended.

Side Effects (Testosterone Suppression):

All anabolic/androgenic steroids when taken in doses sufficient to promote muscle gain are expected to suppress endogenous testosterone production. Without the intervention of testosterone-stimulating substances, testosterone levels should return to normal within 1-4 months of drug secession. Note that prolonged hypogonadotrophic hypogonadism can develop secondary to steroid abuse, necessitating medical intervention.

The above side effects are not inclusive. For more detailed discussion of potential side effects, see the Steroid Side Effects section of this book.

Administration (General):

Studies have shown that taking an oral anabolic steroid with food may decrease its bioavailability.[620] This is caused by the fat-soluble nature of steroid hormones, which can allow some of the drug to dissolve with undigested dietary fat, reducing its absorption from the gastrointestinal tract. For maximum utilization, this steroid should be taken on an empty stomach.

Administration (Men):

Calusterone was not FDA-approved for use in men, although clinical studies with the drug tended to use comparable doses as women. Effective doses for physique- or performance-enhancing purposes have not been determined, but would likely fall in the range of 100-200 mg per day. Note that this drug is not strongly anabolic, and does not offer high value as a muscle-building substance.

Administration (Women):

Calusterone was most commonly used in a clinical dose of 200 mg per day, taken for at least 3 consecutive months. Doses of 150-300 mg per day have also been used. Note that at the recommended therapeutic dose, mild to moderate virilizing side effects, including deepening of the voice, acne, and facial hair growth, occurred in up to 25% of patients. This drug is generally not recommended for women for physique- or performance-enhancing purposes due to its weak anabolic and stronger androgenic nature.

Availability:

Calusterone is no longer produced as a prescription drug, and is unavailable on the black market.

Methyl-1-testosterone (methyldihydroboldenone)

Androgenic	100-220
Anabolic	910-1,600
Standard	Methyltestosterone (oral)
Chemical Name	17alpha methyl-17beta-hydroxy-androst-1-ene-3-one
Estrogenic Activity	none
Progestational Activity	moderate

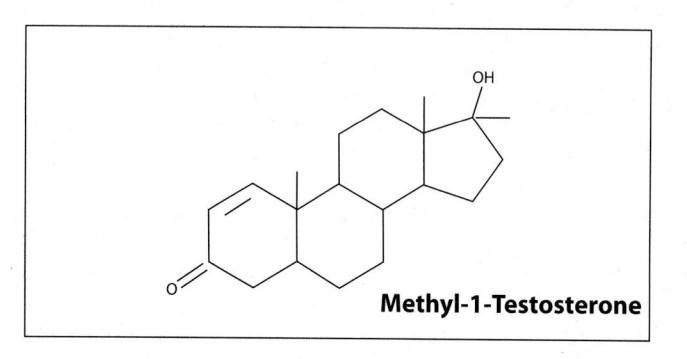

Methyl-1-Testosterone

Description:

Methyl-1-testosterone (methyldihydroboldenone) is an oral anabolic steroid derived from dihydrotestosterone. It is closest in structure to 1-testosterone (dihydroboldenone), differing only by the addition of c-17 alkylation (which does change the activity of this steroid considerably). M1T for short, this agent can be looked at as some kind of amalgamation of Primobolan, Winstrol, and trenbolone. It has the basic 1-ene structure of Primobolan, the bioavailability of a methylated oral steroid like Winstrol, and the high potency of a strong synthetic anabolic and androgenic agent like trenbolone. Based on standard assays, the potency of methyl-1-testosterone actually exceeds that of every prescription anabolic steroid currently sold. It is popular among bodybuilders as a bulking agent, with an ability to promote rapid gains in muscle size and strength, which are often accompanied by some level of water or fat retention.

History:

Methyl-1-testosterone was first described in 1962.[621] This compound was developed during some of the most active years of steroid research, a time when literally hundreds of different effective anabolic agents were being actively studied and pursued by drug companies. Although methyl-1-testosterone did see some favorable assays, displaying a high level of potency and an acceptable ratio of anabolic to androgenic effect, like most agents synthesized during this time period it never actually developed into a medicine. As is common in many areas of pharmaceutical research, a select number of agents were given the dollars for full studies and eventual release, and the rest were ignored. Methyl-1-testosteroe, for whatever reason, was simply not one of the select few drugs to reach pharmacy shelves, and it lay dormant in the medical books for approximately forty years.

Methyl-1-testosterone reemerged sharply in 2003, when it was introduced as an OTC (Over-The-Counter) "nutritional supplement" in the United States, due to the fact that it was unknown when the 1991 law controlling anabolic steroids was written, and therefore not included. The product was introduced to the market by Legal Gear, and was soon extremely popular due to its very high level of effectiveness. It was also soon the subject of many generic copies. Methyl-1-testosterone did not last long in the U.S., and laws were soon passed to include it as a controlled substance. The laws went into effect January 20, 2005, at which point the possession or distribution of this steroid started carrying the same Federal penalties as other anabolic steroids. This effectively ended the market for methyl-1-testosterone, and the agent is again unavailable to bodybuilders worldwide.

How Supplied:

No prescription drug product containing methyl-1-testosterone currently exists. When it was sold as an OTC supplement, it was produced as an oral capsule and tablet in various strengths.

Structural Characteristics:

Methyl-1-Testosterone is a derivative of dihydrotestosterone. It contains 1) the addition of a methyl group at carbon 17-alpha to protect the hormone during oral administration and 2) the introduction of a double bond between carbons 1 and 2, which helps to stabilize the 3-keto group and increase the steroid's anabolic properties.

Side Effects (Estrogenic):

Although not studied, it is believed that the body does not appreciably aromatize methyl-1-testosterone. It is of note, however, that this steroid likely has inherent progestational activity. The side effects associated with progesterone are similar to those of estrogen, including negative feedback inhibition of testosterone production and enhanced rate of fat storage. Progestins also augment the stimulatory effect of estrogens on mammary tissue growth. There appears to be a strong synergy between these two hormones here, such that gynecomastia might even occur with the help of progestins, without excessive estrogen levels. The use of an anti-estrogen, which inhibits the estrogenic component of this disorder, is often sufficient to mitigate gynecomastia caused by progestational anabolic/androgenic steroids.

Side Effects (Androgenic):

Although classified as an anabolic steroid, androgenic side effects are still possible with this substance. This may include bouts of oily skin, acne, and body/facial hair growth. Anabolic/androgenic steroids may also aggravate male pattern hair loss. Women are warned of the potential virilizing effects of anabolic/androgenic steroids. These may include a deepening of the voice, menstrual irregularities, changes in skin texture, facial hair growth, and clitoral enlargement. Its low relative androgenicity could theoretically make this preparation acceptable to women, although (in practice) not its very high potency. Although methyl-1-testosterone is primarily anabolic in nature, strong androgenic side effects are possible with higher doses, and should be carefully considered. Note that the 5-alpha reductase enzyme does not metabolize methyl-1-testosterone, so its relative androgenicity is not affected by finasteride or dutasteride.

Side Effects (Hepatotoxicity):

Methyl-1-testosterone is a c17-alpha alkylated compound. This alteration protects the drug from deactivation by the liver, allowing a very high percentage of the drug entry into the bloodstream following oral administration. C17-alpha alkylated anabolic/androgenic steroids can be hepatotoxic. Prolonged or high exposure may result in liver damage. In rare instances life-threatening dysfunction may develop. It is advisable to visit a physician periodically during each cycle to monitor liver function and overall health. Intake of c17-alpha alkylated steroids is commonly limited to 6-8 weeks, in an effort to avoid escalating liver strain.

The use of a liver detoxification supplement such as Liver Stabil, Liv-52, or Essentiale Forte is advised while taking any hepatotoxic anabolic/androgenic steroids.

Side Effects (Cardiovascular):

Anabolic/androgenic steroids can have deleterious effects on serum cholesterol. This includes a tendency to reduce HDL (good) cholesterol values and increase LDL (bad) cholesterol values, which may shift the HDL to LDL balance in a direction that favors greater risk of arteriosclerosis. The relative impact of an anabolic/androgenic steroid on serum lipids is dependant on the dose, route of administration (oral vs. injectable), type of steroid (aromatizable or non-aromatizable), and level of resistance to hepatic metabolism. Although not extensively studied in humans, the oral route, high relative potency, and poorly or non-aromatizable nature of methyl-1-testosterone suggest that this agent is extremely prone to negatively altering lipid values and increasing atherogenic risk. Anabolic/androgenic steroids may also adversely affect blood pressure and triglycerides, reduce endothelial relaxation, and support left ventricular hypertrophy, all potentially increasing the risk of cardiovascular disease and myocardial infarction.

To help reduce cardiovascular strain it is advised to maintain an active cardiovascular exercise program and minimize the intake of saturated fats, cholesterol, and simple carbohydrates at all times during active AAS administration. Supplementing with fish oils (4 grams per day) and a natural cholesterol/antioxidant formula such as Lipid Stabil or a product with comparable ingredients is also recommended.

Side Effects (Testosterone Suppression):

All anabolic/androgenic steroids when taken in doses sufficient to promote muscle gain are expected to suppress endogenous testosterone production. Without the intervention of testosterone-stimulating substances, testosterone levels should return to normal within 1-4 months of drug secession. Note that prolonged hypogonadotrophic hypogonadism can develop secondary to steroid abuse, necessitating medical intervention.

The above side effects are not inclusive. For more detailed discussion of potential side effects, see the Steroid Side Effects section of this book.

Administration (General):

Studies have shown that taking an oral anabolic steroid with food may decrease its bioavailability.[622] This is caused by the fat-soluble nature of steroid hormones, which can allow some of the drug to dissolve with undigested dietary fat, reducing its absorption from the gastrointestinal tract. For maximum utilization, this steroid should be taken on an empty stomach.

Administration (Men):

Methyl-1-Testosterone was never approved for use in humans. Prescribing guidelines are unavailable. For physique- or performance-enhancing purposes, a typical effective oral daily dose will be in the range of 5-10 mg, taken for no longer than 4-6 weeks. A dose of 20 mg is sometimes used, although this increases the likelihood for side effects. Many users feel they are better served by not exceeding a 10 mg daily dose, and instead stack it with an injectable like testosterone cypionate (200-400 mg per week) when a stronger effect is needed. This may reduce liver toxicity compared to a higher dose of M1T, and also provide a more balanced cycle in terms of anabolic vs. androgenic effect. A common complaint when M1T is taken alone is lethargy, which may be due, in part, to its low androgenic or estrogenic component. Stacking it with an aromatizable androgen like testosterone will usually alleviate this problem. Note that while a small percentage of users exceed 20 mg per day, it should be remembered that even this is a serious dose for a potent steroid like this, and is not to be taken lightly, either for its effectiveness or toxicity. Like Anadrol, methyl-1-testosterone is not necessarily a friendly steroid, but it is definitely an effective one.

Administration (Women):

Methyl-1-Testosterone was never approved for use in humans. Prescribing guidelines are unavailable. This agent is not recommended for women for physique- or performance-enhancing purposes due to its high potency and tendency to produce virilizing side effects.

Availability:

Methyl-1-Testosterone is not produced as a prescription drug. It is presently unavailable, except as an underground product.

Methyl-D (Methyldienolone)

Androgenic	200-300
Anabolic	1,000
Standard	Methyltestosterone (oral)
Chemical Name	17a-methyl-17beta-hydroxyestra-4,9(10)dien-3-one
Estrogenic Activity	none
Progestational Activity	moderate

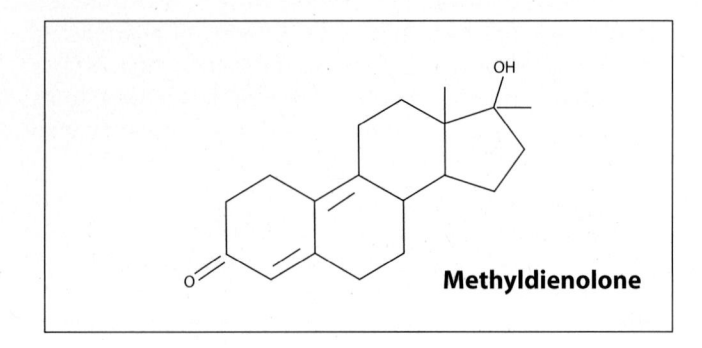

Description:

Methyldienolone is an anabolic steroid that was researched in the early 1960's, but never sold as a prescription drug. It is a nandrolone-based compound, modified to be orally active and to have greatly increased anabolic properties. Methyldienolone is a close chemical cousin of methyltrienolone, one of the strongest steroids profiled in this reference. Methyldienolone is not quite as potent, however it remains quite strong next to most commercial agents. Animal tests find it to be 5 times more potent than Dianabol, 10 times more potent than methyltestosterone, and 13 times more potent than Primobolan® on a milligram for milligram basis. Although the real world relevance of these values may be questionable, methyldienolone is well favored by bodybuilders for its ability to promote lean muscle gains with minimal side effects.

History:

Methyldienolone was first described in 1960.[623] Eli Lilly & Co. (U.S.) developed this steroid, although the firm never released it as an actual medicine. It is of note that Lilly also developed a 17-alpha-ethylated version (ethyldienolone) at the same time, which had an even more favorable anabolic to androgenic ratio in standard assay tests, but was not quite as potent overall. Being that methyldienolone was never sold as a prescription drug, it remained a research steroid of little interest for approximately forty years. The steroid actually came to life not as a prescription agent, but as an OTC "nutritional supplement" in 2004. Bruce Kneller, who had found the old research on methyldienolone and determined it to be a favorable agent to market with Gaspari Nutrition, was actually credited with developing the product. Gaspari sold the agent for a brief time as Methyl-D, before the 2004 amended Anabolic Steroid Control Act was passed, eliminating much of the grey area "prohormone" or "prosteroid" market in the U.S. Today, methyldienolone is again unavailable to athletes.

How Supplied:

Methyldienolone is not available as a commercial agent. When sold as a nutritional supplement, it contained 1mg of steroid per tablet.

Structural Characteristics:

Methyldienolone is a modified form of nandrolone. It differs by: 1) the addition of a methyl group at carbon 17-alpha to protect the hormone during oral administration and 2) the introduction of a double bond at carbon 9, which increases its binding affinity and slows its metabolism. The resulting steroid is significantly more potent than its nandrolone base, and displays a much longer half-life and lower affinity for serum-binding proteins in comparison.

Side Effects (Estrogenic):

Methyldienolone is not aromatized by the body, and is not measurably estrogenic. It is of note, however, that based on its structure methyldienolone likely displays significant binding affinity for the progesterone receptor. The side effects associated with progesterone can be similar to those of estrogen, including negative feedback inhibition of testosterone production and enhanced rate of fat storage. Progestins also augment the stimulatory effect of estrogens on mammary tissue growth. There appears to be a strong synergy between these two hormones here, such that gynecomastia might even occur with the help of progestins, without excessive estrogen levels. The use of an anti-estrogen, which inhibits the estrogenic component of this disorder, is often sufficient to mitigate gynecomastia caused by progestational anabolic/androgenic steroids. Note that significant side effects are not likely unless high doses are taken, or the drug is used with other strongly aromatizable steroids.

Side Effects (Androgenic):

Although classified as an anabolic steroid, androgenic side effects are still common with this substance. This may include bouts of oily skin, acne, and body/facial hair growth. Anabolic/androgenic steroids may also aggravate male pattern hair loss. Women are also warned of the potential virilizing effects of anabolic/androgenic steroids. These may include a deepening of the voice, menstrual irregularities, changes in skin texture, facial hair growth, and clitoral enlargement. Additionally, the 5-alpha reductase enzyme does not metabolize methyldienolone, so its relative androgenicity is not affected by finasteride or dutasteride.

Side Effects (Hepatotoxicity):

Methyldienolone is a c17-alpha alkylated compound. This alteration protects the drug from deactivation by the liver, allowing a very high percentage of the drug entry into the bloodstream following oral administration. C17-alpha alkylated anabolic/androgenic steroids can be hepatotoxic. Prolonged or high exposure may result in liver damage. In rare instances life-threatening dysfunction may develop. It is advisable to visit a physician periodically during each cycle to monitor liver function and overall health. Intake of c17-alpha alkylated steroids is commonly limited to 6-8 weeks, in an effort to avoid escalating liver strain. Note that given its high level of potency and close structural similarity to methyltrienolone, one of the most hepatotoxic steroids known, methyldienolone is likely also very hepatotoxic; liver strain should be carefully monitored with use.

The use of a liver detoxification supplement such as Liver Stabil, Liv-52, or Essentiale Forte is advised while taking any hepatotoxic anabolic/androgenic steroids.

Side Effects (Cardiovascular):

Anabolic/androgenic steroids can have deleterious effects on serum cholesterol. This includes a tendency to reduce HDL (good) cholesterol values and increase LDL (bad) cholesterol values, which may shift the HDL to LDL balance in a direction that favors greater risk of arteriosclerosis. The relative impact of an anabolic/androgenic steroid on serum lipids is dependant on the dose, route of administration (oral vs. injectable), type of steroid (aromatizable or non-aromatizable), and level of resistance to hepatic metabolism. Although not studied in humans, the high relative potency, oral route, and non-aromatizable nature of methydienolone suggests that this agent is extremely prone to negatively altering lipid values and increasing atherogenic risk. Anabolic/androgenic steroids may also adversely affect blood pressure and triglycerides, reduce endothelial relaxation, and support left ventricular hypertrophy, all potentially increasing the risk of cardiovascular disease and myocardial infarction.

To help reduce cardiovascular strain it is advised to maintain an active cardiovascular exercise program and minimize the intake of saturated fats, cholesterol, and simple carbohydrates at all times during active AAS administration. Supplementing with fish oils (4 grams per day) and a natural cholesterol/antioxidant formula such as Lipid Stabil or a product with comparable ingredients is also recommended.

Side Effects (Testosterone Suppression):

All anabolic/androgenic steroids when taken in doses sufficient to promote muscle gain are expected to suppress endogenous testosterone production. Without the intervention of testosterone-stimulating substances, testosterone levels should return to normal within 1-4 months of drug secession. Note that prolonged hypogonadotrophic hypogonadism can develop secondary to steroid abuse, necessitating medical intervention.

The above side effects are not inclusive. For more detailed discussion of potential side effects, see the Steroid Side Effects section of this book.

Administration (General):

Studies have shown that taking an oral anabolic steroid with food may decrease its bioavailability.[624] This is caused by the fat-soluble nature of steroid hormones, which can allow some of the drug to dissolve with undigested dietary fat, reducing its absorption from the gastrointestinal tract. For maximum utilization, this steroid should be taken on an empty stomach.

Administration (Men):

Methyldienolone was never approved for use in humans. Prescribing guidelines are unavailable. Effective oral daily doses for physique- or performance-enhancing purposes fall in the range of 2-10 mg. At this level, one should expect measurable strength and lean tissue gains, which should be accompanied by decent fat loss and minimal side effects. In an effort to reduce liver strain, it is usually recommended to limit drug duration to no longer than 6-8 weeks, after which point a break is taken from all c-17 alkylated steroids. Users often avoid combining this drug with other liver toxic orals, and instead opt to use an injectable base when stacking. A dose of 5 mg per day of methyldienolone combined with 400 mg weekly of testosterone cypionate/enanthate or Equipoise® seems to be a common and effective lean-mass stack. Trenbolone (225 mg) or Primobolan® (300-400 mg) is often used instead for cutting purposes.

Administration (Women):

Methyldienolone was never approved for use in humans. Prescribing guidelines are unavailable. This agent is not recommended for women for physique- or performance-enhancing purposes due to its high level of potency and tendency to produce virilizing side effects. Note that the high anabolic to androgenic ratio of methyldienolone makes use possible without significant virilization, but would likely require measuring very small doses (well below 1mg per day) and respecting a very periodic use schedule (4 weeks or less).

Availability:

Methyldienolone is not produced as a prescription steroid product in any part of the world. This agent was manufactured as a nutritional supplement for a brief period of time before the 2004 amendment to the Anabolic Steroid Act went into effect, although no stock should be left in circulation.

Metribolone (methyltrienolone)

Androgenic	6,000-7,000
Anabolic	12,000-30,000
Standard	Methyltestosterone (oral)
Chemical Names	17alpha-methyl-17beta-hydroxyestra-4,9,11-triene-3-one
	17alpha-methyl-trenbolone
Estrogenic Activity	none
Progestational Activity	no data available

Description:

Methyltrienolone is one of the strongest oral anabolic steroids ever produced. This agent is a derivative of trenbolone (trienolone), which has been c-17 alpha alkylated to allow for oral administration. This modification has created a steroid that is significantly stronger than its non-methylated cousin. Its potency has been measured to be anywhere from 120-300 times greater than that of methyltestosterone, with greater dissociation between anabolic and androgenic effects.[625][626] Milligram for milligram methyltrienolone is a more active steroid than any agent sold on the commercial market, requiring doses as little as .5-1 milligram per day to notice a strong anabolic effect. Its potency is only matched by its relative toxicity, however, which has limited its modern use to that of laboratory research only.

History:

Methyltrienolone was first described in 1965.[627] It was immediately identified as an extremely potent anabolic agent, far more potent than the commercially available agents of the time. In spite of its high relative activity, however, methyltrienolone has seen very limited use in humans. It was used clinically during the late 1960's and early '70's, most notably in the treatment of advanced breast cancer. Here, its exceedingly strong anabolic/androgenic action helps the drug counter the local effects of endogenous estrogens, lending it some efficacy for slowing or even regressing tumor growth. Such application was not long lived, however, as more realistic evaluations of the drug's toxicity soon led to its abandonment in human medicine.

By the mid-1970's, methyltrienolone was becoming an accepted standard in non-human research studies, particularly those pertaining to the study of the androgen receptor activity. For this purpose the agent is very well suited. Its sheer potency and resistance to serum-binding proteins makes it an excellent in-vitro receptor-binding standard to compare other agents to. Being so resistant to metabolism, active methyltrienolone metabolites are also not going to greatly interfere with the results of most experiments. Body tissues can metabolize most steroids fairly easily, which means that even incubation studies can be complicated with the question of what is causing a particular effect, the steroid or one of its unidentified metabolites. This is much less of an issue with methyltrienolone. Today, methyltrienolone remains an agent of research use only.

How Supplied:

Methyltrienolone is not available as a commercial agent.

Structural Characteristics:

Methyltrienolone is a modified form of nandrolone. It differs by: 1) the addition of a methyl group at carbon 17-alpha to protect the hormone during oral administration and 2) the introduction of double bonds at carbons 9 and 11, which increases its binding affinity and slows its metabolism. The resulting steroid is significantly more potent than its nandrolone base, and displays a much longer half-life and lower affinity for serum-binding proteins in comparison. Methyltrienolone chemically differs from trenbolone only by the addition of a methyl group at c-17. This alteration changes the activity of methyltrienolone considerably, however, such that this agent should not simply be considered an oral form of trenbolone.

Side Effects (Estrogenic):

Methyltrienolone is not aromatized by the body, and is not measurably estrogenic. It is of note, however, that methyltrienolone displays significant binding affinity for the progesterone receptor.[628] The side effects associated with progesterone are similar to those of estrogen, including negative feedback inhibition of testosterone production and enhanced rate of fat storage. Progestins also augment the stimulatory effect of estrogens on mammary tissue growth. There appears to be a strong synergy between these two hormones here, such that gynecomastia might even occur with the help of progestins, without excessive estrogen levels. The use of an anti-estrogen, which inhibits the estrogenic component of this disorder, is often sufficient to mitigate gynecomastia caused by progestational anabolic/androgenic steroids.

Side Effects (Androgenic):

Although classified as an anabolic steroid, androgenic side effects are still common with this substance. This may include bouts of oily skin, acne, and body/facial hair growth. Anabolic/androgenic steroids may also aggravate male pattern hair loss. Women are also warned of the potential virilizing effects of anabolic/androgenic steroids. These may include a deepening of the voice, menstrual irregularities, changes in skin texture, facial hair growth, and clitoral enlargement. Additionally, the 5-alpha reductase enzyme does not metabolize methyltrienolone, so its relative androgenicity is not affected by finasteride or dutasteride.

Side Effects (Hepatotoxicity):

Methyltrienolone is a c17-alpha alkylated compound. This alteration protects the drug from deactivation by the liver, allowing a very high percentage of the drug entry into the bloodstream following oral administration. C17-alpha alkylated anabolic/androgenic steroids can be hepatotoxic. Prolonged or high exposure may result in liver damage. In rare instances life-threatening dysfunction may develop. It is advisable to visit a physician periodically during each cycle to monitor liver function and overall health. Intake of c17-alpha alkylated steroids is commonly limited to 6-8 weeks, in an effort to avoid escalating liver strain.

Methyltrienolone is an exceedingly potent oral steroid, with a very high level of resistance to hepatic metabolism. This makes methyltrienolone exceedingly liver-toxic, precluding its use as a prescription agent at this time, in any part of the world. Studies published from the University of Bonn Germany back in 1966 make this very clear.[629] In fact, at this time researchers had deemed this the most liver-toxic steroid to ever be studied in humans, summing up their findings well when stating:

> "Methyltrienolone... which is orally active as an anabolic agent in a dose less than 1.0 mg per day in normal adults, has been tested with regard to its influence on liver function. As measured by multiple parameters (BSP retention; total bilirubin; activities of transaminases, alkaline phosphates and cholinesterase in serum; activity of proaccelerin in plasma) methyltrienolone turned out to be very active as to causing biochemical symptoms of intrahepatic cholestasis. ...thus methyltrienolone at present being the most 'hepatotoxic' steroid."

The use of a liver detoxification supplement such as Liver Stabil, Liv-52, or Essentiale Forte is advised while taking any hepatotoxic anabolic/androgenic steroids.

Side Effects (Cardiovascular):

Anabolic/androgenic steroids can have deleterious effects on serum cholesterol. This includes a tendency to reduce HDL (good) cholesterol values and increase LDL (bad) cholesterol values, which may shift the HDL to LDL balance in a direction that favors greater risk of arteriosclerosis. The relative impact of an anabolic/androgenic steroid on serum lipids is dependant on the dose, route of administration (oral vs. injectable), type of steroid (aromatizable or non-aromatizable), and level of resistance to hepatic metabolism. Although not extensively studied in humans, the oral route, high relative potency, and non-aromatizable nature of methyltrienolone suggest that this agent is extremely prone to negatively altering lipid values and increasing atherogenic risk. Anabolic/androgenic steroids may also adversely affect blood pressure and triglycerides, reduce endothelial relaxation, and support left ventricular hypertrophy, all potentially increasing the risk of cardiovascular disease and myocardial infarction.

To help reduce cardiovascular strain it is advised to maintain an active cardiovascular exercise program and minimize the intake of saturated fats, cholesterol, and simple carbohydrates at all times during active AAS administration. Supplementing with fish oils (4 grams per day) and a natural cholesterol/antioxidant formula such as Lipid Stabil or a product with comparable ingredients is also recommended.

Side Effects (Testosterone Suppression):

All anabolic/androgenic steroids when taken in doses sufficient to promote muscle gain are expected to suppress endogenous testosterone production. Without the intervention of testosterone-stimulating substances, testosterone levels should return to normal within 1-4 months of drug secession. Note that prolonged hypogonadotrophic hypogonadism can develop secondary to steroid abuse, necessitating medical intervention.

The above side effects are not inclusive. For more detailed discussion of potential side effects, see the Steroid Side Effects section of this book.

Administration (General):

Studies have shown that taking an oral anabolic steroid with food may decrease its bioavailability.[630] This is caused by the fat-soluble nature of steroid hormones, which can allow some of the drug to dissolve with undigested dietary fat, reducing its absorption from the gastrointestinal tract. For maximum utilization, methyltrienolone should be taken on an empty stomach.

Administration (Men):

Methyltrienolone is no longer used in clinical medicine due to an unacceptable level of hepatotoxicity. This agent is generally not recommended for physique- or performance-enhancing purposes for the same reason. Those absolutely insisting on its use need to take its level of liver toxicity very seriously. At the very least, routine blood tests should be conducted to ensure the agent is not imparting damage. Drug duration should also be very limited, preferably to 4 weeks of use or less. The relative potency of methyltrienolone is extremely high, requiring doses as little as .5 milligram per day. Its effective and tolerable range is usually considered to be .5 to 2mg per day. Dianabol-type doses of 20-30 mg daily are completely unthinkable, and should never be attempted. Again, this is an extremely toxic steroid, and all good advice would say to avoid it. Any one of the many commercially available steroids would be much safer choices.

Administration (Women):

Methyltrienolone is no longer used in clinical medicine due to an unacceptable level of hepatotoxicity. This agent is not recommended for women for physique- or performance-enhancing purposes due to its extremely strong toxicity and tendency to produce virilizing side effects.

Availability:

Methyltrienolone is not produced as a prescription steroid product in any part of the world. With the rapid expansion of underground steroid manufacturers, this agent has been released as a black market designer compound. Those contemplating the use of underground forms of methyltrienolone should consider that such agents are being released for human use without any government approval or consideration to its safety.

Miotolan® (furazabol)

Androgenic	73-94
Anabolic	270-330
Standard	Methyltestosterone (oral)
Chemical Name	17-Methyl-5alpha-androstano [2,3-c]furazan-17beta-ol
Estrogenic Activity	none
Progestational Activity	no data available (low)

Description:

Furazabol is an oral anabolic steroid derived from dihydrotestosterone. This agent is moderately anabolic, with only mild androgenic properties. This is no doubt due to the modification of the steroid's A-ring, which allows the steroid structure to remain stable and bind receptors in muscle tissue long enough to provide an anabolic benefit. Dihydrotestosterone, in comparison, is a poor anabolic, quickly metabolized in muscle tissue to inactive metabolites. The gains associated with furazabol are not extreme, and would more closely resemble the quality growth of a mild non-aromatizing anabolic like stanozolol or drostanolone, instead of the watery bulk of a testosterone. For this reason, furazabol is most often applied during cutting phases of training, and by athletes in speed and weight-restricted sports.

History:

Furazabol was first described in 1965.[631] The only modern pharmaceutical preparation of record containing furazabol, at least known to researchers in the West, was Miotolan from Daiichi Seiyaku Labs in Japan, which was sold in Japan mainly during the 1970's and '80's. The agent itself is scarcely mentioned in the Western medical literature, and consequently a great deal of myth has come to surround it among athletes. A realistic appraisal sits this agent in a very similar class to stanozolol, however, with both agents being moderately strong anabolics with low androgenic activity. Aside from this, it is difficult to ascribe any drastically unique traits to this drug.

Furazabol was a popular steroid among Olympic athletes during the 1980's, when it was quietly known among certain trainers that testing officials had not yet identified the agent, and therefore could not test for it. Dr. Jamie Astaphan, the physician that accompanied Ben Johnson to the 1988 Olympics in Seoul, reportedly was giving Johnson (and numerous other athletes at the time) furazabol, knowing the drug would not be detectable. It remains uncertain how Johnson ultimately tested positive for stanozolol, which Dr. Astaphan strongly denied giving his athletes. Within two years, methods for the detection of furazabol in urine were published, immediately eliminating any value this agent formerly possessed as a steroid undetectable to drug screeners.

Today, furazabol is very scarcely known to bodybuilders. The Miotolan brand from Japan was discontinued many years ago, and no pharmaceutical preparation containing furazabol has been known to exist since. The drug is occasionally located on the black market, however, due to the fact that is it still produced in bulk (as a raw material for product manufacturing) in Asia. From there it is obtained by underground steroid manufacturing operations in the West, and produced into oral tablets and capsules. Currently the actual number of products containing furazabol is small, although could easily be expanded if market demand for the agent increases. It remains unlikely that an actual prescription product containing this steroid will ever be seen again.

How Supplied:

Furazabol is no longer available as a prescription drug preparation. When sold it came in the form of tablets containing 1mg of steroid.

Structural Characteristics:

Furazabol is a modified form of dihydrotestosterone. It differs by: 1) the addition of a methyl group at carbon 17-alpha, which helps protect the hormone during oral administration, and 2) the attachment of a furazan group to the A-ring, replacing the normal 3-keto group. When viewed in the light of 17-alpha methyldihydrotestosterone, the A-ring modification on furazabol seems to considerably increase its anabolic strength while reducing its relative androgenicity.

Side Effects (Estrogenic):

Furazabol is not aromatized by the body, and is not measurably estrogenic. An anti-estrogen is not necessary when using this steroid, as gynecomastia should not be a concern even among sensitive individuals. Since estrogen is the usual culprit with water retention, this steroid instead produces a lean, quality look to the physique with no fear of excess subcutaneous fluid retention. This makes it a favorable steroid to use during cutting cycles, when water and fat retention are major concerns.

Side Effects (Androgenic):

Although classified as an anabolic steroid, androgenic side effects are still possible with this substance, especially with higher doses. This may include bouts of oily skin, acne, and body/facial hair growth. Anabolic/androgenic steroids may also aggravate male pattern hair loss. Women are warned of the potential virilizing effects of anabolic/androgenic steroids. These may include a deepening of the voice, menstrual irregularities, changes in skin texture, facial hair growth, and clitoral enlargement. Furazabol is a steroid with relatively low androgenic activity relative to its tissue-building actions, making the threshold for strong androgenic side effects comparably higher than with more androgenic agents such as testosterone, methandrostenolone, or fluoxymesterone. Note that furazabol is unaffected by the 5-alpha reductase enzyme, so its relative androgenicity is not affected by the concurrent use of finasteride or dutasteride.

Side Effects (Hepatotoxicity):

Furazabol is a c17-alpha alkylated compound. This alteration protects the drug from deactivation by the liver, allowing a very high percentage of the drug entry into the bloodstream following oral administration. C17-alpha alkylated anabolic/androgenic steroids can be hepatotoxic. Prolonged or high exposure may result in liver damage. In rare instances life-threatening dysfunction may develop. It is advisable to visit a physician periodically during each cycle to monitor liver function and overall health. Intake of c17-alpha alkylated steroids is commonly limited to 6-8 weeks, in an effort to avoid escalating liver strain.

The use of a liver detoxification supplement such as Liver Stabil, Liv-52, or Essentiale Forte is advised while taking any hepatotoxic anabolic/androgenic steroids.

Side Effects (Cardiovascular):

Anabolic/androgenic steroids can have deleterious effects on serum cholesterol. This includes a tendency to reduce HDL (good) cholesterol values and increase LDL (bad) cholesterol values, which may shift the HDL to LDL balance in a direction that favors greater risk of arteriosclerosis. The relative impact of an anabolic/androgenic steroid on serum lipids is dependant on the dose, route of administration (oral vs. injectable), type of steroid (aromatizable or non-aromatizable), and level of resistance to hepatic metabolism. Furazabol has a strong effect on the hepatic management of cholesterol due to its non-aromatizable nature, structural resistance to liver breakdown, and route of administration. Anabolic/androgenic steroids may also adversely affect blood pressure and triglycerides, reduce endothelial relaxation, and support left ventricular hypertrophy, all potentially increasing the risk of cardiovascular disease and myocardial infarction.

Note that furazabol is often mistakenly described as a steroid with unique beneficial cholesterol-lowering effects. Such statements usually make reference of studies conducted in the early 1970's, which examined the lipid-lowering effects of the agent.[632] Such a position, however, lacks a modern perspective of the drug. To draw a parallel, during the early 1970's there was research done on oxandrolone, demonstrating a lipid-lowering effect.[633] Upon closer inspection, however, it was shown that oxandrolone tends to lower HDL (good) cholesterol, increasing the HDL-LDL ratio and atherogenic risk. General cholesterol-lowering applications for the drug never materialized. The same is true for furazabol. Some have gone so far as to recommend this steroid to those with high cholesterol! Such use absolutely should be avoided.

To help reduce cardiovascular strain it is advised to maintain an active cardiovascular exercise program and minimize the intake of saturated fats, cholesterol, and simple carbohydrates at all times during active AAS administration. Supplementing with fish oils (4 grams per day) and a natural cholesterol/antioxidant formula such as Lipid Stabil or a product with comparable ingredients is also recommended.

Side Effects (Testosterone Suppression):

All anabolic/androgenic steroids when taken in doses sufficient to promote muscle gain are expected to suppress endogenous testosterone production. Without the intervention of testosterone-stimulating substances, testosterone levels should return to normal within 1-4 months of drug secession. Note that prolonged hypogonadotrophic hypogonadism can develop secondary to steroid abuse, necessitating medical intervention.

The above side effects are not inclusive. For more detailed discussion of potential side effects, see the Steroid Side Effects section of this book.

Administration (Men):

An effective dosage of furazabol seems to begin in the range of 10-20 mg daily for men, taken for no longer than 6 or 8 weeks. At this level it seems to impart a measurable muscle-building effect, which is usually accompanied by fat loss and increased definition. Doses of 30 mg per day or more considerably increase the anabolic potential of the drug, but at the expense of greater hepatotoxicity. The muscle-building activity of furazabol could, instead, be further enhanced by the addition of an injectable anabolic such as Deca-Durabolin® or Equipoise®. In this case, the combination should provide a noteworthy gain of solid, quality muscle mass without a loss of definition due to water retention. We could alternately use a more potent aromatizable androgen such as testosterone, although here the gains may be accompanies by some level of water retention, and potentially a decrease in muscle definition.

Administration (Women):

In the athletic arena, an effective oral daily dosage would fall in the range of 2-5 mg, taken in cycles lasting no more than 4-6 weeks to minimize the chance for virilization. As with all steroids, virilizing side effects are still possible in women, but remain rare with conservative dosing.

Availability:

Furazabol is no longer produced as a prescription drug product, although underground preparations containing this steroid may be located.

MOHN (methylhydroxynandrolone)

Androgenic	281
Anabolic	1304
Standard	Methyltestosterone (oral)
Chemical Name	4-Hydroxy-17alpha-methyl hydroxyestra-4-ene-3-one
Estrogenic Activity	none
Progestational Activity	none

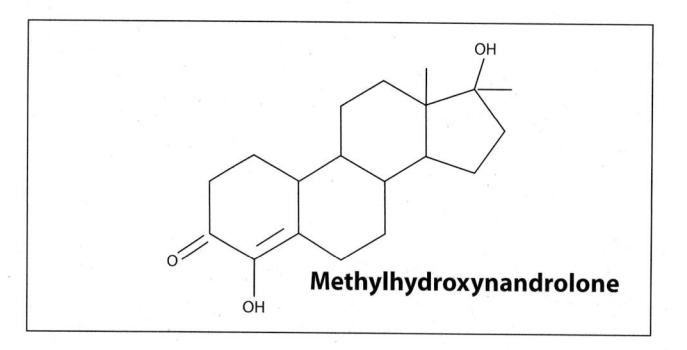

Description:

Methylhydroxynandrolone, or MOHN for short, is a potent derivative of nandrolone. This agent is orally active and non-aromatizable, with a profile somewhat similar to that of Winstrol or Anavar – primarily anabolic, with no discernable estrogenic activity. According to early assay results, methylhydroxynandrolone is 13 times more anabolic than methyltestosterone, with approximately 3 times greater androgenicity. Although animal assay data doesn't translate perfectly to humans, it remains clear that MOHN is considerably stronger on a milligram for milligram basis than the common prescription steroids. MOHN is also a bit more androgenic than the assay data conveys, and behaves slightly more like trenbolone than nandrolone in this regard. Its 4-hydroxyl group, a modification that prevents its 5-alpha reduction in humans to weaker "dihydro" metabolites in the skin, scalp and prostate, intensifies the relative androgenicity of this steroid. Athletes favor it for lean gains in muscle mass, strength, and performance, with minimal side effects.

History:

Methylhydroxynandrolone was first described in 1964, developed during a series of investigations that looked at the effects of 4-hydroxylation on various nandrolone compounds.[634] Being that 4-hydroxylation inhibits 5-alpha reduction, nandrolone derivatives with this alteration tend to be more androgenic. They are, therefore, less likely to cause side effects relating to low libido and reduced androgenicity, common with injectable nandrolone esters. Although early results showed that methylhydroxynandrolone was both effective and retained a favorable ratio of anabolic to androgenic effect, it was ultimately never developed into a medicine. Only MOHN's non-methylated cousin, oxabolone (as oxabolone cypionate), had reached the stage of prescription drug product. For approximately forty years after its synthesis, little mention was made of methylhydroxynandrolone in the medical literature. For all intents and purposes, it was a dead and forgotten anabolic steroid.

MOHN suddenly reemerged in 2004, when it was introduced as a "nutritional product" on the U.S. supplement market. It was being sold OTC, without the restrictions of a synthetic anabolic steroid. This was due primarily to the fact that it was never regulated as a drug in the U.S., and barring a direct listing in the 1991 Anabolic Steroid Control Act, could not be covered by it. Its legality as a supplement may have been questionable, but that was a matter for the FDA to handle, not the DEA (Drug Enforcement Agency). MOHN has since been included in the most recent expansion of U.S. anabolic steroid laws, however, and formally became a controlled anabolic steroid on January 20, 2005. Possession of this agent after this date carries all the same legal risks and consequences as other popular and illegal steroids according to Federal law. Due to the fact that it is not a prescription drug, this law effectively marked the commercial end of methylhydroxynandrolone products.

How Supplied:

Methylhydroxynandrolone is not available as a commercial agent. When sold as a nutritional supplement, it generally contained 3mg of steroid per tablet.

Structural Characteristics:

Methylhydroxynandrolone is a modified form of nandrolone. It differs by: 1) the addition of a methyl group at carbon 17-alpha to protect the hormone during oral administration and 2) the introduction of a hydroxyl group at carbon 4, which inhibits aromatization, progestational activity, and 5-alpha reduction, and reduces relative steroid androgenicity.

Side Effects (Estrogenic):

Methylhydroxynandrolone is not aromatized by the body, and is not measurably estrogenic. Estrogenic side effects such as increased water retention, fat gain, and gynecomastia are not likely to occur with use. The non-estrogenic nature of methylhydroxynandrolone makes this agent favorable during cutting or lean mass phases of training, when muscle definition is favored over raw bulk gains.

Side Effects (Androgenic):

Although classified as an anabolic steroid, androgenic side effects are still common with this substance. This may include bouts of oily skin, acne, and body/facial hair growth. Anabolic/androgenic steroids may also aggravate male pattern hair loss. Women are also warned of the potential virilizing effects of anabolic/androgenic steroids. These may include a deepening of the voice, menstrual irregularities, changes in skin texture, facial hair growth, and clitoral enlargement. Additionally, the 5-alpha reductase enzyme does not metabolize methylhydroxynandrolone, so its relative androgenicity is not affected by finasteride or dutasteride.

Side Effects (Hepatotoxicity):

Methylhydroxynandrolone is a c17-alpha alkylated compound. This alteration protects the drug from deactivation by the liver, allowing a very high percentage of the drug entry into the bloodstream following oral administration. C17-alpha alkylated anabolic/androgenic steroids can be hepatotoxic. Prolonged or high exposure may result in liver damage. In rare instances life-threatening dysfunction may develop. It is advisable to visit a physician periodically during each cycle to monitor liver function and overall health. Intake of c17-alpha alkylated steroids is commonly limited to 6-8 weeks, in an effort to avoid escalating liver strain.

The use of a liver detoxification supplement such as Liver Stabil, Liv-52, or Essentiale Forte is advised while taking any hepatotoxic anabolic/androgenic steroids.

Side Effects (Cardiovascular):

Anabolic/androgenic steroids can have deleterious effects on serum cholesterol. This includes a tendency to reduce HDL (good) cholesterol values and increase LDL (bad) cholesterol values, which may shift the HDL to LDL balance in a direction that favors greater risk of arteriosclerosis. The relative impact of an anabolic/androgenic steroid on serum lipids is dependant on the dose, route of administration (oral vs. injectable), type of steroid (aromatizable or non-aromatizable), and level of resistance to hepatic metabolism. Although not studied in humans, the high relative potency, oral route, and non-aromatizable nature of methylhydroxynandrolone suggest that this agent is extremely prone to negatively altering lipid values and increasing atherogenic risk. Anabolic/androgenic steroids may also adversely affect blood pressure and triglycerides, reduce endothelial relaxation, and support left ventricular hypertrophy, all potentially increasing the risk of cardiovascular disease and myocardial infarction.

To help reduce cardiovascular strain it is advised to maintain an active cardiovascular exercise program and minimize the intake of saturated fats, cholesterol, and simple carbohydrates at all times during active AAS administration. Supplementing with fish oils (4 grams per day) and a natural cholesterol/antioxidant formula such as Lipid Stabil or a product with comparable ingredients is also recommended.

Side Effects (Testosterone Suppression):

All anabolic/androgenic steroids when taken in doses sufficient to promote muscle gain are expected to suppress endogenous testosterone production. Without the intervention of testosterone-stimulating substances, testosterone levels should return to normal within 1-4 months of drug secession. Note that prolonged hypogonadotrophic hypogonadism can develop secondary to steroid abuse, necessitating medical intervention.

The above side effects are not inclusive. For more detailed discussion of potential side effects, see the Steroid Side Effects section of this book.

Administration (General):

Studies have shown that taking an oral anabolic steroid with food may decrease its bioavailability.[635] This is caused by the fat-soluble nature of steroid hormones, which can allow some of the drug to dissolve with undigested dietary fat, reducing its absorption from the gastrointestinal tract. For maximum utilization, this steroid should be taken on an empty stomach.

Administration (Men):

Methylhydroxynandrolone was never approved for use in humans. Prescribing guidelines are unavailable. Effective oral daily doses for physique- or performance-enhancing purposes fall in the range of 2-10 mg. In an effort to reduce liver strain, it is usually recommended to limit drug duration to no longer than 6-8 weeks, after which point a break is taken from all c-17 alkylated steroids. At this level MOHN should provide very solid gains in lean muscle mass and strength, without water retention or increased fat deposition. MOHN is not thought of as a bulking drug itself, although is very versatile for stacking, and mixes well with many other anabolics depending on the individual goals of the user.

Administration (Women):

Methylhydroxynandrolone was never approved for use in humans. Prescribing guidelines are unavailable. The high anabolic to androgenic ratio of methylhydroxynandrolone makes use possible without significant virilization, but would likely require small doses (1-3mg per day) and respecting a very periodic use schedule (4 weeks or less).

Availability:

Methylhydroxynandrolone is not available as a prescription agent at this time, in any part of the world. Since this agent was manufactured as a nutritional supplement for a brief period of time before the 2004 amendment to the Anabolic Steroid Act went into effect, there may be some leftover drug in circulation.

Myagen (bolasterone)

Androgenic	300
Anabolic	575
Standard	Methyltestosterone (oral)

Chemical Names 17beta-Hydroxy-7,17alpha-dimethylandrost-4-en-3-one
7,17-dimethyltestosterone

Estrogenic Activity	high
Progestational Activity	no data available

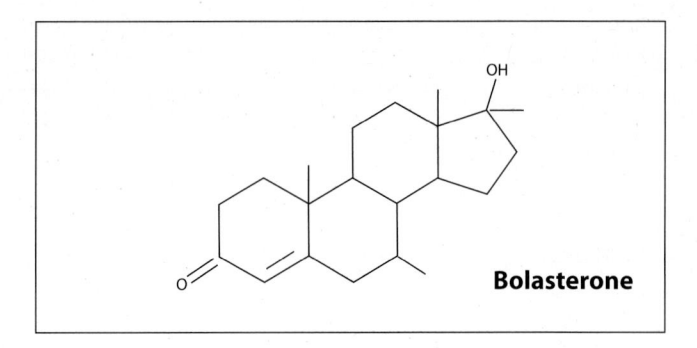

Description:

Bolasterone is an oral anabolic steroid structurally related to methyltestosterone. It differs only by the addition of a methyl group at c-7, which accounts for its given chemical name, 7,17-dimethyltestosterone. The added c-7 methyl group makes the activity of this steroid far removed from methyltestosterone, however, such that any direct comparison is difficult to justify. For starters, bolasterone is a fairly potent steroid, measured in human subjects to have approximately twice the anabolic effect of methandrostenolone.[636] This is in contrast to methyltestosterone, which is considerably less potent than methandrostenolone. Despite being a testosterone derivative, bolasterone is also much more anabolic than androgenic in nature. At a given therapeutic level, it is much less likely to cause androgenic/virilizing side effects. It does have one strong similarity to methyltestosterone, however, which lies in the fact that bolasterone too is quite estrogenic. Both agents are, therefore, most appropriately used during bulking phases or training.

History:

Bolasterone was first described in 1959.[637] It was closely evaluated for anabolic and androgenic effect approximately 3 years later.[638] The drug was developed by Upjohn, and sold in the U.S. during the 1960's under the Myagen brand name. It was mainly indicated for the treatment of advanced breast cancer in women, although the agent was also investigated for its stimulatory effect on blood cells and its general anabolic (lean-tissue sparing) activity. Bolasterone was ultimately a short-lived drug, disappearing from the U.S. market shortly after its release. By the 1980's, bolasterone had been out of commerce for so long that it was all but forgotten among athletes. Although bolasterone is no longer produced, the drug remains listed in the U.S. Pharmacopeias, suggesting it would not be impossible to see this agent for sale (legally) in the U.S. again, perhaps under order by a private compounding pharmacy. The reemergence of an actual commercial bolasterone compound, however, remains very unlikely.

How Supplied:

Bolasterone is no longer available as a prescription drug product.

Structural Characteristics:

Bolasterone is a modified form of testosterone. It differs by: 1) the addition of a methyl group at carbon 17-alpha, which helps protect the hormone during oral administration, and 2) the introduction of a methyl group at carbon 7 (alpha), which inhibits 5-alpha reduction and shifts the anabolic to androgenic ratio in favor of the former. 7,17-dimethylated steroids also tend to be very resistant to metabolism and serum-binding proteins, greatly enhancing their relative biological activity.

Side Effects (Estrogenic):

Bolasterone is aromatized by the body, and is considered a highly estrogenic steroid due to its conversion to 7,17-dimethylestradiol (an estrogen with high biological activity). Gynecomastia may be a concern during treatment, especially when higher than normal therapeutic doses are used. At the same time water retention can become a problem, causing a notable loss of muscle definition as both subcutaneous water retention and fat levels build. To avoid strong estrogenic side effects, it may be necessary to use an anti-estrogen such as Nolvadex®. One may alternately use an aromatase inhibitor like Arimidex® (anastrozole), which is a more effective remedy for estrogen control. Aromatase inhibitors, however, can be quite expensive in comparison to standard estrogen maintenance therapies, and may also have negative effects on blood lipids.

Side Effects (Androgenic):

Although bolasterone is classified as an anabolic steroid, androgenic side effects are still possible with this substance. These may include bouts of oily skin, acne, and body/facial hair growth. Higher doses are more likely to cause such side effects. Anabolic/androgenic steroids may also aggravate male pattern hair loss. Women are additionally warned of the potential virilizing effects of anabolic/androgenic steroids. These may include a deepening of the voice, menstrual irregularities, changes in skin texture, facial hair growth, and clitoral enlargement. Bolasterone is unaffected by the 5-alpha reductase enzyme, so its relative androgenicity is not affected by the concurrent use of finasteride or dutasteride. Note that studies administering 1mg and 2mg of bolasterone per day have shown no outward androgenic side effects in children and hypogonadotrophic males, as would be characterized by public hair growth, genital changes, voice changes, and acne. Higher doses remain likely to induce androgenic effects. Bolasterone is considered to have a comparable ratio of anabolic to androgenic effect as oxymetholone and methandrostenolone.

Side Effects (Hepatotoxicity):

Bolasterone is a c17-alpha alkylated compound. This alteration protects the drug from deactivation by the liver, allowing a very high percentage of the drug entry into the bloodstream following oral administration. C17-alpha alkylated anabolic/androgenic steroids can be hepatotoxic. Prolonged or high exposure may result in liver damage. In rare instances life-threatening dysfunction may develop. It is advisable to visit a physician periodically during each cycle to monitor liver function and overall health. Intake of c17-alpha alkylated steroids is commonly limited to 6-8 weeks, in an effort to avoid escalating liver strain. Studies administering 1mg and 2mg of bolasterone daily for 6 weeks to 27 patients have demonstrated a trend toward increases in serum alkaline phosphatase (a marker of liver stress), although no significant untoward effects on the liver were documented.

The use of a liver detoxification supplement such as Liver Stabil, Liv-52, or Essentiale Forte is advised while taking any hepatotoxic anabolic/androgenic steroids.

Side Effects (Cardiovascular):

Anabolic/androgenic steroids can have deleterious effects on serum cholesterol. This includes a tendency to reduce HDL (good) cholesterol values and increase LDL (bad) cholesterol values, which may shift the HDL to LDL balance in a direction that favors greater risk of arteriosclerosis. The relative impact of an anabolic/androgenic steroid on serum lipids is dependant on the dose, route of administration (oral vs. injectable), type of steroid (aromatizable or non-aromatizable), and level of resistance to hepatic metabolism. Bolasterone has a strong effect on the hepatic management of cholesterol due to its structural resistance to liver breakdown and route of administration. Anabolic/androgenic steroids may also adversely affect blood pressure and triglycerides, reduce endothelial relaxation, and support left ventricular hypertrophy, all potentially increasing the risk of cardiovascular disease and myocardial infarction. Studies administering 1mg and 2mg of bolasterone daily for 6 weeks to 27 patients have demonstrated a trend toward increased serum cholesterol. Although no HDL and LDL breakdown was provided, it can be assumed based on the structure and route of administration that bolasterone significantly shifted the ratio of these two fractions of cholesterol further apart, measurably increasing atherogenic risk.

To help reduce cardiovascular strain it is advised to maintain an active cardiovascular exercise program and minimize the intake of saturated fats, cholesterol, and simple carbohydrates at all times during active AAS administration. Supplementing with fish oils (4 grams per day) and a natural cholesterol/antioxidant formula such as Lipid Stabil or a product with comparable ingredients is also recommended.

Side Effects (Testosterone Suppression):

All anabolic/androgenic steroids when taken in doses sufficient to promote muscle gain are expected to suppress endogenous testosterone production. Without the intervention of testosterone-stimulating substances, testosterone levels should return to normal within 1-4 months of drug secession. Note that prolonged hypogonadotrophic hypogonadism can develop secondary to steroid abuse, necessitating medical intervention.

The above side effects are not inclusive. For more detailed discussion of potential side effects, see the Steroid Side Effects section of this book.

Administration (General):

Studies have shown that taking an oral anabolic steroid with food may decrease its bioavailability.[639] This is caused by the fat-soluble nature of steroid hormones, which can allow some of the drug to dissolve with undigested dietary fat, reducing its absorption from the gastrointestinal tract. For maximum utilization, this steroid should be taken on an empty stomach.

Administration (Men):

Clinical studies have demonstrated that significant nitrogen retention and weight gain can be induced with a daily dosage of 1-2mg per day. In the athletic arena, doses of 2-5 mg daily seem to be most reasonable, taken in cycles lasting no more than 6-8 weeks in length to minimize hepatotoxicity. This level is sufficient for strong increases in muscle size and strength, although such gains will likely be accompanied by significant water retention.

Administration (Women):

Bolasterone was not widely used with women in clinical medicine. When applied, it was most often used as a secondary medication during inoperable breast cancer, when other therapies have failed to produce a desirable effect. The dosage used for this application would be as high as 10 mg per day, a level that has caused significant virilization among patients. Bolasterone is generally not recommended for women for physique- or performance-enhancing purposes due to its very strong nature and tendency to produce virilizing side effects.

Availability:

Bolasterone is no longer produced as a prescription drug, although a handful of underground laboratories have taken to selling this material.

Nandrabolin (nandrolone/methandriol blend)

Androgenic	
Anabolic	
Standard	
Chemical Names	
Estrogenic Activity	
Progestational Activity	

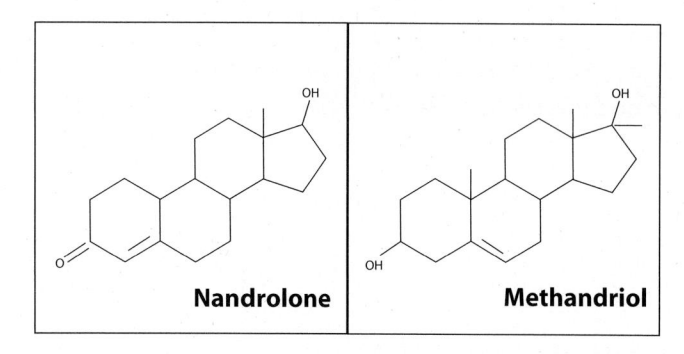

Nandrolone

Methandriol

Description:

Nandrabolin is an injectable veterinary steroid product from Australia. It contains a mixture of methandriol dipropionate and nandrolone cypionate, the two steroids present in a concentration of 45 mg/mL and 30 mg/mL respectively. This adds up to a total of 75 mg per milliliter of steroid, or 750 mg total each 10 mL multi-dose vial. These two agents are primarily anabolic in nature, and tend to provide the user a good ratio of muscle growth to androgenic/estrogenic side effects. Methandriol does carry some inherent estrogenicity, however, which makes this product less than perfectly suited for drastic cutting phases. Athletes do not generally view this steroid preparation as a bulking drug, but instead value its as a lean-tissue-building drug.

History:

The Nandrabolin formulation was originally developed by Jurox, a company with a 30-year history of manufacturing veterinary drugs in Australia. It is designed to improve the muscularity of racehorses, as well as provide benefits of maintaining a proper fluid balance and aid the digestion and assimilation of dietary protein. Jurox voluntarily scaled back its line of steroid products considerably in early 2001 (this formulation included), amidst a great deal of public controversy concerning their exportation of high volumes of steroids to Mexico (known to feed the American black market). Although the exact relationship between the companies is unknown, many of the discontinued Jurox products were registered under the SYD Group label in August 2002. Nandrabolin was among them, and has been sold by SYD Group exclusively ever since. It would be marketed under the new trade name Anabolic NA.

SYD Group had initially marketed many of its products heavily in Mexico, even producing distinct formulations and labeling to compete in the then very competitive market. Anabolic NA did not appear to be one of them, however, likely due to the low concentration and perceived low value. SYD Group had also acquired Grupo Comercial Tarasco around this time, a company that was formed several years ago specifically to import Jurox products into Mexico. Things changed rapidly in December 2005, however, when U.S. authorities spearheaded Operation Gear Grinder, which targeted many companies operating in Mexico (SYD Group included) for providing steroid products to illegal American importers. The firm quickly discontinued the sale of all anabolic steroid products in Mexico, and stated they will no longer produce high-concentration anabolics which entice abuse. The Anabolic NA product remains available in Australia, although given tight controls is not commonly diverted to the black market.

How Supplied:

Anabolic NA is available on the Australian veterinary drug market. It contains 75 mg/mL of steroid in oil in a 10 mL vial.

Structural Characteristics:

For a more comprehensive discussion on the individual steroids nandrolone cypionate and methandriol dipropionate, refer to their respective drug profiles.

Side Effects (Estrogenic):

Methylandrostendiol is not directly aromatized by the body, although one of its known metabolites is methyltestosterone, which can aromatize. Methyandrostenediol is also believed to have some inherent estrogenic activity. Combined with nandrolone, which also weakly aromatizes, this product is considered a weak to moderate estrogenic steroid preparation. Gynecomastia is possible during treatment, but generally only when higher doses are used. Water and fat retention can also become issues, again depending on dose. Sensitive individuals may need to addition an anti-estrogen such as Nolvadex® to minimize related side effects.

Side Effects (Androgenic):

Although classified as an anabolic steroid preparation, androgenic side effects are still common with this substance. This may include bouts of oily skin, acne, and body/facial hair growth. Anabolic/androgenic steroids may also aggravate male pattern hair loss. Women are warned of the potential virilizing effects of anabolic/androgenic steroids. These may include a deepening of the voice, menstrual irregularities, changes in skin texture, facial hair growth, and clitoral enlargement.

Side Effects (Hepatotoxicity):

Methylandrostenediol is a c17-alpha alkylated compound. This alteration protects the drug from deactivation by the liver, allowing a very high percentage of the drug entry into the bloodstream following oral administration. C17-alpha alkylated anabolic/androgenic steroids can be hepatotoxic. Prolonged or high exposure may result in liver damage. In rare instances life-threatening dysfunction may develop. It is advisable to visit a physician periodically during each cycle to monitor liver function and overall health. Intake of c17-alpha alkylated steroids is commonly limited to 6-8 weeks, in an effort to avoid escalating liver strain. Injectable forms of the drug may present slightly less strain on the liver by avoiding the first pass metabolism of oral dosing, although may still present substantial hepatotoxicity.

The use of a liver detoxification supplement such as Liver Stabil, Liv-52, or Essentiale Forte is advised while taking any hepatotoxic anabolic/androgenic steroids.

Side Effects (Cardiovascular):

Anabolic/androgenic steroids can have deleterious effects on serum cholesterol. This includes a tendency to reduce HDL (good) cholesterol values and increase LDL (bad) cholesterol values, which may shift the HDL to LDL balance in a direction that favors greater risk of arteriosclerosis. The relative impact of an anabolic/androgenic steroid on serum lipids is dependant on the dose, route of administration (oral vs. injectable), type of steroid (aromatizable or non-aromatizable), and level of resistance to hepatic metabolism. Methylandrostenediol has a strong effect on the hepatic management of cholesterol due to its structural resistance to liver breakdown and (with the oral) route of administration. Anabolic/androgenic steroids may also adversely affect blood pressure and triglycerides, reduce endothelial relaxation, and support left ventricular hypertrophy, all potentially increasing the risk of cardiovascular disease and myocardial infarction.

To help reduce cardiovascular strain it is advised to maintain an active cardiovascular exercise program and minimize the intake of saturated fats, cholesterol, and simple carbohydrates at all times during active AAS administration. Supplementing with fish oils (4 grams per day) and a natural cholesterol/antioxidant formula such as Lipid Stabil or a product with comparable ingredients is also recommended.

Side Effects (Testosterone Suppression):

All anabolic/androgenic steroids when taken in doses sufficient to promote muscle gain are expected to suppress endogenous testosterone production. Without the intervention of testosterone stimulating substances, testosterone levels should return to normal within 1-4 months of drug secession. Note that prolonged hypogonadotrophic hypogonadism can develop secondary to steroid abuse, necessitating medical intervention.

The above side effects are not inclusive. For more detailed discussion of potential side effects, see the Steroid Side Effects section of this book.

Administration (Men):

Nandrabolin has not been approved for use in humans. Prescribing guidelines for men are unavailable. Typical dosing schedule for physique- or performance-enhancing purposes would be in the range of 225 mg (3cc's) to 450 mg (6cc's) per week, a level that should provide quality lean mass gain without bloating or significant body fat retention. Given the relatively low per ML steroid concentration, this drug is often used in a low dose, and stacked with other agents for a stronger effect. Given the mild estrogenicity already present with methandriol, this is often an agent with low or no estrogenic properties.

Administration (Women):

Nandrabolin has not been approved for use in humans. Prescribing guidelines for women are unavailable. Drugs containing methylandrostenediol are generally not recommended for women for physique- or performance-enhancing purposes due to its androgenic nature and tendency to produce virilizing side effects.

Availability:

Nandrabolin is presently available in Australia under the Anabolic NA trade name (SYD Group), but is not widely available on the black market due to strict controls preventing product diversion.

Nebido (testosterone undecanoate)

Androgenic	100
Anabolic	100
Standard	Standard
Chemical Names	4-androsten-3-one-17beta-ol
	17beta-hydroxy-androst-4-en-3-one
Estrogenic Activity	moderate
Progestational Activity	low

Testosterone

Description:

Nebido® is an injectable steroid that contains testosterone undecanoate, a very slow-acting ester of testosterone. This is the active drug that is used in Andriol, but in that case it is part of an oral medication, not an injectable. Nebido is being marketed as a replacement for established injectable testosterone products like Delatestryl®, Depo-Testosterone®, and Sustanon®, which are actually much faster acting in comparison. It is designed to offer a much less frequent injection schedule, and, therefore, much greater comfort for the patient. Nebido is a drug developed under a similar focus as testosterone buciclate, which is another very slow-acting injectable ester of testosterone.

History:

Nebido® was developed by international giant Schering AG, Germany. It first surfaced as a prescription drug in Finland and Germany in October and November of 2004, respectively. Within a year it had been approved for sale in several other European countries, including France, United Kingdom, Sweden, Denmark, Austria, and Ireland. Schering has since also brought this product to Mexico, Brazil, Argentina, South Africa, Colombia, Korea, Venezuela, and various countries in Eastern Europe. In July 2005, the U.S. pharmaceuticals firm Indevus purchased the rights to Nebido in the U.S., with the intent to push for FDA approval. In March of 2006, Indevus received FDA approval on Phase III pharmacokinetic studies of Nebido, and expects to file an NDA (New Drug Application) on the product sometime in 2007. Ultimate approval in the United States seems likely.

Nebido® is described by Schering as being the, "first long-acting injection for the treatment of male hypogonadism." This may be a matter of perspective, as other slow-acting esters do exist. Schering AG, however, is taking the lead to market in most regions. The applications for Nebido® are extremely narrow, being approved for use in men as a long-term treatment option for low androgen levels only. It is not labeled for use in women, or in males for other uses.

Given the growing acceptance of androgen replacement therapy, and the comfort advantage that Nebido® seems to offer male hormone replacement therapy patients (esters like enanthate and cypionate generally require between 13 and 26 injections per year), it may very well become a dominant testosterone product in the years to come, especially with the marketing support of a pharmaceutical giant like Schering AG.

How Supplied:

Testosterone undecanoate (injection) is available in various human drug markets. All products (Nebido®) contain 250 mg/ml of steroid dissolved in oil; packaged in 4ml ampules containing 1,000 mg of steroid in total.

Structural Characteristics:

Testosterone undecanoate is a modified form of testosterone, where a carboxylic acid ester (undecanoic acid) has been attached to the 17-beta hydroxyl group. Esterified forms of testosterone are less polar than free testosterone, and are absorbed more slowly from the area of injection. Once in the bloodstream, the ester is removed to yield free (active) testosterone. Esterified forms of testosterone are designed to prolong the window of therapeutic effect following administration, allowing for a less frequent injection schedule compared to injections of free (unesterified) steroid. Nebido® is designed to maintain physiological levels of testosterone for up to 14 weeks after injection.[640]

Side Effects (Estrogenic):

Testosterone is readily aromatized in the body to estradiol (estrogen). The aromatase (estrogen synthetase) enzyme is responsible for this metabolism of testosterone. Elevated estrogen levels can cause side effects such as increased water retention, body fat gain, and gynecomastia. Testosterone is considered a moderately estrogenic steroid. An anti-estrogen such as clomiphene citrate or tamoxifen citrate may be necessary to prevent estrogenic side effects. One may alternately use an aromatase inhibitor like Arimidex® (anastrozole), which more efficiently controls estrogen by preventing its synthesis. Aromatase inhibitors can be quite expensive in comparison to anti-estrogens, however, and may also have negative effects on blood lipids.

Estrogenic side effects will occur in a dose-dependant manner, with higher doses (above normal therapeutic levels) of testosterone more likely to require the concurrent use of an anti-estrogen or aromatase inhibitor. Since water retention and loss of muscle definition are common with higher doses of testosterone, this drug is usually considered a poor choice for dieting or cutting phases of training. Its moderate estrogenicity makes it more ideal for bulking phases, where the added water retention will support raw strength and muscle size, and help foster a stronger anabolic environment.

Side Effects (Androgenic):

Testosterone is the primary male androgen, responsible for maintaining secondary male sexual characteristics. Elevated levels of testosterone are likely to produce androgenic side effects including oily skin, acne, and body/facial hair growth. Men with a genetic predisposition for hair loss (androgenetic alopecia) may notice accelerated male pattern balding. Those concerned about hair loss may find a more comfortable option in nandrolone decanoate, which is a comparably less androgenic steroid. Women are warned of the potential virilizing effects of anabolic/androgenic steroids, especially with a strong androgen such as testosterone. These may include deepening of the voice, menstrual irregularities, changes in skin texture, facial hair growth, and clitoral enlargement.

In androgen-responsive target tissues such as the skin, scalp, and prostate, the high relative androgenicity of testosterone is dependant on its reduction to dihydrotestosterone (DHT). The 5-alpha reductase enzyme is responsible for this metabolism of testosterone. The concurrent use of a 5-alpha reductase inhibitor such as finasteride or dutasteride will interfere with site-specific potentiation of testosterone action, lowering the tendency of testosterone drugs to produce androgenic side effects. It is important to remember that anabolic and androgenic effects are both mediated via the cytosolic androgen receptor. Complete separation of testosterone's anabolic and androgenic properties is not possible, even with total 5-alpha reductase inhibition.

Side Effects (Hepatotoxicity):

Testosterone does not have hepatotoxic effects; liver toxicity is unlikely. One study examined the potential for hepatotoxicity with high doses of testosterone by administering 400 mg of the hormone per day (2,800 mg per week) to a group of male subjects. The steroid was taken orally so that higher peak concentrations would be reached in hepatic tissues compared to intramuscular injections. The hormone was given daily for 20 days, and produced no significant changes in liver enzyme values including serum albumin, bilirubin, alanine-amino-transferase, and alkaline phosphatases.[641]

Side Effects (Cardiovascular):

Anabolic/androgenic steroids can have deleterious effects on serum cholesterol. This includes a tendency to reduce HDL (good) cholesterol values and increase LDL (bad) cholesterol values, which may shift the HDL to LDL balance in a direction that favors greater risk of arteriosclerosis. The relative impact of an anabolic/androgenic steroid on serum lipids is dependant on the dose, route of administration (oral vs. injectable), type of steroid (aromatizable or non-aromatizable), and level of resistance to hepatic metabolism. Anabolic/androgenic steroids may also adversely affect blood pressure and triglycerides, reduce endothelial relaxation, and support left ventricular hypertrophy, all potentially increasing the risk of cardiovascular disease and myocardial infarction.

Testosterone tends to have a much less dramatic impact on cardiovascular risk factors than synthetic steroids. This is due in part to its openness to metabolism by the liver, which allows it to have less effect on the hepatic management of cholesterol. The aromatization of testosterone to estradiol also helps to mitigate the negative effects of androgens on serum lipids. In one study, 280 mg per week of testosterone ester (enanthate) had a slight but not statistically significant effect on HDL cholesterol after 12 weeks, but when taken with an aromatase inhibitor a strong (25%) decrease was seen.[642] Studies using 300 mg of testosterone ester (enanthate) per week for twenty weeks without an aromatase inhibitor demonstrated only a 13% decrease in HDL cholesterol, while at 600 mg the reduction reached 21%.[643] The negative impact of aromatase inhibition should be taken into consideration before such drug is added to testosterone therapy.

Due to the positive influence of estrogen on serum lipids, tamoxifen citrate or clomiphene citrate are preferred to aromatase inhibitors for those concerned with cardiovascular health, as they offer a partial estrogenic effect in the liver. This allows them to potentially improve lipid profiles and offset some of the negative effects of androgens. With doses of 600 mg or less per week, the impact on lipid profile tends to be noticeable but not dramatic, making an anti-estrogen (for cardioprotective purposes) perhaps unnecessary. Doses of 600 mg or less per week have also failed to produce statistically significant changes in LDL/VLDL cholesterol, triglycerides, apolipoprotein B/C-III, C-reactive protein, and insulin sensitivity, all indicating a relatively weak impact on cardiovascular risk factors.[644] When used in moderate doses, injectable testosterone esters are usually considered to be the safest of all anabolic/androgenic steroids.

To help reduce cardiovascular strain it is advised to maintain an active cardiovascular exercise program and minimize the intake of saturated fats, cholesterol, and simple carbohydrates at all times during active AAS administration. Supplementing with fish oils (4 grams per day) and a natural cholesterol/antioxidant formula such as Lipid Stabil or a product with comparable ingredients is also recommended.

Side Effects (Testosterone Suppression):

All anabolic/androgenic steroids when taken in doses sufficient to promote muscle gain are expected to suppress endogenous testosterone production. Testosterone is the primary male androgen, and offers strong negative feedback on endogenous testosterone production. Testosterone-based drugs will, likewise, have a strong effect on the hypothalamic regulation of natural steroid hormones. Without the intervention of testosterone stimulating substances, testosterone levels should return to normal within 1-4 months after the drug has fully cleared the body. Note that prolonged hypogonadotrophic hypogonadism can develop secondary to steroid abuse, necessitating medical intervention.

The above side effects are not inclusive. For more detailed discussion of potential side effects, see the Steroid Side Effects section of this book.

Administration (General):

Due to the large injection volume, prescribing guidelines recommend that each injection be given slowly, taking approximately 60 seconds to administer the full 4ml dose. Nebido® should always be injected deep in the gluteal muscle.

Administration (Men):

To treat androgen insufficiency, the prescribing guidelines for testosterone undecanoate (Nebido®) call for a dosage of 1,000 mg (4ml) every twelve weeks. Therapy is usually initiated with a loading phase, which requires that the second injection of 1,000 mg be given at approximately the six-week mark. For bodybuilding purposes, supraphysiological (rather than physiological) hormone levels would require injecting the drug on a more regular basis. The most logical protocol would be to administer a 4ml injection of Nebido every 2-4 weeks, for an approximate average weekly dosage of 250-500 mg of testosterone ester. At this level one could expect results very much in line with other testosterone esters, albeit with a less frequent injection schedule. The onset of action may, however, be much slower with Nebido. Some may opt to begin their cycle with a faster acting ester, such as enanthate or cypionate, which would allow testosterone levels to reach into supraphysiological ranges sooner. Testosterone is ultimately very versatile, and can be combined with many other anabolic/androgenic steroids depending on the desired effect.

Administration (Women):

Testosterone undecanoate is not approved for use with women in clinical medicine. This drug is not recommended for women for physique- or performance-enhancing purposes due to its strong androgenic nature, tendency to produce virilizing side effects, and very slow acting characteristics (making blood levels difficult to control).

Availability:

The availability of Nebido on the black market is currently low, mainly due to the high price of the agent compared to other esters of testosterone like cypionate and enanthate. Its advantages, applications, and price seem to be most properly suited for the hormone replacement therapy market.

Neo-Ponden (androisoxazol)

Androgenic	22
Anabolic	155
Standard	Methyltestosterone (oral)
Chemical Names	17alpha-methylandrostan-17beta-ol[2,3-d]isoxazole
Estrogenic Activity	none
Progestational Activity	no data available

Description:

Androisoxazol is an oral anabolic steroid derived from dihydrotestosterone. It is similar in structure to stanozolol, which carries a 2,3-pyrazole group instead of the 2,3-isoxazole modification used here. Danazol is another commercial 2,3-isoxazole, although this particular agent has minimal anabolic activity. Similar to stanozolol, androisoxazol is non-estrogenic, and displays a highly favorable balance of anabolic to androgenic effect. Depending on the source, it is identified as having an anabolic to androgenic ratio ranging from 7:1, all the way up to 40:1. Although no longer available, this agent possesses strong muscle building and performance enhancing properties, which are accompanied by a low inclination for androgenic side effects. Being a non-estrogenic agent, androisoxazol is well suited for lean mass gains, cutting purposes, and competitive athletics.

History:

Androisoxazol was first described in 1961.[645] The drug was developed into a medicine by Serono, an international pharmaceuticals giant that was originally founded in Italy in 1906 as Ares-Serono. Serono would sell the agent on the Italian drug market under the Neo-Ponden brand name. Androisoxazol was developed subsequent to the successful synthesis of stanozolol a couple of years earlier, which is another heterocyclic steroid with a favorable anabolic/androgenic profile. Numerous other A-ring heterocyclic DHT derivatives were synthesized around the same time as well, including thiazoles, pyridines, oxadiazoles, indoles, and triazoles. The isoxazole androisoxazol was found to be the most potent of this group, and most closely resembled stanozolol in its pharmacological properties.

Given its favorably low androgenic profile, androisoxazol was used clinically in a number of androgen sensitive patient populations including women, children, and the elderly.[646][647] Although human studies on the drug are not extensive, it appears to have been used with success and safety in these populations. In spite of this fact, however, it was ultimately short lived as a commercial product. Serono would discontinue sale of the agent less than a decade after introducing it in Italy, long before there was great controversy surrounding the use of anabolic steroids in sports. Androisoxazol was rarely studied outside of this region, although isolated other products containing the drug (such as the brand Androxan) did exist for a short time. Today, all forms of this agent have been out of commerce for so long that few people have any knowledge of it.

How Supplied:

Androisoxazol is no longer available as a prescription agent. When manufactured, it came in the form of an oral tablet.

Structural Characteristics:

Androisoxazol is a modified form of dihydrotestosterone. It differs by: 1) the addition of a methyl group at carbon 17-alpha to protect the hormone during oral administration and 2) the attachment of an isoxazole group to the A-ring, replacing the normal 3-keto group, which increases anabolic strength while reducing relative androgenicity.

Side Effects (Estrogenic):

Androisoxazol is not aromatized by the body, and is not measurably estrogenic. An anti-estrogen is not necessary when using this steroid, as gynecomastia should not be a concern even among sensitive individuals. Since estrogen is the usual culprit with water retention, this steroid instead produces a lean, quality look to the physique with no fear of excess subcutaneous fluid retention.

Side Effects (Androgenic):

Although classified as an anabolic steroid, androgenic side effects are still possible with this substance. This may include bouts of oily skin, acne, and body/facial hair growth. Anabolic/androgenic steroids may also aggravate male pattern hair loss. Women are also warned of the potential virilizing effects of anabolic/androgenic steroids. These may include a deepening of the voice, menstrual irregularities, changes in skin texture, facial hair growth, and clitoral enlargement. Additionally, the 5-alpha reductase enzyme does not metabolize androisoxazol, so its relative androgenicity is not affected by finasteride or dutasteride. This is a steroid with relatively low androgenic activity in relation to its tissue-building actions, making the threshold for strong androgenic side effects comparably higher than more androgenic agents such as testosterone, methandrostenolone, or fluoxymesterone.

Side Effects (Hepatotoxicity):

Androisoxazol is a c17-alpha alkylated compound. This alteration protects the drug from deactivation by the liver, allowing a very high percentage of the drug entry into the bloodstream following oral administration. C17-alpha alkylated anabolic/androgenic steroids can be hepatotoxic. Prolonged or high exposure may result in liver damage. In rare instances life-threatening dysfunction may develop. It is advisable to visit a physician periodically during each cycle to monitor liver function and overall health. Intake of c17-alpha alkylated steroids is commonly limited to 6-8 weeks, in an effort to avoid escalating liver strain.

The use of a liver detoxification supplement such as Liver Stabil, Liv-52, or Essentiale Forte is advised while taking any hepatotoxic anabolic/androgenic steroids.

Side Effects (Cardiovascular):

Anabolic/androgenic steroids can have deleterious effects on serum cholesterol. This includes a tendency to reduce HDL (good) cholesterol values and increase LDL (bad) cholesterol values, which may shift the HDL to LDL balance in a direction that favors greater risk of arteriosclerosis. The relative impact of an anabolic/androgenic steroid on serum lipids is dependant on the dose, route of administration (oral vs. injectable), type of steroid (aromatizable or non-aromatizable), and level of resistance to hepatic metabolism. Androisoxazol has a strong effect on the hepatic management of cholesterol due to its structural resistance to liver breakdown, non-aromatizable nature, and route of administration. Anabolic/androgenic steroids may also adversely affect blood pressure and triglycerides, reduce endothelial relaxation, and support left ventricular hypertrophy, all potentially increasing the risk of cardiovascular disease and myocardial infarction.

To help reduce cardiovascular strain it is advised to maintain an active cardiovascular exercise program and minimize the intake of saturated fats, cholesterol, and simple carbohydrates at all times during active AAS administration. Supplementing with fish oils (4 grams per day) and a natural cholesterol/antioxidant formula such as Lipid Stabil or a product with comparable ingredients is also recommended.

Side Effects (Testosterone Suppression):

All anabolic/androgenic steroids when taken in doses sufficient to promote muscle gain are expected to suppress endogenous testosterone production. Without the intervention of testosterone stimulating substances, testosterone levels should return to normal within 1-4 months of drug secession. Note that prolonged hypogonadotrophic hypogonadism can develop secondary to steroid abuse, necessitating medical intervention.

The above side effects are not inclusive. For more detailed discussion of potential side effects, see the Steroid Side Effects section of this book.

Administration (General):

Studies have shown that taking an oral anabolic steroid with food may decrease its bioavailability.[648] This is caused by the fat-soluble nature of steroid hormones, which can allow some of the drug to dissolve with undigested dietary fat, reducing its absorption from the gastrointestinal tract. For maximum utilization, this steroid should be taken on an empty stomach.

Administration (Men):

Androisoxazol was used in a clinical dose of .2mg per kg of bodyweight per day (.2mg/kg/d). This would equate to a daily dose of approximately 15 mg for a 175-pound male. It was taken for a maximum period of 60 consecutive days. An effective dosage for physique- or performance-enhancing purposes falls between 15 mg and 40 mg per day. The drug would be taken for no longer than 6-8 weeks to minimize potential hepatic stress. This level is sufficient for solid gains in lean muscle tissue, which may be accompanied by increased hardness and definition.

Administration (Women):

Androisoxazol was used in a clinical dose of .2mg per kg of bodyweight per day (.2mg/kg/d). This would equate to a daily dose of approximately 10 mg for a 120–pound female. In an effort to reduce the chance for virilization, it was recommended to take the drug only for 20 consecutive days, followed by a break of 10 days before resuming drug therapy. A total of no more than three 20-day cycles were recommended. An effective daily dosage for physique- or performance-enhancing purposes falls between 5-10 mg per day. The drug would be taken for no longer than 6-8 weeks to minimize potential hepatic stress. This level is sufficient for solid gains in lean muscle tissue, which may be accompanied by increased hardness and definition. Although this compound is mildly androgenic, the risk of virilization symptoms cannot be excluded.

Availability:

Androisoxazol is no longer produced as a prescription drug product, and is unavailable on the black market.

Neodrol (dihydrotestosterone)

Androgenic	30-260
Anabolic	60-220
Standard	Testosterone, Testosterone Propionate
Chemical Names	5-alpha-androstan-3-one-17beta-ol 5-alpha-androstanolone stanolone
Estrogenic Activity	none
Progestational Activity	none

Dihydrotestosterone

Description:

Neodrol is a prescription steroid preparation (no longer in production) that contains the potent androgenic steroid dihydrotestosterone. Dihydrotestosterone itself is the most active androgen in the human body, displaying an ability to bind and activate the androgen receptor at least three or four times greater than that of its parent steroid testosterone. This trait, however, is not accompanied by equally powerful anabolic tendencies. In the case of dihydrotestosterone, we have a steroid that is almost purely androgenic, with only minimal muscle-building (anabolic) action. Dihydrotestosterone may have very effective uses in areas such as fat loss, hardening, increasing CNS activity, and pure strength gains, but this steroid does not perform well as an anabolic agent, and is not generally used as such among athletes.

History:

Dihydrotestosterone was first synthesized in 1935.[649] Pfizer developed this strong androgenic steroid into an injectable medication during the mid-1950's, sold on the U.S. prescription drug market under the trade name Neodrol. This preparation contained a simple saline solution with dihydrotestosterone (50 mg/ml) in a 10 mL multi-dose vial. The product literature describes the steroid as a new androgen for the treatment of certain cases of inoperable breast cancer in females, or postoperative cases of carcinoma of the breast with metastases. It is also described as a drug effective for promoting protein anabolism in select patients. Given the unesterified nature of the drug, it was to be injected at least three times per week, although it was often required on a daily basis.

Other dihydrotestosterone preparations had also been produced over the years in other markets. Such popular brands included Pesomax (Italy), Anabolex (England, Italy), Anaboleen (England, Switzerland), and Androlone (Italy). Injectable dihydrotestosterone suspensions were ultimately short lived as prescription drug products, made effectively obsolete by newer and more effective anabolic/androgenic steroids that dominated many areas of medicine during the 1960's. Dihydrotestosterone has not disappeared completely from clinical medicine, however, and today remains available, albeit scarcely. It is currently in extremely limited use globally, mainly produced in Europe as a transdermal product for the treatment of gynecomastia and insufficient androgen levels (Andractim).

How Supplied:

Dihydrotestosterone suspension is no longer available. When produced as Neodrol, it contained 50 mg/ml of dihydrotestosterone in saline solution, in a 10 mL multi-dose vial.

Structural Characteristics:

Neodrol contained dihydrotestosterone, a primary androgenic steroid.

Side Effects (Estrogenic):

Dihydrotestosterone is not aromatized by the body, and is not measurably estrogenic. An anti-estrogen is not necessary when using this steroid, as gynecomastia and water retention should not be concerns even among sensitive individuals. DHT also has inherent anti-estrogenic properties, competing with other substrates for binding to the aromatase enzyme. Dihydrotestosterone may be an effective option for the treatment of gynecomastia. Studies have reported a good level of success when treating certain forms of this disorder with Andractim (transdermal dihydrotestosterone), the drug affecting the ratio of androgenic to estrogenic action in the breast area enough that a notable regression of mammary tissue has been achieved in many cases.[650][651]

Side Effects (Androgenic):

Dihydrotestosterone is the strongest natural male

androgen. Higher than normal therapeutic doses are likely to produce androgenic side effects including oily skin, acne, and body/facial hair growth. Men with a genetic predisposition for hair loss (androgenetic alopecia) may notice accelerated male pattern balding. Women are warned of the potential virilizing effects of anabolic/androgenic steroids, especially with a strong androgen such as dihydrotestosterone. These may include deepening of the voice, menstrual irregularities, changes in skin texture, facial hair growth, and clitoral enlargement. Note that the 5-alpha reductase enzyme does not metabolize dihydrotestosterone, so its relative androgenicity is not affected by finasteride or dutasteride.

Side Effects (Hepatotoxicity):

Dihydrotestosterone does not have hepatotoxic effects; liver toxicity is unlikely.

Side Effects (Cardiovascular):

Anabolic/androgenic steroids can have deleterious effects on serum cholesterol. This includes a tendency to reduce HDL (good) cholesterol values and increase LDL (bad) cholesterol values, which may shift the HDL to LDL balance in a direction that favors greater risk of arteriosclerosis. The relative impact of an anabolic/androgenic steroid on serum lipids is dependant on the dose, route of administration (oral vs. injectable), type of steroid (aromatizable or non-aromatizable), and level of resistance to hepatic metabolism. Anabolic/androgenic steroids may also adversely affect blood pressure and triglycerides, reduce endothelial relaxation, and support left ventricular hypertrophy, all potentially increasing the risk of cardiovascular disease and myocardial infarction. Therapeutic doses of dihydrotestosterone used to correct insufficient androgen production in otherwise healthy aging men are unlikely to increase atherogenic risk. Higher doses are likely to increase atherogenic risk, but less dramatically than equivalent doses of synthetic oral anabolic/androgenic steroids.

To help reduce cardiovascular strain it is advised to maintain an active cardiovascular exercise program and minimize the intake of saturated fats, cholesterol, and simple carbohydrates at all times during active AAS administration. Supplementing with fish oils (4 grams per day) and a natural cholesterol/antioxidant formula such as Lipid Stabil or a product with comparable ingredients is also recommended.

Side Effects (Testosterone Suppression):

All anabolic/androgenic steroids when taken in doses sufficient to promote muscle gain are expected to suppress endogenous testosterone production. Without the intervention of testosterone stimulating substances, testosterone levels should return to normal within 1-4 months of drug secession. Note that prolonged hypogonadotrophic hypogonadism can develop secondary to steroid abuse, necessitating medical intervention.

The above side effects are not inclusive. For more detailed discussion of potential side effects, see the Steroid Side Effects section of this book.

Administration (Men):

Early prescribing information for Neodrol recommended an injection of 50 mg given three to seven times per week, for the promotion of protein anabolism. For physique- or performance-enhancing purposes, similar doses are used, but generally on the higher end of the therapeutic spectrum (50 mg daily). Dihydrotestosterone is of little value for building muscle, and is most commonly applied for cutting or pure-strength-promoting purposes.

Administration (Women):

Early prescribing information for Neodrol recommended an injection of 100 mg given three to seven times per week, for the treatment of breast cancer. Dihydrotestosterone is not recommended for women for physique- or performance-enhancing purposes due to its strong androgenic nature and tendency to produce virilizing side effects.

Availability:

Dihydrotestosterone suspension (Neodrol) is no longer manufactured, and is presently unavailable on the black market.

Neotest 250 (testosterone decanoate)

Androgenic	100
Anabolic	100
Standard	Standard
Chemical Names	4-androsten-3-one-17beta-ol
	17beta-hydroxy-androst-4-en-3-one
Estrogenic Activity	moderate
Progestational Activity	low

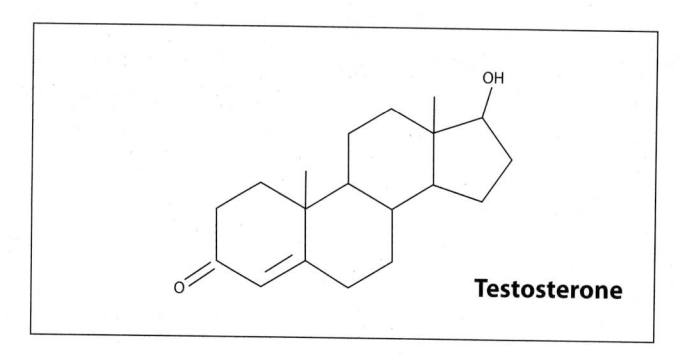

Testosterone

Description:

Testosterone decanoate is a slow-acting injectable form of the primary male androgen testosterone. This steroid is mostly commonly identified as part of the four-ester blend in Sustanon® 250, but here is described as a standalone agent. The long decanoate ester used to make testosterone decanoate creates a drug with pharmacokinetic properties similar to nandrolone decanoate, providing a sustained release of hormone (in this case testosterone) for approximately three weeks following injection. Testosterone decanoate is slightly slower-acting than the commercially available esters cypionate and enanthate, and could provide a slightly less frequent injection schedule in comparison.

History:

Testosterone decanoate was developed decades ago, and offers favorable pharmacokinetics of testosterone release (arguably more balanced than Sustanon® 250). In spite of this, testosterone decanoate was never a commercial success as a single-agent steroid product. The only modern preparation to contain this testosterone ester exclusively has been Neotest 250, a veterinary steroid produced by Loeffler in Mexico. This drug was favored by a small audience of loyal consumers because it offered less frequent injections than testosterone enanthate, and more user comfort than Sustanon® 250 (notorious for pain and soreness at the injection site). Neotest was only sold on the Mexican veterinary market for a short while, however. Political pressures against steroid sales and a U.S. indictment of the company (Operation Gear Grinder) have apparently resulted in Loeffler eliminating Neotest from their product line, as well as many other "controversial" products. No other commercial product using testosterone decanoate as the only active agent is known to exist at this time.

How Supplied:

Testosterone decanoate is no longer available as a standalone commercial drug product. When produced, the Neotest 250 brand contained 250 mg/ml of testosterone decanoate in oil, packaged in a 10 mL multi-dose vial.

Structural Characteristics:

Testosterone decanoate is a modified form of testosterone, where a carboxylic acid ester (decanoic acid) has been attached to the 17-beta hydroxyl group. Esterified forms of testosterone are less polar than free testosterone, and are absorbed more slowly from the area of injection. Once in the bloodstream, the ester is removed to yield free (active) testosterone. Esterified forms of testosterone are designed to prolong the window of therapeutic effect following administration, allowing for a less frequent injection schedule compared to injections of free (unesterified) steroid.

Side Effects (Estrogenic):

Testosterone is readily aromatized in the body to estradiol (estrogen). The aromatase (estrogen synthetase) enzyme is responsible for this metabolism of testosterone. Elevated estrogen levels can cause side effects such as increased water retention, body fat gain, and gynecomastia. Testosterone is considered a moderately estrogenic steroid. An anti-estrogen such as clomiphene citrate or tamoxifen citrate may be necessary to prevent estrogenic side effects. One may alternately use an aromatase inhibitor like Arimidex® (anastrozole), which more efficiently controls estrogen by preventing its synthesis. Aromatase inhibitors can be quite expensive in comparison to anti-estrogens, however, and may also have negative effects on blood lipids.

Estrogenic side effects will occur in a dose-dependant manner, with higher doses (above normal therapeutic levels) of testosterone more likely to require the concurrent use of an anti-estrogen or aromatase inhibitor. Since water retention and loss of muscle definition are common with higher doses of testosterone, this drug is usually considered a poor choice for dieting or cutting phases of training. Its moderate estrogenicity makes it more ideal for bulking phases, where the added water retention will support raw strength and muscle size, and help foster a stronger anabolic environment.

Side Effects (Androgenic):

Testosterone is the primary male androgen, responsible for maintaining secondary male sexual characteristics. Elevated levels of testosterone are likely to produce androgenic side effects including oily skin, acne, and body/facial hair growth. Men with a genetic predisposition for hair loss (androgenetic alopecia) may notice accelerated male pattern balding. Those concerned about hair loss may find a more comfortable option in nandrolone decanoate, which is a comparably less androgenic steroid. Women are warned of the potential virilizing effects of anabolic/androgenic steroids, especially with a strong androgen such as testosterone. These may include a deepening of the voice, menstrual irregularities, changes in skin texture, facial hair growth, and clitoral enlargement.

In androgen-responsive target tissues such as the skin, scalp, and prostate, the high relative androgenicity of testosterone is dependant on its reduction to dihydrotestosterone (DHT). The 5-alpha reductase enzyme is responsible for this metabolism of testosterone. The concurrent use of a 5-alpha reductase inhibitor such as finasteride or dutasteride will interfere with site-specific potentiation of testosterone action, lowering the tendency of testosterone drugs to produce androgenic side effects. It is important to remember that anabolic and androgenic effects are both mediated via the cytosolic androgen receptor. Complete separation of testosterone's anabolic and androgenic properties is not possible, even with total 5-alpha reductase inhibition.

Side Effects (Hepatotoxicity):

Testosterone does not have hepatotoxic effects; liver toxicity is unlikely. One study examined the potential for hepatotoxicity with high doses of testosterone by administering 400 mg of the hormone per day (2,800 mg per week) to a group of male subjects. The steroid was taken orally so that higher peak concentrations would be reached in hepatic tissues compared to intramuscular injections. The hormone was given daily for 20 days, and produced no significant changes in liver enzyme values including serum albumin, bilirubin, alanine-amino-transferase, and alkaline phosphatases.[652]

Side Effects (Cardiovascular):

Anabolic/androgenic steroids can have deleterious effects on serum cholesterol. This includes a tendency to reduce HDL (good) cholesterol values and increase LDL (bad) cholesterol values, which may shift the HDL to LDL balance in a direction that favors greater risk of arteriosclerosis. The relative impact of an anabolic/androgenic steroid on serum lipids is dependant on the dose, route of administration (oral vs. injectable), type of steroid (aromatizable or non-aromatizable), and level of resistance to hepatic metabolism. Anabolic/androgenic steroids may also adversely affect blood pressure and triglycerides, reduce endothelial relaxation, and support left ventricular hypertrophy, all potentially increasing the risk of cardiovascular disease and myocardial infarction.

Testosterone tends to have a much less dramatic impact on cardiovascular risk factors than synthetic steroids. This is due in part to its openness to metabolism by the liver, which allows it to have less effect on the hepatic management of cholesterol. The aromatization of testosterone to estradiol also helps to mitigate the negative effects of androgens on serum lipids. In one study, 280 mg per week of testosterone ester (enanthate) had a slight but not statistically significant effect on HDL cholesterol after 12 weeks, but when taken with an aromatase inhibitor a strong (25%) decrease was seen.[653] Studies using 300 mg of testosterone ester (enanthate) per week for twenty weeks without an aromatase inhibitor demonstrated only a 13% decrease in HDL cholesterol, while at 600 mg the reduction reached 21%.[654] The negative impact of aromatase inhibition should be taken into consideration before such drug is added to testosterone therapy.

Due to the positive influence of estrogen on serum lipids, tamoxifen citrate or clomiphene citrate are preferred to aromatase inhibitors for those concerned with cardiovascular health, as they offer a partial estrogenic effect in the liver. This allows them to potentially improve lipid profiles and offset some of the negative effects of androgens. With doses of 600 mg or less per week, the impact on lipid profile tends to be noticeable but not dramatic, making an anti-estrogen (for cardioprotective purposes) perhaps unnecessary. Doses of 600 mg or less per week have also failed to produce statistically significant changes in LDL/VLDL cholesterol, triglycerides, apolipoprotein B/C-III, C-reactive protein, and insulin sensitivity, all indicating a relatively weak impact on cardiovascular risk factors.[655] When used in moderate doses, injectable testosterone esters are usually considered to be the safest of all anabolic/androgenic steroids.

To help reduce cardiovascular strain it is advised to maintain an active cardiovascular exercise program and minimize the intake of saturated fats, cholesterol, and simple carbohydrates at all times during active AAS administration. Supplementing with fish oils (4 grams per day) and a natural cholesterol/antioxidant formula such as Lipid Stabil or a product with comparable ingredients is also recommended.

Side Effects (Testosterone Suppression):

All anabolic/androgenic steroids when taken in doses sufficient to promote muscle gain are expected to suppress endogenous testosterone production. Testosterone is the primary male androgen, and offers strong negative feedback on endogenous testosterone production. Testosterone-based drugs will, likewise, have a strong effect on the hypothalamic regulation of natural steroid hormones. Without the intervention of testosterone stimulating substances, testosterone levels should return to normal within 1-4 months of drug secession. Note that prolonged hypogonadotrophic hypogonadism can develop secondary to steroid abuse, necessitating medical intervention.

The above side effects are not inclusive. For more detailed discussion of potential side effects, see the Steroid Side Effects section of this book.

Administration (Men):

Although active in the body for longer, testosterone decanoate is usually injected once every 7 to 10 days for bodybuilding purposes. The total weekly dosage is typically 200-600 mg, which is sufficient to provide excellent gains in muscle size and strength. Testosterone drugs are ultimately very versatile, and can be combined with many other anabolic/androgenic steroids depending on the desired effect.

Administration (Women):

Testosterone decanoate is not recommended for women for physique- or performance-enhancing purposes due to its strong androgenic nature, tendency to produce virilizing side effects, and slow-acting characteristics (making blood levels difficult to control).

Availability:

Neotest 250 is no longer available. No other testosterone decanoate product is known to be in circulation.

Nilevar® (norethandrolone)

Androgenic	22-55
Anabolic	100-200
Standard	Methyltestosterone (oral)
Chemical Names	17alpha-Ethyl-17beta-hydroxyestr-4-en-3-one
	17a-ethyl-19-nortestosterone
Estrogenic Activity	high
Progestational Activity	high

Norethandrolone

Description:

Norethandrolone is an anabolic steroid closely related to nortestosterone (nandrolone) in structure. The activity of this steroid is that of a mild to moderate oral anabolic steroid, which is accompanied by distinguishable androgenic and estrogenic components. Although this steroid is essentially nandrolone modified (alkylated) to make oral dosing viable, it cannot be looked at simply as an oral alternative to Deca-Durabolin®. Most notably, the greatly increased estrogenicity caused by 17-alkylation makes norethandrolone much more problematic when trying to build quality (lean) muscle mass. In administering an effective amount of steroid in terms of muscle growth, the user has to deal with much more in terms of estrogenic side effects. The muscle accumulation with norethandrolone is also going to be accompanied by a high level of water and (likely) fat retention, not the quality muscularity normally associated with nandrolone decanoate.

History:

Norethandrolone was first described in 1954.[656] It was developed into a medicine by Searle, which introduced it into the U.S. prescription drug market under the Nilevar brand name during the late 1950's. The drug was originally sold as an oral tablet, an oral solution (with dropper bottle), and an injectable solution (in 25 mg ampules). The latter form of norethandrolone has been out of commerce for so long that few remember it was once also given by injection. Nilevar was prescribed for a variety of illnesses that were benefited by a protein sparing anabolic agent, Listed indications included preparation for and recovery from surgery, severe or prolonged illness, anorexia nervosa, severe burns and trauma, decubitus ulcers, osteoporosis, bone fracture healing, gastrointestinal disease, prolonged corticosteroid administration, and various forms of malnourishment in adults and children.

Norethandrolone ultimately saw only limited success as a prescription anabolic agent. It did make its way to Europe and certain other markets, but not widely. The drug was an early functional anabolic, displaying more tissue-building properties than androgenic effects. But it also remained an agent with a troubling estrogenic side. This eventually led to norethandrolone being passed over clinically for more refined compounds as they became available. Searle decided to discontinue the sale of Nilevar in the U.S. during the 1960's, and instead began focusing energies on its newer, more strongly anabolic, and non-estrogenic steroid oxandrolone (sold as Anavar). Most other markets carrying norethandrolone, either by Searle or other companies, soon began losing this compound as well. Today, this drug is available on a limited basis, most notably in Australia where it remains viable on the veterinary drug market.

How Supplied:

Norethandrolone is available in select veterinary drug markets. Composition and dosage may vary by country and manufacturer, but typically contain 5 or 10 mg of steroid per tablet.

Structural Characteristics:

Norethandrolone is a modified form of nandrolone. It differs by the addition of an ethyl group at carbon 17-alpha to protect the hormone during oral administration.

Side Effects (Estrogenic):

Norethandrolone is aromatized by the body, and converts to a synthetic estrogen with a high level of biological activity (17alpha-ethyl-estradiol). As a result, it is a highly estrogenic steroid. Gynecomastia is often a concern during treatment, and may present itself quite early into a cycle (particularly when higher doses are used). At the same time water retention can become a problem, causing a notable loss of muscle definition as both subcutaneous water retention and fat levels build. Sensitive individuals may want to keep the estrogen under control with the addition of an anti-estrogen such as Nolvadex®. One may alternately use an aromatase inhibitor like Arimidex® (anastrozole), which is a more effective remedy for estrogen control. Aromatase inhibitors, however, can be quite expensive in comparison to standard estrogen maintenance therapies, and may also have negative effects on blood lipids.

It is of note that norethandrolone has some additional activity as a progestin in the body.[657] The side effects associated with progesterone are similar to those of estrogen, including negative feedback inhibition of testosterone production and enhanced rate of fat storage. Progestins also augment the stimulatory effect of estrogens on mammary tissue growth. There appears to be a strong synergy between these two hormones here, such that gynecomastia might even occur with the help of progestins without excessive estrogen levels being present. The use of an anti-estrogen, which inhibits the estrogenic component of this disorder, is often sufficient to mitigate gynecomastia caused by norethandrolone.

Side Effects (Androgenic):

Although classified as an anabolic steroid, androgenic side effects are still common with this substance. This may include bouts of oily skin, acne, and body/facial hair growth. Anabolic/androgenic steroids may also aggravate male pattern hair loss. Individuals sensitive to the androgenic effects of this steroid may find a milder anabolic such as Deca-Durabolin® to be more comfortable. Women are additionally warned of the potential virilizing effects of anabolic/androgenic steroids. These may include a deepening of the voice, menstrual irregularities, changes in skin texture, facial hair growth, and clitoral enlargement.

Note that in androgen-responsive target tissues such as the skin, scalp, and prostate, the relative androgenicity of norethandrolone is reduced by its reduction to dihydronorethandrolone. The 5-alpha reductase enzyme is responsible for this metabolism. The concurrent use of a 5-alpha reductase inhibitor such as finasteride or dutasteride will interfere with site-specific reduction of norethandrolone action, considerably increasing the tendency of the drug to produce androgenic side effects. Reductase inhibitors should be avoided with this steroid if maintaining low relative androgenicity is desired.

Side Effects (Hepatotoxicity):

Norethandrolone is a c17-alpha alkylated compound. This alteration protects the drug from deactivation by the liver, allowing a very high percentage of the drug entry into the bloodstream following oral administration. C17-alpha alkylated anabolic/androgenic steroids can be hepatotoxic. Prolonged or high exposure may result in liver damage. In rare instances life-threatening dysfunction may develop. It is advisable to visit a physician periodically during each cycle to monitor liver function and overall health. Intake of c17-alpha alkylated steroids is commonly limited to 6-8 weeks, in an effort to avoid escalating liver strain. Severe liver complications are rare given the periodic nature in which most people use oral anabolic/androgenic steroids, although cannot be excluded with this steroid, especially with high doses and/or prolonged administration periods.

The use of a liver detoxification supplement such as Liver Stabil, Liv-52, or Essentiale Forte is advised while taking any hepatotoxic anabolic/androgenic steroids.

Side Effects (Cardiovascular):

Anabolic/androgenic steroids can have deleterious effects on serum cholesterol. This includes a tendency to reduce HDL (good) cholesterol values and increase LDL (bad) cholesterol values, which may shift the HDL to LDL balance in a direction that favors greater risk of arteriosclerosis. The relative impact of an anabolic/androgenic steroid on serum lipids is dependant on the dose, route of administration (oral vs. injectable), type of steroid (aromatizable or non-aromatizable), and level of resistance to hepatic metabolism. Norethandrolone has a strong effect on the hepatic management of cholesterol due to its structural resistance to liver breakdown and route of administration. Anabolic/androgenic steroids may also adversely affect blood pressure and triglycerides, reduce endothelial relaxation, and support left ventricular hypertrophy, all potentially increasing the risk of cardiovascular disease and myocardial infarction.

To help reduce cardiovascular strain it is advised to maintain an active cardiovascular exercise program and minimize the intake of saturated fats, cholesterol, and simple carbohydrates at all times during active AAS administration. Supplementing with fish oils (4 grams per day) and a natural cholesterol/antioxidant formula such as Lipid Stabil or a product with comparable ingredients is also recommended.

Side Effects (Testosterone Suppression):

All anabolic/androgenic steroids when taken in doses sufficient to promote muscle gain are expected to suppress endogenous testosterone production. Without the intervention of testosterone stimulating substances, testosterone levels should return to normal within 1-4 months of drug secession. Note that prolonged hypogonadotrophic hypogonadism can develop secondary to steroid abuse, necessitating medical intervention.

The above side effects are not inclusive. For more detailed discussion of potential side effects, see the Steroid Side Effects section of this book.

Administration (General):

Studies have shown that taking an oral anabolic steroid with food may decrease its bioavailability.[658] This is caused by the fat-soluble nature of steroid hormones, which can allow some of the drug to dissolve with undigested dietary fat, reducing its absorption from the gastrointestinal tract. For maximum utilization, this steroid should be taken on an empty stomach.

Administration (Men):

The original prescribing guidelines for Nilevar called for a daily dosage of 20 to 30 mg. This was to be administered on an intermittent basis, with the drug taken for no more than 12 consecutive weeks. Thereafter, a break of at least 1 month was advised before therapy was resumed. When used for physique- or performance-enhancing purposes, the drug is also used intermittently, with cycles usually lasting between 6 and 8 weeks in length followed by 6-8 weeks off. A daily dosage of 20 to 40 mg is most common for such applications. This level is typically sufficient for rapid gains in strength and muscle mass (bulk). The high estrogenicity makes norethandrolone of little value in speed and endurance sports, causing an unwanted retention of water weight. When given by injection, the same milligram dosage is recommended as when the drug is given orally.

Administration (Women):

The original prescribing guidelines for Nilevar made no special dosing recommendations for women, although it did warn that androgenicity is likely on a high dosage. When used by women for physique- or performance-enhancing purposes, a daily dosage of 5-10 mg is most common, taken for no longer than 4 weeks. This level is quite effective for promoting new muscle growth. Note that virilizing side effects are still sometimes noticed at lower doses, and need to be carefully examined for.

Availability:

This steroid is still produced in select markets, but is rarely diverted for black market sale.

William Llewellyn's ANABOLICS, 9th ed.

Omnadren® 250 (testosterone blend)

Androgenic	100
Anabolic	100
Standard	Standard

Chemical Names	4-androsten-3-one-17beta-ol
	17beta-hydroxy-androst-4-en-3-one
Estrogenic Activity	moderate
Progestational Activity	low

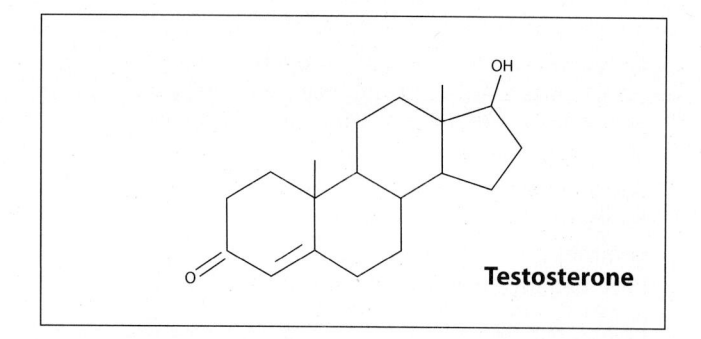

Testosterone

Description:

Omnadren® 250 (in its original formulation), was an oil-based injectable testosterone blend that contained four different testosterone esters: testosterone propionate (30 mg); testosterone phenylpropionate (60 mg); testosterone isocaproate (60 mg); and testosterone caproate (100 mg). Being a four-component testosterone blend, this preparation was most commonly compared to Sustanon® 250. While it did contain testosterone propionate, phenylpropionate, and isocaproate in the same strengths as Sustanon®, the last ester is different. It was a slightly shorter-acting drug, making Omnadren® more analogous to Testoviron® (the caproate ester is one carbon shorter than enanthate) than Sustanon® 250. Please note that there were even older versions of Omnadren® listing isohexanoate and hexanoate as the final two ingredients, which are simply different words for isocaproate and caproate.

History:

Omnadren® 250 was developed in Poland by Polfa during the years of Soviet control. Its formulation (original) is very similar to that of Sustanon® 250, barring the substitution of one of the component esters. This was likely done to avoid patent issues with the international pharmaceutical giant Organon, which exclusively controlled the global supply of Sustanon® 250. In clinical medicine, Omnadren® 250 was used most commonly to treat adult men suffering from low androgen levels, usually noticing symptoms of impotence or hormonal disturbance of spermatogenesis. This drug was also used on occasion to treat adolescents with delayed puberty, and women with advanced breast or endometrial cancer.

The manufacture of Omnadren® 250 under the Polfa label was discontinued in 1994. That year, the newly privatized Polfa firm was renamed Jelfa, mainly to distinguish itself from other firms that use a Polfa prefix as part of their names. Jelfa continued to produce Omnadren® 250 for the domestic market, which remained available without interruption in the same familiar 5-pack of ampules (albeit with a new company label and logo) for years after. Today, Jelfa continues to market Omnadren® 250 in Poland, as well as in many neighboring markets including Russia, Ukraine, Kazakhstan, Uzbekistan, Kurdistan, Kyrgyzstan, Armenia, Moldavia, Latvia, Lithuania, Azerbaijan, Georgia, and Belarus, however the formulation has recently changed. All Omnadren 250 sold today carries the same exact formulation as Sustanon 250. This profile refers to the original formulation only, which is now unavailable worldwide.

How Supplied:

Omnadren® 250 (original formulation) in no longer available. When manufactured, it was supplied in 1 mL glass ampules containing an oily solution; sold in boxes of 5 ampules.

Structural Characteristics:

Omnadren® 250 contains a mixture of four testosterone compounds, which where modified with the addition of carboxylic acid esters (propionic, propionic phenyl ester, isocaproic, and caproic acids) at the 17-beta hydroxyl group. Esterified forms of testosterone are less polar than free testosterone, and are absorbed more slowly from the area of injection. Once in the bloodstream, the ester is removed to yield free (active) testosterone. Esterified forms of testosterone are designed to prolong the window of therapeutic effect following administration, allowing for a less frequent injection schedule compared to injections of free (unesterified) steroid. Omnadren® 250 is designed to provide a rapid peak in testosterone levels (24-48 hours after injection), and maintain physiological concentrations for approximately 14 days.

Side Effects (Estrogenic):

Testosterone is readily aromatized in the body to estradiol

(estrogen). The aromatase (estrogen synthetase) enzyme is responsible for this metabolism of testosterone. Elevated estrogen levels can cause side effects such as increased water retention, body fat gain, and gynecomastia. Testosterone is considered a moderately estrogenic steroid. An anti-estrogen such as clomiphene citrate or tamoxifen citrate may be necessary to prevent estrogenic side effects. One may alternately use an aromatase inhibitor like Arimidex® (anastrozole), which more efficiently controls estrogen by preventing its synthesis. Aromatase inhibitors can be quite expensive in comparison to anti-estrogens, however, and may also have negative effects on blood lipids.

Estrogenic side effects will occur in a dose-dependant manner, with higher doses (above normal therapeutic levels) of testosterone more likely to require the concurrent use of an anti-estrogen or aromatase inhibitor. Since water retention and loss of muscle definition are common with higher doses of testosterone, this drug is usually considered a poor choice for dieting or cutting phases of training. Its moderate estrogenicity makes it more ideal for bulking phases, where the added water retention will support raw strength and muscle size, and help foster a stronger anabolic environment.

Side Effects (Androgenic):

Testosterone is the primary male androgen, responsible for maintaining secondary male sexual characteristics. Elevated levels of testosterone are likely to produce androgenic side effects including oily skin, acne, and body/facial hair growth. Men with a genetic predisposition for hair loss (androgenetic alopecia) may notice accelerated male pattern balding. Those concerned about hair loss may find a more comfortable option in nandrolone decanoate, which is a comparably less androgenic steroid. Women are warned of the potential virilizing effects of anabolic/androgenic steroids, especially with a strong androgen such as testosterone. These may include deepening of the voice, menstrual irregularities, changes in skin texture, facial hair growth, and clitoral enlargement.

In androgen-responsive target tissues such as the skin, scalp, and prostate, the high relative androgenicity of testosterone is dependant on its reduction to dihydrotestosterone (DHT). The 5-alpha reductase enzyme is responsible for this metabolism of testosterone. The concurrent use of a 5-alpha reductase inhibitor such as finasteride or dutasteride will interfere with site-specific potentiation of testosterone action, lowering the tendency of testosterone drugs to produce androgenic side effects. It is important to remember that anabolic and androgenic effects are both mediated via the cytosolic androgen receptor. Complete separation of testosterone's anabolic and androgenic properties is not possible, even with total 5-alpha reductase inhibition.

Side Effects (Hepatotoxicity):

Testosterone does not have hepatotoxic effects; liver toxicity is unlikely. One study examined the potential for hepatotoxicity with high doses of testosterone by administering 400 mg of the hormone per day (2,800 mg per week) to a group of male subjects. The steroid was taken orally so that higher peak concentrations would be reached in hepatic tissues compared to intramuscular injections. The hormone was given daily for 20 days, and produced no significant changes in liver enzyme values including serum albumin, bilirubin, alanine-amino-transferase, and alkaline phosphatases.[659]

Side Effects (Cardiovascular):

Anabolic/androgenic steroids can have deleterious effects on serum cholesterol. This includes a tendency to reduce HDL (good) cholesterol values and increase LDL (bad) cholesterol values, which may shift the HDL to LDL balance in a direction that favors greater risk of arteriosclerosis. The relative impact of an anabolic/androgenic steroid on serum lipids is dependant on the dose, route of administration (oral vs. injectable), type of steroid (aromatizable or non-aromatizable), and level of resistance to hepatic metabolism. Anabolic/androgenic steroids may also adversely affect blood pressure and triglycerides, reduce endothelial relaxation, and support left ventricular hypertrophy, all potentially increasing the risk of cardiovascular disease and myocardial infarction.

Testosterone tends to have a much less dramatic impact on cardiovascular risk factors than synthetic steroids. This is due in part to its openness to metabolism by the liver, which allows it to have less effect on the hepatic management of cholesterol. The aromatization of testosterone to estradiol also helps to mitigate the negative effects of androgens on serum lipids. In one study, 280 mg per week of testosterone ester (enanthate) had a slight but not statistically significant effect on HDL cholesterol after 12 weeks, but when taken with an aromatase inhibitor a strong (25%) decrease was seen.[660] Studies using 300 mg of testosterone ester (enanthate) per week for 20 weeks without an aromatase inhibitor demonstrated only a 13% decrease in HDL cholesterol, while at 600 mg the reduction reached 21%.[661] The negative impact of aromatase inhibition should be taken into consideration before such drug is added to testosterone therapy.

Due to the positive influence of estrogen on serum lipids, tamoxifen citrate or clomiphene citrate are preferred to aromatase inhibitors for those concerned with cardiovascular health, as they offer a partial estrogenic effect in the liver. This allows them to potentially improve lipid profiles and offset some of the negative effects of androgens. With doses of 600 mg or less of testosterone per week, the impact on lipid profile tends to be noticeable but not dramatic, making an anti-estrogen (for cardioprotective purposes) perhaps unnecessary. Doses of 600 mg or less per week have also failed to produce statistically significant changes in LDL/VLDL cholesterol, triglycerides, apolipoprotein B/C-III, C-reactive protein, and insulin sensitivity, all indicating a relatively weak impact on cardiovascular risk factors.[662] When used in moderate doses, injectable testosterone esters are usually considered to be the safest of all anabolic/androgenic steroids.

To help reduce cardiovascular strain it is advised to maintain an active cardiovascular exercise program and minimize the intake of saturated fats, cholesterol, and simple carbohydrates at all times during active AAS administration. Supplementing with fish oils (4 grams per day) and a natural cholesterol/antioxidant formula such as Lipid Stabil or a product with comparable ingredients is also recommended.

Side Effects (Testosterone Suppression):

All anabolic/androgenic steroids when taken in doses sufficient to promote muscle gain are expected to suppress endogenous testosterone production. Testosterone is the primary male androgen, and offers strong negative feedback on endogenous testosterone production. Testosterone-based drugs will, likewise, have a strong effect on the hypothalamic regulation of natural steroid hormones. Without the intervention of testosterone-stimulating substances, testosterone levels should return to normal within 1-4 months of drug secession. Note that prolonged hypogonadotrophic hypogonadism can develop secondary to steroid abuse, necessitating medical intervention.

The above side effects are not inclusive. For more detailed discussion of potential side effects, see the Steroid Side Effects section of this book.

Administration (General):

Testosterone propionate is often regarded as a painful injection. This is due to the very short carbon chain of the propionic acid ester, which can be irritating to tissues at the site of injection. Many sensitive individuals choose to stay away from this steroid completely, their bodies reacting with a pronounced soreness and low-grade fever that may last for a few days after each injection.

Administration (Men):

Depending on the application, the prescribing guidelines for Omnadren® 250 call for a dosage of 250 mg (1 ampule) to be injected every 3 to 4 weeks. Although active in the body for a longer time, Omnadren® 250 is usually administered on a weekly basis for muscle-building purposes. This schedule will allow for the higher doses most commonly applied by athletes, and more stable elevations in hormone level. The usual dosage among male athletes is in the range of 250-750 mg per injection, taken in cycles 6 to 12 weeks in length. This level is sufficient for most users to notice exceptional gains in muscle size and strength. Some bodybuilders have been known to use excessively high dosages of this drug (1,000 mg per week or more), although this practice is generally not advised due to the higher incidence of side effects. Testosterone is ultimately very versatile, and can be combined with many other anabolic/androgenic steroids to tailor the desired effect.

Administration (Women):

Omnadren® 250 is rarely used with women in clinical medicine. When applied, it is most often used to treat inoperable breast or endometrial cancer. Omnadren® 250 is not recommended for women for physique- or performance-enhancing purposes due to its strong androgenic nature, tendency to produce virilizing side effects, and slow- acting characteristics (making blood levels difficult to control).

Availability:

The original Omnadren 250 formulation is no longer available. Jelfa continues to use the trade name to market a steroid product, but it is now equivalent in makeup to Sustanon 250. See the Sustanon 250 profile for more information.

Orabolin® (ethylestrenol)

Androgenic	20-400
Anabolic	200-400
Standard	Methyltestosterone (oral)
Chemical Names	19-Nor-17alpha-pregn-4-en-17b-ol
	17alpha-ethly-estr-4-en-17b-ol
Estrogenic Activity	low
Progestational Activity	high

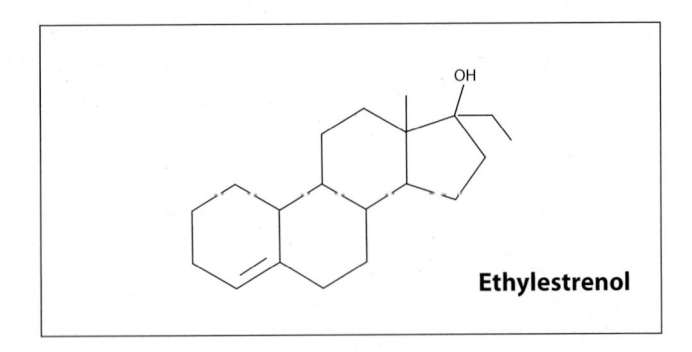

Ethylestrenol

Description:

Ethylestrenol is an oral anabolic steroid derived from nandrolone. As is typical for many 19-nor steroids, this agent exhibits far greater anabolic properties than androgenic, is only weakly estrogenic, and is strongly progestational. Structurally, ethylestrenol most closely resembles Nilevar (norethandrolone). The two differ only by the absence of an oxygen atom at the c3 position of ethylestrenol, and in the body ethylestrenol actually has a notable affinity to convert to norethandrolone.[663] This path of metabolism is responsible for much of the anabolic, androgenic, and estrogenic activity we see with this compound, and in most regards ethylestrenol can be viewed as a pro-drug to norethandrolone. Although ethylestrenol is strongly anabolic relative to its androgenicity, athletes generally find this steroid to be extremely weak. The level of muscle growth obtained with this steroid is generally much less noticeable than that expected with either Nilevar or Deca-Durabolin®, and it is considerably less effective than both stanozolol and oxandrolone on a milligram for milligram basis.

History:

Ethylestrenol was first described in 1959.[664] It was developed into an oral medicine by Organon, appearing in most markets between 1961 and 1964. Organon sold the tablets under the trade name Maxibolin in the U.S., and as Orabolin, Orgabolin, and Durabolin-O in other markets. The latter name is a compressed form of "Durabolin-Oral," noting that the drug is an oral cousin to Durabolin (nandrolone phenylpropionate). Organon also produced oral ethylestrenol solutions, such as Maxibolin Elixir (U.S.) and Fertabolin (India, Philippines). Ethylestrenol was initially indicated for several uses, mainly focused on preserving lean mass. Early U.S. product literature states, "… along with a good dietary regimen, Maxibolin promotes tissue-building and weight gain, stimulation of appetite and sense of wellbeing, renewal of vigor, is an aid in bone matrix reconstruction and in combating the depression and weakness of chronic illness or prolonged convalescence. It can also prevent or reverse certain catabolic effects associated with corticosteroid therapy."

Ethylesterenol became a steroid of great controversy during the early 1980's, when Western media attention was given to the marketing of the drug to malnourished children in Third-World markets such as India, Bangladesh, and the Philippines. Advertising on Fertabolin in India claimed the drug would "help children gain full weight and height," "simulates physiological appetite," and "ensures optimal assimilation of food." It also described a "delicious [raspberry] syrup flavor children love." The main point of contention was the promotion of an anabolic steroid to treat the lack of adequate food supply, the real issue at hand. Many viewed Organon's actions as potentially dangerous and highly unethical, and the company soon discontinued Fertabolin and related marketing practices. Maxibolin and Maxibolin Elixir were voluntarily withdrawn from the U.S. market during the late 1980's as well, and most Western ethylestrenol products from Organon soon followed. Today, Organon retains only a limited interest in the drug. Ethylestrenol is currently a rare find, as it is only manufactured (as a generic drug or under other brand names) is a select few countries.

How Supplied:

Ethylestrenol is available in select human and veterinary drug markets. Composition and dosage may vary by country and manufacturer, but typically contains 2mg of steroid per tablet. Oral solutions have also been produced in the past, such as Maxibolin Elixir, which contained 2mg/5 mL in a 4 ounce bottle. Fertabolin for children contained .2mg/2 mL of solution.

Structural Characteristics:

Ethylestrenol is a modified form of nandrolone. It differs by: 1) the addition of an ethyl group at carbon 17-alpha to protect the hormone during oral administration and 2) the removal of the 3-oxygen.

Side Effects (Estrogenic):

Ethylestrenol is aromatized by the body, and converts to a synthetic estrogen with a high level of biological activity (17alpha-ethyl-estradiol). Rate of aromatization is so low, however, that it remains classified as a weakly estrogenic steroid. Gynecomastia is possible during treatment, but generally only when higher doses are used. Water and fat retention can also become issues, again depending on dose. Sensitive individuals may need to addition an anti-estrogen such as Nolvadex®. One may alternately use an aromatase inhibitor like Arimidex® (anastrozole), which is a more effective remedy for estrogen control. Aromatase inhibitors, however, can be quite expensive in comparison to standard estrogen maintenance therapies, and may also have negative effects on blood lipids.

It is of note that ethylestrenol has strong activity as a progestin in the body.[665] The side effects associated with progesterone are similar to those of estrogen, including negative feedback inhibition of testosterone production and enhanced rate of fat storage. Progestins also augment the stimulatory effect of estrogens on mammary tissue growth. There appears to be a strong synergy between these two hormones here, such that gynecomastia might even occur with the help of progestins without excessive estrogen levels being present. The use of an anti-estrogen, which inhibits the estrogenic component of this disorder, is often sufficient to mitigate gynecomastia caused by this steroid.

Side Effects (Androgenic):

Although classified as an anabolic steroid, androgenic side effects are still common with this substance. This may include bouts of oily skin, acne, and body/facial hair growth. Anabolic/androgenic steroids may also aggravate male pattern hair loss. Individuals sensitive to the androgenic effects of this steroid may find a milder anabolic such as Deca-Durabolin® to be more comfortable. Women are additionally warned of the potential virilizing effects of anabolic/androgenic steroids. These may include a deepening of the voice, menstrual irregularities, changes in skin texture, facial hair growth, and clitoral enlargement.

Note that in androgen-responsive target tissues such as the skin, scalp, and prostate, the relative androgenicity of ethylestrenol is reduced by its reduction to weaker "dihidyo" metabolites. The 5-alpha reductase enzyme is responsible for this metabolism. The concurrent use of a 5-alpha reductase inhibitor such as finasteride or dutasteride will interfere with site-specific reduction of ethylestrenol action, increasing the tendency of the drug to produce androgenic side effects. Reductase inhibitors should be avoided with this steroid if maintaining low relative androgenicity is desired.

Side Effects (Hepatotoxicity):

Ethylestrenol is a c17-alpha alkylated compound. This alteration protects the drug from deactivation by the liver, allowing a very high percentage of the drug entry into the bloodstream following oral administration. C17-alpha alkylated anabolic/androgenic steroids can be hepatotoxic. Prolonged or high exposure may result in liver damage. In rare instances life-threatening dysfunction may develop. It is advisable to visit a physician periodically during each cycle to monitor liver function and overall health. Intake of c17-alpha alkylated steroids is commonly limited to 6-8 weeks, in an effort to avoid escalating liver strain. Severe liver complications are rare given the periodic nature in which most people use oral anabolic/androgenic steroids, although cannot be excluded with this steroid, especially with high doses and/or prolonged administration periods.

The use of a liver detoxification supplement such as Liver Stabil, Liv-52, or Essentiale Forte is advised while taking any hepatotoxic anabolic/androgenic steroids.

Side Effects (Cardiovascular):

Anabolic/androgenic steroids can have deleterious effects on serum cholesterol. This includes a tendency to reduce HDL (good) cholesterol values and increase LDL (bad) cholesterol values, which may shift the HDL to LDL balance in a direction that favors greater risk of arteriosclerosis. The relative impact of an anabolic/androgenic steroid on serum lipids is dependant on the dose, route of administration (oral vs. injectable), type of steroid (aromatizable or non-aromatizable), and level of resistance to hepatic metabolism. Ethylestrenol has a strong effect on the hepatic management of cholesterol due to its structural resistance to liver breakdown and route of administration. Anabolic/androgenic steroids may also adversely affect blood pressure and triglycerides, reduce endothelial relaxation, and support left ventricular hypertrophy, all potentially increasing the risk of cardiovascular disease and myocardial infarction.

To help reduce cardiovascular strain it is advised to maintain an active cardiovascular exercise program and minimize the intake of saturated fats, cholesterol, and simple carbohydrates at all times during active AAS administration. Supplementing with fish oils (4 grams per day) and a natural cholesterol/antioxidant formula such as Lipid Stabil or a product with comparable ingredients is

also recommended.

Side Effects (Testosterone Suppression):

All anabolic/androgenic steroids when taken in doses sufficient to promote muscle gain are expected to suppress endogenous testosterone production. Without the intervention of testosterone-stimulating substances, testosterone levels should return to normal within 1-4 months of drug secession. Note that prolonged hypogonadotrophic hypogonadism can develop secondary to steroid abuse, necessitating medical intervention.

The above side effects are not inclusive. For more detailed discussion of potential side effects, see the Steroid Side Effects section of this book.

Administration (General):

Studies have shown that taking an oral anabolic steroid with food may decrease its bioavailability.[666] This is caused by the fat-soluble nature of steroid hormones, which can allow some of the drug to dissolve with undigested dietary fat, reducing its absorption from the gastrointestinal tract. For maximum utilization, this steroid should be taken on an empty stomach.

Administration (Men):

Original prescribing guidelines recommend a dosage of 4mg to 8mg per day, taken for no more than 6 consecutive weeks. After a break for 4 weeks, the drug is resumed for an additional 6 weeks if indicated. When used for physique- or performance-enhancing purposes, a daily dosage of 20 mg to 40 mg is most common, which equates to ten to twenty 2mg tablets. The drug is typically used in cycles lasting no longer than 6-8 weeks, in an effort to minimize hepatic strain. This level is sufficient for some measurable gains in muscle size and strength, although experienced steroid users are likely to still be disappointed with the results. Instead of increasing the dosage, most opt to add a second steroid to the cycle, usually an injectable such as testosterone cypionate or enanthate, boldenone undecylenate, or methenolone enanthate (usually at a dose of 200-400 mg per week), which do not provide additional liver toxicity.

Administration (Women):

Original prescribing guidelines recommend a dosage of 4mg to 8mg per day, taken for no more than 6 consecutive weeks. After a break for 4 weeks, the drug is resumed for an additional 6 weeks if indicated. When used for physique- or performance-enhancing purposes, a daily dosage of 10 mg to 16mg is most common, taken for no longer than 4 weeks. This level seems to be fairly effective for promoting new muscle growth. Higher doses are likely to produce virilizing side effects, and are not recommended. Note that virilizing side effects are still sometimes noticed at lower doses.

Availability:

Since the demand for Orabolin is so low, it does not make its way to the black market very often. When found it is usually in the form of one of a couple Australian veterinary preparations. The only solid tablet from this country is in fact the .5 mg Nandoral, made by Intervet. When found this can probably be considered a safe buy, but then again its low dose would make it a very poor choice.

Oral Turinabol (4-chlorodehydromethyltestosterone)

Androgenic	no data available
Anabolic	>100
Standard	Methyltestosterone (oral)
Chemical Name	4-chloro-17a-methyl-17b-hydroxyandrosta-1,4-dien-3-one
Estrogenic Activity	none
Progestational Activity	no data available (low)

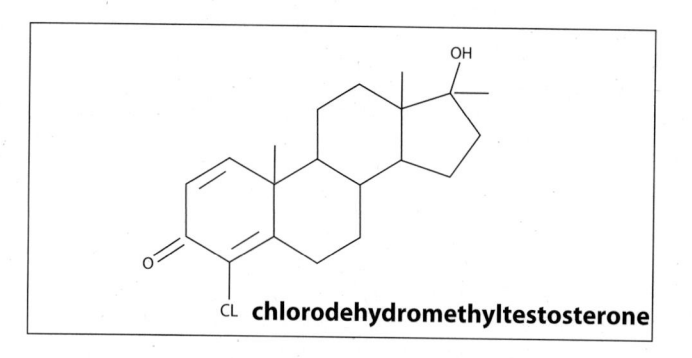

Description:

Chlorodehydromethyltestosterone is a potent derivative of Dianabol. This oral steroid is structurally a cross between methandrostenolone and clostebol (4-chlorotestosterone), having the same base structure as Dianabol with the added 4-chloro alteration of clostebol. This alteration makes chlorodehydromethyltestosterone a milder cousin of Dianabol, the new steroid displaying no estrogenic and a much less androgenic activity in comparison to its more famous counterpart. The anabolic activity of chlorodehydromethyltestosterone is somewhat lower than that of Dianabol as well, but it does maintain a much more favorable balance of anabolic to androgenic effect. This means that at any given level of muscle-building activity, chlorodehydromethyltestosterone will be less likely to produce androgenic side effects.

History:

Chlorodehydromethyltestosterone was first described in 1962.[667] Jenapharm (Jena, Germany) soon after released the drug for sale in the East German prescription drug market, under the brand name Oral Turinabol. The drug was favored by clinicians for its highly anabolic and low anabolic nature, lending itself to use in not only adult males, but women and children as well. The product was manufactured in two strengths, containing 1mg and 5 mg of drug per tablet, so that a lower-dosed version was available for the more sensitive populations. Chlorodehydromethyltestosterone was applied for a number of medical uses; mainly those focusing on the building or preservation of lean muscle tissue and bone mass.

Oral Turinabol became a steroid of infamy during the 1990's, when it was revealed that chlorodehydromethyltestosterone had been one of the closely held secrets inside the "East German Doping Machine." This is referring to the state-sponsored doping program, called "State Plan Research Theme 14.25," that operated in East Germany between 1974 and 1989. It was an aggressive anabolic steroid administration program, designed with one goal in mind: cheating the Olympic drug test. In many cases, the Olympic athletes, both male and female, were unwitting participants, simply told by their trainers and coaches that they were being given "vitamins." Many of these blue vitamins turned out to be Oral Turinabol, a potent and undetectable (at the time) anabolic steroid. As many as 10,000 athletes were given anabolic steroids during the time the program was active, many of them taking Oral Turinabol. For a more in-depth look at this dramatic historic event, including the trials of several former East German officials for their participation, I recommend you look at the book "Faust's Gold: Inside the East German Doping Machine" by Steven Ungerleider.

In spite of an arguably favorable profile of activity and safety record, Jenapharm discontinued Oral Turinabol in 1994. This was at a time when a great deal of negative attention was being given to sports doping, lending credibility to the speculation that this decision was one based on public relations, and not necessarily finances or health concerns over the drug. Regardless, Jenapharm was acquired by Schering AG (Germany) in 1996, a company with no interest in reliving the controversies of the past (Schering had already discontinued many of its controversial anabolic steroid products as well). Before or since, no other brand of chlorodehydromethyltestosterone has existed as a prescription drug product. Today, this agent is still available, but is only produced by a small number of underground manufacturers and export-only suppliers.

How Supplied:

Chlorodehydromethyltestosterone is not available as a prescription drug product. When manufactured, it was found in 1mg and 5 mg tablets, sold in Germany/German Democratic Republic.

Structural Characteristics:

Chlorodehydromethyltestosterone is a modified form of testosterone. It differs by: 1) the addition of a methyl group at carbon 17-alpha, which helps protect the hormone during oral administration, 2) the introduction of a double bond between carbons 1 and 2 (1-ene), which shifts the anabolic to androgenic ratio in favor of the former, and 3) the attachment of a chloro group at carbon 4, which inhibits steroid aromatization and reduces relative androgenicity.

Side Effects (Estrogenic):

Chlorodehydromethyltestosterone is not aromatized by the body, and is not measurably estrogenic. An anti-estrogen is not necessary when using this steroid, as gynecomastia should not be a concern even among sensitive individuals. Since estrogen is the usual culprit with water retention, this steroid instead produces a lean, quality look to the physique with no fear of excess subcutaneous fluid retention. This makes it a favorable steroid to use during cutting cycles, when water and fat retention are major concerns.

Side Effects (Androgenic):

Although chlorodehydromethyltestosterone is classified as an anabolic steroid, androgenic side effects are still possible with this substance. These may include bouts of oily skin, acne, and body/facial hair growth. Doses higher than normally prescribed are more likely to cause such side effects. Anabolic/androgenic steroids may also aggravate male pattern hair loss. Women are additionally warned of the potential virilizing effects of anabolic/androgenic steroids. These may include a deepening of the voice, menstrual irregularities, changes in skin texture, facial hair growth, and clitoral enlargement. Chlorodehydromethyltestosterone is not extensively metabolized by the 5-alpha reductase enzyme, so its relative androgenicity is not greatly altered by the concurrent use of finasteride or dutasteride

Side Effects (Hepatotoxicity):

Chlorodehydromethyltestosterone is a c17-alpha alkylated compound. This alteration protects the drug from deactivation by the liver, allowing a very high percentage of the drug entry into the bloodstream following oral administration. C17-alpha alkylated anabolic/androgenic steroids can be hepatotoxic. Prolonged or high exposure may result in liver damage. In rare instances life-threatening dysfunction may develop. It is advisable to visit a physician periodically during each cycle to monitor liver function and overall health. Intake of c17-alpha alkylated steroids is commonly limited to 6-8 weeks, in an effort to avoid escalating liver strain.

The use of a liver detoxification supplement such as Liver Stabil, Liv-52, or Essentiale Forte is advised while taking any hepatotoxic anabolic/androgenic steroids.

Side Effects (Cardiovascular):

Anabolic/androgenic steroids can have deleterious effects on serum cholesterol. This includes a tendency to reduce HDL (good) cholesterol values and increase LDL (bad) cholesterol values, which may shift the HDL to LDL balance in a direction that favors greater risk of arteriosclerosis. The relative impact of an anabolic/androgenic steroid on serum lipids is dependant on the dose, route of administration (oral vs. injectable), type of steroid (aromatizable or non-aromatizable), and level of resistance to hepatic metabolism. Chlorodehydromethyltestosterone has a strong effect on the hepatic management of cholesterol due to its non-aromatizable nature, structural resistance to liver breakdown, and route of administration. Anabolic/androgenic steroids may also adversely affect blood pressure and triglycerides, reduce endothelial relaxation, and support left ventricular hypertrophy, all potentially increasing the risk of cardiovascular disease and myocardial infarction.

To help reduce cardiovascular strain it is advised to maintain an active cardiovascular exercise program and minimize the intake of saturated fats, cholesterol, and simple carbohydrates at all times during active AAS administration. Supplementing with fish oils (4 grams per day) and a natural cholesterol/antioxidant formula such as Lipid Stabil or a product with comparable ingredients is also recommended.

Side Effects (Testosterone Suppression):

All anabolic/androgenic steroids when taken in doses sufficient to promote muscle gain are expected to suppress endogenous testosterone production. Without the intervention of testosterone-stimulating substances, testosterone levels should return to normal within 1-4 months of drug secession. Note that prolonged hypogonadotrophic hypogonadism can develop secondary to steroid abuse, necessitating medical intervention.

The above side effects are not inclusive. For more detailed discussion of potential side effects, see the Steroid Side Effects section of this book.

Administration (General):

Studies have shown that taking an oral anabolic steroid with food may decrease its bioavailability.[668] This is caused by the fat-soluble nature of steroid hormones, which can allow some of the drug to dissolve with undigested dietary fat, reducing its absorption from the gastrointestinal tract. For maximum utilization, this steroid should be taken on an empty stomach.

Administration (Men):

A common clinical dose of chlorodehydromethyltestosterone is estimated to be 5 mg per day; actual prescribing guidelines are unavailable. In the athletic arena, an effective oral daily dosage falls in the range of 15-40 mg, taken in cycles lasting no more than 6-8 weeks to minimize hepatotoxicity. This level is sufficient for measurable increases in lean muscle mass and strength. This agent is most often applied as a pre-contest or cutting steroid for bodybuilding purposes, and is not viewed as an ideal bulking agent due to its lack of estrogenicity. Athletes in sports where speed tends to be a primary focus also find strong favor in chlorodehydromethyltestosterone, obtaining a strong anabolic benefit without having to carry around any extra water or fat weight.

Administration (Women):

A common clinical dose of chlorodehydromethyltestosterone is estimated to be 1-2.5 mg per day; actual prescribing guidelines are unavailable. In the athletic arena, women would commonly take a single 5 mg tablet per day, taken in cycles lasting no more than 4-6 weeks to minimize hepatotoxicity. Virilizing effects are unlikely at this level of use. Much higher doses were often used with female athletes in the former GDR doping program, but often to detriment of strong virilizing side effects.

Availability:

Chlorodehydromethyltestosterone is no longer available as a prescription drug product. Several export and underground manufacturers do sell this steroid, however.

Oranabol (oxymesterone)

Androgenic	50
Anabolic	330
Standard	Methyltestosterone (oral)
Chemical Names	4-hydroxy-17a-methyltestosterone
	4,17-dihydroxyandrost-4-en-3-one
Estrogenic Activity	none
Progestational Activity	none

Oxymesterone

Description:

Oxymesterone is a potent oral anabolic steroid derived from testosterone. In structure, it is most closely related to 4-hydroxytestosterone, differing only by the addition of a c-17 alpha methyl group, which makes oral dosing viable. Like its non-methylated analog, oxymesterone remains an effective lean-tissue-building steroid with only a minimal to moderate androgenic component. It has no known estrogenic or progestational activity, and no discernable ability to cause side effects related to female sex hormones. Oxymesterone is a "clean" drug among oral steroids: potent, non-aromatizable, and primarily anabolic in nature. According to the standard laboratory assays, oxymesterone is over three times more anabolic than methyltestosterone, with only half the androgenicity. Closer comparisons to methyltestosterone, which may seem structurally logical, do not hold up well in practice, given the sharp contrasts in relative effects between these drugs. The differences are as drastic as their applications, with methyltestosterone being used almost exclusively for bulking phases of training while oxymesterone would fit most comfortably with cutting cycles or competitive athletics.

History:

Oxymesterone was first closely described in 1956.[669] It was developed into a medicine during the early 1960's by Societa Farmaceutici (Italy), which filed for patent protection on this compound in at least three countries including the United Kingdom, the United States, and Italy.[670] This drug saw limited clinical use as a prescription agent under the Oranabol brand name in Spain and Italy, and under the names Anamidol, Balinmax, Sanabol, and Theranabol in other countries including Japan, the UK, and the Netherlands. Oxymesterone ultimately enjoyed little commercial success, and has been unavailable as a prescription drug worldwide for more than three decades now. It was never released in the United States. At very best, only a small handful of U.S. athletes have experimented with this obscure anabolic steroid over the years, and certainly very few in recent times.

By the 1990's, oxymesterone had already become a forgotten relic of early steroid development. In all this time there has been limited mention of its use in the medical literature. The drug did show up in a report released in 1993 by the department of Clinical Pharmacology and Toxicology at St. Vincent's Hospital in New South Wales, concerning two young football players who died of cardiac events in 1988 and 1990. The two men, who had unobstructed arteries and were only 18 and 24 years of age,[671] died during routine training sessions. Despite never being offered for sale in Australia, and having been removed from the global market long before 1988, oxymesterone had been detected in the men during autopsy. No conclusive link between the drug and their deaths could be established, neither discounted. Today, oxymesterone remains unavailable as a prescription agent worldwide.

How Supplied:

Oxymesterone is no longer available as a prescription drug product.

Structural Characteristics:

Oxymesterone is a modified form of testosterone. It differs by: 1) the addition of a methyl group at carbon 17-alpha, which helps protect the hormone during oral administration, and 2) the attachment of a hydroxyl group at carbon 4, which inhibits steroid aromatization and reduces relative androgenicity.

Side Effects (Estrogenic):

Oxymesterone is not aromatized by the body, and is not measurably estrogenic. An anti-estrogen is not necessary when using this steroid, as gynecomastia should not be a concern even among sensitive individuals. Since estrogen is the usual culprit with water retention, this steroid instead produces a lean, quality look to the physique with no fear of excess subcutaneous fluid retention. This makes it a favorable steroid to use during cutting cycles, when water and fat retention are major concerns.

Note that when a 4-hydroxyl group is applied to testosterone (as in hydroxytestosterone) a suicide aromatase inhibitor is created, capable of significantly suppressing serum estrogen levels. It is unknown if this property exists in Oranabol (methylhydroxytestosterone), as this potential aspect of its pharmacology has never been investigated. Its non-estrogenic and non-progestational profile would support, at the very least, this agent being a steroid for increasing muscle density and visibility, regardless of a related aromatase-inhibiting effect, which may indeed also be present.

Side Effects (Androgenic):

Although oxymesterone is classified as an anabolic steroid, androgenic side effects are still possible with this substance. These may include bouts of oily skin, acne, and body/facial hair growth. Doses higher than normally prescribed are more likely to cause such side effects. Anabolic/androgenic steroids may also aggravate male pattern hair loss. Women are additionally warned of the potential virilizing effects of anabolic/androgenic steroids. These may include a deepening of the voice, menstrual irregularities, changes in skin texture, facial hair growth, and clitoral enlargement. Note that oxymesterone is not extensively metabolized by the 5-alpha reductase enzyme, so its relative androgenicity is not greatly altered by the concurrent use of finasteride or dutasteride

Side Effects (Hepatotoxicity):

Oxymesterone is a c17-alpha alkylated compound. This alteration protects the drug from deactivation by the liver, allowing a very high percentage of the drug entry into the bloodstream following oral administration. C17-alpha alkylated anabolic/androgenic steroids can be hepatotoxic. Prolonged or high exposure may result in liver damage. In rare instances life-threatening dysfunction may develop. It is advisable to visit a physician periodically during each cycle to monitor liver function and overall health. Intake of c17-alpha alkylated steroids is commonly limited to 6-8 weeks, in an effort to avoid escalating liver strain. Note that in studies this agent offered slightly less hepatic strain than methandrostenolone and norethandrolone, as measured by bromosulphalein (BSP) retention.

The use of a liver detoxification supplement such as Liver Stabil, Liv-52, or Essentiale Forte is advised while taking any hepatotoxic anabolic/androgenic steroids.

Side Effects (Cardiovascular):

Anabolic/androgenic steroids can have deleterious effects on serum cholesterol. This includes a tendency to reduce HDL (good) cholesterol values and increase LDL (bad) cholesterol values, which may shift the HDL to LDL balance in a direction that favors greater risk of arteriosclerosis. The relative impact of an anabolic/androgenic steroid on serum lipids is dependant on the dose, route of administration (oral vs. injectable), type of steroid (aromatizable or non-aromatizable), and level of resistance to hepatic metabolism. Oxymesterone has a strong effect on the hepatic management of cholesterol due to its structural resistance to liver breakdown and route of administration. Anabolic/androgenic steroids may also adversely affect blood pressure and triglycerides, reduce endothelial relaxation, and support left ventricular hypertrophy, all potentially increasing the risk of cardiovascular disease and myocardial infarction.

To help reduce cardiovascular strain it is advised to maintain an active cardiovascular exercise program and minimize the intake of saturated fats, cholesterol, and simple carbohydrates at all times during active AAS administration. Supplementing with fish oils (4 grams per day) and a natural cholesterol/antioxidant formula such as Lipid Stabil or a product with comparable ingredients is also recommended.

Side Effects (Testosterone Suppression):

All anabolic/androgenic steroids when taken in doses sufficient to promote muscle gain are expected to suppress endogenous testosterone production. Without the intervention of testosterone-stimulating substances, testosterone levels should return to normal within 1-4 months of drug secession. Note that prolonged hypogonadotrophic hypogonadism can develop secondary to steroid abuse, necessitating medical intervention.

The above side effects are not inclusive. For more detailed discussion of potential side effects, see the Steroid Side Effects section of this book.

Administration (General):

Studies have shown that taking an oral anabolic steroid with food may decrease its bioavailability.[672] This is caused by the fat-soluble nature of steroid hormones, which can allow some of the drug to dissolve with undigested dietary fat, reducing its absorption from the gastrointestinal tract. For maximum utilization, this steroid should be taken on an empty stomach.

Administration (Men):

A common clinical dose for oxymesterone was 20-40 mg per day. In the athletic arena, an effective oral daily dosage also falls in the range of 20-40 mg, taken in cycles lasting no more than 6-8 weeks to minimize hepatotoxicity. This level is sufficient for formidable strength gains, increased fat loss, increased muscle definition, and an overall increase in lean muscle mass. This drug would further stack well with a variety of other steroids, especially a 200-400 mg per week dose of an injectable base like testosterone cypionate/enanthate or Equipoise® during bulking phases of training, or a milder anabolic like Deca-Durabolin® or Primobolan® for cutting and defining. All of these stack combinations should work extremely well, and would not add to the liver toxicity already present in oxymesterone.

Administration (Women):

A common clinical dose for oxymesterone was 20-40 mg per day. In the athletic arena, women would likely notice substantial gains on 10 mg per day, taken for no longer than 4 weeks. Virilizing side effects are still possible with a powerful hormone like oxymesterone, especially with higher doses, and should be carefully monitored.

Availability:

Despite being an effective steroid, oxymesterone has never been a widely available one. This agent has not been available as a prescription drug for over 30 years.

Oreton (testosterone propionate)

Androgenic	100
Anabolic	100
Standard	Standard
Chemical Names	4-androsten-3-one-17beta-ol
	17beta-hydroxy-androst-4-en-3-one
Estrogenic Activity	moderate
Progestational Activity	low

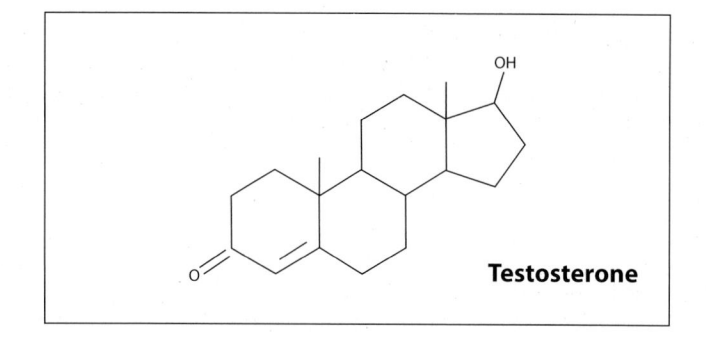

Description:

Testosterone propionate is a commonly manufactured injectable form of the primary male androgen testosterone. The added propionate ester will slow the rate in which testosterone is released from the injection site, but only for a few days. Testosterone propionate is, therefore, comparatively much faster-acting than other testosterone esters such as cypionate or enanthate, and requires a much more frequent dosing schedule. By most accounts testosterone propionate is an older and cruder form of injectable testosterone, made obsolete by the slower-acting and more comfortable esters that were developed subsequent to it. Still, those who are not bothered by the frequent injection schedule find testosterone propionate every bit as acceptable. As an injectable testosterone, it is a powerful mass-building drug, capable of producing rapid gains in both muscle size and strength.

History:

Testosterone propionate was first described in 1935, during a series of experiments that set out to increase the therapeutic usefulness of testosterone by slowing its release into the bloodstream.[673] Two years later, Schering AG in Germany would introduce the first testosterone propionate product under the brand name Testoviron®. Propionate was also the first commercially available injectable ester of testosterone on the U.S. prescription drug market, and remained the dominant form of testosterone globally before 1960. Back during the early 1950's, for example, when steroids were first being experimented with by small numbers of American athletes, the only readily available anabolic/androgenic steroids were methyltestosterone, testosterone propionate, and testosterone suspension. Interesting enough, during this time testosterone propionate was also available in orally administered (Buccal) preparations, but they disappeared from the U.S. market during the 1980's.

Early prescribing guidelines for testosterone propionate called for a number of therapeutic uses. It was mainly applied to cases of male androgen insufficiency, and those issues normally surrounding low testosterone levels such as reduced sex drive and impotence in adults, and cryptorchidism (undescended testicles) in teenagers and young adults. But it also had such other uses as treating menopause, menorrhagia (heavy menstrual bleeding), menstrual tension, chronic cystic mastitis (fibrocystic breasts), endometriosis, and excessive lactation, covering a wide range of situations in which the male hormone testosterone was being applied to female patients. Over the years these wide guidelines were narrowed by the U.S. Food & Drug Administration, however, and by the 1980's, testosterone propionate was being largely applied only to male patients.

Testosterone propionate has a long history of availability in the U.S. and abroad, and remains a very common form of testosterone on the global market to this day. It must be emphasized, however, that its ability to remain on the market is more a product of history than unique application. Testosterone propionate was the first acceptable ester of testosterone, and consequently has many decades of history as a useable therapeutic agent. Many companies have sold it for decades now, and so long as it is still in demand will continue to do so. But other (more modern) forms of testosterone such as enanthate and cypionate are much more popular today, as they are much slower-acting still, and allow for far more comfortable administration schedules. Testosterone propionate is still approved for sale in the United States, although its ultimate market future here remains questionable.

Bodybuilders commonly consider propionate to be the mildest testosterone ester, and the preferred form of this hormone for dieting/cutting phases of training. Some will go so far as to say that propionate will harden the physique, while giving the user less water and fat retention than one typically expects to see with a testosterone like enanthate, cypionate or Sustanon. Realistically, however, these advantages do not hold up to close scrutiny. The propionate ester is actually removed before the testosterone it carries is active in the body, and ultimately has little effect outside of slowing steroid release. It all really boils down to how much testosterone you are getting into your blood with each particular esterified compound. Otherwise, there are no real functional differences between them.

How Supplied:

Testosterone propionate is widely available in human and veterinary drug markets. Composition and dosage may vary by country and manufacturer, but usually contain 25 mg/ml, 50 mg/ml, or 100 mg/ml of steroid dissolved in oil.

Structural Characteristics:

Testosterone propionate is a modified form of testosterone, where a carboxylic acid ester (propionic acid) has been attached to the 17-beta hydroxyl group. Esterified forms of testosterone are less polar than free testosterone, and are absorbed more slowly from the area of injection. Once in the bloodstream, the ester is removed to yield free (active) testosterone. Esterified forms of testosterone are designed to prolong the window of therapeutic effect following administration, allowing for a less frequent injection schedule compared to injections of free (unesterified) steroid. The half-life of testosterone propionate is approximately two days after injection.

Figure 1. Pharmacokinetics of 25 mg labeled testosterone propionate injection. Source: Pharmacokinetic properties of testosterone propionate in normal men. Fujioka M, Shinohara Y, Baba S. et. Al. J Clin Endocrinol Metab 63 (1986):1361-4.

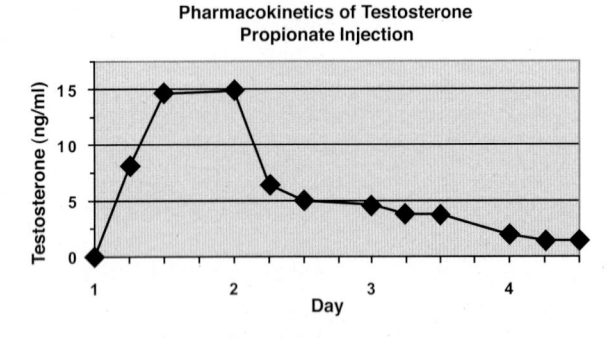

Side Effects (Estrogenic):

Testosterone is readily aromatized in the body to estradiol (estrogen). The aromatase (estrogen synthetase) enzyme is responsible for this metabolism of testosterone. Elevated estrogen levels can cause side effects such as increased water retention, body fat gain, and gynecomastia. Testosterone is considered a moderately estrogenic steroid. An anti-estrogen such as clomiphene citrate or tamoxifen citrate may be necessary to prevent estrogenic side effects. One may alternately use an aromatase inhibitor like Arimidex® (anastrozole), which more efficiently controls estrogen by preventing its synthesis. Aromatase inhibitors can be quite expensive in comparison to anti-estrogens, however, and may also have negative effects on blood lipids.

Estrogenic side effects will occur in a dose-dependant manner, with higher doses (above normal therapeutic levels) of testosterone propionate more likely to require the concurrent use of an anti-estrogen or aromatase inhibitor. Since water retention and loss of muscle definition are common with higher doses of testosterone, this drug is usually considered a poor choice for dieting or cutting phases of training. Its moderate estrogenicity makes it more ideal for bulking phases, where the added water retention will support raw strength and muscle size, and help foster a stronger anabolic environment.

Side Effects (Androgenic):

Testosterone is the primary male androgen, responsible for maintaining secondary male sexual characteristics. Elevated levels of testosterone are likely to produce androgenic side effects including oily skin, acne, and body/facial hair growth. Men with a genetic predisposition for hair loss (androgenetic alopecia) may notice accelerated male pattern balding. Those concerned about hair loss may find a more comfortable option in nandrolone decanoate, which is a comparably less androgenic steroid. Women are warned of the potential virilizing effects of anabolic/androgenic steroids, especially with a strong androgen such as testosterone. These may include deepening of the voice, menstrual irregularities, changes in skin texture, facial hair growth, and clitoral enlargement.

In androgen-responsive target tissues such as the skin, scalp, and prostate, the high relative androgenicity of testosterone is dependant on its reduction to dihydrotestosterone (DHT). The 5-alpha reductase enzyme is responsible for this metabolism of testosterone. The concurrent use of a 5-alpha reductase inhibitor such as finasteride or dutasteride will interfere with site-specific potentiation of testosterone action, lowering the tendency of testosterone drugs to produce androgenic side effects. It is important to remember that both anabolic and androgenic effects are mediated via the cytosolic androgen receptor. Complete separation of testosterone's anabolic and androgenic properties is not possible, even with total 5-alpha reductase inhibition.

Side Effects (Hepatotoxicity):

Testosterone does not have hepatotoxic effects; liver toxicity is unlikely. One study examined the potential for hepatotoxicity with high doses of testosterone by administering 400 mg of the hormone per day (2,800 mg per week) to a group of male subjects. The steroid was taken orally so that higher peak concentrations would be reached in hepatic tissues compared to intramuscular injections. The hormone was given daily for 20 days, and produced no significant changes in liver enzyme values including serum albumin, bilirubin, alanine-amino-transferase, and alkaline phosphatases.[674]

Side Effects (Cardiovascular):

Anabolic/androgenic steroids can have deleterious effects on serum cholesterol. This includes a tendency to reduce HDL (good) cholesterol values and increase LDL (bad) cholesterol values, which may shift the HDL to LDL balance in a direction that favors greater risk of arteriosclerosis. The relative impact of an anabolic/androgenic steroid on serum lipids is dependant on the dose, route of administration (oral vs. injectable), type of steroid (aromatizable or non-aromatizable), and level of resistance to hepatic metabolism. Anabolic/androgenic steroids may also adversely affect blood pressure and triglycerides, reduce endothelial relaxation, and support left ventricular hypertrophy, all potentially increasing the risk of cardiovascular disease and myocardial infarction.

Testosterone tends to have a much less dramatic impact on cardiovascular risk factors than synthetic steroids. This is due in part to its openness to metabolism by the liver, which allows it to have less effect on the hepatic management of cholesterol. The aromatization of testosterone to estradiol also helps to mitigate the negative effects of androgens on serum lipids. In one study, 280 mg per week of testosterone ester (enanthate) had a slight but not statistically significant effect on HDL cholesterol after 12 weeks, but when taken with an aromatase inhibitor a strong (25%) decrease was seen.[675] Studies using 300 mg of testosterone ester (enanthate) per week for twenty weeks without an aromatase inhibitor demonstrated only a 13% decrease in HDL cholesterol, while at 600 mg the reduction reached 21%.[676] The negative impact of aromatase inhibition should be taken into consideration before such drug is added to testosterone therapy.

Due to the positive influence of estrogen on serum lipids, tamoxifen citrate or clomiphene citrate are preferred to aromatase inhibitors for those concerned with cardiovascular health, as they offer a partial estrogenic effect in the liver. This allows them to potentially improve lipid profiles and offset some of the negative effects of androgens. With doses of 600 mg or less of testosterone per week, the impact on lipid profile tends to be noticeable but not dramatic, making an anti-estrogen (for cardioprotective purposes) perhaps unnecessary. Doses of 600 mg or less per week have also failed to produce statistically significant changes in LDL/VLDL cholesterol, triglycerides, apolipoprotein B/C-III, C-reactive protein, and insulin sensitivity, all indicating a relatively weak impact on cardiovascular risk factors.[677] When used in moderate doses, injectable testosterone esters are usually considered to be the safest of all anabolic/androgenic steroids.

To help reduce cardiovascular strain it is advised to maintain an active cardiovascular exercise program and minimize the intake of saturated fats, cholesterol, and simple carbohydrates at all times during active AAS administration. Supplementing with fish oils (4 grams per day) and a natural cholesterol/antioxidant formula such as Lipid Stabil or a product with comparable ingredients is also recommended.

Side Effects (Testosterone Suppression):

All anabolic/androgenic steroids when taken in doses sufficient to promote muscle gain are expected to suppress endogenous testosterone production. Testosterone is the primary male androgen, and offers strong negative feedback on endogenous testosterone production. Testosterone-based drugs will, likewise, have a strong effect on the hypothalamic regulation of natural steroid hormones. Without the intervention of testosterone-stimulating substances, testosterone levels should return to normal within 1-4 months of drug secession. Note that prolonged hypogonadotrophic hypogonadism can develop secondary to steroid abuse, necessitating medical intervention.

The above side effects are not inclusive. For more detailed discussion of potential side effects, see the Steroid Side Effects section of this book.

Administration (General):

Testosterone propionate is often regarded as a painful injection. This is due to the very short carbon chain of the propionic acid ester, which can be irritating to tissues at the site of injection. Many sensitive individuals choose to stay away from this steroid completely, their bodies reacting with a pronounced soreness and low-grade fever that may last for a few days after each injection. Even the mild soreness that is experienced by most users can be quite uncomfortable, especially when you take into account that the drug is being administered multiple times each week for a number of consecutive weeks.

Administration (Men):

To treat androgen insufficiency, early prescribing guidelines recommended a dosage of 25 mg given two to three times per week. Modern product literature usually recommends 25 mg to 50 mg given two to three times per week for the same purpose. The usual dosage among male athletes is in the range of 50-100 mg per injection, which is given every second or third day. Similar to other esters of testosterone, testosterone propionate is commonly used at a weekly cumulative dosage between 200 mg to 400 mg. This level is sufficient for most users to notice exceptional gains in muscle size and strength.

Testosterone propionate is usually incorporated into bulking phases of training, when added water retention will be of little consequence, the user more concerned with raw mass than definition. Some do incorporate this drug into cutting cycles as well, but typically in lower doses (100-200 mg per week) and/or when accompanied by an aromatase inhibitor to keep estrogen levels under control. Testosterone propionate is a very effective anabolic drug, and is often used alone with great benefit. Some, however, find a need to stack it with other anabolic/androgenic steroids for a stronger effect, in which case an additional 200-400 mg per week of boldenone undecylenate, methenolone enanthate, or nandrolone decanoate should provide substantial results with no significant hepatotoxicity. Testosterone is ultimately very versatile, and can be combined with many other anabolic/androgenic steroids to tailor the desired effect.

Administration (Women):

Testosterone propionate is rarely used with women in clinical medicine. When applied, it is most often used as a secondary medication during inoperable breast cancer, when other therapies have failed to produce a desirable effect and suppression of ovarian function is necessary. Testosterone propionate is not recommended for women for performance-enhancing purposes due to its strong androgenic nature and tendency to produce virilizing side effects. Female bodybuilders who insist on using testosterone, however, often choose propionate, as blood levels are easier to control with this ester compared to cypionate or enanthate. Should virilization symptoms develop, hormone levels will decline in a matter of days, instead of weeks, following drug cessation. The administration schedule is often more conservative as well, with a small injection (25 mg at most) given every 5 to 7 days, and cycle duration limited to 6-8 weeks or less.

Availability:

Testosterone propionate is common on the black market, although less so than testosterone enanthate or cypionate. In going over some of the more popular items circulating the black market at this time, the following observations can be made.

Brovel in Mexico makes a testosterone propionate in a 50 mg/mL dosage for veterinary use. Counterfeits are not known to be a problem.

No testosterone propionate products are being manufactured in the U.S. at this time, so avoid all such products on the black market.

Alpha-Pharma in India makes a testosterone propionate product called Testorapid. It comes in 1 mL dark amber glass ampules. Note that this product is sold for export only.

Testolic is made by T.P. Drug Laboratories in Thailand, and distributed by Body Research. Counterfeits are not known to be a significant problem.

Balkan Pharmaceuticals in Moldova makes a propionate product called Testosterona P. It comes in 1 mL glass ampules. Counterfeits are not known to be an issue.

Testosteron is a popular brand from Bulgaria, and is commonly exported to other markets in high volume. It comes in the form of 1 mL glass ampules containing 50 mg/mL of steroid.

A generic made by the company Farmak is popularly exported from the Ukraine. This also comes in the form of 1 mL glass ampules containing 50 mg of steroid.

Jelfa makes Testosteronum Propionicum in Poland, which makes its way most often to the European black market (rarely to the U.S.). However, it only contains 25 mg of steroid in each 1 mL ampule.

Virormone is still manufactured in the UK, most recently by the firm Nordic. These 2 mL 100 mg ampules are not extremely popular in the U.S., but do circulate here from time to time. The UK has been taking steroid distribution more seriously as of late, limiting greatly the supply of domestic drugs making it to the international black market.

Vetoquinol sells a propionate in Canada, called Anatest. It contains 100 mg/ml of testosterone propionate in a 10 mL vial, giving it a dosage and volume comparable to many of the higher dosed veterinary items on the black market. Combine this with the rigid standards of Canadian drug manufacturing (if you find a legitimate product), and Anatest starts looking like an excellent product if you come across it. Unfortunately, the firm doesn't use any hologram or sophisticated security measures. Shop carefully.

Orgasteron (normethandrolone)

Androgenic	110-125
Anabolic	325-580
Standard	Methyltestosterone (oral)
Chemical Names	17a-methyl-19-nor-delta4-androsten-17b-ol-3-one
Estrogenic Activity	moderate
Progestational Activity	high

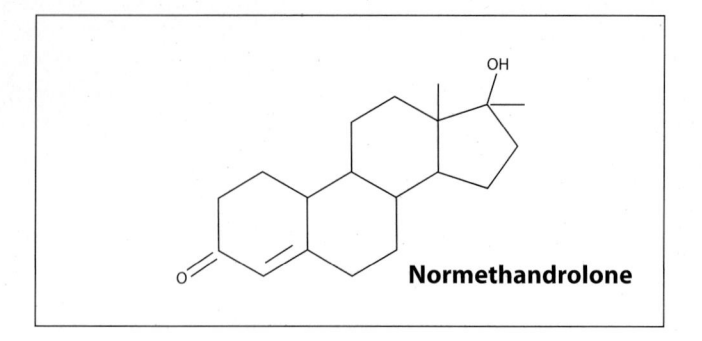

Description:

Normethandrolone is a potent oral anabolic steroid derived from nandrolone. Also called methylnandrolone or methylnortestosterone, normethandrolone can crudely be looked at as the "methyltestosterone of nandrolone." It differs from its parent hormone nandrolone only by the addition of c-17 alpha methyl group, the same alteration that creates methyltestosterone from testosterone. This, of course, was added to make oral dosing viable. Animal studies looking at the oral potency of this steroid rate it to be roughly 3-6 times more anabolic than methyltestosterone, while possessing only roughly 10-25% more androgenicity.[678][679] The overall anabolic-androgenic ratio of this steroid falls somewhere between 3:1 and 5.5:1. Although it is effective orally, normethandrolone is not the most ideal steroid for bodybuilders and athletes, at least where lean mass or sports performance are concerned (something for which nandrolone is highly favored). In this case methylation has amplified the estrogenic and progestational activity of the steroid considerably, which means that muscle gains are likely to be accompanied by considerable water and fat retention.

History:

Normethandrolone was first described in 1954.[680] Shortly after, it was developed into a medicine by Organon, which introduced it under the Orgasterone brand name in Belgium and Switzerland, and as Orga-steron in the Netherlands. This steroid had also been sold by other manufacturers in various parts of Europe as Methalutin, Lutenin, and Matdonal. Although a simple oral methylated nandrolone, with strong properties as an anabolic steroid, normethandrolone exhibits such strong progestational activity that it was marketed as an oral progestin. Its anabolic effects were more looked at as secondary applications for the drug, and accounted for very little medical interest. It was also mainly sold under the trivial name methylestrenolone, which again seems to visibly separate the drug from the anabolic steroid category.

Given the unobvious naming and unrelated marketing of normethandrolone, it was ultimately given very little interest by athletes. Even during the 1960's, a time when many new and exotic agents were appearing on the black market, normethandrolone was essentially unheard of. The various normethandrolone preparations soon began drying up, as newer and more targeted oral progestins became available to clinicians. The drug quietly disappeared from the various international markets before bodybuilders ever made any type of substantial connection with it. Normethandrolone is now discontinued worldwide. Note that in spite of its current obscurity in the U.S., normethandrolone was added to the Federal controlled substances laws in 2004 as a schedule III anabolic steroid.

How Supplied:

Normethandrolone is no longer available as a prescription drug product.

Structural Characteristics:

Normethandrolone is a modified form of nandrolone. It differs by the addition of a methyl group at carbon 17-alpha to protect the hormone during oral administration.

Side Effects (Estrogenic):

Normethandrolone is aromatized by the body, and converts to a synthetic estrogen with a high level of biological activity (17alpha-methyl-estradiol). As a result, it is a highly estrogenic steroid. Gynecomastia is often a concern during treatment, and may present itself quite early into a cycle (particularly when higher doses are used). At the same time water retention can become a problem, causing a notable loss of muscle definition as both subcutaneous water retention and fat levels build. Sensitive individuals may want to keep the estrogen under control with the addition of an anti-estrogen such as

Nolvadex®. One may alternately use an aromatase inhibitor like Arimidex® (anastrozole), which is a more effective remedy for estrogen control. Aromatase inhibitors, however, can be quite expensive in comparison to standard estrogen maintenance therapies, and may also have negative effects on blood lipids.

It is also of note that normethandrolone has very strong activity as a progestin in the body.[681] In fact, it was assayed to be more active than progesterone itself.[682] Studies usually refer to this agent as a progestogenic (progestational) compound with anabolic action, not directly as an anabolic/androgenic steroid. The side effects associated with progesterone are similar to those of estrogen, including negative feedback inhibition of testosterone production and enhanced rate of fat storage. Progestins also augment the stimulatory effect of estrogens on mammary tissue growth. There appears to be a strong synergy between these two hormones here, such that gynecomastia might even occur with the help of progestins without excessive estrogen levels being present. The use of an anti-estrogen, which inhibits the estrogenic component of this disorder, may be sufficient to mitigate gynecomastia caused by normethandrolone.

Side Effects (Androgenic):

Although classified as an anabolic steroid, androgenic side effects are still possible with this substance. This may include bouts of oily skin, acne, and body/facial hair growth. Anabolic/androgenic steroids may also aggravate male pattern hair loss. Individuals sensitive to the androgenic effects of this steroid may find a milder anabolic such as Deca-Durabolin® to be more comfortable. Women are additionally warned of the potential virilizing effects of anabolic/androgenic steroids. These may include a deepening of the voice, menstrual irregularities, changes in skin texture, facial hair growth, and clitoral enlargement.

Note that in androgen-responsive target tissues such as the skin, scalp, and prostate, the relative androgenicity of normethandrolone is reduced by its reduction to dihydronormethandrolone. The 5-alpha reductase enzyme is responsible for this metabolism. The concurrent use of a 5-alpha reductase inhibitor such as finasteride or dutasteride will interfere with site-specific reduction of normethandrolone action, considerably increasing the tendency of the drug to produce androgenic side effects. Reductase inhibitors should be avoided with this steroid if maintaining low relative androgenicity is desired.

Side Effects (Hepatotoxicity):

Normethandrolone is a c17-alpha alkylated compound. This alteration protects the drug from deactivation by the liver, allowing a very high percentage of the drug entry into the bloodstream following oral administration. C17-alpha alkylated anabolic/androgenic steroids can be hepatotoxic. Prolonged or high exposure may result in liver damage. In rare instances life-threatening dysfunction may develop. It is advisable to visit a physician periodically during each cycle to monitor liver function and overall health. Intake of c17-alpha alkylated steroids is commonly limited to 6-8 weeks, in an effort to avoid escalating liver strain. Jaundice (bile duct obstruction) was reported as early as 1958 with this steroid,[683] so this possibility definitely should not be disregarded. Severe liver complications are rare given the periodic nature in which most people use oral anabolic/androgenic steroids, although cannot be excluded with this steroid, especially with high doses and/or prolonged administration periods.

The use of a liver detoxification supplement such as Liver Stabil, Liv-52, or Essentiale Forte is advised while taking any hepatotoxic anabolic/androgenic steroids.

Side Effects (Cardiovascular):

Anabolic/androgenic steroids can have deleterious effects on serum cholesterol. This includes a tendency to reduce HDL (good) cholesterol values and increase LDL (bad) cholesterol values, which may shift the HDL to LDL balance in a direction that favors greater risk of arteriosclerosis. The relative impact of an anabolic/androgenic steroid on serum lipids is dependant on the dose, route of administration (oral vs. injectable), type of steroid (aromatizable or non-aromatizable), and level of resistance to hepatic metabolism. Normethandrolone has a strong effect on the hepatic management of cholesterol due to its structural resistance to liver breakdown and route of administration. Anabolic/androgenic steroids may also adversely affect blood pressure and triglycerides, reduce endothelial relaxation, and support left ventricular hypertrophy, all potentially increasing the risk of cardiovascular disease and myocardial infarction.

To help reduce cardiovascular strain it is advised to maintain an active cardiovascular exercise program and minimize the intake of saturated fats, cholesterol, and simple carbohydrates at all times during active AAS administration. Supplementing with fish oils (4 grams per day) and a natural cholesterol/antioxidant formula such as Lipid Stabil or a product with comparable ingredients is also recommended.

Side Effects (Testosterone Suppression):

All anabolic/androgenic steroids when taken in doses sufficient to promote muscle gain are expected to suppress endogenous testosterone production. Without the intervention of testosterone-stimulating substances, testosterone levels should return to normal within 1-4 months of drug secession. Note that prolonged hypogonadotrophic hypogonadism can develop secondary to steroid abuse, necessitating medical intervention.

The above side effects are not inclusive. For more detailed discussion of potential side effects, see the Steroid Side Effects section of this book.

Administration (General):

Studies have shown that taking an oral anabolic steroid with food may decrease its bioavailability.[684] This is caused by the fat-soluble nature of steroid hormones, which can allow some of the drug to dissolve with undigested dietary fat, reducing its absorption from the gastrointestinal tract. For maximum utilization, this steroid should be taken on an empty stomach.

Administration (Men):

For bodybuilding purposes, this drug would typically be taken at a dosage of 10 mg to 30 mg per day, taken in cycles lasting 6 to 8 weeks. This level is sufficient for rapid gains in strength and muscle mass (bulk). This compound is used almost exclusively for bulking phases of training, as its progestational and estrogenic nature will undoubtedly work against fat loss and muscle definition when trying to cut. Used alone, one can expect to see decent gains, something perhaps in line with a Dianabol cycle, but with a seemingly more noteworthy estrogenic side to it. The high progestational and estrogenic activities of normethandrolone also make it of little value in speed and endurance sports, causing an unwanted retention of water weight.

Administration (Women):

When used by women for physique- or performance-enhancing purposes, a daily dosage of 2.5-10 mg is most common, taken for no longer than 4 weeks. This level is quite effective for promoting new muscle growth. Note that virilizing side effects are still possible with primarily anabolic substances, and need to be carefully monitored.

Availability:

Orgasteron is long gone now and no commercial preparations containing normethandrolone are known to exist. Still, normethandrolone is being synthesized overseas, and undoubtedly is circulating in the U.S. in small amounts. Underground versions of the drug are likely. Given that this is still a relatively "crude" steroid with virtually no demand for it, however, a big future for this agent on the black market is not expected.

Parabolan® (trenbolone hexahydrobenzylcarbonate)

Androgenic	500
Anabolic	500
Standard	Nandrolone acetate
Chemical Name	17beta-Hydroxyestra-4,9,11-trien-3-one
Estrogenic Activity	none
Progestational Activity	moderate

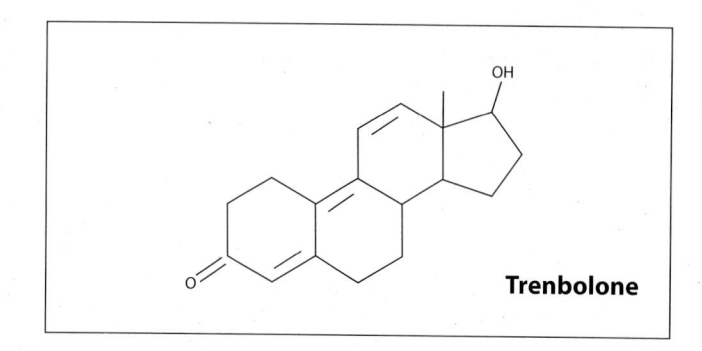

Trenbolone

Description:

Trenbolone hexahydrobenzylcarbonate is a slow-acting injectable ester of the potent anabolic steroid trenbolone. Trenbolone appears most commonly as trenbolone acetate, which is a much faster-acting form of the drug (see: Finajet). The hexahydrobenzylcarbonate ester used here extends the release of trenbolone for more than 2 weeks, which has always been thought of as more suitable for human use due to the less frequent injection schedule. The base steroid trenbolone is roughly three times more androgenic than testosterone, making it a fairly potent androgen. It also displays about 3 times greater tissue-building activity in comparison to its androgenic properties, making its official classification as that of an anabolic steroid. The muscle-building effect of trenbolone is often compared to such popular bulking agents as testosterone or Dianabol, but without the same estrogen-related side effects. It is most commonly identified as a lean-mass-building drug, and is extremely popular with athletes for its ability to promote the rapid buildup of strength, muscle size, and definition.

History:

The first long-acting trenbolone ester (undecanoate) was studied in 1967, described during a series of experiments into synthetic anabolic steroids by Roussel-UCLAF.[685] Trenbolone hexahydrobenzylcarbonate was a subsequent and uniquely French slant to this long-acting anabolic steroid, possessing an unusual but roughly equivalent compound. Trenbolone hexahydrobenzylcarbonate was developed into a medicine by Negma Laboratoires in France, which sold the drug under the Parabolan trade name. It was also sold for a period of time as Hexabolan, a name that referred to the unusual ester it possesses. Trenbolone hexahydrobenzylcarbonate is the only known form of trenbolone ever produced as a medicine for human consumption. The most notable appearance of trenbolone comes as trenbolone acetate, which is used widely and exclusively in veterinary medicine.

Parabolan was prescribed in France as a protein-sparing anabolic agent in cases of cachexia (lean body mass wasting) and malnutrition, as well as to combat certain forms of osteoporosis. Its prescribing guidelines included recommendations for the treatment of androgen-sensitive populations, such as women and the elderly. Owing to its moderate androgenic properties, however, the drug was contraindicated in children, especially young females. Parabolan remained on the French market for a very long time, although it was finally discontinued (voluntarily) by Negma in 1997. For a brief period of time it seemed that the demise of Parabolan would mark the end of human-use trenbolone preparations, as no other medicine approved for human use was known to exist worldwide at the time. A very small number of Parabolan preparations have been brought to market since, however, so while the drug is still poorly available, it is not completely defunct.

How Supplied:

Trenbolone hexahydrobenzylcarbonate is no longer produced as a prescription drug product. When manufactured in France it came in the form of a 1.5 mL ampule containing 76mg of steroid (product information lists this as equivalent to 50 mg of base trenbolone).

Structural Characteristics:

Trenbolone is a modified form of nandrolone. It differs by the introduction of double bonds at carbons 9 and 11, which inhibit aromatization (9-ene), increase androgen-binding affinity,[686] and slows its metabolism. The resulting steroid is significantly more potent as both an anabolic and an androgen than its nandrolone base. The trenbolone here is modified with a hexahydrobenzylcarbonate ester at the 17-beta hydroxyl group, so that the free steroid is released more slowly from the area of injection.

Side Effects (Estrogenic):

Trenbolone is not aromatized by the body, and is not measurably estrogenic. It is of note, however, that this steroid displays significant binding affinity for the progesterone receptor (slightly stronger than progesterone itself).[687][688] The side effects associated with progesterone are similar to those of estrogen, including negative feedback inhibition of testosterone production and enhanced rate of fat storage. Progestins also augment the stimulatory effect of estrogens on mammary tissue growth. There appears to be a strong synergy between these two hormones here, such that gynecomastia might even occur with the help of progestins, without excessive estrogen levels. The use of an anti-estrogen, which inhibits the estrogenic component of this disorder, is often sufficient to mitigate gynecomastia caused by progestational anabolic/androgenic steroids. Note that progestational side effects are more common when trenbolone is being taken with other aromatizable steroids.

Side Effects (Androgenic):

Although classified as an anabolic steroid, trenbolone is sufficiently androgenic. Androgenic side effects are still common with this substance, and may include bouts of oily skin, acne, and body/facial hair growth. Anabolic/androgenic steroids may also aggravate male pattern hair loss. Women are also warned of the potential virilizing effects of anabolic/androgenic steroids. These may include a deepening of the voice, menstrual irregularities, changes in skin texture, facial hair growth, and clitoral enlargement. Additionally, the 5-alpha reductase enzyme does not metabolize trenbolone[689], so its relative androgenicity is not affected by finasteride or dutasteride.

Side Effects (Hepatotoxicity):

Trenbolone is not c-17 alpha alkylated, and is generally not considered a hepatotoxic steroid; liver toxicity is unlikely. This steroid does have a strong level of resistance to hepatic breakdown, however, and severe liver toxicity has been noted in bodybuilders abusing trenbolone.[690] Although unlikely, hepatotoxicity cannot be completely excluded, especially with high doses.

Side Effects (Cardiovascular):

Anabolic/androgenic steroids can have deleterious effects on serum cholesterol. This includes a tendency to reduce HDL (good) cholesterol values and increase LDL (bad) cholesterol values, which may shift the HDL to LDL balance in a direction that favors greater risk of arteriosclerosis. The relative impact of an anabolic/androgenic steroid on serum lipids is dependant on the dose, route of administration (oral vs. injectable), type of steroid (aromatizable or non-aromatizable), and level of resistance to hepatic metabolism. Due to its non-aromatizable nature and strong resistance to metabolism, trenbolone has a moderate to strong (negative) impact on lipid values and atherogenic risk. Anabolic/androgenic steroids may also adversely affect blood pressure and triglycerides, reduce endothelial relaxation, and support left ventricular hypertrophy, all potentially increasing the risk of cardiovascular disease and myocardial infarction.

To help reduce cardiovascular strain it is advised to maintain an active cardiovascular exercise program and minimize the intake of saturated fats, cholesterol, and simple carbohydrates at all times during active AAS administration. Supplementing with fish oils (4 grams per day) and a natural cholesterol/antioxidant formula such as Lipid Stabil or a product with comparable ingredients is also recommended.

Side Effects (Testosterone Suppression):

All anabolic/androgenic steroids when taken in doses sufficient to promote muscle gain are expected to suppress endogenous testosterone production. Without the intervention of testosterone-stimulating substances, testosterone levels should return to normal within 1-4 months of drug secession. Note that prolonged hypogonadotrophic hypogonadism can develop secondary to steroid abuse, necessitating medical intervention. In experimental studies, trenbolone was determined to be approximately three times stronger at suppressing gonadotropins than testosterone on a milligram for milligram basis.

The above side effects are not inclusive. For more detailed discussion of potential side effects, see the Steroid Side Effects section of this book.

Administration (Men):

Trenbolone hexahydrobenzylcarbonate was generally administered in a clinical dosage of 3 ampules per month. Therapy was initiated the first month with all 3 ampules given over the first 15 days. During the subsequent 3 months, one injection (76 mg) was given every 10 days. For physique- or performance-enhancing purposes, trenbolone hexahydrobenzylcarbonate is most often administered at a dosage of 152-220 mg per week. The drug would be taken in cycles ranging from 6 to 12 weeks. Although a weekly administration schedule would be more than sufficient, athletes usually injected a single ampule (76mg) at a time, and the total amount would be spread evenly throughout the week. Although not necessary, this type of schedule helps to reduce injection volume per application. The results with the use of trenbolone hexahydrobenzylcarbonate should be a visibly more muscular physique (larger, leaner), and, if body fat levels are low enough, that hard ripped look most valued by dieting and competitive bodybuilders.

While this drug is quite potent when used alone, it is sometimes combined with other steroids for an even greater effect. Leading up to a show one could successfully add a non-aromatizing anabolic such as Winstrol® or Primobolan®. Such combinations will elicit a greater level of density and hardness to the build, often proving dramatic for a stage appearance. We could also look for bulk with this drug, and addition stronger compounds like Dianabol or Testosterone. While the mass gain would be quite formidable with such a stack, some level of water retention would probably also accompany it. Moderately effective anabolics such Deca-Durabolin® or Equipoise® would be somewhat of a halfway point, providing extra strength and mass but without the same level of water bloat we see with more readily aromatized steroids.

Administration (Women):

Trenbolone hexahydrobenzylcarbonate was generally administered in a clinical dosage of 3 ampules per month. Therapy was initiated the first month with all 3 ampules given over the first 15 days. During the subsequent 3 months, one injection (76mg) was given every 10 days. Given the risk of virilization, lower doses were likely used by physicians with many female patients. This agent is generally not recommended for women for physique- or performance-enhancing purposes due to strong androgenic nature and tendency to produce virilizing side effects.

Availability:

Trenbolone hexahydrobenzylcarbonate is no longer made as a prescription drug product. It is presently only manufactured by underground laboratories.

Perandren (testosterone phenylacetate)

Androgenic	100
Anabolic	100
Standard	Standard
Chemical Names	4-androsten-3-one-17beta-ol
	17beta-hydroxy-androst-4-en-3-one
Estrogenic Activity	moderate
Progestational Activity	low

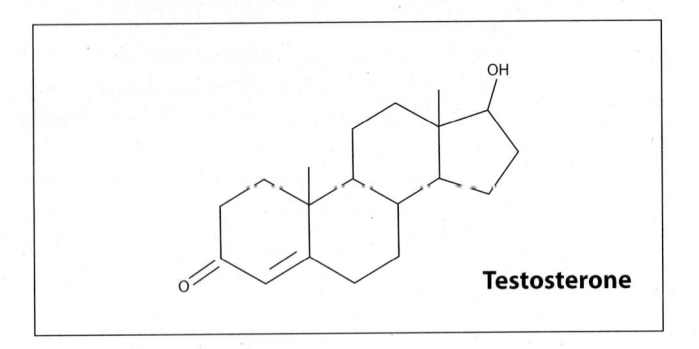

Description:

Testosterone phenylacetate is an injectable form of the primary male androgen testosterone. This compound uses a phenylacetate ester to extend the biological activity of testosterone, which is very similar in structure to phenylpropionate. It is a short chain ester of testosterone, although was designed in this case to have a protracted effect in the body similar to testosterone cypionate or enanthate. As an injectable testosterone, testosterone phenylacetate is a powerful mass-building drug, capable of producing rapid gains in both muscle size and strength.

History:

Testosterone phenylacetate was developed by Ciba during the 1960's, the same company to introduce Dianabol (methandrostenolone) to the world. This steroid was sold in the U.S. under the brand name of Perandren® phenylacetate, which incidentally had used the same Perandren name that Ciba had designated for its testosterone propionate years earlier (Perandren® propionate). At the time of its release, Perandren phenylacetate was intended to offer improvements over other esters of testosterone, most notably a longer window of therapeutic effect following each injection. Product information on the drug from 1967 reads, "[Perandren phenylacetate] Has a more prolonged action than other androgens and a markedly greater intensity of effect; in adequate dosage, a single injection per month suffices for many patients."

Early prescribing guidelines for testosterone phenylacetate called for a number of therapeutic uses. It was mainly applied to cases of male androgen insufficiency, and those issues normally surrounding low testosterone levels such as reduced sex drive and impotence in adults, and cryptorchidism (undescended testicles) in teenagers and young adults. But it also had such other uses as treating osteoporosis, menorrhagia (heavy menstrual bleeding), metrorrhagia (abnormal bleeding of the uterus), and breast cancer. It was also used to offset the catabolic effects of corticosteroids, to heal fractures, to promote wellness following surgery or convalescence, and as a general tissue-repairing anabolic when needed.

The life of Perandren phenylacetate on the U.S. prescription drug market was ultimately a short one. By the late 1960's, other "new" esters of testosterone were also widely available, namely testosterone cypionate and enanthate, and Ciba's slow-acting creation was quickly losing market share to these agents. These esters of testosterone offered a similar period of therapeutic benefit to Perandren phenylacetate, but with considerably more patient comfort (they did not need to be mixed with anesthetic for injections to be semi-tolerable like Perandren phenylacetate). As a result of this shift in consumer interest, Ciba withdrew this product from market. By 1970, Perandren phenylacetate was no longer available.

How Supplied:

Testosterone phenylacetate is no longer commercially available. When produced, it contained 50 mg/ml of steroid in a water-based solution.

Structural Characteristics:

Testosterone phenylacetate is a modified form of testosterone, where a carboxylic acid ester (acetic acid phenyl ester) has been attached to the 17-beta hydroxyl group. Esterified forms of testosterone are less polar than free testosterone, and are absorbed more slowly from the area of injection. Once in the bloodstream, the ester is removed to yield free (active) testosterone. Esterified forms of testosterone are designed to prolong the window of therapeutic effect following administration, allowing for a less frequent injection schedule compared to injections of free (unesterified) steroid.

Side Effects (Estrogenic):

Testosterone is readily aromatized in the body to estradiol (estrogen). The aromatase (estrogen synthetase) enzyme is responsible for this metabolism of testosterone. Elevated estrogen levels can cause side effects such as increased water retention, body fat gain, and gynecomastia. Testosterone is considered a moderately estrogenic steroid. An anti-estrogen such as clomiphene citrate or tamoxifen citrate may be necessary to prevent estrogenic side effects. One may alternately use an aromatase inhibitor like Arimidex® (anastrozole), which more efficiently controls estrogen by preventing its synthesis. Aromatase inhibitors can be quite expensive in comparison to anti-estrogens, however, and may also have negative effects on blood lipids.

Estrogenic side effects will occur in a dose-dependant manner, with higher doses (above normal therapeutic levels) of testosterone more likely to require the concurrent use of an anti-estrogen or aromatase inhibitor. Since water retention and loss of muscle definition are common with higher doses of testosterone, this drug is usually considered a poor choice for dieting or cutting phases of training. Its moderate estrogenicity makes it more ideal for bulking phases, where the added water retention will support raw strength and muscle size, and help foster a stronger anabolic environment.

Side Effects (Androgenic):

Testosterone is the primary male androgen, responsible for maintaining secondary male sexual characteristics. Elevated levels of testosterone are likely to produce androgenic side effects including oily skin, acne, and body/facial hair growth. Men with a genetic predisposition for hair loss (androgenetic alopecia) may notice accelerated male pattern balding. Those concerned about hair loss may find a more comfortable option in nandrolone decanoate, which is a comparably less androgenic steroid. Women are warned of the potential virilizing effects of anabolic/androgenic steroids, especially with a strong androgen such as testosterone. These may include deepening of the voice, menstrual irregularities, changes in skin texture, facial hair growth, and clitoral enlargement.

In androgen-responsive target tissues such as the skin, scalp, and prostate, the high relative androgenicity of testosterone is dependant on its reduction to dihydrotestosterone (DHT). The 5-alpha reductase enzyme is responsible for this metabolism of testosterone. The concurrent use of a 5-alpha reductase inhibitor such as finasteride or dutasteride will interfere with site-specific potentiation of testosterone action, lowering the tendency of testosterone drugs to produce androgenic side effects. It is important to remember that anabolic and androgenic effects are both mediated via the cytosolic androgen receptor. Complete separation of testosterone's anabolic and androgenic properties is not possible, even with total 5-alpha reductase inhibition.

Side Effects (Hepatotoxicity):

Testosterone does not have hepatotoxic effects; liver toxicity is unlikely. One study examined the potential for hepatotoxicity with high doses of testosterone by administering 400 mg of the hormone per day (2,800 mg per week) to a group of male subjects. The steroid was taken orally so that higher peak concentrations would be reached in hepatic tissues compared to intramuscular injections. The hormone was given daily for 20 days, and produced no significant changes in liver enzyme values including serum albumin, bilirubin, alanine-amino-transferase, and alkaline phosphatases.[691]

Side Effects (Cardiovascular):

Anabolic/androgenic steroids can have deleterious effects on serum cholesterol. This includes a tendency to reduce HDL (good) cholesterol values and increase LDL (bad) cholesterol values, which may shift the HDL to LDL balance in a direction that favors greater risk of arteriosclerosis. The relative impact of an anabolic/androgenic steroid on serum lipids is dependant on the dose, route of administration (oral vs. injectable), type of steroid (aromatizable or non-aromatizable), and level of resistance to hepatic metabolism. Anabolic/androgenic steroids may also adversely affect blood pressure and triglycerides, reduce endothelial relaxation, and support left ventricular hypertrophy, all potentially increasing the risk of cardiovascular disease and myocardial infarction.

Testosterone tends to have a much less dramatic impact on cardiovascular risk factors than synthetic steroids. This is due in part to its openness to metabolism by the liver, which allows it to have less effect on the hepatic management of cholesterol. The aromatization of testosterone to estradiol also helps to mitigate the negative effects of androgens on serum lipids. In one study, 280 mg per week of testosterone ester (enanthate) had a slight but not statistically significant effect on HDL cholesterol after 12 weeks, but when taken with an aromatase inhibitor a strong (25%) decrease was seen.[692] Studies using 300 mg of testosterone ester (enanthate) per week for 20 weeks without an aromatase inhibitor demonstrated only a 13% decrease in HDL cholesterol, while at 600 mg the reduction reached 21%.[693] The negative impact of aromatase inhibition should be taken into consideration before such drug is added to testosterone therapy.

Due to the positive influence of estrogen on serum lipids, tamoxifen citrate or clomiphene citrate are preferred to aromatase inhibitors for those concerned with cardiovascular health, as they offer a partial estrogenic effect in the liver. This allows them to potentially improve lipid profiles and offset some of the negative effects of androgens. With doses of 600 mg or less of testosterone per week, the impact on lipid profile tends to be noticeable but not dramatic, making an anti-estrogen (for cardioprotective purposes) perhaps unnecessary. Doses of 600 mg or less per week have also failed to produce statistically significant changes in LDL/VLDL cholesterol, triglycerides, apolipoprotein B/C-III, C-reactive protein, and insulin sensitivity, all indicating a relatively weak impact on cardiovascular risk factors.[694] When used in moderate doses, injectable testosterone esters are usually considered to be the safest of all anabolic/androgenic steroids.

To help reduce cardiovascular strain it is advised to maintain an active cardiovascular exercise program and minimize the intake of saturated fats, cholesterol, and simple carbohydrates at all times during active AAS administration. Supplementing with fish oils (4 grams per day) and a natural cholesterol/antioxidant formula such as Lipid Stabil or a product with comparable ingredients is also recommended.

Side Effects (Testosterone Suppression):

All anabolic/androgenic steroids when taken in doses sufficient to promote muscle gain are expected to suppress endogenous testosterone production. Testosterone is the primary male androgen, and offers strong negative feedback on endogenous testosterone production. Testosterone-based drugs will, likewise, have a strong effect on the hypothalamic regulation of natural steroid hormones. Without the intervention of testosterone-stimulating substances, testosterone levels should return to normal within 1-4 months of drug secession. Note that prolonged hypogonadotrophic hypogonadism can develop secondary to steroid abuse, necessitating medical intervention.

The above side effects are not inclusive. For more detailed discussion of potential side effects, see the Steroid Side Effects section of this book.

Administration (General):

The design of testosterone phenylacetate (as Perandren phenylacetate) was slightly different than that of most testosterone esters, which are usually made as oily solutions. Phenylacetate instead contained a microcrystalline aqueous suspension. The crystals would form a repository in the muscle following injection, where they would slowly dissolve over time. Product information on Perandren phenylacetate stated that injections could result in local irritation, pain, and redness. To help offset the discomfort associated with injection, each vial contained 1% procaine by weight, which acted as a local anesthetic. Although this was an effective method of delivering testosterone over time, patient comfort was likely not ideal with this formulation.

Administration (Men):

To treat androgen insufficiency, early prescribing guidelines recommended a dosage of 50 mg to 200 mg given every 3 to 5 weeks. An adequate dosage among male athletes would be in the range of 200 mg to 400 mg per week. Although active for longer periods of time, weekly injections would be preferred due to the low dosage and tendency for pain at the site of injection (large injection volumes would not be advised). The total weekly dosage may need to be further subdivided into two or more separate injections. A 200-400 mg per week dosage level would be sufficient for most users to notice exceptional gains in muscle size and strength.

Administration (Women):

Product information for Perandren phenylacetate recommended no more than 150 mg per month for women, so as to avoid virilizing side effects. In modern clinical medicine, testosterone compounds are rarely used with women. Testosterone phenylacetate is not recommended for women for physique- or performance-enhancing purposes due to its strong androgenic nature and tendency to produce virilizing side effects.

Availability:

Testosterone phenylacetate is no longer commercially available. The raw material is available from certain manufacturers, and may turn up in black market (underground) preparations.

Primobolan® (methenolone acetate)

Androgenic	44-57
Anabolic	88
Standard	Testosterone
Chemical Names	17beta-Hydroxy-1-methyl-5alpha-androst-1-en-3-one
	1-methyl-1(5-alpha)-androsten-3-one-17b-ol
Estrogenic Activity	none
Progestational Activity	no data available (low)

Methenolone

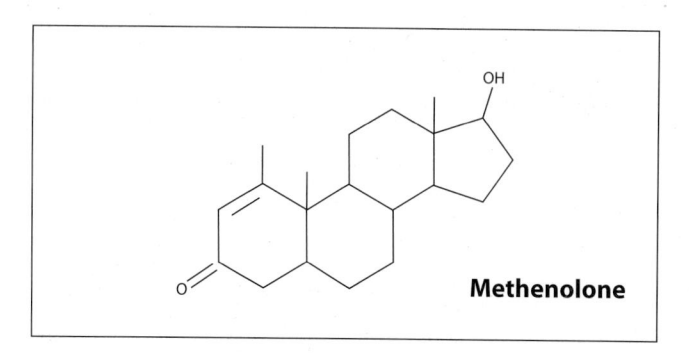

Description:

Primobolan® is a brand name for the anabolic steroid methenolone acetate. This agent is very similar in action to Primobolan® Depot (methenolone enanthate), except here the drug is designed for oral administration instead of injection. Methenolone acetate is a non-c17-alpha-alkylated oral steroid, one of only a few commercially available oral agents that presents limited liver toxicity to the user. It is also highly favored for its properties as a moderately effective anabolic with low androgenic and no estrogenic properties. It is, likewise, commonly used during cutting phases of training, when lean tissue growth and solid muscularity, not raw bulk, are the key objectives.

History:

Methenolone was first described in 1960.[695] Squibb would introduce the drug (as methenolone acetate) to the United States in 1962.[696] This agent was sold for a very short time as a 20 mg tablet, under the brand name of Nibal®. Schering in West Germany would be granted rights to the drug that same year, and would sell it under the Primobolan® name. Nibal® was soon removed from the U.S. market, never to return as a commercial product. Schering now had exclusive patent rights to produce methenolone acetate, and would continue to sell the drug uninterrupted since 1962, and consumers had naturally come to identify methenolone acetate as a product of Schering.

Primobolan® has always been identified as a European steroid, and during the 1960's and '70's was being offered for sale in such countries as Germany, Austria, Belgium, France, the Netherlands, and Finland. At one time Schering also manufactured a 20 mg/ml oil-based injectable of methenolone acetate in limited markets (called Primobolan® Acetate), but it has been out of manufacture since 1993. Injectable methenolone acetate proved to be very popular for pre-contest cutting use, and was gravely missed among European competitors when discontinued. Although we still have the acetate in oral form, it is a close, but not equal, substitute (injection is a much more efficient form of delivery for this steroid).

Primobolan® is prescribed as a lean tissue building anabolic agent, often used in cases where body wasting has occurred secondary to major surgery, infection, wasting disease, aggressive corticosteroid administration, or malnutrition. (Some clinicians also prescribe this agent for treating osteoporosis and sarcopenia, or the natural loss of muscle mass with aging). This steroid has also been used to promote weight gain in underweight premature infants and children in clinical studies, and was able to do so effectively and without signs of toxicity or undesirable effects.[697] Athletes have long favored the combined strong anabolic, weak androgenic, and non-estrogenic nature of this drug, which makes it very desirable for building lean muscularity without side effects.

Although Primobolan® demonstrated a good record of clinical safety, Schering has since withdrawn this drug from most of the markets it was originally sold in. No 50 mg versions are still in manufacture, and all but a select couple of products containing 5 mg and 25 mg are left in circulation. The only confirmed sources for oral Primobolan in recent years were in Japan and South Africa. In spite of its almost nonexistent availability, Schering remains the sole producer of methenolone acetate in the human drug business worldwide, perhaps due to the fact that it had defended its patent rights so well for so many years.

How Supplied:

All forms of Schering Primobolan® contain 5 mg, 25 mg, or 50 mg (no longer available) of methenolone acetate per tablet. Composition and dosage of other brands may vary by country and manufacturer.

Structural Characteristics:

Methenolone is a derivative of dihydrotestosterone. It

contains one additional double bond between carbons 1 and 2, which helps to stabilize the 3-keto group and increase the steroid's anabolic properties, and an additional 1-methyl group, which protects the steroid against hepatic metabolism. Primobolan makes use of methenolone with a carboxylic acid ester (acetic acid) attached to the 17-beta hydroxyl group to further help protect it from oxidation during oral administration. Studies have demonstrated the methenolone is an effective oral anabolic agent in both the acetate and unesterified forms.[698][699]

Side Effects (Estrogenic):

Methenolone is not aromatized by the body,[700] and is not measurably estrogenic. Estrogen-linked side effects should not be seen when administering this steroid. Sensitive individuals need not worry about developing gynecomastia, nor should they be noticing any appreciable water retention with this drug. The increase seen with methenolone should be quality muscle mass, not the smooth bulk that often accompanies steroids open to aromatization. During a cycle, the user should additionally not notice strong elevations in blood pressure, as this effect is also related (generally) to estrogen and water retention. Methenolone is a steroid most favored during cutting phases of training, when water and fat retention are major concerns, and sheer mass not the central objective.

Side Effects (Androgenic):

Although classified as an anabolic steroid, androgenic side effects are still possible with this substance. This may include bouts of oily skin, acne, and body/facial hair growth. Anabolic/androgenic steroids may also aggravate male pattern hair loss. Women are warned of the potential virilizing effects of anabolic/androgenic steroids. These may include a deepening of the voice, menstrual irregularities, changes in skin texture, facial hair growth, and clitoral enlargement. Methenolone is still a very mild steroid, however, and strong androgenic side effects are typically related to higher doses. Women often find this preparation an acceptable choice, observing it to be a very comfortable and effective anabolic.

Side Effects (Hepatotoxicity):

Methenolone is not considered a hepatotoxic steroid; liver toxicity is unlikely. Studies have failed to produce appreciable changes in markers of hepatic stress when the drug was given in therapeutic levels.[701] This steroid does have some resistance to hepatic breakdown, however, and liver toxicity, failure, and death was reported in one elderly patient receiving oral methenolone acetate.[702] Although unlikely, hepatotoxicity cannot be completely excluded, especially with very high oral doses.

Side Effects (Cardiovascular):

Anabolic/androgenic steroids can have deleterious effects on serum cholesterol. This includes a tendency to reduce HDL (good) cholesterol values and increase LDL (bad) cholesterol values, which may shift the HDL to LDL balance in a direction that favors greater risk of arteriosclerosis. The relative impact of an anabolic/androgenic steroid on serum lipids is dependant on the dose, route of administration (oral vs. injectable), type of steroid (aromatizable or non-aromatizable), and level of resistance to hepatic metabolism. Methenolone should have a stronger negative effect on the hepatic management of cholesterol than testosterone or nandrolone due to its non-aromatizable nature, but a much weaker impact than c-17 alpha alkylated steroids. Due to the route of delivery, oral methenolone will have a slightly stronger negative effect on lipids compared to methenolone enanthate injections. Anabolic/androgenic steroids may also adversely affect blood pressure and triglycerides, reduce endothelial relaxation, and support left ventricular hypertrophy, all potentially increasing the risk of cardiovascular disease and myocardial infarction.

To help reduce cardiovascular strain it is advised to maintain an active cardiovascular exercise program and minimize the intake of saturated fats, cholesterol, and simple carbohydrates at all times during active AAS administration. Supplementing with fish oils (4 grams per day) and a natural cholesterol/antioxidant formula such as Lipid Stabil or a product with comparable ingredients is also recommended.

Side Effects (Testosterone Suppression):

All anabolic/androgenic steroids when taken in doses sufficient to promote muscle gain are expected to suppress endogenous testosterone production. Without the intervention of testosterone-stimulating substances, testosterone levels should return to normal within 1-4 months of drug secession. Note that prolonged hypogonadotrophic hypogonadism can develop secondary to steroid abuse, necessitating medical intervention. Primobolan® is generally described as having a low impact on endogenous testosterone production. While this may be true in small clinical doses (20-25 mg daily), this may not be a major distinction when used for physique- or performance-enhancing purposes. In one study, more than half of the patients receiving only 30-45 mg per day noticed a 15-65% suppression of gonadotropin levels.[703] While this is far from having no hormonal impact, the suppression caused by methenolone acetate may still be less pronounced than with many other agents. If Primobolan® is used at moderate doses for less than 8 weeks, hormonal recovery should not be a protracted experience.

The above side effects are not inclusive. For more detailed discussion of potential side effects, see the Steroid Side Effects section of this book.

Administration (General):

Studies have shown that taking an oral anabolic steroid with food may decrease its bioavailability.[704] This is caused by the fat-soluble nature of steroid hormones, which can allow some of the drug to dissolve with undigested dietary fat, reducing its absorption from the gastrointestinal tract. For maximum utilization, this steroid should be taken on an empty stomach.

Administration (Men):

The prescribing guidelines for Primobolan® recommend a maximum daily dosage of 100-150 mg per day. The usual administration protocols for physique- or performance-enhancing purposes call for 75-150 mg daily, which is taken for 6 to 8 weeks. This level is sufficient to impart a measurable anabolic effect, although one usually doesn't expect to achieve great gains in muscle mass with this drug. Instead, Primobolan® is utilized when the athlete has a specific need for a mild anabolic agent, most notably in cutting phases of training.

Due to its mild nature, Primobolan® is often used in conjunction with other steroids for a stronger effect. In such cases, a slightly lower dose is often used (50-100 mg per day). During a dieting or cutting phase, thought to be its primary application, a non-aromatizing androgen like Halotestin® or trenbolone is often added. Such combinations would enhance the physique without water retention, and help bring out a harder and more defined look of muscularity. Non-aromatizing androgen/anabolic stacks like this are very popular among competing bodybuilders, and prove quite reliable for rapidly improving the contest form. This compound is also occasionally used with more potent androgens during bulking phases of training. The addition of testosterone, Dianabol or Anadrol 50® is common, although the gains are often accompanied by some level of smoothness due to the added estrogenic component, as well as hepatotoxicity in the case of the latter two agents.

Administration (Women):

The prescribing guidelines for Primobolan® do not offer separate dosing recommendations for women, although it is indicated that women who are pregnant, or may become pregnant, should not use the drug. Female athletes generally respond well to 50-75 mg daily, with no signs of virilization symptoms. One would not expect a tremendous amount of muscle mass with this drug, and instead find a slow and steady (quality) increase. Some women choose to further add-in other anabolics such as Winstrol® or oxandrolone, in an effort to increase the muscle-building effectiveness of a cycle. While both of these compounds are quite tolerable, one must be sure not to use too high an accumulated dosage. Taken at too high a dosage, these weak anabolics can quickly cause masculinizing side effects.

Availability:

Methenolone acetate is scarcely produced as a legitimate pharmaceutical product. It is presently only sold in a select number of markets.

The only legitimate version of note comes from Balkan Pharmaceuticals in Moldova. It comes packaged in foil and plastic strips of 20 tablets each. Counterfeits are not known to be a problem.

Primobolan® Depot (methenolone enanthate)

Androgenic	44-57
Anabolic	88
Standard	Testosterone
Chemical Names	17beta-Hydroxy-1-methyl-5alpha-androst-1-en-3-one
	1-methyl-1(5-alpha)-androsten-3-one-17b-ol
Estrogenic Activity	none
Progestational Activity	no data available (low)

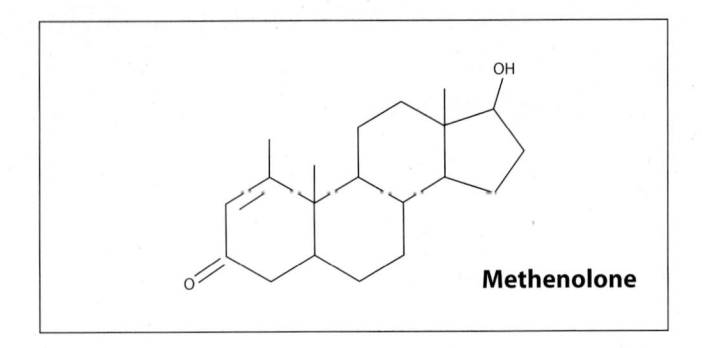

Methenolone

Description:

Primobolan® Depot is an injectable version of the steroid methenolone. This is the same constituent in Primobolan® orals (methenolone acetate), although here an enanthate ester is used to slow the steroid's release from a site of injection. Methenolone enanthate offers a similar pattern of steroid release as testosterone enanthate, with blood hormone levels remaining markedly elevated for approximately 2 weeks. Methenolone itself is a moderately strong anabolic steroid with very low androgenic properties. Its anabolic effect is considered to be slightly less than Deca-Durabolin® (nandrolone decanoate) on a milligram for milligram basis. Methenolone enanthate is most commonly used during cutting cycles, when lean mass gain, not a raw mass increase, is the main objective.

History:

Methenolone was first described in 1960.[705] Squibb introduced the drug (as methenolone enanthate) to the U.S. prescription drug market in 1962,[706] sold for a very short time in the U.S. under the brand name of Nibal® Depot. Rights to the drug were given to Schering in West Germany that same year, and Nibal® Depot soon disappeared from the U.S. market. Schering would sell methenolone enanthate under its new and ultimately most recognizable brand name, Primobolan® Depot. During the 1960's and '70's Primobolan® Depot was available mainly in Europe, including such countries as Switzerland, Italy, Germany, Austria, Belgium, France, Portugal, and Greece.

Schering maintained patent control over methenolone enanthate until the late 1970's. Before its patents expired, Schering had rigorously protected its intellectual property rights against any potential infringement, even in the U.S. market, where the company had not been marketing Primobolan Depot. Although methenolone enanthate has not been available for commercial sale in the United States for decades, it has technically retained its status as an FDA-approved drug. This has allowed some U.S. doctors to import Primobolan Depot for their patients, and at least one U.S. private compounding pharmacy to resume the production of a generic form, which is now obtainable on special order from a licensed doctor.

Primobolan Depot is typically prescribed as a lean tissue building anabolic agent, often used in cases where body wasting has occurred secondary to an operation, prolonged infection, wasting disease, aggressive corticosteroid administration, or convalescence. Some clinicians also prescribe this agent for treating osteoporosis, sarcopenia (the natural loss of muscle mass with aging), certain cases of chronic hepatitis, and breast carcinoma (usually as a secondary medication following other therapies). The steroid has also been used to promote weight gain in underweight premature infants and children in clinical studies, and was able to do so effectively and without signs of toxicity or undesirable effects.[707] Athletes have long favored the combined strong anabolic, weak androgenic, and non-estrogenic nature of this drug, which makes it very desirable for building lean muscularity without side effects.

Although Primobolan Depot demonstrated a good record of clinical safety, by the 1990's Schering had grown to be a multinational pharmaceutical giant, and was inevitably forced to reexamine its global steroid offerings in light of public concerns about sports doping. Primobolan Depot would be voluntarily withdrawn from most of the countries that had originally sold it. Today, the brand is sold in just a handful of countries including Spain, Turkey, Japan, Paraguay, and Ecuador. In spite of its limited supply, Schering remains the sole producer of methenolone enanthate in the human drug business worldwide. In recent years, however, methenolone enanthate has shown up in a small number of veterinary, export, and underground steroid preparations.

How Supplied:

All forms of Schering Primobolan® Depot are packaged in 1 mL glass ampules and contain 100 mg of methenolone enanthate. Composition and dosage of other brands may vary by country and manufacturer.

Structural Characteristics:

Methenolone is a derivative of dihydrotestosterone. It contains one additional double bond between carbons 1 and 2, which helps to stabilize the 3-keto group and increase the steroid's anabolic properties, and an additional 1-methyl group, which gives the steroid some protection against hepatic metabolism. Primobolan Depot makes use of methenolone with a carboxylic acid ester (enanthoic acid) attached to the 17-beta hydroxyl group. Esterified steroids are less polar than free steroids, and are absorbed more slowly from the area of injection. Once in the bloodstream, the ester is removed to yield free (active) methenolone. Esterified steroids are designed to prolong the window of therapeutic effect following administration, allowing for a less frequent injection schedule compared to injections of free (unesterified) steroid.

Side Effects (Estrogenic):

Methenolone is not aromatized by the body,[708] and is not measurably estrogenic. Estrogen-linked side effects should not be seen when administering this steroid. Sensitive individuals need not worry about developing gynecomastia, nor should they be noticing any appreciable water retention with this drug. The increase seen with methenolone should be quality muscle mass, not the smooth bulk that often accompanies steroids open to aromatization. During a cycle, the user should additionally not notice strong elevations in blood pressure, as this effect is also related (generally) to estrogen and water retention. Methenolone is a steroid most favored during cutting phases of training, when water and fat retention are major concerns, and sheer mass not the central objective.

Side Effects (Androgenic):

Although classified as an anabolic steroid, androgenic side effects are still possible with this substance. This may include bouts of oily skin, acne, and body/facial hair growth. Anabolic/androgenic steroids may also aggravate male pattern hair loss. Women are warned of the potential virilizing effects of anabolic/androgenic steroids. These may include a deepening of the voice, menstrual irregularities, changes in skin texture, facial hair growth, and clitoral enlargement. Methenolone is still a very mild steroid, however, and strong androgenic side effects are typically related to higher doses. Women often find this preparation an acceptable choice, observing it to be a very comfortable and effective anabolic.

Side Effects (Hepatotoxicity):

Methenolone is not considered a hepatotoxic steroid; liver toxicity is unlikely. Studies have failed to produce appreciable changes in markers of hepatic stress when the drug was given in therapeutic levels.[709]

Side Effects (Cardiovascular):

Anabolic/androgenic steroids can have deleterious effects on serum cholesterol. This includes a tendency to reduce HDL (good) cholesterol values and increase LDL (bad) cholesterol values, which may shift the HDL to LDL balance in a direction that favors greater risk of arteriosclerosis. The relative impact of an anabolic/androgenic steroid on serum lipids is dependant on the dose, route of administration (oral vs. injectable), type of steroid (aromatizable or non-aromatizable), and level of resistance to hepatic metabolism. Methenolone should have a stronger negative effect on the hepatic management of cholesterol than testosterone or nandrolone due to its non-aromatizable nature, but a much weaker impact than c-17 alpha alkylated steroids. Anabolic/androgenic steroids may also adversely affect blood pressure and triglycerides, reduce endothelial relaxation, and support left ventricular hypertrophy, all potentially increasing the risk of cardiovascular disease and myocardial infarction.

To help reduce cardiovascular strain it is advised to maintain an active cardiovascular exercise program and minimize the intake of saturated fats, cholesterol, and simple carbohydrates at all times during active AAS administration. Supplementing with fish oils (4 grams per day) and a natural cholesterol/antioxidant formula such as Lipid Stabil or a product with comparable ingredients is also recommended.

Side Effects (Testosterone Suppression):

All anabolic/androgenic steroids when taken in doses sufficient to promote muscle gain are expected to suppress endogenous testosterone production. Without the intervention of testosterone-stimulating substances, testosterone levels should return to normal within 1-4 months of drug secession. Note that prolonged hypogonadotrophic hypogonadism can develop secondary to steroid abuse, necessitating medical intervention. At a moderate dosage of 100-200 mg weekly, methenolone should offer measurably less testosterone suppression than an equal dose of nandrolone or testosterone, due to its non-aromatizable nature. If used for less than eight weeks, hormonal recovery should not be a protracted experience.

The above side effects are not inclusive. For more detailed discussion of potential side effects, see the Steroid Side Effects section of this book.

Administration (Men):

The prescribing guidelines for Primobolan Depot recommend a maximum dosage of 200 mg at the onset of therapy, and a continuing dosage of 100 mg every week. Prolonged administration protocols generally call for a 100 mg dosage every 1-2 weeks, or 200 mg every 2-3 weeks. The usual administration protocols among male athletes call for a 200-400 mg per week dosage, which is taken for 6 to 12 weeks, which is sufficient to promote very noticeable increases in lean muscle tissue. It is, however, not unusual to see the drug taken in doses as high as 600 mg per week or more, although such amounts are likely to highlight a more androgenic side of methenolone, as well as exacerbate its negative effects on serum lipids.

Methenolone enanthate is often stacked with other (typically stronger) steroids in order to obtain a faster and more enhanced effect. During a dieting or cutting phase, a non-aromatizing androgen like Halotestin® or trenbolone can be added. The stronger androgenic component here should help to bring about an added density and hardness to the muscles. On the other hand, one might add another mild anabolic steroid such as stanozolol. The result of such a combination should again be a notable increase in muscle mass and hardness, which still should not be accompanied by greatly increased side effects. Methenolone enanthate is also used effectively during bulking phases of training. In such a scenario, the addition of testosterone or boldenone would prove quite effective for adding new muscle mass without presenting any notable hepatotoxicity to the user.

Administration (Women):

The prescribing guidelines for Primobolan® Depot do not offer separate dosing recommendations for women, although it was indicated that women who were pregnant, or may become pregnant, should not use the drug. Female athletes generally respond well to a dosage of 50-100 mg per week. If both oral and injectable versions are available, the oral is often given preference, as it allows for greater control over blood hormone levels. Additionally, some women choose to include Winstrol® Depot (25 mg twice per week) or Oxandrolone (7.5-10 mg daily), and with it receive a greatly enhanced anabolic effect. Androgenic activity can be a concern with such dosing, however, and should be monitored closely. If stacking, it would be best to use a much lower starting dosage for each drug than if they were to be used alone. This is especially good advice if you are unfamiliar with the effect such a combination may have on you. A popular recommendation would also be to first experiment by stacking with oral Primobolan®, and later venture into the injectable if this is still necessary.

Availability:

The situation with injectable Primobolan® Depot is similar to that of the oral Primobolan® tablets. The drug is available, but not as abundantly as it was a few years ago. Schering has been actively discontinuing this drug in most of the markets around the world. The only major source countries for genuine Schering Primobolan Depot right now are Spain and Turkey. There are many counterfeits of both items, so be cautious to purchase these products only after careful examination.

To help differentiate real Turkish Primobolan® Depot from the many counterfeits, here are a couple of things to look at. First, open the bottom flap of the box. It should be cut at an unusual angle, and will not be even left to right like a normal box flap. Many of the more popular fakes missed this, probably for lack of a proper cutting dye. However, at least one counterfeiter has correctly copied this. Another good point of detail to look at is the Schering logo, which is found on the box and product insert. The counterfeiters tend to show the ribbon in the center of the Schering logo as one filled block < symbol. The correct logo has this ribbon with a small cut where the top and bottom lines intersect, as if to show that the top ribbon is resting on the bottom. This small detail is probably lost when the original box and insert were scanned into a computer by the illicit operation. Looking towards the ampule, first take notice of the lot number and manufacture date (not the expiration date). The first number in the lot always corresponds with the year the drug was made. Many of the fakes thus far have missed this trait, and these digits do not match.

In regards to Spanish Primobolan® Depot, this is also a high-profile item for counterfeiters. There have been many fakes circulating the past several years, often in large numbers. Be sure to purchase this product only if you can verify it was dispensed by a pharmacy.

Balkan Pharmaceuticals from Moldova makes a 100 mg/mL methenolone enanthate called Primobol. It comes in 1 mL ampules. Counterfeiting is not known to be a problem.

Promagnon (chloromethylandrostenediol)

Androgenic	no data available
Anabolic	no data available
Standard	Methyltestosterone (oral)
Chemical Name	4-chloro-17alpha-methyl-4-androstene-3,17beta-diol
Estrogenic Activity	none
Progestational Activity	no data available (low)

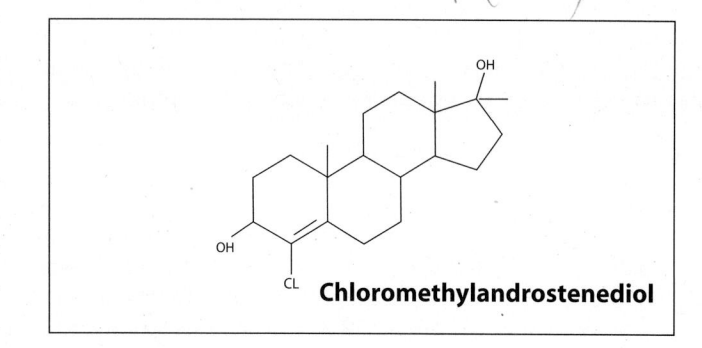

Description:

Chloromethylandrostenediol (CMA) is an oral anabolic steroid derived from testosterone. This agent is closest in structure to chloromethyltestosterone, which is a non-aromatizable and milder analog of methyltestosterone. In animal assays chloromethyltestosterone displayed about 30-50% of the anabolic activity of methyltestosterone, with about 10% of the accompanying androgenic activity. CMA, however, carries a 3-beta hydroxyl group instead of the common 3-keto that facilitates receptor binding, which makes it somewhat weaker than chloromethyltestosterone in comparison. Normal metabolic pathways should yield some amount of chloromethyltestosterone after ingestion, although most of the activity we see with this steroid is expected to be intrinsic. Chloromethylandrostenediol is a primarily anabolic but fairly weak steroid milligram for milligram, although it does possess enough potency to be an effective lean mass building drug.

History:

Chloromethylandrostenediol appears to be a new chemical entity, although its structure is fairly basic in light of other similar steroids. The drug was first described in 2005, when a new company called Peak Performance Laboratories introduced it to the U.S. supplement market under the brand name Promagnon. This steroid product was designed by Bruce Kneller, the same person that developed the widely selling and highly regarded designer compound Halodrol. Like Halodrol, Promagnon was considered a "grey market" product because it contained a steroid that was not specifically listed as a controlled substance in the U.S. It would, however, be considered an unapproved new drug in the eyes of the Food and Drug Administration, which by law cannot be sold. Although no specific action was taken against Peak Performance Laboratories for their sale of chloromethylandrostenediol, the company likely recognized that an FDA response would eventually come, and voluntarily discontinued the sale of Promagnon in late 2006.

How Supplied:

Chloromethylandrostenediol is not available as a prescription drug product. When manufactured as a supplement, it contained 25 mg of steroid per tablet.

Structural Characteristics:

Chloromethylandrostenediol is a modified form of testosterone. It differs by: 1) the addition of a methyl group at carbon 17-alpha, which helps protect the hormone during oral administration, 2) the attachment of a chloro group at carbon 4, which inhibits steroid aromatization and reduces relative androgenicity, and 3) the substitution of 3-keto with 3-hydroxyl, which reduces relative steroid activity.

Side Effects (Estrogenic):

Chloromethylandrostenediol is not aromatized by the body, and is not measurably estrogenic. An anti-estrogen is not necessary when using this steroid, as gynecomastia should not be a concern even among sensitive individuals. Since estrogen is the usual culprit with water retention, this steroid instead produces a lean, quality look to the physique with no fear of excess subcutaneous fluid retention. This makes it a favorable steroid to use during cutting cycles, when water and fat retention are major concerns.

Side Effects (Androgenic):

Although chloromethylandrostenediol is classified as an anabolic steroid, androgenic side effects are still possible with this substance. These may include bouts of oily skin, acne, and body/facial hair growth. Higher doses are more likely to cause such side effects. For those with a genetic predisposition, anabolic/androgenic steroids may also aggravate male pattern hair loss. Women are additionally warned of the potential virilizing effects of anabolic/androgenic steroids. These may include a deepening of the voice, menstrual irregularities, changes in skin texture, body and facial hair growth, and clitoral enlargement. Note that chloromethylandrostenediol is not extensively metabolized by the 5-alpha reductase enzyme, so its relative androgenicity is not greatly altered by the concurrent use of finasteride or dutasteride.

Side Effects (Hepatotoxicity):

Chloromethylandrostenediol is a c17-alpha alkylated compound. This alteration protects the drug from deactivation by the liver, allowing a very high percentage of the drug entry into the bloodstream following oral administration. C17-alpha alkylated anabolic/androgenic steroids can be hepatotoxic. Prolonged or high exposure may result in liver damage. In rare instances life-threatening dysfunction may develop. It is advisable to visit a physician periodically during each cycle to monitor liver function and overall health. Intake of c17-alpha alkylated steroids is commonly limited to 6-8 weeks, in an effort to avoid escalating liver strain.

The use of a liver detoxification supplement such as Liver Stabil, Liv-52, or Essentiale Forte is advised while taking any hepatotoxic anabolic/androgenic steroids.

Side Effects (Cardiovascular):

Anabolic/androgenic steroids can have deleterious effects on serum cholesterol. This includes a tendency to reduce HDL (good) cholesterol values and increase LDL (bad) cholesterol values, which may shift the HDL to LDL balance in a direction that favors greater risk of arteriosclerosis. The relative impact of an anabolic/androgenic steroid on serum lipids is dependant on the dose, route of administration (oral vs. injectable), type of steroid (aromatizable or non-aromatizable), and level of resistance to hepatic metabolism. Chloromethylandrostenediol has a strong effect on the hepatic management of cholesterol due to its non-aromatizable nature, structural resistance to liver breakdown, and route of administration. Anabolic/androgenic steroids may also adversely affect blood pressure and triglycerides, reduce endothelial relaxation, and support left ventricular hypertrophy, all potentially increasing the risk of cardiovascular disease and myocardial infarction.

To help reduce cardiovascular strain it is advised to maintain an active cardiovascular exercise program and minimize the intake of saturated fats, cholesterol, and simple carbohydrates at all times during active AAS administration. Supplementing with fish oils (4 grams per day) and a natural cholesterol/antioxidant formula such as Lipid Stabil or a product with comparable ingredients is also recommended.

Side Effects (Testosterone Suppression):

All anabolic/androgenic steroids when taken in doses sufficient to promote muscle gain are expected to suppress endogenous testosterone production. Without the intervention of testosterone stimulating substances, testosterone levels should return to normal within 1-4 months of drug secession. Note that prolonged hypogonadotrophic hypogonadism can develop secondary to steroid abuse, necessitating medical intervention.

The above side effects are not inclusive. For more detailed discussion of potential side effects, see the Steroid Side Effects section of this book.

Administration (General):

Studies have shown that taking an oral anabolic steroid with food may decrease its bioavailability . This is caused by the fat-soluble nature of steroid hormones, which can allow some of the drug to dissolve with undigested dietary fat, reducing its absorption from the gastrointestinal tract. For maximum utilization, this steroid should be taken on an empty stomach.

Administration (Men):

Chloromethylandrostenediol was never approved for use in humans. Prescribing guidelines are unavailable. When used for physique- or performance-enhancing purposes, an effective oral daily dosage falls in the range of 50-100 mg, taken in cycles lasting no more than 6-8 weeks to minimize hepatotoxicity. This level is sufficient for noticeable increases in lean muscle mass and strength. Higher doses will impart a stronger effect, but are also more likely to present significant hepatotoxicity.

Administration (Women):

Chloromethylandrostenediol was never approved for use in humans. Prescribing guidelines are unavailable. Although this drug is primarily anabolic in nature, safe dosage recommendations for women have not been established. This steroid is, therefore, generally not recommended to women for physique- or performance-enhancing purposes.

Availability:

Promagnon Is no longer available, although old lots may circulate on the black market. Several other generics or spin-off brands may also still be in circulation.

Prostanozol (demethylstanozolol tetrahydropyranyl)

Androgenic	no data available
Anabolic	no data available
Standard	no data available
Chemical Names	17beta-Hydroxy-5alpha-androstano[3,2-c]pyrazole
Estrogenic Activity	none
Progestational Activity	no data available

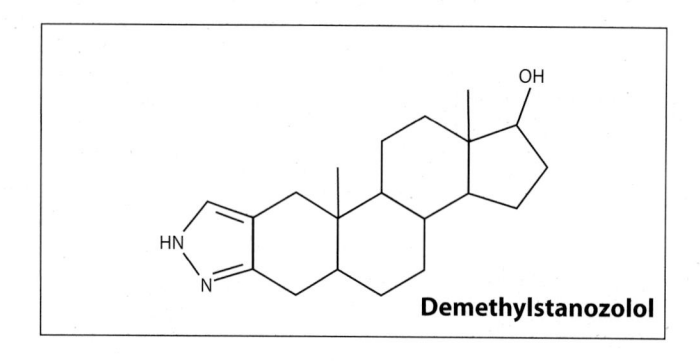

Description:

Prostanozol (demethylstanozolol THP) is an oral anabolic steroid closely related to Winstrol (stanozolol) in structure. It differs from stanozolol only by the removal of the c-17 alpha alkyl group, which undoubtedly hurts the oral bioavailability of this steroid. In an attempt to compensate for this, an ether group has been added. The ether increases oil solubility and the likelihood of lymphatic delivery with dietary fats, which bypass the first pass through the liver. This is the same principle on which Anabolicum Vister (quinbolone) was developed. In the case of Prostanozol, however, there is no oil carrier, which significantly lowers the chance for lymphatic delivery. This will necessitate a much higher oral dosage than would be needed otherwise. Among athletes, the drug is valued as a non-liver-toxic oral anabolic with properties qualitatively (although not quantitatively) similar to those of stanozolol.

History:

Demethylstanozolol appears to be a new chemical entity. If a non-methylated stanozolol were synthesized and assayed in the past, it could not be located. This steroid was introduced to the U.S. sports nutrition market in 2005 as a "post-ban" hormone, distributed openly as a "dietary supplement" instead of being regulated as a prescription drug. This is stemming from the fact that it was unknown to lawmakers at the time the 1991 and 2004 anabolic steroid laws were enacted, and as such simply could not be included in them. Although its legal status as a nutritional supplement may be in question (it is technically not found in the food supply, and therefore not a dietary food supplement), there are no U.S. criminal laws against its possession or use (yet).

Prostanozol is one of several legitimate synthetic anabolic/androgenic steroid products that hit the market in 2005. Later that year, however, the FDA and others in the government angrily acknowledged that there were new "designer steroids" on the supplement market, and made clear their intentions on investigating and even prosecuting those misbranding steroid products (drugs) as supplements. The original manufacturer (ALRI) quickly discontinued the sale of Prostanozol, anticipating FDA action. Other versions, such as Orastane-E by Gaspari Nutrition, have been discontinued as well. Given the threats of prosecution, it is unlikely that a major supplement manufacturer will risk introducing demethylstanozolol to market again. As such, this likely ended the commercial availability of this steroid.

How Supplied:

Demethylstanozolol is not available as a prescription drug product. When produced in the U.S. as a dietary supplement, it came in the form of a 25 mg capsule.

Structural Characteristics:

Demethylstanozolol is a modified form of dihydrotestosterone. It differs by the attachment of a pyrazol group to the A ring, replacing the normal 3-keto group (this gives demethylstanozolol the chemical classification of a heterocyclic steroid). Prostanozol contains demethylstanozolol with an ether (tetrahydropyranyl) attached to the 17-beta hydroxyl group, which slightly increases its oral bioavailability by facilitating absorption via the lymphatic route.

Side Effects (Estrogenic):

Demethylstanozolol is not aromatized by the body, and is not measurably estrogenic. An anti-estrogen is not necessary when using this steroid, as gynecomastia should not be a concern even among sensitive individuals. Since estrogen is the usual culprit with water retention, this steroid instead produces a lean, quality look to the physique with no fear of excess subcutaneous fluid retention. This makes it a favorable steroid to use during cutting cycles, when water and fat retention are major concerns.

Side Effects (Androgenic):

Although classified as an anabolic steroid, androgenic side effects are still common with this substance. This may include bouts of oily skin, acne, and body/facial hair growth. Anabolic/androgenic steroids may also aggravate male pattern hair loss. Women are also warned of the potential virilizing effects of anabolic/androgenic steroids. These may include a deepening of the voice, menstrual irregularities, changes in skin texture, facial hair growth, and clitoral enlargement. Additionally, the 5-alpha reductase enzyme does not metabolize demethylstanozolol, so its relative androgenicity is not affected by finasteride or dutasteride. Note that this steroid is relatively mild as an androgen, and much less likely to produce androgenic side effects than therapy with testosterone, methandrostenolone, or fluoxymesterone.

Side Effects (Hepatotoxicity):

Demethylstanozolol is not a c17-alpha alkylated compound, and is not known to have hepatotoxic effects; liker toxicity is unlikely.

Side Effects (Cardiovascular):

Anabolic/androgenic steroids can have deleterious effects on serum cholesterol. This includes a tendency to reduce HDL (good) cholesterol values and increase LDL (bad) cholesterol values, which may shift the HDL to LDL balance in a direction that favors greater risk of arteriosclerosis. The relative impact of an anabolic/androgenic steroid on serum lipids is dependant on the dose, route of administration (oral vs. injectable), type of steroid (aromatizable or non-aromatizable), and level of resistance to hepatic metabolism. Demethylstanozolol should have a stronger effect on the hepatic management of cholesterol than testosterone or nandrolone due to its non-aromatizable nature and route of administration. Anabolic/androgenic steroids may also adversely affect blood pressure and triglycerides, reduce endothelial relaxation, and support left ventricular hypertrophy, all potentially increasing the risk of cardiovascular disease and myocardial infarction.

To help reduce cardiovascular strain it is advised to maintain an active cardiovascular exercise program and minimize the intake of saturated fats, cholesterol, and simple carbohydrates at all times during active AAS administration. Supplementing with fish oils (4 grams per day) and a natural cholesterol/antioxidant formula such as Lipid Stabil or a product with comparable ingredients is also recommended.

Side Effects (Testosterone Suppression):

All anabolic/androgenic steroids when taken in doses sufficient to promote muscle gain are expected to suppress endogenous testosterone production. Without the intervention of testosterone-stimulating substances, testosterone levels should return to normal within 1-4 months of drug secession. Note that prolonged hypogonadotrophic hypogonadism can develop secondary to steroid abuse, necessitating medical intervention.

The above side effects are not inclusive. For more detailed discussion of potential side effects, see the Steroid Side Effects section of this book.

Administration (Men):

Demethylstanozolol was never approved for use in humans. Prescribing guidelines are unavailable. An effective dosage for physique- or performance-enhancing purposes seems to begin in the range of 100 mg-150 mg per day, taken for 6-8 weeks. This level seems to impart a decent effect on lean tissue gain and strength, although higher doses would be needed for a very strong anabolic effect.

Administration (Women):

Demethylstanozolol was never approved for use in humans. Prescribing guidelines are unavailable. An effective dosage for physique- or performance-enhancing purposes seems to be 25 mg per day, taken for no longer than 4-6 weeks. For most users, this level seems to impart a decent effect on lean tissue gain and strength without side effects. Higher doses would increase the likelihood of virilizing effects, however, and should be carefully monitored.

Availability:

Demethylstanozolol was never produced as a prescription drug product. It has been sold as a nutritional supplement in the U.S.

Proviron® (mesterolone)

Androgenic	30-40
Anabolic	100-150
Standard	Testosterone propionate
Chemical Names	17beta-hydroxy-1alpha-methyl-5alpha-androstan-3-one
	1-methyl-5alpha-dihydrotestosterone
Estrogenic Activity	none
Progestational Activity	not significant

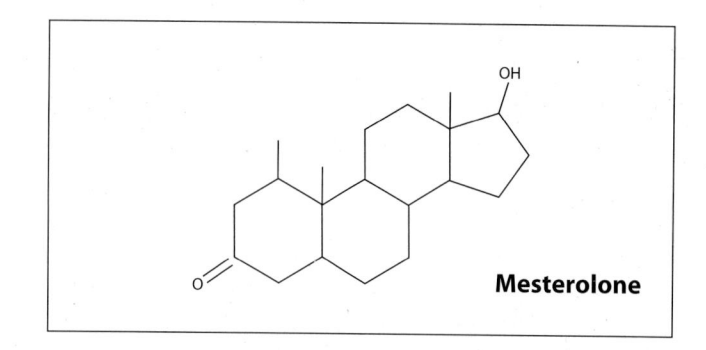

Description:

Proviron® is Schering's brand name for the oral androgen mesterolone (1-methyl dihydrotestosterone). Similar to dihydrotestosterone, mesterolone is a strong androgen with only a weak level of anabolic activity. This is due to the fact that like dihydrotestosterone, mesterolone is rapidly reduced to inactive diol metabolites in muscle tissue where concentrations of the 3-hydroxysteroid dehydrogenase enzyme are high. The belief that the weak anabolic nature of this compound indicates a tendency to block the androgen receptor in muscle tissue, thereby reducing the gains of other more potent muscle-building steroids, should likewise not be taken seriously. In fact, due to its extremely high affinity for plasma binding proteins such as SHBG, mesterolone may actually work to potentate the activity of other steroids by displacing a higher percentage into a free, unbound state. Among athletes, mesterolone is primarily used to increase androgen levels when dieting or preparing for a contest, and as an anti-estrogen due to its intrinsic ability to antagonize the aromatase enzyme.

History:

According to company literature, Schering developed Proviron® in 1934, making this is an extremely old medication as far as anabolic/androgenic steroids. Schering also states that it was the first medication put into clinical practice for the treatment of "hormone-related diseases and complaints in men." Accordingly, mesterolone would have been developed around the same time as methyltestosterone (1935) and testosterone propionate (1937), which are both very old agents generally considered obsolete by today's standards. In spite of its age, Proviron has a long history of clinical effectiveness and safety, and remains in widespread clinical use today. It is generally prescribed to males for the treatment of declining physical and mental capacity caused by age and subnormal androgen levels, low libido caused by insufficient androgen levels, hypogonadism (in pre- and post- pubescent males), and infertility (in certain situations mesterolone increases the quality and quantity of sperm).

The use of mesterolone as a fertility aid is perhaps one of the most controversial indications for this drug considering that anabolic/androgenic steroids are generally linked to infertility. It is also a use of mesterolone that is quite often misunderstood by athletes. Mesterolone is applicable here because it is an effective androgen that offers minimal suppression of gonadotropins in normal therapeutic doses, not because it increases LH output. Absent gonadotropin suppression, the drug may supplement androgenicity necessary for sperm production. It is well understood that androgens have direct stimulatory effects on spermatogenesis, and also influence the transportation and maturation of sperm via effects on the epididymis, ductus deferens, and seminal vesicles. So the role of these hormones is not entirely suppressive. Mesterolone seems to have a unique positive influence on certain cases of male fertility because its potential stimulatory effects on sperm quantity and quality are not overridden by the suppression of gonadotropins.

Mesterolone is widely manufactured by Schering, which currently sells the drug in more than thirty countries worldwide. The most common brand name used for its sale is Proviron, although Schering has sold the agent under other names in certain markets, including Mestoranum and Provironum. Additionally, other manufacturers have sold mesterolone over the years, appearing under such brand names as Pluriviron (Asche, Germany), Vistimon (Jenepharm, Germany), and Restore (Brown & Burke, India). In spite of its long track record of safety and efficacy, mesterolone was never approved for sale in the United States. It remains available in many Western nations, however. Schering remains the major (almost exclusive) global supplier of mesterolone today, although on rare occasion other brands of the drug can be located.

How Supplied:

Mesterolone is widely available in human drug markets. Composition and dosage may vary by country and manufacturer; preparations generally contain 25 mg or 50 mg of steroid per tablet.

Structural Characteristics:

Mesterolone is a modified form of dihydrotestosterone. It differs by the addition of a methyl group at carbon 1, which helps protect the hormone from hepatic metabolism during oral administration. The same structural modification is also used with oral Primobolan® (methenolone) tablets. Alkylation at the one position slows hepatic metabolism of the steroid during the first pass, although much less profoundly than c-17 alpha alkylation. Mesterolone is resistant enough to breakdown to allow therapeutically beneficial blood levels to be achieved, although the overall bioavailability remains much lower than c-17 alpha alkylated oral steroids. Mesterolone also has a very strong binding affinity for Sex Hormone Binding Globulin.[710] This may act to displace other steroids more weakly bound to SHBG into a free (active) state.

Side Effects (Estrogenic):

Mesterolone is not aromatized by the body, and is not measurably estrogenic. An anti-estrogen is not necessary when using this steroid, as the drug is unlikely to induce gynecomastia, water retention, or other estrogen-related side effects.

Mesterolone is actually believed to act as an anti-aromatase in the body, preventing or slowing the conversion of steroids into estrogen. The result is somewhat comparable to Arimidex®, although less profound. The anti-estrogenic properties of mesterolone are not unique, and a number of other steroids have demonstrated similar activity. Dihydrotestosterone and Masteron (2-methyl-dihydrotestosterone), for example, have been successfully used as therapies for gynecomastia and breast cancer due to their strong androgenic and potentially anti-estrogenic effect. It has also been suggested that nandrolone may even lower aromatase activity in peripheral tissues where it is more resistant to estrogen conversion (the most active site of nandrolone aromatization seems to be the liver). The anti-estrogenic effect of all of these compounds is presumably caused by their ability to compete with other substrates for binding to the aromatase enzyme. With the aromatase enzyme bound to the steroid, yet being unable to alter it, an inhibiting effect is achieved as it is temporarily blocked from interacting with other hormones.

Side Effects (Androgenic):

Mesterolone is classified as an androgenic steroid. Androgenic side effects are common with this substance, especially with higher doses. This may include bouts of oily skin, acne, and body/facial hair growth. Anabolic/androgenic steroids may also aggravate male pattern hair loss. Women are also warned of the potential virilizing effects of anabolic/androgenic steroids. These may include a deepening of the voice, menstrual irregularities, changes in skin texture, facial hair growth, and clitoral enlargement. Additionally, the 5-alpha reductase enzyme does not metabolize mesterolone, so its relative androgenicity is not affected by finasteride or dutasteride.

Side Effects (Hepatotoxicity):

Mesterolone is not c17-alpha alkylated, and not known to produce hepatotoxic effects; liver toxicity is unlikely.

Side Effects (Cardiovascular):

Anabolic/androgenic steroids can have deleterious effects on serum cholesterol. This includes a tendency to reduce HDL (good) cholesterol values and increase LDL (bad) cholesterol values, which may shift the HDL to LDL balance in a direction that favors greater risk of arteriosclerosis. The relative impact of an anabolic/androgenic steroid on serum lipids is dependant on the dose, route of administration (oral vs. injectable), type of steroid (aromatizable or non-aromatizable), and level of resistance to hepatic metabolism. Mesterolone is an oral non-aromatizable androgen, and expected to have a notable negative effect on lipids. Studies administering 100 mg of mesterolone per day to hypogonadal men for approximately 6 months demonstrated a significant increase in total cholesterol (18.8%) and LDL cholesterol (65.2%), accompanied by a significant decrease in HDL cholesterol (-35.7%).[711]

Mesterolone should not be used when cardiovascular risk factors preclude the use of other oral steroids.

To help reduce cardiovascular strain it is advised to maintain an active cardiovascular exercise program and minimize the intake of saturated fats, cholesterol, and simple carbohydrates at all times during active AAS administration. Supplementing with fish oils (4 grams per day) and a natural cholesterol/antioxidant formula such as Lipid Stabil or a product with comparable ingredients is also recommended.

Side Effects (Testosterone Suppression):

Mesterolone has a very weak suppressive effect on gonadotropins and serum testosterone. Studies show that when given in moderate doses (150 mg per day or less), significant suppression of testosterone levels does not occur.[712] In studies with higher doses (300 mg per day and above), the agent strongly suppressed serum testosterone.[713]

The above side effects are not inclusive. For more detailed discussion of potential side effects, see the Steroid Side Effects section of this book.

Administration (Men):

To treat androgen insufficiency, mesterolone is usually given in a dose of 1 tablet (25 mg) three times per day at the initiation of therapy. The drug is later continued at a lower maintenance dose, which usually consists of taking 1 tablet (25 mg) one to two times per day. Similar doses are used to support male fertility, usually in conjunction with other fertility drugs like injectable FSH. The usual dosage among male athletes is between 50 mg and 150 mg of mesterolone per day, or two to six 25 mg tablets. The drug is typically taken in cycles of 6-12 weeks in length, which is usually a sufficient period of time to notice the benefits of drug therapy.

Many bodybuilders favor the use of mesterolone during dieting phases or contest preparation, when low estrogen and high androgen levels are particularly desirable. This is especially beneficial when anabolics like Winstrol®, Anavar, or Primobolan® are being used alone, as the androgenic content of these drugs is relatively low. Mesterolone can be effectively used here to adjust the androgen to estrogen ratio upwards, bringing about an increase in the hardness and density of the muscles, supporting libido and general sense of well being, and increasing the tendency to burn body fat. It is also commonly used (at a similar dosage) to prevent gynecomastia when other aromatizable steroids are being administered, often in conjunction with 10-20 mg per day of Nolvadex.

Administration (Women):

Mesterolone is not approved for use in women. This agent is not recommended for women for physique- or performance-enhancing purposes due to its strong androgenic nature and tendency to produce virilizing side effects. Some women do favor the drug, however, and find a single 25 mg tablet enough to efficiently shift the hormone balance in the body, greatly impacting the look of definition to the physique. Intake is usually limited to no longer than four or five weeks in such situations to minimize the chance of developing lasting virilizing effects. One tablet used in conjunction with 10 or 20 mg of Nolvadex® can be even more efficient for muscle hardening, creating an environment where the body is much more inclined to burn off extra body fat, especially in female trouble areas like the hips and thighs. Extreme caution should be taken with such use, however.

Availability:

Most versions of mesterolone are manufactured by, or under license from, Schering. These are packaged in both push-through strips and small glass vials, depending on the market. Counterfeits are not currently known to be a problem.

Roxilon (dimethazine)

Androgenic	96
Anabolic	210
Standard	Methyltestosterone (oral)
Chemical Name	17beta-hydroxy-2alpha,17alpha-dimethyl-5alpha-androstan-3-one azine mebolazine
Estrogenic Activity	none
Progestational Activity	none

Methyldrostanolone

Description:

Dimethazine, also known as mebolazine, is a potent oral anabolic steroid derived from dihydrotestosterone. The dimethazine molecule is fairly unique in structure, being made from two methyldrostanolone molecules bonded together with an azine bridge. The body breaks this bond, however, so that the drug actually provides free methyldrostanolone (Superdrol) to the user. Dimethazine is strongly anabolic, moderately androgenic, and not appreciably estrogenic or progestational. Although presently unavailable, this drug was once highly favored by athletes for its ability to promote solid gains in lean muscle tissue without excess water retention or fat gain. Qualitatively, the drug behaves in a very similar manner to drostanolone propionate (Masteron), although as an oral c-17alpha alkylated steroid it presents considerably more toxicity.

History:

Dimethazine was first described in 1962.[714] It was developed into a medicine by Ormonoterapia Richter in Milan, Italy. The firm sold it under the Roxilon brand name in Italy, and as Dostalon in Mexico. The Roxilon brand was also reportedly sold under license by Lepetit. Dimethazine has been evaluated clinically for a number of treatments, often including use with women, the elderly, and children. Such applications have included the promotion of growth in underweight children and adolescents, the retention of lean body mass with chronic pulmonary tuberculosis, the treatment of osteoporosis, and as a general anabolic in conditions necessitating the use of such an agent. In spite of a favorable record of efficacy and safety, dimethazine was ultimately a drug that saw only limited success as a prescription agent. It was discontinued many years ago, and has been unavailable worldwide for so long that few even recognize the active ingredient as a once-marketed commercial steroid.

How Supplied:

Dimethazine is no longer sold as a prescription drug preparation.

Structural Characteristics:

Methyldrostanolone is a modified form of dihydrotestosterone. It differs by: 1) the addition of a methyl group at carbon 17-alpha, which helps protect the hormone during oral administration, and 2) the introduction of a methyl group at carbon-2 (alpha), which considerably increases the anabolic strength of the steroid by heightening its resistance to metabolism by the 3-hydroxysteroid dehydrogenase enzyme in skeletal muscle tissue. Dimethazine consists of two methyldrostanolone molecules bonded together with an azine bridge. These molecules are metabolically separated, yielding free methyldrostanolone.

Side Effects (Estrogenic):

Dimethazine is not aromatized by the body, and is not measurably estrogenic or progestational.[715] An anti-estrogen is not necessary when using this steroid, as gynecomastia should not be a concern even among sensitive individuals. Since estrogen is the usual culprit with water retention, this steroid instead produces a lean, quality look to the physique with no fear of excess subcutaneous fluid retention. This makes it a favorable steroid to use during cutting cycles, when water and fat retention are major concerns.

Side Effects (Androgenic):

Although classified as an anabolic steroid, androgenic side effects are still possible with this substance, especially with higher doses. This may include bouts of oily skin, acne, and body/facial hair growth. Anabolic/androgenic steroids may also aggravate male pattern hair loss. Women are warned of the potential virilizing effects of anabolic/androgenic steroids. These may include a deepening of the voice, menstrual irregularities, changes in skin texture, facial hair growth, and clitoral enlargement. Dimethazine is a steroid with relatively low androgenic activity relative to its tissue-building actions, making the threshold for strong androgenic side effects comparably higher than with more androgenic agents such as testosterone, methandrostenolone, or fluoxymesterone. Note that the 5-alpha reductase enzyme does not metabolize dimethazine, so its relative androgenicity is not affected by the concurrent use of finasteride or dutasteride.

Side Effects (Hepatotoxicity):

Dimethazine is a c17-alpha alkylated compound. This alteration protects the drug from deactivation by the liver, allowing a very high percentage of the drug entry into the bloodstream following oral administration. C17-alpha alkylated anabolic/androgenic steroids can be hepatotoxic. Prolonged or high exposure may result in liver damage. In rare instances life-threatening dysfunction may develop. It is advisable to visit a physician periodically during each cycle to monitor liver function and overall health. Intake of c17-alpha alkylated steroids is commonly limited to 6-8 weeks, in an effort to avoid escalating liver strain. Note that in studies administering 20 mg per day to patients for 45-95 days, dimethazine was shown to induce modest to moderate bilirubinemia (excess bilirubin in the blood, indicative of hepatic stress) in close to 50% of patients.[716] Approximately 25% of the patients noticed substantial increases in serum transaminases. These results suggest this steroid has a significant level of hepatotoxicity.

The use of a liver detoxification supplement such as Liver Stabil, Liv-52, or Essentiale Forte is advised while taking any hepatotoxic anabolic/androgenic steroids.

Side Effects (Cardiovascular):

Anabolic/androgenic steroids can have deleterious effects on serum cholesterol. This includes a tendency to reduce HDL (good) cholesterol values and increase LDL (bad) cholesterol values, which may shift the HDL to LDL balance in a direction that favors greater risk of arteriosclerosis. The relative impact of an anabolic/androgenic steroid on serum lipids is dependant on the dose, route of administration (oral vs. injectable), type of steroid (aromatizable or non-aromatizable), and level of resistance to hepatic metabolism. Dimethazine has a strong effect on the hepatic management of cholesterol due to its non-aromatizable nature, structural resistance to liver breakdown, and route of administration. Anabolic/androgenic steroids may also adversely affect blood pressure and triglycerides, reduce endothelial relaxation, and support left ventricular hypertrophy, all potentially increasing the risk of cardiovascular disease and myocardial infarction.

To help reduce cardiovascular strain it is advised to maintain an active cardiovascular exercise program and minimize the intake of saturated fats, cholesterol, and simple carbohydrates at all times during active AAS administration. Supplementing with fish oils (4 grams per day) and a natural cholesterol/antioxidant formula such as Lipid Stabil or a product with comparable ingredients is also recommended.

Side Effects (Testosterone Suppression):

All anabolic/androgenic steroids when taken in doses sufficient to promote muscle gain are expected to suppress endogenous testosterone production. Without the intervention of testosterone-stimulating substances, testosterone levels should return to normal within 1-4 months of drug secession. Note that prolonged hypogonadotrophic hypogonadism can develop secondary to steroid abuse, necessitating medical intervention.

The above side effects are not inclusive. For more detailed discussion of potential side effects, see the Steroid Side Effects section of this book.

Administration (Men):

An effective dosage of dimethazine for physique- or performance-enhancing purposes begins in the range of 10-20 mg per day, taken for no longer than 6 or 8 weeks. At this level it seems to impart a measurable muscle-building effect, which is usually accompanied by fat loss and increased definition. Higher doses are usually avoided due to potential hepatotoxicity.

Administration (Women):

An effective dosage of dimethazine for physique- or performance-enhancing purposes would fall around 2.5 mg per day, taken in cycles lasting no more than 4-6 weeks to minimize the chance for virilization. As with all anabolic/androgenic steroids, virilization is still possible.

Availability:

Dimethazine is no longer commercially produced, and is unavailable on the black market.

Roxilon Inject (bolazine caproate)

Androgenic	25-40
Anabolic	62-130
Standard	Testosterone
Chemical Names	17beta-Hydroxy-2alpha-methyl-5alpha-androstan-3-one azine
Estrogenic Activity	none
Progestational Activity	no data available (low)

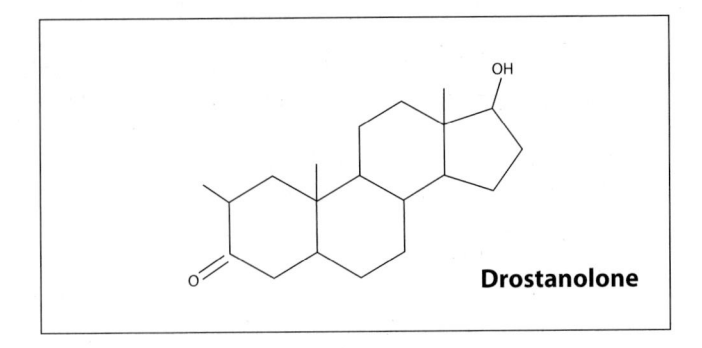

Drostanolone

Description:

Bolazine caproate is an injectable anabolic steroid derived from dihydrotestosterone. This agent is a close chemical cousin of dimethazine, which is also known as mebolazine (for methyl bolazine). Bolazine is a unique steroid that is made from two molecules of drostanolone bonded together. This bond is broken once in the body, however, so this drug ultimately provides the same active drostanolone as Masteron. Bolazine is a strong anabolic agent with moderate androgenicity and no estrogenic or progestational properties. This drug, although no longer produced, was once highly favored by athletes for its ability to promote solid muscle tissue gains without unnecessary water or fat retention. The results from bolazine are qualitatively identical to those of Masteron, and for all intents and purposes the two agents are interchangeable.

History:

Bolazine caproate first appeared in Europe in the 1960's. It was developed into a medicine by Ormonoterapia Richter in Milan, Italy, which sold it under the brand name Roxilon Inject. As the name implies, the drug was intended to be an injectable (non-alkylated) version of the firm's oral Roxilon medication (dimethazine; mebolazine). Although c-17 methylated and non-methylated analogs often tend to have very different activities from one another, here the separation between the two agents is not great, and therefore the comparison is somewhat appropriate. Owing to their high relative anabolic to androgenic ratios, Roxilon and Roxilon Inject were both used clinically to treat a variety of androgen-sensitive populations, including women, the elderly, and children. Although clinically effective, both steroids saw limited financial success, and Richter discontinued them many years ago. There is currently no legitimate prescription drug product worldwide containing bolazine caproate.

How Supplied:

Bolazine caproate is no longer available as a prescription drug preparation.

Structural Characteristics:

Drostanolone is a modified form of dihydrotestosterone. It differs by the introduction of a methyl group at carbon-2 (alpha), which considerably increases the anabolic strength of the steroid by heightening its resistance to metabolism by the 3-hydroxysteroid dehydrogenase enzyme in skeletal muscle tissue. Bolazine consists of two drostanolone molecules bonded together with an azine bridge. These molecules are metabolically separated, yielding free drostanolone. Bolazine caproate is a modified form of bolazine, where a carboxylic acid ester (caproic acid) has been attached to the 17-beta hydroxyl group to slow its release from the site of injection (depot).

Side Effects (Estrogenic):

Bolazine is not aromatized by the body, and is not measurably estrogenic. An anti-estrogen is not necessary when using this steroid, as gynecomastia should not be a concern even among sensitive individuals. Since estrogen is the usual culprit with water retention, this steroid instead produces a lean, quality look to the physique with no fear of excess subcutaneous fluid retention. This makes it a favorable steroid to use during cutting cycles, when water and fat retention are major concerns. As a non-aromatizable DHT derivative, this steroid may also impart an anti-estrogenic effect, the drug competing with other (aromatizable) substrates for binding to the aromatase enzyme.

Side Effects (Androgenic):

Although classified as an anabolic steroid, androgenic side effects are still possible with this substance, especially with higher doses. This may include bouts of oily skin, acne, and body/facial hair growth. Anabolic/androgenic steroids may also aggravate male pattern hair loss. Women are warned of the potential virilizing effects of anabolic/androgenic steroids. These may include a deepening of the voice, menstrual irregularities, changes in skin texture, facial hair growth, and clitoral enlargement. Bolazine is a steroid with relatively low androgenic activity relative to its tissue-building actions, making the threshold for strong androgenic side effects comparably higher than with more androgenic agents such as testosterone, methandrostenolone, or fluoxymesterone. Note that bolazine is unaffected by the 5-alpha reductase enzyme, so its relative androgenicity is not affected by the concurrent use of finasteride or dutasteride.

Side Effects (Hepatotoxicity):

Bolazine is not c17-alpha alkylated, and not known to have hepatotoxic properties. Liver toxicity is unlikely.

Side Effects (Cardiovascular):

Anabolic/androgenic steroids can have deleterious effects on serum cholesterol. This includes a tendency to reduce HDL (good) cholesterol values and increase LDL (bad) cholesterol values, which may shift the HDL to LDL balance in a direction that favors greater risk of arteriosclerosis. The relative impact of an anabolic/androgenic steroid on serum lipids is dependant on the dose, route of administration (oral vs. injectable), type of steroid (aromatizable or non-aromatizable), and level of resistance to hepatic metabolism. Bolazine should have a stronger negative effect on the hepatic management of cholesterol than testosterone or nandrolone due to its non-aromatizable nature, but a weaker impact than c-17 alpha alkylated steroids. Anabolic/androgenic steroids may also adversely affect blood pressure and triglycerides, reduce endothelial relaxation, and support left ventricular hypertrophy, all potentially increasing the risk of cardiovascular disease and myocardial infarction.

To help reduce cardiovascular strain it is advised to maintain an active cardiovascular exercise program and minimize the intake of saturated fats, cholesterol, and simple carbohydrates at all times during active AAS administration. Supplementing with fish oils (4 grams per day) and a natural cholesterol/antioxidant formula such as Lipid Stabil or a product with comparable ingredients is also recommended.

Side Effects (Testosterone Suppression):

All anabolic/androgenic steroids when taken in doses sufficient to promote muscle gain are expected to suppress endogenous testosterone production. Without the intervention of testosterone-stimulating substances, testosterone levels should return to normal within 1-4 months of drug secession. Note that prolonged hypogonadotrophic hypogonadism can develop secondary to steroid abuse, necessitating medical intervention.

The above side effects are not inclusive. For more detailed discussion of potential side effects, see the Steroid Side Effects section of this book.

Administration (Men):

An effective dose for physique- or performance-enhancing purposes falls in the range of 150-400 mg per week, taken for 6-12 weeks. This level is sufficient to provide measurable gains in lean muscle mass and strength, which (depending on diet and metabolic factors) may be accompanied by increased hardness and definition to the physique. Due to the slow-acting nature of this drug, injections are typically given once per week.

Administration (Women):

When used for physique- or performance-enhancing purposes, a dosage of 50-100 mg per week is most common, taken for 4 to 6 weeks. Virilization symptoms are rare in doses of 100 mg per week or below. This level is sufficient to provide measurable gains in lean muscle mass and strength, which (depending on diet and metabolic factors) may be accompanied by increased hardness and definition to the physique.

Availability:

Bolazine caproate is no longer available as a prescription drug product. It was discontinued many years ago, so no old lots should still be circulating.

Spectriol (testosterone/nandrolone/methandriol blend)

Androgenic	
Anabolic	
Standard	
Chemical Names	
Estrogenic Activity	
Progestational Activity	

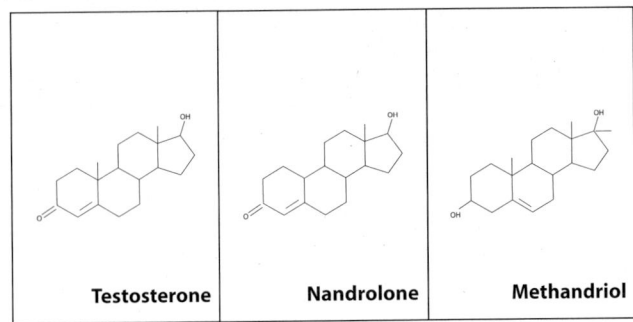

Description:

Spectriol is an injectable veterinary steroid preparation from Australia that contains five different steroid ingredients. More specifically, each milliliter contains 10 mg of testosterone cypionate, 10 mg of testosterone propionate, 10 mg of testosterone hexahydrobenzoate, 15 mg of nandrolone phenylpropionate, and 20 mg of methandriol dipropionate, for a total steroid concentration is 65 mg/mL. Given the nature of its components, the product mixture provides a moderately strong anabolic and androgenic effect. The product is also moderately estrogenic, given its testosterone and methandriol content. This agent is most commonly valued for its ability to promote strong gains in muscle size and strength, often with some level of accompanied water retention.

History:

Spectriol is a product of RWR Veterinary Products (formerly a subsidiary of Nature Vet), sold only on the Australian veterinary drug market. The drug is used to treat horses, mainly as an anabolic and tonic aid to improve muscle tone, enhance recovery, aid protein assimilation, and maintain a favorable water balance in the animal. To treat an adult horse, a dosage of 5 mL (325 mg) is generally administered once every 2 weeks for a set duration. Although never marketed or intended for human use, the product has historically piqued the interest of bodybuilders, due to the fact that it is an unusual preparation that contains 5 different steroids in a blend. Prior to the year 2000, multi-component products like this were rarely seen, especially legitimate pharmaceutical preparations. As such, the ingredients were a key marketing point for Spectriol, even if unintended by its manufacturer. Given its relatively low per-milliliter steroid concentration, however, as well as diverse competition in today's international steroid market from export and veterinary manufacturers, this product is much less desirable than it used to be.

How Supplied:

Spectriol is available on the Australian veterinary drug market. It contains 65 mg/mL of steroid in oil in a 10 mL vial.

Structural Characteristics:

For a more comprehensive discussion of the individual steroids testosterone, nandrolone, and methandriol, refer to some of their respective profiles.

Side Effects (Estrogenic):

Testosterone is readily aromatized in the body to estradiol (estrogen). Methylandrostendiol is not directly aromatized by the body, but one of its known metabolites is methyltestosterone, which can aromatize. Methlyandrostenediol is also believed to have some inherent estrogenic activity.[717] Nandrolone is aromatized weakly compared to testosterone. With such a blend, Spectriol is considered a moderately estrogenic steroid. Gynecomastia is possible during treatment, as well as significant water and fat retention, depending on the dose used and individual sensitivity. Estrogenic side effects may necessitate the use of an anti-estrogen during therapy.

Side Effects (Androgenic):

Although technically classified as an anabolic steroid preparation due to its nandrolone content (which offsets the androgenicity of testosterone and methylandrostenediol slightly), this steroid is still markedly androgenic. Androgenic side effects are, therefore, common with this substance. This may include bouts of oily skin, acne, and body/facial hair growth. Anabolic/androgenic steroids may also aggravate male pattern hair loss. Women are warned of the potential virilizing effects of anabolic/androgenic steroids. These may include a deepening of the voice, menstrual irregularities, changes in skin texture, facial hair growth, and clitoral enlargement.

Side Effects (Hepatotoxicity):

Methylandrostenediol is a c17-alpha alkylated compound. This alteration protects the drug from deactivation by the liver, allowing a very high percentage of the drug entry into the bloodstream following oral administration. C17-alpha alkylated anabolic/androgenic steroids can be hepatotoxic. Prolonged or high exposure may result in liver damage. In rare instances life-threatening dysfunction may develop. It is advisable to visit a physician periodically during each cycle to monitor liver function and overall health. Intake of c17-alpha alkylated steroids is commonly limited to 6-8 weeks, in an effort to avoid escalating liver strain. Injectable forms of the drug may present slightly less strain on the liver by avoiding the first pass metabolism of oral dosing, although may still present substantial hepatotoxicity. Given the relatively low dose of methylandrostenediol in Spectriol, liver toxicity is not likely with this drug unless high doses are taken, or it is used for prolonged durations.

Side Effects (Cardiovascular):

Anabolic/androgenic steroids can have deleterious effects on serum cholesterol. This includes a tendency to reduce HDL (good) cholesterol values and increase LDL (bad) cholesterol values, which may shift the HDL to LDL balance in a direction that favors greater risk of arteriosclerosis. The relative impact of an anabolic/androgenic steroid on serum lipids is dependant on the dose, route of administration (oral vs. injectable), type of steroid (aromatizable or non-aromatizable), and level of resistance to hepatic metabolism. Methylandrostenediol has a strong effect on the hepatic management of cholesterol due to its structural resistance to liver breakdown and (with the oral) route of administration. Testosterone and nandrolone have a weaker negative impact on cholesterol, but still do tend to alter lipid values unfavorably. Anabolic/androgenic steroids may also adversely affect blood pressure and triglycerides, reduce endothelial relaxation, and support left ventricular hypertrophy, all potentially increasing the risk of cardiovascular disease and myocardial infarction.

To help reduce cardiovascular strain it is advised to maintain an active cardiovascular exercise program and minimize the intake of saturated fats, cholesterol, and simple carbohydrates at all times during active AAS administration. Supplementing with fish oils (4 grams per day) and a natural cholesterol/antioxidant formula such as Lipid Stabil or a product with comparable ingredients is also recommended.

The use of a liver detoxification supplement such as Liver Stabil, Liv-52, or Essentiale Forte is advised while taking any hepatotoxic anabolic/androgenic steroids.

Side Effects (Testosterone Suppression):

All anabolic/androgenic steroids when taken in doses sufficient to promote muscle gain are expected to suppress endogenous testosterone production. Without the intervention of testosterone-stimulating substances, testosterone levels should return to normal within 1-4 months of drug secession. Note that prolonged hypogonadotrophic hypogonadism can develop secondary to steroid abuse, necessitating medical intervention.

The above side effects are not inclusive. For more detailed discussion of potential side effects, see the Steroid Side Effects section of this book.

Administration (Men):

Spectriol has not been approved for use in humans. Prescribing guidelines are unavailable. Typical dosing schedule for physique- or performance-enhancing purposes is in the range of 195 mg (3mL) to 390 mg (6mL) per week, a level that should provide significant muscle and strength gains. To reduce injection volume, the total weekly dosage is commonly divided into 2-3 smaller applications.

Administration (Women):

Spectriol has not been approved for use in humans. Prescribing guidelines are unavailable. Drugs containing testosterone and methylandrostenediol are generally not recommended for women for physique- or performance-enhancing purposes due their strong androgenic nature and tendency to produce virilizing side effects.

Availability:

Spectriol is found only in 10 mL multi-dose vials, and is made only by RWR (formerly a subsidiary of Nature Vet Pty, but now an independent company) in Australia. This item does not circulate on the international black market in much volume, as Australia is no longer considered a major source country for steroids. Australian prescription drugs are not easily diverted to the black market in high volumes, and the steroid market especially has been scrutinized in recent years. Add this to the fact that the packaging for Spectriol is easy to duplicate, most product located on the black market is met with suspicion.

Sten (testosterone cypionate & propionate)

Androgenic	100
Anabolic	100
Standard	Standard

Chemical Names	4-androsten-3-one-17beta-ol
	17beta-hydroxy-androst-4-en-3-one
Estrogenic Activity	moderate
Progestational Activity	low

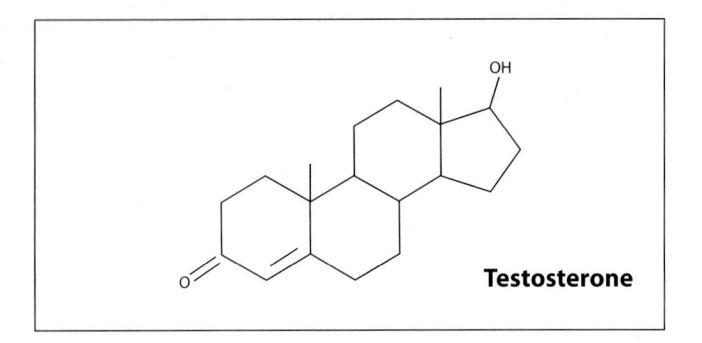

Description:

Sten is a two-component testosterone blend from Mexico that contains a mixture of testosterone propionate (25 mg), testosterone cypionate (75 mg), and DHEA (dehydroepiandrosterone; 20 mg) in a 2 mL ampule. Some references incorrectly list this product as containing 20 mg of DHT (dihydrotestosterone), which would be a third androgen. This is, however, just a confusion of the Spanish word for DHEA (dehidroisoandrosterona), which at a quick glance looks similar to "dihidrotestosterona." More recent packaging lists this ingredient as the less confusing "prasterona" (prasterone; another accepted term for DHEA). Holding the DHEA irrelevant at the moment, this steroid product contains a simple 50 mg/ml mixture of two common testosterone esters.

Many consider Sten to be a low-budget alternative to Sustanon® 250. While it does contain a blend of two testosterone esters, Sten is not as slow-acting in comparison. The longest ester of testosterone it uses is cypionate, which allows testosterone levels to return to baseline approximately 2 weeks after injection. Testosterone cypionate is also not a delayed-onset drug, so Sten doesn't offer much advantage in regards to a "sustained-release" effect. The testosterone propionate only compounds the initial testosterone spike, making its pharmacokinetic profile more uneven than if testosterone cypionate were used alone. Of course Sten and Sustanon® are both testosterone products, so given equivalently dosed weekly injections the end result should not be very different between the two.

History:

Sten is made in Mexico by the pharmaceutical firm Atlantis, S.A. de C.V. This agent is used primarily to correct low androgen levels in males, for the treatment of hypogonadism, andropause, and impotence. It is also sometimes prescribed to women for excessive lactation, advanced breast cancer, and low sex drive. Sten has a long history of sale on the Mexican market, where it is one of the country's more inexpensive human-use testosterone products. It has consequently remained a somewhat popular item there, even if its formulation may not be the most properly suited for the higher-dosed requirements of athletic use.

How Supplied:

Sten is available on the human drug market in Mexico. It contains a blend of 25 mg/75 mg testosterone propionate and testosterone cypionate (respectively) per 2-milliliter ampule.

Structural Characteristics:

Sten contains a mixture of two testosterone compounds, which where modified with the addition of carboxylic acid esters (propionic and cyclopentylpropionic acids) at the 17-beta hydroxyl group. Esterified forms of testosterone are less polar than free testosterone, and are absorbed more slowly from the area of injection. Once in the bloodstream, the ester is removed to yield free (active) testosterone. Esterified forms of testosterone are designed to prolong the window of therapeutic effect following administration, allowing for a less frequent injection schedule compared to injections of free (unesterified) steroid. Sten is designed to provide a rapid peak in testosterone levels (24-48 hours after injection), and maintain physiological concentrations for approximately 14 days.

Side Effects (Estrogenic):

Testosterone is readily aromatized in the body to estradiol (estrogen). The aromatase (estrogen synthetase) enzyme is responsible for this metabolism of testosterone. Elevated estrogen levels can cause side effects such as increased water retention, body fat gain, and gynecomastia. Testosterone is considered a moderately estrogenic steroid. An anti-estrogen such as clomiphene citrate or tamoxifen citrate may be necessary to prevent estrogenic side effects. One may alternately use an aromatase inhibitor like Arimidex® (anastrozole), which more efficiently controls estrogen by preventing its synthesis. Aromatase inhibitors can be quite expensive in comparison to anti-estrogens, however, and may also have negative effects on blood lipids.

Estrogenic side effects will occur in a dose-dependant manner, with higher doses (above normal therapeutic levels) of testosterone more likely to require the concurrent use of an anti-estrogen or aromatase inhibitor. Since water retention and loss of muscle definition are common with higher doses of testosterone, this drug is usually considered a poor choice for dieting or cutting phases of training. Its moderate estrogenicity makes it more ideal for bulking phases, where the added water retention will support raw strength and muscle size, and help foster a stronger anabolic environment.

Side Effects (Androgenic):

Testosterone is the primary male androgen, responsible for maintaining secondary male sexual characteristics. Elevated levels of testosterone are likely to produce androgenic side effects including oily skin, acne, and body/facial hair growth. Men with a genetic predisposition for hair loss (androgenetic alopecia) may notice accelerated male pattern balding. Those concerned about hair loss may find a more comfortable option in nandrolone decanoate, which is a comparably less androgenic steroid. Women are warned of the potential virilizing effects of anabolic/androgenic steroids, especially with a strong androgen such as testosterone. These may include deepening of the voice, menstrual irregularities, changes in skin texture, facial hair growth, and clitoral enlargement.

In androgen-responsive target tissues such as the skin, scalp, and prostate, the high relative androgenicity of testosterone is dependant on its reduction to dihydrotestosterone (DHT). The 5-alpha reductase enzyme is responsible for this metabolism of testosterone. The concurrent use of a 5-alpha reductase inhibitor such as finasteride or dutasteride will interfere with site-specific potentiation of testosterone action, lowering the tendency of testosterone drugs to produce androgenic side effects. It is important to remember that anabolic and androgenic effects are both mediated via the cytosolic androgen receptor. Complete separation of testosterone's anabolic and androgenic properties is not possible, even with total 5-alpha reductase inhibition.

Side Effects (Hepatotoxicity):

Testosterone does not have hepatotoxic effects; liver toxicity is unlikely. One study examined the potential for hepatotoxicity with high doses of testosterone by administering 400 mg of the hormone per day (2,800 mg per week) to a group of male subjects. The steroid was taken orally so that higher peak concentrations would be reached in hepatic tissues compared to intramuscular injections. The hormone was given daily for 20 days, and produced no significant changes in liver enzyme values including serum albumin, bilirubin, alanine-amino-transferase, and alkaline phosphatases.[718]

Side Effects (Cardiovascular):

Anabolic/androgenic steroids can have deleterious effects on serum cholesterol. This includes a tendency to reduce HDL (good) cholesterol values and increase LDL (bad) cholesterol values, which may shift the HDL to LDL balance in a direction that favors greater risk of arteriosclerosis. The relative impact of an anabolic/androgenic steroid on serum lipids is dependant on the dose, route of administration (oral vs. injectable), type of steroid (aromatizable or non-aromatizable), and level of resistance to hepatic metabolism. Anabolic/androgenic steroids may also adversely effect blood pressure and triglycerides, reduce endothelial relaxation, and support left ventricular hypertrophy, all potentially increasing the risk of cardiovascular disease and myocardial infarction.

Testosterone tends to have a much less dramatic impact on cardiovascular risk factors than synthetic steroids. This is due in part to its openness to metabolism by the liver, which allows it to have less effect on the hepatic management of cholesterol. The aromatization of testosterone to estradiol also helps to mitigate the negative effects of androgens on serum lipids. In one study, 280 mg per week of testosterone ester (enanthate) had a slight but not statistically significant effect on HDL cholesterol after 12 weeks, but when taken with an aromatase inhibitor a strong (25%) decrease was seen.[719] Studies using 300 mg of testosterone ester (enanthate) per week for twenty weeks without an aromatase inhibitor demonstrated only a 13% decrease in HDL cholesterol, while at 600 mg the reduction reached 21%.[720] The negative impact of aromatase inhibition should be taken into consideration before such drug is added to testosterone therapy.

Due to the positive influence of estrogen on serum lipids, tamoxifen citrate or clomiphene citrate are preferred to aromatase inhibitors for those concerned with cardiovascular health, as they offer a partial estrogenic effect in the liver. This allows them to potentially improve lipid profiles and offset some of the negative effects of androgens. With doses of 600 mg or less per week, the impact on lipid profile tends to be noticeable but not dramatic, making an anti-estrogen (for cardioprotective purposes) perhaps unnecessary. Doses of 600 mg or less per week have also failed to produce statistically significant changes in LDL/VLDL cholesterol, triglycerides, apolipoprotein B/C-III, C-reactive protein, and insulin sensitivity, all indicating a relatively weak impact on cardiovascular risk factors.[721] When used in moderate doses, injectable testosterone esters are usually considered to be the safest of all anabolic/androgenic steroids.

To help reduce cardiovascular strain it is advised to maintain an active cardiovascular exercise program and minimize the intake of saturated fats, cholesterol, and simple carbohydrates at all times during active AAS administration. Supplementing with fish oils (4 grams per day) and a natural cholesterol/antioxidant formula such as Lipid Stabil or a product with comparable ingredients is also recommended.

Side Effects (Testosterone Suppression):

All anabolic/androgenic steroids when taken in doses sufficient to promote muscle gain are expected to suppress endogenous testosterone production. Testosterone is the primary male androgen, and offers strong negative feedback on endogenous testosterone production. Testosterone-based drugs will, likewise, have a strong effect on the hypothalamic regulation of natural steroid hormones. Without the intervention of testosterone-stimulating substances, testosterone levels should return to normal within 1-4 months of drug secession. Note that prolonged hypogonadotrophic hypogonadism can develop secondary to steroid abuse, necessitating medical intervention.

The above side effects are not inclusive. For more detailed discussion of potential side effects, see the Steroid Side Effects section of this book.

Administration (General):

Testosterone propionate is often regarded as a painful injection. This is due to the very short carbon chain of the propionic acid ester, which can be irritating to tissues at the site of injection. Many sensitive individuals choose to stay away from this steroid completely, their bodies reacting with a pronounced soreness and low-grade fever that may last for a few days after each injection.

Administration (Men):

For the treatment of low androgen levels, the prescribing guidelines for Sten recommend one injection of one 2 mL ampule (100 mg testosterone esters; 20 mg DHEA) every 15-30 days. For bodybuilding purposes, this drug is usually injected on a weekly basis, in a dosage of 2-4 ampules (200-400 mg of testosterone esters in total). This level is sufficient to provide excellent gains in muscle size and strength. Higher doses are possible, but even the injection volume needed with 4 ampules per week (8ml) can become too uncomfortable for many. Testosterone drugs are ultimately very versatile, and can be combined with many other anabolic/androgenic steroids depending on the desired effect.

Administration (Women):

The prescribing guidelines for Sten do not make special dosing recommendations for women, except to say that androgenic symptoms may occur, and in certain scenarios therapy should be suspended until symptoms resolve, and after a lower dose used. This drug is not recommended for women for physique- or performance-enhancing purposes due to its strong androgenic nature, tendency to produce virilizing side effects, and slow acting characteristics (making blood levels difficult to control).

Availability:

Sten is commonly found on the black market. In Mexico, 2 pre-loaded syringes are packaged in a box and sell for about $10 in the pharmacy.

Steranabol Ritardo (oxabolone cypionate)

Androgenic	20-60
Anabolic	50-90
Standard	Testosterone
Chemical Names	19-norandrost-4-en-4,17b-ol-3-one
	4,17beta-dihydroxyestr-4-en-3-one
Estrogenic Activity	none
Progestational Activity	none

Oxabolone

Description:

Oxabolone cypionate is an injectable anabolic steroid that is a close structural derivative of 19-nortestosterone (nandrolone). The base steroid differs from nandrolone only by the addition of a 4-hydroxyl group, the same alteration that is used to make hydroxytestosterone from testosterone. As a nandrolone-based compound, oxabolone is more anabolic than androgenic in nature, although it is comparably more androgenic than its parent due to differences in metabolism. Oxabolone is also non-aromatizable, and less likely to produce estrogenic side effects. In terms of muscle-building potency, oxabolone is weaker than nandrolone, but it seems to produce an even harder, tighter look in comparison, probably owing to the fact that it does not have the same low level of estrogenic activity. For those who find nandrolone to be a failure during cutting/hardening cycles, or prefer purer strength and lean muscle gains without water/fat retention, this nandrolone derivative is often a valuable find.

History:

Oxabolone was first described in 1934.[722] It was finally developed into a long-acting injectable medication during the 1960's, sold by Farmitalia Carlo Erba in Italy and Germany as Steranabol-Ritardo and Steranabol-Depot, respectively. This relatively mild nandrolone derivative was used mainly to treat osteoporosis, although it has also been indicated when there was a need for a protein-sparing anabolic agent. It appears to have exhibited a very favorable clinical record, having been used effectively in men, women, the elderly, and children with minimal side effects for several decades. By all accounts, the drug was very safe. There is a great lack of information on this agent in the medical literature, however, being that it was used in a small number of markets only. As such, there is much less data to draw from than with many of the more widely used compounds.

Pharmacia acquired Farmitalia in 1993, at the time one of the largest pharmaceutical conglomerates in the world. Two years later, Pharmacia would go on to merge with Upjohn, another long-standing giant in the drug business. The Steranabol-Depot brand from Germany had been discontinued years earlier, but the Italian product remained on the market well after this corporate transition. For several years it was sold in Italy as a Pharmacia & Upjohn product. Steranabol Ritardo too was eventually discontinued, however, and would be gone by the time Pfizer acquired Pharmacia in 2003. The drug has been out of commerce for long enough now that it has been effectively removed from the black market. The dosage of this product was considerably low anyway (12.5 mg/ml), and as such was never very popular among athletes. Since this was the last remaining prescription drug product to contain oxabolone cypionate worldwide, this marked the commercial end to this steroid. Note that although this agent was unknown to U.S. Federal lawmakers before, it was added to the Anabolic Steroid Control Act in 2005.

How Supplied:

Oxabolone cypionate is no longer available as a commercial agent. When produced (Steranabol Ritardo) it contained 12.5 mg/ml of steroid in a 2 mL glass ampule.

Structural Characteristics:

Oxabolone is a modified form of nandrolone. It differs by the introduction of a hydroxyl group at carbon 4, which inhibits aromatization, reduces relative steroid androgenicity, and eliminates progestational activity. Oxabolone cypionate contains boldenone modified with the addition of carboxylic acid ester (cyclopentylpropionic acid) at the 17-beta hydroxyl group, so that the free steroid is released more slowly from the area of injection. Oxabolone cypionate is designed to provide a peak release of oxabolone within a few days after injection, and sustain hormone release for approximately 14-21 days.

Side Effects (Estrogenic):

Oxabolone is not aromatized by the body, and is not measurably estrogenic. Estrogenic side effects such as increased water retention, fat gain, and gynecomastia are not likely with use. Note that as a 4-hydroxy steroid, this agent may actually inhibit the aromatase enzyme by competitively inhibiting the binding and conversion of other aromatizable substrates. As such, it may actually impart a measurable anti-estrogenic effect. This trait is unconfirmed with oxabolone, but well understood with 4-hydroxyandrostendione. It is of note that in spite of it being a 19-nortestosterone analog, oxabolone has no significant progestational activity.

Side Effects (Androgenic):

Although classified as an anabolic steroid, androgenic side effects are still possible with this substance. This may include bouts of oily skin, acne, and body/facial hair growth. Anabolic/androgenic steroids may also aggravate male pattern hair loss. Women are also warned of the potential virilizing effects of anabolic/androgenic steroids. These may include a deepening of the voice, menstrual irregularities, changes in skin texture, facial hair growth, and clitoral enlargement. Additionally, oxabolone is not extensively metabolized by the 5-alpha reductase enzyme, so its relative androgenicity is not greatly altered by the concurrent use of finasteride or dutasteride. Note that oxabolone is primarily anabolic in nature, and is comparably less likey to produce androgenic side effects than more androgenic agents such as testosterone, methandrostenolone, and fluoxymesterone.

Side Effects (Hepatotoxicity):

Oxabolone is not a c17-alpha alkylated compound, and not known to have hepatotoxic effects. Liver toxicity is unlikely.

Side Effects (Cardiovascular):

Anabolic/androgenic steroids can have deleterious effects on serum cholesterol. This includes a tendency to reduce HDL (good) cholesterol values and increase LDL (bad) cholesterol values, which may shift the HDL to LDL balance in a direction that favors greater risk of arteriosclerosis. The relative impact of an anabolic/androgenic steroid on serum lipids is dependant on the dose, route of administration (oral vs. injectable), type of steroid (aromatizable or non-aromatizable), and level of resistance to hepatic metabolism. Oxabolone should have a stronger negative effect on the hepatic management of cholesterol than testosterone or nandrolone due to its non-aromatizable nature, but a much weaker impact than c-17 alpha alkylated steroids. Anabolic/androgenic steroids may also adversely affect blood pressure and triglycerides, reduce endothelial relaxation, and support left ventricular hypertrophy, all potentially increasing the risk of cardiovascular disease and myocardial infarction.

To help reduce cardiovascular strain it is advised to maintain an active cardiovascular exercise program and minimize the intake of saturated fats, cholesterol, and simple carbohydrates at all times during active AAS administration. Supplementing with fish oils (4 grams per day) and a natural cholesterol/antioxidant formula such as Lipid Stabil or a product with comparable ingredients is also recommended.

Side Effects (Testosterone Suppression):

All anabolic/androgenic steroids when taken in doses sufficient to promote muscle gain are expected to suppress endogenous testosterone production. Without the intervention of testosterone-stimulating substances, testosterone levels should return to normal within 1-4 months of drug secession. Note that prolonged hypogonadotrophic hypogonadism can develop secondary to steroid abuse, necessitating medical intervention.

The above side effects are not inclusive. For more detailed discussion of potential side effects, see the Steroid Side Effects section of this book.

Administration (Men):

Oxabolone cypionate is generally used in clinical doses ranging from 25-50 mg per application, given once every 1 to 3 weeks. Effective doses for physique- or performance-enhancing purposes fall in the range of 100-300 mg per week, taken for 6-12 weeks. At 25 mg per 2 mL ampule, however, reaching the higher (more effective) doses is difficult. Instead, many would use this steroid as more of an adjunct to an already running stack. At 3-4 ampules per week, or 75-100 mg in total, this steroid is generally strong enough for the user to notice some level of hardening and fat loss on top of the effects of other agents.

Administration (Women):

Oxabolone cypionate is used in clinical doses ranging from 25-50 mg per application, given once every 1 to 3 weeks. An ideal dosage of .5 mg/kg of bodyweight has been determined for the stimulation of growth in children. Effective doses for physique- or performance-enhancing purposes fall in the range of 25-50 mg per week, taken for no longer than 6-8 weeks.

Availability:

Oxabolone cypionate is not available as a prescription agent at this time, in any part of the world.

Sterandryl Retard (testosterone hexahydrobenzoate)

Androgenic	100
Anabolic	100
Standard	Standard
Chemical Names	4-androsten-3-one-17beta-ol
	17beta-hydroxy-androst-4-en-3-one
Estrogenic Activity	moderate
Progestational Activity	low

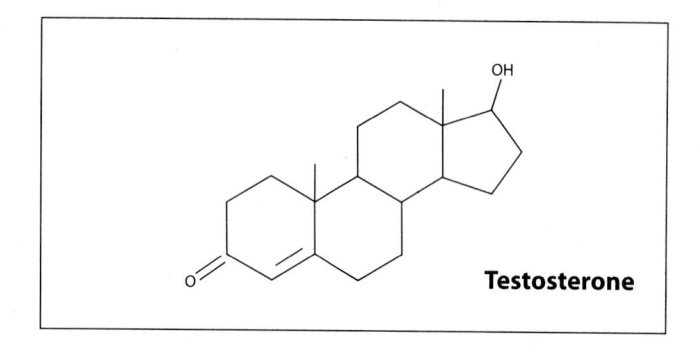

Description:

Testosterone hexahydrobenzoate is an injectable ester of the primary male androgen testosterone. The hexahydrobenzoate ester used here is a short-acting one, maintaining steady blood levels of testosterone for only several days. It, therefore, requires a much more frequent injection schedule than testosterone enanthate or cypionate. Testosterone hexahydrobenzoate is very similar to testosterone propionate in duration of effect, though perhaps slightly longer acting. For all intents and purposes, these two steroids could be used interchangeably. As with all testosterone injectables, testosterone hexahydrobenzoate is capable of promoting strong increases in muscle mass and strength.

History:

Testosterone hexahydrobenzoate is an ester of testosterone that was first closely studied in Europe during the mid-1950's. It was subsequently sold as a prescription drug item during the 1960's and '70's, most notably under the brand names of Sterandryl Retard (France) and Testormon Depositum (Portugal). Testosterone hexahydrobenzoate was used clinically to treat insufficient androgen levels in males, and menorrhagia (heavy menstrual bleeding), metrorrhagia (abnormal bleeding of the uterus), excessive lactation, and breast cancer in females. It was also used with both sexes to treat certain skin conditions (associated with itching), psychoneurosis, and asthenia (abnormal physical weakness or lack of energy). In spite of the numerous accepted medical uses for this drug, testosterone hexahydrobenzoate was ultimately only a minor testosterone ester in clinical medicine, and was withdrawn from the world market (as a standalone item) before the 1980's. This ester can still be found as a constituent of Spectriol, an Australian veterinary steroid.

How Supplied:

Testosterone hexahydrobenzoate is no longer available as a standalone drug item. When available, it usually contained 50 mg/ml, 100 mg/ml, or 125 mg/ml of steroid dissolved in oil. Packaging was generally as a 1 mL or 2 mL glass ampule.

Structural Characteristics:

Testosterone hexahydrobenzoate is a modified form of testosterone, where a carboxylic acid ester (hexahydrobenzoic acid, also known as cyclohexanecarboxylic acid) has been attached to the 17-beta hydroxyl group. Esterified forms of testosterone are less polar than free testosterone, and are absorbed more slowly from the area of injection. Once in the bloodstream, the ester is removed to yield free (active) testosterone. Esterified forms of testosterone are designed to prolong the window of therapeutic effect following administration, allowing for a less frequent injection schedule compared to injections of free (unesterified) steroid.

Side Effects (Estrogenic):

Testosterone is readily aromatized in the body to estradiol (estrogen). The aromatase (estrogen synthetase) enzyme is responsible for this metabolism of testosterone. Elevated estrogen levels can cause side effects such as increased water retention, body fat gain, and gynecomastia. Testosterone is considered a moderately estrogenic steroid. An anti-estrogen such as clomiphene citrate or tamoxifen citrate may be necessary to prevent estrogenic side effects. One may alternately use an aromatase inhibitor like Arimidex® (anastrozole), which more efficiently controls estrogen by preventing its synthesis. Aromatase inhibitors can be quite expensive in comparison to anti-estrogens, however, and may also have negative effects on blood lipids.

Side Effects (Androgenic):

Testosterone is the primary male androgen, responsible for maintaining secondary male sexual characteristics. Elevated levels of testosterone are likely to produce androgenic side effects including oily skin, acne, and body/facial hair growth. Men with a genetic predisposition for hair loss (androgenetic alopecia) may notice accelerated male pattern balding. Those concerned about hair loss may find a more comfortable option in nandrolone decanoate, which is a comparably less androgenic steroid. Women are warned of the potential virilizing effects of anabolic/androgenic steroids, especially with a strong androgen such as testosterone. These may include deepening of the voice, menstrual irregularities, changes in skin texture, facial hair growth, and clitoral enlargement.

In androgen-responsive target tissues such as the skin, scalp, and prostate, the high relative androgenicity of testosterone is dependant on its reduction to dihydrotestosterone (DHT). The 5-alpha reductase enzyme is responsible for this metabolism of testosterone. The concurrent use of a 5-alpha reductase inhibitor such as finasteride or dutasteride will interfere with site-specific potentiation of testosterone action, lowering the tendency of testosterone drugs to produce androgenic side effects. It is important to remember that anabolic and androgenic effects are both mediated via the cytosolic androgen receptor. Complete separation of testosterone's anabolic and androgenic properties is not possible, even with total 5-alpha reductase inhibition.

Side Effects (Hepatotoxicity):

Testosterone does not have hepatotoxic effects; liver toxicity is unlikely. One study examined the potential for hepatotoxicity with high doses of testosterone by administering 400 mg of the hormone per day (2,800 mg per week) to a group of male subjects. The steroid was taken orally so that higher peak concentrations would be reached in hepatic tissues compared to intramuscular injections. The hormone was given daily for 20 days, and produced no significant changes in liver enzyme values including serum albumin, bilirubin, alanine-amino-transferase, and alkaline phosphatases.[723]

Side Effects (Cardiovascular):

Anabolic/androgenic steroids can have deleterious effects on serum cholesterol. This includes a tendency to reduce HDL (good) cholesterol values and increase LDL (bad) cholesterol values, which may shift the HDL to LDL balance in a direction that favors greater risk of arteriosclerosis. The relative impact of an anabolic/androgenic steroid on serum lipids is dependant on the dose, route of administration (oral vs. injectable), type of steroid (aromatizable or non-aromatizable), and level of resistance to hepatic metabolism. Anabolic/androgenic steroids may also adversely effect blood pressure and triglycerides, reduce endothelial relaxation, and support left ventricular hypertrophy, all potentially increasing the risk of cardiovascular disease and myocardial infarction.

Testosterone tends to have a much less dramatic impact on cardiovascular risk factors than synthetic steroids. This is due in part to its openness to metabolism by the liver, which allows it to have less effect on the hepatic management of cholesterol. The aromatization of testosterone to estradiol also helps to mitigate the negative effects of androgens on serum lipids. In one study, 280 mg per week of testosterone ester (enanthate) had a slight but not statistically significant effect on HDL cholesterol after 12 weeks, but when taken with an aromatase inhibitor a strong (25%) decrease was seen.[724] Studies using 300 mg of testosterone ester (enanthate) per week for 20 weeks without an aromatase inhibitor demonstrated only a 13% decrease in HDL cholesterol, while at 600 mg the reduction reached 21%.[725] The negative impact of aromatase inhibition should be taken into consideration before such drug is added to testosterone therapy.

Due to the positive influence of estrogen on serum lipids, tamoxifen citrate or clomiphene citrate are preferred to aromatase inhibitors for those concerned with cardiovascular health, as they offer a partial estrogenic effect in the liver. This allows them to potentially improve lipid profiles and offset some of the negative effects of androgens. With doses of 600 mg or less per week, the impact on lipid profile tends to be noticeable but not dramatic, making an anti-estrogen (for cardioprotective purposes) perhaps unnecessary. Doses of 600 mg or less per week have also failed to produce statistically significant changes in LDL/VLDL cholesterol, triglycerides, apolipoprotein B/C-III, C-reactive protein, and insulin sensitivity, all indicating a relatively weak impact on cardiovascular risk factors.[726] When used in moderate doses, injectable testosterone esters are usually considered to be the safest of all anabolic/androgenic steroids.

To help reduce cardiovascular strain it is advised to maintain an active cardiovascular exercise program and minimize the intake of saturated fats, cholesterol, and simple carbohydrates at all times during active AAS administration. Supplementing with fish oils (4 grams per day) and a natural cholesterol/antioxidant formula such as Lipid Stabil or a product with comparable ingredients is also recommended.

Side Effects (Testosterone Suppression):

All anabolic/androgenic steroids when taken in doses sufficient to promote muscle gain are expected to suppress endogenous testosterone production. Testosterone is the primary male androgen, and offers strong negative feedback on endogenous testosterone production. Testosterone-based drugs will, likewise, have a strong effect on the hypothalamic regulation of natural steroid hormones. Without the intervention of testosterone-stimulating substances, testosterone levels should return to normal within 1-4 months of drug secession. Note that prolonged hypogonadotrophic hypogonadism can develop secondary to steroid abuse, necessitating medical intervention.

The above side effects are not inclusive. For more detailed discussion of potential side effects, see the Steroid Side Effects section of this book.

Administration (Men):

To treat androgen insufficiency, the prescribing guidelines for testosterone hexahydrobenzoate (Testormon Depot) called for a dosage of 25 mg given daily, or every second or third day. An effective dosage among male athletes would be in the range of 50-100 mg three times per week, taken in cycles 6 to 12 weeks in length. This level is sufficient for most users to notice exceptional gains in muscle size and strength. Testosterone is usually incorporated into bulking phases of training, when added water retention will be of little consequence, the user more concerned with raw mass than definition. Testosterone is ultimately very versatile, and can be combined with many other anabolic/androgenic steroids to tailor the desired effect.

Administration (Women):

Testosterone hexahydrobenzoate was used with women in clinical medicine when available, typically at a dosage of 5-25 mg given three times per week. The recommended applications for testosterone with females have been reduced in most areas of modern medicine, and this hormone is no longer widely used. Testosterone hexahydrobenzoate is not recommended for women for physique- or performance-enhancing purposes due to its strong androgenic nature and tendency to produce virilizing side effects.

Availability:

Testosterone hexahydrobenzoate is no longer available as a commercial standalone drug product.

Striant® (testosterone)

Androgenic	100
Anabolic	100
Standard	Standard
Chemical Names	4-androsten-3-one-17beta-ol
	17beta-hydroxy-androst-4-en-3-one
Estrogenic Activity	moderate
Progestational Activity	low

Testosterone

Description:

Striant® is a mucoadhesive buccal testosterone delivery system. It is prepared in the form of a small (aspirin-sized) tablet, which contains 30 mg of (free) testosterone. The tablet is not taken orally, but is affixed to the gums, where it transfers testosterone across the inner lining of the cheek and into the bloodstream. The buccal delivery of anabolic/androgenic steroids is not new, and has been used in the past (with limited success) on agents like methyltestosterone and testosterone propionate. The adhesive Striant system, however, is an improvement over the old rapidly dissolving buccal tablets, as it is much more stable in the mouth (it stays affixed for 12 hours and needs to be removed). As such, it provides a much more prolonged and efficacious delivery of hormone in comparison. Twice daily dosing is enough to maintain physiological hormone levels over a 24-hour period.

History:

Striant® was developed in the United States by Columbia Laboratories. It was approved by the FDA for sale as a prescription drug in June of 2003, and is indicated for use in men with conditions associated with a deficiency or absence of endogenous testosterone. With this product, Columbia was likely trying to target those hormone replacement therapy (HRT) consumers that do not welcome biweekly injections, and find patches and gels uncomfortable or cosmetically objectionable. Striant was shipped to pharmacies in late 2003, and quickly met with mixed reviews. Some patients find it a very convenient option for HRT, while others find the oral tablets too uncomfortable to use for long periods of time. Striant was released in the UK in 2004 under the Striant SR (Sustained Release) brand name, licensed and sold by Ardana Bioscience. Columbia's partnership with Ardana expects to see sale of Straint in 18 European markets.

How Supplied:

Striant® mucoadhesive buccal testosterone delivery system is available in various human drug markets. Product comes in the form of a small buccal tablet; usually packaged in strips of 10 tablets, 6 strips to a box.

Structural Characteristics:

Striant® mucoadhesive buccal testosterone delivery system is a buccal tablet containing 30 mg of (free) testosterone. The system is adhered to the inside of the mouth, where the gum meets the upper lip above the incisor teeth. With exposure to saliva the tablet softens into a gel-like consistency, which can stay in place for 12 hours. The product delivers physiological concentrations of testosterone through the mucous membrane, where it is absorbed into the bloodstream via the superior vena cava (major blood vessel), bypassing the liver.

Side Effects (Estrogenic):

Testosterone is readily aromatized in the body to estradiol (estrogen). The aromatase (estrogen synthetase) enzyme is responsible for this metabolism of testosterone. Elevated estrogen levels can cause side effects such as increased water retention, body fat gain, and gynecomastia. Testosterone is considered a moderately estrogenic steroid. Exceeding therapeutic doses will increase the likelihood of estrogenic side effects. In such cases, an anti-estrogen such as clomiphene citrate or tamoxifen citrate is commonly applied to prevent estrogenic side effects. One may alternately use an aromatase inhibitor like Arimidex® (anastrozole), which more efficiently controls estrogen by preventing its synthesis. Aromatase inhibitors can be quite expensive in comparison to anti-estrogens, however, and may also have negative effects on blood lipids.

Side Effects (Androgenic):

Testosterone is the primary male androgen, responsible for maintaining secondary male sexual characteristics.

Exceeding normal therapeutic doses is likely to produce androgenic side effects including oily skin, acne, and body/facial hair growth. Men with a genetic predisposition for hair loss (androgenetic alopecia) may notice accelerated male pattern balding. Women are warned of the potential virilizing effects of anabolic/androgenic steroids, especially with a strong androgen such as testosterone. These may include deepening of the voice, menstrual irregularities, changes in skin texture, facial hair growth, and clitoral enlargement.

In androgen-responsive target tissues such as the skin, scalp, and prostate, the high relative androgenicity of testosterone is dependant on its reduction to dihydrotestosterone (DHT). The 5-alpha reductase enzyme is responsible for this metabolism of testosterone. The concurrent use of a 5-alpha reductase inhibitor such as finasteride or dutasteride will interfere with site-specific potentiation of testosterone action, lowering the tendency of testosterone drugs to produce androgenic side effects. It is important to remember that anabolic and androgenic effects are both mediated via the cytosolic androgen receptor. Complete separation of testosterone's anabolic and androgenic properties is not possible, even with total 5-alpha reductase inhibition.

Side Effects (Hepatotoxicity):

Testosterone does not have hepatotoxic effects; liver toxicity is unlikely. One study examined the potential for hepatotoxicity with high doses of testosterone by administering 400 mg of the hormone per day (2,800 mg per week) to a group of male subjects. The steroid was taken orally so that higher peak concentrations would be reached in hepatic tissues compared to intramuscular injections. The hormone was given daily for 20 days, and produced no significant changes in liver enzyme values including serum albumin, bilirubin, alanine-amino-transferase, and alkaline phosphatases.[727]

Side Effects (Cardiovascular):

Anabolic/androgenic steroids can have deleterious effects on serum cholesterol. This includes a tendency to reduce HDL (good) cholesterol values and increase LDL (bad) cholesterol values, which may shift the HDL to LDL balance in a direction that favors greater risk of arteriosclerosis. The relative impact of an anabolic/androgenic steroid on serum lipids is dependant on the dose, route of administration (oral vs. injectable), type of steroid (aromatizable or non-aromatizable), and level of resistance to hepatic metabolism. Anabolic/androgenic steroids may also adversely affect blood pressure and triglycerides, reduce endothelial relaxation, and support left ventricular hypertrophy, all potentially increasing the risk of cardiovascular disease and myocardial infarction. Therapeutic doses of testosterone used to correct insufficient androgen production in otherwise healthy aging men are unlikely to increase atherogenic risk, and may actually reduce the risk of cardiovascular mortality.[728]

To help reduce cardiovascular strain it is advised to maintain an active cardiovascular exercise program and minimize the intake of saturated fats, cholesterol, and simple carbohydrates at all times during active AAS administration. Supplementing with fish oils (4 grams per day) and a natural cholesterol/antioxidant formula such as Lipid Stabil or a product with comparable ingredients is also recommended.

Side Effects (Testosterone Suppression):

All anabolic/androgenic steroids when taken in doses sufficient to promote muscle gain are expected to suppress endogenous testosterone production. Testosterone is the primary male androgen, and offers strong negative feedback on endogenous testosterone production. Testosterone-based drugs will, likewise, have a strong effect on the hypothalamic regulation of natural steroid hormones. Without the intervention of testosterone-stimulating substances, testosterone levels should return to normal within 1-4 months of drug secession. Note that prolonged hypogonadotrophic hypogonadism can develop secondary to steroid abuse, necessitating medical intervention.

The above side effects are not inclusive. For more detailed discussion of potential side effects, see the Steroid Side Effects section of this book.

Administration (General):

The Striant mucoadhesive buccal testosterone delivery system is placed on the gums just above the incisor tooth. It is left affixed for 12 hours, at which point it is carefully removed. The product is usually administered twice daily. The application site should be rotated between left and right sides of the mouth with each dose.

Administration (Men):

To treat androgen insufficiency, the prescribing guidelines for Striant recommend administering one buccal tablet twice daily. Doses are given once in the morning and once at night, 12 hours apart. For physique- or performance-enhancing purposes, higher doses would be necessary to achieve supraphysiological levels of testosterone. This will be difficult, if not impractical, given the method of delivery. Such use would require a minimum of 4 systems per day, a level sufficient for most users to notice significant gains in muscle size and strength, but not much comfort. Lower (therapeutic) doses may be effective when accompanied by other anabolic/androgenic steroids. Testosterone is ultimately very versatile, and can be combined with many other anabolic/androgenic steroids to tailor the desired effect.

Administration (Women):

The Striant mucoadhesive buccal testosterone delivery system is not FDA-approved for use in women. Testosterone is not recommended for women for physique- or performance-enhancing purposes due to its strong androgenic nature and tendency to produce virilizing side effects.

Availability:

Given its high relative price and low delivery of testosterone, Striant is not commonly traded on the black market. Counterfeits have not yet been reported.

Superdrol (methyldrostanolone)

Androgenic	20
Anabolic	400
Standard	Methyltestosterone (oral)
Chemical Names	2a, 17a-dimethyl-5a-androstane-17b-ol-3-one
Estrogenic Activity	none
Progestational Activity	no data available

Description:

Methyldrostanolone, also known as methasteron, is a potent oral anabolic steroid that was never sold as a prescription drug. In structure, this steroid is a close derivative of drostanolone (Masteron). The only difference in this case is the addition of a c-17 alpha methyl group, a modification that gives this steroid high oral bioavailability. The two agents remain very comparable, however. Both methyldrostanolone and drostanolone are non-aromatizable, so there is no difference in the estrogenicity of these two steroids, and both steroids retain favorable anabolic to androgenic ratios. Lab assays do put Superdrol ahead here, however, showing it to possess 4 times the anabolic potency of oral methyltestosterone while displaying only 20% of the androgenicity (a 20:1 ratio, compared to 3:1). The exact real-world relevance of these figures remains to be seen, however. Methyldrostanolone is favored by athletes for its moderate anabolic properties, which are usually accompanied by fat loss and minimal androgenic side effects.

History:

Methyldrostanolone was first described in 1959.[729] This steroid was developed by the international pharmaceuticals giant Syntex, alongside such other well-known anabolic agents as drostanolone propionate and oxymetholone. Unlike drostanolone and oxymetholone, however, this steroid (at least in its basic form) was never released as a medicinal product. It was only sold for a brief period of time as a modified hormone called dimethazine. Dimethazine is made from two molecules of methyldrostanolone that are bonded together, which are later metabolically separated to yield free methyldrostanolone. So while technically methyldrostanolone itself was never sold as a prescription agent, we can say that the drug was one utilized medicinally (for more information see the Roxilon drug profile). Otherwise, the methyldrostanolone molecule remained an obscure research steroid only, and was never itself approved for use in humans.

Methyldrostanolone was released in early 2005 as an over the counter "grey market" anabolic steroid in the United States. The drug was being sold without restrictions as a nutritional supplement product, barring some minimum age disclaimers by the manufacturer. No State or Federal laws identify this drug as an anabolic steroid, which remove the legalities associated with being a Class III controlled substance like other steroids. This is simply due to the fact that methyldrostanolone was not in commerce at the time such laws were written, and was unknown to lawmakers. It was never legal to sell as a dietary supplement, however, and in late 2005 the FDA angrily acknowledged methyldrostanolone was being sold on the sports supplement market. In early 2006, the FDA sent letters to the manufacturer and a distributor demanding it be pulled from commerce. Superdrol has since been discontinued.

How Supplied:

Methyldrostanolone was never sold as a prescription drug preparation. When sold as a nutritional supplement, it was generally in the form of capsules containing 10 mg of steroid each.

Structural Characteristics:

Methyldrostanolone is a modified form of dihydrotestosterone. It differs by: 1) the addition of a methyl group at carbon 17-alpha, which helps protect the hormone during oral administration, and 2) the introduction of a methyl group at carbon-2 (alpha), which considerably increases the anabolic strength of the steroid by heightening its resistance to metabolism by the 3-hydroxysteroid dehydrogenase enzyme in skeletal muscle tissue.

Side Effects (Estrogenic):

Methyldrostanolone is not aromatized by the body, and is not measurably estrogenic. An anti-estrogen is not necessary when using this steroid, as gynecomastia should not be a concern even among sensitive individuals. Since estrogen is the usual culprit with water retention, methyldrostanolone instead produces a lean, quality look to the physique with no fear of excess subcutaneous fluid retention. This makes it a favorable steroid to use during cutting cycles, when water and fat retention are major concerns.

Side Effects (Androgenic):

Although classified as an anabolic steroid, androgenic side effects are still possible with this substance, especially with higher doses. This may include bouts of oily skin, acne, and body/facial hair growth. Anabolic/androgenic steroids may also aggravate male pattern hair loss. Women are warned of the potential virilizing effects of anabolic/androgenic steroids. These may include a deepening of the voice, menstrual irregularities, changes in skin texture, facial hair growth, and clitoral enlargement. Methyldrostanolone is a steroid with relatively low androgenic activity relative to its tissue-building actions, making the threshold for strong androgenic side effects comparably higher than with more androgenic agents such as testosterone, methandrostenolone, or fluoxymesterone. Note that methyldrostanolone is unaffected by the 5-alpha reductase enzyme, so its relative androgenicity is not affected by the concurrent use of finasteride or dutasteride.

Side Effects (Hepatotoxicity):

Methyldrostanolone is a c17-alpha alkylated compound. This alteration protects the drug from deactivation by the liver, allowing a very high percentage of the drug entry into the bloodstream following oral administration. C17-alpha alkylated anabolic/androgenic steroids can be hepatotoxic. Prolonged or high exposure may result in liver damage. In rare instances life-threatening dysfunction may develop. It is advisable to visit a physician periodically during each cycle to monitor liver function and overall health. Intake of c17-alpha alkylated steroids is commonly limited to 6-8 weeks, in an effort to avoid escalating liver strain. Note that although no human data can be found to make reference of, doses of 10 mg and 20 mg per day have been sufficient to produce high elevations of liver enzymes in consumers, as reported by private lab test results. Also, a small number of serious adverse events relating to liver toxicity have been reported with the use of this substance.

The use of a liver detoxification supplement such as Liver Stabil, Liv-52, or Essentiale Forte is advised while taking any hepatotoxic anabolic/androgenic steroids.

Side Effects (Cardiovascular):

Anabolic/androgenic steroids can have deleterious effects on serum cholesterol. This includes a tendency to reduce HDL (good) cholesterol values and increase LDL (bad) cholesterol values, which may shift the HDL to LDL balance in a direction that favors greater risk of arteriosclerosis. The relative impact of an anabolic/androgenic steroid on serum lipids is dependant on the dose, route of administration (oral vs. injectable), type of steroid (aromatizable or non-aromatizable), and level of resistance to hepatic metabolism. Methyldrostanolone has a strong effect on the hepatic management of cholesterol due to its non-aromatizable nature, structural resistance to liver breakdown, and route of administration. Anabolic/androgenic steroids may also adversely affect blood pressure and triglycerides, reduce endothelial relaxation, and support left ventricular hypertrophy, all potentially increasing the risk of cardiovascular disease and myocardial infarction.

To help reduce cardiovascular strain it is advised to maintain an active cardiovascular exercise program and minimize the intake of saturated fats, cholesterol, and simple carbohydrates at all times during active AAS administration. Supplementing with fish oils (4 grams per day) and a natural cholesterol/antioxidant formula such as Lipid Stabil or a product with comparable ingredients is also recommended.

Side Effects (Testosterone Suppression):

All anabolic/androgenic steroids when taken in doses sufficient to promote muscle gain are expected to suppress endogenous testosterone production. Without the intervention of testosterone-stimulating substances, testosterone levels should return to normal within 1-4 months of drug secession. Note that prolonged hypogonadotrophic hypogonadism can develop secondary to steroid abuse, necessitating medical intervention.

The above side effects are not inclusive. For more detailed discussion of potential side effects, see the Steroid Side Effects section of this book.

Administration (Men):

Methydrostanolone was never approved for use in humans. Prescribing guidelines are unavailable. An effective dosage of methyldrostanolone for physique- or performance-enhancing purposes seems to begin in the range of 10-20 mg per day, taken for no longer than 6 or 8 weeks. At this level it seems to impart a measurable muscle-building effect, which is usually accompanied by fat loss and increased definition. Don't expect to gain 30 pounds on this agent (its name, which is short for "Super Anadrol," is more marketing than reality), but many do walk away with more than 10 pounds of solid muscle gain when using this agent alone.

In determining an optimal daily dosage, some do find the drug to be measurably more effective when venturing up to the 30 mg range. Potential hepatotoxicity should definitely be taken into account with such use, however. To avoid further escalating liver strain, 20 mg daily of methyldrostanolone is sometimes stacked with a non-toxic injectable steroid, such as testosterone for mass-building phases of training, or nandrolone or boldenone for more lean tissue gain and definition, instead of simply increasing the dosage. The drug also works well in cutting cycles, where its lack of estrogenicity is highly favored. Often it is combined here with a non-aromatizable injectable steroid like Primobolan or Parabolan.

Administration (Women):

Methyldrostanolone was never approved for use in humans. Prescribing guidelines are unavailable. In the athletic arena, an effective oral daily dosage would fall around 2.5 mg per day, taken in cycles lasting no more than 4-6 weeks to minimize the chance for virilization. The main point of contention with females is probably going to be the 10 mg per capsule dosage, which is far too high to use. Application would require opening each capsule and splitting the powdered contents up into 4 separate doses. As with all steroids, virilization is still possible.

Availability:

Superdrol is no longer commercially produced, although some clone products may still be located.

Sustanon® 100 (testosterone blend)

Androgenic	100
Anabolic	100
Standard	Standard
Chemical Names	4-androsten-3-one-17beta-ol
	17beta-hydroxy-androst-4-en-3-one
Estrogenic Activity	moderate
Progestational Activity	low

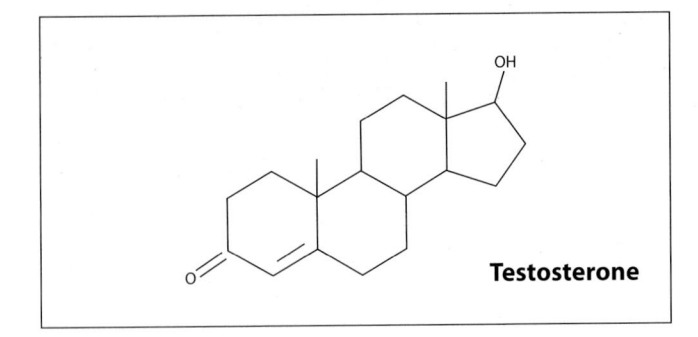

Testosterone

Description:

Sustanon® 100 is an oil-based injectable testosterone blend that contains three different testosterone esters: testosterone propionate (20 mg); testosterone phenylpropionate (40 mg); and testosterone isocaproate (40 mg). This product is manufactured by Organon, and is essentially a lower dosed version of their Sustanon® 250. Like Sustanon® 250, Sustanon® 100 makes use of multiple esters of testosterone to produce a desired slow-acting effect. The different esters have different levels of oil solubility, and likewise rates of release from the site of injection. The design is such that the rapid distribution of testosterone is followed by a sustained release of hormone. Sustanon® 100 is shorter acting than Sustanon® 250, as it lacks the longer decanoate ester, and is usually administered on a biweekly basis. This drug is ultimately very similar to testosterone cypionate or enanthate, but with a slightly shorter window of therapeutic effect.

History:

Sustanon® 100 is a modern adaptation of the well-known injectable testosterone blend Sustanon® 250, both of which were developed by the international pharmaceutical giant Organon. Sustanon® 100 is essentially a lower dosed equivalent of Sustanon® 250, supplying the same hormone in a similar (though not exact) time-released fashion. Sustanon® 100 is recommended for the same medical uses as Sustanon® 250, namely treating male androgen insufficiency, which can manifest itself with such symptoms as reduced sex drive, impotence, infertility, and bone loss. Increased adiposity (fat mass) and reduced lean mass are also common with patients suffering from low androgen levels. In addition to these uses, Sustanon® 100 is also recommended to induce masculinization in female-to-male transsexuals. Sustanon® 100 is produced only in a handful of countries at this time, and is not widely available.

How Supplied:

Sustanon® 100 is available in select human drug markets. All products are supplied in 1 mL glass ampules containing an oily solution; sold by or under license from Organon.

Structural Characteristics:

Sustanon® 100 contains a mixture of three testosterone compounds, which where modified with the addition of carboxylic acid esters (propionic, propionic phenyl ester, and isocaproic acids) at the 17-beta hydroxyl group. Esterified forms of testosterone are less polar than free testosterone, and are absorbed more slowly from the area of injection. Once in the bloodstream, the ester is removed to yield free (active) testosterone. Esterified forms of testosterone are designed to prolong the window of therapeutic effect following administration, allowing for a less frequent injection schedule compared to injections of free (unesterified) steroid. Sustanon 100 is designed to provide a rapid peak in testosterone levels (24-48 hours after injection), and maintain physiological concentrations for approximately 14 days.

Side Effects (Estrogenic):

Testosterone is readily aromatized in the body to estradiol (estrogen). The aromatase (estrogen synthetase) enzyme is responsible for this metabolism of testosterone. Elevated estrogen levels can cause side effects such as increased water retention, body fat gain, and gynecomastia. Testosterone is considered a moderately estrogenic steroid. An anti-estrogen such as clomiphene citrate or tamoxifen citrate may be necessary to prevent estrogenic side effects. One may alternately use an aromatase inhibitor like Arimidex® (anastrozole), which more efficiently controls estrogen by preventing its synthesis. Aromatase inhibitors can be quite expensive in comparison to anti-estrogens, however, and may also have negative effects on blood lipids.

Estrogenic side effects will occur in a dose-dependant manner, with higher doses (above normal therapeutic levels) of testosterone more likely to require the concurrent use of an anti-estrogen or aromatase inhibitor. Since water retention and loss of muscle definition are common with higher doses of testosterone, this drug is usually considered a poor choice for dieting or cutting phases of training. Its moderate estrogenicity makes it more ideal for bulking phases, where the added water retention will support raw strength and muscle size, and help foster a stronger anabolic environment.

Side Effects (Androgenic):

Testosterone is the primary male androgen, responsible for maintaining secondary male sexual characteristics. Elevated levels of testosterone are likely to produce androgenic side effects including oily skin, acne, and body/facial hair growth. Men with a genetic predisposition for hair loss (androgenetic alopecia) may notice accelerated male pattern balding. Those concerned about hair loss may find a more comfortable option in nandrolone decanoate, which is a comparably less androgenic steroid. Women are warned of the potential virilizing effects of anabolic/androgenic steroids, especially with a strong androgen such as testosterone. These may include deepening of the voice, menstrual irregularities, changes in skin texture, facial hair growth, and clitoral enlargement.

In androgen-responsive target tissues such as the skin, scalp, and prostate, the high relative androgenicity of testosterone is dependant on its reduction to dihydrotestosterone (DHT). The 5-alpha reductase enzyme is responsible for this metabolism of testosterone. The concurrent use of a 5-alpha reductase inhibitor such as finasteride or dutasteride will interfere with site-specific potentiation of testosterone action, lowering the tendency of testosterone drugs to produce androgenic side effects. It is important to remember that anabolic and androgenic effects are both mediated via the cytosolic androgen receptor. Complete separation of testosterone's anabolic and androgenic properties is not possible, even with total 5-alpha reductase inhibition.

Side Effects (Hepatotoxicity):

Testosterone does not have hepatotoxic effects; liver toxicity is unlikely. One study examined the potential for hepatotoxicity with high doses of testosterone by administering 400 mg of the hormone per day (2,800 mg per week) to a group of male subjects. The steroid was taken orally so that higher peak concentrations would be reached in hepatic tissues compared to intramuscular injections. The hormone was given daily for 20 days, and produced no significant changes in liver enzyme values including serum albumin, bilirubin, alanine-aminotransferase, and alkaline phosphatases.[730]

Side Effects (Cardiovascular):

Anabolic/androgenic steroids can have deleterious effects on serum cholesterol. This includes a tendency to reduce HDL (good) cholesterol values and increase LDL (bad) cholesterol values, which may shift the HDL to LDL balance in a direction that favors greater risk of arteriosclerosis. The relative impact of an anabolic/androgenic steroid on serum lipids is dependant on the dose, route of administration (oral vs. injectable), type of steroid (aromatizable or non-aromatizable), and level of resistance to hepatic metabolism. Anabolic/androgenic steroids may also adversely affect blood pressure and triglycerides, reduce endothelial relaxation, and support left ventricular hypertrophy, all potentially increasing the risk of cardiovascular disease and myocardial infarction.

Testosterone tends to have a much less dramatic impact on cardiovascular risk factors than synthetic steroids. This is due in part to its openness to metabolism by the liver, which allows it to have less effect on the hepatic management of cholesterol. The aromatization of testosterone to estradiol also helps to mitigate the negative effects of androgens on serum lipids. In one study, 280 mg per week of testosterone ester (enanthate) had a slight but not statistically significant effect on HDL cholesterol after 12 weeks, but when taken with an aromatase inhibitor a strong (25%) decrease was seen.[731] Studies using 300 mg of testosterone ester (enanthate) per week for 20 weeks without an aromatase inhibitor demonstrated only a 13% decrease in HDL cholesterol, while at 600 mg the reduction reached 21%.[732] The negative impact of aromatase inhibition should be taken into consideration before such drug is added to testosterone therapy.

Due to the positive influence of estrogen on serum lipids, tamoxifen citrate or clomiphene citrate are preferred to aromatase inhibitors for those concerned with cardiovascular health, as they offer a partial estrogenic effect in the liver. This allows them to potentially improve lipid profiles and offset some of the negative effects of androgens. With doses of 600 mg or less of testosterone per week, the impact on lipid profile tends to be noticeable but not dramatic, making an anti-estrogen (for cardioprotective purposes) perhaps unnecessary. Doses of 600 mg or less per week have also failed to produce statistically significant changes in LDL/VLDL cholesterol, triglycerides, apolipoprotein B/C-III, C-reactive protein, and insulin sensitivity, all indicating a relatively weak impact on cardiovascular risk factors.[733] When used in moderate doses, injectable testosterone esters are usually considered to be the safest of all anabolic/androgenic steroids.

To help reduce cardiovascular strain it is advised to maintain an active cardiovascular exercise program and minimize the intake of saturated fats, cholesterol, and simple carbohydrates at all times during active AAS administration. Supplementing with fish oils (4 grams per day) and a natural cholesterol/antioxidant formula such as Lipid Stabil or a product with comparable ingredients is also recommended.

Side Effects (Testosterone Suppression):

All anabolic/androgenic steroids when taken in doses sufficient to promote muscle gain are expected to suppress endogenous testosterone production. Testosterone is the primary male androgen, and offers strong negative feedback on endogenous testosterone production. Testosterone-based drugs will, likewise, have a strong effect on the hypothalamic regulation of natural steroid hormones. Without the intervention of testosterone-stimulating substances, testosterone levels should return to normal within 1-4 months of drug secession. Note that prolonged hypogonadotrophic hypogonadism can develop secondary to steroid abuse, necessitating medical intervention.

The above side effects are not inclusive. For more detailed discussion of potential side effects, see the Steroid Side Effects section of this book.

Administration (General):

Testosterone propionate is often regarded as a painful injection. This is due to the very short carbon chain of the propionic acid ester, which can be irritating to tissues at the site of injection. Many sensitive individuals choose to stay away from this steroid completely, their bodies reacting with a pronounced soreness and low-grade fever that may last for a few days after each injection.

Administration (Men):

To treat androgen insufficiency, the prescribing guidelines for Sustanon® 100 call for a dosage of 100 mg (1 ampule) every 2 weeks. Although active in the body for a longer time, Sustanon® 100 is usually injected every 7 to 10 days for muscle-building purposes. This schedule will allow for the higher doses most commonly applied by athletes, and more stable elevations in hormone level. The usual dosage among male athletes is in the range of 200-600 mg per week, taken in cycles 6 to 12 weeks in length. This level is sufficient for most users to notice exceptional gains in muscle size and strength. Testosterone is ultimately very versatile, and can be combined with many other anabolic/androgenic steroids depending on the desired effect.

Administration (Women):

Sustanon® 100 is rarely used with women in clinical medicine. When applied, it is most often used to induce masculinization in female to male transsexuals. Sustanon® 100 is not recommended for women for physique- or performance-enhancing purposes due to its strong androgenic nature, tendency to produce virilizing side effects, and slow-acting characteristics (making blood levels difficult to control).

Availability:

Sustanon® 100 is less widely distributed on the black market than Sustanon® 250, due to the fact that source countries producing this drug are limited. The moderate total amount of drug contained in each ampule (100 mg) also makes this product far less desirable to consumers than Sustanon® 250. Sustanon® 100 is mainly located in the Netherlands, Egypt, and the United Kingdom.

Sustanon® 250 (testosterone blend)

Androgenic	100
Anabolic	100
Standard	Standard
Chemical Names	4-androsten-3-one-17beta-ol
	17beta-hydroxy-androst-4-en-3-one
Estrogenic Activity	moderate
Progestational Activity	low

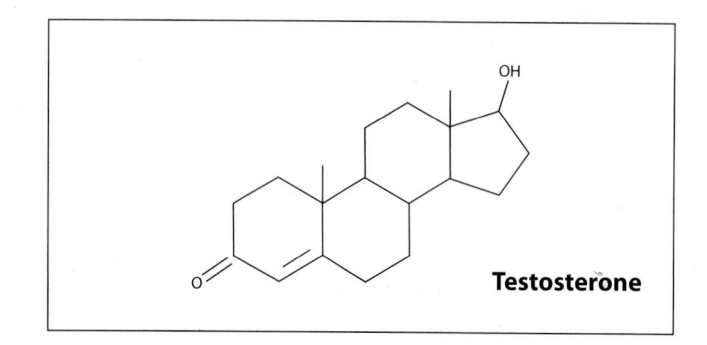

Description:

Sustanon® 250 is an oil-based injectable testosterone blend that contains four different testosterone esters: testosterone propionate (30 mg); testosterone phenylpropionate (60 mg); testosterone isocaproate (60 mg); and testosterone decanoate (100 mg). Sustanon® is designed to provide a fast yet extended release of testosterone, usually requiring injections once every 3 to 4 weeks in a clinical setting. This is an improvement from standard testosterones such as cypionate or enanthate, which provide a shorter duration of activity. As with all testosterone products, Sustanon® 250 is a very strong anabolic drug with pronounced androgenic activity. It is most commonly used in bulking cycles, providing exceptional gains in strength and muscle mass. A shorter-acting version of Sustanon®, called Sustanon® 100, is also made in certain areas (see: Sustanon 100).

History:

Sustanon® 250 first appeared on international drug markets during the early 1970's. It was developed by the international pharmaceutical giant Organon, also responsible for such steroids as Durabolin®, Deca-Durabolin®, and Andriol®. Sustanon® 250 was designed to offer a therapeutic advantage over existing single esters of testosterone, which need to be injected more frequently (cited advantages in hormone stability are probably not valid). In spite of this advantage, however, Sustanon® 250 has never been approved for sale in the United States, although around the world it is one of the most popular brands of testosterone available. The lack of U.S. availability is probably due to the high costs associated with the FDA approval process and the availability of other somewhat comparable agents, as Organon has a history of working in the U.S. market when it is financially feasible.

Over the past 25 years, Sustanon® 250 has probably been the most sought-after injectable testosterone among athletes. It must be emphasized, however, that this is not due to an unusual potency of this testosterone combination (esters really only affect the release of testosterone). This is simply due to the fact that a stack of four different testosterone compounds is a very good selling point; it is perceived to have more value. In most instances you will actually get a lot more for your money with testosterone enanthate or cypionate. The advantages to be found in Sustanon® 250 are for the medical user only. If you were tied to your doctor for regular injections, then Sustanon® 250 would allow you to visit him or her less frequently. This equates to a clear improvement in patient comfort. But if you are a bodybuilder injecting the drug every week, blood levels will build to the same extremes with either type of testosterone, and the added expense is probably not warranted.

How Supplied:

Sustanon® 250 is widely available in human and (select) veterinary drug markets. Packaging volume may vary by country and manufacturer; the majority of products are supplied as 1 mL glass ampules containing an oily solution; sold by or under license from Organon.

Structural Characteristics:

Sustanon® 250 contains a mixture of four testosterone compounds, which where modified with the addition of carboxylic acid esters (propionic, propionic phenyl ester, isocaproic, and decanoic acids) at the 17-beta hydroxyl group. Esterified forms of testosterone are less polar than free testosterone, and are absorbed more slowly from the area of injection. Once in the bloodstream, the ester is removed to yield free (active) testosterone. Esterified forms of testosterone are designed to prolong the window of therapeutic effect following administration, allowing for a less frequent injection schedule compared to injections of free (unesterified) steroid. Sustanon 250 is designed to provide a rapid peak in testosterone levels (24-48 hours after injection), and maintain physiological concentrations for approximately 21 days.[734] Each 250 mg ampule provides 176mg of testosterone.

Side Effects (Estrogenic):

Testosterone is readily aromatized in the body to estradiol (estrogen). The aromatase (estrogen synthetase) enzyme is responsible for this metabolism of testosterone. Elevated estrogen levels can cause side effects such as increased water retention, body fat gain, and gynecomastia. Testosterone is considered a moderately estrogenic steroid. An anti-estrogen such as clomiphene citrate or tamoxifen citrate may be necessary to prevent estrogenic side effects. One may alternately use an aromatase inhibitor like Arimidex® (anastrozole), which more efficiently controls estrogen by preventing its synthesis. Aromatase inhibitors can be quite expensive in comparison to anti-estrogens, however, and may also have negative effects on blood lipids.

Estrogenic side effects will occur in a dose-dependant manner, with higher doses (above normal therapeutic levels) of Sustanon® 250 more likely to require the concurrent use of an anti-estrogen or aromatase inhibitor. Since water retention and loss of muscle definition are common with higher doses of testosterone, this drug is usually considered a poor choice for dieting or cutting phases of training. Its moderate estrogenicity makes it more ideal for bulking phases, where the added water retention will support raw strength and muscle size, and help foster a stronger anabolic environment.

Side Effects (Androgenic):

Testosterone is the primary male androgen, responsible for maintaining secondary male sexual characteristics. Elevated levels of testosterone are likely to produce androgenic side effects including oily skin, acne, and body/facial hair growth. Men with a genetic predisposition for hair loss (androgenetic alopecia) may notice accelerated male pattern balding. Those concerned about hair loss may find a more comfortable option in nandrolone decanoate, which is a comparably less androgenic steroid. Women are warned of the potential virilizing effects of anabolic/androgenic steroids, especially with a strong androgen such as testosterone. These may include deepening of the voice, menstrual irregularities, changes in skin texture, facial hair growth, and clitoral enlargement.

In androgen-responsive target tissues such as the skin, scalp, and prostate, the high relative androgenicity of testosterone is dependant on its reduction to dihydrotestosterone (DHT). The 5-alpha reductase enzyme is responsible for this metabolism of testosterone. The concurrent use of a 5-alpha reductase inhibitor such as finasteride or dutasteride will interfere with site-specific potentiation of testosterone action, lowering the tendency of testosterone drugs to produce androgenic side effects. It is important to remember that anabolic and androgenic effects are both mediated via the cytosolic androgen receptor. Complete separation of testosterone's anabolic and androgenic properties is not possible, even with total 5-alpha reductase inhibition.

Side Effects (Hepatotoxicity):

Testosterone does not have hepatotoxic effects; liver toxicity is unlikely. One study examined the potential for hepatotoxicity with high doses of testosterone by administering 400 mg of the hormone per day (2,800 mg per week) to a group of male subjects. The steroid was taken orally so that higher peak concentrations would be reached in hepatic tissues compared to intramuscular injections. The hormone was given daily for 20 days, and produced no significant changes in liver enzyme values including serum albumin, bilirubin, alanine-amino-transferase, and alkaline phosphatases.[735]

Side Effects (Cardiovascular):

Anabolic/androgenic steroids can have deleterious effects on serum cholesterol. This includes a tendency to reduce HDL (good) cholesterol values and increase LDL (bad) cholesterol values, which may shift the HDL to LDL balance in a direction that favors greater risk of arteriosclerosis. The relative impact of an anabolic/androgenic steroid on serum lipids is dependant on the dose, route of administration (oral vs. injectable), type of steroid (aromatizable or non-aromatizable), and level of resistance to hepatic metabolism. Anabolic/androgenic steroids may also adversely affect blood pressure and triglycerides, reduce endothelial relaxation, and support left ventricular hypertrophy, all potentially increasing the risk of cardiovascular disease and myocardial infarction.

Testosterone tends to have a much less dramatic impact on cardiovascular risk factors than synthetic steroids. This is due in part to its openness to metabolism by the liver, which allows it to have less effect on the hepatic management of cholesterol. The aromatization of testosterone to estradiol also helps to mitigate the negative effects of androgens on serum lipids. In one study, 280 mg per week of testosterone ester (enanthate) had a slight but not statistically significant effect on HDL cholesterol after 12 weeks, but when taken with an aromatase inhibitor a strong (25%) decrease was seen.[736] Studies using 300 mg of testosterone ester (enanthate) per week for 20 weeks without an aromatase inhibitor demonstrated only a 13% decrease in HDL cholesterol, while at 600 mg the reduction reached 21%.[737] The negative impact of aromatase inhibition should be taken into consideration before such drug is added to testosterone therapy.

Due to the positive influence of estrogen on serum lipids, tamoxifen citrate or clomiphene citrate are preferred to aromatase inhibitors for those concerned with cardiovascular health, as they offer a partial estrogenic effect in the liver. This allows them to potentially improve lipid profiles and offset some of the negative effects of androgens. With doses of 600 mg or less of testosterone per week, the impact on lipid profile tends to be noticeable but not dramatic, making an anti-estrogen (for cardioprotective purposes) perhaps unnecessary. Doses of 600 mg or less per week have also failed to produce statistically significant changes in LDL/VLDL cholesterol, triglycerides, apolipoprotein B/C-III, C-reactive protein, and insulin sensitivity, all indicating a relatively weak impact on cardiovascular risk factors.[738] When used in moderate doses, injectable testosterone esters are usually considered to be the safest of all anabolic/androgenic steroids.

To help reduce cardiovascular strain it is advised to maintain an active cardiovascular exercise program and minimize the intake of saturated fats, cholesterol, and simple carbohydrates at all times during active AAS administration. Supplementing with fish oils (4 grams per day) and a natural cholesterol/antioxidant formula such as Lipid Stabil or a product with comparable ingredients is also recommended.

Side Effects (Testosterone Suppression):

All anabolic/androgenic steroids when taken in doses sufficient to promote muscle gain are expected to suppress endogenous testosterone production. Testosterone is the primary male androgen, and offers strong negative feedback on endogenous testosterone production. Testosterone-based drugs will, likewise, have a strong effect on the hypothalamic regulation of natural steroid hormones. Without the intervention of testosterone-stimulating substances, testosterone levels should return to normal within 1-4 months of drug secession. Note that prolonged hypogonadotrophic hypogonadism can develop secondary to steroid abuse, necessitating medical intervention.

The above side effects are not inclusive. For more detailed discussion of potential side effects, see the Steroid Side Effects section of this book.

Administration (General):

Testosterone propionate is often regarded as a painful injection. This is due to the very short carbon chain of the propionic acid ester, which can be irritating to tissues at the site of injection. Many sensitive individuals choose to stay away from this steroid completely, their bodies reacting with a pronounced soreness and low-grade fever that may last for a few days after each injection.

Administration (Men):

To treat androgen insufficiency, the prescribing guidelines for Sustanon® 250 call for a dosage of 250 mg every 3 weeks. Although active in the body for a longer time, Sustanon® 250 is usually injected every 7 to 10 days for muscle-building purposes. This schedule will allow for the higher doses most commonly applied by athletes, and more stable elevations in hormone level. The usual dosage among male athletes is in the range of 250-750 mg per injection, taken in cycles 6 to 12 weeks in length. This level is sufficient for most users to notice exceptional gains in muscle size and strength.

Sustanon® 250 is usually incorporated into bulking phases of training, when added water retention will be of little consequence, the user more concerned with raw mass than definition. Some do incorporate this drug into cutting cycles as well, but typically in lower doses (125-250 mg every 7-10 days) and/or when accompanied by an aromatase inhibitor to keep estrogen levels under control. Sustanon® 250 is a very effective anabolic drug, and is often used alone with great benefit. Some, however, find a need to stack it with other anabolic/androgenic steroids for a stronger effect, in which case an additional 200-400 mg per week of boldenone undecylenate, methenolone enanthate, or nandrolone decanoate should provide substantial results with no significant hepatotoxicity. Testosterone is ultimately very versatile, and can be combined with many other anabolic/androgenic steroids to tailor the desired effect.

Some bodybuilders have been known to use excessively high dosages of this drug (1,000 mg per week or more), although this practice is generally not advised. At dosages above 750 mg per week, water retention will likely account for more of the additional weight gain than new muscle tissue. The practice of "megadosing" is inefficient (not to mention potentially dangerous), especially when we take into account the typical high cost of Sustanon 250. Such use is usually not justified outside of aggressive bodybuilding regimens.

Administration (Women):

Sustanon® 250 is rarely used with women in clinical medicine. When applied, it is most often used to induce masculinization in female to male transsexuals. Sustanon® 250 is not recommended for women for physique- or performance-enhancing purposes due to its strong androgenic nature, tendency to produce virilizing side effects, and slow- acting characteristics (making blood levels difficult to control).

Availability:

Despite being much more costly than other esters, Sustanon® remains very abundant on the U.S. black market.

Intervet, makers of Laurabolin, manufactures a 5 mL vial in Australia called Durateston. Don't expect it to circulate the black market very much though, as these drugs are tightly controlled in Australia.

BM Pharmaceuticals is an India export company that produces Sustaretard 250. This product comes in the form of 1 mL ampules, each containing the 250 mg blend of esters. This product is very reminiscent of Russian Sustanon by Infar (see below) in its packaging (see pictures in the photo section)

Russian Sustanon, manufactured under license by Infar in India (for export to former Soviet countries), may still be in circulation. This product comes packaged in plastic strips that hold five ampules, sealed on the face with white paper label. Each ampule is enclosed in a separate compartment, and the packaging is scored so as to break off individual ampule sections. One standout characteristic is that the ampule labels and packaging bear a big green "250" imprint under the lettering.

Organon Sustanon is marketed directly in Russia. The product looks very much like European forms of Sustanon, with clear glass ampules, colored bands, and paper labels. Note that the product name is written in Cyrillic as "CYCTAHOH."

Omnadren® 250 from Poland now carries the Sustanon 250 formulation, and is readily exported and made available on the black market. Counterfeits are a concern, so be careful when shopping. Best advice would be to purchase this product only when it is properly packaged in its 5-ampule box. This will weed out a good majority of the fake loose ampules in circulation. Also, measure one of the ampules. Real Omnadren® 250 uses an ampule that measures 5 centimeters in height. There are some very nice fakes (currently circulating in high volume) that measure about 4.5cm, a half centimeter too short.

Sostenon 250 redi-jects manufactured by Organon in Mexico are also still found, although much less commonly in recent years in light of the less expensive products now coming out of this country. The price for a Sostenon redi-ject is about $7-8 in Mexico, $10 in some more expensive tourist areas. In the United States they can sell for as high as $25 each. Note that Organon has embedded a watermark of their logo around the surface of the box. This is a difficult trait to copy without spending quite a bit of money, although probably unnecessary given that the syringes and foil-sealed trays are already too costly for underground labs to consider duplicating. If you want a guaranteed safe buy, the Mexican "Pre-load" has always been one.

Less common, but still seen on the U.S. black market, are the European versions of Sustanon from countries like Italy, Portugal, Belgium, and England. All of these products use ampules that are scored, carry colored (yellow and red) rings on the tip, and have white paper labels.

Durateston, the brand name Organon uses to market this multi-component testosterone blend in Brazil, is also seen in the U.S. on occasion. Be sure your product has the accompanying box and paperwork, which will weed out some of the cheaper counterfeits.

Two versions of this steroid have been made in Egypt by the Nile Co in recent years. The first is called Testonon, and the second Sustanon. The fact that two different versions exist may have to do with licensing issues with Organon, as only the latter product is seen to bear the Organon logo. Fakes are known to exist, so be careful when shopping. In particular, make sure the Nile logo is genuine on the box (both products), which will help you identify one of the most common fakes in circulation at this time (see photo section for comparison photographs). Also, the Nile Sustanon is highly counterfeited, but there are a couple of things you can look for to weed out most of them. For one, make sure the "/" in "250 mg / ML" touches or almost touches the Organon logo. Many of the fakes have a larger than normal space here. Also, look at the letter "X" in "Exp." closely. The real product doesn't really have a normal "Western" letter X. The two halves of the letter do not intersect perfectly in the middle, and the letter actually looks more like a K or N upon close examination. Fakes are normally printed with the help of Western computer equipment with more familiar typestyles. If your X looks like a perfect X, the product you have is fake.

Sustanon 250 from Karachi Pakistan is also popular as of late. These ampules are clear glass with yellow silk-screen printing. This is one of the few versions of this steroid product sold by Organon globally that does not carry a paper label. Fakes are circulating in high volume at this time, so be careful. Note that the current real product has its lot numbers printed on with electronic equipment, and are not silk-screened on the glass at the same time as the rest of the lettering.

Balkan Pharmaceuticals manufactures a Sustanon clone in Moldova called Sustamed. It comes in 1 mL glass ampules. Counterfeits are not known to be a problem.

Synovex® (testosterone propionate & estradiol)

Androgenic	100
Anabolic	100
Standard	standard
Chemical Names	4-androsten-3-one-17beta-ol
	17beta-hydroxy-androst-4-en-3-one
Estrogenic Activity	moderate
Progestational Activity	low

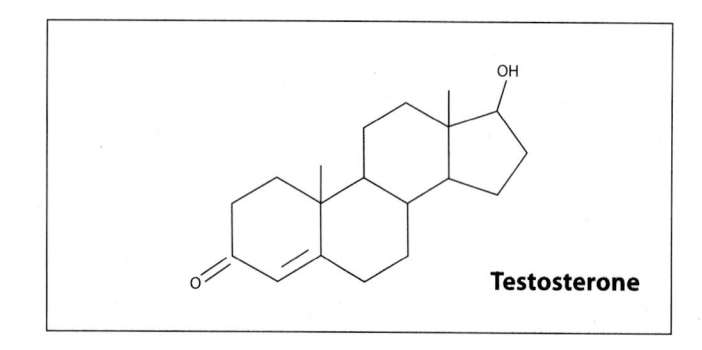

Description:

Synovex is a blended-ingredient steroid implant preparation, which is available only as a veterinary item for use in cattle. The implant comes in the form of small pellets, which are pushed into the ear of an animal with a very large implant gun. Once implanted, the pellets slowly dissolve, providing an extended release of steroids for many weeks. The hormone content of Synovex is mixed, with each pellet containing 25 mg testosterone propionate and 2.5 mg estradiol benzoate. This 10:1 ratio has been demonstrated to provide an added anabolic/weight gaining effect in feed animals, improving the value of the livestock. Given its estrogen content, Synovex is clearly not an ideal steroid for humans. Most athletes have only become attracted to this product out of sheer desperation for legitimate anabolics, as cattle implants like this are not regulated as controlled substances in the U.S. to spite their steroid content. Otherwise, a pure testosterone propionate product would be much more appropriate.

History:

Testosterone propionate plus estrogen implant pellets were first approved by the U.S. Food and Drug administration for use in heifers in 1958.[739] Diethylstilbestrol, a potent estrogen often used to increase animal carcass weight, had been approved four years earlier for use in cattle, however, and would remain the leading product for many years. Syntex introduced their version of testosterone/estrogen pellets (Synovex) during the early 1970's, as part of the company's new Animal Health division. This was during a time a time when diethylstilbestrol was getting a great deal of negative publicity. Synovex became a huge seller when the FDA banned the use of diethylstilbestrol in 1973, the product quickly capturing more than 50% of the market for growth-promoting implants. The popularity of Synovex soon caught the attention of other companies, a number of which soon started making their own blended testosterone/estrogen implants. Popular brand names in the U.S. have included F-TO (Upjohn), Heifer-oid (Boehringer), and Implus (Upjohn). Synovex and other testosterone/estrogen pellets remain widely available in the U.S. and abroad today, although are not highly popular with athletes given their estrogen content.

How Supplied:

Synovex contains 25 mg of testosterone propionate and 2.5 mg of estradiol benzoate in a small sterile implantation pellet. The number of pellets in each cartridge dose will vary depending on the intended target animal. Implants denoted "H" for heifer will carry the most; in the case of U.S. Synovex-H it is 80 pellets (10 doses consisting each of 8 pellets). We will see a slightly lower pellet count in the "S" implants (steer) and "C" (calf) cartridges.

Structural Characteristics:

Testosterone propionate is a modified form of testosterone, where a carboxylic acid ester (propionic acid) has been attached to the 17-beta hydroxyl group to slow the release of testosterone from the area of implantation. This preparation also contains an ester (benzoic acid) of estradiol.

Side Effects (Estrogenic):

Testosterone is readily aromatized in the body to estradiol (estrogen). Additionally, this preparation contains an active estrogen. Elevated estrogen levels can cause side effects such as increased water retention, body fat gain, and gynecomastia. This steroid preparation is considered to be highly estrogenic. An anti-estrogen such as clomiphene citrate or tamoxifen citrate may be necessary to prevent estrogenic side effects. One may alternately use an aromatase inhibitor like Arimidex® (anastrozole), although it will not have an affect on the additional estrogen present in the preparation. Since water retention and loss of muscle definition are common with highly estrogenic steroid products, this drug is usually considered a poor choice for dieting or cutting phases of training. It would only be appropriate during bulking phases, where the added water retention will support raw strength and muscle size, and help foster a stronger anabolic environment.

Side Effects (Androgenic):

Testosterone is the primary male androgen, responsible for maintaining secondary male sexual characteristics. Elevated levels of testosterone are likely to produce androgenic side effects including oily skin, acne, and body/facial hair growth. Men with a genetic predisposition for hair loss (androgenetic alopecia) may notice accelerated male pattern balding. Those concerned about hair loss may find a more comfortable option in nandrolone decanoate, which is a comparably less androgenic steroid. Women are warned of the potential virilizing effects of anabolic/androgenic steroids, especially with a strong androgen such as testosterone. These may include deepening of the voice, menstrual irregularities, changes in skin texture, facial hair growth, and clitoral enlargement.

Side Effects (Hepatotoxicity):

Testosterone and estrogen do not have hepatotoxic effects; liver toxicity is unlikely.

Side Effects (Cardiovascular):

Anabolic/androgenic steroids can have deleterious effects on serum cholesterol. This includes a tendency to reduce HDL (good) cholesterol values and increase LDL (bad) cholesterol values, which may shift the HDL to LDL balance in a direction that favors greater risk of arteriosclerosis. The relative impact of an anabolic/androgenic steroid on serum lipids is dependant on the dose, route of administration (oral vs. injectable), type of steroid (aromatizable or non-aromatizable), and level of resistance to hepatic metabolism. Testosterone tends to have a much less dramatic impact on cardiovascular risk factors than synthetic steroids. This is due in part to its openness to metabolism by the liver, which allows it to have less effect on the hepatic management of cholesterol. The aromatization of testosterone to estradiol also helps to mitigate the negative effects of androgens on serum lipids. The added estrogen in this product may further help to offset some of the androgenic effect on lipid values, and the preparation may, therefore, have a weaker impact on cholesterol than a comparably dosed straight testosterone product. Anabolic/androgenic steroids may also adversely affect blood pressure and triglycerides, reduce endothelial relaxation, and support left ventricular hypertrophy, all potentially increasing the risk of cardiovascular disease and myocardial infarction.

Side Effects (Testosterone Suppression):

All anabolic/androgenic steroids when taken in doses sufficient to promote muscle gain are expected to suppress endogenous testosterone production. Testosterone is the primary male androgen, and offers strong negative feedback on endogenous testosterone production. The added estrogen will also provide negative-feedback suppression. This preparation should have a strong effect on the hypothalamic regulation of natural steroid hormones. Without the intervention of testosterone stimulating substances, testosterone levels should return to normal within 1-4 months of drug secession. Note that prolonged hypogonadotrophic hypogonadism can develop secondary to steroid abuse, necessitating medical intervention.

To help reduce cardiovascular strain it is advised to maintain an active cardiovascular exercise program and minimize the intake of saturated fats, cholesterol, and simple carbohydrates at all times during active AAS administration. Supplementing with fish oils (4 grams per day) and a natural cholesterol/antioxidant formula such as Lipid Stabil or a product with comparable ingredients is also recommended.

The above side effects are not inclusive. For more detailed discussion of potential side effects, see the Steroid Side Effects section of this book.

Administration (General):

Synovex implant pellets were not designed for human consumption. To make use of these pellets, they must be converted into another (more suitable) delivery form. To do this, an athlete will typically grind them up and rub them on the skin in a 50/50 mixture of DMSO and water to facilitate transdermal delivery. Alternately, one may mix up a homebrew injection with the pellets. This is done by grinding them into a fine powder and introducing the powder into filtered oil or an oil-based steroid. One should remember that the practice of preparing Synovex for injection is not going to be sterile, and as such could be potentially dangerous. Note that some methods have additionally been published for removing the estrogen from the pellets, to make the drug more comfortable to use. They generally involve the use of highly flammable materials, take a number of different steps to complete, and leave some estrogen when the process is over, however, usually making the process more trouble than it is worth.

Administration (Men):

Synovex is not approved for use in humans. Prescribing

guidelines are unavailable. When used for physique- or performance-enhancing purposes (very rarely), the dose is calculated based on the route of administration. When given by transdermal delivery, a bioavailability rate of no more than 10% is assumed. A daily dosage of 4 pellets (100 mg) would, therefore, provide the equivalent of 70 mg per week of testosterone propionate (as given by injection). When given by injection a dose of 100 mg every second or third day is most common. The drug is generally taken for no more than 8 weeks, and is used almost exclusively during bulking phases of training. Those who have experimented with this product have been generally disappointed with the results, as the added estrogen has often resulted in rapid gynecomastia, noticeable body fat accumulation, and severe water retention. In many cases the water retained has caused an unsightly bloated look (extreme loss of definition).

Administration (Women):

Synovex is not approved for use in humans. Prescribing guidelines are unavailable. Synovex is not recommended for women for physique- or performance-enhancing purposes due to its strong androgenic nature and tendency to produce virilizing side effects.

Availability:

Synovex is rarely found on the black market, given that the product is in poor demand and generally can be obtained through legitimate Agricultural or Veterinary supply stores. No counterfeits have ever been known to exist.

Test® 400 (testosterone propionate/cypionate/enanthate)

Androgenic	100
Anabolic	100
Standard	Standard
Chemical Names	4-androsten-3-one-17beta-ol
	17beta-hydroxy-androst-4-en-3-one
Estrogenic Activity	moderate
Progestational Activity	low

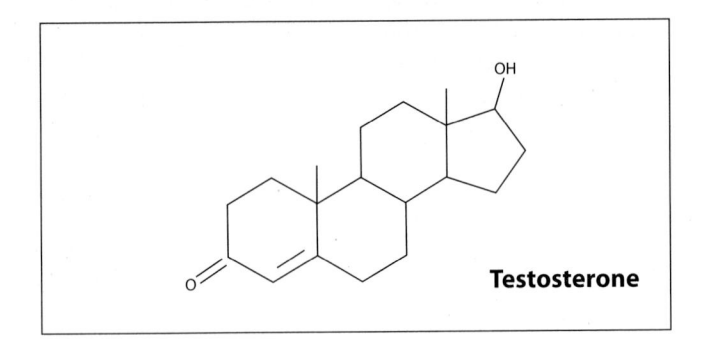

Testosterone

Description:

Test 400 is an injectable preparation containing a blend of three testosterone esters. According to the product labeling, each milliliter contains 25 milligrams of testosterone propionate, 187 milligrams of testosterone cypionate, and 188 milligrams of testosterone enanthate, for a total steroid concentration of 400 mg/ml. The design of this steroid most closely resembles that of Testoviron®, the only differences between the two being the concentrations of the esters, and the addition of testosterone cypionate in the case of Test 400. The pharmacokinetics of testosterone enanthate and cypionate are virtually identical, so there should be little functional difference between this preparation and the propionate/enanthate blend of Testoviron®. Like Testoviron®, Test 400® offers the disadvantage of having a rapid onset of action, and very unbalanced pharmacokinetics compared to testosterone enanthate or cypionate alone.

History:

Test 400® was developed in Mexico by the veterinary drug manufacturer Denkall. The product was popular during the early 2000's, its high dosage a big selling point for dealers. Test 400® was developed at a time when the Mexican veterinary steroid market had an abundance of steroids, purportedly for animal treatment, but with obvious appeal to bodybuilders. In December 2005, the U.S. DEA arrested Denkall's owner Albert Saltiel-Cohen, charging him with illegally distributing anabolic steroids in the U.S. The arrest was part of Operation Gear-Grinder, a 21-month investigation into the robust U.S.-Mexican steroid trade that effectively closed Denkall and Cohen's other operations, Animal Power and Quality Vet. Gear-Grinder also resulted in the voluntary withdrawal of the SYD Group steroid line, and many other individual products from other manufacturers.

How Supplied:

Test 400® contained 25 mg of testosterone propionate, 187mg of testosterone cypionate, and 188mg of testosterone enanthate per milliliter of oil; packaged in a 10 mL multi-dose vial.

Structural Characteristics:

Test 400® contains a mixture of three testosterone compounds, which where modified with the addition of carboxylic acid esters (propionic, cyclopentylpropionic, and enanthoic acids) at the 17-beta hydroxyl group. Esterified forms of testosterone are less polar than free testosterone, and are absorbed more slowly from the area of injection. Once in the bloodstream, the ester is removed to yield free (active) testosterone. Esterified forms of testosterone are designed to prolong the window of therapeutic effect following administration, allowing for a less frequent injection schedule compared to injections of free (unesterified) steroid. Test 400® is designed to provide a rapid peak in testosterone levels (24-48 hours after injection), and maintain physiological concentrations for approximately 14 days.

Side Effects (Estrogenic):

Testosterone is readily aromatized in the body to estradiol (estrogen). The aromatase (estrogen synthetase) enzyme is responsible for this metabolism of testosterone. Elevated estrogen levels can cause side effects such as increased water retention, body fat gain, and gynecomastia. Testosterone is considered a moderately estrogenic steroid. An anti-estrogen such as clomiphene citrate or tamoxifen citrate may be necessary to prevent estrogenic side effects. One may alternately use an aromatase inhibitor like Arimidex® (anastrozole), which more efficiently controls estrogen by preventing its synthesis. Aromatase inhibitors can be quite expensive in comparison to anti-estrogens, however, and may also have negative effects on blood lipids.

Estrogenic side effects will occur in a dose-dependant manner, with higher doses (above normal therapeutic levels) of testosterone more likely to require the concurrent use of an anti-estrogen or aromatase inhibitor. Since water retention and loss of muscle definition are common with higher doses of testosterone, this drug is usually considered a poor choice for dieting or cutting phases of training. Its moderate estrogenicity makes it more ideal for bulking phases, where the added water retention will support raw strength and muscle size, and help foster a stronger anabolic environment.

Side Effects (Androgenic):

Testosterone is the primary male androgen, responsible for maintaining secondary male sexual characteristics. Elevated levels of testosterone are likely to produce androgenic side effects including oily skin, acne, and body/facial hair growth. Men with a genetic predisposition for hair loss (androgenetic alopecia) may notice accelerated male pattern balding. Those concerned about hair loss may find a more comfortable option in nandrolone decanoate, which is a comparably less androgenic steroid. Women are warned of the potential virilizing effects of anabolic/androgenic steroids, especially with a strong androgen such as testosterone. These may include deepening of the voice, menstrual irregularities, changes in skin texture, facial hair growth, and clitoral enlargement.

In androgen-responsive target tissues such as the skin, scalp, and prostate, the high relative androgenicity of testosterone is dependant on its reduction to dihydrotestosterone (DHT). The 5-alpha reductase enzyme is responsible for this metabolism of testosterone. The concurrent use of a 5-alpha reductase inhibitor such as finasteride or dutasteride will interfere with site-specific potentiation of testosterone action, lowering the tendency of testosterone drugs to produce androgenic side effects. It is important to remember that anabolic and androgenic effects are both mediated via the cytosolic androgen receptor. Complete separation of testosterone's anabolic and androgenic properties is not possible, even with total 5-alpha reductase inhibition.

Side Effects (Hepatotoxicity):

Testosterone does not have hepatotoxic effects; liver toxicity is unlikely. One study examined the potential for hepatotoxicity with high doses of testosterone by administering 400 mg of the hormone per day (2,800 mg per week) to a group of male subjects. The steroid was taken orally so that higher peak concentrations would be reached in hepatic tissues compared to intramuscular injections. The hormone was given daily for 20 days, and produced no significant changes in liver enzyme values including serum albumin, bilirubin, alanine-aminotransferase, and alkaline phosphatases.[740]

Side Effects (Cardiovascular):

Anabolic/androgenic steroids can have deleterious effects on serum cholesterol. This includes a tendency to reduce HDL (good) cholesterol values and increase LDL (bad) cholesterol values, which may shift the HDL to LDL balance in a direction that favors greater risk of arteriosclerosis. The relative impact of an anabolic/androgenic steroid on serum lipids is dependant on the dose, route of administration (oral vs. injectable), type of steroid (aromatizable or non-aromatizable), and level of resistance to hepatic metabolism. Anabolic/androgenic steroids may also adversely affect blood pressure and triglycerides, reduce endothelial relaxation, and support left ventricular hypertrophy, all potentially increasing the risk of cardiovascular disease and myocardial infarction.

Testosterone tends to have a much less dramatic impact on cardiovascular risk factors than synthetic steroids. This is due in part to its openness to metabolism by the liver, which allows it to have less effect on the hepatic management of cholesterol. The aromatization of testosterone to estradiol also helps to mitigate the negative effects of androgens on serum lipids. In one study, 280 mg per week of testosterone ester (enanthate) had a slight but not statistically significant effect on HDL cholesterol after 12 weeks, but when taken with an aromatase inhibitor a strong (25%) decrease was seen.[741] Studies using 300 mg of testosterone ester (enanthate) per week for 20 weeks without an aromatase inhibitor demonstrated only a 13% decrease in HDL cholesterol, while at 600 mg the reduction reached 21%.[742] The negative impact of aromatase inhibition should be taken into consideration before such drug is added to testosterone therapy.

Due to the positive influence of estrogen on serum lipids, tamoxifen citrate or clomiphene citrate are preferred to aromatase inhibitors for those concerned with cardiovascular health, as they offer a partial estrogenic effect in the liver. This allows them to potentially improve lipid profiles and offset some of the negative effects of androgens. With doses of 600 mg or less per week, the impact on lipid profile tends to be noticeable but not dramatic, making an anti-estrogen (for cardioprotective purposes) perhaps unnecessary. Doses of 600 mg or less per week have also failed to produce statistically significant changes in LDL/VLDL cholesterol, triglycerides, apolipoprotein B/C-III, C-reactive protein, and insulin sensitivity, all indicating a relatively weak impact on cardiovascular risk factors.[743] When used in moderate doses, injectable testosterone esters are usually considered to be the safest of all anabolic/androgenic steroids.

To help reduce cardiovascular strain it is advised to maintain an active cardiovascular exercise program and minimize the intake of saturated fats, cholesterol, and simple carbohydrates at all times during active AAS administration. Supplementing with fish oils (4 grams per day) and a natural cholesterol/antioxidant formula such as Lipid Stabil or a product with comparable ingredients is also recommended.

Side Effects (Testosterone Suppression):

All anabolic/androgenic steroids when taken in doses sufficient to promote muscle gain are expected to suppress endogenous testosterone production. Testosterone is the primary male androgen, and offers strong negative feedback on endogenous testosterone production. Testosterone-based drugs will, likewise, have a strong effect on the hypothalamic regulation of natural steroid hormones. Without the intervention of testosterone-stimulating substances, testosterone levels should return to normal within 1-4 months of drug secession. Note that prolonged hypogonadotrophic hypogonadism can develop secondary to steroid abuse, necessitating medical intervention.

The above side effects are not inclusive. For more detailed discussion of potential side effects, see the Steroid Side Effects section of this book.

Administration (General):

Testosterone propionate is often regarded as a painful injection. This is due to the very short carbon chain of the propionic acid ester, which can be irritating to tissues at the site of injection. This irritation may be amplified by higher than normal amounts of alcohol, which would be required to solubilize the high concentration of steroid labeled to be in Test 400. Sensitive individuals may choose to stay away from this steroid completely, their bodies reacting with a pronounced soreness and low-grade fever that may last for a few days after each injection. Diluting the Test 400® dosage with an equal volume of a low concentration steroid may lessen injection discomfort.

Administration (Men):

For bodybuilding purposes, Test 400® is usually injected on a weekly basis, in a dosage of 200-600 mg. Cycles are generally between 6 and 12 weeks in length. This level is sufficient to provide excellent gains in muscle size and strength. Testosterone drugs are ultimately very versatile, and can be combined with many other anabolic/androgenic steroids depending on the desired effect.

Administration (Women):

Test 400® is not recommended for women for physique- or performance-enhancing purposes due to its strong androgenic nature, tendency to produce virilizing side effects, and slow acting characteristics (making blood levels difficult to control).

Availability:

Test 400® from Denkall is no longer being manufactured. Some underground preparations may be found with similar blends of testosterone propionate, cypionate, and enanthate.

Testoderm® (testosterone)

Androgenic	100
Anabolic	100
Standard	Standard
Chemical Names	4-androsten-3-one-17beta-ol
	17beta-hydroxy-androst-4-en-3-one
Estrogenic Activity	moderate
Progestational Activity	low

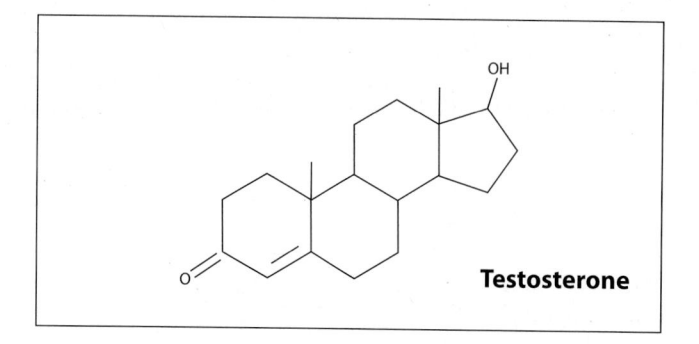

Description:

Testoderm® and Testoderm® TTS are testosterone delivery systems that utilize a "patch" to deliver the hormone transdermally. Both products were designed to deliver an approximate 5 mg dose of testosterone to the body over a 24-hour period, after which point the patch is replaced with a fresh one. Testoderm is an older matrix-type skin patch, which uses no penetration enhancers, so it must be applied on the scrotum, where the skin is much more permeable to testosterone. Testoderm TTS is a newer reservoir-type skin patch containing an alcoholic gel of testosterone, which can be placed on the arm, back, or upper buttocks. Testoderm and Testoderm TTS are designed to mimic the natural circadian rhythm of testosterone release in healthy young men, higher during the first 12 hours and lower during the next 12 hours of each day. The clinical significance of this, if any, is not known.

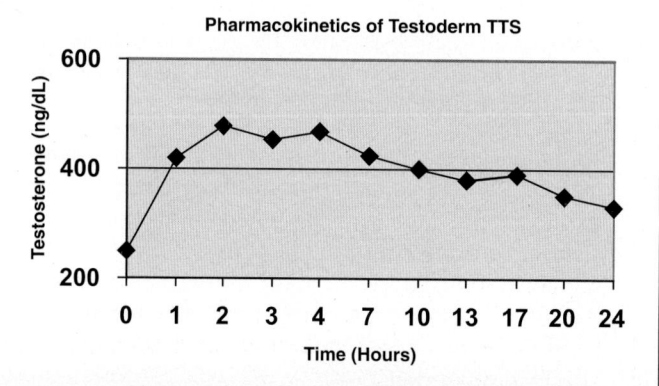

Figure 1. Mean serum testosterone concentrations (ng/dL) measured during application of Testoderm TTS to 32 hypogonadal men. Source: Transdermal testosterone administration in hypogonadal men: comparison of pharmacokinetics at different sites of application and at the first and 5ths days of application. J Clin Pharmacol 37: 1129-38.

History:

Testoderm® was developed in the United States by Alza Corporation, and introduced for sale in 1998. The drug is FDA-approved for testosterone replacement therapy in men with a deficiency or absence of endogenous testosterone. The Testoderm system itself did not make use of any penetration enhancers, and consequently is applied to an area of shaved scrotal skin, which is about 5 times more permeable to testosterone than normal body skin. Lacking an integrated adhesive, Alza soon released an updated version of Testoderm called simply Testoderm With Adhesive. Testoderm was an effective androgen replacement product, but did have the slight disadvantage of elevating DHT levels in many patients due to the prominence of 5-alpha reductase in the scrotum.[744]

Testoderm was ultimately the first testosterone patch to be developed for commercial sale. While it was deemed a success initially, it was soon obsolete next to the newer and less intrusive Androderm patch (FDA approved in 1995). Alza released Testoderm TTS in 1998, in an effort to retain its share of the male androgen replacement market. The new updated patch can be placed on three types of skin (back, arms, and upper buttocks), and has the advantage of causing less skin irritation next to Androderm. It also does not require that the patient rotate application sites each day. Since its approval in the U.S., Testoderm TTS has also been approved in select markets abroad, although not widely.

How Supplied:

Testoderm, Testoderm With Adhesive, and Testoderm TTS transdermal testosterone systems are available in select human drug markets. Each comes in the form of a transdermal patch system, which delivers approximately 5 mg of testosterone each.

Structural Characteristics:

Testoderm® is a matrix-type transdermal drug delivery system that contains testosterone (free) enclosed in a skin-applied patch. Testoderm® TTS is reservoir-type transdermal drug delivery system that contains testosterone (free) enclosed in a skin-applied adhesive patch. Both are designed to provide steady but varying levels of testosterone transdermally during each 24-hour period of application.

Side Effects (Estrogenic):

Testosterone is readily aromatized in the body to estradiol (estrogen). The aromatase (estrogen synthetase) enzyme is responsible for this metabolism of testosterone. Elevated estrogen levels can cause side effects such as increased water retention, body fat gain, and gynecomastia. Testosterone is considered a moderately estrogenic steroid. Exceeding therapeutic doses will increase the likelihood of estrogenic side effects. In such cases, an anti-estrogen such as clomiphene citrate or tamoxifen citrate is commonly applied to prevent estrogenic side effects. One may alternately use an aromatase inhibitor like Arimidex® (anastrozole), which more efficiently controls estrogen by preventing its synthesis. Aromatase inhibitors can be quite expensive in comparison to anti-estrogens, however, and may also have negative effects on blood lipids.

Side Effects (Androgenic):

Testosterone is the primary male androgen, responsible for maintaining secondary male sexual characteristics. Exceeding therapeutic doses is likely to produce androgenic side effects including oily skin, acne, and body/facial hair growth. Men with a genetic predisposition for hair loss (androgenetic alopecia) may notice accelerated male pattern balding. Women are warned of the potential virilizing effects of anabolic/androgenic steroids, especially with a strong androgen such as testosterone. These may include deepening of the voice, menstrual irregularities, changes in skin texture, facial hair growth, and clitoral enlargement.

In androgen-responsive target tissues such as the skin, scalp, and prostate, the high relative androgenicity of testosterone is dependant on its reduction to dihydrotestosterone (DHT). The 5-alpha reductase enzyme is responsible for this metabolism of testosterone. The concurrent use of a 5-alpha reductase inhibitor such as finasteride or dutasteride will interfere with site-specific potentiation of testosterone action, lowering the tendency of testosterone drugs to produce androgenic side effects. It is important to remember that anabolic and androgenic effects are both mediated via the cytosolic androgen receptor. Complete separation of testosterone's anabolic and androgenic properties is not possible, even with total 5-alpha reductase inhibition.

Side Effects (Hepatotoxicity):

Testosterone does not have hepatotoxic effects; liver toxicity is unlikely. One study examined the potential for hepatotoxicity with high doses of testosterone by administering 400 mg of the hormone per day (2,800 mg per week) to a group of male subjects. The steroid was taken orally so that higher peak concentrations would be reached in hepatic tissues compared to intramuscular injections. The hormone was given daily for 20 days, and produced no significant changes in liver enzyme values including serum albumin, bilirubin, alanine-amino-transferase, and alkaline phosphatases.[745]

Side Effects (Cardiovascular):

Anabolic/androgenic steroids can have deleterious effects on serum cholesterol. This includes a tendency to reduce HDL (good) cholesterol values and increase LDL (bad) cholesterol values, which may shift the HDL to LDL balance in a direction that favors greater risk of arteriosclerosis. The relative impact of an anabolic/androgenic steroid on serum lipids is dependant on the dose, route of administration (oral vs. injectable), type of steroid (aromatizable or non-aromatizable), and level of resistance to hepatic metabolism. Anabolic/androgenic steroids may also adversely affect blood pressure and triglycerides, reduce endothelial relaxation, and support left ventricular hypertrophy, all potentially increasing the risk of cardiovascular disease and myocardial infarction. Therapeutic doses of testosterone used to correct insufficient androgen production in otherwise healthy aging men are unlikely to increase atherogenic risk, and may actually reduce the risk of cardiovascular mortality.[746]

To help reduce cardiovascular strain it is advised to maintain an active cardiovascular exercise program and minimize the intake of saturated fats, cholesterol, and simple carbohydrates at all times during active AAS administration. Supplementing with fish oils (4 grams per day) and a natural cholesterol/antioxidant formula such as Lipid Stabil or a product with comparable ingredients is also recommended.

Side Effects (Testosterone Suppression):

All anabolic/androgenic steroids when taken in doses sufficient to promote muscle gain are expected to suppress endogenous testosterone production. Testosterone is the primary male androgen, and offers strong negative feedback on endogenous testosterone production. Testosterone-based drugs will, likewise, have a strong effect on the hypothalamic regulation of natural steroid hormones. Without the intervention of testosterone-stimulating substances, testosterone levels should return to normal within 1-4 months of drug secession. Note that prolonged hypogonadotrophic hypogonadism can develop secondary to steroid abuse, necessitating medical intervention.

The above side effects are not inclusive. For more detailed discussion of potential side effects, see the Steroid Side Effects section of this book.

Administration (General):

Testoderm is applied daily (in the morning) to intact, clean, shaven dry skin of the scrotum. Testoderm TTS is applied daily (in the morning) to intact, clean, dry skin of the back, arms, or upper buttocks. Many OTC ointments will significantly reduce the penetration of testosterone when applied to the skin before use, and should be avoided.

Administration (Men):

To treat androgen insufficiency, the prescribing guidelines for Testoderm and Testoderm TTS recommend the application of one patch daily, which delivers approximately 5 mg of testosterone systemically. For physique- or performance-enhancing purposes, higher doses would be necessary to achieve supraphysiological levels of testosterone. This would require at least three or four patches per day, delivering approximately 15-20 mg of testosterone. This level is sufficient for most users to notice gains in muscle size and strength, although this is not a very realistic idea in a practical sense. Lower doses may be used, but typically when accompanied by other anabolic/androgenic steroids. Testosterone is ultimately very versatile, and can be combined with many other anabolic/androgenic steroids to tailor the desired effect.

Administration (Women):

Testoderm and Testoderm TTS are not FDA-approved for use in women. Testosterone is not recommended for women for physique- or performance-enhancing purposes due to its strong androgenic nature and tendency to produce virilizing side effects.

Availability:

Given their high relative price and low delivery of testosterone, Testoderm and Testoderm TTS are not commonly traded on the black market. Counterfeits have not yet been reported. These preparations can probably be considered real if located.

Testolent (testosterone phenylpropionate)

Androgenic	100
Anabolic	100
Standard	Standard
Chemical Names	4-androsten-3-one-17beta-ol
	17beta-hydroxy-androst-4-en-3-one
Estrogenic Activity	moderate
Progestational Activity	low

Testosterone

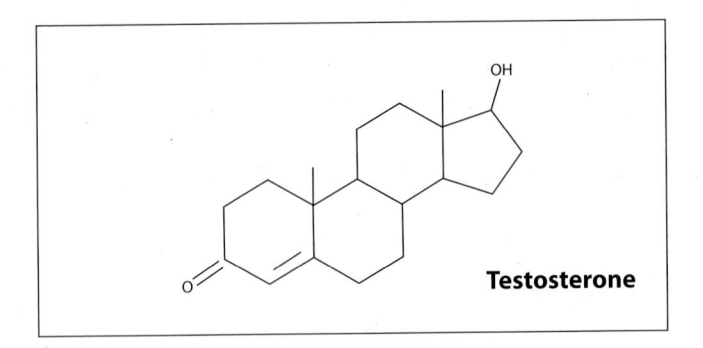

Description:

Testolent is an injectable testosterone preparation containing the fast-acting phenylpropionate ester of testosterone. Testosterone phenylpropionate is one of the constituents in Sustanon®, although this profile concerns its use as a stand-alone ingredient. The activity of Testolent is ultimately very similar to testosterone propionate, supplying the same hormone over at best a slightly longer duration of release. While propionate is injected every second or third day, phenylpropionate might be stretched out to every fourth day. Testolent might be more comfortable to use, as testosterone propionate is notoriously very painful at the site of injection, but otherwise there is really no strong advantage to this preparation in comparison.

History:

Testosterone phenylpropionate was first described in a French medical journal in 1955.[747] A few isolated commercial products containing testosterone phenylpropionate were developed in the years following, although this never was a popular item. Testolent was the most recent preparation of testosterone phenylpropionate known to be on the global steroid market, and was marketed in Romania by Sicomed. This agent was used primarily to correct low androgen levels in males, but as also occasionally prescribed in females for the treatment of advanced breast cancer, osteoporosis, uterine neoplasm, and low sex drive. Sicomed recently discounted its sale, however, and no other products containing only testosterone phenylpropionate are currently known to exist.

How Supplied:

Testosterone phenylpropionate is no longer available as a stand-alone commercial drug product. When produced in Romania, the Testolent brand contained 100 mg of testosterone phenylpropionate in a 1-milliliter ampule.

Structural Characteristics:

Testosterone phenylpropionate is a modified form of testosterone, where a carboxylic acid ester (propionic acid phenyl ester) has been attached to the 17-beta hydroxyl group. Esterified forms of testosterone are less polar than free testosterone, and are absorbed more slowly from the area of injection. Once in the bloodstream, the ester is removed to yield free (active) testosterone. Esterified forms of testosterone are designed to prolong the window of therapeutic effect following administration, allowing for a less frequent injection schedule compared to injections of free (unesterified) steroid.

Side Effects (Estrogenic):

Testosterone is readily aromatized in the body to estradiol (estrogen). The aromatase (estrogen synthetase) enzyme is responsible for this metabolism of testosterone. Elevated estrogen levels can cause side effects such as increased water retention, body fat gain, and gynecomastia. Testosterone is considered a moderately estrogenic steroid. An anti-estrogen such as clomiphene citrate or tamoxifen citrate may be necessary to prevent estrogenic side effects. One may alternately use an aromatase inhibitor like Arimidex® (anastrozole), which more efficiently controls estrogen by preventing its synthesis. Aromatase inhibitors can be quite expensive in comparison to anti-estrogens, however, and may also have negative effects on blood lipids.

Estrogenic side effects will occur in a dose-dependant manner, with higher doses (above normal therapeutic levels) of testosterone more likely to require the concurrent use of an anti-estrogen or aromatase inhibitor. Since water retention and loss of muscle definition are common with higher doses of testosterone, this drug is usually considered a poor choice for dieting or cutting phases of training. Its moderate estrogenicity makes it more ideal for bulking phases, where the added water retention will support raw strength and muscle size, and help foster a stronger anabolic environment.

Side Effects (Androgenic):

Testosterone is the primary male androgen, responsible for maintaining secondary male sexual characteristics. Elevated levels of testosterone are likely to produce androgenic side effects including oily skin, acne, and body/facial hair growth. Men with a genetic predisposition for hair loss (androgenetic alopecia) may notice accelerated male pattern balding. Those concerned about hair loss may find a more comfortable option in nandrolone decanoate, which is a comparably less androgenic steroid. Women are warned of the potential virilizing effects of anabolic/androgenic steroids, especially with a strong androgen such as testosterone. These may include deepening of the voice, menstrual irregularities, changes in skin texture, facial hair growth, and clitoral enlargement.

In androgen-responsive target tissues such as the skin, scalp, and prostate, the high relative androgenicity of testosterone is dependant on its reduction to dihydrotestosterone (DHT). The 5-alpha reductase enzyme is responsible for this metabolism of testosterone. The concurrent use of a 5-alpha reductase inhibitor such as finasteride or dutasteride will interfere with site-specific potentiation of testosterone action, lowering the tendency of testosterone drugs to produce androgenic side effects. It is important to remember that anabolic and androgenic effects are both mediated via the cytosolic androgen receptor. Complete separation of testosterone's anabolic and androgenic properties is not possible, even with total 5-alpha reductase inhibition.

Side Effects (Hepatotoxicity):

Testosterone does not have hepatotoxic effects; liver toxicity is unlikely. One study examined the potential for hepatotoxicity with high doses of testosterone by administering 400 mg of the hormone per day (2,800 mg per week) to a group of male subjects. The steroid was taken orally so that higher peak concentrations would be reached in hepatic tissues compared to intramuscular injections. The hormone was given daily for 20 days, and produced no significant changes in liver enzyme values including serum albumin, bilirubin, alanine-aminotransferase, and alkaline phosphatases.[748]

Side Effects (Cardiovascular):

Anabolic/androgenic steroids can have deleterious effects on serum cholesterol. This includes a tendency to reduce HDL (good) cholesterol values and increase LDL (bad) cholesterol values, which may shift the HDL to LDL balance in a direction that favors greater risk of arteriosclerosis. The relative impact of an anabolic/androgenic steroid on serum lipids is dependant on the dose, route of administration (oral vs. injectable), type of steroid (aromatizable or non-aromatizable), and level of resistance to hepatic metabolism. Anabolic/androgenic steroids may also adversely affect blood pressure and triglycerides, reduce endothelial relaxation, and support left ventricular hypertrophy, all potentially increasing the risk of cardiovascular disease and myocardial infarction.

Testosterone tends to have a much less dramatic impact on cardiovascular risk factors than synthetic steroids. This is due in part to its openness to metabolism by the liver, which allows it to have less effect on the hepatic management of cholesterol. The aromatization of testosterone to estradiol also helps to mitigate the negative effects of androgens on serum lipids. In one study, 280 mg per week of testosterone ester (enanthate) had a slight but not statistically significant effect on HDL cholesterol after 12 weeks, but when taken with an aromatase inhibitor a strong (25%) decrease was seen.[749] Studies using 300 mg of testosterone ester (enanthate) per week for 20 weeks without an aromatase inhibitor demonstrated only a 13% decrease in HDL cholesterol, while at 600 mg the reduction reached 21%.[750] The negative impact of aromatase inhibition should be taken into consideration before such drug is added to testosterone therapy.

Due to the positive influence of estrogen on serum lipids, tamoxifen citrate or clomiphene citrate are preferred to aromatase inhibitors for those concerned with cardiovascular health, as they offer a partial estrogenic effect in the liver. This allows them to potentially improve lipid profiles and offset some of the negative effects of androgens. With doses of 600 mg or less per week, the impact on lipid profile tends to be noticeable but not dramatic, making an anti-estrogen (for cardioprotective purposes) perhaps unnecessary. Doses of 600 mg or less per week have also failed to produce statistically significant changes in LDL/VLDL cholesterol, triglycerides, apolipoprotein B/C-III, C-reactive protein, and insulin sensitivity, all indicating a relatively weak impact on cardiovascular risk factors.[751] When used in moderate doses, injectable testosterone esters are usually considered to be the safest of all anabolic/androgenic steroids.

To help reduce cardiovascular strain it is advised to maintain an active cardiovascular exercise program and minimize the intake of saturated fats, cholesterol, and simple carbohydrates at all times during active AAS administration. Supplementing with fish oils (4 grams per day) and a natural cholesterol/antioxidant formula such as Lipid Stabil or a product with comparable ingredients is

also recommended.

Side Effects (Testosterone Suppression):

All anabolic/androgenic steroids when taken in doses sufficient to promote muscle gain are expected to suppress endogenous testosterone production. Testosterone is the primary male androgen, and offers strong negative feedback on endogenous testosterone production. Testosterone-based drugs will, likewise, have a strong effect on the hypothalamic regulation of natural steroid hormones. Without the intervention of testosterone-stimulating substances, testosterone levels should return to normal within 1-4 months of drug secession. Note that prolonged hypogonadotrophic hypogonadism can develop secondary to steroid abuse, necessitating medical intervention.

The above side effects are not inclusive. For more detailed discussion of potential side effects, see the Steroid Side Effects section of this book.

Administration (Men):

For the treatment of low androgen levels, the prescribing guidelines for Testolent recommend administering a dose of 100 mg every 25 days. For physique- or performance-enhancing purposes, this drug is usually injected twice per week. The total weekly dosage is typically 200-600 mg, which is sufficient to provide excellent gains in muscle size and strength. Testosterone drugs are ultimately very versatile, and can be combined with many other anabolic/androgenic steroids depending on the desired effect.

Administration (Women):

The prescribing guidelines for Testolent do not make special dosing recommendations for women. This drug is not recommended for women for physique- or performance-enhancing purposes due to its strong androgenic nature, tendency to produce virilizing side effects, and slow acting characteristics (making blood levels difficult to control).

Availability:

Testolent is no longer available, although residual stock may still be located. Counterfeits are not known to be a problem.

Testopel® (testosterone)

Androgenic	100
Anabolic	100
Standard	Standard
Chemical Names	19-norandrost-4-en-3-one-17beta-ol
	17beta-hydroxy-estr-4-en-3-one
Estrogenic Activity	moderate
Progestational Activity	low

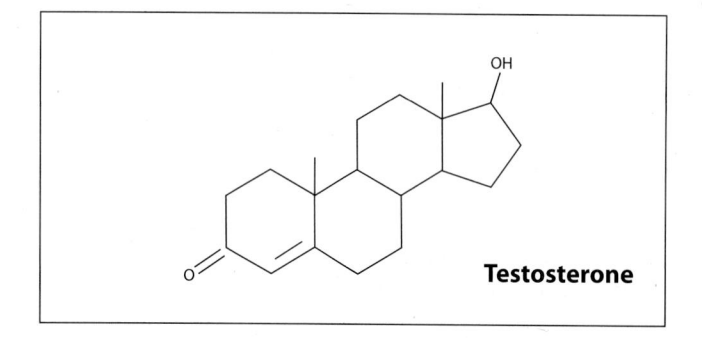

Description:

Testopel® is a testosterone delivery system comprised of small cylindrical pellets of pressed testosterone. The pellets are sterile, and are comprised almost purely of testosterone, barring a small amount of added binders for stability. These pellets are implanted subcutaneously, and provide the patient a continuous and very even release of hormone for several months. Testosterone pellets have the advantage of allowing the patient to not think about their hormone replacement therapy on a daily, weekly, or monthly basis as with many other hormone delivery systems, and provide a much more even release of hormone (less highs and lows) than popular injections. Testosterone implant pellets, however, have the disadvantage of requiring that the patient undergo minor office surgery twice to several times per year.

History:

Soon after the oral delivery of testosterone was deemed impractical due to rapid first pass metabolism, it was realized that pressed pellets of surgically implanted sterile testosterone could provide physiological androgen levels for extended periods of time to patients in need of such therapy. Implanted testosterone pellets were accepted very early as viable options for delivering testosterone, and various such commercial preparations have been introduced and prescribed over the years (although historically injectable esters and suspensions of testosterone have been the norm in this field of medicine).

Currently, Bartor Pharmacal produces the only commercially available brand of testosterone pellet in the U.S., sold as Testopel. Each pellet contains 75 mg of (free) testosterone. It is FDA-approved for use in adult males with conditions associated with a deficiency or absence of endogenous testosterone. This includes cases of primary hypogonadism caused by cryptorchidism, bilateral torsion, orchitis, vanishing testis syndrome, orchiectomy, Klinefelter's syndrome, chemotherapy, or alcohol/heavy metal toxicity. It is also prescribed to treat hypogonadotrophic hypogonadism caused by tumors, injury, or radiation. FDA laws also allow certain private compounding pharmacies to manufacture generic testosterone implant pellet preparations. Testosterone implant pellets are not commonly made outside the U.S., but can be located in certain markets.

How Supplied:

Testosterone implant pellets are available in select human drug markets. Composition and dosage may vary by country or manufacturer, but generally contain approximately 98.5% pure testosterone (along with some inert binders) in a small cylindrical pressed pellet.

Structural Characteristics:

Sterile testosterone pellets for implantation contain (free) testosterone in a pressed pellet. The pellets are implanted subcutaneously with a minor surgical procedure, and slowly dissolve over time, releasing testosterone into the blood. Testosterone pellets are designed to provide testosterone for approximately 4-6 months following implantation.

Side Effects (Estrogenic):

Testosterone is readily aromatized in the body to estradiol (estrogen). The aromatase (estrogen synthetase) enzyme is responsible for this metabolism of testosterone. Elevated estrogen levels can cause side effects such as increased water retention, body fat gain, and gynecomastia. Testosterone is considered a moderately estrogenic steroid. Exceeding therapeutic doses will increase the likelihood of estrogenic side effects. In such cases, an anti-estrogen such as clomiphene citrate or tamoxifen citrate is commonly applied to prevent estrogenic side effects. One may alternately use an aromatase inhibitor like Arimidex® (anastrozole), which more efficiently controls estrogen by preventing its synthesis. Aromatase inhibitors can be quite expensive in comparison to anti-estrogens, however, and may also have negative effects on blood lipids.

Side Effects (Androgenic):

Testosterone is the primary male androgen, responsible for maintaining secondary male sexual characteristics. Exceeding normal therapeutic doses is likely to produce androgenic side effects including oily skin, acne, and body/facial hair growth. Men with a genetic predisposition for hair loss (androgenetic alopecia) may notice accelerated male pattern balding. Women are warned of the potential virilizing effects of anabolic/androgenic steroids, especially with a strong androgen such as testosterone. These may include deepening of the voice, menstrual irregularities, changes in skin texture, facial hair growth, and clitoral enlargement.

In androgen-responsive target tissues such as the skin, scalp, and prostate, the high relative androgenicity of testosterone is dependant on its reduction to dihydrotestosterone (DHT). The 5-alpha reductase enzyme is responsible for this metabolism of testosterone. The concurrent use of a 5-alpha reductase inhibitor such as finasteride or dutasteride will interfere with site-specific potentiation of testosterone action, lowering the tendency of testosterone drugs to produce androgenic side effects. It is important to remember that anabolic and androgenic effects are both mediated via the cytosolic androgen receptor. Complete separation of testosterone's anabolic and androgenic properties is not possible, even with total 5-alpha reductase inhibition.

Side Effects (Hepatotoxicity):

Testosterone does not have hepatotoxic effects; liver toxicity is unlikely. One study examined the potential for hepatotoxicity with high doses of testosterone by administering 400 mg of the hormone per day (2,800 mg per week) to a group of male subjects. The steroid was taken orally so that higher peak concentrations would be reached in hepatic tissues compared to intramuscular injections. The hormone was given daily for 20 days, and produced no significant changes in liver enzyme values including serum albumin, bilirubin, alanine-amino-transferase, and alkaline phosphatases.[752]

Side Effects (Cardiovascular):

Anabolic/androgenic steroids can have deleterious effects on serum cholesterol. This includes a tendency to reduce HDL (good) cholesterol values and increase LDL (bad) cholesterol values, which may shift the HDL to LDL balance in a direction that favors greater risk of arteriosclerosis. The relative impact of an anabolic/androgenic steroid on serum lipids is dependant on the dose, route of administration (oral vs. injectable), type of steroid (aromatizable or non-aromatizable), and level of resistance to hepatic metabolism. Anabolic/androgenic steroids may also adversely affect blood pressure and triglycerides, reduce endothelial relaxation, and support left ventricular hypertrophy, all potentially increasing the risk of cardiovascular disease and myocardial infarction. Therapeutic doses of testosterone used to correct insufficient androgen production in otherwise healthy aging men are unlikely to increase atherogenic risk, and may actually reduce the risk of cardiovascular mortality.[753]

To help reduce cardiovascular strain it is advised to maintain an active cardiovascular exercise program and minimize the intake of saturated fats, cholesterol, and simple carbohydrates at all times during active AAS administration. Supplementing with fish oils (4 grams per day) and a natural cholesterol/antioxidant formula such as Lipid Stabil or a product with comparable ingredients is also recommended.

Side Effects (Testosterone Suppression):

All anabolic/androgenic steroids when taken in doses sufficient to promote muscle gain are expected to suppress endogenous testosterone production. Testosterone is the primary male androgen, and offers strong negative feedback on endogenous testosterone production. Testosterone-based drugs will, likewise, have a strong effect on the hypothalamic regulation of natural steroid hormones. Without the intervention of testosterone-stimulating substances, testosterone levels should return to normal within 1-4 months of the drug leaving the body. Note that prolonged hypogonadotrophic hypogonadism can develop secondary to steroid abuse, necessitating medical intervention.

The above side effects are not inclusive. For more detailed discussion of potential side effects, see the Steroid Side Effects section of this book.

Administration (General):

Sterile testosterone pellets are implanted subdermally in the lower abdominal wall. Prior to insertion, the skin is cleaned with alcohol and draped with a 2% xylocaine solution. A 2-cm incision is made through anaesthetized skin, and the pellets administered with the aid of a cannula. The incision site is covered with a sterile Band-Aid and a waterproof dressing for 1 week, and should not require stitching.

Administration (Men):

To treat androgen insufficiency, the prescribing guidelines

for Testopel recommend implanting a row of 4-6 pellets (300-450 mg of testosterone) once every 4-6 months. For physique- or performance-enhancing purposes, higher doses would be necessary to achieve supraphysiological levels of testosterone. This would be in the range of 12-18 pellets per application, which is not highly practical given the higher volume and surgical requirements for implantation.

Administration (Women):

Testopel is not FDA-approved for use in women. Testosterone implant pellets are not recommended for women for physique- or performance-enhancing purposes due to their strong androgenic nature, tendency to produce virilizing side effects, and very slow-acting characteristics.

Availability:

Due to the relative impracticality of general private use, Testopel is not commonly traded on the black market.

William Llewellyn's ANABOLICS, 9th ed.

Testoviron® (testosterone propionate/enanthate blend)

Androgenic	100
Anabolic	100
Standard	Standard
Chemical Names	4-androsten-3-one-17beta-ol 17beta-hydroxy-androst-4-en-3-one
Estrogenic Activity	moderate
Progestational Activity	low

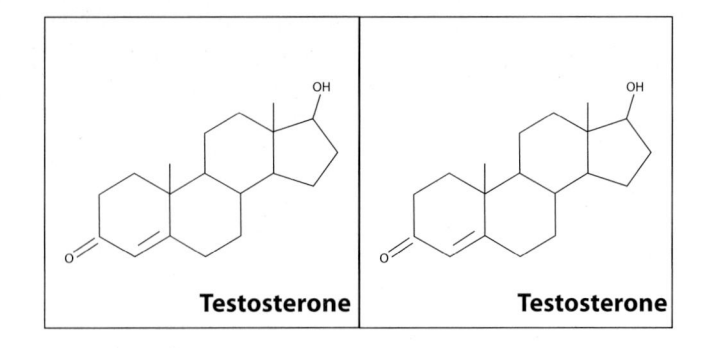

Description:

Testoviron® is a mixed testosterone injectable, containing varying amounts of testosterone propionate and testosterone enanthate. The faster-acting propionate ester is included to support testosterone release during the early days of therapy, while the longer-acting ester is included to support the latter part of the therapeutic window. Together, the two are supposed to result in a rapid increase in testosterone level, followed by a sustained hormone elevation for approximately 2 weeks. The design of this steroid is therefore very similar to Sustanon®, although lacking the decanoate ester Testoviron® will remain active in the body for a shorter duration. Testoviron® was originally marketed as an improvement over single-ester preparations like testosterone enanthate, said to provide a much more balanced release of hormone in comparison.

Upon close analysis, the pharmacokinetic properties of Testoviron® are not as ideal as initially described. The problem lies in the fact that testosterone enanthate is not a delayed-onset drug, but actually provides a sharp spike in testosterone levels 24-48 hours after administration. Adding a fast-acting ester like testosterone propionate to a formulation of testosterone enanthate only compounds the initial testosterone spike. See the provided computer simulation of the release pattern. It shows an even sharper early testosterone peak compared to the use of testosterone enanthate alone, providing the user with a greater imbalance between the early and latter days of the administration window. A study administering a blend of 115.7mg of testosterone enanthate and 20 mg of testosterone propionate confirms this tendency; demonstrating maximal increases in serum testosterone the first day following injection.[754]

History:

Testoviron® was developed by international pharmaceutical giant Schering in Germany, and marketed at one time in many of the European markets including Germany, Austria, Italy, Spain, Ireland, Greece, Switzerland, Netherlands, Denmark, and Sweden. This product is, likewise, usually identified as a European item, although it was produced scarcely in Eastern Europe and the Caribbean as well. Schering also uses the Testoviron® brand for its pure testosterone enanthate products, which are generally used for the same medical applications (generally male androgen replacement therapy), and have always been much more widely distributed.

The Schering Testoviron® products first surfaced in Europe during the early 1950's, and have since been duplicated in one form or another by numerous different drug manufacturers in many different parts of the world. Although scarcely remembered, blended enanthate and propionate products were once even available commercially in the U.S. Most notable was the brand Testoject E.P. from Mayrand, which contained 200 mg of testosterone enanthate and 25 mg of testosterone propionate in a 1 mL vial. Today, however, no such commercial product exists. Blended ester products like this are still prescribed in the United States, but lack of a commercial item means they are only dispensed by private compounding pharmacies.

Schering has been refining its steroid product line a great deal since the 1990's, eliminating many unprofitable or controversial items. This has resulted in their discontinuing the sale of blended ester Testoviron® compounds in most markets. At this time these products remain in extremely limited production globally. The only known product left on the European market is Testoviron® Depot 100, which contains 110 mg of testosterone enanthate and 25 mg testosterone propionate, for a 100 mg total dose of (free) testosterone. As mentioned earlier, blended testosterone enanthate and propionate products are produced by many other companies, and can still be located in a wide variety of human and veterinary drug markets.

How Supplied:

Testosterone propionate and testosterone enanthate blends are available in various human and veterinary drug markets. Composition and dosage may vary by country and manufacturer. Schering Testoviron® products contained a blend of 20 mg/55 mg, 25 mg/110 mg, or 50 mg/200 mg of testosterone propionate and enanthate (respectively) per milliliter; packaged in 1 mL ampules.

Structural Characteristics:

Testoviron® contains a mixture of two testosterone compounds, which where modified with the addition of carboxylic acid esters (propionic and enanthoic acids) at the 17-beta hydroxyl group. Esterified forms of testosterone are less polar than free testosterone, and are absorbed more slowly from the area of injection. Once in the bloodstream, the ester is removed to yield free (active) testosterone. Esterified forms of testosterone are designed to prolong the window of therapeutic effect following administration, allowing for a less frequent injection schedule compared to injections of free (unesterified) steroid. Testoviron® is designed to provide a rapid peak in testosterone levels (24-48 hours after injection), and maintain physiological concentrations for approximately 14 days.

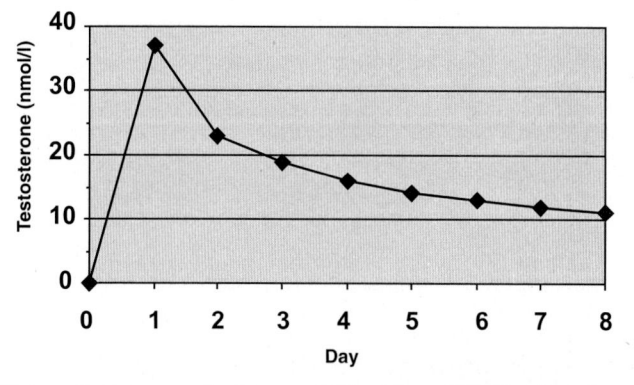

Figure 1. Proposed pharmacokinetics of Testoviron® injection (110 mg testosterone enanthate, 25 mg testosterone propionate) based on an analysis of the published properties of testosterone propionate and enanthate. Source: Testosterone Action Deficiency Substitution 2nd Edition. E. Nieschlag H.M. Behre (Eds.) Springer-Verlag Berlin Heidelberg New York (1998)

Side Effects (Estrogenic):

Testosterone is readily aromatized in the body to estradiol (estrogen). The aromatase (estrogen synthetase) enzyme is responsible for this metabolism of testosterone. Elevated estrogen levels can cause side effects such as increased water retention, body fat gain, and gynecomastia. Testosterone is considered a moderately estrogenic steroid. An anti-estrogen such as clomiphene citrate or tamoxifen citrate may be necessary to prevent estrogenic side effects. One may alternately use an aromatase inhibitor like Arimidex® (anastrozole), which more efficiently controls estrogen by preventing its synthesis. Aromatase inhibitors can be quite expensive in comparison to anti-estrogens, however, and may also have negative effects on blood lipids.

Estrogenic side effects will occur in a dose-dependant manner, with higher doses (above normal therapeutic levels) of testosterone more likely to require the concurrent use of an anti-estrogen or aromatase inhibitor. Since water retention and loss of muscle definition are common with higher doses of testosterone, this drug is usually considered a poor choice for dieting or cutting phases of training. Its moderate estrogenicity makes it more ideal for bulking phases, where the added water retention will support raw strength and muscle size, and help foster a stronger anabolic environment.

Side Effects (Androgenic):

Testosterone is the primary male androgen, responsible for maintaining secondary male sexual characteristics. Elevated levels of testosterone are likely to produce androgenic side effects including oily skin, acne, and body/facial hair growth. Men with a genetic predisposition for hair loss (androgenetic alopecia) may notice accelerated male pattern balding. Those concerned about hair loss may find a more comfortable option in nandrolone decanoate, which is a comparably less androgenic steroid. Women are warned of the potential virilizing effects of anabolic/androgenic steroids, especially with a strong androgen such as testosterone. These may include deepening of the voice, menstrual irregularities, changes in skin texture, facial hair growth, and clitoral enlargement.

In androgen-responsive target tissues such as the skin, scalp, and prostate, the high relative androgenicity of testosterone is dependant on its reduction to dihydrotestosterone (DHT). The 5-alpha reductase enzyme is responsible for this metabolism of testosterone. The concurrent use of a 5-alpha reductase inhibitor such as finasteride or dutasteride will interfere with site-specific potentiation of testosterone action, lowering the tendency of testosterone drugs to produce androgenic side effects. It is important to remember that anabolic and androgenic effects are both mediated via the cytosolic androgen receptor. Complete separation of testosterone's anabolic and androgenic properties is not possible, even with total 5-alpha reductase inhibition.

Side Effects (Hepatotoxicity):

Testosterone does not have hepatotoxic effects; liver toxicity is unlikely. One study examined the potential for hepatotoxicity with high doses of testosterone by administering 400 mg of the hormone per day (2,800 mg per week) to a group of male subjects. The steroid was taken orally so that higher peak concentrations would be reached in hepatic tissues compared to intramuscular injections. The hormone was given daily for 20 days, and produced no significant changes in liver enzyme values including serum albumin, bilirubin, alanine-aminotransferase, and alkaline phosphatases.[755]

Side Effects (Cardiovascular):

Anabolic/androgenic steroids can have deleterious effects on serum cholesterol. This includes a tendency to reduce HDL (good) cholesterol values and increase LDL (bad) cholesterol values, which may shift the HDL to LDL balance in a direction that favors greater risk of arteriosclerosis. The relative impact of an anabolic/androgenic steroid on serum lipids is dependant on the dose, route of administration (oral vs. injectable), type of steroid (aromatizable or non-aromatizable), and level of resistance to hepatic metabolism. Anabolic/androgenic steroids may also adversely affect blood pressure and triglycerides, reduce endothelial relaxation, and support left ventricular hypertrophy, all potentially increasing the risk of cardiovascular disease and myocardial infarction.

Testosterone tends to have a much less dramatic impact on cardiovascular risk factors than synthetic steroids. This is due in part to its openness to metabolism by the liver, which allows it to have less effect on the hepatic management of cholesterol. The aromatization of testosterone to estradiol also helps to mitigate the negative effects of androgens on serum lipids. In one study, 280 mg per week of testosterone ester (enanthate) had a slight but not statistically significant effect on HDL cholesterol after 12 weeks, but when taken with an aromatase inhibitor a strong (25%) decrease was seen.[756] Studies using 300 mg of testosterone ester (enanthate) per week for 20 weeks without an aromatase inhibitor demonstrated only a 13% decrease in HDL cholesterol, while at 600 mg the reduction reached 21%.[757] The negative impact of aromatase inhibition should be taken into consideration before such drug is added to testosterone therapy.

Due to the positive influence of estrogen on serum lipids, tamoxifen citrate or clomiphene citrate are preferred to aromatase inhibitors for those concerned with cardiovascular health, as they offer a partial estrogenic effect in the liver. This allows them to potentially improve lipid profiles and offset some of the negative effects of androgens. With doses of 600 mg or less per week, the impact on lipid profile tends to be noticeable but not dramatic, making an anti-estrogen (for cardioprotective purposes) perhaps unnecessary. Doses of 600 mg or less per week have also failed to produce statistically significant changes in LDL/VLDL cholesterol, triglycerides, apolipoprotein B/C-III, C-reactive protein, and insulin sensitivity, all indicating a relatively weak impact on cardiovascular risk factors.[758] When used in moderate doses, injectable testosterone esters are usually considered to be the safest of all anabolic/androgenic steroids.

To help reduce cardiovascular strain it is advised to maintain an active cardiovascular exercise program and minimize the intake of saturated fats, cholesterol, and simple carbohydrates at all times during active AAS administration. Supplementing with fish oils (4 grams per day) and a natural cholesterol/antioxidant formula such as Lipid Stabil or a product with comparable ingredients is also recommended.

Side Effects (Testosterone Suppression):

All anabolic/androgenic steroids when taken in doses sufficient to promote muscle gain are expected to suppress endogenous testosterone production. Testosterone is the primary male androgen, and offers strong negative feedback on endogenous testosterone production. Testosterone-based drugs will, likewise, have a strong effect on the hypothalamic regulation of natural steroid hormones. Without the intervention of testosterone-stimulating substances, testosterone levels should return to normal within 1-4 months of drug secession. Note that prolonged hypogonadotrophic hypogonadism can develop secondary to steroid abuse, necessitating medical intervention.

The above side effects are not inclusive. For more detailed discussion of potential side effects, see the Steroid Side Effects section of this book.

Administration (General):

Testosterone propionate is often regarded as a painful injection. This is due to the very short carbon chain of the propionic acid ester, which can be irritating to tissues at the site of injection. Many sensitive individuals choose to stay away from this steroid completely, their bodies reacting with a pronounced soreness and low-grade fever that may last for a few days after each injection.

Administration (Men):

For the treatment of low androgen levels, prescribing guidelines for Testoviron® call for a dosage of 250 mg once every 3-6 weeks. For bodybuilding purposes, this drug is usually injected on a weekly basis, in a dosage of 250-500 mg. Cycles are generally between 6 and 12 weeks in length. This level is sufficient to provide excellent gains in muscle size and strength. Given the poor pharmacokinetics and higher price of Testoviron® and related products, testosterone enanthate or cypionate are often given preference. Testosterone drugs are ultimately very versatile, and can be combined with many other anabolic/androgenic steroids depending on the desired effect.

Administration (Women):

Testoviron® is not commonly prescribed to women in clinical medicine. It is occasionally used to treat a declining sex drive with age, in which case a low dose (50 mg) may be given every 5-6 weeks. It is also sometimes used to treat advanced inoperable breast cancer, at a dose of 250 mg every 2-4 weeks (virilizing effects are expected at such dosing). This drug is not recommended for women for physique- or performance-enhancing purposes due to its strong androgenic nature, tendency to produce virilizing side effects, and slow-acting characteristics (making blood levels difficult to control).

Availability:

Schering has discontinued manufacture of its blended Testoviron product in most parts of the world.

Testoprim-D from Mexico is most likely to show up in the U.S. Counterfeits of this item are not known to be a problem. This item comes in a light resistant ampule that is packaged in a red box bearing white print. The writing is printed directly on the glass surface of the ampule. The ink used is a white/grayish color that does not smear with a good thumb rub. By the time this item is found in the United States, these boxes have usually been discarded (the ampules are easier to smuggle loose).

Aratest from Aranda (Mexico) appears to still be circulating.

BM Pharmaceuticals in India (this is an export company) makes Testenon, which contains a 135 mg/mL Testoviron blend in a 2 mL multi-dose vial.

Bi Testo is made by Cimol in Argentina. This product comes in a multi-dose vial. There are no security features to deter counterfeiting, although copies are not known to be a problem.

THG (tetrahydrogestrinone)

Androgenic	no data available
Anabolic Standard	no data available
Chemical Name	18a-Homo-pregna-4,9,11-trien-17b-ol-3-one
Estrogenic Activity	none
Progestational Activity	very high

Tetrahydrogestrinone

Description:

Tetrahydrogestrinone (THG) is an oral anabolic steroid derived from nandrolone. This agent is a designer steroid, meaning that it was never commercialized, but developed specifically for use by athletes due to the fact that it was once unknown (and therefore unidentifiable) to drug screening. THG is most similar in structure to the European prescription anti-gonadotropic agent gestrinone.[759] Gestrinone is not an active anabolic steroid itself, but does have a close structural relationship to trenbolone. Adding four hydrogen atoms (tetra-hydro) to gestrinone breaks down its 17-alpha ethynyl group (a trait that greatly interferes with binding to the androgen receptor) to an ethyl, creating a steroid capable of strong anabolic and androgenic action. THG is simply 17-alpha-ethylated gestrinone, a novel offshoot of the powerful anabolic steroid trenbolone. The resulting steroid is highly anabolic, moderately androgenic, non-estrogenic, and highly progestational.

History:

Tetrahydrogestrinone was first described in 2004.[760] It was brought to light in what was called "the biggest organized bust for steroid use in the history of competitive sports." These were the words of Terry Madden, Chief Executive Officer of the U.S. Anti-Doping Agency (USADA), when addressing a group of newspaper and television reporters in a press conference disclosing the international doping scandal. His accompanying press release spoke of an anonymous Olympic coach, who turned over a syringe containing the designer steroid and implicated Victor Conte of BALCO Labs in California, then credited with coaching many of the world's top athletes, as the source for the agent. The anonymous source was later identified as track coach Trevor Graham. USADA was soon amidst media frenzy, with many big names fingered for testing positive for the use of THG.

For a short period of time, THG was an ideal steroid for athletes in drug-tested sports, being both extremely effective and undetectable on a urine screen. It was also technically legal to own in the U.S., being that it was unknown to lawmakers at the time the Anabolic Steroid Control Act was written. But with the international doping scandal that would come to surround BALCO Laboratories, any value that THG held as a "designer steroid" has since disappeared. This steroid was also added to the U.S. controlled substance list in January 2005. Victor Conte would serve several months in prison for his role in the BALCO scandal, due to the fact that an unknown drug like THG may have been legal to own, but it was not legal to sell. Patrick Arnold, the chemist behind THG, pled guilty to criminal charges as well, and is scheduled to begin serving a 3-month prison term in late 2006.

Tetrahydrogestrinone was a designer steroid of opportunity, created from a readily available and unregulated intermediary chemical with a simple synthesis method. It would arise from the doping scandal fallout as the world's famous superstar of designer steroids. The existence of THG would be a constant reminder that the determination of athletes to utilize all available tools to win goes far beyond the abilities of the governing athletic bodies to police them. Until much more effective drug-testing methods are developed, which rely not on structural and metabolic knowledge of the various substances but can actually determine if a new previously unidentified steroid is being used, THG will also be a reminder that it is possible, if not highly likely, that many other designer steroids are out in the field of use at this very moment.

How Supplied:

Tetrahydrogestrinone is not available as a prescription drug product.

Structural Characteristics:

Tetrahydrogestrinone is a modified form of nandrolone. It differs by: 1) the addition of an ethyl group at carbon 17-alpha to protect the hormone during oral administration, 2) the introduction of double bonds at carbons 9 and 11, which greatly increase relative steroid activity, and 3) the possession of an 18a-homo group, which gives the steroid strong progestational activity.

Side Effects (Estrogenic):

Tetrahydrogestrinone is not aromatized by the body, and is not believed to be measurably estrogenic. Gynecomastia remains a concern during treatment, however, due to its progestational nature (see below), especially when combined with other estrogenic drugs. At the same time water retention can become a problem, causing a notable loss of muscle definition as both subcutaneous water retention and fat levels build. To avoid such strong side effects, it may be necessary to use an anti-estrogen such as Nolvadex®.

Note that tetrahydrogestrinone is an extremely active progestin.[761] In assays it was shown to have stronger progestational activity than nandrolone, trenbolone, and even gestrinone, a synthetic progestin. THG was actually shown to be 7 times more potent than progesterone itself. The side effects associated with progesterone are similar to those of estrogen, including negative feedback inhibition of testosterone production and enhanced rate of fat storage. Progestins also augment the stimulatory effect of estrogens on mammary tissue growth. There appears to be a strong synergy between these two hormones here, such that gynecomastia might even occur with the help of progestins without excessive estrogen levels being present. The use of an anti-estrogen, which inhibits the estrogenic component of this disorder, is often sufficient to mitigate gynecomastia caused by progestational steroids.

Side Effects (Androgenic):

Although classified as an anabolic steroid, androgenic side effects are still common with this substance. This may include bouts of oily skin, acne, and body/facial hair growth. Anabolic/androgenic steroids may also aggravate male pattern hair loss. Women are additionally warned of the potential virilizing effects of anabolic/androgenic steroids. These may include a deepening of the voice, menstrual irregularities, changes in skin texture, facial hair growth, and clitoral enlargement. Note that THG does not appear to be subject to 5-alpha reduction, so its relative androgenicity is not affected by the concurrent use of finasteride or dutasteride.

Side Effects (Hepatotoxicity):

Tetrahydrogestrinone is a c17-alpha alkylated compound. This alteration protects the drug from deactivation by the liver, allowing a very high percentage of the drug entry into the bloodstream following oral administration. C17-alpha alkylated anabolic/androgenic steroids can be hepatotoxic. Prolonged or high exposure may result in liver damage. In rare instances life-threatening dysfunction may develop. It is advisable to visit a physician periodically during each cycle to monitor liver function and overall health. Intake of c17-alpha alkylated steroids is commonly limited to 6-8 weeks, in an effort to avoid escalating liver strain. Severe liver complications are rare given the periodic nature in which most people use oral anabolic/androgenic steroids, although cannot be excluded with this steroid, especially with high doses and/or prolonged administration periods.

The use of a liver detoxification supplement such as Liver Stabil, Liv-52, or Essentiale Forte is advised while taking any hepatotoxic anabolic/androgenic steroids.

Side Effects (Cardiovascular):

Anabolic/androgenic steroids can have deleterious effects on serum cholesterol. This includes a tendency to reduce HDL (good) cholesterol values and increase LDL (bad) cholesterol values, which may shift the HDL to LDL balance in a direction that favors greater risk of arteriosclerosis. The relative impact of an anabolic/androgenic steroid on serum lipids is dependant on the dose, route of administration (oral vs. injectable), type of steroid (aromatizable or non-aromatizable), and level of resistance to hepatic metabolism. Tetrahydrogestrinone has a strong effect on the hepatic management of cholesterol due to its structural resistance to liver breakdown, non-aromatizable nature, and route of administration. Anabolic/androgenic steroids may also adversely affect blood pressure and triglycerides, reduce endothelial relaxation, and support left ventricular hypertrophy, all potentially increasing the risk of cardiovascular disease and myocardial infarction.

To help reduce cardiovascular strain it is advised to maintain an active cardiovascular exercise program and minimize the intake of saturated fats, cholesterol, and simple carbohydrates at all times during active AAS administration. Supplementing with fish oils (4 grams per day) and a natural cholesterol/antioxidant formula such as Lipid Stabil or a product with comparable ingredients is also recommended.

Side Effects (Testosterone Suppression):

All anabolic/androgenic steroids when taken in doses sufficient to promote muscle gain are expected to suppress endogenous testosterone production. Without the intervention of testosterone-stimulating substances, testosterone levels should return to normal within 1-4 months of drug secession. Note that prolonged hypogonadotrophic hypogonadism can develop secondary to steroid abuse, necessitating medical intervention.

The above side effects are not inclusive. For more detailed discussion of potential side effects, see the Steroid Side Effects section of this book.

Administration (General):

Studies have shown that taking an oral anabolic steroid with food may decrease its bioavailability.[762] This is caused by the fat-soluble nature of steroid hormones, which can allow some of the drug to dissolve with undigested dietary fat, reducing its absorption from the gastrointestinal tract. For maximum utilization, this steroid should be taken on an empty stomach.

Administration (Men):

Tetrahydrogestrinone was never approved for use in humans. Prescribing guidelines are unavailable. Methyltrienolone is its closest chemical relative, and known to be effective in doses lower than 1mg per day. THG should also require very small doses, perhaps in the range of 2-5 mg per day. We can also note that THG minus its delta-11 modification (a di-ene instead of a tri-ene) has been documented to be over 14 times more active than methyltestosterone.[763] There is no reason to think that the jump to THG would be anything but an improvement. Although exact figures don't exist, this designer steroid should be far more potent than any anabolic steroid commercially available, and would probably fall slightly short of methyltrienolone. For those athletes who use THG, the results should be measurable improvements in strength, muscle size, and performance.

Administration (Women):

Tetrahydrogestrinone was never approved for use in humans. Prescribing guidelines are unavailable. THG is generally not recommended for women for physique- or performance-enhancing purposes due to its very strong nature and tendency to produce virilizing side effects. This compound could be used with success, but only with a commercial preparation that makes measuring out the very low (microgram) amounts needed with females possible.

Availability:

THG is presently unavailable on the black market.

Thioderon (mepitiostane)

Androgenic	25
Anabolic	100
Standard	Methyltestosterone (oral)
Chemical Names	17beta-(1-methoxycyclopentyloxy)-2alpha,3alpha,-epithio-5alpha-androstane
Estrogenic Activity	none
Progestational Activity	none

Epitiostane

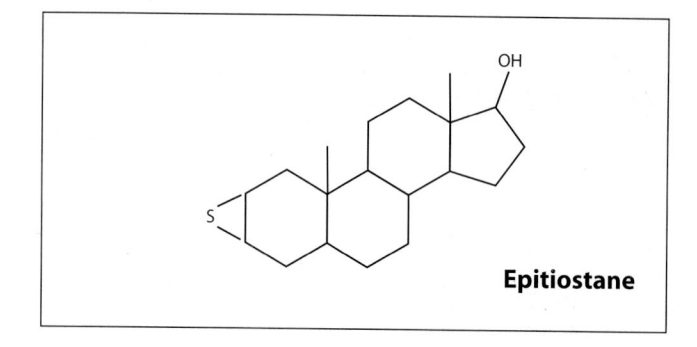

Description:

Mepitiostane is a 17-beta etherified derivative of epitiostane. The ether is necessary to facilitate oral dosing,[764] which occurs via the lymphatic system very similar to Anabolicum Vister (quinbolone). As such, epitiostane is actually the active steroid that is provided to the user once the ether is removed metabolically, which is a non-methylated (non-hepatotoxic) derivative of dihydrotestosterone. Mepitiostane is a moderately anabolic steroid, which displays roughly the same anabolic effect as methyltestosterone on a milligram for milligram basis, at least according to standard animal assays. This activity is accompanied by only a mild androgenic component, however, which makes this steroid primarily anabolic in nature. It is also non-aromatizable, and possesses antiestrogenic properties. Although this steroid is not widely used by athletes and bodybuilders, it exhibits favorable lean muscle building properties, which tend to be accompanied by fat loss and increased definition.

History:

Mepitiostane was first described in 1966, during investigations into a series of A-ring modified androstane derivatives.[765] The only modern pharmaceutical preparation of record containing mepitiostane is Thioderon, which is sold in Japan by Shinogi. The active drug seemed to enter extensive studies in Japan in 1974, which saw the bulk of mepitiostane research. The drug is used in Japanese medicine as an anabolic agent, and is mainly given to patients (twice daily) for the treatment of breast carcinoma and anemia associated with renal failure. In clinical trials where the agent was compared to an equal dose of fluoxymesterone (also used to treat breast carcinoma), mepitiostane was shown to offer a similar level of efficacy, but without the unwanted hepatotoxicity of a c-17alpha alkylated agent.[766] Mepitiostane was never widely experimented with outside of Japan, and newer medicines to treat the associated conditions make it less useful today than in the past. Still, the drug remains available for sale, though it is not widely found outside of Japan.

How Supplied:

Mepitiostane is available as a prescription drug preparation in Japan. It is supplied in the form of capsules containing 5 mg of steroid.

Structural Characteristics:

Mepitiostane is a modified form of dihydrotestosterone. It differs by 1) the addition of a 17-beta methoxycyclopentyl ether, which helps facilitate lymphatic delivery (bioavailability) during oral administration, and 2) the replacement of 3-keto with 2,3alpha-epithio, which increases its anabolic strength while reducing its relative androgenicity.

Side Effects (Estrogenic):

Mepitiostane is not aromatized by the body, and is not measurably estrogenic. Furthermore, the drug is used clinically for its inherent antiestrogenic effect. An antiestrogen is not necessary when using this steroid, as gynecomastia should not be a concern even among sensitive individuals. Since estrogen is the usual culprit with water retention, this steroid instead produces a lean, quality look to the physique with no fear of excess subcutaneous fluid retention. This makes it a favorable steroid to use during cutting cycles, when water and fat retention are major concerns.

Side Effects (Androgenic):

Although classified as an anabolic steroid, androgenic side effects are still possible with this substance, especially with higher doses. This may include bouts of oily skin, acne, and body/facial hair growth. Anabolic/androgenic steroids may also aggravate male pattern hair loss. Women are warned of the potential virilizing effects of anabolic/androgenic steroids. These may include a deepening of the voice, menstrual irregularities, changes in skin texture, facial hair growth, and clitoral enlargement. Mepitiostane is a steroid with relatively low androgenic activity relative to its tissue-building actions, making the threshold for strong androgenic side effects comparably higher than with more androgenic agents such as testosterone, methandrostenolone, or fluoxymesterone. Note that mepitiostane is unaffected by the 5-alpha reductase enzyme, so its relative androgenicity is not affected by the concurrent use of finasteride or dutasteride.

Side Effects (Hepatotoxicity):

Mepitiostane is not a c17-alpha alkylated compound, and is not known to have hepatotoxic effects. Liver toxicity is unlikely.

Side Effects (Cardiovascular):

Anabolic/androgenic steroids can have deleterious effects on serum cholesterol. This includes a tendency to reduce HDL (good) cholesterol values and increase LDL (bad) cholesterol values, which may shift the HDL to LDL balance in a direction that favors greater risk of arteriosclerosis. The relative impact of an anabolic/androgenic steroid on serum lipids is dependant on the dose, route of administration (oral vs. injectable), type of steroid (aromatizable or non-aromatizable), and level of resistance to hepatic metabolism. Mepitiostane should have a stronger effect on the hepatic management of cholesterol than testosterone due to its non-aromatizable nature and route of administration, but a weaker effect than c-17 alpha alkylated agents. Anabolic/androgenic steroids may also adversely effect blood pressure and triglycerides, reduce endothelial relaxation, and support left ventricular hypertrophy, all potentially increasing the risk of cardiovascular disease and myocardial infarction.

To help reduce cardiovascular strain it is advised to maintain an active cardiovascular exercise program and minimize the intake of saturated fats, cholesterol, and simple carbohydrates at all times during active AAS administration. Supplementing with fish oils (4 grams per day) and a natural cholesterol/antioxidant formula such as Lipid Stabil or a product with comparable ingredients is also recommended.

Side Effects (Testosterone Suppression):

All anabolic/androgenic steroids when taken in doses sufficient to promote muscle gain are expected to suppress endogenous testosterone production. Without the intervention of testosterone stimulating substances, testosterone levels should return to normal within 1-4 months of drug secession. Note that prolonged hypogonadotrophic hypogonadism can develop secondary to steroid abuse, necessitating medical intervention.

The above side effects are not inclusive. For more detailed discussion of potential side effects, see the Steroid Side Effects section of this book.

Administration (Men):

When used clinically, this drug is most commonly administered at a dose of 10 mg twice daily (20 mg total). An effective dosage of mepitiostane for physique- or performance-enhancing purposes falls in the range of 20-50 mg daily. This is usually taken for 8-12 weeks. At this level it should to impart a measurable but moderate lean-mass-building effect, which is usually accompanied by fat loss. The result is usually an increase in definition, and what is often referred to as a very "dry" look to the physique.

Administration (Women):

When used clinically, this drug is most commonly administered at a dose of 10 mg twice daily (20 mg total). An effective dosage of mepitiostane for physique- or performance-enhancing purposes falls around 10 mg per day, taken for 4-6 weeks. Note that virilizing side effects including hoarseness, male-pattern hair growth, and acne were commonly reported in patients taking the recommended clinical dose of 20 mg per day.[767]

Availability:

Mepitiostane is currently only produced in Japan under the Thioderon trade name. This agent is not commonly diverted for use outside of clinical settings, nor is it a known target for counterfeiting. On the rare occasion it may be located, the Shinogi product can likely be trusted.

Trenabol® (trenbolone enanthate)

Androgenic	500
Anabolic	500
Standard	Nandrolone acetate
Chemical Names	17beta-Hydroxyestra-4,9,11-trien-3-one
Estrogenic Activity	none
Progestational Activity	moderate

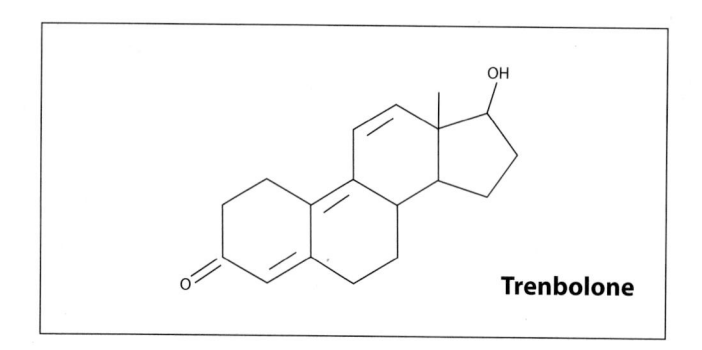

Description:

Trenbolone enanthate is an injectable form of the strong anabolic steroid trenbolone. Given the use of an enanthate ester, this drug will exhibit virtually identical pharmacokinetics to testosterone enanthate, providing a peak release of its steroid within the first several days after injection, followed by declining levels for approximately 2 weeks. The base steroid here (trenbolone) is a derivative of nandrolone, and exhibits strong anabolic and androgenic properties. On a milligram for milligram basis it is considerably more potent than testosterone as both an anabolic and androgenic agent, though it does carry a more favorable balance (toward anabolism). Trenbolone is also unable to convert to estrogen, however it does exhibit notable progestational activity, which may mimic estrogenic side effects given the right physiological conditions. Trenbolone enanthate is virtually interchangeable with Parabolan (trenbolone hexahydrobenzylcarbonate), capable of promoting strong gains in lean muscle mass, often with an accompanying increase in relative hardness and definition.

History:

Slow-acting trenbolone esters were first studied in 1967, during a series of experiments into synthetic anabolic steroids by Roussel-UCLAF.[768] Roussel did not specifically investigate Trenbolone enanthate, although the drug would have remained an obvious possibility once trenbolone was released given the widespread application of steroid esters (including enanthate) by the 1960's. The drug would not see the light of day for many decades, however, and was only first released for commercial sale in 2004. It was introduced by British Dragon, a Thai company that manufactured products for export only. British Dragon would sell it under the trade name Trenabol, in 200 mg/mL strength. The firm would go on to develop a line of several trenbolone products under the Trenabol label, including a trenbolone acetate product, a Parabolan clone (trenbolone hexahydrobenzylcarbonate), and a three-ester blended injectable called Tri-Trenabol.

Although it was not for sale through pharmacies nor approved for human or veterinary use, Trenabol was widely distributed throughout the world, and became an extremely popular product with athletes and bodybuilders. Much of this had to do with the fact that it was unique, in that it was one of but a few options for injectable trenbolone that used slow-acting esters. At the time of its introduction, trenbolone acetate products were by and large the dominant form of trenbolone, and remain the dominant form of the drug to this day. Although British Dragon was perhaps the largest and most well known export-only steroid manufacturer in the world, the company abruptly collapsed at the end of 2006. It appears that disagreements arose among partners that could not be fixed, and the company was subsequently dissolved. The future of the British Dragon trade name remains uncertain. In spite of this loss, trenbolone enanthate continues to be sold by a number of underground labs, and will likely be reintroduced by other registered facilities before long, ensuring its continued availability.

How Supplied:

Trenbolone enanthate is not available as a prescription drug product.

Structural Characteristics:

Trenbolone is a modified form of nandrolone. It differs by the introduction of double bonds at carbons 9 and 11, which inhibit aromatization (9-ene), increase androgen-binding affinity,[769] and slows its metabolism. The resulting steroid is significantly more potent as both an anabolic and an androgen than its nandrolone base. The trenbolone here is modified with an enanthate ester at the 17-beta hydroxyl group, so that the free steroid is released more slowly from the area of injection.

Side Effects (Estrogenic):

Trenbolone is not aromatized by the body, and is not measurably estrogenic. It is of note, however, that this steroid displays significant binding affinity for the progesterone receptor (slightly stronger than progesterone itself).[770,771] The side effects associated with progesterone are similar to those of estrogen, including negative feedback inhibition of testosterone production and enhanced rate of fat storage. Progestins also augment the stimulatory effect of estrogens on mammary tissue growth. There appears to be a strong synergy between these two hormones, such that gynecomastia might even occur with the help of progestins, without excessive estrogen levels. The use of an anti-estrogen, which inhibits the estrogenic component of this disorder, is often sufficient to mitigate gynecomastia caused by progestational anabolic/androgenic steroids. Note that progestational side effects are more common when trenbolone is being taken with other aromatizable steroids.

Side Effects (Androgenic):

Although classified as an anabolic steroid, trenbolone is sufficiently androgenic. Androgenic side effects are still common with this substance, and may include bouts of oily skin, acne, and body/facial hair growth. Anabolic/androgenic steroids may also aggravate male pattern hair loss. Women are also warned of the potential virilizing effects of anabolic/androgenic steroids. These may include a deepening of the voice, menstrual irregularities, changes in skin texture, facial hair growth, and clitoral enlargement. Additionally, the 5-alpha reductase enzyme does not metabolize trenbolone,[772] so its relative androgenicity is not affected by finasteride or dutasteride.

Side Effects (Hepatotoxicity):

Trenbolone is not c-17 alpha alkylated, and is generally not considered a hepatotoxic steroid; liver toxicity is unlikely. This steroid does have a strong level of resistance to hepatic breakdown, however, and severe liver toxicity has been noted in bodybuilders abusing trenbolone.[773] Although unlikely, hepatotoxicity cannot be completely excluded, especially with high doses.

Side Effects (Cardiovascular):

Anabolic/androgenic steroids can have deleterious effects on serum cholesterol. This includes a tendency to reduce HDL (good) cholesterol values and increase LDL (bad) cholesterol values, which may shift the HDL to LDL balance in a direction that favors greater risk of arteriosclerosis. The relative impact of an anabolic/androgenic steroid on serum lipids is dependant on the dose, route of administration (oral vs. injectable), type of steroid (aromatizable or non-aromatizable), and level of resistance to hepatic metabolism. Due to its non-aromatizable nature and strong resistance to metabolism, trenbolone has a moderate to strong (negative) impact on lipid values and atherogenic risk. Anabolic/androgenic steroids may also adversely affect blood pressure and triglycerides, reduce endothelial relaxation, and support left ventricular hypertrophy, all potentially increasing the risk of cardiovascular disease and myocardial infarction.

To help reduce cardiovascular strain it is advised to maintain an active cardiovascular exercise program and minimize the intake of saturated fats, cholesterol, and simple carbohydrates at all times during active AAS administration. Supplementing with fish oils (4 grams per day) and a natural cholesterol/antioxidant formula such as Lipid Stabil or a product with comparable ingredients is also recommended.

Side Effects (Testosterone Suppression):

All anabolic/androgenic steroids when taken in doses sufficient to promote muscle gain are expected to suppress endogenous testosterone production. Without the intervention of testosterone-stimulating substances, testosterone levels should return to normal within 1-4 months of drug secession. Note that prolonged hypogonadotrophic hypogonadism can develop secondary to steroid abuse, necessitating medical intervention. In experimental studies, trenbolone was determined to be approximately three times stronger at suppressing gonadotropins than testosterone on a milligram for milligram basis.

The above side effects are not inclusive. For more detailed discussion of potential side effects, see the Steroid Side Effects section of this book.

Administration (Men):

Trenbolone enanthate was never approved for use in humans. Prescribing guidelines are unavailable. Common doses for physique- and performance-enhancing purposes fall in the range of 150-300 mg per week, which is usually taken for 6-10 consecutive weeks. This level is sufficient to produce considerable increases in lean muscle mass and strength, which are usually combined with notable fat loss and increased muscle definition. As with all trenbolone injectables, this product is fairly versatile, and can be combined with many other agents depending on the desired results.

Administration (Women):

Trenbolone enanthate was never approved for use in humans. Prescribing guidelines are unavailable. This agent is generally not recommended for women for physique- or performance-enhancing purposes due to strong androgenic nature and tendency to produce virilizing side effects.

Availability:

All forms of trenbolone enanthate currently available on the black market are made by underground manufacturers. They are of unverifiable quality.

William Llewellyn's ANABOLICS, 9th ed.

Tri-Trenabol 150 (trenbolone blend)

Androgenic	500
Anabolic	500
Standard	Nandrolone acetate

Chemical Names	17beta-Hydroxyestra-4,9,11-trien-3-one

Estrogenic Activity	none
Progestational Activity	moderate

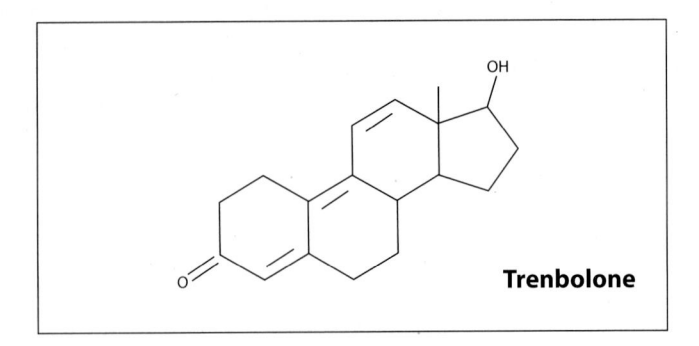

Trenbolone

Description:

Tri-Trenabol is an injectable blend of three different trenbolone esters: acetate, hexahydrobenzylcarbonate, and enanthate. These compounds are provided in equal parts, 50 mg each. The preparation provides a total duration of effect very similar to what we would see with Parabolan (trenbolone hexahydrobenzylcarbonate). The short-acting acetate ester, however, exaggerates the initial release peak. In crude terms, this steroid is a form of Parabolan that is slightly more front heavy than normal. In regards to bodybuilding applications, for all intents and purposes it is interchangeable with regular Parabolan. This formulation offers advantages over pure trenbolone acetate products, however, as the 2-3 times per week injection schedule needed for the faster-acting drug can be very uncomfortable. As a trenbolone injectable, this steroid is favored by athletes for its ability to promote rapid gains in muscle size and strength, often with accompanying increases in fat loss and muscle definition.

History:

Tri-Trenabol was developed by British Dragon, a now defunct underground company allegedly with roots to British Dispensary (makers of Anabol and Androlic). British Dragon was reportedly formed by one of the principles of British Dispensary, with the intent to branch off and sell a wider variety of products for export sale only. Tri-Trenabol was introduced to market in 2004, and originally sold under the trade name Trinabol 150. It was changed to the Tri-Trenabol 150 name in 2006, which reflected that it was a triple ester addition to their popular Trenabol (trenbolone) line. With a mix of short- and long-acting esters, this product was essentially designed to be the trenbolone equivalent of Sustanon 250. As we have learned with Sustanon, however, such designs tend to offer no real advantages to single-ester (long acting) preparations. Trenbolone enanthate and hexahydrobenzylcarbonate both have strong initial peaks of release, making the addition of a short-acting ester like acetate superfluous. Regardless of this fact, Tri-Trinabol remained an effective product. The preparation was finally discontinued in 2006, however, with the close of British Dragon.

How Supplied:

Tri-Trenabol is not available as a prescription drug product.

Structural Characteristics:

Trenbolone is a modified form of nandrolone. It differs by the introduction of double bonds at carbons 9 and 11, which inhibit aromatization (9-ene), increase androgen-binding affinity,[774] and slows its metabolism. The resulting steroid is significantly more potent as both an anabolic and an androgen than its nandrolone base. Tri-Trenabol contains trenbolone modified with the addition of carboxylic acid esters (acetic, enanthoic, hexahydrobenzylcarbonic acids) at the 17-beta hydroxyl group. Esterified steroids are less polar than free steroids, and are absorbed more slowly from the area of injection. Once in the bloodstream, the ester is removed to yield free (active) trenbolone. Esterified steroids are designed to prolong the window of therapeutic effect following administration, allowing for a less frequent injection schedule compared to injections of free (unesterified) steroid. Tri-Trenabol is designed to provide a peak release of trenbolone approximately 24-48 hours after injection, and sustain hormone release for approximately 21 days.

Side Effects (Estrogenic):

Trenbolone is not aromatized by the body, and is not measurably estrogenic. It is of note, however, that this steroid displays significant binding affinity for the progesterone receptor (slightly stronger than progesterone itself).[775,776] The side effects associated with progesterone are similar to those of estrogen, including negative feedback inhibition of testosterone production and enhanced rate of fat storage. Progestins also augment the stimulatory effect of estrogens on mammary tissue growth. There appears to be a strong synergy between these two hormones here, such that gynecomastia might even occur with the help of progestins, without excessive estrogen levels. The use of an anti-estrogen, which inhibits the estrogenic component of this disorder, is often sufficient to mitigate gynecomastia caused by progestational anabolic/androgenic steroids. Note that progestational side effects are more common when trenbolone is being taken with other aromatizable steroids.

Side Effects (Androgenic):

Although classified as an anabolic steroid, trenbolone is sufficiently androgenic. Androgenic side effects are still common with this substance, and may include bouts of oily skin, acne, and body/facial hair growth. Anabolic/androgenic steroids may also aggravate male pattern hair loss. Women are also warned of the potential virilizing effects of anabolic/androgenic steroids. These may include a deepening of the voice, menstrual irregularities, changes in skin texture, facial hair growth, and clitoral enlargement. Additionally, the 5-alpha reductase enzyme does not metabolize trenbolone,[777] so its relative androgenicity is not affected by finasteride or dutasteride.

Side Effects (Hepatotoxicity):

Trenbolone is not c-17 alpha alkylated, and is generally not considered a hepatotoxic steroid; liver toxicity is unlikely. This steroid does have a strong level of resistance to hepatic breakdown, however, and severe liver toxicity has been noted in bodybuilders abusing trenbolone.[778] Although unlikely, hepatotoxicity cannot be completely excluded, especially with high doses.

Side Effects (Cardiovascular):

Anabolic/androgenic steroids can have deleterious effects on serum cholesterol. This includes a tendency to reduce HDL (good) cholesterol values and increase LDL (bad) cholesterol values, which may shift the HDL to LDL balance in a direction that favors greater risk of arteriosclerosis. The relative impact of an anabolic/androgenic steroid on serum lipids is dependant on the dose, route of administration (oral vs. injectable), type of steroid (aromatizable or non-aromatizable), and level of resistance to hepatic metabolism. Due to its non-aromatizable and strong resistance to metabolism, trenbolone is prone to negatively altering lipid values and increasing atherogenic risk. Anabolic/androgenic steroids may also adversely affect blood pressure and triglycerides, reduce endothelial relaxation, and support left ventricular hypertrophy, all potentially increasing the risk of cardiovascular disease and myocardial infarction.

To help reduce cardiovascular strain it is advised to maintain an active cardiovascular exercise program and minimize the intake of saturated fats, cholesterol, and simple carbohydrates at all times during active AAS administration. Supplementing with fish oils (4 grams per day) and a natural cholesterol/antioxidant formula such as Lipid Stabil or a product with comparable ingredients is also recommended.

Side Effects (Testosterone Suppression):

All anabolic/androgenic steroids when taken in doses sufficient to promote muscle gain are expected to suppress endogenous testosterone production. Without the intervention of testosterone-stimulating substances, testosterone levels should return to normal within 1-4 months of drug secession. Note that prolonged hypogonadotrophic hypogonadism can develop secondary to steroid abuse, necessitating medical intervention. In experimental studies, trenbolone was determined to be approximately three times stronger at suppressing gonadotropins than testosterone on a milligram for milligram basis.

The above side effects are not inclusive. For more detailed discussion of potential side effects, see the Steroid Side Effects section of this book.

Administration (Men):

Tri-Trenabol was never approved for use in humans. Prescribing guidelines are unavailable. Typical dosages for physique- or performance-enhancing purposes are in the range of 1-2 mL per week, or 150-300 mg of trenbolone ester. Being that trenbolone is significantly more potent than testosterone on a milligram for milligram basis, the 1-2 mL weekly injection should provide a very substantial benefit. Often one will make significant progress with the use of this agent alone. In many cases, however, trenbolone is combined with another base steroid. You will commonly see stacks with testosterone or boldenone during bulking phases of training, or Winstrol, Primobolan, or Anavar during cutting cycles. In such situations, a single 150 mg dose per week will usually sufficient on the trenbolone side. As a trenbolone injectable, Tri-Trenabol is a potent lean mass building and cutting steroid. The gains produced by this drug tend to be of very high quality, often accompanied by fat loss and increased definition.

Administration (Women):

Tri-Trenabol was never approved for use in humans. Prescribing guidelines are unavailable. This agent is generally not recommended for women for physique- or performance-enhancing purposes due to strong androgenic nature and tendency to produce virilizing side effects.

Availability:

Tri-Trenabol blends are made by underground manufacturers, but are of unverifiable quality.

Tribolin (nandrolone/methandriol blend)

Androgenic	
Anabolic	
Standard	
Chemical Names	
Estrogenic Activity	
Progestational Activity	

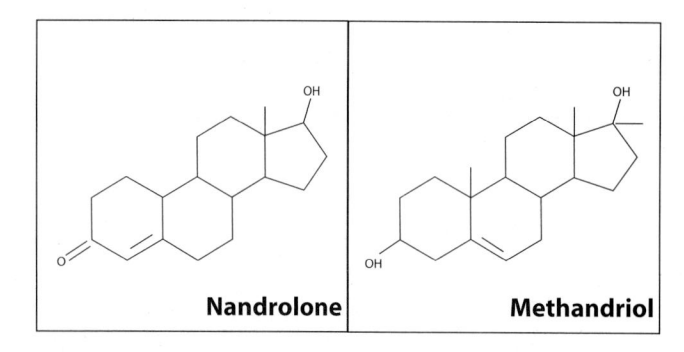

Description:

Tribolin is an Australian veterinary steroid preparation that contains a blend of methandriol dipropionate and nandrolone decanoate, in a dose of 40 mg/mL and 35 mg/mL respectively. This adds up to a total steroid concentration of 75 mg/mL. The manufacturer also makes a similar formulation called Filybol Forte, which contains the same steroid blend but with a 5 mg/mL lower dose on the nandrolone decanoate. With its blend of methandriol and nandrolone, Tribolin is considerably more anabolic than androgenic in nature. Its estrogenic effect should also be minimal, barring the methandriol content, which is intrinsically slightly estrogenic. Although not widely available, Tribolin (and Filybol Forte) is favored by athletes as a mild anabolic agent with low androgenic activity.

History:

Tribolin was developed by the Ranvet Company, a popular veterinary drug and vitamin manufacturer in Australia. It is used specifically in horses, usually racehorses or other animals subject to strenuous straining or performance periods. Ranvet advertises it as a "powerful, triple acting anabolic combination… possessing marked anabolic properties and only a minimal amount of androgenic activity." The "triple action" and Tri in the name are not referring to the formula, as it only contains two active steroids, not three. They refer to the purported benefits of its use. The three points of drug action are stated to be the facilitation of muscular development, the offsetting of dehydration, and the aiding of protein digestion. It is commonly applied to an overworked or debilitated animal in an attempt to aid recovery, and is also used to assist in the repair of muscle, tendon, and ligament injuries. For a horse weighing approximately 1,100 pounds (500kg), a dosage of 5 ml (350 mg) is usually given every 4 to 5 weeks. Treatment would often run for 3 to 4 months. The drug is presently still available, as is the very similar Ranvet preparation Filybol Forte. Due to strict controls in Australia it is not widely available for use by athletes.

How Supplied:

Tribolin is available on the Australian veterinary drug market. It contains 75 mg/mL of steroid in oil in a 10 mL and 20 mL vial. Filybol Forte contains 70 mg/mL of steroid in the same vial sizes.

Structural Characteristics:

For a more comprehensive discussion of the individual steroids nandrolone decanoate and methandriol dipropionate, refer to their respective drug profiles.

Side Effects (Estrogenic):

Methylandrostendiol is not directly aromatized by the body, although one of its known metabolites is methyltestosterone, which can aromatize. Methyandrostenediol is also believed to have some inherent estrogenic activity. Combined with nandrolone, which also weakly aromatizes, Tribolin is considered a weakly to moderately estrogenic steroid. Gynecomastia is possible during treatment, but generally only when higher doses are used. Water and fat retention can also become issues, again depending on dose. Sensitive individuals may need to addition an anti-estrogen such as Nolvadex® to minimize related side effects.

Side Effects (Androgenic):

Although classified as an anabolic steroid preparation, androgenic side effects are still common with this substance. This may include bouts of oily skin, acne, and body/facial hair growth. Anabolic/androgenic steroids may also aggravate male pattern hair loss. Women are warned of the potential virilizing effects of anabolic/androgenic steroids. These may include a deepening of the voice, menstrual irregularities, changes in skin texture, facial hair growth, and clitoral enlargement.

Side Effects (Hepatotoxicity):

Methylandrostenediol is a c17-alpha alkylated compound. This alteration protects the drug from deactivation by the liver, allowing a very high percentage of the drug entry into the bloodstream following oral administration. C17-alpha alkylated anabolic/androgenic steroids can be hepatotoxic. Prolonged or high exposure may result in liver damage. In rare instances life-threatening dysfunction may develop. It is advisable to visit a physician periodically during each cycle to monitor liver function and overall health. Intake of c17-alpha alkylated steroids is commonly limited to 6-8 weeks, in an effort to avoid escalating liver strain. Injectable forms of the drug may present slightly less strain on the liver by avoiding the first pass metabolism of oral dosing, although may still present substantial hepatotoxicity.

The use of a liver detoxification supplement such as Liver Stabil, Liv-52, or Essentiale Forte is advised while taking any hepatotoxic anabolic/androgenic steroids.

Side Effects (Cardiovascular):

Anabolic/androgenic steroids can have deleterious effects on serum cholesterol. This includes a tendency to reduce HDL (good) cholesterol values and increase LDL (bad) cholesterol values, which may shift the HDL to LDL balance in a direction that favors greater risk of arteriosclerosis. The relative impact of an anabolic/androgenic steroid on serum lipids is dependant on the dose, route of administration (oral vs. injectable), type of steroid (aromatizable or non-aromatizable), and level of resistance to hepatic metabolism. Methylandrostenediol has a strong effect on the hepatic management of cholesterol due to its structural resistance to liver breakdown and (with the oral) route of administration. Anabolic/androgenic steroids may also adversely affect blood pressure and triglycerides, reduce endothelial relaxation, and support left ventricular hypertrophy, all potentially increasing the risk of cardiovascular disease and myocardial infarction.

To help reduce cardiovascular strain it is advised to maintain an active cardiovascular exercise program and minimize the intake of saturated fats, cholesterol, and simple carbohydrates at all times during active AAS administration. Supplementing with fish oils (4 grams per day) and a natural cholesterol/antioxidant formula such as Lipid Stabil or a product with comparable ingredients is also recommended.

Side Effects (Testosterone Suppression):

All anabolic/androgenic steroids when taken in doses sufficient to promote muscle gain are expected to suppress endogenous testosterone production. Without the intervention of testosterone-stimulating substances, testosterone levels should return to normal within 1-4 months of drug secession. Note that prolonged hypogonadotrophic hypogonadism can develop secondary to steroid abuse, necessitating medical intervention.

The above side effects are not inclusive. For more detailed discussion of potential side effects, see the Steroid Side Effects section of this book.

Administration (Men):

Tribolin has not been approved for use in humans. Prescribing guidelines for men are unavailable. Typical dosing schedule for physique- or performance-enhancing purposes would be in the range of 225 mg (3cc's) to 450 mg (6cc's) per week, a level that should provide quality lean mass gain without bloating or significant body fat retention.

Administration (Women):

Tribolin has not been approved for use in humans. Prescribing guidelines for women are unavailable. Drugs containing methylandrostenediol are generally not recommended for women for physique- or performance-enhancing purposes due to its androgenic nature and tendency to produce virilizing side effects.

Availability:

Due to tight controls on drug products in Australia, Tribolin and Filybol do not make it to the black market very often. The packaging is also fairly plain on both items, inviting counterfeiting. For these reasons, it is advisable to be suspicious of any Tribolin or Filybol bottle (or any Australian vet steroids for that matter) that may be found outside of legitimate channels. It is highly uncommon for volume sales of this product to be made. Unless you can personally trace these back to a legitimate supplier in Australia, they should be considered of unverified authenticity.

Triolandren (testosterone blend)

Androgenic	100
Anabolic	100
Standard	Standard

Chemical Names	4-androsten-3-one-17beta-ol
	17beta-hydroxy-androst-4-en-3-one
Estrogenic Activity	moderate
Progestational Activity	low

Description:

Triolandren is an injectable testosterone preparation that contains a mixture of three different esters of testosterone. Each milliliter specifically contains 20 mg of testosterone propionate, 80 mg of testosterone valerianate, and 150 mg of testosterone undecylenate, for a total steroid concentration of 250 mg/mL. With its mix of fast- and long-acting esters, Triolandren is very much like Sustanon® 250 in design, intended to deliver testosterone slowly to a patient over a period of several weeks. In this case the slowest-releasing ester used is undecylenate, whereas Sustanon® uses decanoate. This would make Triolandren the longer-acting agent between the two, also with a softer initial peak of testosterone release. As a testosterone drug, Triolandren is capable of promoting rapids gains in muscle size and strength.

History:

The Triolandren testosterone formulation was first described in the medical literature in 1957.[779] It was marketed commercially by Ciba in 1965, and sold as a human prescription drug in various parts of Europe. It was used primarily to treat anemia, androgen deficiency in males, breast cancer in females, and excessive growth in adolescents. During the 1980's, Ciba began trimming their global steroid offerings in light of the new public interest towards sports doping. By the mid-1990's, the last of the Triolandren preparations were withdrawn from continental Europe. Key markets such as Switzerland, Sweden, and Norway, which once were very active in its supply, no longer carried the drug, and it soon began to fade from the memory of most athletes. In 1996, Sandoz and Ciba officially merged to form Novartis. Any remaining Triolandren products made by Ciba-Geigy in other parts of the world were subsequently produced under the Novartis label. Triolandren remains available on the Egyptian drug market, although it is not commonly an item of export.

How Supplied:

Triolandren® from Novartis is available in select human pharmaceutical markets. The product contains 250 mg/mL of steroid; packaged in 1 mL ampules.

Structural Characteristics:

Triolandren® contains a mixture of three testosterone compounds, which are modified with the addition of carboxylic acid esters (propionic, valerianic, and undecanoic acids) at the 17-beta hydroxyl group. Esterified forms of testosterone are less polar than free testosterone, and are absorbed more slowly from the area of injection. Once in the bloodstream, the ester is removed to yield free (active) testosterone. Esterified forms of testosterone are designed to prolong the window of therapeutic effect following administration, allowing for a less frequent injection schedule compared to injections of free (unesterified) steroid.

Side Effects (Estrogenic):

Testosterone is readily aromatized in the body to estradiol (estrogen). The aromatase (estrogen synthetase) enzyme is responsible for this metabolism of testosterone. Elevated estrogen levels can cause side effects such as increased water retention, body fat gain, and gynecomastia. Testosterone is considered a moderately estrogenic steroid. An anti-estrogen such as clomiphene citrate or tamoxifen citrate may be necessary to prevent estrogenic side effects. One may alternately use an aromatase inhibitor like Arimidex® (anastrozole), which more efficiently controls estrogen by preventing its synthesis. Aromatase inhibitors can be quite expensive in comparison to anti-estrogens, however, and may also have negative effects on blood lipids.

Estrogenic side effects will occur in a dose-dependant manner, with higher doses (above normal therapeutic levels) of testosterone more likely to require the concurrent use of an anti-estrogen or aromatase inhibitor. Since water retention and loss of muscle definition are common with higher doses of testosterone, this drug is usually considered a poor choice for dieting or cutting phases of training. Its moderate estrogenicity makes it more ideal for bulking phases, where the added water retention will support raw strength and muscle size, and help foster a stronger anabolic environment.

Side Effects (Androgenic):

Testosterone is the primary male androgen, responsible for maintaining secondary male sexual characteristics. Elevated levels of testosterone are likely to produce androgenic side effects including oily skin, acne, and body/facial hair growth. Men with a genetic predisposition for hair loss (androgenetic alopecia) may notice accelerated male pattern balding. Those concerned about hair loss may find a more comfortable option in nandrolone decanoate, which is a comparably less androgenic steroid. Women are warned of the potential virilizing effects of anabolic/androgenic steroids, especially with a strong androgen such as testosterone. These may include deepening of the voice, menstrual irregularities, changes in skin texture, facial hair growth, and clitoral enlargement.

In androgen-responsive target tissues such as the skin, scalp, and prostate, the high relative androgenicity of testosterone is dependant on its reduction to dihydrotestosterone (DHT). The 5-alpha reductase enzyme is responsible for this metabolism of testosterone. The concurrent use of a 5-alpha reductase inhibitor such as finasteride or dutasteride will interfere with site-specific potentiation of testosterone action, lowering the tendency of testosterone drugs to produce androgenic side effects. It is important to remember that anabolic and androgenic effects are both mediated via the cytosolic androgen receptor. Complete separation of testosterone's anabolic and androgenic properties is not possible, even with total 5-alpha reductase inhibition.

Side Effects (Hepatotoxicity):

Testosterone does not have hepatotoxic effects; liver toxicity is unlikely. One study examined the potential for hepatotoxicity with high doses of testosterone by administering 400 mg of the hormone per day (2,800 mg per week) to a group of male subjects. The steroid was taken orally so that higher peak concentrations would be reached in hepatic tissues compared to intramuscular injections. The hormone was given daily for 20 days, and produced no significant changes in liver enzyme values including serum albumin, bilirubin, alanine-amino-transferase, and alkaline phosphatases.[780]

Side Effects (Cardiovascular):

Anabolic/androgenic steroids can have deleterious effects on serum cholesterol. This includes a tendency to reduce HDL (good) cholesterol values and increase LDL (bad) cholesterol values, which may shift the HDL to LDL balance in a direction that favors greater risk of arteriosclerosis. The relative impact of an anabolic/androgenic steroid on serum lipids is dependant on the dose, route of administration (oral vs. injectable), type of steroid (aromatizable or non-aromatizable), and level of resistance to hepatic metabolism. Anabolic/androgenic steroids may also adversely affect blood pressure and triglycerides, reduce endothelial relaxation, and support left ventricular hypertrophy, all potentially increasing the risk of cardiovascular disease and myocardial infarction.

Testosterone tends to have a much less dramatic impact on cardiovascular risk factors than synthetic steroids. This is due in part to its openness to metabolism by the liver, which allows it to have less effect on the hepatic management of cholesterol. The aromatization of testosterone to estradiol also helps to mitigate the negative effects of androgens on serum lipids. In one study, 280 mg per week of testosterone ester (enanthate) had a slight but not statistically significant effect on HDL cholesterol after 12 weeks, but when taken with an aromatase inhibitor a strong (25%) decrease was seen.[781] Studies using 300 mg of testosterone ester (enanthate) per week for 20 weeks without an aromatase inhibitor demonstrated only a 13% decrease in HDL cholesterol, while at 600 mg the reduction reached 21%.[782] The negative impact of aromatase inhibition should be taken into consideration before such a drug is added to testosterone therapy.

Due to the positive influence of estrogen on serum lipids, tamoxifen citrate or clomiphene citrate are preferred to aromatase inhibitors for those concerned with cardiovascular health, as they offer a partial estrogenic effect in the liver. This allows them to potentially improve lipid profiles and offset some of the negative effects of androgens. With doses of 600 mg or less per week, the impact on lipid profile tends to be noticeable but not dramatic, making an anti-estrogen (for cardioprotective purposes) perhaps unnecessary. Doses of 600 mg or less per week have also failed to produce statistically significant changes in LDL/VLDL cholesterol, triglycerides, apolipoprotein B/C-III, C-reactive protein, and insulin sensitivity, all indicating a relatively weak impact on cardiovascular risk factors.[783] When used in moderate doses, injectable testosterone esters are usually considered to be the safest of all anabolic/androgenic steroids.

To help reduce cardiovascular strain it is advised to maintain an active cardiovascular exercise program and minimize the intake of saturated fats, cholesterol, and simple carbohydrates at all times during active AAS administration. Supplementing with fish oils (4 grams per day) and a natural cholesterol/antioxidant formula such as Lipid Stabil or a product with comparable ingredients is also recommended.

Side Effects (Testosterone Suppression):

All anabolic/androgenic steroids when taken in doses sufficient to promote muscle gain are expected to suppress endogenous testosterone production. Testosterone is the primary male androgen, and offers strong negative feedback on endogenous testosterone production. Testosterone-based drugs will, likewise, have a strong effect on the hypothalamic regulation of natural steroid hormones. Without the intervention of testosterone-stimulating substances, testosterone levels should return to normal within 1-4 months of drug secession. Note that prolonged hypogonadotrophic hypogonadism can develop secondary to steroid abuse, necessitating medical intervention.

The above side effects are not inclusive. For more detailed discussion of potential side effects, see the Steroid Side Effects section of this book.

Administration (General):

Testosterone propionate is often regarded as a painful injection. This is due to the very short carbon chain of the propionic acid ester, which can be irritating to tissues at the site of injection. Many sensitive individuals choose to avoid this steroid, their bodies reacting with a pronounced soreness and low-grade fever that may last for a few days after each injection.

Administration (Men):

Although active for longer periods, this drug is usually injected on a weekly basis for bodybuilding purposes. The dosage used per injection is typically 250-500 mg (1-2 ampules). Cycles are generally between 6 and 12 weeks in length. This level is sufficient to provide excellent gains in muscle size and strength. Testosterone drugs are ultimately very versatile, and can be combined with many other anabolic/androgenic steroids depending on the desired effect.

Administration (Women):

This drug is not recommended for women for physique- or performance-enhancing purposes due to its strong androgenic nature, tendency to produce virilizing side effects, and very-slow acting characteristics (making blood levels difficult to control).

Availability:

Triolandren is not commonly found on the black market, due to limited supply. It appears to currently be available only in Egypt and Taiwan (under the Novartis label).

Winstrol® (stanozolol)

Androgenic	30
Anabolic	320
Standard	Methyltestosterone (oral)

Chemical Name	17beta-Hydroxy-17-methyl-5alpha-androstano[3,2-c]pyrazole
Estrogenic Activity	none
Progestational Activity	not significant

Description:

Winstrol is the most widely recognized trade name for the drug stanozolol. Stanozolol is a derivative of dihydrotestosterone, chemically altered so that the hormone's anabolic (tissue-building) properties are greatly amplified and its androgenic activity minimized. Stanozolol is classified as an "anabolic" steroid, and exhibits one of the strongest dissociations of anabolic to androgenic effect among commercially available agents. It also cannot be aromatized into estrogens. Stanozolol is the second most widely used oral steroid, succeeded in popularity only by Dianabol (methandrostenolone). It is favored for its ability to promote muscle growth without water-retention, making it highly valued by dieting bodybuilders and competitive athletes.

History:

Stanozolol was first described in 1959.[784] It was developed into a medicine by Winthrop Laboratories in Great Britain. Parent firm (Sterling) filed for U.S. patent on the agent in 1961.[785] Stanozolol was officially released to the U.S. prescription drug market in 1962 under the brand name Winstrol. Stanozolol was initially prescribed for a variety of medical purposes, including the induction of appetite and lean tissue gain in cases of weight loss associated with many malignant and non-malignant diseases, the preservation of bone mass during osteoporosis, the promotion of liner growth in children with growth failure, as an anti-catabolic during prolonged corticosteroid therapy or for post-operative and post-trauma (burns, fractures) patients, and even to treat debility in the elderly.

The FDA's control over the prescription drug market had tightened by the mid-1970's, and the indicated uses for Winstrol were soon narrowed. During this time the FDA officially supported that Winstrol was "Probably Effective" as an adjunct therapy for treating osteoporosis, and for promoting growth in pituitary-deficient dwarfism. With this position, Winthrop was given more time to sell and study the agent. Winthrop was able to continually satisfy the FDA regarding Winstrol's validity as a therapeutic agent, and it remained in the U.S. throughout the 1980's and 1990's, a time when many other anabolic steroids were disappearing from the marketplace. Stanozolol was also showing some promise during this period for improving red blood cell concentrations, combating breast cancer, and (more recently) treating angioedema, a disorder characterized by the swelling of subdermal tissues, often with hereditary causes.

Winthrop went through a number of corporate changes during the 1990's, including a 1991 merger with Elf Sanofi to form Sanofi Winthrop. Sanofi Winthrop continued on to sell Winstrol in the U.S. for approximately 10 more years, before finally discontinuing the medication because of "manufacturing issues" (Searle was actually making the product for Sanofi at the time, and had reportedly ceased production). In 2003, the rights to Winstrol were officially transferred to Ovation Pharmaceuticals. Winstrol remains an approved drug on the U.S. pharmaceutical market, although is not under active production by Ovation label. All forms of Winstrol are presently unavailable in the U.S., although the Winstrol brand remains available in Spain. Numerous other brands and generic forms of the drug are produced in other countries, in both human and veterinary drug markets.

How Supplied:

Stanozolol is widely available in both human and veterinary drug markets. Composition and dosage may vary by country and manufacturer. Stanozolol was originally designed as an oral anabolic steroid, containing 2mg of drug per tablet (Winstrol). Other brands commonly contain 5 mg or 10 mg per tablet. Stanozolol can also be found in injectable preparations. These are most commonly water-based suspensions carrying 50 mg/ml of steroid.

Structural Characteristics:

Stanozolol is a modified form of dihydrotestosterone. It differs by: 1) the addition of a methyl group at carbon 17-alpha to protect the hormone during oral administration and 2) the attachment of a pyrazol group to the A-ring, replacing the normal 3-keto group (this gives stanozolol the chemical classification of a heterocyclic steroid). When viewed in the light of 17-alpha methyldihydrotestosterone, the A-ring modification on stanozolol seems to considerably increase its anabolic strength while reducing its relative androgenicity.

Stanozolol has a much weaker relative binding affinity for the androgen receptor than testosterone or dihydrotestosterone. At the same time it displays a much longer half-life and lower affinity for serum binding proteins in comparison. These features (among others) allow stanozolol to be a very potent anabolic steroid in spite of a weaker affinity for receptor binding. Recent studies have additionally confirmed that its primary mode if action involves interaction with the cellular androgen receptor.[786] Although not fully elucidated, stanozolol may have additional (some potentially unique) properties with regard to antagonism of the progesterone receptor, Low Affinity Glucocorticoid-binding Site interaction, and AR/PR/GR independent activities.[787,788,789] In therapeutic doses stanozolol does not have significant progestational activity.[790]

Stanozolol is known to strongly suppress levels of SHBG (sex hormone-binding globulin). This trait is characteristic of all anabolic/androgenic steroids, although its potency and form of administration make oral Winstrol® particularly effective in this regard. One study with a group of 25 normal males demonstrated a 48.4% reduction in SHBG after only 3 days of use.[791] The dose administered was .2mg/kg, or roughly 18mg for a person weighing 200lbs. Plasma binding proteins such as SHBG act to temporarily constrain steroid hormones from exerting activity in the body, and effectively reduce the available percentage of free (active) steroid. Oral stanozolol may be useful for providing a greater percentage of unbound steroid in the body, especially when taken in combination with a hormone that is more avidly bound by SHBG, such as testosterone.

Side Effects (Estrogenic):

Stanozolol is not aromatized by the body, and is not measurably estrogenic. An anti-estrogen is not necessary when using this steroid, as gynecomastia should not be a concern even among sensitive individuals. Since estrogen is the usual culprit with water retention, stanozolol instead produces a lean, quality look to the physique with no fear of excess subcutaneous fluid retention. This makes it a favorable steroid to use during cutting cycles, when water and fat retention are major concerns. Stanozolol is also very popular among athletes in combination strength/speed sports such as Track and Field. In such disciplines one usually does not want to carry around excess water weight, and may find the raw muscle-growth brought about by stanozolol to be quite favorable over the lower quality mass gains of aromatizable agents.

Side Effects (Androgenic):

Although classified as an anabolic steroid, androgenic side effects are still common with this substance. This may include bouts of oily skin, acne, and body/facial hair growth. Anabolic/androgenic steroids may also aggravate male pattern hair loss. Women are also warned of the potential virilizing effects of anabolic/androgenic steroids. These may include a deepening of the voice, menstrual irregularities, changes in skin texture, facial hair growth, and clitoral enlargement. Additionally, the 5-alpha reductase enzyme does not metabolize stanozolol, so its relative androgenicity is not affected by finasteride or dutasteride. Stanozolol is a steroid with relatively low androgenic activity in relation to its tissue-building actions, making the threshold for strong androgenic side effects comparably higher than more androgenic agents such as testosterone, methandrostenolone, or fluoxymesterone.

Side Effects (Hepatotoxicity):

Stanozolol is a c17-alpha alkylated compound. This alteration protects the drug from deactivation by the liver, allowing a very high percentage of the drug entry into the bloodstream following oral administration. C17-alpha alkylated anabolic/androgenic steroids can be hepatotoxic. Prolonged or high exposure may result in liver damage. In rare instances life-threatening dysfunction may develop. It is advisable to visit a physician periodically during each cycle to monitor liver function and overall health. Intake of c17-alpha alkylated steroids is commonly limited to 6-8 weeks, in an effort to avoid escalating liver strain.

Stanozolol appears to offer less hepatic stress than an equivalent dose of Dianabol (methandrostenolone). Studies giving 12mg of stanozolol per day for 27 weeks failed to demonstrate clinically-significant changes in markers of liver function, including serum aspartate aminotransferase, alanine aminotransferase, gamma-glutamyltransferase, bilirubin, and alkaline phosphatase.[792] Relative hepatotoxicity increases as the dosage escalates, so hepatic dysfunction should still be a concern. In rare instances, high doses (alone or in combination with other steroids) have been implicated in cases of serious life-threatening hepatotoxicity in bodybuilders. Injectable stanozolol has also been implicated in severe hepatotoxicity in an otherwise healthy bodybuilder,[793] and should not be used as an alternative medication when liver toxicity precludes oral stanozolol use.

The use of a liver detoxification supplement such as Liver Stabil, Liv-52, or Essentiale Forte is advised while taking any hepatotoxic anabolic/androgenic steroids.

Side Effects (Cardiovascular):

Anabolic/androgenic steroids can have deleterious effects on serum cholesterol. This includes a tendency to reduce HDL (good) cholesterol values and increase LDL (bad) cholesterol values, which may shift the HDL to LDL balance in a direction that favors greater risk of arteriosclerosis. The relative impact of an anabolic/androgenic steroid on serum lipids is dependant on the dose, route of administration (oral vs. injectable), type of steroid (aromatizable or non-aromatizable), and level of resistance to hepatic metabolism. Stanozolol has a strong effect on the hepatic management of cholesterol due to its structural resistance to liver breakdown, non-aromatizable nature, and route of administration. Studies using an oral dose of 6mg per day for six weeks demonstrated a mean serum HDL reduction of 33% in healthy male weight-training subjects, which was combined with a 29% increase in serum LDL.[794] Anabolic/androgenic steroids may also adversely affect blood pressure and triglycerides, reduce endothelial relaxation, and support left ventricular hypertrophy, all potentially increasing the risk of cardiovascular disease and myocardial infarction.

Injectable stanozolol has also been documented to produce strong negative changes in serum lipids. One study was carried out on a group of 12 healthy male subjects, and demonstrated a measurable reduction in HDL cholesterol values, as well as an increase in LDL and total cholesterol values, following a single injection of 50 mg.[795] These changes persisted for 4 weeks after the drug was administered, and represent a potential increased risk for developing arteriosclerosis. Injectable stanozolol should not be used as an alternative medication when cardiovascular risk factors preclude oral stanozolol use.

To help reduce cardiovascular strain it is advised to maintain an active cardiovascular exercise program and minimize the intake of saturated fats, cholesterol, and simple carbohydrates at all times during active AAS administration. Supplementing with fish oils (4 grams per day) and a natural cholesterol/antioxidant formula such as Lipid Stabil or a product with comparable ingredients is also recommended.

Side Effects (Testosterone Suppression):

All anabolic/androgenic steroids when taken in doses sufficient to promote muscle gain are expected to suppress endogenous testosterone production. Stanozolol is no exception, and is noted for its strong influence on the hypothalamic-pituitary-testicular axis. Clinical studies giving 10 mg per day to healthy male subjects for 14 days caused the mean plasma testosterone level to fall by 55%.[796] Without the intervention of testosterone-stimulating substances, testosterone levels should return to normal within 1-4 months of drug secession. Note that prolonged hypogonadotrophic hypogonadism can develop secondary to steroid abuse, necessitating medical intervention.

The above side effects are not inclusive. For more detailed discussion of potential side effects, see the Steroid Side Effects section of this book.

Administration (General):

Studies have shown that taking an oral anabolic steroid with food may decrease its bioavailability.[797] This is caused by the fat-soluble nature of steroid hormones, which can allow some of the drug to dissolve with undigested dietary fat, reducing its absorption from the gastrointestinal tract. For maximum utilization, oral forms of stanozolol should be taken on an empty stomach.

There can be large discrepancies in the steroid particle size between injectable stanozolol preparations. For example, Winstrol from Zambon (Spain) was designed for human use, and uses a refined powder that will pass through a 27-gauge needle. Winstrol®-V is a veterinary product in the U.S. and Canada, and has larger particles that will jam in needles smaller than 22-gauge. Solutions that utilize a larger particle size may also cause more discomfort at the site of injection. Injectable forms of stanozolol can be taken in measured oral doses should injection prove intolerable.

Administration (Men):

The original prescribing guidelines for Winstrol called for a daily dosage of 6mg, which was administered on a schedule of one 2mg tablet three times per day. The usual dosage for physique- or performance-enhancing purposes is between 15 mg and 25 mg per day, or three to five 5 mg tablets, taken for no longer than 6-8 weeks. Injectable Winstrol is generally recommended at a clinical dosage of one 50 mg injection every 2-3 weeks. When used for physique- or performance-enhancing purposes, a dosage of 50 mg every other day is most commonly applied. Veterinary stanozolol preparations with a larger particle size will be more slowly dispersed by the body, and are commonly given at 75 mg every third day. Doses of 50 mg per day with injectable stanozolol are not uncommon, although probably not advised. Note that injectable forms of the drug are expected to have, milligram for milligram, a greater anabolic effect than oral.[798]

Stanozolol is often combined with other steroids for a more dramatic result. For example, while bulking one might opt to add in 200-400 mg of a testosterone ester (cypionate, enanthate, or propionate) per week. The result should be a considerable gain in new muscle mass, with a more comfortable level of water and fat retention than if taking a higher dose of testosterone alone. For dieting phases, one might alternately combine stanozolol with a non-aromatizing steroid such as 150 mg per week of a trenbolone ester or 200-300 mg of Primobolan® (methenolone enanthate). Such stacks are highly favored for increasing definition and muscularity. An in-between (lean mass gain) might be to add in 200-400 mg of a low estrogenic compound like Deca-Durabolin® (nandrolone decanoate) or Equipoise® (boldenone undecylenate).

Administration (Women):

The original prescribing guidelines for Winstrol called for a daily dosage of 4mg (one 2mg tablet twice daily) with young women particularly susceptible to the androgenic effects of anabolic steroids. This dosage was increased to 6mg (the same as the recommended dose for males) when necessary. When used for physique- or performance-enhancing purposes, a dosage of 5 mg to 10 mg daily is most common, taken for no longer than 4-6 weeks. Injectable Winstrol is generally recommended at a clinical dose of 50 mg every 2-3 weeks. The injectable is usually not advised with women for physique- or performance-enhancing purposes, as it allows for less control over blood hormone levels. Those women who absolutely must use the injectable commonly administer 25 mg every 3 or 4 days. Although this compound is weakly androgenic, the risk of virilization symptoms cannot be completely excluded, even at therapeutic doses.

Availability:

Winstrol is an extremely popular steroid, and the fact that it is found in abundance on the black market reflects this. It is also a popular target for counterfeit steroid manufacturers. In going over the popular brands circulating right now, the following observations have been made.

British Dispensary in Thailand makes a stanozolol product. Their trade name for the drug is Azolol, and it contains 5 mg of steroid in a 400 tablet bottle. The bottle itself looks very similar to that of Androlic, with dark plastic and a shiny chrome top. Be sure to look for the company's holographic sticker when shopping.

Stanol tablets from Thailand appear to be in production again, under a new license held under T.P. Drug Laboratories (1969) CO. LTD. Note that counterfeits are very common, so be sure to compare your product to the photographs included in this book very closely. The current popular fake is very close in appearance, but has deviant lot number printings (done with the rest of the label) and a slightly "off" overall appearance. The firm is likely also marketing its injectable Stanol product again.

Acdhon in Thailand makes Stanozodon, which comes in the old industry standard of 2 mg of steroid per tablet. It is packaged in bottles of 1,000. Counterfeits are not known to be a problem at this time although the product is not widely distributed on the black market either.

Xelox, an export company from the Philippines, sells a brand of stanozolol called Anazol. It comes in both an oral and injectable form. The injectable, Anazol Depot, carries 50 mg/mL of steroid in a 5 mL multi-dose vial. The formulation includes 5 mg/mL of added lidocaine, to reduce injection discomfort. The oral comes as a 2mg tablet, with 100 coming per plastic bottle. Both forms of the drug will carry the Xelox security sticker to deter counterfeiting.

Winstrol® tablets and injectable ampules are still produced in Spain, by Desma. This remains the most popular stanozolol injectable in Europe. All boxes are protected with a holographic sticker, which carries the company logo embedded into the image. Thus far counterfeiters have not yet duplicated these stickers.

The Greek generic by Genepharm is still in production. This item does not appear to be a big target for counterfeiters as of yet, and can usually be trusted. Remember to look for a Greek drug ID sticker on the box to assure legitimacy. This will show a hidden mark under UV light, and provides a very reliable detection method.

Chinfield makes a 50 mg/mL injectable stanozolol in Argentina called Nabolic Strong. This is the same firm that makes regular Nabolic, a very low dosed (2 mg/mL) version of the same drug. This new product is now much more popular on the black market than the first, due to the more useable dosage. Note that Chinfield prints their logo on the inside of the vial carton, which offers somewhat of a simple security check (obviously one very easy to duplicate). Your box is definitely counterfeit if it is blank on the inside.

Anabolico Cimol is an injectable form of stanozolol from Argentina. It comes in multi-dose vials containing 50 mg/mL of the steroid. This item has not been subject to widescale counterfeiting, but also bears no security features that would deter this practice.

Balkan Pharmaceuticals in Moldova makes both a 10 mg and 50 mg oral tablet of stanozolol, which it sells under the Strombafort trade name. Counterfeits are not known to be a problem.

Stanozoland from Landerlan in Paraguay is common on the black market, particularly in South America. It comes in the form of a 10 mg tablets, packaged in bottles of 100 tablets each. The company also makes a 50 mg/mL injectable.

Also from Paraguay is a generic stanozolol injectable from Indufar. It contains 50 mg/mL of steroid in a 1 mL glass ampule. Three ampules are packaged per box.

ANABOLIC AGENTS (NON-STEROID) Drug Profiles

Arachidonic Acid (eicosa-5,8,11,14-enoic acid)

Description:

Arachidonic acid is an omega-6 essential fatty acid that serves as the principle building block for the synthesis of dienolic prostaglandins (such as PGE2 and PGF2a). These prostaglandins are integral to protein turnover and muscle accumulation, and have such important activities as increasing blood flow to the muscles (pumps), increasing local IGF-1 and insulin sensitivity (corresponding receptor levels), supporting satellite cell activation, proliferation, and differentiation, and increasing the overall rate of protein synthesis and muscle growth. Arachidonic acid release serves as the main thermostat for prostaglandin turnover in skeletal muscle tissue, and is responsible for initiating many of the immediate biochemical changes during resistance exercise that will ultimately produce muscle hypertrophy. As such, it is a highly anabolic nutrient. Among the large variety of nutrients available to athletes and bodybuilders for supplementation, next to protein, arachidonic acid is the most integral to muscle growth, as it sits at the very center of the anabolic response.

Clinical Studies:

In 2005, the Exercise & Sport Nutrition Laboratory at Baylor University conducted a double-blind placebo-controlled study to determine if 50 days of resistance training and arachidonic acid (X-Factor™) supplementation would affect training adaptations in 31 experienced (>1 year) resistance-trained males. The results were presented at the International Society of Sports Nutrition conference on June 15, 2006. All subjects ingested a total of four capsules each day (one 250 mg capsule of AA or placebo every four hours). Subjects taking X-Factor added an average of 25lbs to their bench press maximum weight in 50 days, which was an increase of nearly 45% greater than the placebo group. The X-Factor group outperformed the placebo group on Average Power (225% > placebo), Peak Anaerobic Power (600% > placebo), and Total Work Capacity (250% > placebo). No side effects were reported during the investigation.

Pharmacology:

Arachidonic acid begins to display its anabolic activity early during exercise. This nutrient is released from your muscle fibers as they are damaged during intense training, triggering a localized inflammatory and anabolic response. This is part of the same biological process that causes you to be sore a day or two following a good workout, and reminds us that the old adage "no pain, no gain" is a fundamentally true one. Arachidonic acid liberation from damaged muscle fibers is, similarly, the very first anabolic trigger in a long cascade that will control the rebuilding and strengthening of muscle tissue after exercise.[799][800][801] Among other things, by increasing local IGF-1 and insulin receptor density, arachidonic acid supports the anabolic actions of these hormones, making the repair process both faster and more intense. As a crude explanation, arachidonic acid helps direct the body to where it needs muscle tissue repair by facilitating the localized actions of anabolic hormones.

The availability of arachidonic acid, and our ability to liberate it during exercise, is important to the anabolic productivity of our workouts. We also need to be aware of the fact that regular exercise significantly lowers the content of arachidonic acid in skeletal muscle tissue.[802][803][804] Since dienolic prostaglandin synthesis is tied to the amount of available arachidonic acid, lower levels result in less arachidonic acid being released during exercise, and a less intense anabolic response. The depletion of arachidonic acid in skeletal muscle tissue is also one of the key reasons we find it harder to get sore the more regularly we exercise. With lower levels of arachidonic acid, you need to work more vigorously to receive the same level of release and anabolic stimulation. On the same note, when you change up your routine and hit your muscles from new angles, arachidonic acid is the reason you may find yourself more sore than usual. You have called upon new muscle fibers, which have higher stores of arachidonic acid to work with. Dan Duchaine once said, "The best exercise is the one you are not doing." This may have a lot to do with what he was talking about.

History:

The arachidonic acid supplementation protocols, and the concept of using this nutrient to improve muscle mass, strength, and performance, were first developed by William Llewellyn, author of this book series. Llewellyn filed patent on the technology on November 27, 2002, and released an arachidonic acid supplement under the X-Factor trademark (Molecular Nutrition) shortly after. Although the product was initially met with a great deal of skepticism and criticism by industry peers, it has since been proven effective both in the marketplace and in clinical trials, and established itself as a powerful supplement for body recomposition goals. The U.S. Patent & Trademark Office granted Llewellyn's patent application for arachidonic acid on January 11, 2005 (U.S. Patent # 6,841,573), and the product has since been offered for license to other companies in the industry. The original X-Factor product remains widely available in the U.S. and abroad, and rapid expansion in the arachidonic acid category is expected as more companies license the technology. Note that any officially licensed arachidonic acid product sold in the sports nutrition marketplace will carry the original X-Factor trademark on its packaging.

Structural Characteristics:

Arachidonic acid (eicosa-5,8,11,14-enoic acid) is an essential polyunsaturated fatty acid found in animal fats. Supplemental arachidonic acid is commonly produced in two forms, triglyceride and ethyl ester. As with other fatty acid supplements such as fish oils, the natural triglyceride form (as present in X-Factor and licensed products) offers up to 400% greater absorption than the ethyl ester, and is the preferred form for supplementation.

How Supplied:

Arachidonic acid is sold under the X-Factor trademark by Molecular Nutrition, and is supplied in 250 mg capsules. Arachidonic acid may also be found in a number of licensed products; all will display the patent number (#6,841,573) on the packaging.

Administration (Short-Term Anabolic):

As a short-term anabolic agent, arachidonic acid is supplemented at a dose of 500 mg to 1,000 mg per day (2-4 250 mg capsules). The full 1,000 mg dose is most commonly used, regardless of bodyweight. The nutrient is cycled in the same way steroids commonly are, and is taken for a period of 7-8 weeks followed by an equal amount of time off. This level is sufficient to notice measurable increases in lean muscle mass, strength, and anaerobic power. Depending on dietary and individual metabolic factors, these gains may be accompanied by a decrease in body fat. Gains of 1-2lbs of lean muscle mass per week are fairly consistent, with total accrued weight gain often measuring approximately 10lbs during a cycle. There is also no hormonal disruption with arachidonic acid supplementation, so the retention of gains after the product is discontinued is generally high. Note that arachidonic acid also has some effect as a vasodilator, and may produce increased pumps in response to intense training. This often occurs within two weeks of initiating supplementation at anabolic levels.

Administration (Normal Supplementation):

Arachidonic acid may also be an important nutrient to consider in regular supplemental doses, particularly if you do not consume animal products (red meat, organ meat, eggs) on a regular basis. Studies have shown that given somewhat comparable amounts of protein, those who consume animal products will make more progress with resistance exercise than those that do not (vegetarians).[805] Arachidonic acid may be the missing component in such diets, too integral to the anabolic response for lower dietary levels not to be noticed. There is also empirical evidence suggesting that an arachidonic acid deficiency exists in many experienced bodybuilders, given that training depletes AA stores. On a number of cases, tissue tests for the content of phospholipids have revealed unusually low levels of arachidonic acid in highly trained athletes. For those who find their intake of animal products inadequate, or feel that they may have insufficient tissue stores of AA, a single capsule of 250 mg provides about the equivalent of a day's supply of arachidonic acid within a normal western diet with animal products. Taken every day or two, the capsule should provide a necessary supply of this essential omega-6 fatty acid.

Safety:

In clinical studies involving the supplementation of 1,500-1,700 mg of arachidonic acid per day, general markers of health were also unaffected with 50 days of continuous use. This includes no notable change in HDL, LDL, or total cholesterol values, immune system response functioning, or platelet aggregation values.[806][807][808] Furthermore, the investigation at Baylor University demonstrated safety on all of the basic markers of health including lipids, blood pressure, blood cell counts, immune system mediators, and liver enzymes. The study also produced a strong trend for reduced IL-6 in the X-Factor supplemented group, which is a principle inflammatory cytokine and stimulus for the hepatic production of C-reactive protein. High levels of IL-6 are correlated with poor health and mortality, and are deemed undesirable. The results suggest that while arachidonic acid may be "pro-inflammatory" in the sedentary (inactive) state, when combined with resistance training, a reduction in systemic inflammation may actually be noticed. It is speculated that an amplification of some of the health-beneficial aspects of resistance exercise, namely the improved management of insulin, may be responsible for reducing this inflammatory marker.

Side Effects:

Arachidonic acid (X-Factor) often produces an amplification of residual post-workout (Delayed Onset) muscle soreness. Often recovery is slightly prolonged (perhaps an additional day of rest is required), and the user may need to adjust their schedule accordingly. This is due to an intensification of the normal physiological response to training, and represents increased intensity of the anabolic cascade (and rate of muscle growth). Those with existing minor muscle, connective tissue, or joint injuries may notice more pain, due to the greater prostaglandin signaling caused by supplementation.

While arachidonic acid should not exacerbate the injury, if greater soreness interferes with one's ability to train comfortably, the supplement should be discontinued until the injury is healed. Arachidonic acid supplementation may also produce a greater incidence of headaches in a small percentage of users, which may be due to its effect as a vasodilator. Increasing daily water consumption often alleviates this side effect. Additionally, arachidonic acid seems to produce a very weak androgenic effect in some users, often producing minor oily skin. This may be caused by a slight amplification of testosterone's effect. It should not be strong enough to concern females about virilizing side effects.

Contraindications:

Those with an existing medical condition related to inflammation may find that the added arachidonic acid exacerbates symptoms of their disorder, and should avoid supplementation. This supplement should only be used after the approval of a physician if someone is taking medication, has an existing medical condition, or has a familial predisposition for cardiovascular disease, high blood pressure, or any other disorder that may require the limiting of dietary arachidonic acid. Also, as a potent growth-promoting agent, arachidonic acid joins androgens (testosterone, anabolic steroids), growth hormone, IGF-1, estrogens, and many other growth factors as potentially supporting the growth rate of certain cancer cells if you have the disease. Dietary arachidonic acid intake has been generally eliminated as a causative factor in cancer,[809][810] just as testosterone level has been eliminated as predictive of prostate cancer risk, however these types of growth-promoting agents should be avoided in such diseased states unless approved by a physician. If you have prostate cancer, for example, the last thing you want to start taking is a growth promoter like testosterone. The same goes for arachidonic acid. The bottom line is that if you are in poor health, you should probably not be taking this supplement. If you are healthy, you should be able to use it with great safety.

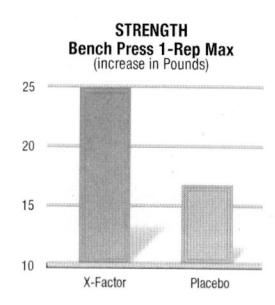

STRENGTH
Bench Press 1-Rep Max
(increase in Pounds)

During the clinical study, subjects taking X-Factor added an average of 25lbs to their bench press maximum weight in 50 days. This increase was nearly 45% greater than that noted in the exercise-only (placebo) group. Some subjects gained more than 50 lbs on their bench press 1-rep max over the 50-day period.

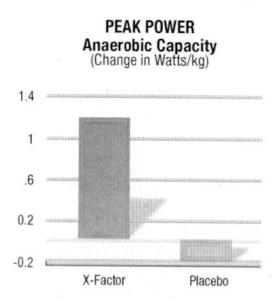

PEAK POWER
Anaerobic Capacity
(Change in Watts/kg)

Using the standard Wingate cycle ergometer test to measure relative peak anaerobic power, subjects taking X-Factor increased leg power by 1.2 Watts·kg-1. This represents a net increase of more than 600% over the placebo group (-.2 Watts·kg-1).

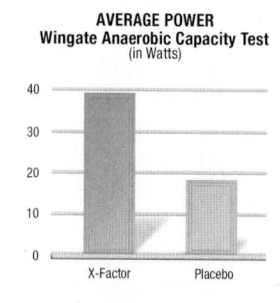

AVERAGE POWER
Wingate Anaerobic Capacity Test
(in Watts)

In the standard Wingate cycle ergometer test to measure anaerobic power and performance, the X-Factor group outperformed the placebo group on Average Power by an amazing 21 watts (AA: 37.9W P: 17.0W). That's a net increase of nearly 225% compared to placebo.

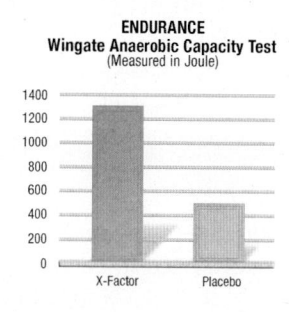

ENDURANCE
Wingate Anaerobic Capacity Test
(Measured in Joule)

Total Work, as recorded in the standard energy unit Joules, increased by 1,292J in the group taking X-Factor, while Total Work increased 510J in the placebo group. This is more than a 250% increase compared to placebo.

Kynoselen®

Description:

Kynoselen is an injectable veterinary drug, currently produced by the international firm Vetoquinol. It contains a mixture of heptaminol, AMP (adenosine monophosphate), vitamin B-12, sodium selenite, magnesium aspartate, and potassium aspartate. This blend makes for a restorative "tonic" type drug, administered to protect an animal's muscle mass and overall wellness after illness, injury, or trauma. It is most often used on horses, and is typically applied as an anti-catabolic after strenuous activity, or to help get an animal back on its feet after a debilitating infection/illness. At other times it is simply used to support the vitality of an animal that is otherwise healthy, but at the moment less than vigorous in its daily activities. In some cases it is even used for the very basic purpose of remedying a deficiency in vitamin B-12 or selenium intake. Bodybuilders are attracted to Kynoselen for its mild anabolic and lipolytic properties.

The principle active ingredient in Kynoselen is heptaminol, which is classified as an amino alcohol with myocardial stimulant and vasodilatory properties. It is also identified as an inotropic compound, which increases contractile strength, and minimizes fatigue, of skeletal muscles.[811] It has demonstrated a specific ability to increase the differentiation of satellite muscle cells,[812] a process that helps generate new muscle tissue (skeletal muscle growth). This same ingredient is also known to affect the release and uptake of norepinephrine (noradrenalin), increasing levels of this hormone/neurotransmitter in the blood.[813] Since noradrenalin is an important regulator of lipolysis in humans, this allows heptaminol to impart some fat-loss effect. Adenosine triphosphate is also regarded as a key component of the product, and plays a role in the storage and release of energy. Overall, both the anabolic and lipolytic properties of Kynoselen are measurable when used in humans, but not dramatic. It is capable of imparting some increases in strength, muscle mass, and fat loss, but the results will not rival those of anabolic steroids. Still, being that this drug is legal in most jurisdictions, it remains an attractive alternative to anabolic steroids for many individuals.

History:

Heptaminol, the principle active ingredient in Kynoselen, was first heavily investigated in clinical medicine during the early 1950s. It was soon developed into a prescription drug, and has since been sold by a series of drug manufacturers in many different parts of the world. Currently its most common therapeutic use is to treat orthostatic hypotension, which is a sudden drop in blood pressure upon standing. Various preparations containing heptaminol have been produced over the years, the most notable of which have included Amidrina (Italy), Cortensor (Belgium and Switzerland), Hept-A-Myl (USA), Heptamyl (Belgium and Switzerland), and Heptylon (France). Although a variety of human medications containing heptaminol have been in commerce for decades, these preparations were rarely of interest to athletes. Years later, under a far different medical setting, Western athletes were first introduced to the drug.

The French veterinary preparation Kynoselen would be the first heptaminol-containing drug to grab large-scale international attention, becoming popular among American bodybuilders and athletes during the latter part of the 1990s. This was some years subsequent to laws being passed that had increased the penalties for dealing in anabolic steroids. During this time, availability of the drugs had shifted, and for some buyers scarce supply and high legal risk made the drugs less attractive. Many athletes were becoming increasingly resourceful in finding other non-scheduled performance-enhancing drugs that could be purchased and used with less legal risk. Kynoselen was already known to athletes in Europe, and would quickly cross the Atlantic. By the year 2000, a number of exporters had set up operation to market the drug directly to American athletes. Today, Kynoselen remains unscheduled and widely available in the United States and many areas abroad.

How Supplied:

Kynoselen is most commonly supplied in a 100 mL multi-dose vial for injection. Active ingredients are heptaminol, disodic adenosine monophosphate, vitamin B12, selenium (sodium selenite), magnesium aspartate, and potassium aspartate.

Structural Characteristics:

Heptaminol (supplied as heptaminol hydrochloride) is an amino alcohol with a structure of 6-amino-2-methyl-heptan-2-ol.

Administration:

Kynoselen is not approved for use in humans. Prescribing guidelines are unavailable. An effective dosage for physique- or performance-enhancing purposes generally falls in the range of 1 mL weekly for every 25 pounds of bodyweight. This would mean that a 200lb bodybuilder would use around 8 mL per week. Due to high injection volume, some opt to take a lower dosage, injecting at the very least a 2 mL three times per week. At this dose, a single

100 mL vial would last about 16 weeks. At 8-10 mL per week a 100 mL bottle would last for 10 to 12 weeks. It is generally recommended to use the entire bottle once it has been opened, or discard any remaining drug that was not used during the cycle. As with all injectable drugs packaged in multi-dosed vials, contaminants will be introduced into the solution immediately once the seal is broken for the first injection.

Because it tends to increase noradrenalin levels, Kynoselen is also a mild stimulant. It is likely for this specific reason that its use has been banned by certain horseracing organizations. This means that one can expect certain stimulant-related side effects, especially when taking this drug in higher dosages. This includes rapid heartbeat, sweating, jitters, restlessness, increased blood pressure, or insomnia. A good rule of thumb used by bodybuilders to try and keep such side effects from becoming a problem is to never inject more than 2 mL per day. They may also want to start with an amount lower than the recommended dosage (determined by bodyweight), perhaps even half of this. The dose is then slowly increased, so that the peak level is reached only after three to four weeks of slow incremental increases.

Warnings:

Individuals with high blood pressure or cardiovascular disease should not use Kynoselen.

Availability:

Kynoselen usually sells for $75 to $100 per bottle at the retail level. It is not a controlled substance in the United States, and is likewise pretty easy to obtain locally or via mail order. Currently no significant fakes are known to exist. Given its abundance and low cost, counterfeits are not expected to be a significant problem anytime soon. It is also important to note that legitimate Kynoselen is a veterinary drug only, and has never been manufactured for human use.

Lutalyse® (diniprost tromethamine)

Description:

Dinoprost tromethamine is a pharmaceutical form of the natural prostaglandin PGF2alpha. Prostaglandins are a series of natural oxygenated unsaturated cyclic fatty acids, which have a variety of hormone-like actions in the body. Among other things, PGF2alpha is involved in vasoconstriction, increasing protein synthesis in skeletal muscle tissue, and reducing adipose tissue mass. This hormone-like chemical also stimulates smooth muscle contraction, and is involved in pain, inflammation, fever, ovulation, gastric motility, and fluid absorption in the gastrointestinal tract. In veterinary medicine dinoprost tromethamine is most commonly used in estrus synchronization/fertility timing, for treating chronic endometriosis, and to induce abortion or labor. Dinoprost is not widely used in human medicine, but is sometimes applied to terminate pregnancy or induce labor.

Athletes and bodybuilders are attracted to dinoprost tromethamine for its strong thermogenic and muscle-building properties. The anabolic effect of this drug has been substantiated by clinical studies, which have shown PGF2a to be a strong stimulator of protein synthesis, and key to both the immediate and long-term physiological adaptations to resistance training.[814][815][816][817] Reports from athletes who have experimented with this agent generally support this compound being an excellent promoter of localized muscle growth, usually resulting in both increases in muscle size and definition. Dinoprost is also reported to be a very fast acting drug, with many claiming it has caused noticeable effect after being injected in a particular muscle group for only a couple of weeks. Clinical data also supports it being a substantially potent fat-loss drug, with PGF2a shown in studies to inhibit the stimulation of lipogenesis in fat cells.[818] Again there is a great deal of anecdotal support for this property of dinoprost tromethamine among athletes and bodybuilders, with many claiming they notice a slight temperature elevation and marked fat loss during therapy.

History:

Dinoprost tromethamine was first introduced into clinical medicine in the early 1970s. The first approved use of the drug in human patients was to stimulate abortion during the second trimester. It has since remained of use for this purpose, but is most commonly associated these days with veterinary medicine. Here, it is widely applied to help farmers regulate the estrous cycle and fertility of various livestock. Interest in dinoprost tromethamine as an anabolic/thermogenic drug for athletes and bodybuilders did not appear until the late 1990s. This likely occurred subsequent to the release of numerous medical studies linking PGF2alpha to muscle hypertrophy. Early theoretical concepts stemming from this research evolved into modern application protocols for the drug, which in spite of a high propensity to generate side effects, have proven to be highly successful for many athletes and bodybuilders.

Over the years dinoprost tromethamine has appeared as a human medicine under a wide number of trade names, including such popular drug products as Amoglandin (Sweden), Prostin (Sweden), Prostin F2 alpha (U.S., Australia, Israel, Italy, New Zealand, South Africa, and the United Kingdom), Minprostin F2a (Germany), Enzaprost (Greece, Poland) and Prostarmon (Japan). Prostin F2 is no longer sold in the U.S., however, and there is presently no FDA approved replacement available for human use. Veterinary versions are more widely available and tend to provide significantly more active drug for less money than their human counterpart medicines, and as a result have been the products most commonly associated with the physique- or performance-enhancing use of dinoprost tromethamine. Popular veterinary brands have included Lutalyse (Pharmacia Animal Health), Prostamate (Pfizer), Panacelan (Daiichi Pharmaceutical Co.) and Dinolytic (Upjohn). Several corporate mergers have taken place in this segment of the market, and the (now larger) conglomerate Pharmacia has emerged as the worldwide leader in dinoprost sales. Lutalyse is consequently the most common form of dinoprost tromethamine of use among the athletic/bodybuilding community.

How Supplied:

Dinoprost tromethamine is most commonly supplied in a multi-dose vial (5 mL-100 mL) in a dose of 5 mg per mL. It is prepared in a sterile solution of water with benzyl alcohol added as a preservative and sodium hydroxide and/or hydrochloric acid to adjust pH.

Structural Characteristics:

Dinoprost tromethamine is the tromethamine salt of

prosta,5,13-dien-1-oic acid (PGF2alpha).

Side Effects:

Possible side effects or signs of dinoprost tromethamine overexposure may include such respiratory effects as bronchoconstriction, wheezing, coughing, lung irritation, rapid breathing, and anaphylaxis. Asthmatic individuals may be particularly susceptible to these effects. Dinoprost may also cause gastrointestinal disturbances such as abdominal cramping, diarrhea, vomiting and nausea. Other effects may include increased pulse rate, elevated blood pressure, chills, fever, and anorexia, and in women uterine contractions, vaginal bleeding, and uterine or urinary infections. Pregnant women should not take or handle dinoprost. Reports of side effects among athletes using dinoprost for physique- or performance-enhancing purposes are common, and often extreme. This includes pronounced soreness at the site of injection; often beginning with a dull burning almost immediately after the shot is given. Chills and flu-like feelings are also commonly reported during cycles, as are bouts of shortness of breath. Injections are also commonly followed by uncontrollable urges to urinate or defecate, including strong spasmodic contractions of the muscles involved in the control of these functions. Nausea and vomiting have also been commonly reported. For many, the cramping, diarrhea, pain, and general feelings of upset stomach, malaise, and discomfort make dinoprost a drug they experiment with only briefly. Others, however, continue on with the drug, and often report that side effects become more tolerable over time.

Administration:

As a human medication, dinoprost tromethamine is most commonly given intra-amniotically at a dose of 40 mg for the termination of pregnancy. It is also sometimes given orally to pregnant women at a dose of 30-100 mg to induce labor, although this tends to produce more side effects than other, more recently adopted, medications. When used for physique- or performance-enhancing purposes, dinoprost tromethamine is generally given by intramuscular injection. Most noted for its ability to generate localized growth, common sites of injection include the shoulders, biceps, triceps, calves, chest, back, and legs. The user will typically inject in only one site per day at the start of therapy, but this may be increased to 2 or more injections per day as they become more accustomed to the drug and its side effects. Therapy begins slowly, and is initiated with a low starting dose of approximately .5 milligram per injection. If the first injection were given without significant side effects, the next injection would be increased to 1 milligram. This is slowly increased by .5-1mg per application until a peak dose is reached. This might be a maximum of 5 mg per injection site. Injection sites are also regularly rotated so that several days separate administration in the same muscle group. Note that for some, the pain after injection is so severe that training for that specific muscle group must be delayed for at least a few days. Individual sensitivity to the drug may, therefore, require modifications of their injection and training schedule to maximize results and comfort.

Availability:

Dinoprost tromethamine is available in the U.S. and many other nations as a prescription drug product. It is also found infrequently on the black market.

ANTI-ACNE Drug Profiles

Accutane (isotretinoin)

Description:

Isotretinoin is an anti-acne medication that is chemically related to retinoic acid and retinol (Vitamin A). Although its exact mode of action is unknown, this agent works by inhibiting sebaceous gland functioning, which diminishes oil production in the skin and hinders acne development. Isotretinoin is sold in many countries throughout the world, and is largely regarded as one of the most effective medications for treating severe acne. Studies also support it having an excellent success rate with even some of the strongest cases of clinical acne (acne vulgaris). For example, an investigation published in 2005 involved the treatment of 160 patients with isotretinoin.[819] They took the drug for a 2-28 week treatment period, which was followed an additional one-year observation period. Of the 133 patents that finished the study, 127 noticed partial or complete clearance of acne during treatment. This was a success rate of over 95%. Nearly 60% of these patients were free of relapse a full year after isotretinoin therapy had been discontinued. Given that acne is one of the most common side effects of anabolic/androgenic steroid use, isotretinoin is utilized by bodybuilders and athletes to reduce or eliminate this cosmetic issue during steroid therapy.

History:

Isotretinoin was developed by Hoffmann-La Roche, and was first introduced as a drug product in 1982. The firm marketed it under the brand name Accutane, and retained U.S. patent rights on the drug until 2002. Upon expiration, a number of other drug products containing isotretinoin were approved for sale by the FDA. Isotretinoin is presently available under many trade names including Accutane (Roche), Amnesteem (Mylan), Claravis (Barr), Decutan (Actavis), Isotane (Pacific Pharmaceuticals), Sotret (Ranbaxy), and Roaccutane (Roche). Topical versions are also sold including Isotrex/Isotrexin (Stiefel).

Isotretinoin is not a controlled substance, but has been regulated by the FDA in recent years due to potential risks (see: Side Effects). It became part of a national patient database dubbed iPLEDGE in 2005, which was initiated to guard against potential birth defects and other health risks. The iPLEDGE requirements to receive and fill a prescription for isotretinoin are substantial, especially for female patients. The process involves not only an extensive education about the potential side effects of the drug and a signed contract acknowledging this education, but also agreements to maintain the use of birth control while taking the drug, and proof of at least two negative pregnancy test results. All this must be done prior to a prescription ever being written. On top of that, special yellow stickers must be taken to the pharmacy by the patient so the pharmacist can further verify that the patient has a valid script for current use and is educated about the side effect potential. Each script also must be filled in a very limited time frame or it is voided, which is done to avoid use at a later date.

How Supplied:

Isotretinoin is most commonly supplied in soft gelatin capsules of 10 mg, 20 mg, or 40 mg.

Structural Characteristics:

Isotretinoin is a derivative of retinoic acid, specifically 13-cis-retinoic acid.

Side Effects:

Isotretinoin is a powerful medication with many potential side effects. In fact, by some accounts this drug is a highly controversial one. Isotretinoin made front-page news on a number of occasions, where it was linked to birth defects, depression, and a string of patient suicides. As a result of identified potential health risks, the warnings on this product are numerous and very strong. This is especially important because any woman who potentially might become pregnant should not use the drug. Even small exposure has been linked to very serious complications with fetal development. It also displays some level of hepatotoxicity, and can lead to inflammatory bowel disease, pancreatitis, suppressed HDL cholesterol levels, elevated triglyceride values, and visual impairment. It may also be linked to a number of other peculiar side effects including psychosis,[820] heart palpitations,[821] hoarseness,[822] intracranial hypertension,[823] and even nasal tip deformities when taken following cosmetic surgery.[824]

The FDA approved literature on Accutane has warned of depression and suicide risks for many years. In support of this concern, it appears that isotretinoin does indeed directly affect brain function to some degree. This was demonstrated in a study published in early 2005.[825] Here, scientists began with the premise that in order for isotretinoin to induce depression and thoughts of suicide it must affect brain chemistry in some definable way. They set out to examine what changes, if any, the drug would have on the various regions of the brain. Twenty-eight people participated in total, approximately half being treated with isotretinoin and the other half a topical antibiotic. Examinations were conducted before the drug was initiated, and after it had been used for 4 weeks. Using positron emission tomography, they were able to demonstrate a 21% reduction in brain metabolism in the orbitofrontal cortex with isotretinoin use (there was a 2% increase with the antibiotic). This is a brain area known to mediate symptoms of depression, which suddenly gives claims of depression and suicide linked to isotretinoin a lot more validity and understanding. More work will need to be done in this area before any definitive conclusions are made.

Administration:

The typical method of using Isotretinoin involves taking a dosage of .5 to 1mg/kg of bodyweight per day. This would equate to a maximum daily dosage of 100 mg for a 220lb person. Very severe adult cases (with scarring perhaps) may require upwards adjustments in dosage later on, reaching as high as 2mg/kg/day. The daily dose itself is divided into two equal doses, which are to be given at two separate times of the day. Roche is very clear about this, stating that the safety of once daily dosing has not been established and, therefore, is not recommended. Isotretinoin also should be taken with meals, not on an empty stomach, as food significantly aids in the absorption of this drug (high fat meals have the strongest benefit on bioavailability). One course of therapy lasting 15-20 weeks is usually sufficient to clear up or at least control a patient's condition. If necessary, however, a second course may be initiated by the doctor. This must follow a break from the first course of therapy of at least 2 months.

Among athletes and bodybuilders taking the drug without the oversight of a physician, doses are often reduced as compared to the standard medical guidelines. This is done in an effort to minimize the chance of health damage or other unwanted side effects often linked to the drug. In many instances a dosage of 10-20 mg per day is used for this purpose. Intake duration is often much shorter than the prescription recommendations of 15-20 weeks as well, usually lasting only 6-8 weeks in length. Many athletes prone to steroid-induced acne, however, will take more than one course of therapy in a given year. The potential health risks of taking isotretinoin in lower doses, but periodically for longer total cumulative periods of time, are unknown.

Availability:

Isotretinoin is not a controlled substance in the United States, but is still tightly regulated. Most use among bodybuilders and athletes comes from black market sources, which make the drug readily available in most regions.

ANTI-ESTROGENS Drug Profiles

Arimidex® (anastrozole)

Description:

Anastrozole is an anti-estrogenic drug developed for the treatment of advanced breast cancer in women. Specifically, this agent is the first in a newer class of third-generation selective oral aromatase inhibitors.[826] It acts by blocking the enzyme aromatase, subsequently blocking the production of estrogen in the body. Since many forms of breast cancer cells are stimulated by estrogen, reducing levels of this hormone in the body may retard the progression of the disease. This is also the fundamental use of tamoxifen citrate (Nolvadex®), except Nolvadex blocks the action of estrogen at the receptor, not its actual endogenous production. The effects of anastrozole can be very substantial, with a daily dose of 1mg (commonly 1 tablet) capable of producing estrogen suppression greater than 80% in treated patients. With the powerful effect this drug has on hormone levels, it is usually only prescribed to post-menopausal women. Side effects like hot flashes and hair thinning can present themselves during therapy, and would be much more severe in pre-menopausal patients. For the steroid-using male athlete, anastrozole is applied to minimize the side effects associated with elevated estrogen levels secondary to anabolic/androgenic steroid use. In comparison with traditional methods such as Nolvadex and Proviron, anastrozole is significantly more effective at controlling estrogen.

History:

Anastrozole was developed by Zeneca Pharmaceuticals, and approved for use in the United States at the end of 1995. The drug was developed as a new adjunct treatment for operable breast cancer in postmenopausal female patients, an area of medicine that had a long history of tamoxifen use. Substantial data was needed to shift prescribing trends away from such an established medication treatment. Shortly after its release, anastrozole was investigated as part of an extremely large multicenter double blind trial based out of Rome (ATAC). The study evaluated the use of anastrozole and tamoxifen, alone or in combination, in 9,366 postmenopausal women following breast cancer surgery. The results favored anastrozole over tamoxifen at promoting disease regression and improving overall survival rates. Upon publication of this trial in 2002, anastrozole emerged as a new contender for the adjunctive treatment of postmenopausal breast cancer.[827][828] Around this same time the drug was also gained popularity with male bodybuilders and athletes who began taking notice of the strong estrogen suppression caused by anastrozole, both in the anecdotal reports of others and in clinical trials.

How Supplied:

Anastrozole is most commonly supplied in tablets of 1mg.

Structural Characteristics:

Anastrozole is classified as a selective non-steroidal aromatase inhibitor. It has the chemical designation 1,3-benzenediacetonitrile,a,a,a',a'-tetramethyl-5-(1H-1,2,4-triazol-1-ylmethyl).

Side Effects:

Common side effects associated with the use of an aromatase inhibitor include hot flashes, joint pain, weakness, fatigue, mood changes, depression, high blood pressure, swelling of the arms/legs, and headache. Aromatase inhibitors may also decrease bone mineral density, which may lead to osteoporosis and an increase in fractures in susceptible patients. Some individuals may also respond to the medication with gastrointestinal side effects including nausea and vomiting. Aromatase inhibitors can harm the development of an unborn fetus, and should never be taken or handled during pregnancy. When taken by men (as an off-label use) to reduce estrogenicity during prolonged periods of steroid treatment, aromatase inhibitors may increase cardiovascular disease (CVD) risk by retarding some beneficial properties of estrogen on cholesterol values. Studies have demonstrated that when an aromatizable steroid such as testosterone enanthate is taken in conjunction with an aromatase inhibitor, suppression of HDL (good) cholesterol levels become significantly more pronounced. Since the estrogen receptor agonist/antagonist Nolvadex® generally does not display the same anti-estrogenic (negative) effect on cholesterol values, it is usually favored over aromatase inhibitors for estrogen maintenance by male bodybuilders and athletes concerned with cardiovascular health.

Administration:

Anastrozole is FDA approved for adjunctive treatment of postmenopausal women with hormone receptor-positive early breast cancer, first-line treatment of postmenopausal women with hormone receptor-positive or receptor unknown locally advanced metastatic breast cancer, and treatment of advanced breast cancer in postmenopausal women with disease progression following tamoxifen therapy. The dosage prescribed in all instances is 1mg per day until disease progression has halted. When used to mitigate the estrogenic side effects of anabolic/androgenic steroid use, male athletes and bodybuilders will commonly take .5 mg to 1mg of anastrozole per day. In some instances a half of a tablet (.5 mg) taken every other day is sufficient to mitigate the buildup of estrogen. When used with readily aromatizing androgens such as methandrostenolone or testosterone, gynecomastia and water retention are often effectively blocked. Additionally, the use of anastrozole may decrease fat mass, which can also be tied to estrogen levels. The result can be a harder and much more defined appearance to the muscles and physique, which makes this agent of interest for dieting/cutting purposes as well.

It is of note that food does not appear to affect the absorption of anastrozole, so the drug may be taken with or between meals.

Availability:

Anastrozole is widely available in the U.S. and many other nations as a prescription drug product. It is also found readily on the black market.

Aromasin® (exemestane)

Description:

Exemestane is a steroidal suicide aromatase inhibitor. It is very similar in structure and action to formestane, although it is significantly more potent in comparison. As a class of drugs, aromatase inhibitors offer an anti-estrogenic effect by blocking the enzyme responsible for synthesizing estrogens. Exemestane is approved by the FDA for the treatment of breast cancer in women, specifically in postmenopausal patients whose cancer has progressed following therapy with tamoxifen. Male bodybuilders and athletes often use the drug for non-approved purposes, namely to counter the estrogenic side effects associated with the use of aromatizable anabolic/androgenic steroids. This may include gynecomastia, fat buildup, and water retention. In some instances aromatase inhibitors may also assist this group with the loss of body fat and increases in muscular definition. Exemestane is one of the most potent aromatase inhibitors presently available. The most commonly cited data (found in the Aromasin packaging insert) reports a lowering of serum estrogen levels by 85% on average in clinical studies with women.

History:

Exemestane was developed by Pharmacia & Upjohn (Pharmacia), which gained FDA approval for sale of the drug in late 1999. They introduced it under the Aromasin brand name in early 2000. Although the drug proved to be effective in doses as low as 2.5 mg per day in some patients, the company developed it in a standard and near universally effective dosage of 25 mg per tablet. The company has since introduced the drug to many other nations under the same trade name. Due to various patents and general market dominance, Aromasin is the only brand name of exemestane one is likely to come across in general commerce at the present time. It is currently available in over three dozen countries including Argentina, Australia, Austria, Belgium, Brazil, Canada, Czech Republic, Chile, Denmark, Finland, France, Germany, Greece, Hong Kong, Hungary, Ireland, Israel, Italy, Malaysia, Netherlands, Norway, New Zealand, Philippines, Poland, Portugal, Russia, South Africa, Singapore, Spain, Sweden, Switzerland, Thailand, Turkey, United Kingdom, United States, and Venezuela.

How Supplied:

Exemestane is most commonly supplied in tablets of 25 mg.

Structural Characteristics:

Exemestane is classified as an irreversible steroidal aromatase inhibitor. It has the chemical designation 6-methyl-enandrosta-1,4-diene-3,17-dione.

Side Effects:

Common side effects associated with the use of an aromatase inhibitor include hot flashes, joint pain, weakness, fatigue, mood changes, depression, high blood pressure, swelling of the arms/legs, and headache. Aromatase inhibitors may also decrease bone mineral density, which may lead to osteoporosis and an increase in fractures in susceptible patients. Some individuals may also respond to the medication with gastrointestinal side effects including nausea and vomiting. Aromatase inhibitors can harm the development of an unborn fetus, and should never be taken or handled during pregnancy. When taken by men (as an off-label use) to reduce estrogenicity during prolonged periods of steroid treatment, aromatase inhibitors may increase cardiovascular disease (CVD) risk by retarding some beneficial properties of estrogen on cholesterol values. Studies have demonstrated that when an aromatizable steroid such as testosterone enanthate is taken in conjunction with an aromatase inhibitor, suppression of HDL (good) cholesterol levels become significantly more pronounced. Since the estrogen receptor agonist/antagonist Nolvadex® generally does not display the same anti-estrogenic (negative) effect on cholesterol values, it is usually favored over aromatase inhibitors for estrogen maintenance by male bodybuilders and athletes concerned with cardiovascular health.

Administration:

Exemestane is FDA approved for adjunctive treatment of postmenopausal women with estrogen- receptor positive early breast cancer with disease progression following tamoxifen. Therapy is initiated 2-3 years after tamoxifen has failed to elicit a desirable response, at which point tamoxifen is discontinued. Treatment with exemestane is continued for 2-3 additional years, and is completed after 5 years of cumulative adjunctive drug therapy (tamoxifen and exemestane treatment combined). The dosage prescribed in all instances is one 25 mg tablet per day, taken after a meal. When used to mitigate the estrogenic side effects of anabolic/androgenic steroid use or increase muscle definition, male athletes and bodybuilders will commonly take 12.5 mg to 25 mg of exemestane per day. In some instances a half of a tablet (12.5 mg) taken every other day is sufficient to prevent the onset of estrogenic side effects.

Availability:

Exemestane is available in the U.S and in more than three dozen other nations under the Aromasin brand name (Pharmacia). Aromasin, likewise, dominates the global market, and is presently the only exemestane product one is likely to encounter.

Clomid® (clomiphene citrate)

Description:

Clomiphene citrate is an anti-estrogenic drug that is prescribed to women to treat anovulatory infertility (inability to ovulate). In clinical medicine it is specifically referred to as a nonsteroidal ovulatory stimulant. The drug works by interacting with estrogen receptors, often in an antagonistic manner, in various tissues of the body including the hypothalamus, pituitary, ovary, endometrium, vagina, and cervix. One main focus is that the drug will oppose the negative feedback of estrogens on the hypothalamic-pituitary-ovarian axis, enhancing the release of gonadotropins (LH and FSH). This surge in gonadotropins may cause egg release (follicular rupture), ideally leading to conception. Clomiphene citrate is chemically a synthetic estrogen with both agonist/antagonist properties, and in this regard is very similar in structure and action to Nolvadex®. It is believed that both the estrogenic and anti-estrogenic properties of clomiphene citrate play a role in its ability to support female fertility.

In men, clomiphene citrate also acts as a partial anti-estrogen, and may be used to counter some of the side effects of aromatizable steroid use including gynecomastia and increased water retention. As an anti-estrogenic drug, clomiphene citrate may also produce an elevation of follicle stimulating hormone, and luteinizing hormone levels, which can elevate testosterone production. This effect is especially beneficial at the conclusion of a steroid cycle, when endogenous testosterone levels are depressed. Here, clomiphene citrate is most often applied in combination with HCG and tamoxifen, in an effort to restore endogenous testosterone production more quickly (see PCT: Post-Cycle Therapy). If testosterone levels are not brought back to normal in a short period of time, a significant loss in size and strength may occur. This is due to the fact that without testosterone (or other anabolic/androgenic steroids) to impart an ongoing anabolic message, the catabolic hormone cortisol becomes the dominant force affecting muscle protein synthesis. Often referred to as the post-steroid crash, when not corrected this state of imbalance in the endocrine system can quickly reduce muscle mass levels, diminishing the long-term return on anabolic/androgenic steroid therapy.

Note that the triphenylethylene compounds (toremifene citrate, tamoxifen citrate, clomiphene citrate) tend to be somewhat intrinsically estrogenic in the liver. This means that while they can block estrogenic activity in some areas of the body, they can actually act as estrogens in this other key area. Estrogenic action in the liver is important in the regulation of serum cholesterol (it tends to support HDL synthesis and LDL reductions). Since steroid-using bodybuilders are already dealing with the negative cardiovascular effects of these drugs, compounding the issue with aromatase inhibitors (which will lower total serum estrogen levels) may not always be the best option. Using a drug that blocks gynecomastia, for example, while at the same time supporting improved cholesterol values, might be much more ideal.

History:

Clomiphene citrate is a fertility drug with a substantial history of use in the United States. It first gained widespread acceptance during the early 1970s, and has been a drug common to the fertility practice ever since. The drug is now considered a standard medication for certain forms of fertility therapy, and has been adopted as such far outside U.S. border. Clomiphene citrate is presently available in most nations worldwide. The two most popular brand names one is likely to encounter are Clomid and Serofene, although the drug can be found under numerous other trade names as well including (but not limited to) Sepafar, Omifin, Pergotime, Gonaphene, Duinum, Clostil, Ova-Mit, and Clostibegyt. Clomiphene citrate is generally a very inexpensive medication compared to stronger anti-estrogens such as the newer selective third-generation aromatase inhibitors. It, likewise, remains a very popular agent of use among bodybuilders and athletes.

How Supplied:

Clomiphene citrate is most commonly supplied in tablets of 50 mg.

Structural Characteristics:

Clomiphene citrate is classified as a selective estrogen receptor modulator, with both agonist and antagonist properties. It has the chemical designation 2-[4-(2-chloro-1,2-diphenylvinyl)phenoxy]triethylamine dihydrogen citrate.

Warnings (Visual Symptoms):

Some patients using clomiphene citrate notice blurring or other visual disturbances such as spots or flashes. These symptoms occur more frequently at higher doses or longer durations of therapy, and often disappear within a few days or weeks of use. Prolonged visual disturbances have been reported after the discontinuation of clomiphene citrate therapy, however, and in some cases may be irreversible. Those taking clomiphene citrate should be warned that these symptoms might make activities like driving a car or operating heavy machinery more hazardous than usual. While the exact cause of these visual symptoms is not yet understood, it is advisable to discontinue treatment and have a thorough medical/opthalmological examination should they occur.

Side Effects:

Clomiphene citrate appears to be well tolerated, with a low incidence of significant side effects. Common adverse reactions during clinical trails included ovarian enlargement (13.6%), vasomotor flushes (10.4%), abdominal discomfort (5.5%), nausea/vomiting (2.2%), breast discomfort (2.1%), visual symptoms (1.5%), headache (1.3%), and abnormal uterine bleeding (1.3%). Data also suggests that the prolonged use of clomiphene citrate may increase the chance of ovarian tumor. Clomiphene citrate is occasionally associated with a serious and potentially life threatening side effect called ovarian hyperstimulation syndrome (OHSS). Early warning signs of OHSS include abdominal pain and distention, nausea, diarrhea, and weight gain.

Administration:

Clomiphene citrate is FDA approved for the treatment of women with ovulatory dysfunction preventing pregnancy. The recommended dosage is 50 mg daily for 5 days, which is initiated approximately 5 days into the menstrual cycle. If ovulation does not occur, follow up cycles may use a dosage of 100 mg per day for 5 days. Many clinicians recommend a limit of 6 courses of therapy. When used by men (off-label) to mitigate the estrogenic side effects of anabolic/androgenic steroid use, a daily dosage of 50-100 mg (1-2 tablets) is usually administered while any offending steroids are taken. Note, however, that tamoxifen is usually given preference over clomiphene citrate for this purpose. More commonly, clomiphene citrate is used by men at a dosage of 50-100 mg per day for 30 days at the conclusion of a steroid cycle, in an effort to bring natural testosterone production back to normal levels. Here, it is usually deemed most appropriate to use as part of a multi-component post-cycle recovery program (see PCT: Post-Cycle Therapy). Female athletes occasionally use clomiphene citrate for the reduction of estrogenicity near the time of a bodybuilding contest. In some instances this may aid in increasing fat loss and muscularity, particularly in female trouble areas such as the hips and thighs. The drug, however, often produces very troubling side effects in pre-menopausal women, and is likewise not in very high demand among this group.

Availability:

Clomiphene citrate is widely available on the international market in a variety of brand names. It generally sells for a reasonable price, and is of low interest to counterfeiters.

Cytadren® (aminoglutethimide)

Description:

Aminoglutethimide is mainly identified as an inhibitor of adrenocortical steroid synthesis. Its primary function is to block the conversion of cholesterol to pregnenolone, which is required for the biosynthesis of adrenal glucocorticoids, mineralocorticoids, estrogens, and androgens. Aminoglutethimide is a nonspecific inhibitor, and also blocks several other steps in steroid synthesis including hydroxylation at C-11, C-18, and C-21, and the aromatization of androgens to estrogens. The drug may be used clinically to treat estrogen dependent breast cancer, and to treat Cushing's syndrome, which is a condition where the body overproduces the hormone cortisol. The effect that aminogluthethimide can have on cortisol and estrogen production is what makes this a drug of interest to athletes and bodybuilders.

Cortisol Inhibition: While cortisol is an essential hormone for life, its levels may also vary greatly within "normal" ranges depending on the individual, their training and dietary status, and many other personal metabolic factors. It has been a common pursuit in the sports community to find ways to control (limit) cortisol production. This is because while androgens give your muscle cells a message to increase protein synthesis, cortisol (a catabolic hormone) imparts a message to breakdown and release amino acids. If one can limit this catabolic message, net protein synthesis should, in theory, be increased. Aminoglutethimide has been used by a number of athletes and bodybuilders for this purpose, usually in combination with anabolic/androgenic steroids because it has a low level of androgen inhibition. Together with even a relatively small dose, it was thought one could shift the ratio of anabolic to catabolic hormones in favor of the former, the goal being new muscle growth. The results for this use have been mixed.

When first looked at in the realm of athletics, however, research was bare as to the best way to use aminoglutethimide as a cortisol lowering anti-catabolic. Dubbed the "adrenal escape phenomenon", it has been noted that after a short period of regular use your body often reacts to lowered cortisol levels by increasing the release of another hormone, ACTH (adrenocorticotropic hormone). Increased ACTH could overcome the activity of aminoglutethimide, resulting in your body resuming its original levels of cortisol production (negating the benefits of cortisol inhibition)[829]. A moderate amount of hydrocortisone (20-30 mg daily) is given to patients when this occurs. This can keep glucocorticoid activity from completely diminishing, preventing the ACTH response and allowing the drug to retain its effect. For athletes, however, supplementing glucocorticoids would probably be counterproductive given the desired goal. A 2-day-on 2-day-off regime of administration was, therefore, implemented as a way to delay or even avoid the adrenal escape phenomenon. This strategy is based on theory and experimentation, however, and no clinical studies have evaluated aminiglutethimide as an anti-catabolic agent.

It is important to note that while many people believe they have used this drug as an anti-catabolic, few have actually taken the correct dosage. Four tablets per day, or 1,000 mg, appears necessary to significantly inhibit the demolase enzyme (the enzyme responsible for converting cholesterol to pregnenolone, and the target when reduced cortisol is desired). Those who do venture this high commonly report fatigue and discomfort, stating that the drug is intolerable for any type of prolonged use. Today, many athletes and bodybuilders are accepting that the original proposed use of aminogluthethimide as a non-steroidal muscle-building agent does not seem to be a plausible one. The only instances this author has really heard of this drug ever being used at such doses consistently with any type of positive response were competitive bodybuilders partaking in high-dosed Cytadren shortly before a contest. They claimed the short-term rise in androgen to corticosteroid ratio greatly aided their abilities to bring out a show-ready hard and dense physique, and credit the drug as genuinely being a very effective pre-contest agent. In speaking with the late Paul Borresen he summed up the pre-contest use of Cytadren by stating, *"I have had considerable experience with the high dose use. It makes athletes sleepy and weak. It seems to help the last ten days before a show, and this is tried and tested."*

Aromatase Inhibition: Aminoglutethimide is an efficient aromatase inhibitor, and tends to inhibit the activity of this enzyme at a much lower dosage from that what is required for inhibition of corticosteroid production.[830][831] While a daily dosage of 1000 mg is typically needed to inhibit cortisol, maximum suppression of aromatase and estrogen levels is typically achieved at a dosage between 250 mg and 500 mg, a point where strong adrenal steroid blockage is not noted. There also seems to be no added benefit by adding cortisol in terms of survival/response rate among breast cancer patients, pointing to the fact that the "adrenal escape phenomenon" bears little relation to its abilities as an aromatase inhibitor. Ultimately, it appears that not only do we need a higher dose (1,000 mg or 4 tablets per day minimum) to really inhibit cortisol production, but also that there is no need for an athlete to implement a rotating dose schedule if the drug is being used as an anti-estrogen.

Aminoglutethimide is usually regarded highly among athletes and bodybuilders as an estrogen maintenance agent. Studies have shown it to be capable of decreasing aromatase activity by as much as 92% after administration of 250 mg per day. Patient response rates also show aminoglutethimide to be at least as effective as tamoxifen therapy in treating estrogen dependent cancer cells, and more effective under certain conditions. Due to its discussed broad range of non-specific activity, however, including the potential inhibition of not only estrogens, but corticosteroids, aldosterone, and androgens as well, it is not regarded as highly as newer (second and third generation) aromatase inhibitors in terms of patient comfort and efficacy, and is not widely used for this purpose today. Athletes, however, still tend to consider it to be an effective remedy for estrogenic side effects like gynecomastia, increased water retention, and fat gain.

History:

Aminoglutethimide was FDA approved as an anticonvulsant drug in 1960. Side effects were common with treatment, however, including drowsiness, dizziness, and partial loss of motor control. In 1966 reports of adrenal insufficiency subsequent to aminoglutethimide use were reported. The drug was withdrawn from the U.S. market as an anticonvulsant that same year due to its recently understood effects on the adrenal gland. By 1967, however, the drug was reintroduced for a new purpose, namely inhibition of aromatase activity and the treatment of breast cancer. It was one of the first aromatase inhibitors sold, and is identified alongside testolactone as a "first-generation" agent of this type. Given its novel effects on adrenal steroid production, the U.S. FDA also granted approval for the use of aminoglutethimide for the treatment of Cushing's syndrome.

At one time aminoglutethimide was available under numerous brand names and in more than 2-dozen countries. Ciba's Cytadren and Orimeten preparations were by far the most common, and could be found in such nations as Argentina, Australia, Austria, Brazil, Canada, Chile, Czech Republic, France, Germany, Hong Kong, Ireland, Israel, Italy, Malaysia, Netherlands, Norway, New Zealand, Russia, South Africa, Spain, Sweden, Switzerland, United Kingdom, and the United States. Additionally, the drug could be found on occasion under other names including Aminoblastin, Rodazol, and Mamomit. The vast majority of original aminoglutethimide preparations have since been discontinued, however. Today, the drug remains available in a very small number of countries, most notably the United States (Cytadren), Russia (Mamomit), Hong Kong (Orimetene), and Australia (Cytadren).

How Supplied:

Aminoglutethimide is most commonly supplied in tablets of 250 mg.

Structural Characteristics:

Aminoglutethimide is an analog of glutethimide. It has the chemical designation 2-(4-Aminophenyl)-2-ethylglutarimide;3-(4-Aminophenyl)-3-ethylpiperidine-2,6-dione.

Side Effects:

Frequent side effects associated with aminoglutethimide include fatigue, dizziness, skin rashes, fever, and nausea. Other side effects may include sleep disorder, apathy, depression, vomiting, stomach upset, thyroid dysfunction, virilization, jaundice, elevated cholesterol levels, changes in blood cell counts, and high blood pressure. Additionally, those bodybuilders and athletes taking it at a dosage high enough to promote cortisol suppression often note that reduced levels of this hormone bring about more aches and pains in the joints when trying to lift heavy weights. It seems logical that this might lead to an increased susceptibility to injury. Users should be careful not to overexert themselves during the short periods in which this drug is used in high doses. Most of the listed side effects listed here are most common with higher dosed regimens that inhibit the adrenal production of cortisol, and are less common with athletes taking one or two tablets per day as an anti-estrogen. Even in low doses aminoglutethimide may cause birth defects, and should never be taken during pregnancy.

Administration:

Aminoglutethimide is medically indicated for the treatment of Cushing's syndrome, metastatic breast cancer in postmenopausal women, and palliative treatment in men with advanced prostate cancer. When used to treat Cushings syndrome, the dosage used may range from 1,000 mg to 2,000 mg per day, often in conjunction with 20-30 mg of hydrocortisone to avoid the aforementioned adrenal escape phenomenon. Athletes and bodybuilders using aminoglutethimide for cortisol inhibition will commonly take a dosage of 1,000 mg per day, usually for brief periods of 2-3 weeks or less (10 days of use pre-contest is reported with some bodybuilders). A schedule of 2-days on, 2-days off may be used in an attempt to extend the effectiveness of aminoglutethimide for longer periods, but such use is usually discarded in place of daily short-term administration. The dosage most commonly used for mitigating the estrogenic side effects of anabolic/androgenic steroid use ranges from 125 mg to 500 mg per day (1/2 to 2 tablets), with 1 tablet (250 mg) per day appearing to be the most common dosage selected.

Availability:

Aminoglutethimide is produced in a small number of countries, and is a fairly expensive pharmaceutical. As such, it may sell for as much as $2 per tablet on the black market. This, combined with limited availability, has severely limited its more widespread use.

Evista (raloxifene hydrochloride)

Description:

Raloxifene hydrochloride is a second-generation Selective Estrogen Receptor Modulator (SERM) of the benzothiophene family. This drug is similar in effect to tamoxifen, exhibiting estrogen receptor antagonist (blocking) properties in some tissues while acting as an estrogen receptor agonist (activator) in others. The main point of variation between these two agents is their tissue selectivity. While raloxifene hydrochloride is a strong anti-estrogen in breast and uterine tissues, it appears to be estrogenic in bone. This allows it to protect bone density, mimicking the beneficial effects of endogenous estradiol. This is quite different from tamoxifen, which is anti-estrogenic in both breast and bone. In a role that was novel for an anti-estrogen, raloxifene hydrochloride was approved by the FDA for the prevention and treatment of osteoporosis in post-menopausal women. It is also being investigated for several other potential uses, including the treatment and prevention of cardiovascular disease, breast cancer, gynecomastia, prostate cancer, acromegaly, and uterine cancer.

As an anti-estrogen, athletes and bodybuilders may use this compound to combat the estrogenic side effects caused by aromatizable or estrogenic steroids. The principle among these side effects is gynecomastia, a purpose for which raloxifene hydrochloride seems better suited than tamoxifen. This was demonstrated in a July 2004 study in the *Journal of Pediatrics*, which looked at how these two agents compared in the treatment of persistent pubertal gynecomastia.[832] The investigation involved a group of 38 patients, averaging 15 years of age and suffering from gynecomastia for a little over 2 years. Treatment for 3 to 9 months with either agent had a high success rate for seeing "some improvement" (91% for raloxifene and 86% for Nolvadex). However, a significant reduction of gynecomastia was seen in more than twice as many patients with raloxifene hydrochloride (86% compared to 41%). Given its relative potency, raloxifene hydrochloride may offer an alternative to surgery for some cases of gynecomastia.

Typical of an anti-estrogen, raloxifene hydrochloride should also offer some benefit as a testosterone-stimulating compound. We see this effect demonstrated in studies on a group of older men (aged 60-70 years), where daily doses of 120 mg were able to increase serum and bioavailable (unbound) testosterone by 20%.[833] Though these figures are not dramatic, they do demonstrate an anti-estrogenic effect instead of an estrogenic (negative) one when it comes to testosterone production. This drug may, therefore, be of some value when utilized as an adjunct to HCG injections during a post-cycle testosterone recovery program. This same study above also showed raloxifene hydrochloride to have at least a partial estrogenic effect on serum lipids, exhibiting a trend toward decreases in all cholesterol values (total, LDL, and HDL). It is difficult to discern if there are any real benefits to male bodybuilders when it comes to using raloxifene hydrochloride to counteract the negative cardiovascular side effects of steroid use. As discussed in its respective profile, this may be a notable benefit with the use of Nolvadex, a first-generation SERM agent shown to improve HDL (good) cholesterol levels in many patients.

There are some negatives to inhibiting the actions of estrogen that should be addressed. For one, estrogen is a beneficial hormone when it comes to IGF-1 levels. In studies with acromegaly patients that suffer from GH hypersecretion, 60 mg of raloxifene hydrochloride twice daily was able to reliably suppress IGF-1 levels by an average of 16%.[834] Estrogen is also understood to exert positive anabolic effects in regards to increasing androgen receptor concentrations in certain tissues, and enhancing enzymes involved in the utilization of glucose for tissue growth and repair. This is further support for the belief that anti-estrogens should not be used unless there is a defined reason for doing so. When used for simple side-effect prevention (without visible side effects occurring), the drug may inadvertently lessen the total anabolic potency of steroid therapy.

History:

Raloxifene hydrochloride was developed by Eli Lilly & Company, and FDA approved for U.S. sale in 1997. Its first indicated use was as that of an osteoporosis treatment, owing to its ability to increase bone density. In 2007, the FDA expanded the indicated uses for the drug to include reducing the risk of invasive breast cancer in two populations: postmenopausal women with osteoporosis and postmenopausal women at high risk for invasive breast cancer. Today, raloxifene hydrochloride is a fairly popular drug in clinical medicine, and is approved for sale in over 50 countries. The Evista brand from Eli Lilly & Company dominates the global market, although a small number of other brands can be found including Ketidin, Oseofem, and Raxeto (Argentina), Bonmax, Estroact, and Ralista (India), and Optruma (Spain, France, Italy).

How Supplied:

Raloxifene hydrochloride is most commonly supplied in tablets of 60 mg.

Structural Characteristics:

Raloxifene hydrochloride is classified a selective estrogen receptor modulator, with both agonist and antagonist properties. It has the chemical designation 6-Hydroxy-2-(p-hydroxyphenyl)benzo[b]thien-3-yl-p-(2-piperidinoethoxy)phenyl ketone hydrochloride.

Warnings (Stroke):

The FDA mandates that the following warning be present on the prescribing information for Evista (raloxifene hydrochloride): "WARNING: INCREASED RISK OF VENOUS THROMBOEMBOLISM AND DEATH FROM STROKE. Increased risk of deep vein thrombosis and pulmonary embolism have been reported with Evista. Women with active or past history of venous thromboembolism should not take Evista. Increased risk of death due to stroke occurred in a trial in postmenopausal women with documented coronary heart disease or at increased risk for major coronary events. Consider risk-benefit balance in women at risk for stroke."

Side Effects:

Common side effects associated with the use of raloxifene hydrochloride include hot flashes/flushing, headache, malaise, weakness, cramping, edema, sweating, depression, weight gain, and gastrointestinal disturbances such as nausea, vomiting, indigestion, and diarrhea. Less common side effects include breast pain, vaginal bleeding, thrombophlebitis (inflammation of vein associated with blood clot), and visual disturbances. In rare cases raloxifene hydrochloride use has been associated with stroke, narrowing of the arteries (transient ischaemic attack), pulmonary embolus, deep-vein thrombosis, low white blood cell or platelet count, upper gastrointestinal hemorrhage, or ulcer. Antiestrogens may harm the developing fetus, and should never be used during pregnancy.

Administration:

Raloxifene hydrochloride is FDA approved for the treatment and prevention of osteoporosis in postmenopausal women, reducing the risk of invasive breast cancer in postmenopausal women with osteoporosis, and reducing the risk of invasive breast cancer in postmenopausal women at high risk for invasive breast cancer. The recommended dose is one 60 mg tablet administered once per day, without regard to meals. When used (off-label) to mitigate the estrogenic side effects of anabolic/androgenic steroid use, male athletes and bodybuilders often take 30 mg to 60 mg per day.

Availability:

Raloxifene hydrochloride is available in over 50 countries. Aside from a small number of other brands, the Evista product from Eli Lilly & Company is most likely to be encountered. Price is often a concern, as raloxifene hydrochloride is considerably more expensive than some of the anti-estrogens bodybuilders and athletes are already accustomed to such as Nolvadex and Clomid. The price per individual daily dose of raloxifene hydrochloride (1 tablet) can exceed $2. That would add up to $200 or more per 100 doses. A hundred tablets of generic tamoxifen (20 mg) often sell for approximately $50. This is about 50 cents per dose, or 1/4th the price of raloxifene hydrochloride. Thus far, price, not availability, seem to be preventing the more widespread diversion of raloxifene hydrochloride for black market sale.

Fareston® (toremifene citrate)

Description:

Toremifene citrate is an anti-estrogenic drug, specifically classified as a Selective Estrogen-Receptor Modulator (SERM) with mixed agonist and antagonist properties. It is a non-steroidal triphenylethylene derivative, similar in structure and action to both Nolvadex (tamoxifen citrate) and Clomid (clomiphene citrate). Toremifene citrate is used for the treatment of breast cancer in postmenopausal women with estrogen-receptor positive or estrogen-receptor unknown (unsure if the cancer is estrogen responsive) tumors. It works by attaching to the estrogen receptor in various tissues in a competitive manner, blocking endogenous estrogen from exerting biological activity. As an anti-estrogen in many tissues, male bodybuilders and athletes may use toremifene citrate to counter some of the side effects associated with the use of aromatizable or estrogenic anabolic/androgenic steroids. This may include gynecomastia, body fat gain, and increased water retention.

The triphenylethylene compounds (toremifene citrate, tamoxifen citrate, clomiphene citrate) tend to be somewhat intrinsically estrogenic in the liver. This means that while they can block estrogenic activity in some areas of the body, they can actually act as estrogens in this other key area. Estrogenic action in the liver is important in the regulation of serum cholesterol (it tends to support HDL synthesis and LDL reductions). Since steroid-using bodybuilders are already dealing with the negative cardiovascular effects of these drugs, compounding the issue with aromatase inhibitors (which will lower total serum estrogen levels) may not always be the best option. Using a drug that blocks gynecomastia, for example, while at the same time supporting improved cholesterol values, might be much more ideal. In terms of which triphenylethylene agent is most effective in this regard, evidence suggests that the positive lipid altering benefits of toremifene are significantly stronger than those of tamoxifen, a drug normally favored for this purpose. Toremifene citrate may, therefore, be the preferred anti-estrogen among those concerned about their lipid profiles.

History:

Toremifene citrate was approved by the FDA as a prescription drug in 1997. It is sold in the U.S. under the Fareston brand name, which is made by GTx, Inc. Fareston is also available in over two dozen other countries including Australia, Austria, Belgium, Czech Republic, Finland, France, Germany, Greece, Hungary, Ireland, Italy, Mexico, Netherlands, New Zealand, Portugal, Russia, South Africa, Spain, Sweden, Switzerland, Thailand, Turkey, and the United Kingdom.

How Supplied:

Toremifene citrate is most commonly supplied in tablets of 88.4mg, which are labeled as (and equate to) 60 mg of toremifene base.

Structural Characteristics:

Toremifene citrate is classified as a selective estrogen receptor modulator, with both agonist and antagonist properties. It has the chemical designation 2-{p-[(Z)-4-chloro-1,2-diphenyl-1-butenyl]phenoxy}-N,N-dimethylethylamine citrate (1:1).

Side Effects:

Toremifene citrate appears to be well tolerated, with a low incidence of serious side effects. In clinical trials, common side effects associated with its use included hot flashes (35%), sweating (20%), elevated liver enzymes (19%), nausea (14%), vaginal discharge (13%), dizziness (95%), edema (5%), vomiting (4%), and vaginal bleeding (2%). Other observed rare adverse events that may or may not be linked to toremifene citrate administration include low white blood cell and platelet counts, skin discoloration or dermatitis, constipation, difficulty breathing, partial motor paralysis, tremor, vertigo, itching, anorexia, visual disturbances, loss of strength, hair loss, depression, jaundice, and rigors (stiffening of the muscles). Antiestrogens may harm the developing fetus and should never be used during pregnancy.

Administration:

Toremifene citrate is FDA approved for the treatment of metastatic breast cancer in postmenopausal women with estrogen-receptor positive or unknown tumors. The recommended dose is one 60 mg tablet administered once per day. When used (off-label) to mitigate the estrogenic side effects of anabolic/androgenic steroid use, male athletes and bodybuilders may use 30 mg to 60 mg per day during steroid treatment.

Availability:

Toremifene citrate is widely available under the Fareston brand name. It is not commonly sold on the black market, nor is it a high profile item for counterfeiters.

Faslodex® (fulvestrant)

Description

Fulvestrant is a highly selective estrogen receptor antagonist (also classified as an estrogen receptor downregulator). It exerts its action in the body not by targeting the production of estrogen, but by preventing it from exerting activity in the body. It does this by binding available estrogen receptors in a competitive manner, making them unavailable for circulating estrogens. This mode of action is very similar to Nolvadex (tamoxifen citrate) and Clomid (clomiphene citrate), although unlike these two agents fulvestrant does not have mixed agonist/antagonist properties. It is a pure estrogen receptor antagonist. This agent also stands out as the first injectable estrogen antagonist to catch the attention of the athletic/bodybuilding world. Although not widely used here, when applied it may be an effective drug for mitigating the side effects of excess estrogen caused by anabolic/androgenic steroid use such as gynecomastia, fat buildup, and increased water retention.

Fulvestrant is very potent as an anti-estrogen, significantly more so than earlier medications like Nolvadex and Clomid. Although it targets estrogen at its receptor and not its production, it can still produce an environment of low estrogenicity on par with strong aromatase inhibition. One study, for example, shows fulvestrant to be as effective in Arimidex in treating breast cancer patients who have already failed with first line endocrine treatments.[835] Another shows the drug prevents tumor cell turnover and growth significantly more effectively than tamoxifen citrate.[836] Studies investigating the physiological response to fulvestrant note that the drug actually downregulates estrogen receptor concentrations. Furthermore, it also tends to downregulate progesterone receptor concentrations.[837] Fulvestrant does not cross the blood brain barrier, and for this reason is believed to produce fewer neurological side effects related to estrogen antagonism such as hot flashes, mood alterations, and low energy.

History:

Fulvestrant was developed by AstraZeneca. It was approved as a prescription drug in the U.S. in 2002, and is sold under the Faslodex brand name. The drug is indicated for the treatment of estrogen receptor positive breast cancer with disease progression following traditional anti-estrogen therapy (such as tamoxifen). AstraZeneca has since expanded the market for Faslodex to include over one dozen countries, including Argentina, Belgium, Brazil, Denmark, Finland, France, Germany, Greece, Ireland, Israel, Italy, Netherlands, Norway, Poland, Portugal, Spain, Sweden, Switzerland, United Kingdom, and Venezuela.

How supplied:

Faslodex (fulvestrant) is supplied in pre-filled syringes containing 50-mg/mL fulvestrant, either as a single 5 mL or two 2.5 mL injections. The product must be refrigerated for storage.

Structural Characteristics:

Fulvestrant is an estrogen receptor antagonist. It has the chemical designation 7-alpha-[9-(4,4,5,5,5-penta fluoropentylsulphinyl)nonyl]estra-1,3,5-(10)- triene-3,17-beta-diol.

Side Effects:

The most common side effects associated with fulvestrant include gastrointestinal disturbances such as nausea, vomiting, constipation, abdominal pain, and diarrhea. Other common adverse effects include headache, back pain, hot flashes, and sore throat. Less common side effects include rash, loss of strength, urinary-tract infections, venous thromboembolism, liver enzyme elevations, vaginal bleeding, muscle pain, and low white blood cell count. Injection side reactions may also occur. Anti-estrogens can harm the development of an unborn fetus, and should never be taken during pregnancy. When taken by men (as an off-label use) to reduce estrogenicity during prolonged periods of steroid treatment, a pure estrogen antagonist may increase cardiovascular disease (CVD) risk by retarding some beneficial properties of estrogen on cholesterol values. This may include a suppression of HDL (good) cholesterol values greater than that induced by steroid therapy alone.

Administration:

Fulvestrant is FDA approved for the treatment of hormone receptor positive metastatic breast cancer in postmenopausal women with disease progression following anti-estrogen therapy. The recommended dose is 250 mg administered intramuscularly (buttock) per month, as either a single 5 mL injection or two 2.5 mL injections. When used (off-label) to mitigate the estrogenic side effects of anabolic/androgenic steroid use, male athletes and bodybuilders may find a similar dose to be beneficial.

Availability:

Fulvestrant is available in more than one dozen countries. At the present time, all fulvestrant in circulation is likely to be of the Faslodex brand name. The drug itself is exceedingly expensive, and as a result is not widely traded on the black market.

Femara® (letrozole)

Description:

Letrozole is a non-steroidal selective third generation aromatase inhibitor. The structure and activity of this compound are very similar to that of Arimidex (anastrozole), and it is prescribed for similar medical purposes. More specifically, U.S. prescribing guidelines for letrozole recommend it be used for the treatment of postmenopausal women with estrogen receptor-positive or estrogen receptor-unknown (unsure if the cancer is responsive to estrogen) breast cancer. It is typically used as a second line of treatment after an estrogen-receptor antagonist like tamoxifen has failed to elicit a desirable response, although it is sometimes initiated as the first course of therapy depending on the circumstances. Male bodybuilders and athletes find value in letrozole for its ability to mitigate the estrogenic side effects associated with the use of aromatizable anabolic/androgenic steroids, such as gynecomastia, fat buildup, and visible water retention.

Letrozole represents one of the newer achievements in a long line of drugs targeting aromatase inhibition. It is among the most potent estrogen-lowering drugs developed to date, and has an effect significantly stronger than non-selective first generation aromatase inhibitors like Teslac and Cytadren. The dosage of each tablet of Femara is 2.5 milligrams, which according to product information was sufficient to lower estrogen levels by an average of 78% during clinical trails. The drug, however, appears to often remain quite effective in lower doses. The package insert for the product itself comments that during clinical studies doses as low as .1 and .5 milligrams produced 75 and 78% estrogen inhibition, respectively in many patients. The recommended dose, likewise, reflects a level that seems to elicit a desired level of inhibition in nearly all patients. A large number of people may, therefore, respond well to lower doses of the drug.

History:

The U.S. Food & Drug Administration approved letrozole for prescription sale in 1997, where it is sold by Novartis under the Femara trade name. Novartis also extensively markets the drug in other nations, and more than 70 nations now carry letrozole as an approved drug. The Femara brand is by far the dominant preparation worldwide, and is found in such nations as Argentina, Australia, Belgium, Brazil, Canada, Chile, Czech Republic, France, Germany, Greece, Hong Kong, India, Netherlands, New Zealand, Italy, South Africa, Switzerland, and Russia. Novartis also markets the drug under the Femar trade name in some other nations including Finland, Denmark, Norway, and Sweden. Additionally, letrozole products can also be found under such other brand names as Fempro (India), Oncolet (India), Trozet (India), Insegar (Spain), Aromek (Poland), Lametta (Poland), Cendalon (Argentina), Fecinole (Argentina), and Kebirzol (Argentina). Given its high level of efficacy and strong marketing support, Femara, and Femar, remain the most popular letrozole product currently available.

How Supplied:

Letrozole is most commonly supplied in tablets of 2.5 mg.

Structural Characteristics:

Letrozole is classified as a non-steroidal selective third generation aromatase inhibitor. It has the chemical designation 4,4'(1H-1,2,4-Triazol-1-ylmethylene)dibenzonitrile.

Side Effects:

Common side effects associated with the use of an aromatase inhibitor include hot flashes, joint pain, weakness, fatigue, mood changes, depression, high blood pressure, swelling of the arms/legs, and headache. Aromatase inhibitors may also decrease bone mineral density, which may lead to osteoporosis and an increase in fractures in susceptible patients. Some individuals may also respond to the medication with gastrointestinal side effects including nausea and vomiting. Aromatase inhibitors can harm the development of an unborn fetus, and should never be taken or handled during pregnancy. When taken by men (as an off-label use) to reduce estrogenicity during prolonged periods of steroid treatment, aromatase inhibitors may increase cardiovascular disease (CVD) risk by retarding some beneficial properties of estrogen on cholesterol values. Studies have demonstrated that when an aromatizable steroid such as testosterone enanthate is taken in conjunction with an aromatase inhibitor, suppression of HDL (good) cholesterol levels become significantly more pronounced. Since the estrogen receptor agonist/antagonist Nolvadex® generally does not display the same anti-estrogenic (negative) effect on cholesterol values, it is usually favored over aromatase inhibitors for estrogen maintenance by male bodybuilders and athletes concerned with cardiovascular health.

Administration:

Letrozole is FDA approved for 1) adjuvant treatment of postmenopausal women with hormone receptor positive early breast cancer; 2) the extended adjuvant treatment of early breast cancer in postmenopausal women who have received 5 years of adjuvant tamoxifen therapy; 3) first-line treatment of postmenopausal women with hormone receptor positive or hormone receptor unknown locally advanced or metastatic breast cancer; and 4) the treatment of advanced breast cancer in postmenopausal women with disease progression following anti-estrogen therapy. The recommended dose of letrozole is one 2.5 mg tablet administered once per day, without regard to meals. When used (off-label) to mitigate the estrogenic side effects of anabolic/androgenic steroid use or increase muscle definition, male athletes and bodybuilders often take 1.25 mg to 2.5 mg per day. In some cases a dosage of a half of a tablet (1.25 mg) taken every other day is sufficient to prevent the onset of estrogenic side effects.

Availability:

Letrozole is most commonly sold under the brand name Femara by the international drug-manufacturing firm Novartis. It is widely available at the present time.

Fertodur® (cyclofenil)

Description:

Cyclofenil is a non-steroidal anti-estrogen that is used in the treatment of menstrual disturbances and anovualtory infertility (an inability to ovulate). It is very similar in structure to Clomid® and Nolvadex®, and also works in the body as a mixed estrogen agonist/antagonist. This drug is commonly used for off-label purposes by male bodybuilders and athletes, typically at the conclusion of a steroid cycle for the purpose of increasing endogenous testosterone levels. This is in an attempt to minimize the negative impact that a period of low androgen levels may have on the physique, which can include significant muscle loss. The drug HCG is also commonly used for this purpose, but it works by mimicking the action of luteinizing hormone, not as an anti-estrogen. HCG is typically looked at as a rapid acting drug, used in the first couple of weeks after the steroids are withdrawn. Anti-estrogens like cyclofenil, Clomid® and/or Nolvadex® are often used in conjunction with HCG, but may be continued for several weeks after the HCG has been removed (see PCT: Post-Cycle Therapy).

Cyclofenil stimulates the release of testosterone via its anti-estrogenic action. The hypothalamus is one target site of this. By interfering with the binding of estrogen to its receptor in this area of the body, cyclofenil blocks the negative feedback inhibition brought fourth by this sex hormone. The enhanced release of gonadotropin releasing hormone (GnRH) may result, which in turn would stimulate the pituitary to heighten the release of luteinizing hormone. LH is the primary signal for the testes to increase the production of testosterone, so its increased release (provided the testes are properly sensitive to LH) leads to an elevation in the androgen level. The anti-estrogenic effect of this drug in breast tissue has also led to its use during a steroid cycle to prevent gynecomastia, similar to how Nolvadex® might be used. Cyclofenil, however, is reported to be somewhat weaker than Nolvadex®, which is usually preferred as an estrogen maintenance drug. Women do occasionally find a use for anti-estrogens, most often around contest time when the management of endogenous estrogens can help increase fat loss and definition. The side effects that can be brought about by a lowering of estrogen activity in the female body are usually strong and uncomfortable, however, making this approach less than ideal.

History:

Cyclofenil was developed during the early 1960s, a time when other agents of the same class (such as tamoxifen and clomiphene) were being thoroughly investigated. Cyclofenil was soon released as a prescription drug agent, sold mainly to increase the chance of conception and to counter certain menopausal symptoms. Although the drug seemed to offer a good clinical effect without significant health concerns, it did not see extensive success on the global market. Instead, Nolvadex and Clomid dominated this drug category for many decades. Still, cyclofenil did not completely disappear, and remained available in certain nations. The most popular brand was Fertodur, produced by Schering. It was sold in a few countries, including Brazil, Germany, Italy, Mexico, Switzerland, and Turkey. Other popular brands have included Rehibin (U.K.), Menopax (Brazil), Neoclym (Italy), Sexovid (Japan), and Ondogyne (France). Today, although most original cyclofenil products have been discontinued, the drug can still be found in some areas including Turkey, Italy, and Brazil.

How Supplied:

Cyclofenil is most commonly supplied in tablets of 200 mg.

Structural Characteristics:

Cyclofenil is classified as a selective estrogen receptor modulator, with both agonist and antagonist properties. It has the chemical designation 4,4'-(Cyclohexylidenemethylene)bis(phenyl acetate).

Side Effects:

Cyclofenil appears to be well tolerated, with a low incidence of significant side effects. Common adverse reactions include liver enzyme elevations, vasomotor flushes (hot flashes), abdominal discomfort, nausea/vomiting, breast discomfort, headache, and abnormal uterine bleeding. Premenopausal women may be more susceptible to hot flashes due to the stronger effect estrogenic disruption can have on this population. In males, the testosterone boosting properties of cyclofenil may result in some androgenic side effects including oily skin, acne, and increased libido.

Administration:

Cyclofenil is most commonly used (medically) to treat anovulatory infertility. Therapeutic protocols recommend a dose of 200 mg three times per day for 5 days, which is initiated near the start of the menstrual cycle. If pregnancy is not achieved with the first cycle, it may be used for 3 or 4 cycles in total. In some instances the drug is also given in lower doses to treat menopausal symptoms. When used after steroid administration (off-label) to increase natural testosterone production, a dosage 400-600 mg per day is the most common. It is often used for a period of 4 to 5 weeks as part of a comprehensive post-cycle recovery program in place of Clomid (see PCT: Post-Cycle Therapy). Similar doses are used for estrogen maintenance purposes while on-cycle, although Nolvadex is usually given preference for this purpose. Some athletes have experimented with using cyclofenil as a standalone anabolic, finding its ability to increase testosterone levels beneficial. The dosage used for this purpose is typically 400-600 mg per day for 6-8 weeks. While some have reported this approach to be effective, many others find the drug too mild, especially in light of the effects of exogenous testosterone.

Availability:

Cyclofenil is not widely produced. Availability is presently low on the international market. When located in the U.S., the drug is usually found in the form of Fertodur, made by Schering in Turkey. Counterfeits of cyclofenil drugs have not been a significant problem.

Lentaron® (formestane)

Description:

Formestane is classified as a selective irreversible steroidal aromatase inhibitor. This agent is structurally a derivative of androstenedione, differing from this well known prohormone only by the addition of a 4-hydroxyl group. This group, however, is responsible for causing an irreversible attachment between formestane and aromatase when the two come into contact with each other. This means that formestane will bond with the enzyme and never let it go, permanently deactivating it as a result. The enzyme will need to be replaced, through normal attrition, before the body will recover its lost estrogen synthesizing capacity. This may take several days or more following cessation of therapy. Given this mode of action, formestane is also referred to as a "suicide" aromatase inhibitor, as the drug essentially sacrifices itself in the process of blocking estrogen conversion. As a class of drugs, aromatase inhibitors are used (off-label) by male bodybuilders and athletes to prevent the estrogenic side effects of certain anabolic/androgenic steroids, and to increase fat loss and muscle definition while dieting.

Because of its potent estrogen-suppressing action, formestane has been used clinically to treat breast cancer patients in a number of countries including England, Germany, Switzerland, Spain, Australia, New Zealand, Italy, and Malaysia . It has been shown to be an effective option as a second line of defense after tamoxifen, an estrogen receptor antagonist, has failed to elicit a positive response with patients, and produces an overall response statistically similar to tamoxifen when administered as the first-line therapy . In terms of overall potency, formestane is not as strong as the selective third generation inhibitors like Arimidex (anastrozole) or Femara (letrozole). One study, for example, notes a 79% level of suppression of estrogen levels with 4 weeks use of Arimidex 1 mg daily (on par with levels noted with Femara use), but only a 58% level of suppression with intramuscular formestane injections (250 mg every two weeks) . But next to estrogen receptor antagonists like Clomid (clomiphene citrate) and Nolvadex (tamoxifen citrate), formestane is significantly more effective at blocking the effects of estrogen in the body.

History:

Formestane was the first selective aromatase inhibitor to be developed as a prescription drug, first appearing in Europe during the mid-1990s under the Lentaron Depot brand name. It was sold by Novartis, which marketed Lentaron Depot in two-dozen countries including Argentina, Austria, Belgium, Brazil, Canada, Chile, Czech Republic, Denmark, France, Germany, Greece, Hong Kong, Ireland, Israel, Italy, Malaysia, Netherlands, Portugal, South Africa, Spain, Switzerland, Turkey, and the United Kingdom. With the emergence of newer and more effective aromatase inhibitors, however, formestane soon lost market presence at a rapid rate. Most of the initial Lentaron Depot preparations have since been discontinued. The drug remains available today, but only in a small number of nations. This includes Austria, Brazil, Czech Republic, Hong Kong, and Turkey.

How Supplied:

Formestane is most commonly supplied in a sterile solution containing 125 mg/mL of drug in a 2 mL ampule.

Structural Characteristics:

Formestane is classified a steroidal selective irreversible aromatase inhibitor. It has the chemical designation 4-Hydroxyandrost-4-ene-3,17-dione.

Side Effects:

Common side effects associated with the use of an aromatase inhibitor include hot flashes, joint pain, weakness, fatigue, mood changes, depression, high blood pressure, swelling of the arms/legs, and headache. Aromatase inhibitors may also decrease bone mineral density, which may lead to osteoporosis and an increase in fractures in susceptible patients. Some individuals may also respond to the medication with gastrointestinal side effects including nausea and vomiting. Aromatase inhibitors can harm the development of an unborn fetus, and should never be taken or handled during pregnancy. When taken by men (as an off-label use) to reduce estrogenicity during prolonged periods of steroid treatment, aromatase inhibitors may increase cardiovascular disease (CVD) risk by retarding some beneficial properties of estrogen on cholesterol values. Studies have demonstrated that when an aromatizable steroid such as testosterone enanthate is taken in conjunction with an aromatase inhibitor, suppression of

HDL (good) cholesterol levels becomes significantly more pronounced. Since the estrogen receptor agonist/antagonist Nolvadex® generally does not display the same anti-estrogenic (negative) effect on cholesterol values, it is usually favored over aromatase inhibitors for estrogen maintenance by male bodybuilders and athletes concerned with cardiovascular health.

Administration:

Formestane is indicated for the treatment of advanced breast cancer in postmenopausal women. The recommended dosage is 250 mg by intramuscular injection (buttock) every two weeks. Although not a medically approved form of the drug, studies have demonstrated that a similar level of estrogen suppression can also be achieved with oral use of formestane. Due to poor bioavailability, however, the dose needed is around 250 mg per day . When used (off-label) to mitigate the estrogenic side effects of anabolic/androgenic steroid use or increase muscle definition, male athletes and bodybuilders often take 250 mg every two weeks by injection, or 250 mg per day orally.

Availability:

Formestane is not widely available as a prescription drug, and consequently is rarely circulated in the athletic community. Note that a small number of oral preparations can be found in the United States, where they are occasionally marketed as nutritional supplements.

Nolvadex® (tamoxifen citrate)

Description:

Tamoxifen citrate is a non-steroidal anti-estrogenic drug, used widely in clinical medicine. It is specifically a Selective Estrogen-Receptor Modulator (SERM) of the triphenylethylene family, and possesses both estrogen agonist and antagonist properties. As such, it may act as an estrogen in some tissues while blocking the action of estrogen in others. In breast tissue tamoxifen citrate is a strong anti-estrogen, and as a result it is commonly used in the treatment of hormone-responsive breast cancer in women. In some cases it is even utilized as a preventative measure, taken by women with an extremely high familial tendency for breast cancer. In male bodybuilders and athletes, tamoxifen citrate is commonly used (off-label) to counter the side effects caused by elevated estrogens subsequent to the use of certain anabolic/androgenic steroids.

The primary worry among the athletic/bodybuilding population is gynecomastia, or the very unsightly development of female breast tissue in men. This can be first noticed by the appearance of swelling or a small lump under the nipple. If left to progress, this can develop into a large hard-tissue gynecomastia that may be an irreversible occurrence without surgery. The estrogen can also lead to an increase in the level of water retained in the body, resulting in a notable loss of definition as the muscles begin to look smooth (even bloated) due to the retention of subcutaneous fluid. Fat storage may also be increased as estrogen levels rise in men. In fact, differences in the estrogen/androgen ratio are one of the reasons women have a higher body fat percentage, and different fat distribution (hips/thighs), than men.

Tamoxifen citrate also possesses the ability to increase production of FSH (follicle stimulating hormone) and LH (luteinizing hormone). This is accomplished by blocking negative feedback inhibition caused by estrogen at the hypothalamus and pituitary, which fosters the release of the mentioned pituitary hormones. This is very similar to the function of Clomid® and cyclofenil. Since a higher release of LH can stimulate the Leydig's cells in the testes (men) to produce more testosterone, tamoxifen citrate can have a positive impact on one's serum testosterone level. This "testosterone stimulating" effect is an added benefit when preparing to conclude a steroid cycle. Since anabolic/androgenic steroids tend to suppress endogenous testosterone production, tamoxifen citrate can help restore a balance in hormone levels. It is most commonly used as part of a comprehensive post cycle recovery program (see PCT: Post-Cycle Recovery).

Note that like some other triphenylethylene compounds, tamoxifen citrate can act as an estrogen in the liver. Estrogenic action in the liver is important in the regulation of serum cholesterol, and tends to support HDL (good) cholesterol synthesis and LDL (bad) cholesterol reductions. Since steroid-using bodybuilders are already dealing with the negative cardiovascular effects of these drugs, compounding the issue with aromatase inhibitors (which will lower total serum estrogen levels) may not always be the best option. Using a drug that blocks gynecomastia, for example, while at the same time supporting improved cholesterol values, might be much more ideal. It is important to note that tamoxifen citrate is not sufficient to stabilize serum cholesterol at healthy levels with the use of c-17alpha alkylated orals or high doses of steroids in general. The effect it would have on cholesterol values would likely be one of degrees, and cannot be relied upon to eliminate cardiovascular disease risk from anabolic/androgenic steroid use.

History:

Tamoxifen citrate was first synthesized in 1962 by ICI. It was made commercially available in the U.S. not long after, but was initially used to treat certain forms of female infertility, a purpose for which tamoxifen citrate does not seemed ideally suited. In 1971, the first clinical trials evaluating the effectiveness of tamoxifen citrate in breast cancer patients were undertaken. Two years later, noting the link between estrogen and breast cancer and the success of early trials, ICI pursued marketing the drug in the U.S. to treat breast cancer. It was not until 1977 that FDA approval for this use would finally be granted. Tamoxifen citrate was sold by ICI in a wide number of countries under the Nolvadex brand name (the company would later become known as AstraZeneca). A number of generics and other brands followed, presently too numerous to list. In 1998, the FDA approved expanding the indicated uses of tamoxifen citrate to include breast cancer prevention for women at high risk for developing the disease. In spite of continued clinical success with the drug for both cancer treatment and prevention, in June 2006 AstraZenica finally discontinued the sale of Nolvadex in the U.S. A number of generic versions are still available in this country, however, ensuring easy patient access to the drug. Tamoxifen citrate is presently the most popular anti-estrogen used by athletes and bodybuilders.

How Supplied:

Tamoxifen citrate is most commonly supplied in tablets of 10 mg or 20 mg.

Structural Characteristics:

Tamoxifen citrate is classified as a selective estrogen receptor modulator, with both agonist and antagonist properties (also known as an estrogen agonist/angagonist). It has the chemical designation (Z)2-[4-(1,2-diphenyl-1-butenyl) phenoxy]-N, N-dimethylethanamine 2- hydorxy-1,2,3-propanetricarboxylate (1:1).

Side Effects:

Common side effects associated with the administration of tamoxifen citrate include hot flashes, vaginal bleeding, vaginal discharge, vaginal itching, upset stomach, headache, light-headedness, edema, and hair loss. Other listed adverse reactions include skin rash, reduced platelet or white blood cell count, visual disturbances, uterine fibroids, endometriosis and other endometrial changes, deep vein thrombosis and pulmonary embolism, changes in liver enzyme levels, and increased triglyceride levels. An increased incidence of endometrial cancer and uterine sarcoma has been reported in association with tamoxifen citrate. Tamoxifen citrate may cause birth defects and should not be taken during pregnancy.

Administration:

Tamoxifen citrate is indicated for 1) the treatment of metastatic breast cancer in women and men; 2) adjuvant treatment of node-negative breast cancer following breast surgery and radiation; 3) adjuvant treatment of node-positive breast cancer in postmenopausal women following breast surgery and radiation; 4) reduction in incidence of contralateral breast cancer (in the other breast) in the adjuvant setting; 5) reduction in incidence of invasive breast cancer in women with DCIS (Ductal Carcinoma in Situ) following breast surgery and radiation; and 6) reduction in incidence of breast cancer in women at high risk for breast cancer. In women and men with metastatic breast cancer, a dose of 10-20 mg is administered twice a day (morning and evening). When used by men (off-label) to mitigate the estrogenic effects of anabolic/androgenic steroid use, a daily dosage of 10-30 mg (1-3 tablets) is usually administered while any offending steroids are taken, or as part of a comprehensive post-cycle hormone recovery program.

It is important to note that anti-estrogen use may slightly reduce gains made during a steroid cycle, as many androgenic/anabolic steroids seem to exhibit their most powerful anabolic effects when accompanied by a sufficient level of estrogen (See: Estrogen Aromatization). This may be one reason why gains made with a strong aromatizable androgen like testosterone are usually more pronounced than those achieved with anabolic steroids that aromatizes to a lower (or no) degree. Therefore, it is usually advised to identify a specific need for tamoxifen citrate before committing to its use during a cycle. Many people, in fact, find the use of an anti-estrogen unnecessary, even when utilizing problematic compounds such as testosterone or methandrostenolone. Others, however, find they are troubled by water retention and gynecomastia even with milder (less estrogenic) drugs like Deca-Durabolin® and Equipoise®. The estrogenic response to steroid use is very individual, and may be influenced by factors such as age and body fat percentage (adipose tissue is a primary site of aromatization).

Availability:

Tamoxifen citrate is widely manufactured, and can be found in virtually every developed nation of the world. The drug is also commonly circulated on the black market. Given its relatively low price and high availability, counterfeit product do not appear to be a large issue.

Teslac® (testolactone)

Description:

Testolactone is a first generation non-selective steroidal aromatase inhibitor, used clinically to treat estrogen-dependent breast cancer. Its exact mode of action is unknown, but it is believed to inhibit the aromatase enzyme in a noncompetitive and irreversible manner. If so, this would be an activity that is very similar to that of Lentaron (formestane). This might also explain why cessation of the drug does not provide an immediate restoration of normal estrogen production. Like formestane, it takes several days after ceasing use for the body to recover its normal estrogen synthesizing capacity, which is the time required by the body to replenish its enzyme levels. It seems logical based on structure and action that the same thing occurs with testolactone.

Although testolactone is technically steroidal in structure, it offers no anabolic or androgenic effect to its user. This is because it does not possess the traits necessary to bind and activate the androgen receptor, namely an active 17-beta-hydroxyl group. In fact, its D ring is an unusual six-membered lactone ring, and not the normal five-membered carboxylic ring that testosterone and its derivatives normally possess. This is likely where testolactone got its name, which may be short for testosterone-lactone. Studies actually suggest this steroidal drug possesses some level of anti-androgenic action, which likely occurs via competitive inhibition of the cellular androgen receptor . Regardless of this, testolactone has been included in the U.S. controlled substance list as an anabolic/androgenic steroid. For the purposes of this reference book it will remain classified as an anti-estrogenic drug. Likewise, testolactone is used by athletes and bodybuilders not to increase muscle mass and performance, but to mitigate the estrogenic side effects caused by certain anabolic/androgenic steroids.

Note that the level of aromatase inhibition produced with testolactone is significantly lower than that produced by the newer selective third generation inhibitors such as anastrozole, letrozole, and exemestane. For example, one study conducted in 1985 showed that 1,000 mg of testolactone per day given to nine normal men for a period of ten days suppressed serum estradiol levels by 25% . Another using the same 1,000 mg dose noted a 50% reduction after six days of use . These numbers are lower than what would be expected of the newer third-generation agents given the substantial estrogen suppression figures they have produced during clinical trials with women.

History:

Testolactone was first approved as a prescription drug by the FDA back in 1970. It was an early anti-estrogenic drug, exhibiting a moderately pronounced effect but failing to reach levels of high clinical success. As other more effective medications began to surface for the treatment of breast cancer, testolactone would not see the success its developers likely planned for it. It would see production in a small number of countries outside the U.S., most notably Brazil, Germany, and Chile. It has since been discontinued in all countries but the U.S., where the Teslac brand is still available.

How Supplied:

Testolactone is most commonly supplied in tablets of 50 mg.

Structural Characteristics:

Testolactone is classified as a steroidal noncompetitive irreversible steroidal aromatase inhibitor. It has the chemical designation 13-hydroxy-3-oxo-13,17-secoandrosta-1,4-dien-17-oic acid [dgr]-lactone.

Side Effects:

Common side effects associated with the use of an aromatase inhibitor include hot flashes, joint pain, weakness, fatigue, mood changes, depression, high blood pressure, swelling of the arms/legs, and headache. In 1999, the FDA officially added malaise to the list of possible side effects from this drug, reflecting something bodybuilders had noticed for some time: low estrogen levels can lead to lethargy, as this sex hormone plays an important role in the functioning of the central nervous system. Aromatase inhibitors may also decrease bone mineral density, which may lead to osteoporosis and an increase in fractures in susceptible patients. Some individuals may also respond to the medication with gastrointestinal side effects including nausea and vomiting. Aromatase inhibitors can harm the development of an unborn fetus, and should never be taken or handled during pregnancy. When taken by men (as an off-label use) to reduce estrogenicity during prolonged periods of steroid treatment, aromatase inhibitors may increase cardiovascular disease (CVD) risk by retarding some beneficial properties of estrogen on cholesterol values. Studies have demonstrated that when an aromatizable steroid such as testosterone enanthate is taken in conjunction with testolactone, suppression of HDL (good) cholesterol levels becomes significantly more pronounced. Since the estrogen receptor agonist/antagonist Nolvadex® generally does not display the same anti-estrogenic (negative) effect on cholesterol values, it is usually favored over aromatase inhibitors for estrogen maintenance by male bodybuilders and athletes concerned with cardiovascular health.

Administration:

Testolactone is FDA approved as adjunctive therapy in the palliative treatment of advanced or disseminated breast cancer in postmenopausal women when hormonal therapy is indicated. It may also be used in women who were diagnosed as having had disseminated breast carcinoma when premenopausal, in whom ovarian function has been subsequently terminated. The recommended dosage is 250 mg taken 4 times per day. When used (off-label) for estrogen suppression in male steroid users, a dosage of 250 mg (five tablets) is usually taken per day.

Availability:

Testolactone is no longer commonly used in clinical medicine, and consequently is not manufactured on a large sale globally. Presently a small number of testolactone preparations still exist, but are not commonly diverted for sale on the black market given the very low demand for the drug in this population.

ANTI-PROLACTIN Drug Profiles

Dostinex (cabergoline)

Description:

Cabergoline is a selective dopamine receptor agonist. This agent is highly specific in its actions, with a strong affinity for the dopamine D2 receptor, and a low affinity for dopamine D1, A1-adrenergic, A2-adrenergic, 5-HT1-serotonin, and 5-HT2-serotonin receptors. Its main clinical use is for the treatment of hyperprolactinemia, or the hypersecretion of prolactin from lactotropes in the anterior pituitary (pituitary tumor is a common cause of this disorder). It is also applied in the management of Parkinson's disease. Cabergoline effectively inhibits prolactin secretion, which it does by mimicking the actions of dopamine on the D2 receptor (dopamine normally serves as negative feedback for prolactin release). As a targeted agonist of the dopamine D2 receptor, cabergoline should not affect other pituitary hormones like growth hormone (GH), luteinizing hormone (LH), corticotrophin (ACTH), or thyroid stimulating hormone (TSH).

Prolactin is a somatotropic hormone, in the same family as human growth hormone (somatropin). It is a single peptide hormone, containing a chain of 199 amino acids. This makes it similar to (though slightly larger than) growth hormone, which is made of 192 amino acids. Any similarity between these two hormones, however, ends at structure. Prolactin is not an anabolic agent (at least not to skeletal muscle) but a lactation hormone. Most of its physiological value is in women, and becomes apparent during pregnancy when it aids in milk production. Cabergoline, likewise, is sometimes used to suppress lactation postpartum if there is a particular medical need for it. In men, prolactin has no known therapeutic value, and high levels are associated with impotence, infertility, and sometimes even gynecomastia (whether or not it has a causative role here remains the subject of much debate).

Although this is almost never associated with males, high levels of prolactin have actually been related to lactating gynecomastia in a very small percentage of steroid-using athletes. This disorder is often characterized by small fluid discharge that becomes noticeable with the squeezing of one's gynecomastic nipple. Although the situation can become worse, the first sign of this is often enough to scare the individual away from their current regimen of steroids. Gynecomastia is not automatically (or even normally) associated with lactation, so this is a somewhat rare phenomenon. It is probably caused by an unusual imbalance of hormones (androgens, estrogens, and progestins can all be involved and play varying roles), and/or a particular personal sensitivity to the disorder. When it does occur, however, cabergoline has been looked at as a remedy for the potentially embarrassing situation.

High prolactin levels (as would be associated with the need for cabergoline) are not regularly documented in steroid-using athletes, further underscoring the relative uncommon nature of this disorder. We do know that estrogen plays a stimulatory role here, and likely is the key to increasing prolactin secretion in males.[838][839][840] Other studies, however, show suppressive actions toward prolactin from other hormones including androgens.[841] This is perhaps why an actual hormonal imbalance, and not necessarily high estrogen, may be the cause of lactating gynecomastia. Scanning the medical books, there are few studies even looking at prolactin levels and steroid use, and those few are relatively inconclusive. One study analyzed the effects of testosterone enanthate and propionate in men and noted a significant prolactin increase 4 days after injection.[842] Yet another noted a 7-fold increase in estrogen (to values typical for women) in 5 power athletes self-administering testosterone and other steroids, yet no consistent effect on prolactin secretion.[843] A third self-administration study with athletes,[844] and a fourth clinical with nandrolone,[845] failed to show an increase in prolactin levels.

History:

Cabergoline was developed during the 1980s. The most popular trade name for this agent is Dostinex, which is produced in the U.S. and many other countries by the giant pharmaceutical conglomerate Pharmacia. Dostinex retained market exclusivity on cabergoline in the U.S. for many years, but between 2005 and 2007 several generic versions were approved for sale by the FDA. This includes products from Barr, Ivax, and Par Pharm. Cabergoline is widely available internationally, and can be found in more than 3-dozen different countries. Outside the U.S. the Dostinex trade name still dominates most markets, and can be found in Argentina, Australia, Austria, Belgium, Brazil, Canada, Chile, Czech Republic, Denmark, Finland, France, Germany, Greece, Hong Kong, Ireland, Israel, Italy, Malaysia, Mexico, Netherlands, Norway, New Zealand, Poland,

Portugal, Russia, South Africa, Singapore, Spain, Sweden, Switzerland, Turkey, United Kingdom, and Venezuela. In addition to Dostinex, cabergoline is marketed under at least 1-dozen other trade names.

How Supplied:

Cabergoline is most commonly supplied in tablets of 500mcg.

Structural Characteristics:

Cabergoline is an ergot derivative with the chemical designation 1-[(6-allylergolin-8beta-yl)carbonyl]-1-[3-(dimethylamino)propyl]-3-ethylurea.

Side Effects:

The most common side effects reported with cabergoline use include headache, nausea, and vomiting, which occurred in 26, 27, and 2% of patients (respectively) receiving the medication during one clinical trial.[846] Other potential side effects include (but are not limited to) constipation, dry mouth, abdominal pain, diarrhea, dizziness, vertigo, fatigue, anxiety, anorexia, malaise, depression, insomnia, hot flashes, heart palpitations, hypotension, breast pain, and acne, however nausea and headache were the most prominent side effects. Many side effects are dose related, further reason for starting off with the lowest possible therapeutic dose and working up. The prescribing information does not mention death as a clear consequence of an overdose, but it does list hallucinations, low blood pressure, and nasal congestion. Note that overdose patients may need supportive measures to raise blood pressure.

Administration:

When used medically to inhibit prolactin secretion, cabergoline is given in an initial dosage of 500mcg per week. This may be taken in one single dose or divided into 2 or more doses on separate days. The dose may be increased by 500mcg per week at monthly intervals until a desired physiological response is achieved. Dosage is most commonly maintained at 1mg per week, although doses up to 4.5 mg may be used in some cases. When used by athletes/bodybuilders to inhibit prolactin secretion (as with lactating gynecomastia), doses on the lower end of the therapeutic range are most commonly used. The user typically starts with a dosage of 250mcg per application (a half tablet) twice per week. This is used for four weeks, at which point the dosage might be adjusted upwards to a full tablet if needed (1 mg per week). In clinical medicine this drug may be taken for 6 months or longer, although athletes/bodybuilders usually find a 4-6 week course of therapy (combined with an intelligent rearrangement of the offending drugs) most appropriate.

Availability:

Cabergoline is not widely used by bodybuilders and athletes, and consequently is not commonly traded in black market commerce. The drug itself is widely available in legitimate medical commerce.

Parlodel® (bromocriptine mesylate)

Description:

Bromocriptine mesylate is a dopaminomimetic ergot derivative with D2 dopamine receptor agonist and D1 dopamine receptor antagonist activities. It is used most commonly as a prolactin inhibitor in cases of hyperprolactinemia, a growth hormone suppressant in acromegaly (high doses are required), and as an adjunctive medication to levodopa in the management of Parkinson's disease. The structure and activity of this drug are very similar to that of cabergoline (Dostinex). In the athletic/bodybuilding communities, bromocriptine is sometimes used to induce fat loss or combat elevated prolactin levels subsequent to anabolic/androgenic steroid use (a rare occurrence, sometimes marked by lactating gynecomastia).

The most vocal proponent of bromocriptine use for fat loss is probably Lyle McDonald, author of the online e-Book *Bromocriptine: An Old Drug With New Uses*. In this book McDonald describes how the drug can be used to normalize the metabolism, such that some of the normal physiological responses to dieting (which begin to slow the loss of body fat as the duration of dieting increases) are hindered. A lot of this focuses on leptin, a hormone looked at as sort of a fat thermostat, telling your brain how much adipose tissue you have on your body and how many calories you are regularly consuming (an "anti-starvation" hormone). Dieting tends to lower leptin levels significantly, which causes your body to respond in an appropriate way for survival (it tries to hold on to its nutrient stores as much as possible). Maintaining normal leptin stimulation could be key to keeping any diet productive, and bromocriptine may indeed allow us to do that.

The human medical data concerning the potential role this drug might play in supporting ongoing fat loss is encouraging. In cases where it was given while dieting, bromocriptine was capable of increasing total fat loss by a statistically significant degree, and seemed to extend the duration in which the diet was most effective. In one case, both placebo and treatment groups were noticing a measurable fat loss during the first 6 weeks of calorie restriction. Only the bromocriptine group, however, continued to lose significant amounts of weight for the remaining 12 weeks of intervention. Dieting plateau, or a point in which continued fat loss drastically slows or stops, is a common issue among those undertaking a calorie-restricted diet for the purpose of reducing body fat mass. A drug that can prevent or delay this plateau may logically be able to increase the overall effectiveness of dieting for many individuals.

History:

Bromocriptine has been used widely in clinical medicine for its indicated used since the 1970s. It is also much more widely distributed than its counterpart medication cabergoline, which is used for a similar set of clinical indications. In the U.S., the most common brand name is Parlodel, which is sold by Novartis. The drug is available in dozens of countries, and is sold under a similarly large number of different trade names including (but not limited to) Bromed, Criten, Grifocriptina, Bromo-Kin, Pavidel, and Gynodel. Bromocriptine remains a common medication today in most developed nations for its intended therapeutic uses.

How Supplied:

Bromocriptine mesylate is most commonly supplied in tablets of 2.5 mg and 5 mg. The doses are expressed in terms of base bromocriptine, so each 2.5 mg tablet contains 2.87mg of bromocriptine mesylate.

Structural Characteristics:

Bromocriptine mesylate is an ergot derivative with the chemical designation (5'S)-2-bromo-12'-hydroxy-2'-(1-methylethyl)-5'-(2-methylpropyl)-ergotaman-3',6',18-trione methanesulphonate.

Side Effects:

Bromocriptine can produce a number of unwanted side effects, the most notable being low blood pressure, dizziness, confusion and nausea. These side effects do tend to be dose related, with the low recommended doses used in bodybuilding are not likely to be much trouble for many. Further, initial nausea sometimes goes away after a couple of applications, once the user becomes accustomed to the drug. However, the strong incidence of any unwelcome side effects should warrant discontinuing therapy, especially if blood pressure is becoming negatively affected (too low a drop). Less common adverse reactions include anxiety, dry mouth, edema, seizures, fatigue, headache, lethargy, nasal congestion, rash, elevated liver enzymes, and changes in urinary frequency.

Administration:

When used medically to treat disorders marked by hyperprolactinaemia (hyper secretion of prolactin), an initial dosage of 1.25 mg to 2.5 mg per day is usually recommended. This may be increased by 2.5 mg every 2-7 days until an acceptable therapeutic dosage is established. This may require taking as much as 20-30 mg per day. When used (off-label) to support fat loss, dieting individuals commonly take between 2.5 mg and 5 mg per day. This is given in a single morning dose, due to the relatively long half-life of the drug. This may be used in short dieting cycles, and should not be considered for long-term weight management. Similar dosing schedules are common when used by athletes and bodybuilders to counter lactating gynecomastia, although higher doses may be required in some instances. A 4-6 week course of therapy, combined with a rearrangement of offending steroids, is usually undertaken.

Availability:

Bromocriptine is produced in most developed countries, including the United States where it is sold as a generic drug and under the Parlodel brand name. The brand name product comes in the form of both 2.5 mg tablets and 5 mg capsules, with 100 doses per bottle. At the pharmacy, 100 5 mg capsules may cost nearly $400. In some nations, this price may be as low as $50 to 200 ($.50 to $1.00 per dose) for generic and other brands of bromocriptine. Bromocriptine is not widely diverted for sale on the black market, but can be found circulating on occasion.

APPETITE STIMULANTS Drug Profiles

Periactin (cyproheptadine hydrochloride)

Description:

Cyproheptadine hydrochloride is a first-generation prescription histamine and serotonin antagonist. This drug is most often given in the U.S. for the treatment of allergy-related symptoms, including hay fever, runny nose, irritated eyes, hives, and swelling. It is also FDA approved for the treatment of anaphylactic reactions caused by allergens, often as an adjunct to injectable epinephrine (adrenalin). The serotonin inhibiting effect of this drug also gives it a unique ability to increase appetite. This has led to a considerable amount of off-label use as a weight-gain medication, particularly with patients who are suffering from a lean tissue wasting associated with AIDS infection, cancer, or other debilitating diseases. Cyproheptadine hydrochloride is also used on occasion as an adjunct to growth hormone therapy in children, to foster greater nutrient uptake and increases in linear growth beyond what is normally achieved with rHGH alone.[847] Bodybuilders and athletes use the drug on occasion to help increase caloric intake, usually during periods of bulking training where increased mass is desired, and often used in conjunction with anabolic/androgenic steroids.

Although this is a controversial use of the drug, references to the appetite stimulating properties of cyproheptadine hydrochloride are abundant in the medical literature. One of the more detailed papers compares the appetite increasing effects of cyproheptadine hydrochloride to megestrol acetate[848] in a group of 14 men with weight loss associated with HIV infection. The other agent, megestrol, is a progestin that was approved by the FDA in 1993 for the treatment of anorexia, cachexia, or weight loss in patients with AIDS. In this investigation, cyproheptadine hydrochloride was shown to have a similar level of benefit to FDA approved agent megestrol, with patients consuming about 500 extra calories per day, and gaining a moderate amount of weight with either medications. While the benefits were similar, the side effects were not. The investigators reported that more than 50% of the patients taking megestrol suffered impotence during the investigation, while the cyproheptadine hydrochloride group had no such side effects. Cyproheptadine hydrochloride may offer an effective alternative to megestrol therapy for many patients, especially those prone to negative side effects associated with this type of hormone manipulation.

History:

Cyproheptadine hydrochloride is an early anti-histamine drug, and has been sold as a prescription medication in most developed nations for decades. It was introduced to the U.S. in 1961 under the Periactin® brand name by Merck & Co. This brand of cyproheptadine hydrochloride was sold for many years in the U.S, but was voluntarily discontinued by Merck in 2003 (in both the U.S. and Canada). While Merck & Co. has withdrawn Periactin from a number of other nations (likely due to low financial interest), the brand is still sold in more than one dozen countries including Australia, Austria, Belgium, Ireland, Italy, Netherlands, New Zealand, South Africa, Spain, Sweden, Thailand, and the United Kingdom. It is also sold under dozens of other brand names around the world, in both single- and multi-ingredient preparations. A number of generic products are still sold in both the U.S. and Canada as well. Subsequent to studies questioning the long-term weight gaining value of cyproheptadine hydrochloride therapy, in 1994 the World Health Organization warned against using the drug for this purpose.[849] Regardless of this report, many still support the value of cyproheptadine hydrochloride as a short-term appetite stimulant.

How Supplied:

Cyproheptadine hydrochloride is most commonly supplied in tablets of 4 mg.

Structural Characteristics:

Cyproheptadine hydrochloride is antihistaminic and antiserotonergic agent with the chemical designation 4-(5H-dibenzo[a,d]cyclohepten-5-ylidene)-1-methylpiperidine hydrochloride sesquihydrate.

Side Effects:

As a first-generation anti-histamine, cyproheptadine hydrochloride may be prone to producing a number of side effects in its users. The most common of which is sedation or the classic "anti-histamine lethargy", which is common to these types of drugs. For some users, the tiredness that cyproheptadine hydrochloride will produce will outweigh any potential as a weight-gaining/performance-enhancing agent. For most, this side effect of cyproheptadine hydrochloride is not very noticeable, and perhaps a nuisance (not strong enough to necessitate discontinuation) at best. Other less common side effects of concern include, but are not limited to, dizziness, disturbed coordination, muscular weakness, nausea, vomiting, diarrhea, constipation, dryness of the mouth, difficulty urinating, vertigo, blurred vision, tightness of the chest, wheezing, stuffed nose, sweating, early period, headaches, and faintness. Any strong incidence of unwelcome side effects would immediately warrant discontinuing the drug, or even seeking immediate medical attention if severe.

Administration:

The dosage required for medical purposes may vary depending on the individual and their particular needs. The established therapeutic range for cyproheptadine hydrochloride is 4mg to 20 mg per day, with most adults requiring 12mg to 16mg daily. The total daily dosage is usually divided into three separate applications. When used (off-label) as an appetite stimulant, a dosage of 4mg is commonly taken 2-3 times per day (8-12mg). Above this level, side effects may become more noticeable (most notably sleepiness), often interfering with the benefit of the drug. This may be used during a steroid cycle focused on bulking, with the intake of cyproheptadine hydrochloride usually lasting no more than 4-8 weeks. For those who tolerate this anti-histamine's side effects (mainly tiredness), cyproheptadine hydrochloride is often reported to offer significant value as an appetite stimulant during weight gaining cycles. This is especially so in individuals that have trouble eating enough food to meet the high calorie/protein requirements for optimal muscle growth.

Availability:

Cyproheptadine hydrochloride is produced in a wide number of countries. Although it is not commonly traded on the black market, high supply and the relatively benign nature of this drug (loose controls) make it easily diverted for sale when needed. Given its low demand, counterfeiting of cyproheptadine hydrochloride preparations is not common.

It is interesting to also note that the Dominican steroid product, Anabolex, actually includes 1.5 mg of cyproheptadine hydrochloride in each 3 mg methandrostenolone tablet, which was added by its developers to facilitate increased caloric intake and weight gain during anabolic therapy. The 2:1 ratio provided is optimal for a daily dose of 24 mg Dianabol (a very common amount), as it would provide 12 mg of cyproheptadine hydrochloride (the maximum common daily dose). This is the only common anabolic steroid product that includes cyproheptadine hydrochloride as an ingredient.

Cardiovascular Support Product Profiles

Lipid Stabil™

Description:

Lipid Stabil is a cholesterol and cardiovascular health support supplement. It was specifically designed to be a foundation supplement for steroid users, and is especially useful during on-cycle periods. The formula specifically focuses on supporting four separate areas of cardiovascular health: 1) reducing LDL (low-density lipoprotein) "bad" cholesterol; 2) increasing beneficial HDL (high-density lipoprotein) cholesterol; 3) reducing serum triglycerides; and 4) reducing oxidative stress and arterial plaque formation. Antioxidant supplementation is an important and often overlooked part of managing cardiovascular health during anabolic/androgenic steroid use, as AAS are known to increase homocysteine levels and oxidative stress. Although no supplement can completely eliminate the cardiovascular risks of AAS abuse, a supplement such as Lipid Stabil (or one with a similar ingredient profile) is highly recommended, as it may help reduce the lasting negative health impact of these medications.

Lipid Stabil contains a comprehensive blend of nearly one dozen natural ingredients. Each component in known to play an important role in cardiovascular health, and many have significant clinical support demonstrating beneficial effects on key health markers. For example, garlic powder is one of the backbone ingredients, and has been shown in studies to increase HDL cholesterol, reduce LDL cholesterol, and improve the antioxidant response.[850][851] Green tea extract (standardized for EGCG and high polyphenol content) is another backbone ingredient, and like garlic, is also shown to improve cholesterol and reduce oxidative stress/LDL oxidation.[852][853] Several other clinically studied ingredients known to improve cholesterol levels, serum triglycerides, and/or systemic antioxidant capacity round out the Lipid Stabil formula including resveratrol,[854] phytosterols,[855] policosanol,[856] selenium,[857] and inositol hexanicotinate (no-flush niacin).[858]

History:

Lipid Stabil was developed in 2008 by Molecular Nutrition (U.S.). The focus was specifically on designing a supplement that can help support cardiovascular health in anabolic/androgenic steroid users. The product can be found through international distribution, although it may possibly be considered a drug product in some regions with strict controls on herbal supplement products.

How Supplied:

Each serving of Lipid Stabil is supplied in 3 capsules, and contains a blend of green tea extract (750 mg), garlic powder (600 mg), inositol hexanicotinate (400 mg), polygonum cuspidatum standardized for resveratrol (200 mg), pantothenic acid (100 mg), phytosterol complex (100 mg), policosanol (10 mg), and selenium (200 mcg).

Side Effects:

Lipid Stabil is a natural dietary supplement and is not expected to have notable side effects.

Administration:

For general cholesterol and lipid support or as an adjunct to anabolic/androgenic steroid use, Lipid Stabil is generally taken at a dosage of 3 capsules per day. Note that a natural product such as Lipid Stabil may help reduce cardiovascular toxicity, but cannot be relied upon to completely eliminate potential cardiovascular damage from the abuse of anabolic/androgenic steroid drugs. Care should always be taken to monitor all aspects of health when taking AAS substances.

Availability:

Lipid Stabil is produced in the U.S. by Molecular Nutrition. It is available for export, and may be found in Canada, Europe, and other international markets.

Lovaza® (omega-3 ethyl esters)

Description:

Lovaza is a prescription omega-3-acid supplement which contains ethyl esters of eicosapentaenoic acid (EPA) and docosahexaenoic acid (DHA). It is fundamentally similar to most over-the-counter fish oil supplements, except that Lovaza is highly purified to drug quality standards, is made with a high (90%) concentration of omega-3 acids, and has gone through extensive clinical trials for a specified therapeutic use. Otherwise, the benefits of EPA/DHA should be reproducible with any quality mercury-free fish oil supplement. In the U.S., Lovaza is approved to lower triglycerides in patients with very high triglyceride levels (>500 mg/dL). Clinical studies showed triglyceride reductions by as much as 45% with its use.[859][860] In addition, this prescription supplement has been shown to increase HDL (good) cholesterol levels, improve lipoprotein particle size and subclass distribution,[861] and reduce cardiovascular mortality in some patients by 30%.[862] EPA/DHA supplements are commonly taken by anabolic/androgenic steroid users in an effort to reduce the negative cardiovascular effects of AAS.

The mechanism of action of eicosapentaenoic acid (EPA) and docosahexaenoic acid (DHA) is not fully understood. These omega-3 acids appear to exert their favorable properties over serum lipids through a number of different but complimentary pathways. For one, EPA and DHA appear to be effective at increasing the enzyme hepatic lipoprotein lipase,[863] which can increase the excretion of LDL cholesterol and triglycerides. These omega-3 acids may also increase mitochondrial and peroxisomal beta-oxidation, reducing the availability of fatty acids for lipid synthesis.[864] They may also suppress nuclear SREBP-1, which reduces hepatic lipogenesis.[865] EPA and DHA also appear to decrease the activity of the triglyceride-synthesizing enzyme diacylgylcerol acyltranferase.[866] The lipid reducing actions of EPA and DHA, therefore, appear to be several fold, including reduced substrate availability, reduced lipid synthesis, and increased lipid breakdown.

History:

The first prescription drug product containing omega-3 acids was approved by the U.S. Food and Drug Administration in 2004. It was sold in this market under the Omacor brand name until 2007, when the manufacturer, Reliant Pharmaceuticals, changed the name of the product to Lovaza. This was done to eliminate any confusion with the blood clotting medication Amicar (aminocaproic acid). Lovaza is presently distributed in the U.S. by the international drug manufacturer GlaxoSmithKline.

How Supplied:

Lovaza is supplied in soft gelatin capsules containing approximately 900 mg of omega-3-acids each. The doage consists mainly of eicosapentaenoic acid (465 mg) and docosahexaenoic acid (375 mg).

Side Effects:

Lovaza is a natural dietary product and is not expected to have notable side effects. A small percentage of patients reported mild adverse reactions during clinical trials, including back pain (2.2%), flu symptoms (3.5%), infection (4.4%), pain (1.8%), angina pectoris (1.3%), indigestion (4.9%), burping (4.9%), rash (1.8%), and altered taste (2.7%).

Administration:

Lovaza is prescribed in a dosage of 4 capsules per day for the treatment of very high triglycerides. Given high cost and limited access, Lovaza is not commonly taken by AAS users. Instead, most steroid users will administer 4-6 grams per day of a quality fish oil supplement for general cholesterol and lipid support. Note that a supplement or prescription drug containing the omega-3-acids EPA and DHA may help reduce cardiovascular toxicity, but cannot be relied upon to completely eliminate potential damage from the abuse of anabolic/androgenic steroid drugs. Care should always be taken to monitor all aspects of health when taking AAS substances.

Availability:

High concentration omega-3 acid is marketed as a prescription drug product in the U.S. under the Lovaza brand name. Lovaza is also sold in select European and Asian markets. High quality fish oil supplements containing EPA and DHA are widely available over-the-counter in most markets.

DIURETICS Drug Profiles

Aldactone® (spironolactone)

Description:

Spironolactone is an antagonist of aldosterone and is pharmaceutically classified as a diuretic. It acts by competitively inhibiting aldosterone binding to receptor sites, especially in the renal tubes where aldosterone is involved in sodium-potassium exchange. The drug causes increased amounts of sodium and water to be excreted and potassium to be retained. This is different from some other agents of this class, such as a loop diuretic like furosemide, which can significantly increase the excretion of sodium, water, and potassium. In this light, spironolactone is commonly referred to as a "potassium sparing" diuretic. It is used medically for a number of conditions including the treatment of high blood pressure, edema related to congestive heart failure, hyeraldosteronism (the over production of aldosterone), and hypokalemia (drop of potassium, often associated with other medical interventions). Spironolactone is often used (off-label) by competitive athletes and bodybuilders to make short-term adjustments in water weight. The primary focus is to bring about increased muscle definition by shedding subcutaneous water (bodybuilders), or to make category adjustments during the weigh-in procedure in sports with restricted weight classes (athletes).

History:

Spironolactone was developed during the late 1950s, and first saw widespread use in clinical medicine during the early 1960s. The drug filled an important need for a diuretic that does not deplete potassium, and therefore has a less dramatic impact on electrolyte balance in the body. In many regards it is looked at as a "safer" and "milder" diuretic compared to other agents in this general category, such as loop diuretics or thiazides, allowing this agent room for market stability and success. Today, spironolactone is widely distributed throughout most of the developed world. It is available in dozens of brand names, the most commonly identified is probably Aldactone from Searle. It is also widely sold in mixed-ingredient preparations alongside other diuretics. This includes furosemide, as seen in the product Lasilacton, or hydrochlorothiazide, in Searle's (also widely distributed) mixed diuretic product Aldactazide.

How Supplied:

Spironolactone is most commonly supplied in tablets of 25 mg.

Structural Characteristics:

Spironolactone is an aldosterone antagonist and diuretic. It has the chemical designation 17-hydroxy-7alpha-mercapto-3-oxo-17alpha-pregn-4-ene-21-carboxylic acid y-lactone acetate.

Warnings (Dehydration, Elevated Potassium, Death):

The misuse of diuretic drugs for physique- or performance-enhancing purposes is characterized as a high-risk practice. Diuretics may produce a life-threatening level of dehydration and electrolyte imbalance when administered without proper medical supervision. Many deaths have been associated with the misuse of these drugs. It is also important to note that the supplementation of potassium, either through pharmaceuticals or a diet rich in potassium, is generally not advised while taking a potassium-sparing diuretic like spironolactone. Excessive potassium intake may cause hyperkalemia, which may lead to cardiac irregularities and possibly death.

Side Effects:

Adverse reactions associated with spironolactone administration may include gynecomastia, cramping, diarrhea, drowsiness, lethargy, headache, skin irritation, rash, mental confusion, fever, impotence, loss of muscle coordination, menstrual irregularities, virilization, and deepening of the voice. Spironolactone has also been shown to cause tumors in rats. Breast cancer has been reported in some patients receiving spironolactone, but no causal relationship has yet been established. Additionally, this compound may exhibit anti-androgenic properties, as both a weak inhibitor of androgen/receptor binding and testosterone biosynthesis.

Administration:

When used medically to treat hypertension, the initial recommended dosage in adults is 50 mg to 100 mg per day in divided doses. It may take two weeks for a maximum response to be achieved. The dosage may be adjusted later depending on the individual needs of the patient. When used (off-label) by male bodybuilders to increase muscle definition or athletes to reduce weight before a weigh-in, a dosage of 100 mg per day in a single morning application, is most common. This may be continued for 3 to 5 days prior to the event, and will often result in a harder and more defined appearance to the muscles (or substantial reduction in body weight prior to rehydration).

Women are occasionally attracted to spironolactone for its effect as an anti-androgen. It is sometimes used as a safety net at a point when androgen levels have become problematic during a cycle, and is used in an effort to reduce the risk of permanent virilization symptoms. A dosage of 25-75 mg daily for 1 to 2 weeks is often used for this purpose, and may be enough to ward off side effects while androgen levels decline (the steroid regimen terminated). Since spironolactone is more effective at lowering endogenous androgen levels than inhibiting androgen action, it is certainly not to be considered a cure-all remedy for adventurous steroid-using female athletes.

Since this compound is one of the mildest (prescription) diuretic options, it is a common starting point for an early competitor. Once familiar with its effects, many attempt to achieve a stronger level of water loss by mixing spironolactone with a thiazide or furosemide (Lasix). The goal is to provide strong water excretion with less calcium/potassium loss than using the stronger diuretics alone. When mixed with hydrochlorothiazide, for example, the 100 mg spironolactone dosage is often cut in half, and an equal amount of the thiazide is taken. The 50 mg/50 mg combination is reported to noticeably increase water excretion without dramatic side effects. The potassium re-absorption seen with spironolactone should be balanced out with the thiazide so potassium levels will not be as greatly affected. On the other hand, Lasix (furosemide) should make an even stronger addition to spironolactone. In this case, dropping the spironolactone dosage to 50 mg and adding 20 mg oral Lasix is a popular choice, and is often said to provide the water-shedding effect that is roughly equivalent to a 40 mg Lasix tablet. Again, the potassium depleting effect of Lasix may be offset to some degree by the potassium sparing effect of spironolactone, so additional potassium supplements are not likely necessary. Many such combination diuretics are widely available, and appear to be well regarded in clinical circles.

It is important to note that while Lasix and Hydrodiuril appear to be more effective at inducing short-term water loss, they also have increased risks as compared to potassium-sparing diuretics, and should be approached with caution.

Availability:

Spironolactone is widely manufactured in both single ingredient and multi-ingredient drug preparations. Low cost and wide scale availability make this a poor financial target for counterfeiting.

Dyrenium® (triamterene)

Description:

Triamterene is an oral diuretic used medically to treat edema. Edema may occur without known cause (idiopathic edema), or be associated with liver or kidney disease, congestive heart failure, corticosteroid/progestin use, or the overproduction of aldosterone. Triamterene is classified as a potassium sparing diuretic, increasing the rate of water and sodium excretion but preserving potassium levels. As the name suggests, this drug produces a pronounced diuretic effect without the potassium loss associated with thiazides/loop diuretics. The need for potassium supplementation is, therefore, eliminated with this agent. The diuretic activity following a single dose of triamterene is usually evident within 2 to 4 hours, reaching peak effect at approximately 3 hours in most cases. Its diuretic effect lasts for a total of 7-9 hours following administration.

Triamterene is utilized (off-label) by bodybuilders and athletes to shed subcutaneous water prior to a bodybuilding competition, or to make weight class adjustments in certain competitive sports. Bodybuilders in particular rely heavily on the increased definition that can result when water retention is reduced. The highly defined "shredded" physique common to bodybuilding today is nearly impossible to achieve without the use of diuretics. At the same time, diuretics are the reason weight class competitors like wrestlers and boxers often appear much heavier during an event than they do at the weigh-in. A considerable amount of bodyweight (in the form of water) can be removed with diuretic use, often resulting in a drop of one or more weight categories. This practice is very common in sports where the user is not drug tested and has ample time to rehydrate following a weigh-in, resulting in the athlete competing at a significantly heavier weight than his or her weight class would dictate.

History:

Triamterene first saw extensive clinical use during the 1960s. It was used largely as a standalone agent at first, but went on to become a widely used agent in clinical medicine in combination products with other diuretic drugs. Today this usually includes other, more potent diuretics like thiazides and loop agents. Here, the potassium loss of the stronger diuretic is balanced to some degree by the potassium sparing triamterene, which often results in a reduced or even eliminated need for potassium supplementation during therapy. Single ingredient preparations of triamterene are still sold, however, and can be found in several countries including Belgium (Dytac), United Kingdom (Dytac), and the United States (Dyrenium).

How Supplied:

Triamterene is most commonly supplied in capsules of 50 mg and 100 mg.

Structural Characteristics:

Triamterene is a potassium-sparing diuretic. It has the chemical designation 2,4,7-triamino-6-phenyl-pteridine.

Warnings (Dehydration, Death):

The misuse of diuretic drug(s) for physique- or performance-enhancing purposes is characterized as a high-risk practice. Diuretics may produce a life-threatening level of dehydration and electrolyte imbalance when administered without proper medical supervision. Many deaths have been associated with the misuse of these drugs. It is also important to note that the supplementation of potassium, either through pharmaceuticals or a diet rich in potassium, is generally not advised while taking a potassium-sparing diuretic like triamterene. Excessive potassium intake may cause hyperkalemia, which may lead to cardiac irregularities and possibly death.

Side Effects:

Triamterene use may be associated with electrolyte imbalance, including elevated or decreased potassium levels. Signs of electrolyte imbalance include dry mouth, thirst, weakness, lethargy, drowsiness, restlessness, muscle pain, muscle cramping, seizures, reduced urine volume, low blood pressure, and gastrointestinal disturbances. Other side effects may include nausea, vomiting, jaundice, blood platelet deficiency, anemia, azotemia (buildup of metabolic waste products in the blood), renal stones, and other kidney disturbances. Additionally, some rare side effects characterized as hypersensitivity reactions have been reported including skin rash, photosensitivity, and anaphylaxis (an extreme and potentially life threatening allergic reaction).

Administration:

When used medically to treat hypertension, the usual initial dosage in adults is 100 mg twice daily after meals (200 mg per day). This may be increased, but should never exceed 300 mg per day in total. Among bodybuilders, this drug is commonly used for only a few days prior to a competition, adjusting the dosage over the course to elicit the best level of diuretic effect. Since it has a long lasting action, it is generally administered once per day. One capsule (100 mg) is usually taken the first thing in the morning with a meal, and the effect judged over the next several hours. The dosage is usually increased by one capsule per day for 2-3 days at most, until the user is noticing the proper water loss for competition. When looking for a stronger diuretic effect, many bodybuilders and athletes will opt to combine triamterene with another stronger diuretic such as hydrochlorthiazide or furosemide. The dosage of both agents would be adjusted downward to compensate for their combined effects. The goal here is usually to increase short-term diuresis, without causing the extreme potassium loss that can be associated with the use of thiazides or loop diuretics alone at higher doses.

Availability:

Triamterene is widely sold throughout the developed world. Although single-ingredient preparations containing triamterene are available, this drug is most commonly sold in multi-ingredient preparations targeting edema and/or high blood pressure. Low cost, modest demand, and high availability make this drug a low-profit target for counterfeiting.

Hydrodiuril® (hydrochlorthiazide)

Description:

Hydrochlorothiazide is a diuretic from the thiazide family, used medically for the treatment of edemas and hypertension. This drug acts by reducing the reabsorption of electrolytes, thereby increasing the excretion of sodium, potassium, chloride, and consequently water. In comparison to other diuretics, Hydrodiuril is stronger than the potassium sparing agent Aldactone® (spironolactone), but weaker then the loop agent Lasix (furosemide). While potassium excretion is much less pronounced than that seen with Lasix, the use of a potassium supplement (or a potassium rich diet) may still be necessary with this product. This is usually dependent on the dose and duration in which the drug is administered. Calcium excretion may also be pronounced with thiazides, but again, are weaker in this regard than Lasix.

The use of diuretics has been increasingly popular in a number of athletic disciplines. For starters, these drugs are very popular among bodybuilders who use them to shed subcutaneous water before a competition. The ability to have a winning physique often relies heavily on the definition that can result from diuretic use. The highly defined, super hard and shredded look common today in this sport is nearly impossible to achieve without the use of these drugs. Many athletes competing in sports with weight categories also utilize diuretics. Wrestlers and boxers, for example, might use diuretics to compete in a heavier weight class than would be dictated by an earlier weigh-in measurement. Given that the weigh-in is usually done a day (or many hours) before a competition, the athlete can reduce water weight with diuretics, yet have enough time to restore fluids and bodyweight before the event. The result can be a shift of one or more weight categories, which can be a formidable advantage in these types sports.

History:

Hydrochlorothiazide was developed during the 1950s. Given the widespread nature of diseases associated with high blood pressure and edema, the drug found a very large market, and quickly achieved large-scale acceptance and distribution. Hydrochlorothiazide became a fundamental form of therapy in this area of medicine, where it remains widely available today. Hydrochlorothiazide preparations are available in virtually all developed nations, and appear in literally hundreds of different brand name and generic products. Single-ingredient preparations (where hydrochlorothiazide is the only active drug) are far outnumbered by multi-ingredient preparations, where the drug is often mixed with other actives that focus on diuresis or blood pressure management.

How Supplied:

Hydrochlorothiazide is most commonly supplied in tablets of 25 mg and 50 mg.

Structural Characteristics:

Hydrochlorothiazide is a diuretic and antihypertensive. It is the 3,4-dihydro derivative of chlorothiazide, and has the chemical designation 6-chloro-3,4-dihydro-2H-1,2,4-benzothiadiazine-7-sulfonamide 1,1-dioxide.

Warnings (Dehydration, Death):

The misuse of diuretic drugs for physique- or performance-enhancing purposes is characterized as a high-risk practice. Diuretics may produce a life-threatening level of dehydration and electrolyte imbalance when administered without proper medical supervision. Many deaths have been associated with the misuse of these drugs.

Side Effects:

Hydrochlorthiazide use may be associated with electrolyte imbalance. This may include potassium and sodium deficiency, as well as hypochloremic alkalosis (an increase in blood bicarbonate due to significant chloride loss). Signs of electrolyte imbalance include dry mouth, thirst, weakness, lethargy, drowsiness, restlessness, muscle pain, muscle cramping, seizures, reduced urine volume, low blood pressure, and gastrointestinal disturbances. Other side effects may include reduced appetite, nausea, vomiting, constipation, diarrhea, inflammation of salivary gland(s), headache, dizziness, sensitivity to light, low blood pressure upon standing, skin irritation, impotence, visual disturbances, jaundice, pancreatitis, and inflammation of the lung(s). Additionally, some rare side effects characterized as hypersensitivity reactions have been reported including skin rash, fever, shock, pulmonary edema, and respiratory distress.

Administration:

When used medically to treat hypertension, the usual initial dose in adults is 25 mg daily given as a single dose. The dose may be increased to 50 mg daily, often in two doses of 25 mg. Note that daily doses above 50 mg are often associated with marked reductions in serum potassium. Athletes and bodybuilders typically use this drug (off-label) for very brief periods (several days) of water adjustment. A common practice is to administer this drug once per day, after the morning meal. The athlete will monitor the level of water lost throughout the day, and adjust the dosage for the following day if necessary. The usual starting dosage is one 50 mg tablet. The user will adjust the effect by adding a 25 mg or 50 mg tablet each subsequent day. This practice is only followed for three or four days, until an optimal dosage is calculated. The total daily dosage will rarely exceed 100-200 mg (doses above 100 mg per day in a clinical setting are not commonly recommended).

If the application of hydrochlorothiazide is not producing the desired effect, many bodybuilders/athletes will choose to add another diuretic (mild) before moving to the stronger loop agents. A combination of a potassium sparing diuretic like Aldactone® (spironolactone) and Hydrodiuril is regarded as particularly useful by many, and is believed to slightly balance out the calcium and potassium loss associated with the use of hydrochlorothiazide. The dosage of each agent would be reduced considerably, usually starting with a 25 mg/25 mg application and working upwards.

It is important to note that the overuse of diuretics, aside from being potentially very dangerous, may result in too much water loss. This can lead to flat, "deflated" looking muscles. A higher diuretic dosage, likewise, does not always equate to increased definition and muscularity. It is usually regarded as good advice by those in the athletic community to become familiar with the practice of using diuretics before using them during competition time. Otherwise, the user may be left to make frantic dosage adjustments at the last minute, which can be a dangerous and ineffective practice.

Availability:

Hydrochlorothiazide is widely manufactured in both single ingredient and multi-ingredient drug preparations. Low cost and wide scale availability make this a poor financial target for counterfeiting.

Lasix® (furosemide)

Description:

Furosemide belongs to a class of drugs known as loop diuretics, which cause the body to excrete water as well as potassium, sodium, magnesium, calcium, and chloride. They are used most commonly to treat edema and high blood pressure. Like other agents of this type, furosemide works by inhibiting the Na-K-2Cl symporter in the thick ascending loop of Henle, which is a carrier protein that pulls sodium, potassium, and chloride inside cells. This mode of action is independent of any inhibition towards aldosterone. Loop diuretics are among the strongest diuretics available, and can have an extremely dramatic effect on fluid and electrolyte levels in the body. Potassium levels need to be closely watched in particular, and patients may require a prescription potassium supplement. If the proper levels of potassium and other electrolytes are not maintained, serious heart complications may develop. Mistakes in potassium dosage have equally serious consequences; so it is of note that furosemide can be a particularly risky item to use without proper medical supervision.

Athletes and bodybuilders use diuretics for a couple of specific purposes, and usually for only brief periods. Competitive athletes in sports with weight class restrictions may use these drugs to drop water weight, in an effort to make adjustments in their weight class standings. Since the weigh-in procedure is often a day or days before a competition, one can drop their bodyweight considerably with diuretics, and be back to normal within hours after drug cessation and rehydration. This may provide a strong competitive advantage, allowing the athlete to compete at a heavier weight than his or her category would dictate. This advantage is only offset to some degree by the now near universal nature of some form of "dropping weight" practice in these sports. Bodybuilders may rely heavily on diuretics when preparing for a contest. Here, a drug like furosemide can efficiently lower subcutaneous water concentrations, helping to produce a more defined ("ripped") look common to competitive bodybuilding.

History:

Furosemide was developed during the early 1960s. Much of the initial research on this diuretic was conducted in Europe, mainly Germany and Italy. The drug proved to be quite successful, however, and within a matter of years gained worldwide attention and acceptance as a treatment for edema and high blood pressure. Over the years, furosemide preparations have become among the most popular medications in their area of medicine. Single- and multi-ingredient preparations making use of this diuretic can presently be found in virtually all corners of the world. The most recognized brand name is Lasix, presently sold in the U.S. and many other nations under the Sanofi Aventis label. The actual number of different brand and generic forms of furosemide would be difficult to calculate and list, but would probably measure in the hundreds.

How Supplied:

Furosemide is most commonly supplied in oral tablets of 20 mg, 40 mg, and 80 mg, and injectable solutions containing 10 mg/ml.

Structural Characteristics:

Furosemide is an anthranilic acid derived loop diuretic. It has the chemical designation 4-chloro-N-furfuryl-5-sulfamoylanthranilic acid.

Warnings (Dehydration, Death):

Furosemide is a highly potent diuretic, which can profoundly increase water excretion (diuresis) and lead to electrolyte depletion. The misuse of diuretic drug(s) like furosemide for physique- or performance-enhancing purposes is characterized as a high-risk practice. Diuretics may produce a life-threatening level of dehydration and electrolyte imbalance when administered without proper medical supervision. Many deaths have been associated with the misuse of these drugs.

Side Effects:

Furosemide use may be associated with electrolyte imbalance. This may include the depletion of potassium (hypokalemia), sodium (hyponatremia), magnesium (hypomagnesemia), and calcium (hypocalcemia), as well as hypochloremic alkalosis, an increase in blood bicarbonate due to significant chloride loss. Signs of electrolyte imbalance include dry mouth, thirst, weakness, lethargy, drowsiness, restlessness, muscle pain, muscle cramping, seizures, reduced urine volume, low blood pressure, and gastrointestinal disturbances. Other side effects may include pancreatitis, jaundice, anorexia, oral and stomach irritation, cramping, diarrhea, constipation, nausea, vomiting, hearing loss, numbness or tingling of the extremities, vertigo, dizziness, headache, blurred vision or other visual disturbances, anemia, decreased white cell or blood platelet count, dermatitis, rash, skin itching and sensitivity to light, low blood pressure, high blood sugar levels (hyperglycemia), muscle spasm, weakness, restlessness, urinary bladder spasm, fever, blood clot, and excess uric acid in the blood (hyperuricemia). Additionally, some rare side effects characterized as hypersensitivity reactions have been reported including inflammation of blood vessels, kidney inflammation, and inflammation of blood vessels or lymph ducts (angiitis).

Administration:

When used medically to treat edema, it is often given orally in a dose of 20 mg to 80 mg per day, which is taken in one single application. For the treatment of hypertension, it is generally recommended to administer 80 mg per day, which is given in two separate 40 mg applications spaced 12 hours apart. Athletes and bodybuilders typically use this drug (off-label) for very brief periods (several days) of water adjustment. The dosage and method of administration is tailored to the individual, dependent on the desired goals and condition of the athlete. Oral tablets are the most common form of administration. The athlete will usually start with a low dose, and increase the amount slightly on subsequent days. The main focus is to calculate the optimal dosage, as well as to determine the best intake schedule, in relation to a show or competition. The initial dosage is usually 20 mg to 40 mg, and the maximum daily intake rarely exceeds 80 mg. In order to minimize the side effects associated with this drug, it is generally used for no longer than 4-5 days.

Note that since furosemide has such a strong effect on electrolyte levels, it is generally considered much safer to add a potassium sparing agent like Aldactone® (spironolactone) than it is to keep increasing the amount of furosemide used. Combination diuretics like this are widely produced as prescription medicines for this reason. The use of 50 mg Aldactone® and 20 mg furosemide is a common starting point, and is believed to have a roughly similar diuretic effect to 40 mg of furosemide, but without the same level of potassium loss. This dosage may be adjusted on subsequent days in order to determine the optimal amount and intake schedule, but should rarely exceed 100 mg/40 mg per day. It is important to remember that these drugs can be active for many hours. It can become difficult to control the dehydrating effect with an overlapping schedule, therefore one should be careful not to administer diuretics on multiple occasions during the same day.

Injectable furosemide solutions are considered to be significantly more powerful forms of the drug milligram for milligram. Furosemide solutions can be administered intramuscularly or intravenously, depending on the individual needs of the patient. The IV method is much more rapid acting, and produces significantly higher peak blood levels of the drug. Given that the action of furosemide can be noticed in a matter of seconds or minutes when given by injection, the effect is actually easier to judge and control with this method of use, at least under normal conditions. Since the injection is much more powerful than the oral, however, is important to emphasize that the dosage must be considerably reduced in comparison. Intramuscular injection is most common with bodybuilders and athletes, and is usually given at a dosage of 10-20 mg. Doses in excess of 40 mg per day are rarely used in the bodybuilding/athletic population.

Availability:

Furosemide is widely available, and is manufactured and sold under many different brand names, in many countries. No version of Lasix (or any other diuretic) is currently being counterfeited on any large scale. Although it is doubtful these will circulate, make sure to never purchase the drug in 500 mg tablets. These are used only in severe medical conditions, and contain a dosage that would likely prove fatal to a healthy person.

ENDURANCE / ERYTHROPOIETIC DRUGS Drug Profiles

Aranesp® (darbepoetin alfa)

Description:

Darbepoetin alfa is a synthetic derivative of the human erythropoietin protein. It also has the same pharmacological action as recombinant human erythropoietin (epoetin alfa). In the body, erythropoietin is normally released by the kidneys in response to hypoxia (low blood oxygen levels). This in turn triggers bone marrow to increase red blood cell production. As such, this hormone is vital to the regulation of normal red blood cell concentrations in humans. With a similar mode of action to recombinant erythropoietin, darbepoetin alfa can be used to augment erythropoiesis when the body is not maintaining adequate red blood cell levels on its own. It is FDA approved for the treatment of anemia (low red blood cell count) associated with chronic renal failure or chemotherapy.

Darbepoetin alfa differs from recombinant human erythropoietin (epoetin alfa) mainly in its duration of activity. This new protein maintains its levels in the blood for approximately three times longer, causing it to have a much longer therapeutic window. This means that with darbepoetin alfa patients are required to administer the product much less frequently than they would epoetin alfa. While epoetin alfa is usually injected on a schedule of three times per week, darbepoetin alfa requires only one injection in the same time frame. This may enhance patient comfort considerably, especially when the patient is visiting the physician for routine drug administration.

Endurance athletes are highly attracted to darbepoetin alfa for the effect it has on red blood cell production. It is no secret that the practice of blood doping has been popular with endurance sports. This procedure involves removing, concentrating, and storing a quantity of red blood cells from your own body to be transfused later. By adding the stored cells before an event (by then the body has restored the lost blood volume), the athlete has a much greater concentration of red blood cells. The blood should, likewise, transport oxygen more efficiently, and the athlete may be given a significant endurance boost. This procedure can be quite risky, however, as blood products can be difficult to store and administer correctly. Darbepoetin alfa is a drug that basically equates to chemical blood doping, and can achieve the same end result (higher red cell concentrations) with the use of a simple medication.

History:

Darbeopetin alfa was developed as a prescription drug by Amgen. The U.S. Food & Drug Administration first approved it for sale in 2001. Amgen is the world's largest biotechnologies company, and the same firm that first brought recombinant erythropoietin (epoetin alfa) to the U.S. market in 1984. The main focus with darbepoetin alfa appears to have been the development of a much longer acting erythropoietic protein in comparison to their earlier recombinant erythropoietin, which is commonly injected on a schedule of three times per week. The prescribing guidelines for darbepoetin alfa recommend a once per week schedule, which seems to offer strong comfort advantages to epoetin alfa for patients that do not like receiving frequent injections. Darbepoetin alfa has not yet reached the level of market success that has been noted with epoetin alfa preparations, but has been a strong selling drug for Amgen ever since its release.

How Supplied:

Darbepoetin alfa is most commonly found in single-dose vials and prefilled syringes containing 25, 40, 60, 100, 150, 200, 300, or 500 mcg of drug.

Structural Characteristics:

Darbepoetin alfa is a 165-amino acid protein that differs from human erythropoietin by the substitution of amino acids on the erythropoietin peptide backbone, which allows the addition of two additional N-linked oligosaccharide chains.

Warnings (Death, Viral Disease):

The misuse of darbepoetin alfa for physique- or performance-enhancing purposes is characterized as a high-risk practice. Like traditional blood doping methods, darbepoetin alfa can produce an abnormally high concentration of hemoglobin in the blood (polycythemia), which may result in heart attack, stroke, seizure, or death.

Some forms of darbepoetin alfa contain albumin, a purified human blood product. Although effective donor screening and product manufacturing procedures are in place, it still carries a risk, though extremely remote, for transmission of viral disease.

Side Effects:

Side effects associated with the use of darbepoetin alfa may include flu-like symptoms such as fever, chills, headache, muscle pain, weakness, or dizziness. Such effects tend to be more pronounced at the initiation of therapy. Other adverse reactions may include infection, rash, swelling of the skin, nausea, vomiting, diarrhea, high blood pressure, low blood pressure, cough, bronchitis, or edema. In some instances darbepoetin alfa has been associated with thromboembolism, deep-vein thrombosis, pulmonary embolism, heart attack, and cerebrovascular accidents.

Administration:

Darbepoetin alfa is indicated for the treatment of anemia associated with chronic renal failure (CRF) and chemotherapy. The recommended starting dose for the treatment of anemia in adult CRF patients is .45 mcg/kg body weight, administered once per week as a single IV or SC injection. The dosage is subsequently adjusted based on changes in hematocrit. Healthy athletes using darbepoetin alfa for performance-enhancing purposes generally start on the very low end of the therapeutic spectrum, and adjust according to changes in hematocrit. This may entail initiating therapy with as little as .05 mcg/kg of body weight once per week. Note that it is considered very important to monitor blood cell counts closely during the entire intake of darbepoetin alfa to help ensure hematocrit is not allowed to increase to an unhealthy level.

Availability:

Darbepoetin alfa is not widely sold on the black market. Yet because of the high cost for erythropoiesis stimulating agents like darbepoetin alfa, it is a high profile target for counterfeit drug manufacturing operations. Counterfeit drugs of this class have even infiltrated legitimate pharmaceutical distribution channels, suggesting that care should be taken when purchasing this and similar drug products.

Epogen® (epoetin alfa)

Description:

Erythropoietin is a glycoprotein that is produced in the kidneys, and is responsible for stimulating red blood cell production. Epoetin alfa is a pharmaceutical form of erythropoietin, which was manufactured using recombinant DNA technology. The compound is produced from animal cells into which the gene coding for human erythropoietin has been inserted. The biological activity and structure of epoetin alfa are indistinguishable from that of human erythropoietin. Epoetin alfa is used to treat many forms of anemia, effectively stimulating and maintaining erythropoiesis in a large percentage of patients treated. The efficiency of this drug quickly made it a ready replacement for older (less effective) therapies such as Anadrol 50®.

Endurance athletes are highly attracted to epoetin alfa for the effect it has on red blood cell production. It is no secret that the practice of blood doping has been popular with endurance sports. This procedure involves removing, concentrating, and storing a quantity of red blood cells from your own body to be transfused later. By adding the stored cells before an event (by then the body has restored the lost blood volume), the athlete has a much greater concentration of red blood cells. The blood should, likewise, transport oxygen more efficiently, and the athlete may be given a significant endurance boost. This procedure can be quite risky, however, as blood products can be difficult to store and administer correctly. Epoetin alfa is a drug that basically equates to chemical blood doping, and can achieve the same end result (higher red cell concentrations) with the use of a simple medication.

History:

Epoetin alfa was developed by the biotechnologies firm Amgen, and first introduced to the U.S. market in 1984. The release of the drug is regarded as a breakthrough in the treatment of anemia, which beforehand was being addressed mainly with agents that indirectly or nonspecifically targeted red cell production, such as oxymetholone, which may present a number of unwanted side effects to the patient. Epoetin alfa marked the development of the first drug that specifically and effectively stimulated the process of erythropoiesis (red blood cell production). Its success was rapid and far reaching. Epoetin alfa has since been introduced to a wide number of different countries. The most popular trade names include Procrit (distributed by Ortho, manufactured by Amgen), Epogen (Amgen), and Eprex (Johnson & Johnson). In addition to these, more than one dozen other trade names are also used to market epoetin alfa.

In 2002 the subcutaneous use of Eprex, which is sold only outside the United States, was linked to a rare disease called pure red-cell aplasia. This is a condition where the body loses its ability to produce red blood cells. Those that suffer from pure red-cell aplasia usually become dependant on continual blood transfusions for survival. Close to 200 people taking Eprex were identified as developing this rare condition, far in excess of normal expected numbers. Internal investigations by Johnson & Johnson linked the high numbers to changes in the product that were made to satisfy European regulations limiting the use of albumin. According to a company spokesperson, a chemical reaction between the new stabilizer that replaced albumin and the rubber stopper allowed organic compounds to leech into the vials. The company subsequently replaced its original stoppers with coated rubber to prevent this reaction. The incidence of pure-red cell anemia in patients receiving erythropoietin seems to have been reduced as a result, although warnings about this reaction remain on the prescribing information for all products sold in the U.S.

How Supplied:

Epoetin alfa is supplied as a dry sterile powder that requires reconstitution with sterile diluent before injection. It is most commonly found in single- and multi-dose ampules and vials containing 2,000-40,000 Units/ml.

Structural Characteristics:

Epoetin alfa is a single chain polypeptide hormone containing 165 amino acids. It is identical in structure to the alpha glycoform of human erythropoietin.

Warnings (Death, Viral Disease):

The misuse of epoetin alfa for physique- or performance-enhancing purposes is characterized as a high-risk practice. Like traditional blood doping methods, epoetin alfa can produce an abnormally high concentration of hemoglobin in the blood (polycythemia), which may result in heart attack, stroke, seizure, or death.

Many forms of epoetin alfa contain albumin, a purified human blood product. Although effective donor screening and product manufacturing procedures are in place, it still carries an extremely remote risk for transmission of viral disease.

Side Effects:

Side effects associated with the use of epoetin alfa may include flu-like symptoms such as fever, chills, headache, muscle pain, weakness, or dizziness. Such effects tend to be more pronounced at the initiation of therapy. Other side effects include rash, swelling of the skin, nausea, vomiting, diarrhea, high blood pressure, hyperkalemia (excess potassium in the blood), and irritation at the site of injection. In some instances epoetin alfa has been associated with thromboembolism, deep-vein thrombosis, pulmonary embolism, heart attack, and cerebrovascular accidents.

Administration:

Epoetin alfa injectable solution is given by subcutaneous or intravenous injection. The two paths of administration have greatly different effects on the blood level of the drug. When given by IV infusion, peak blood levels of the drug are reached within 15 minutes, and the elimination half-life ranges from 4 or 13 hours. When administered via the subcutaneous route, peak blood levels are reached between 5 and 24 hours, and the elimination half-life is approximately 24 hours. Given an equal dose, the peak plasma concentration of epoetin alfa will be significantly lower than the intravenous method. When used medically to treat severe anemia associated with chronic renal failure, the recommended starting dosage range is 50 to 100 Units/kg of bodyweight, given 3 times per week. The dosage is subsequently adjusted based on changes in hematocrit. Healthy athletes using epoetin alfa for performance-enhancing purposes generally start on the very low end of the therapeutic spectrum, and adjust according to changes in hematocrit. This may entail initiating therapy with as little as 5 to 10 Units/kg of bodyweight, taken 3 times per week. Note that it is considered very important to monitor blood cell counts closely during the entire intake of epoetin alfa to help ensure hematocrit is not allowed to increase to an unhealthy level.

Availability:

Epoetin alfa is a very expensive compound, and its use is additionally isolated to certain athletic fields. As such, it is not widely traded on the black market. Given the high cost of this drug, however, it is a lucrative target for counterfeiters.

Provigil® (modafinil)

Description:

Modafinil, known chemically as benzhydrylsulphinylacetamide, is a central stimulant (psychostimulant). It is FDA approved for the treatment of narcolepsy (a disorder characterized by sudden and uncontrollable attacks of deep sleep, mental fatigue, or excessive sleepiness), sleep apnea, and SWSD (Shift Work Sleep Disorder). It is being investigated for a number of other uses, including the treatment of Alzheimer's disease, depression, and attention deficit disorder. Modafinil belongs to a group of drugs known as Eugeroics ("good arousal"), designed to promote a mental state of vigilance and alertness. One of its known mechanisms is to work as an alpha-1 adrenoceptor agonist, exerting its mood and energy enhancing effects through the increased release of dopamine in the CNS. It also results in alterations in local GABA and glutamate levels.

The use of modafinil as a stimulant has been shown in studies to have many advantages over amphetamines. To begin with, it is believed to have a much lower potential for abuse due to the fact that it produces a lower sense of euphoria. It also displays lower peripheral CNS stimulation (less side effects), has minimal effects on blood pressure, produces no interruptions in normal sleeping patterns (no hangover or needing "catch-up" sleep), and has an overall greater safety profile according to clinical trials. This drug is of interest even to the U.S. military, which is looking at it as an energy enhancer for pilots and combat soldiers that need to operate for long periods of time without sleep. This is not as unusual as it may seem at first, as military combat pilots and soldiers have used Dexedrine (an amphetamine) extensively in the past when sleep was inconvenient. Soldiers on modafinil often report that they maintain excellent cognitive functioning for up to 40 hours without sleep, and have fewer side effects than Dexedrine. Modafinil has been tested in recent combat situations such as in Afghanistan and Iraq, and seems poised for official acceptance as a battlefield drug.

Recently, modafinil has become a popular drug among competitive athletes. They use it not simply to "stay awake", but as a performance enhancing agent with both stimulant and endurance-increasing properties. This type of use probably comes as a surprise to those who developed this drug, as early reports suggested that this was a "mild" alertness drug, without strong stimulant properties that would improve athletic performance. Recent studies contradict this determination. A study conducted in Canada shows a very strong athletic benefit inherent in modafinil.[867] During this double-blind investigation, a dose of 4 mg per kg of bodyweight (this equates to 200 mg for a 220lb man) of modafinil, or placebo, was given to a group of 15 male volunteers. Three hours after ingestion, aerobic exercise was conducted on a cycle ergometer at 85% VO2max (maximum aerobic power), and the amount of time until exhaustion was determined. While taking modafinil, the men were able to exercise for significantly longer periods of time (~30%), and had greater oxygen intake at exertion. They also reported lower subjective ratings of perceived exertion (RPE), which suggests that the increased performance was in part due to a significantly less pronounced sensation of fatigue during exercise.

History:

Modafinil was developed by Lafon Laboratories in France. It was approved for sale in the United States by the FDA in 1998, where it was introduced under the Provigil® brand name. Modafinil is also found internationally under this and several additional trade names including Modiodal®, Vigil®, Alertec®, and Modasomil®. Although the drug appears to have a favorable safety record and profile, it was quickly considered a drug of potential abuse in the U.S. It is presently classified as a schedule IV controlled substance, which places modafinil in the same category as Valium and Xanax. This is intended to limit its diversion for nonmedical purposes by placing considerable legal penalties on its possession and importation. The medical applications for the drug are fairly broad, however, including SWSD, which refers to sleep disturbances caused by changing- or late-shift work. Prescriptions for the drug are, likewise, commonly granted by physicians in general medical practice.

Modafinil quietly became popular among competitive athletes between 2000 and 2004, before the athletic bodies were aware of the drug. Its use as a performance-enhancing agent was revealed to the public during the designer steroid (BALCO) doping scandal of 2004, however, when it was disclosed that many of the same athletes who tested positive for THG also used modafinil. The IOC quickly banned its use, and with the help of a number of researchers a methodology for detecting this chemical in the urine was developed. This test is now implemented as part of the standard Olympic level drug screening process. Most of the other international athletic bodies have followed the IOC's lead in banning and testing for modafinil. The drug has since lost all appeal as an "invisible" performance-enhancing agent, although is still being used by many athletes that are not subject to random urine testing.

How Supplied:

Modafinil is most commonly supplied in tablets of 100 mg and 200 mg each.

Structural Characteristics:

Modafinil is a central nervous system stimulant related to adrafinil. It has the chemical designation 2-[(diphenylmethyl)sulfinyl]acetamide.

Side Effects:

Side effects associated with modafinil are commonly the result of its central nervous system stimulating activities, and may include nervousness, insomnia, shakiness, euphoria, personality changes, and excitation. The drug may also produce gastrointestinal disturbances such as nausea, vomiting, abdominal pain, dry mouth, anorexia, and headache. Hypertension, heart palpitations, or abnormal heart rate may also be noticed. In rare instances allergic rash, increases in alkaline phosphatase, or impaired voluntary movement have been reported.

Administration:

When used clinically to treat excessive daytime sleepiness associated with narcolepsy or obstructive sleep apnea, the recommended dose is typically 200 to 400 mg per day. This may be given in a single morning application, or in two divided doses (morning and at midday). When used to enhance physical performance, the typical effective dose is in the range of 100-400 mg. This is often given at least 2-3 hours prior to athletic competition. Note that side effects can be dose dependant. It is often advised to start using modafinil on the low end of the effective dosage range, and increase by 50-100 mg per application until an optimal level is determined.

The arenas in which this drug is applied are vast, and essentially include any sport focused on aerobic activity or endurance. It may also work well with those athletes focused on short repeat bursts of strength or speed (anaerobic activities), such as shot-putting, pole-vaulting, or long-jumping. Modafinil is not a popular drug among bodybuilders, as it holds little direct value for building muscle or reducing body fat levels. Some, however, do find it to be an effective pre-workout stimulant, especially during periods when fatigue or loss of physical drive may be noticed subsequent to a busy work or personal schedule.

Availability:

Modafinil is presently available in more than two dozen countries. The drug is not highly diverted for black market sale, however, and is not a lucrative target for drug counterfeiting operations.

FAT LOSS AGENTS - SYMPATHOMIMETICS Drug Profiles

Adipex-P® (phentermine hydrochloride)

Description:

Phentermine hydrochloride is a sympathomimetic stimulant of the amphetamine family. Like other amphetamine derivatives, it is categorized as an anorectic (appetite suppressing) agent. Phentermine is commonly prescribed as a weight loss aid in obese patients. It is typically used for short periods of time (less than 12 weeks), and as an adjunct to support an ongoing exercise and dieting regimen. The main focus is to curb the desire to eat, thereby reducing the total caloric intake. Although the data seems to vary from trial to trial, much of it supports at least a modest additional loss of fat mass with the use of phentermine hydrochloride.[868] Athletes and bodybuilders use phentermine hydrochloride for the same purpose, typically when weight loss is required for physique remodeling or competition.

History:

Phentermine hydrochloride was first introduced to the U.S. drug market in the 1970s. Base phentermine was available in the U.S. as far back as 1959. Phentermine had long been used as an appetite suppressant, although the most notable attention to it came in the early 1990s, when the drug was successfully paired with fenfluramine during diet studies. Investigators had shown that this type of drug combination was actually more effective at promoting weight loss than diet and exercise, results that quickly catapulted Fen-Phen into top place in the prescription weight loss drug market. By 1997, however, it had become apparent that a very high percentage of Fen-Phen users were noticing heart valve defects as a result of the drugs. Fenfluramine was identified as the principle cause, and was withdrawn from the U.S. market that same year. Phentermine remains available in the U.S. and many nations abroad today. Popular trade names include Adipex, Ionamin, Anoxine, Phentrol, and Obenix. Note that as an amphetamine derivative, this medication has a tendency to be habit forming. For this reason it has been added to the U.S. controlled substances list as a schedule IV medication.

How Supplied:

Phentermine hydrochloride is most commonly supplied in tablets and capsules of 18.75 mg and 37.5 mg each.

Structural Characteristics:

Phentermine hydrochloride is a central stimulant and indirect-acting sympathomimetic of the amphetamine family. It has the chemical designation 2-methyl-1-phenylpropan-2-amine (2-methyl-amphetamine).

Side Effects:

Common side effects associated with phentermine hydrochloride include insomnia, increased blood pressure, irritability, nervousness, and euphoria. Less common side effects include vision disturbances, reduced libido, confusion, diarrhea, dizziness, dry mouth, headache, irregular heartbeat, nausea, vomiting, rash, and tiredness. Phentermine is a CNS stimulant with potential for fatal overdose. Signs of overdose may include rapid breathing, fever, hallucinations, blood pressure irregularities, irregular heartbeat, unconsciousness, trembling, shaking, panic, extreme restlessness, and severe nausea, vomiting, or diarrhea.

Administration:

For optimal effectiveness, phentermine hydrochloride should not be taken with food. The usual adult dose is one capsule or tablet (37.5 mg) daily, administered before or 1-2 hours after breakfast. For some patients a half of a tablet (18.75 mg) daily may be adequate, while in other cases it may be advisable to give a half of a tablet (18.75 mg) twice daily. When taken more than once per day, the second dose should never be taken within 4-6 hours of sleep. The drug is typically used for 3-4 weeks at a time, with longer durations of therapy rarely exceeding 12 weeks. Bodybuilders and athletes typically use the prescribed amount of drug in a similar short-term fashion, due to the high likelihood of side effects as the dose escalates beyond the normal therapeutic range.

Availability:

Phentermine hydrochloride is available in a number of different countries. It is not widely counterfeited. U.S. residents would not be advised to order the drug from overseas, however, since phentermine is a schedule IV controlled substance and carries similar legal restrictions as Valium and anabolic steroids. Many U.S. doctors who specialize in weight loss medications will readily dispense phentermine for controlled periods of weight loss.

Albuterol (albuterol sulfate)

Description:

Albuterol sulfate is a selective beta-2 adrenergic agonist, very similar in structure and action to clenbuterol. Unlike clenbuterol, however, albuterol is readily available as a prescription drug in the United States. It is also sold as salbutamol in a number of other countries, which is another generic name for the drug. Albuterol is most commonly found in the form of a rescue inhaler, which is designed to disperse a measured amount of the drug immediately and directly to the bronchial tubes in times of crisis (asthma attack). This form provides the least amount of systemic drug activity possible, which is great for minimizing unwanted cardiovascular side effects. Albuterol oral tablets are also available, however, and provide a systemic dose of the drug. These are the subject of interest in the bodybuilding and athletic communities, and they can provide significant beta-2 stimulation and measurable fat loss throughout the body given the right conditions. Note that a more comprehensive discussion of the benefits, activities, and side effects of beta-2 agonist drugs can be found under the clenbuterol drug profile.

History:

Albuterol sulfate was introduced to the U.S. drug market in 1980, sold under the Ventolin brand name. Albuterol sulfate has grown to be one of the most popular drugs in history for the management of acute asthma attacks. As a result, many other companies have invested in the market. The Ventrolin brand name is still available in the U.S., however, the FDA has also approved a variety of other generic and brand name forms of the drug. Albuterol sulfate is also presently sold in both inhalation and oral preparations in most developed countries. Popular trade names include Aerolin, Airomir, Asmasal, Asthalin, Asthavent, Asmol, Butahale, Buventol, ProAir, Proventil, Salamol, Sultanol, and Volmax.

How Supplied:

Albuterol sulfate is most commonly supplied in oral metered dose inhalers and tablets of 2 mg, 4 mg, or 8 mg each.

Structural Characteristics:

Albuterol sulfate (salbutamol sulphate) is a short-acting ,2-adrenergic receptor agonist. It is a racemic drug with the chemical designation (±) a1-[(tert-butylamino)methyl]-4-hydroxy-m-xylene-a,a1-diol sulfate (2:1)(salt).

Side Effects:

Common side effects associated with albuterol sulfate include headache, dizziness, lightheadedness, insomnia, tremor, nervousness, sweating, nausea, vomiting, diarrhea, and dry mouth. Less common but more serious adverse events include allergic reactions (rash, hives, swelling of the lips, tongue, or face, or difficulty breathing), chest pain, high blood pressure, and irregular heartbeat. Albuterol sulfate is a CNS stimulant with potential for fatal overdose. Signs of overdose may include rapid breathing, blood pressure irregularities, irregular heartbeat, unconsciousness, trembling, shaking, panic, extreme restlessness, and severe nausea, vomiting, or diarrhea.

Administration:

The usual starting dosage for adults and children 12 years and older for the management of asthma is 2-4 mg three or four times per day. When used (off-label) for fat loss, an effective dose of albuterol usually starts in the range of one to two 4 mg tablets per day (1 tablet X 1-2 applications). This is often increased slightly as the user becomes accustomed to the drug, perhaps to 4 mg three to four times per day. Individuals very sensitive to the stimulant side effects of beta agonists usually start with the lower-dose 2mg tablets first. The administration intervals are spread out as evenly as possible, so as to prevent overlap and sustain active concentrations in the blood for as much of the day as possible. Athletes and bodybuilders will often use their body temperature as a marker of drug efficacy. A degree or two elevation in temperature with use of the drug may indicate that lipolysis (the removal of stored fatty acids in adipose tissue) is being effectively stimulated.

As is noted with all beta agonists, tolerance to the thermogenic benefits of this drug tends to develop quickly. This is usually noticed by the body temperature returning to normal pretreated levels. Due to the potential side effects of these drugs, it is not advised to continually increase the dosage in order to chase down a diminishing effect. Instead, the user will usually opt to discontinue the drug for some time (4 weeks or longer) to let the body restore its normal beta-adrenergic receptor concentrations. More recently, the antihistamine Zaditen (ketotifen) has become popular, which is a potent upregulator of beta-adrenergic receptors, especially beta-2 receptors. This medication may enhance the thermogenic potency of this beta agonist, but might also increase drug potency and the incidence of side effects.

Availability:

Albuterol is a widely available and very cheap medicine. Counterfeiting is not a strong concern with this medication.

Clenasma (clenbuterol hydrochloride)

Description:

Clenbuterol hydrochloride is an anti-asthma medication that belongs to a broad group of drugs knows as sympathomimetics. These drugs affect that sympathetic nervous system in a wide number of ways, largely mediated by the distribution of adrenoceptors. There are actually nine different types of these receptors in the body, which are classified as either alpha or beta and further subcategorized by type number. Depending on the specific affinities of these agents for the various receptors, they can potentially be used in the treatment of conditions such as asthma, hypertension, cardiovascular shock, arrhythmias, migraine headaches and anaphylactic shock. The text *Goodman and Gillman's The Pharmacological Basis of Therapeutics 9th edition* does a good job of describing the diverse nature in which these drugs affect the body:

Most of the actions of catecholamines and sympathomimetic agents can be classified into seven broad types: (1) peripheral excitatory action on certain types of smooth muscles such as those in blood vessels supplying the skin, kidney, and mucous membranes, and on the gland cells, such as those of the salivary and sweat glands; (2) a peripheral inhibitory action on certain other types of smooth muscle, such as those in the wall of the gut, in the bronchial tree, and in blood vessels supplying skeletal muscle; (3) a cardiac excitatory action, responsible for an increase in heart rate and force of contraction; (4) metabolic actions, such as an increase in the rate of glycogenolysis in liver and muscle and liberation of free fatty acids from adipose tissue; (5) endocrine actions, such as modulation of the secretion of insulin, rennin, and pituitary hormones; (6) CNS actions, such as respiratory stimulation and, with some of the drugs, an increase in wakefulness and psychomotor activity and a reduction in appetite; and (7) presynaptic actions that result in either inhibition or facilitation of the release of the neurotransmitters such as such as norepinephrine and acetylcholine.

Clenbuterol hydrochloride is specifically a selective beta-2 sympathomimetic, primarily affecting only one of the three subsets of beta-receptors. Of particular interest is the fact that this drug has little beta-1 stimulating activity. Since beta-1 receptors are closely tied to the cardiac effects of these agents, this allows clenbuterol hydrochloride to reduce reversible airway obstruction (an effect of beta-2 stimulation) with much less cardiovascular side effects compared to non-selective beta agonists. Clinical studies with this drug show it is extremely effective as a bronchodilator, with a low level of user complaints and high patient compliance . Clenbuterol hydrochloride also exhibits an extremely long half-life in the body, which is measured to be approximately 34 hours long . This makes steady blood levels easy to achieve, requiring only a single or twice daily dosing schedule at most . This of course makes it much easier for the patient to use, and may tie in to its high compliance rate.

In animal studies clenbuterol hydrochloride is shown to exhibit anabolic activity , obviously an attractive trait to a bodybuilder or athlete. This compound is additionally a known thermogenic , with beta-2 agonists like clenbuterol hydrochloride shown to directly stimulate fat cells and accelerate the breakdown of triglycerides to form free fatty acids. Its efficacy in this area makes clenbuterol hydrochloride a very popular fat loss drug among the bodybuilding community. Those interested in this drug are often hoping it will produce a little of both benefits, promoting the loss of body fat while imparting increases in strength and muscle mass. But as was well pointed out by a review published in the August 1995 issue of *Medicine and Science in Sports and Exercise*, the possible anabolic results in humans are very questionable, and based only on animal data using much larger doses than would be required for bronchodilation . With such reports there has been a lot of debate as to whether or not clenbuterol hydrochloride is really anabolic in humans at all. Some seem to swear by the fact that it builds muscle, and use clenbuterol hydrochloride regularly as an off-season or adjunct anabolic. To others, the MSSE report is confirmation that athletes have wasted valuable time and money on drugs that do not build muscle. The debate over clenbuterol hydrochloride's potential anabolic activity continues today.

History:

Clenbuterol hydrochloride has been available as a bronchodilator for decades and is widely used in many parts of the world. Although it has a good safety record and approval in a wide number of other countries, this compound has never been made available for human use in the United States. The fact that there are a number of similar effective asthma medications already approved by the FDA and available may have something to do with this, as a prospective drug firm would likely not find it a profitable enough product to warrant undergoing the expense of the new drug approval process. Regardless of this fact, foreign clenbuterol hydrochloride preparations are popular among U.S. bodybuilders and athletes, and today are widely available on the black market. Note that in recent years, clenbuterol overdose/poisoning has been reported in a number of people, striking up a great deal of controversy about the safety of this drug and its off-label use for physique- and performance-enhancing purposes.

How Supplied:

Clenbuterol hydrochloride is most commonly supplied in oral tablets of 20mcg each. It is also supplied in oral syrups, injectable solutions, and for inhalation use.

Structural Characteristics:

Clenbuterol hydrochloride is a long-acting selective ,2-adrenergic receptor agonist. It has the chemical designation 1-(4-amino-3,5-dichloro-phenyl)-2-(tert-butylamino)ethanol.

Side Effects:

The possible side effects of clenbuterol hydrochloride include those of other CNS stimulants, and include such occurrences as shaky hands, insomnia, sweating, increased blood pressure, and nausea. These side effects will generally subside after a week or so of use, once the user becomes accustomed to the drug. Clenbuterol hydrochloride is a CNS stimulant with potential for fatal overdose. Signs of overdose may include rapid breathing, blood pressure irregularities, irregular heartbeat, unconsciousness, trembling, shaking, panic, extreme restlessness, and severe nausea, vomiting, or diarrhea.

Administration:

When used for the management of asthma, the most common clinical dose for adults is 20mcg (1 tablet) twice per day. Some patients require up to 40mcg (2 tablets) twice per day. When using the drug (off-label) for physique- or performance-enhancing purposes, bodybuilders and athletes generally tailor their dosage and cycling of this product based on personal sensitivity to its benefits and side effects. To accomplish this, one often begins a cycle by taking one or two tablets per day, and gradually increasing the dosage every third day by one half to 1 tablet until a desired dosage range is established. At peak therapy some users can tolerate as many as 6-8 tablets per day (120-160mcg). Given the potency and potential for serious side effects, however, any dosage outside of the normal therapeutic range should be approached with an even greater level of caution.

The drug will usually elevate the body temperature shortly after therapy is initiated. The rise in temperature is commonly .5 to 1 degree, sometimes a little more. This elevation is due to one's body burning excess energy (largely from fat), and is usually not uncomfortable. The number of consecutive days clenbuterol hydrochloride is now used is usually dependent on the response of the individual. To be clear, the athletic benefits of this drug will only last for a limited time and then diminish, largely due to beta-receptor downregulation. By most accounts clenbuterol hydrochloride seems to work well for approximately 4 to 6 weeks. During this period, users generally monitor their body temperature on a regular basis. We are given some level of assurance that clenbuterol hydrochloride is working by the temperature elevation. Once the temperature drops back to normal, receptor downregulation has probably diminished the efficacy of the drug. At this point increasing the dosage is usually not regarded as effective, and instead clenbuterol hydrochloride is discontinued for a period of no less than 4-6 weeks.

Many bodybuilding competitors enhance the fat burning effect of clenbuterol hydrochloride with the use of additional substances. Many have commented that when the drug is combined with thyroid hormones, specifically the powerful Cytomel®, the thermogenic effect can become extremely dramatic. Such a mix is often further used during a steroid cycle, helping the individual elicit a much more toned physique from the drugs. A clenbuterol/thyroid mix is also common when using growth hormone, which is believed to enhance the thermogenic and anabolic effect of HGH therapy. Lastly, ketotifen has also been a popular adjunct to clenbuterol hydrochloride, which is an antihistamine that upregulates beta-2 receptor density. It seems capable of not only increasing the potency of each dose of clenbuterol hydrochloride (allowing the user to take less clenbuterol), but also of perhaps even slowing receptor downregulation (see the Ketotifen profile for a more comprehensive discussion).

Availability:

Clenbuterol hydrochloride is readily available on the international market. Although it is usually a very cheap drug in common source countries, allowing black market dealers ample opportunity to obtain legitimate drugs to divert for sale, clenbuterol hydrochloride has been the subject of low-level counterfeiting. A few things are important to note:

Clenbuterol hydrochloride is not produced in the U.S., so

avoid anything bearing a U.S. company name.

Clenbuterol hydrochloride should only be trusted when found with a proper brand name from a foreign drug maker. Spiropent, Novegam and Oxyflux from Mexico are the most common products in the U.S.

From Europe, the brand names of Spiropent, Broncoterol, Clenasma, Monores, Contraspasmin and Ventolase are popular.

Bulgarian clenbuterol hydrochloride is also found commonly, but so are counterfeits. This is a slightly higher risk item.

Ephedrine (ephedrine hydrochloride)

Description:

Ephedrine is a stimulant drug that belongs to the group of medicines known as sympathomimetics. Specifically, it is both an alpha and beta adrenergic agonist (you may remember clenbuterol is a selective beta-2 agonist). In addition, ephedrine enhances the release of norepinephrine, a strong endogenous alpha agonist. The action of this compound is notably similar to that of the body's primary adrenergic hormone epinephrine (adrenaline), which also exhibits action toward both alpha and beta receptors. When administered, ephedrine will notably increase the activity of the central nervous system, as well as have a stimulatory effect on other target cells. This may produce some effects that can be beneficial to a bodybuilder or athlete. For starters, the user's body temperature should rise slightly as more free fatty acids are produced from the breakdown of triglycerides in adipose tissue (stimulating metabolism). This may aid in body fat reductions and increased vascularity. It is also believed that the anabolic effectiveness of steroids might be increased with this substance (mildly), as an increase in metabolic rate may equate to an increase in fat, protein and carbohydrate conversion by the body. The stimulant effect of this drug will also increase the force of skeletal muscle contractions.

History:

Ephedrine is a fairly old medication, and has been used in the United States for a number of medical applications over the years including that of a stimulant, appetite suppressant, decongestant, and hypotension treatment associated with anesthesia. Today, it is approved as an over-the-counter medicine, and sales are largely found in this sector. Controls over ephedrine in the United States are growing in recent years, however, due to the fact that it can be used as a primary base for the manufacture of methamphetamine. With ephedrine available as an over-the-counter product, underground manufacturers have been able to easily obtain it. A trend involving large volume retail purchases for OTC ephedrine products had been developing, and many states have responded with legislation controlling the sale of precursor materials like ephedrine. In 2006, a federal law was passed further restricting the record keeping requirements and available sale channels for ephedrine in the Unites States. With the widespread increase of methamphetamine addiction (and related crime), some speculate ephedrine may soon join the list of federally controlled substances. In spite of tighter regulations, it is still presently available for over-the-counter sale.

How Supplied:

Ephedrine (as ephedrine hydrochloride or ephedrine sulfate) is most commonly supplied in tablets of 25 mg or 50 mg each.

Structural Characteristics:

Ephedrine is a sympathomimetic amine related in structure to amphetamine and methamphetamine. It has the chemical designation (1R,2S)-2-(methylamino)-1-phenylpropan-1-ol.

Side Effects:

Ephedrine can produce a number of unwelcome side effects that the user should be aware of. For starters, the stimulant effect can produce shaky hands, tremors, sweating, rapid heartbeat, dizziness, and feelings of inner unrest. Often these effects subside as the user becomes more accustomed to the effect of this drug, or perhaps the dosage is lowered. In general, those negatively impacted by caffeine would probably not like the stronger effects of ephedrine. The mental and physical state produced by this drug is also quite similar to that seen with clenbuterol, so those who find little discomfort with that treatment should (presumably) be fine with this item (and vice versa). While taking this drug one may also endure a notable loss of appetite, usually a welcome effect when dieting. Ephedrine is in fact a popular ingredient in combination (prescription) appetite suppressants. The user may further notice headaches and an increase in blood pressure with regular use of ephedrine. Those suffering from thyroid dysfunctions, high blood pressure, or cardiac irregularities should also not be taking this drug, as it will certainly not mix well with such conditions. Ephedrine is a CNS stimulant with potential for fatal overdose. Signs of overdose may include rapid breathing, blood pressure irregularities, irregular heartbeat, unconsciousness, trembling, shaking, panic, extreme restlessness, and severe nausea, vomiting or diarrhea.

Administration:

The primary application for ephedrine among bodybuilders and athletes (off-label) is that of a cutting (fat-loss) agent. Here, the individual will generally take this drug a few times per day during a dieting phase of training, at a dosage of 25 to 50 mg per application. The widely touted stack of ephedrine (25-50 mg), caffeine (200 mg), and aspirin (300 mg) (E/C/A) is shown to be extremely potent for fat loss, and is more commonly applied than ephedrine alone. In this combination, the ephedrine and caffeine both act as notable thermogenic stimulants. The added aspirin also helps to inhibit lipogenesis by blocking the incorporation of acetate into fatty acids. The athlete may use an increase in body temperature as a marker that the drug combination is working. This is usually a degree or so (not an uncomfortable raise). This combination is taken 2 to 3 times daily, for several consecutive weeks. It is discontinued once the user's body temperature drops back to normal, a clear sign these drugs are no longer working as desired. A break of at least 4-6 weeks is usually taken so that this stack may once again work at an optimal level.

Ephedrine is also used by some competitive athletes (including powerlifters) as a stimulant before workouts or competitions. The resulting (slight) strength and energy increase may improve anaerobic performance and weight totals on major lifts. On this same note, it is also believed by some to provide a mental edge, making the user more energetic and better able to concentrate on the tasks ahead. A pre-event dose of 25-50 mg of ephedrine is typically used for this purpose. It is important to note that this compound is not used continuously as a pre-workout or pre-event stimulant, as its effect will diminish as the body becomes accustomed to the drug. In most instances, the user will take the drug only 2 or 3 times per week, usually on those days personally "important". The individual would also be wise to take a break (at least 1 to 2 months) from ephedrine after several weeks have passed, so as to continue receiving the optimal effect from this drug.

Availability:

Ephedrine is widely available in the U.S. and in a number of countries abroad. It is not commonly a target of counterfeiting operations.

Meridia® (sibutramine hydrochloride)

Description:

Sibutramine hydrochloride is a selective serotonin and noradrenalin re-uptake inhibitor used for the medical management of obesity. This pharmaceutical is intended to be an adjunct to a reduced calorie diet, which will help increase weight loss compared to that achieved with modifying food intake alone. Sibutramine hydrochloride is not advertised as a rapid acting drug, but instead one that fosters slow, safe, and steady losses in fat mass which are maintained long-term.

Sibutramine hydrochloride exerts a weight-loss effect through two distinct mechanisms. It has a marked ability to suppress appetite. During some studies, patients would reduce their daily energy intake by as much as 1,300 calories while taking this drug.[869] In addition to its effects on caloric intake, sibutramine also stimulates metabolism and daily caloric expenditure. A single 10 mg dose has been demonstrated to increase basal metabolic rate by up to 30%, an effect that is maintained for at least six hours. This thermogenic action is known to occur via the adrenergic system, mainly through the indirect support of beta 3 receptor activation. With the use of this drug, we are specifically seeing a strong increase in brown adipose tissue thermogenesis (BAT), which is accompanied by body temperature increases of .5 – 1 degree Celsius.[870] Elevated body temperature is a good indicator that thermogenesis is being triggered, which you may recall as one of the key things we are looking for when taking clenbuterol.

To get a better idea of exactly how well sibutramine hydrochloride works, we refer to some of the clinical studies on this agent. One investigation was conducted at the Kansas Foundation for Clinical Pharmacology in 2001. Here, a group of 322 obese patients were given either 20 mg of sibutramine or placebo once daily for 24 weeks. By the conclusion of this study, 42% of patients in the sibutramine group lost 5% or more of their initial body weight, while 12% noticed a 10% or greater loss in body weight. Sibutramine was also associated with significant improvements in serum triglyceride and HDL cholesterol levels, which were displaying poor values at the onset of the study. Another detailed investigation was completed in China by the Department of Endocrinology for Rui-jin Hospital this same year, and involved giving only 10 mg per day of sibutramine to a group of 120 men and women.[871] This investigation also faired extremely well, with patients losing an average of 15 pounds by the 24th week of use.

History:

Sibutramine hydrochloride is one of the more recent weight loss medications to reach the commercial drug market in the U.S., receiving Food and Drug Administration approval in 1998. It is sold here under the brand name Meridia. This pharmaceutical was developed by Abbott Laboratories, which also sells it in many international markets under the name Reductil. Sibutramine is classified as a schedule IV controlled substance in this market, which imparts some important legal consequences for its distribution or possession. The drug is not currently extremely popular with athletes, although it does show up in related circles from time to time.

How Supplied:

Sibutramine hydrochloride is most commonly supplied in capsules of 5 mg, 10 mg, and 15 mg.

Structural Characteristics:

Sibutramine hydrochloride is a centrally-acting serotonin-norepinephrine reuptake inhibitor structurally related to amphetamine. It is chemically a racemic mixture of (+) and (-) enantiomers of 1-(4-chlorophenyl)-N,N-dimethyl-a-(2-methylpropyl)-cyclobutanemethanamine.

Side Effects:

The most common side effect with sibutramine is an increase in blood pressure, a trait that contraindicates its use in patents with high blood pressure or other cardiovascular issues. Other common side effects include dry mouth, sleeplessness, irritability, back pain, stomach upset, and constipation, all of which tend to become reduced in magnitude as the user becomes accustomed to the drug. Sibutramine hydrochloride should be discontinued immediately if any of the more serious side effects or symptoms of toxicity occur, including excitement, restlessness, loss of consciousness, confusion, agitation, weakness, shivering, clumsiness, rapid heartbeat, large pupils, vomiting, difficulty breathing, chest pains, swelling of feet, ankles or legs, fainting, disorientation, depression, high fever, eye pain, tremor, or excessive sweating.

Administration:

Sibutramine hydrochloride is FDA approved for the management of obesity, including weight loss and maintenance and should be used in conjunction with a reduced-calorie diet. This drug may be used with patients who have additional weight-related risk factors including controlled hypertension, diabetes, and dyslipidemia (high cholesterol). The recommended starting dosage for most patients is 10 mg once daily, which is to be adjusted upwards to 15 mg after 4 weeks if weight loss has not been sufficiently initiated. Higher doses are usually not recommended.

Availability:

Being that obesity is a ubiquitous problem in the United States, the numbers of prescriptions written for this drug every year are quite high. There are many doctors and clinics that specialize in weight loss therapy, some of which may dispense the drug through the mail (depending on local laws).

Zaditen® (ketotifen fumarate)

Description:

Ketotifen is an antihistamine drug that is used for the treatment of general allergy symptoms, certain allergic conditions (including conjunctivitis), and the management of asthma. When used for asthma, the drug is not regarded as effective for treating an immediate attack (it is not a rapid bronchodilator). Instead, over time its use is associated with a reduction in the frequency, duration, and severity of attacks. It is usually prescribed as a way to increase the efficacy of other asthma medications. Likewise, ketotifen fumarate will usually supplement an existing asthma medication program, and not replace the prescribing of immediate rescue devices such as an asthma inhaler or nebuliser.

Ketotifen fumarate alleviates allergy symptoms by blocking histamine H1 receptors, a property that is common to drugs of the antihistamine class. Its second and very unique mode of action, however, makes it useful in the treatment asthma. Ketotifen fumarate increases the concentration of beta-adrenergic receptors in the body (especially beta-2 receptors). Drugs that stimulate beta-2 receptors are commonly prescribed as bronchodilators, used to increase airflow to the lungs and counter the constriction caused by asthma. While potentially efficacious alone, one key therapeutic effect of ketotifen fumarate is to increase the sensitivity of the body to drugs of the beta agonist class.

The beta-2 receptor upregulating properties of ketotifen fumarate make this drug of interest to the bodybuilding and athletic communities. This is due to the strong role of the beta-2 receptor in supporting fat loss. Although not a strong fat loss compound by itself, when taken with a beta-2 agonist thermogenic like clenbuterol, ketotifen fumarate may increase thermogenic potency and noticeably extend the window of active lipolysis. Clenbuterol and other beta-2 agonists normally have a limited duration of usefulness here because beta-2-adrenergic receptors decrease in number with regular stimulation. Within several weeks of initiating therapy with such a drug, it usually begins to diminish in effectiveness. Ketotifen may extend this time period considerably.

The ability of ketotifen to potentiate the effects of beta-2 agonist drugs has been demonstrated in a number of clinical studies. For example, one study published in 1990 demonstrated that when ketotifen and clenbuterol were taken together, there was a significant increase in beta-adrenergic receptor density compared to the use of clenbuterol alone, which again decreases beta adrenoceptor density fairly quickly.[872] Other studies with salbutamol (also referred to generically as albuterol) showed that beta adrenoceptor downregulation caused by long-term use of this beta-adrenergic agent could be rapidly reversed with as little as 2mg of ketotifen fumarate per day.[873]

History:

Ketotifen was globalized as a prescription medication by Novartis. It is presently prescribed for allergies, allergic conditions, and (most commonly) the management of asthma in more than three-dozen countries around the world. The most widely available brand name is Novartis' Zaditen, which is sold throughout most parts of Europe and Asia. In addition to generic forms of the medication, dozens of other brand names can be found in many different markets as well. Ketotifen fumarate is approved for sale in the United States, but currently only as an ophthalmic anti-allergy solution (Zaditor), not an oral allergy/asthma medication. The dosage of ketotifen fumarate in this product is also too low for it to be considered useful for any other (off label) purpose. Given the ready availability of ketotifen fumarate in other countries, the drug is easily diverted for black market sale. As of now, it is not extremely popular with bodybuilders and athletes.

The UK guidelines on the clinical management of asthma consider ketotifen to be ineffective for the management of this disease. There is admittedly conflicting data on the potential usefulness of ketotifen fumarate for this purpose, with some studies reporting positive results and others showing an insignificant effect. A thorough review of the data published on the Cochrane Database of systematic Reviews in 2004 concluded that it appeared to have some usefulness in controlling asthma and wheezing in many children, but the variability of the disease and response to the drug meant that these positive results could not be generalized for all asthma patients.[874]

How Supplied:

Ketotifen fumarate is most commonly supplied in tablets

of 1mg. This dosage is usually expressed in terms of the base, so each tablet actually contains 1.38mg of ketotifen fumarate.

Structural Characteristics:

Ketotifen fumarate is selective histamine H1 antagonist, anti-allergic, and anti-asthmatic agent. It has the chemical designation 4-(1-Methyl-4-piperidylidene-4H-benzo[4,5]cyclohepta[1,2-b]thiphene-1-(9H)-one fumarate.

Side Effects:

Common side effects include dry mouth, appetite stimulation, weight gain, dizziness, CNS stimulation, and drowsiness. These side effects are all commonly associated with strong antihistamine compounds. In rare cases severe allergic reaction on the skin or a urinary bladder inflammation called cystitis may occur.

Administration:

When used to reduce the frequency, duration, and severity of asthma attacks, ketotifen fumarate is usually initiated at a dosage of 1mg twice per day (2mg total). If necessary, this may be increased to a maximum dosage of 2mg twice per day (4mg total). Bodybuilders and athletes will commonly use a dosage of 1mg twice per day (2mg total) for the (off-label) use of preventing receptor downregulation with clenbuterol or other beta-agonists. This may allow an individual to obtain a strong thermogenic effect from, and run longer cycles with, beta-2 agonist drugs. Note that given its ability to increase drug sensitivity, the dosage of beta-2 agonist medications may need to be reduced upon ketotifen fumarate administration.

Availability:

Ketotifen fumarate is widely available, and is sold under numerous brand names in many countries. Large scale counterfeiting of this medication is currently not known to be a problem.

FAT LOSS AGENTS - THYROID Drug Profiles

Cytomel® (liothyronine sodium)

Description:

Liothyronine sodium is a synthetically manufactured prescription thyroid hormone. It specially consists of the L-isomer of the natural thyroid hormone triiodothyronine (T3). Thyroid hormones stimulate basal metabolic rate, and are involved with many cellular functions including protein, fat, and carbohydrate metabolism. Liothyronine sodium is used medically to treat hypothyroidism, a condition where the thyroid gland does not produce sufficient levels of thyroid hormone. Hypothyroidism is usually diagnosed with a serum hormone profile (T3, T4, & TSH), and may manifest itself with symptoms including loss of energy, lethargy, weight gain, hair loss, and changes in skin texture. T3 is the most active thyroid hormone in the body, and consequently liothyronine sodium is considered to be a more potent thyroid medication than levothyroxine sodium (T4).

Bodybuilders and athletes are attracted to liothyronine sodium for its ability to increase metabolism and support the breakdown of body fat. Most often utilized during contest preparation or periods of "cutting", the drug is usually said to significantly aid in the loss of fat, often on higher levels of caloric intake than would normally be permissive of such fat loss. To this end, the drug is also commonly used in conjunction with other fat loss agents such as human growth hormone or beta agonists. Some users also ascribe an ability of thyroid hormones like liothyronine sodium to increase the anabolic effect of steroids. While in theory these drugs may support the greater utilization of protein and carbohydrates for muscle growth, they are not widely proven or accepted for this purpose.

History:

The first medication that included T3 was technically a thyroid extract, first given to a patient with myxedema (a skin disorder associated with hypothyroidism) in 1891.[875] Natural thyroid extracts contained therapeutically viable levels of the thyroid hormones T3 and T4, and were widely used in medical practice for more than 60 years. In the 1950s, however, these drugs slowly start giving way to new synthetic thyroid medications, namely liothyronine sodium and levothyroxine sodium, which were consistent in dosage and effect, and more desirable to consumers than prepared animal extracts. Although liothyronine sodium and levothyroxine sodium are both widely available in the U.S. and abroad to this day, liothyronine retains a significantly smaller portion of the global thyroid market. Given its more potent and fast acting effect, however, liothyronine sodium remains a popular thyroid drug with bodybuilders and athletes. Cytomel® is the most recognized trade name for the drug in the U.S, where it is presently sold under the King Pharmaceuticals brand name.

How Supplied:

Liothyronine sodium is most commonly supplied in oral tablets of 5 mcg, 25 mcg, and 50 mcg.

Structural Characteristics:

Liothyronine sodium is a synthetic form of T3 thyroid hormone. It has the chemical designation l-tyrosine,o-(4-hydroxy-3-iodophenyl)-3,5-diiodo-,monosodium salt.

Warnings:

FDA requires the following black box warning accompany prescription liothyronine sodium products sold in the U.S.: "Drugs with thyroid hormone activity, alone or together with other therapeutic agents, have been used for the treatment of obesity. In euthyroid patients, doses within the range of daily hormonal requirements are ineffective for weight reduction. Larger doses may produce serious or even life-threatening manifestations of toxicity, particularly when given in association with sympathomimetic amines such as those used for their anorectic effects."

Side Effects:

Side effects are generally associated with overdosage, and may include headache, irritability, nervousness, sweating, irregular heartbeat, increased bowel motility, or menstrual irregularities. Overdosage may also induce shock, and may aggravate or trigger angina or congestive heart failure. Chronic overexposure to liothyronine sodium will produce symptoms normally associated with hyperthyroidism or the overproduction of natural thyroid hormones in the body. The occurrence of overexposure-linked side effects is normally cause to immediately reduce or discontinue therapy with liothyronine sodium. Acute massive overdose may be life threatening.

Administration:

When used to treat mild hypothyroidism, the typical recommended starting dosage is 25 mcg daily. The daily dosage then may be increased by no more than 25 mcg every 1 to 2 weeks. The established maintenance dose is usually 25-75 mcg per day. Once a day administration of the full daily dose is usually recommended. Although liothyronine sodium is fast acting, its effects may persist in the body for several days after discontinuance.

The usual protocol among bodybuilders and athletes taking liothyronine sodium to accelerate fat loss involves initiating its use with a dosage of 25 mcg per day. This dosage may be increased by 25 mcg every 4 to 7 days, usually reaching a maximum of no more than 75 mcg per day. As in a medical setting, the intent of this slow buildup is to help the body become adjust to the increasing thyroid hormone levels, and avoid sudden changes that may initiate side effects.

Cycles of liothyronine sodium usually last no longer than 6 weeks, and administration of the drug should not be halted abruptly. Instead, it is discontinued in the same slow manner in which it was initiated. This usually entails reducing the dosage by 25 mcg every 4 to 7 days. This tapering is done so that the body has time to readjust its endogenous hormone production at the conclusion of therapy, and to avoid the onset of side effects.

Availability:

Liothyronine is an old and widely prescribed medication. It can be found readily in most areas of the world, and is sold in a variety of different brand and generic forms. Counterfeiting is not a large-scale problem. It is important to note than one should never purchase an injectable form of this drug. These are generally used as emergency room products only, with potentially very dangerous side effects if misused.

Synthroid® (levothyroxine sodium)

Description:

Levothyroxine sodium is a synthetically manufactured form of the natural thyroid hormone tetraiodothyronine (T-4). Thyroid hormones are primarily responsible for regulating the body's metabolic rate, and play a vital role in the body's utilization of protein, fat, and carbohydrates. Levothyroxine sodium is used medically to treat cases of hypothyroidism, which is characterized by insufficient natural production of thyroid hormones. This may manifest itself with a number of symptoms including loss of energy, lethargy, weight gain, hair loss, and changes in skin texture. Levothyroxine sodium is considered a slow-acting medication, and may take up to 4 to 6 weeks before full therapeutic levels are reached in the blood. It is also the most commonly prescribed thyroid medication in the world, and is considered to be the standard form of treatment for most cases of hypothyroidism.

The action of levothyroxine sodium is very similar to that of the popular thyroid preparation Cytomel® (liothyronine sodium). Cytomel® is slightly different in structure, however, being a synthetic form of the thyroid hormone triiodothyronine (T-3). A healthy individual with have sufficient levels of both T-3 and T-4 thyroid hormones present in their body. T-3 is considered the primary active form of thyroid hormone, while T4 serves mainly as a reserve for T3, exerting most of its metabolic activity via conversion to T3 in peripheral tissues. T3 is regarded as having an effect that is roughly four times stronger than that of T-4 on a milligram-for-milligram basis. Likewise, Cytomel® is considered to be a more potent form of thyroid medication, both with regard to activity and side effect potential.

Levothyroxine sodium is valued by many drug-using athletes and bodybuilders for its ability to stimulate the metabolic rate and support the breakdown of body fat stores. It is usually taken during a period of calorie restriction ("cutting"), when the individual is focused on fat loss or increasing muscle definition. It is often thought that the use of thyroid drugs can support fat loss at a higher level of caloric intake than would otherwise be possible without the drugs, adding to their perceived value among the communities. Anabolic steroids are generally used in conjunction with these hormones, and many believe that the metabolism boosting effect of these drugs may produce faster gains in muscle mass. The drugs, however, have yet to be widely proven or accepted for this purpose.

History:

Levothyroxine sodium was the first synthetic thyroid medication to be sold in the U.S., and was first introduced to market in 1955 by Flint Laboratories as Synthroid. The drug has a long history of therapeutic use in the U.S. and internationally, and for decades has been the most widely prescribed medication for the treatment of hypothyroid. The Synthroid brand has historically been the most successful, with figures estimating that it retained 85% of total levothyroxine sales and $600 million in annual revenues (1990 estimates). In the bodybuilding and athletic communities, however, the faster acting and more powerful drug Cytomel (liothyronine sodium) is most popular. Since Synthroid is weaker and slower acting, athletes need to take the drug for a longer duration to achieve similar results.

The Synthroid brand itself has a long and at times controversial history.[876] For many years after its inception by Flint Laboratories, Synthroid enjoyed a virtual monopoly on the levothyroxine sodium market. Generic medications finally began taking a large share of levothyroxine sodium sales going in to the 1980s. In response, Flint Laboratories funded a study at the University of California in 1986 which attempted to demonstrate that Synthroid had a higher therapeutic value than its generic counterparts. The study was completed in 1990, and, in fact, proved that the generic drugs had equal efficacy to Synthroid.[877] Flint exercised a clause in its contract requiring company approval before the university could publish its study. A legal battle over its publication ensued. Even after Flint Laboratories was sold to Boots, and thereafter Boots sold to Knoll, publication of the study was vigorously opposed. It was eventually ordered into publication in 1997. A class action lawsuit followed, alleging that misconduct over the publication and marketing claims forced consumers to pay 2 to 3 times more for a brand name drug than an equivalent generic counterpart. Knoll eventually settled for $135 million.

How Supplied:

Levothyroxine sodium is most commonly supplied in oral tablets of 25 mcg, 50 mcg, 75 mcg, 100 mch, 125 mcg, 150 mcg, 200 mcg, and 300 mcg.

Structural Characteristics:

Levothyroxine sodium is a synthetic form of T4 thyroid hormone. It has the chemical designation L-3,3',5,5'-tetraiodothyronine sodium salt.

Warnings:

FDA requires that the following black box warning accompany prescription liothyronine sodium products sold in the U.S. "Thyroid hormones, including levothyroxine sodium, either alone or with other therapeutic agents, should not be used for the treatment of obesity or for weight loss. In euthyroid patients, doses within the range of daily hormonal requirements are ineffective for weight reduction. Larger doses may produce serious or even life threatening manifestations of toxicity, particularly when given in association with sympathomimetic amines such as those used for their anorectic effects."

Side Effects:

Side effects are generally associated with overdosage, and may include headache, irritability, nervousness, sweating, irregular heartbeat, increased bowel motility, or menstrual irregularities. Overdosage may also induce shock, and may aggravate or trigger angina or congestive heart failure. Chronic overexposure to levothyroxine sodium will produce symptoms normally associated with hyperthyroidism, or the overproduction of natural thyroid hormones in the body. The occurrence of overexposure-linked side effects is normally cause to immediately reduce or discontinue therapy with levothyroxine sodium. Acute massive overdose may be life threatening.

Administration:

When used to treat mild to moderate hypothyroidism, the average replacement dose of levothyroxine sodium is approximately 1.7 mcg/kg/day. This equates to 100-125 mcg/day per day for a 154lb adult. The full therapeutic dose may be given from the onset of therapy in otherwise healthy adult patients. Note that due to the long half-life of levothyroxine, the peak therapeutic effect at a given dose may not be achieved for 4 to 6 weeks.

When used (off-label) to accelerate fat loss by bodybuilders and athletes, the typical protocol involves slow buildup of the dosage so that the body has ample time to adjust to the changing thyroid hormone levels. An individual will generally start with a low dosage of 25-50 mcg, and will slowly increase the amount 25-50 mcg each day or two. The final dosage will usually be in the range of 100-150 mcg, and will rarely exceed 250 mcg. It is important to remember that thyroid drugs are strong medications with significant side effect potential. Cautious individuals will be sure not to use excessive amounts of levothyroxine sodium, nor continue treatment for longer than eight weeks. It is also generally advised to also reduce the Synthroid dosage gradually at the conclusion of each cycle. This is usually accomplished by dropping the dosage by 25 mcg every second or third day. The focus here, again, is to help avoid any sudden change in hormone levels that might otherwise trigger side effects. Note that due to the slow acting nature of levothyroxine sodium, it may take several weeks or longer for the active drug to be fully eliminated from the body.

Availability:

Although levothyroxine sodium is a widely manufactured drug, it is not as common on the black market as the stronger thyroid drug Cytomel®. Large scale counterfeiting does not appear to be a problem.

FAT LOSS AGENTS - OTHER Drug Profiles

DNP (2,4-Dinitrophenol)

Description:

DNP is one of the most controversial drugs in use by bodybuilders. This agent is not sold for human use anywhere in the world at this time, but is readily available as an industrial chemical. Among other things, it is used as an intermediary for the production of certain dyes, for photographic development, as a fungicide, in wood pressure-treatment to prevent rotting, and as an insecticide. It is technically classified as a poison. Although quite incongruous with this list of strong industrial/chemical uses, this chemical was sold during the era of patent medicine as a diet drug for humans. It is this property of dinitrophenol that remains of interest to some bodybuilders today.

Dinitrophenol induces weight loss by uncoupling oxidative phosphorylation, thereby markedly increasing the metabolic rate and body temperature. While this is an extremely effective way of producing rapid weight loss, there seems to be no ceiling to DNP's temperature increasing effect. Herein lies perhaps its most dangerous trait; it may allow body temperature to rise to level that can be damaging, even fatal. Writer Carl Malmberg made perhaps one of the earliest and most famous quotes about this danger back in the 1930s when he told of a physician who was "literally cooked to death" from using it. This was far from an isolated case, and deaths associated with DNP have continued over the decades. For example, a recent highly publicized story concerns a man that died on Long Island, NY in 2001 after taking DNP for only four days. The dose used was reported to be 600 mg per day, just three 200 mg capsules.

History:

The fat-loss properties of DNP were reportedly first noticed during World War I, when overweight men working with DNP in munitions plants started losing substantial amounts of weight. It did not take very long for this chemical to be identified as the cause. Soon after, it was packaged as a drug product. By 1935, more than 100,000 Americans had already used "patent medicine" remedies that included DNP. In fact, DNP was the first synthetic drug that was ever used for weight reduction in this country. While it was available, it was being widely advertised as a new, safe, and effective way to get thin. Popular brand names for DNP included Dinitriso, Nitromet, Dinitrenal and Alpha Dinitrophenol. At the peak of DNP's popularity, the drug could be found in pharmacies all across the country.

While the drug may have worked for the intended purpose, it was also introduced at a time before government review and approval of drug safety. In this regard DNP had some very strong shortcomings, and it didn't take long for reports of side effects to began pouring in. One such incident involved a dozen women in California who were temporarily blinded by the drug. Numerous reports of DNP-linked cataracts began coming in from as far away as France and Italy. It was said to be happening with doses as little as 100 mg daily when taken for long periods. Reports of more serious injury, even death, from DNP use followed. With such highly unfavorable safety reports, the drug was soon pulled. By 1938 it was off the market for good. It has never returned as a medicine for human or animal consumption. Even so, reports of death associated with DNP use continue to this day.

Author's Note: I was hesitant to even include a profile of dinitrophenol in this book, for fear it might entice someone who otherwise may not have known about it to use it. But ultimately I decided it would be better to include the historical information about the drug. The true story of DNP is a scary one and needs to be remembered. Bodybuilders must understand that the reemergence of underground DNP in the late 1990s was not a revolutionary new achievement in fat loss, but a scary repitition of one of the biggest mistakes of the patent medicine era. It is a drug from a time when an unregulated market was allowing dangerous chemicals like this to harm the public. The Food and Drug Administration (FDA) exists today to protect the public from such scenarios. Almost all experts today agree that DNP is a dangerous drug, and is not recommended for weight loss.

How Supplied:

DNP is not supplied in a form prepared for human or veterinary consumption. It is available as a research or industrial chemical only.

Structural Characteristics:

DNP (2,4-Dinitrophenol) is a cellular metabolic poison with the chemical designation 1-hydroxy-2,4-dinitrobenzene.

Side Effects:

There are many potential side effects associated with DNP use including increased heart rate, increased breathing rate, nausea, elevated body temperature, insomnia, profuse sweating, rash, skin lesions, decreased white blood cell count, cataracts, coma, and death.

Administration:

DNP is not approved for use in humans. Prescribing guidelines are unavailable. A common dose used among bodybuilders is reportedly 2mg per kg of bodyweight per day. This calculates to a dosage of 200 mg per day for a person of approximately 220 pounds of bodyweight. Note that this population tends to retain more lean muscle mass than the average (sedentary) person of the same bodyweight, which may substantially alter the results and side effects of a given dosage. Admittedly, fat loss due to DNP use is highly rapid and extreme, with some people losing as much as .5 to 1 pound of fat weight per day. This can equate to a drop of 15 or 20 pounds in only a few weeks. Given the high risks associated with DNP use, however, it is usually taken for only a few weeks at a time. The strong incidence of side effects is also regarded as an indicator that the drug should be discontinued immediately. Note that most experts regard DNP as a drug with inherent dangers that far outweigh its potential benefits.

Availability:

DNP is not available as a human or veterinary medication in any part of the world. Availability of products intended for human use is entirely in the underground realm, where products, dosages, and safety are not the subject of government approval.

Lipostabil N (phosphatidylcholine/sodium deoxycholate)

Description:

Lipostabil N is an injectable medication that contains phosphatidylcholine (PPC), a natural phospholipid. Sodium deoxycholate (a bile salt) is also added (among other ingredients) to solubilize PPC in water. It was originally developed as an intravenous solution for the improvement of serum lipids, reduction of arterial plaque, improving liver values, and the prevention or treatment of blood vessel blockages by fat particles (fat embolism). It is approved as an intravenous drug in a number of countries, mainly in Europe. Lipostabil has also had a very popular off-label use over the past several years, namely as a localized fat loss agent. Clinics in many areas of the world including Brazil, Europe, and the United States have actually marketed this as a nonsurgical alternative to liposuction. In recent years, bodybuilders have been paying some attention to this drug as well, using it as a cutting or finishing agent.

The mechanism behind Lipostabil's lipolytic (fat loss promoting) effect is unique. Upon injection, the solution acts as a detergent, causing nonspecific lysis (breakdown) of cell membranes.[878] The bile salt sodium deoxycholate is actually believed to play an important role here, and is therefore considered an active constituent of Lipostabil for the context of this profile (it is normally considered an inactive ingredient). During this process the fatty acids stored in the cell membrane are released, which includes arachidonic acid. This will trigger the inflammatory cascade, benefiting lipolysis (the inflammatory system can be a powerful remodeler of body composition) but also causing unwelcome pain and swelling. Phosphatidylcholine itself also triggers the release of lipases used in the removal of fat.[879] All of this works together to dismantle localized fat stores, which are removed via the liver in the form of gall acids.

History:

Lipostabil first appeared as a medication during the 1950s. Although not approved for prescription use in the U.S., it is approved for medical use in a number of other countries. The most popular brand name is Lipostabil N by Nattermann, although it is also found as Lipostabil Forte and simply as Lipostabil. The application of this drug for fat loss is generally viewed as an "off-label" use of the medication, although it undoubtedly remains a highly popular factor in its sales. Some doctors do believe that using Lipostabil for cosmetic purposes is controversial, and advise against using it for cosmetic reasons. When you look at the available data, however, its safety profile appears to be admittedly very high. Lipostabil has been widely used as an intravenous drug for more than 40 years, and has displayed very few clinically significant side effects during that time. Injecting the same drug subcutaneously is not likely to present any significant new or serious risks to the patient.

Network Lipolysis (an organization of some 350 doctors worldwide that supports this use of Lipostabil) reports over 18,000 cosmetic treatments without unexpected adverse events. Additionally, Dr. Hasengschwandtner, the medical director of the Austrian clinic Therapy Centre Bad Loefelden, has reported on bilirubin and gamma glutamyl transferases (markers of liver stress) values after subcutaneous Lipostabil use,[880] to see if this new method of fat remodeling is causing liver strain. The results were in line with IV use, showing no abnormal change in these values. Although we do not have a great deal of data on this off-label use of Lipostabil, what can be found is generally very positive, and suggests this drug (or natural drug, if you will) is quite safe. Lipostabil is presently sold in Germany, Spain, Italy, Czech Republic, Hong Kong, and South Africa

How Supplied:

Lipostabil is most commonly supplied in injectable ampules containing 5 mL of solution each.

Structural Characteristics:

The primary active ingredients in Lipostabil are phosphatidylcholine (phosphatidyl-N-trimethylethanolamine) and sodium deoxycholate (cholan-24-oic acid, 3,12-dihydroxy-, monosodium salt).

Side Effects:

Potential side effects associated with subcutaneous Lipostabil injections include localized swelling, redness of the skin, burning, pain, tenderness, and bruising. Systemic side effects are reported in approximately 3% of users and may include diarrhea, nausea, dizziness, and intermenstrual bleeding.[881]

Administration:

The typical practice for using this drug to promote localized fat loss involves a series of subcutaneous injections. A total dosage of 1250-2500 mg is often used, which equates to 25-50 mL of injectable solution. This dosage is divided into 20 or more separate smaller injections. These are spaced throughout the problematic area (quite commonly the abdominals or thighs), and are all given during the same office visit or application period. The drug is not administered on a daily basis.

Lipostabil injections usually cause a significant amount of inflammation in the area, which may take a week or longer to fully subside. When the inflammation does subside, however, it usually unveils a noticeable amount of fat loss. In a clinical setting, this procedure is often repeated a few times, so as to sculpt the area and achieve the desired level of fat reduction. The current guidelines set forth by Network Lipolysis call for an 8-week break between treatment periods. When taken outside of a clinical setting, it is usually advised to apply the first course at a much lower dosage in order to judge individual sensitivity to the drug. Some find it simply too painful to use, while others seem to tolerate the whole procedure extremely well.

As for the ultimate question of how well it works, it is difficult to give exact numbers, as few clinical studies have been conducted on this use of the drug. The anecdotal feedback is mixed. Many people who try it report positive results, particularly for the removal of those last stubborn areas of fat interfering with muscle definition. There do not seem to be many reports of dramatic weight loss, however, nor does it seem to be the "pharmaceutical liposuction" that some clinics describe it to be. Regardless, the reports of visible improvements in fat loss and muscle definition are consistent and compelling enough to be given credit. For those extremely overweight, this product is not likely to perform well, but as a finishing touch it may hold value.

Availability:

Lipostabil is not a controlled drug in the U.S. or Europe, and as such is fairly easy to obtain on the black market or via mail order drug distributors. "Mesotherapy" clinics selling procedures with Lipostabil are also fairly common.

GROWTH HORMONES & RELATED Drug Profiles

Human Growth Hormone (somatropin)

Description:

As its name suggests, human growth hormone is an important mediator of the human growth process. This hormone is produced endogenously by the anterior pituitary gland, and exists at especially high levels during childhood. Its growth-promoting effects are broad, and can be separated into three distinct areas: bone, skeletal muscle, and internal organs. It also supports protein, carbohydrate, lipid, and mineral metabolism, and can stimulate the growth of connective tissues. Although vital to early development, human growth hormone is produced throughout adulthood. Its levels and biological role decline with age, but continue to support metabolism, muscle tissue growth/maintenance, and the management (reduction) of adipose tissue throughout life. Somatropin specifically describes pharmaceutical human growth hormone that was synthesized with the use of recombinant DNA technology. Somatropin (rhGH) is biologically equivalent to human growth hormone (hGH) of pituitary origin.

In a medical setting, somatropin is used to treat a number of distinct health conditions. It is most notably associated with pituitary deficient dwarfism, a disease where linear growth is hindered due to insufficient endogenous growth hormone production. The drug is often given to these patients throughout childhood, and while not fully corrective, it is capable of substantially increasing linear growth before it is halted in adolescence. Somatropin is also commonly used in cases of adult-onset growth hormone deficiency, commonly associated with pituitary cancer or its treatment. It may also be prescribed to otherwise healthy individuals who are aging. The intent here is to maintain youthful levels of growth hormone, and impart an anti-aging effect. While not medically supported, the use of somatropin for this purpose is common in North America, South America, and Europe. Additionally, somatropin is used to combat muscle wasting associated with HIV infection or other diseases, and may be prescribed to treat several other conditions including Burns, Short Bowel Syndrome, and Prader-Willi syndrome.

Somatropin may be given by either subcutaneous or intramuscular injection. During clinical studies, the pharmacokinetic properties of somatropin following both methods of use were determined. When given by subcutaneous injection, somatropin has a similar but moderately higher level of bioavailability (75% vs. 63%). The rate of drug metabolism following both routes was also very similar, with somatropin displaying a half-life of approximately 3.8 hours and 4.9 hours after subcutaneous and intramuscular injection, respectively. Baseline hormone levels are usually reached between 12 hours and 18 hours following injection, with the slower times seen with intramuscular use. Given the delayed rise in IGF-1 levels, however, which can remain elevated 24 hours after hGH injection, the metabolic activity of human growth hormone will outlast its actual levels in the body. Although drug absorption is acceptable by both methods of use, daily subcutaneous administration is generally regarded as the preferred method of using somatropin.

A specific analysis of somatropin activity shows a hormone with a diverse set of effects. It is anabolic to skeletal muscle, shown to increase both the size and number of cells (processes referred to as hypertrophy and hyperplasia, respectively). The hormone also seems to have growth-promoting effects on all organs of the body excluding the eyes and brain. Somatropin has a diabetogenic effect on carbohydrate metabolism, which means that it causes blood sugar levels to rise (a process normally associated with diabetes). Excessive administration of somatropin over time may induce a state of type-2 (insulin resistant) diabetes. This hormone also supports triglyceride hydrolysis in adipose tissue, and may reduce body fat stores. Coinciding with this tends to be a reduction in serum cholesterol. The drug also tends to reduce levels of potassium, phosphorous, and sodium, and may cause a decrease in levels of the thyroid hormone triiodothyronine (T3). The latter effect marks a reduction in thyroid-supported metabolism, and can interfere with the effectiveness of extended therapy with somatropin.

Growth hormone has both direct and indirect effects. On the direct side, the hGH protein attaches to receptors in muscle, bone, and adipose tissues, sending messages to support anabolism and lipolysis (fat loss). Growth hormone also directly increases glucose synthesis (gluconeogenesis) in the liver, and induces insulin resistance by blocking its activity in target cells. The indirect effects of growth hormone are largely mediated by IGF-1 (insulin-like growth factor), which is produced in the liver and virtually all other tissues in response to growth hormone. IGF-1 is also anabolic to both muscle and bone, augmenting growth hormone's activity. IGF-1, however, also has effects that are strongly antagonistic to growth hormone. This includes increased lipogenesis (fat retention), increased glucose consumption, and decreased gluconeogenesis. The synergistic and antagonists effects of these two hormones combine to form the character of hGH. Likewise, they also dictate the effects of somatropin administration, which include the support lipolysis, increased serum glucose levels, and reduced insulin sensitivity.

Somatropin is considered to be a controversial anabolic and performance-enhancing drug in the realm of bodybuilding and athletics. The main issue of debate is the exact level of potential benefit this substance carries. While studies with HIV+ patients in a wasting state tend to support potentially strong anabolic and anticatabolic properties, studies demonstrating these same effects in healthy adults and athletes are lacking. During the 1980s, a large body of myth surrounded discussions of hGH in bodybuilding circles, which may have been fueled by the high cost of the drug and its very name ("growth hormone"). It was once thought to be the most powerful anabolic substance you could buy. Today, recombinant human growth hormone is much more affordable and readily obtained. Most experienced individuals now tend to agree that it is the fat-loss-promoting properties of somatropin that are most obvious. The drug can support muscle growth, strength gains, and increased athletic performance, but its effects are generally milder than those of anabolic/androgenic steroids. For a highly advanced athlete or bodybuilder, however, somatropin can help push body and performance further than might have been possible with steroids alone.

History:

The first human growth hormone preparations to be used in medicine were made from pituitary extracts of human origin. These are now commonly referred to as cadaver growth hormone preparations. Approximately 1 mg of hGH (a 1 day dose) could be obtained from each cadaver. The first successful treatment with human cadaver GH was reported in 1958.[882] Soon after these medicines were introduced to market, and were sold in the U.S. until 1985. The Food and Drug Administration banned them that year after they had been linked to the development of Creutzfeldt-Jakob's disease (CJD), a highly degenerative and ultimately fatal brain disorder, in a number of patients. The disease can be transmitted from one person to another under exceptional circumstances (usually blood transfusion or organ implantation are involved), and was likely caused by the extraction of hGH from infected cadavers. CJD has a very slow incubation period, and has been diagnosed anywhere from 4 to 30 years after therapy with growth hormone of cadaver origin. As of 2004 estimates, at least 26 patients that received cadaver GH drugs in the United States have been diagnosed with the disease.[883] The overall incidence of this disease is less than 1%, as approximately 6,000 patients are documented to have received the medication.

The FDA approved the first synthetic human growth hormone drug in 1985. Synthesis produced a pure hormone without biological contamination, eliminating the possibility of CJD transmission. The drug approved was called somatrem (Protropin), and was based on a manufacturing technology developed by Genentech in 1979.[884] Somatrem came at an important time given the removal of cadaver GH by the FDA that same year. This hormone is actually a slight variant of the hGH protein, but displays the same biological properties of the natural hormone. Protropin was initially very successful being it was the first synthetic GH product. By 1987, however, Kabi Vitrum (Sweden) had published methods for the production of pure synthetic somatropin with the exact amino acid sequence of endogenous growth hormone.[885] It was also discovered that the unnatural structure of somatrem causes a much higher incidence of antibody reactions in patients, which can reduce drug efficacy.[886] Somatropin would come to be viewed as a more reliable drug, and would dominate the global market within several years. Today, although somatrem products are still sold, somatropin retains the vast majority of hGH sales worldwide.

How Supplied:

Somatropin is most commonly supplied in multi-dose vials containing a white lyophilized powder that requires reconstitution with sterile or bacteriostatic water before use. Dosage may vary widely from 1mg to 24mg or more per vial. Somatropin is also available as a stabile pre-mixed solution (Nutropin AQ) that is biologically equivalent to reconstituted somatropin.

Structural Characteristics:

Somatropin is human growth hormone protein manufactured by recombinant DNA technology. It has 191 amino acid residues and a molecular weight of 22,125 daltons. It is identical in structure to human growth hormone of pituitary origin.

Storage:

Do not freeze. Follow package insert for storage information. Refrigeration (2º to 8ºC, 35º to 46º F) may be required before and after reconstitution.

Side Effects (General):

The most common adverse reactions to somatropin therapy are joint pain, headache, flu-like symptoms, peripheral edema (water retention), and back pain. Less common adverse reactions include inflammation of mucous membranes in the nose (rhinitis), dizziness, upper respiratory infection, bronchitis, tingling or numbness on the skin, reduced sensitivity to touch, general edema, nausea, sore bones, carpal tunnel syndrome, chest pain, depression, gynecomastia, hypothyroidism, and insomnia. The abuse of somatropin may cause diabetes, acromegaly (a visible thickening of the bones, most notably the feet, forehead, hands, jaw, and elbows), and enlargement of the internal organs. Due to the growth promotion effects of human growth hormone, this drug should not be used by individuals with active or recurring cancer.

Side Effects (Impaired glucose tolerance):

Somatropin may reduce sensitivity to insulin and raise blood sugar levels. This may occur in individuals without preexisting diabetes or impaired glucose tolerance.

Side Effects (Injection site):

The subcutaneous administration of somatropin may cause redness, itching, or lumps at the site of injection. It may also cause a localized decrease of adipose tissue, which may be compounded by the repeated administration at the same site of injection.

Administration:

Somatropin is designed for subcutaneous or intramuscular administration. One milligram of somatropin is equivalent to approximately 3 International Units (3 IU). When used to treat adult onset growth hormone deficiency, the drug is commonly applied at a dosage of .005/mg/kg per day to .01mg/kg per day. This equates to roughly 1 IU to 3 IU per day for person of approximately 180-220 lbs. A long-term maintenance dosage is established after reviewing the patient's IGF-1 levels and clinical response over time.

When used for physique- or performance-enhancing purposes, somatropin is usually administered at a dosage between 1 IU and 6 IU per day (2-4 IU being most common). The drug is commonly cycled in a similar manner to anabolic/androgenic steroids, with the length of intake generally being between 6 weeks and 24 weeks. The anabolic effects of this drug are less apparent than its lipolytic (fat loss) properties, and generally take longer periods of time and higher doses to manifest themselves.

Other drugs are commonly used in conjunction with somatropin in order to elicit a stronger response. Thyroid drugs (usually T3) are particularly common given the known effects of somatropin on thyroid levels, and may significantly enhance fat loss during therapy. Insulin is also commonly used with somatropin. Aside from countering some of the effects somatropin has on glucose tolerance, insulin can increase receptor sensitivity to IGF-1, and reduce levels of IGF binding protein-1, allowing for more IGF-1 activity[887] (growth hormone itself also lowers IGF binding protein levels).[888] Anabolic/androgenic steroids are also commonly taken with somatropin, in an effort to maximize potential muscle-building effects. Anabolic steroids may also further increase free IGF-1 levels via a lowering of IGF binding proteins.[889] Note that the stacking of somatropin with thyroid drugs and/or insulin is usually approached with great care and caution, given that these are particularly strong medications with potentially serious or life threatening acute side effects.

Availability:

Somatropin is produced by many different drug companies, and is distributed in virtually all developed countries. The most common brand names include Serostim (Serono), Saizen (Serono), Humatrope (Eli Lilly), Norditropin (novo nodisk), Omnitrope (Sandoz), and Genotropin (Pharmacia).

Somatropin products are high value targets for drug counterfeiting operations. Many counterfeits are highly deceptive in nature, and have been found in both illicit and legitimate drug distribution channels. Some counterfeit growth hormone products are made by relabeling vials of hCG, which bear a very close visual resemblance to somatropin. A home pregnancy test is sometimes used to help determine if hCG has been used to make a counterfeit hGH product. This test works by detecting hCG in the urine. A few days into a cycle with somatropin, the individual will take a 3-4 IU injection prior to bed. Upon rising, the pregnancy test will be used, and a positive result will indicate that an hCG counterfeit has been used. The powder in the vial of somatropin should also be in the form of a solid (lyophilized) disc. Do not take any product that contains loose powder.

Increlex® (mecasermin)

Description:

Mecasermin is human insulin-like growth factor-1 (IGF-1) manufactured by recombinant DNA technology (rhIGF-1). IGF-1 is the primary mediator of the growth promoting effects of human growth hormone. As such, mecasermin also can stimulate the growth of bone, muscle, and internal organs. Its effects on skeletal muscle are also strongly hyperplasic, meaning it causes an increase in cell number. Unlike hGH, however, mecasermin has very strong insulin-like effects. It can support growth by increasing the uptake of amino acids, glucose, and fatty acids, but lowers blood sugar levels so efficiently that it can induce severe hypoglycemia if too high a dosage is taken. The increased uptake of fatty acids also means that mecasermin may promote lipogenesis, or an increase in the storage of body fat. This agent is of interest to bodybuilders and athletes for its potential to support the growth of skeletal muscle and connective tissue.

Mecasermin is most commonly prescribed for the treatment of severe primary IGF-1 deficiency (Primary IGFD). This disease is characterized by a failure to produce normal levels of IGF-1 due to insufficiencies in the growth hormone / IGF-1 axis (usually involving GH receptor, signaling pathway, or IGF-1 gene defects). Such patients typically have normal or even high levels of growth hormone, but their bodies do not respond to it with the sufficient production of IGF-1. Mecasermin may also be used for the treatment of patients who have developed antibodies to growth hormone therapy. In both instances the patient is not GH deficient, but does not respond properly to growth hormone therapy, making IGF-1 an effective alternative medication. Given its differing effects on metabolism, however, mecasermin is not considered to be a medical substitute for hGH therapy, and retains a narrow field of FDA approved uses.

History:

The U.S. Food and Drug Administration approved Mecasermin in August 2005. It is sold under the brand name Increlex, manufactured by Tercica Inc. of Brisbane ,California. Tercica licenses this technology from Genentech, which was the first company to sell a synthetically manufactured human growth hormone product in the United States (Protropin). Tercica's rhIGF-1 is produced by a similar recombinant DNA technology. The process involves inserting the gene encoding for the human IGF-1 protein into E. coli bacteria, which then synthesize the protein. In October 2006, Tercia licensed the European rights to Increlex to the specialties pharmaceutical firm Ipsen. Ipsen received approval to market Increlex in the European Union in August 2007.

How Supplied:

Mecasermin (Increlex) is supplied in 4mL multi-dose vials containing 10 mg/mL.

Structural Characteristics:

Mecasermin is human IGF-1 protein manufactured by recombinant DNA technology. It consists of a string of 70 amino acids and has a molecular weight of 7,649 daltons. Its amino acid sequence is identical to that of endogenous human IGF-1.

Storage:

Do not freeze. Refrigeration (2° to 8°C, 35° to 46° F) required before and after reconstitution.

Side Effects (Hypoglycemia):

The most common adverse reaction to mecasermin therapy is hypoglycemia, which occurred on at least one occasion in 42% of patients receiving the drug during clinical trials. Approximately 7% of patients noticed severe hypoglycemia, and 5% noticed hypoglycemic seizure or loss of consciousness. Signs of mild to moderate hypoglycemia include hunger, drowsiness, blurred vision, depressive mood, dizziness, sweating, palpitation, tremor, restlessness, tingling in the hands, feet, lips, or tongue, lightheadedness, inability to concentrate, headache, sleep disturbances, anxiety, slurred speech, irritability, abnormal behavior, unsteady movement, and personality changes. If any of these warning signs should occur, one should immediately consume a food or drink containing simple sugars such as a candy bar or carbohydrate drink. Signs of severe hypoglycemia include disorientation, seizure, and unconsciousness. Severe hypoglycemia can lead to death and requires immediate emergency medical attention. Note that in some cases the symptoms of hypoglycemia can be mistaken for drunkenness.

Mecasermin should never be taken before sleep or in higher than recommended doses. A meal or snack must be consumed within 20 minutes (before or after) of administration.

Side Effects (Injection site):

The subcutaneous administration of mecasermin may cause bruising at the site of injection. It may also cause a localized increase of adipose tissue, which may be compounded by the repeated administration at the same site of injection. Rotation of the injection sites is recommended.

Side Effects (General):

Other potential adverse reactions to mecasermin therapy include joint pain, growth of the tonsils, snoring, headache, dizziness, convulsions, vomiting, ear pain, hearing loss, and hypertrophy of the thymus gland. Mild elevations in serum AST, ALT, and LDH levels were found in a significant number of patients, but they were not associated with hepatotoxicity. Mecasermin can stimulate the growth of internal organs. Kidney and spleen hypertrophy was particularly pronounced in the first years of long-term therapy in clinical trials, without declining renal function. Elevations in cholesterol and triglycerides were also observed, but remained within the upper limit of normal values. Evidence of heart enlargement was observed in a few patients, but this appeared without any apparent clinical significance. The overall relationship between mecasermin use and cardiac changes has not yet been fully assessed. Thickening of facial soft tissues was observed in several patients, and should be monitored during therapy. The abuse of mecasermin may cause acromegaly, which is characterized by a visible thickening of the bones, most notably the feet, forehead, hands, jaw, and elbows. Due to the growth promotion effects of hIGF-1, this drug should not be used by individuals with active or recurring cancer.

Administration:

Mecasermin is intended for subcutaneous administration. The initiation of therapy involves close monitoring of blood glucose levels until a proper maintenance dose is established. The recommended starting dose is .04 to .08 mg/kg (40 to 80 mcg/kg) twice daily. The dose may be increased by .04 mg/kg per injection, reaching a maximum of .12 mg/kg twice daily. Doses greater than .12 mg/kg are not advised due to potential hypoglycemic effects. Mecasermin should always be administered within 20 minutes (before or after) a meal or snack.

Mecasermin is not widely used for physique- or performance-enhancing purposes. Common protocols of administration have not yet been established. Due to the potential for severe hypoglycemia, maximum doses among bodybuilders and athletes are not likely to measurably exceed those supplied by therapeutic guidelines. This drug will most likely by taken in cycles lasting no longer than 8-12 weeks in an effort to minimize unwanted organ growth or fat gain.

Availability:

Mecasermin is approved for sale in the United States and Europe under the Increlex brand name.

Protropin® (somatrem)

Description:

Somatrem is a synthetically manufactured form of human growth hormone (hGH). It is actually a variant of endogenous hGH protein, containing the same sequence of 191 amino acids, but with the addition of an extra amino acid, methionine. For this reason somatrem is commonly described as methionyl human growth hormone. As an hGH medication, somatrem supports the growth of bone, skeletal muscle, connective tissues, and internal organs. It also plays a role in protein, carbohydrate, lipid, and mineral metabolism. In a medical setting, somatrem is used to treat children with growth failure caused by endogenous growth hormone deficiency. When administered as a long-term treatment before linear growth is stopped due to closed epiphyses, the drug may impart a significant positive effect on linear growth. Somatrem is considered to be therapeutically equivalent to growth hormone of pituitary origin. As an hGH drug, somatrem is valued by bodybuilders and athletes for its ability to promote fat loss and muscle and connective tissue growth.

Although somatrem is considered equivalent to human growth hormone, it is not a natural protein to the human body. This may increase the chance for developing antibodies to growth hormone during treatment. The antibodies work by binding with the growth hormone molecule, interfering with its ability to bind receptors and exert activity. In one clinical investigation, 2/3rd of the children treated with somatrem developed antibodies to growth hormone after one year.[890] In a similarly configured investigation involving the administration of somatropin for one year, only 1 in 7 patients produced serum antibodies to growth hormone.[891] It is important to note that in both studies the antibody reactions were not strong, and did not appear to substantially diminish the ability of the drugs to be therapeutically effective. Diminishment activity (as determined by antibody levels) appears in an very small percentage (<1%) of patients taking somatrem. Still, the correct 191 amino acid configuration of somatropin is considered more desirable to use.

History:

Somatrem was approved for sale in the U.S. in 1985. It was the first synthetic growth hormone medication available worldwide, produced via a manufacturing process called Inclusion Body Technology.[892] The technology involves inserting the DNA encoding for the hGH protein into escherichia coli (E.coli) bacteria, which assemble and synthesize the pure protein. Prior to the advent of synthetic growth hormone, hGH was made into a medication only by extracting the natural protein from human corpses. Biological or cadaver hGH, as it was called, was banned in the U.S. in 1985 due to the high prevalence of a rare neurological disease in patients. Somatrem was approved for sale that same year, giving Genentech a short monopoly on the growth hormone market. Within several years, however, other biotechnology companies began selling a form of hGH that was identical to the endogenous protein, called somatropin. Although somatrem remains available in a number of markets including the United States, somatropin is much more widely distributed.

How Supplied:

Somatrem is most commonly supplied in multi-dose vials containing a white lyophilized powder that requires reconstitution with sterile or bacteriostatic water before use. Dosage may vary from 1mg to 10 mg per vial.

Structural Characteristics:

Somatrem is a polypeptide (methionyl human growth hormone) manufactured by recombinant DNA technology. It has 192 amino acid residues and a molecular weight of 22,256 daltons.

Storage:

Do not freeze. Refrigeration (2° to 8°C, 35° to 46° F) required before and after reconstitution.

Side Effects (General):

The most commonly reported adverse reactions to somatrem therapy include carpal tunnel syndrome, increased growth of nevi (moles and birthmarks), gynecomastia, and pancreatitis. Note that the side effects of somatrem will generally mirror those of somatropin therapy. The abuse of somatrem may cause diabetes, acromegaly (a visible thickening of the bones, most notably the feet, forehead, hands, jaw, and elbows), and enlargement of the internal organs. Due to the growth promotion effects of human growth hormone, this drug should not be used by individuals with active or recurring cancer.

Side Effects (Impaired glucose tolerance):

Somatrem may reduce sensitivity to insulin and raise blood sugar levels. This may occur in individuals without preexisting diabetes or impaired glucose tolerance.

Side Effects (Injection site):

The subcutaneous administration of somatrem may cause redness, itching, or lumps at the site of injection. It may also cause a localized decrease of adipose tissue, which may be compounded by the repeated administration at the same site of injection.

Administration:

Somatrem is given by subcutaneous or intramuscular injection. One milligram of somatrem is equivalent to approximately 3 International Units (3IU). When used to treat children with growth failure due to growth hormone deficiency, the drug is applied at a dosage up to .04/mg/kg per day. This equates to a maximum of roughly 10IU per day for a person of approximately 180 lbs. A long-term maintenance dosage is established after reviewing the patient's IGF-1 levels and clinical response over time, and may be substantially lower than 10IU.

When used for physique- or performance-enhancing purposes, somatrem is usually administered at a dosage between 1IU and 6 IU per day (2-4 IU being most common). The drug is commonly cycled in a similar manner to anabolic/androgenic steroids, with the length of intake generally being between 6 weeks and 24 weeks. The anabolic effects of this drug are less apparent than its lipolytic (fat loss) properties, and generally take longer periods of time and higher doses to manifest themselves.

Availability:

Somatrem is available in the United States under the Protropin brand name which is distributed by Roche. In Europe and most nations the vast majority of hGH is the correct 191 amino acid sequence somatropin. Somatrem can be found in some markets, however, most commonly in Asia, where it tends to sells for a substantially lower price than somatropin.

HYPOGLYCEMICS Drug Profiles

Insulin (rDNA Origin)

Description:

Insulin is peptide hormone produced in the Islets of Langerhans in the pancreas. The release of this hormone in the human body is most closely tied to blood glucose levels, although a number of other factors including pancreatic and gastrointestinal hormones, amino acids, fatty acids, and ketone bodies are also involved. The main biological role of insulin is to promote the intracellular utilization and storage of amino acids, glucose, and fatty acids, while simultaneously inhibiting the breakdown of glycogen, protein, and fat. It is most notably identified with the control of blood sugar levels, and insulin medications are typically prescribed to people with diabetes, a metabolic disorder characterized by hyperglycemia (high blood sugar). While insulin targets many different organs in the body, this hormone is both anabolic and anti-catabolic to skeletal muscle tissue,[893][894][895] a fact that explains the inclusion of pharmaceutical insulin in the realm of athletics and bodybuilding.

The use of insulin to improve performance and body composition can be a little tricky because this hormone can also promote nutrient storage in fat cells. This, however, is an activity of insulin that can be somewhat managed by the user. Athletes have found that a strict regimen of intense weight training and a diet without excess caloric and fat intake can enable insulin to show a much higher affinity for protein and glucose storage in muscle (as opposed to fatty acid storage in adipose) cells. This is especially true in the post-exercise enhanced-absorptive state, where insulin sensitivity in skeletal muscle has been shown to increase significantly over baseline (rested) levels.[896] When used during the post-training window, the hormone is, likewise, capable of producing rapid and noticeable muscle gains. The muscles often begin to look fuller (and even sometimes more defined) very soon after initiating insulin therapy, and the overall results of therapy are often described as dramatic.

The fact that insulin use cannot be detected by urinalysis has ensured it a place in the drug regimens of many athletes and professional bodybuilders. Note that there has been some progress in drug detection, especially with the analogs, but to date regular insulin is still considered a "safe" drug. Insulin is often used in combination with other "contest safe" drugs like human growth hormone, thyroid medications, and low dose testosterone injections, and together can have a dramatic effect on the user's physique and performance without fear of a positive urinalysis result. Those who do not have to worry about drug testing, however, often find that insulin combined with anabolic/androgenic steroids can be a very synergistic combination. This is because the two actively support an anabolic state through different mechanisms. Insulin strongly enhances the transport of nutrients into muscle cells and inhibits protein breakdown, and the anabolic steroids (among other things) strongly increase the rate of protein synthesis.

As mentioned, the usual medical purpose for insulin is to treat different forms of diabetes. More specifically, the human body may not be producing enough insulin (Type-I diabetes), or may not recognize insulin well at the cell site although some level is present in the blood (Type-II diabetes). Type-I diabetics are, therefore, required to inject insulin on a regular basis, as they are left without a sufficient level of this hormone. Along with medication, the individual will need to constantly monitor blood glucose levels and regulate their sugar intake. Together with lifestyle modifications such as regular exercise and developing a balanced diet, insulin dependent individuals can live a healthy and full life. When left untreated, however, diabetes can be a fatal disease.

History:

Insulin first became available as a medicine during the 1920s. Credit for the discovery is most appropriately given to Canadian physician Fred Banting and Canadian physiologist Charles Best, who worked together to produce the first insulin preparations, and the world's first effective treatment of diabetes. Their work stemmed from an idea initially proposed by Banting, who as a young doctor theorized that an active extract could be made from animal pancreases to regulate blood sugar in human patients. He needed help to try and actualize his idea, and he sought out world-renowned physiologist J.J.R. Macleod at the University of Toronto. Macleod, initially less than impressed with the unusual concept (but likely impressed with Banting's conviction and tenacity), assigned a couple of graduate students to assist him in his work. A coin flip determined who would work with Banting, and he was eventually paired with graduate student Best. Together they made medical history.

The first insulin preparations they produced were made of crude pancreatic extracts taken from dogs. At one point the supply of laboratory animals was exhausted, and desperate to continue their research, the pair actually began taking stray dogs to supplement their pancreas supply. Shortly after, the two found that they could work with the pancreases of slaughtered cows and pigs, making their work much easier (and ethically acceptable). They successfully treated their first diabetic patient with insulin in January 1922. By August of that year, they had been successful in treating a group of clinical patients, including 15-year-old Elizabeth Hughes, daughter of former presidential candidate Charles Evans Hughes. Elizabeth was diagnosed with diabetes in 1918, and her dramatic fight for life with the disease gained national attention. Elizabeth would be saved by insulin on the doorstep of starvation, as severe calorie restriction was the only remedy known to slow the disease at the time. Banting and Macleod swiftly won the Nobel Prize for their discovery, which was presented to them approximately a year later in 1923. Shortly after, dispute over credit arose, and ultimately Banting shared his prize with Best, and Macleod shared his prize with J. B. Collip, a chemist that assisted in the extraction and purification process.

After initially declining the assistance in the hopes that they could work out production issues on their own, Banting and his team worked with Eli Lilly & Co. to develop the first mass-produced insulin medicines using their animal extraction techniques. Their production success was extreme and rapid, and the drug became commercially available on a wide scale in 1923, the same year Banting and Macleod won the Nobel prize. That same year, Nordisk Insulinlaboratorium was founded by Danish scientist Augusta Krogh, who desperately wanted to bring back an insulin manufacturing technique to Denmark to treat his wife, who was ill with diabetes. This Denmark firm eventually became Novo Nordisk, the world's second leading producer of insulin next to Eli Lilly & Co.

The early insulin medications were fairly impure by today's standards. They typically contained 40 units of animal insulin per milliliter, in contrast to today's accepted standard concentration of 100 units. The large doses needed with these early low-concentration drugs were not very comfortable for patients, and injection-site reactions were not uncommon. They also contained significant protein impurities that would sometimes cause allergic reactions in users. Despite these faults, the drugs saved the lives of countless individuals who beforehand were faced with a sure death sentence following a diagnosis of diabetes. Eli Lilly and Novo Nordisk improved the purity of their products in the coming years, but no major improvements in insulin technology developed until the mid-1930s, when the first longer-acting insulin preparations began to surface.

The first longer-acting drug made use of protamine and zinc to delay the action of insulin in the body, extending the activity curve and reducing the number of daily injections required for many patients. Dubbed Protamine Zinc Insulin (PZI), the preparation would have an effect lasting as long as 24-36 hours. Neutral Protamine Hagedorn (NPH) Insulin, also known as Isophane insulin, followed, reaching market by 1950. This preparation was very similar to PZI insulin except that it could be mixed with regular insulin without disturbing the release curve of the respective insulins. In other words, a regular insulin drug could be mixed in the same syringe with NPH insulin, providing a biphasic release pattern characterized by an early peak effect due to the regular insulin, and an extended action brought on by the NPH.

In 1951 the Lente insulins began to surface, which included semilente, lente, and ultra-lente preparations. The amount of zinc used in each varied, producing preparations with distinct and long-acting pharmacokinetics. Unlike previous Insulins, this was also achieved without the use of protamine. Many physicians were soon able to successfully switch their patients from NPH insulin over to a single morning dose of Lente insulin, often heralding the release of the new drugs as a big advance in insulin medications (though some would still require an evening dose with a Lente insulin to maintain full control over blood glucose levels during the 24-hour period). Up to this point the insulin drugs made by the large pharmaceutical companies worked very well. No substantial step forward in the development of new insulin delivery technologies would come for another 23 years.

In 1974, chromatographic purification techniques allowed the manufacture of animal insulin with extremely low impurity levels (less than 1 pmol/l of protein impurities). Novo was the first to release a drug made with this technology, which it called monocomponent (MC) Insulin. Eli Lilly also released a version called "Single Peak" Insulin, likely referring to the single protein peak noticed upon chemical analysis. This advance, though significant, would be short lived. In 1975, Ciba-Geigy produced the first synthetic insulin preparation (CGP 12831). And just three years later, scientists at Genentech were able to produce insulin using modified E. coli bacteria, the first synthetic insulin with an identical amino acid sequence as human insulin (although the animal insulins work fine in humans their structures are slightly different). The U.S. Food and Drug administration approved the first such medicines in 1982, with the acceptance of Humulin R (Regular) and Humulin NPH from Eli Lilly & Co. The name Humulin is a contraction of the words "human" and "insulin", of course. Novo would follow with semi-synthetic insulins Actrapid HM and Monotard HM.

The FDA has approved a variety of other insulin drug combinations over the years, including various biphasic insulin blends that use differing amounts of rapid and longer-acting insulins. More recently, we have also seen the FDA approval of Eli Lilly's rapid-acting insulin analog Humalog. Several other analogs are also now available including Lantus and Apidra from Aventis, and Levemir and Novorapid from Novo Nordisk. A number of additional analogs are also under investigation at this time. With the large variety of different insulin medications approved and sold in the U.S. and other nations, it is important to understand that "insulin" represents an extremely broad class of medicines. As a class, these drugs are likely to continue to expand as new agents are developed and successfully tested. Today, it is estimated that 55 million people use some form of injectable insulin on a regular basis to manage their diabetes, making this an extremely important and lucrative area of human medicine.

How Supplied:

Pharmaceutical insulin comes from one of two basic origins, animal or synthetic. With animal source insulin, the hormone is extracted from the pancreas of either pigs or cows (or both) and prepared for medical use. These preparations are further divided into the categories "standard" and "purified", dependent on the level of purity and non-insulin content of the solution. With such products there is always the slight possibility of pancreatic contaminants making their way into the prepared drug. Specifically called biosynthetic, synthetic insulin is produced by a recombinant DNA procedure similar to the process used to manufacture human growth hormone. The result is a polypeptide hormone consisting of one 21-amino acid "A-chain" coupled by two disulfide bonds with one 30-amino acid "B-chain". The biosynthetic process will produce a drug free of the pancreatic protein contaminants possible with animal insulin, and that is structurally and biologically identical to human pancreatic insulin. With the innate (remote) risk of contamination involved with animal insulin, coupled with the fact that the structure is (very slightly) different from human insulin, synthetic human insulin drugs dominate the market today. Biosynthetic human insulin/insulin analogs are also the most common insulins of use among athletes, and the main focus of this profile.

There are a variety of synthetic insulins available, with each possessing unique properties relating to speed of onset, peak and duration of activity, and concentration of dose. This therapeutic variety may allow physicians to tailor a treatment program for insulin-dependant diabetics that allows for the least amount of daily injections and the greatest level of patient comfort. It is important that one should be aware of the individual activity of any insulin drug before attempting its use. Due to the differences between preparations, it is also medically advised that extreme care be taken whenever a physician attempts to switch an insulin-dependant diabetic patient from one form of insulin medication to another.

Below is a list showing the distinctions between popular forms of biosynthetic insulin.

Short-acting Insulins:

Humalog® (Insulin Lispro): Humalog® is a short-acting analog of human insulin, specifically the Lys(B28) Pro(B29) analog of insulin created when the amino acids at positions 28 and 29 are reversed. It is considered equipotent to regular soluble insulin on a unit-to-unit basis, but with more rapid activity.[897] The onset of drug action following subcutaneous administration is approximately 15 minutes, and its peak effect is reached in 30 to 90 minutes. It has a total duration of action between 3 and 5 hours. Insulin lispro is usually used as a supplement to a longer acting insulin product, providing a fast-acting medication that can be taken before or immediately after meals to mimic the body's natural insulin response. Many athletes believe that its short window of effect makes it an ideal insulin medication for physique- or performance-enhancing purposes, as most of its action can be concentrated in the post-training enhanced-nutrient-uptake window.

Novolog® (Insulin Aspart): Novolog is a short-acting analog of human insulin created when the amino acid proline at position B28 is replaced with aspartic acid. The onset of drug action following subcutaneous administration is approximately 15 minutes, and its peak effect is reached in 1-3 hours. It has a total duration of action between 3 and 5 hours. Insulin lispro is usually used as a supplement to a longer acting insulin product, providing a fast-acting medication that can be taken before or immediately after meals to mimic the body's natural insulin response. Many athletes believe that its short window of effect makes it an ideal insulin medication for physique- or performance-enhancing purposes, as most of its action can be concentrated in the post-training enhanced-nutrient-uptake window.

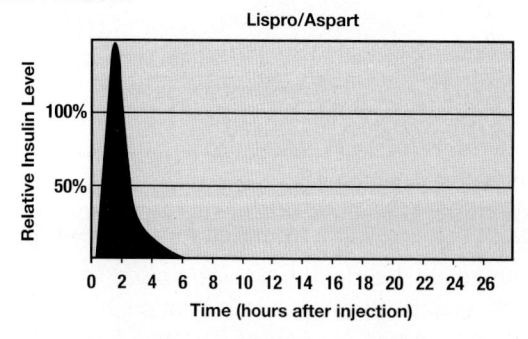

Humulin®-R "Regular" (insulin Inj): Identical to human insulin. Also sold as Humulin-S® (Soluble) in some markets, this product consists of zinc-insulin crystals dissolved in clear fluid. There is nothing added to slow the release of this product, so it is generically referred to as soluble human Insulin. This drug works rapidly and has a short duration of effect. The onset of drug action following subcutaneous administration is 20-30 minutes, and its peak effect is reached in 1-3 hours. It has a total duration of action between 5 and 8 hours. Together with Humalog, these two forms of insulin are the most popular (almost exclusive) choices among athletes and bodybuilders for physique- or performance-enhancement purposes.

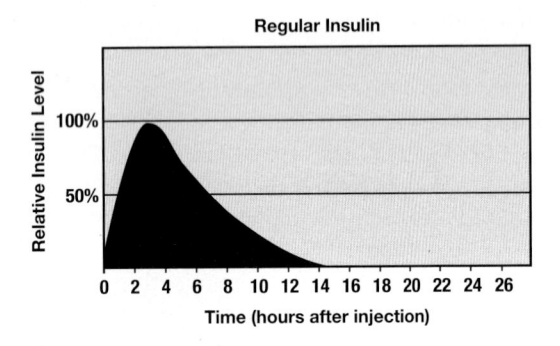

Intermediate- and Long-acting Insulins:

Humulin®-N, NPH (insulin isophane): A crystalline suspension of insulin with protamine and zinc to delay its release and extend its action. Insulin isophane is considered intermediate length insulin. The onset of drug action following subcutaneous administration is approximately 1-2 hours, and its peak effect is reached in 4-10 hours. It has a total duration of activity lasting more than 14 hours. This type of insulin is not commonly used for physique- or performance-enhancement purposes.

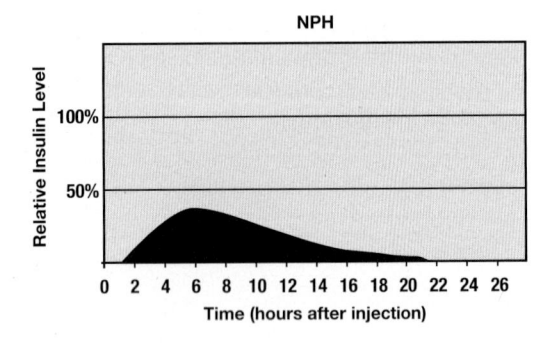

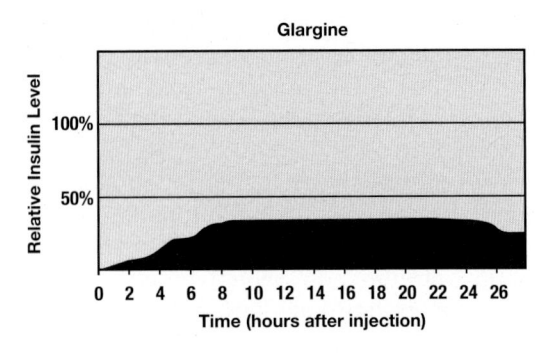

Humulin®-L, Lente (medium zinc suspension): A crystalline suspension of insulin with zinc to delay its release and extend its action. Humulin-L is considered an intermediate length insulin. The onset of drug action following subcutaneous administration is approximately 1-3 hours, and its peak effect is reached in 6-14 hours. It has a total duration of activity lasting more than 20 hours. This type of insulin is not commonly used for physique- or performance-enhancement purposes.

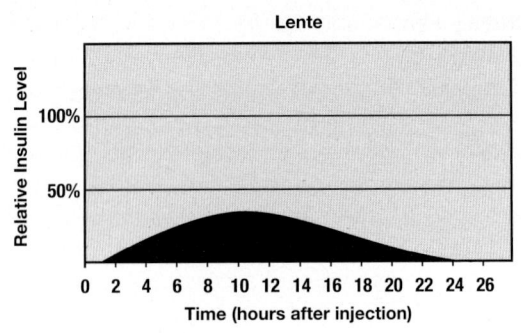

Humulin®-U, Ultralente (prolonged zinc suspension): A crystalline suspension of insulin with zinc to delay its release and extend its action. Humulin-U is considered a long-acting insulin. The onset of drug action following subcutaneous administration is approximately 6 hours, and its peak effect is reached in 14-18 hours. It has a total duration of activity lasting 18-24 hours. This type of insulin is not commonly used for physique- or performance-enhancement purposes.

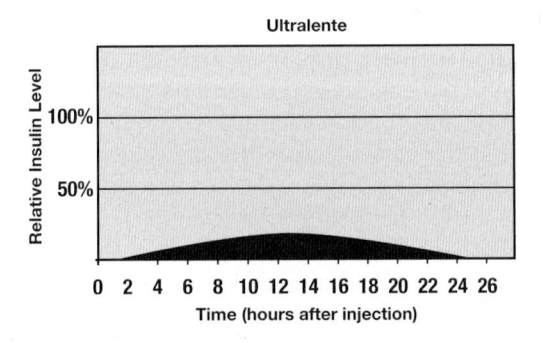

Lantus (insulin glargine): A long-acting analog of human insulin. Insulin glargine is created when the amino acid asparagine at position A21 is replaced by glycine, and two arginines are added to the C-terminus of the insulin B chain. The onset of drug action following subcutaneous administration is approximately 1-2 hours, and the drug is considered to have no significant peak (it is designed to have a very stable release pattern throughout the duration of activity). Insulin glargine lasts between 20-24 hours in the body following subcutaneous injection. This type of insulin is not commonly used for physique- or performance-enhancement purposes.

Biphasic Insulins:

Humulin® Mixtures: These are mixtures of regular soluble insulin for a fast onset of action, and a long- or intermetiate-acting insulin for a prolonged effect. These are labeled by the mixture percentage, commonly 10/90, 20/80, 30/70, 40/60, and 50/50. Mixtures using Humalog as the rapid-acting insulin are also available.

Warning: Concentrated Insulin

The most common forms of insulin come in a concentration of 100 IU of hormone per milliliter. These are identified as "U-100" preparations in the U.S. and many other regions. In addition to this, however, there are also concentrated forms of insulin available for patients that require higher doses and a more economical or comfortable option to U-100 preparations. In the U.S., products containing as much as 5 times the normal concentration, or 500 IU per milliliter, are also sold. These are identified as "U-500" preparations, and are available by prescription only. It can be extremely dangerous or life threatening to replace a U-100 insulin product with a U-500 product without making the necessary dosing adjustments to compensate for the greater drug concentration. Given the general difficulty in accurately measuring athletic doses (2-15 IU) with a drug of such high concentration, U-100 preparations are used almost exclusively for physique- and performance-enhancing purposes.

Side Effects (Hypoglycemia):

Hypoglycemia is the primary danger with the use of insulin. This is a dangerous condition that occurs when blood glucose levels fall too low. It is a common and potentially fatal reaction experienced at some time or another by most medical and nonmedical insulin users, so it needs to be taken seriously. It is, therefore, critical to understand the warning signs of hypoglycemia. The following is a list of symptoms that may indicate mild to moderate hypoglycemia: hunger, drowsiness, blurred vision, depressive mood, dizziness, sweating, palpitation, tremor, restlessness, tingling in the hands, feet, lips, or tongue, lightheadedness, inability to concentrate, headache, sleep disturbances, anxiety, slurred speech, irritability, abnormal behavior, unsteady movement, and personality changes. If any of these warning signs should occur, one should immediately consume a food or drink containing simple sugars such as a candy bar or carbohydrate drink. This will hopefully raise blood glucose levels sufficiently enough to ward off mild to moderate hypoglycemia. There is always a possibility of severe hypoglycemia, which is very serious and requires immediate emergency medical attention. Symptoms of this include disorientation, seizure, unconsciousness, and death. Note that in some cases the symptoms of hypoglycemia are mistaken for drunkenness.

It is also very important to note that you may notice a tendency to get sleepy after injecting insulin. This is an early symptom of hypoglycemia, and a clear sign the user should be consuming more carbohydrates. One should absolutely avoid the temptation to go to sleep at this point, as the insulin may take its peak effect during rest, and blood glucose levels could be left to drop significantly. Unaware of this condition during sleep, the athlete may be at a high risk for going into a state of severe hypoglycemia. The serious dangers of such a state have already been discussed, and unfortunately consuming more carbohydrates during sleep will not be an option. Those experimenting with insulin would, therefore, be wise to always stay awake for the duration of the drug's effect, and also avoid using insulin in the early evening to ensure the drug will not be inadvertently active when retiring for the night. It is also important to make sure others are aware of your use of the drug so that they may inform emergency medical technicians should you lose consciousness or the ability to inform others of your condition due to hypoglycemia. This information can spare valuable (perhaps life saving) time in helping medical professionals establish a diagnosis and provide supportive treatment.

Side Effects (Lipodystrophy):

The subcutaneous administration of insulin may cause a localized increase in adipose tissue at the site of injection. This may be compounded by the repeated administration of insulin at the same site of injection.

Side Effects (Allergy to Insulin):

In a small percentage of users, the administration of insulin may cause a localized allergy. This may include irritation, swelling, itching, and/or redness at the site of injection. This often subsides as therapy continues. In some instances it may be due to an allergy to an ingredient, or in the case of animal insulin, a protein contaminant. Less common, but potentially more serious, is a systemic allergic reaction to insulin administration. This may include a rash on the whole body, wheezing, shortness of breath, fast pulse, sweating, and/or a reduction in blood pressure. In rare instances this may be life threatening. Any adverse reaction should be reported to a medical authority.

Administration (General):

Given that there are varying forms of insulin available for medical use with differing pharmacokinetic patterns, as well as products with different drug concentrations, it is extremely important that the user be familiar with the dosage and actions of any specific insulin preparation they intend to use so that peak-effect, total time of effect, total dosage, and carbohydrate intake can be closely monitored. Rapid-acting insulin preparations (Novolog, Humalog, and Humulin-R) are the most popular choices for physique- or performance-enhancing purposes, and the subject of the dosing information presented in this book. It is also important to stress that before one considers using insulin they should also become very familiar with using a glucometer. This is a medical device that can give you a quick and accurate reading of your blood glucose level. This device can be indispensable in helping one manage and optimize their insulin/carbohydrate intake.

Administration (Short-acting Insulin):

Short acting forms of insulin (Novolog, Humalog, Humulin-R) are designed for subcutaneous injection. Following subcutaneous injection, the injection site should be left alone and not rubbed, to prevent the drug from releasing into circulation too quickly. It is also advised to rotate subcutaneous injection sites regularly to avoid the localized buildup of subcutaneous fat that may develop due to the lipogenic properties of this hormone (see Adverse Reactions: Lipodystrophy). The medical dosage will vary depending on the individual requirements of the patient. Furthermore, changes in such things as diet, activity level, or work/sleep schedule may affect the required insulin dose. Although not recommended medically, it is possible to administer some short-acting insulins via intramuscular injection. This, however, may create more variability (and potential risk) with regard to drug dissipation and hypoglycemic effect.

Insulin dosages can vary slightly among athletes, and are often dependent upon factors like body weight, insulin sensitivity, activity level, diet, and the use of other drugs. Most users choose to administer insulin immediately after a workout, which is the most opportunistic time of the day to use this drug. Among bodybuilders, dosages of regular insulin (Humulin-R) used are usually in the range of 1IU per 15-20 pounds of lean bodyweight; 10IU is perhaps the most common dosage. This amount may be adjusted downward slightly for users of the more rapid-acting Humalog and Novolog preparations, which provide a higher and faster peak effect. First-time cautious users usually ignore bodyweight guidelines, and instead start at a low dosage with the intention of gradually working up to a normal dosage. For example, on the first day of insulin therapy one may begin with a dose as low as 2 IU. Each consecutive post-workout application this dosage might be increased by 1IU, until the user determines a comfortable range. Many feel this is safer and much more tailored to the individual than simply calculating and injecting a dose, as some find they tolerate slightly more or less insulin than weight guidelines would dictate. Athletes using growth hormone in particular often have slightly higher insulin requirements, as HGH therapy is shown to both lower secretion of, and induce cellular resistance to, insulin.

One must also remember that it is very important to consume carbohydrates for several hours following insulin use. One should generally follow the rule-of-thumb of ingesting at least 10-15 grams of simple carbohydrates per IU of insulin injected (with a minimum immediate intake of 100 grams regardless of dose). This is timed 10 to 30 minutes after subcutaneous injection of Humulin-R, or immediately after using Novolog or Humalog. The use of a carbohydrate replacement drink is often used as a fast carbohydrate source. Properly cautious insulin users will always have a source for simple sugars on-hand in case an unexpected drop in glucose levels is noticed. Many athletes will also take creatine monohydrate with their carbohydrate drink, since the insulin may help force more creatine into the muscles. 30-60 minutes after injecting insulin, one should also eat a good meal and consume a protein shake. The carbohydrate drink and meal/protein shake are absolutely necessary, as without them blood sugar levels may drop dangerously low and the athlete may enter a state of hypoglycemia (see Adverse Reactions: Hypoglycemia). Carbohydrates and proteins are continually provided in sufficient amounts to meet glucose requirements throughout the entire window of insulin effect.

Administration (Intermediate-acting, Long-acting, and Biphasic Insulins):

Intermediate-acting, long-acting, and biphasic insulins are designed for subcutaneous injection. Intramuscular injection will cause the drug to be released too rapidly, potentially resulting in hypoglycemia. Following subcutaneous injection, the injection site should be left alone and not rubbed, to prevent the drug from releasing into circulation too quickly. It is also advised to rotate subcutaneous injection sites regularly to avoid the localized buildup of subcutaneous fat due to the lipogenic properties of this hormone (see Adverse Reactions: Lipodystrophy). The medical dosage will vary depending on the individual requirements of the patient. Furthermore, changes in such things as diet, activity level, or work/sleep schedule may affect the required insulin dose. Intermediate-acting, long-acting, and biphasic insulins are not widely used for physique- or performance-enhancing purposes due to their longer acting nature, which makes them poorly suited for concentrating the nutrient partitioning effect of insulin during the short post-workout enhanced-nutrient-uptake window.

Availability:

U-100 insulins may be dispensed from pharmacies in the United States without a prescription. This is so that an insulin-dependent diabetic will have easy access to this life-saving medication. Concentrated (U-500) insulin is sold by prescription only. In most regions of the world, high medical use of the drug leads to easy access and low prices on the black market.

LIVER DETOXIFICATION Product Profiles

Essentiale forte N (Compound N)

Description:

Essentiale forte N is the trade name for a liver-support supplement distributed in Europe by Aventis Pharma. While this is regarded as a medication in some regions, it actually contains a selection of natural vitamins and phospholipids. Likewise, in many areas, including the United States, Essentiale forte N is sold over the counter. The product specifically contains a complex of B vitamins, vitamin E, and phospholipid forms of linoleic, linolinec, and oleic acid. Essentiale forte N is used widely in Europe to treat cases of hepatic dysfunction, such as those caused by chronic infection, allergy, drug toxicity, or other disease. Essential forte N is of interest to steroid using bodybuilders and athletes for its ability to reduce the level of liver strain caused by anabolic/androgenic steroids (particularly those compounds that are c-17 alpha alkylated).

The main mechanism of action with Essential forte N appears to be focused on the supply of antioxidants and building blocks necessary for the repair of damaged cells. This product contains mainly polyunsaturated phospholipids (mostly phosphatidylcholine), and a complex of B and E vitamins. Phosphatidylcholine is identified as a membrane lipid, and is a key component of the Essential forte N formula. This phospholipid is important to the integrity of cells, adding both flexibility and strength. Phosphatidylcholine has long been identified as an important supplement for the liver, supporting normal hepatic fat metabolism and overall liver health. It is also believed to be an important antioxidant for liver and pancreatic wellness. The additional vitamins in the Essential forte N formula are likely included to increase the antioxidant and regenerative properties of the medication.

Essentiale forte N was the first product shown to mitigate the hepatotoxic effects of anabolic steroid use in a clinical study.[898] The investigation looked at the effects of steroid abuse (with or without Essential forte N), and compared them to controls (non-steroid-using subjects). A full panel of liver enzymes was used to determine the level of relative hepatic strain. As expected, the steroid-only group noticed a significant elevation in liver enzymes that were well above the normal range. Liver enzymes were also elevated in the steroid users taking Essential forte N, however, they were similar to controls and remained within the normal range. The researchers concluded: "The positive association of the abuse severity with the increased hepatic enzymes' levels suggest a relationship between abused AAS and hepatic cell damage. However, when AAS were taken with [Essentiale forte N], ... the hepatotoxic effect appears to be attenuated." While this one study does not assure that steroid liver toxicity can be completely eliminated, it does lend strong support for the use of Essential forte N with hepatotoxic anabolic steroids.

History:

Essentiale forte N has been sold in Western and Eastern Europe for many years, where it is distributed by Aventis (formerly Rhone-Poulenc Rorer). This compound has been approved for the treatment of hepatic liver steatosis and other hepatic dysfunction. European bodybuilders have used this medication for years owing to its understood general value with regard to liver health. It did not catch the attention of athletes in the United States and Canada until 2008, however, when the investigation into its effects with steroid abusers was published in the *Clinical Toxicology* journal. Since then, this natural medication has been noting increased popularity with North American consumers.

How Supplied:

Essentiale forte N is supplied in soft gelatin capsules containing vitamin B1 (6mg), vitamin B2 (6mg), vitamin B6 (6mg), vitamin B12 (6mcg), vitamin E (6 mg), niacin (15 mg), and a phospholipid complex [polyene phosphatidylcholine] (diglyceride esters of choline-phosphoric acid and unsaturated fatty acids linoleic, linoliec, and oleic acids) (300 mg).

Side Effects:

Essential forte N is a natural vitamin and supplement medication and is not expected to have notable side effects.

Administration:

When used medically to treat hepatic dysfunction, the most common recommended dosage is 2 capsules 3 times daily with meals. Bodybuilders and athletes using this medication to reduce the hepatic stress of oral steroid use will typically follow the same medical prescribing guidelines, and will taken the product for as long as the hepatotoxic steroids are administered.

Availability:

Essential forte N is widely available in Western and Eastern Europe. It is a relatively inexpensive supplement, and is not a high interest target of counterfeit manufacturing operations.

LIV-52®

Description:

Liv-52 is an herbal medicine used widely in Europe and Asia to support metabolic and liver health. While in some countries this product is regarded as a drug, it contains all natural ingredients including capparis spinosa, terminalia arjuna, cichorium intybus, achillea millefolium, solanum nigrum, tamarix gallica, and cassia occidentalis. It is specifically used in the prevention or treatment of hepatitis, alcoholic liver disease, early liver cirrhosis, protein energy malnutrition, loss of appetite, radiation and chemotherapy-induced liver damage, as an adjunct to hepatotoxic drugs, and to support metabolism during convalescence or prolonged illness. As the first three letters of its name would suggest, overall liver health is the primary focus of this product. Bodybuilders and athletes use Liv-52 as a way to reduce the level of strain placed on the liver by hepatotoxic anabolic/androgenic steroids.

Numerous medical studies have been conducted on Liv-52 in recent years, many of which involve its ability to protect the liver from damage by alcohol or other toxins.[899,900,901,902] One investigation in particular looked at how the herbal medication affected the breakdown of alcohol in the body, showing that it notably increased its excretion, even to the point of being able to reduce next day hangover symptoms after binge drinking.[903] Another study investigated what underlying mechanism might be involved in Liv-52's ability to protect the liver against alcohol toxicity. It demonstrated that one mechanism involved a specific ability to slow the rate of glutathione depletion.[904] This may be very important to the steroid-using athlete, as glutathione depletion is looked at as a direct marker of liver stress with c-17 alpha alkylated orals. Note that while these studies lend support for the use of a natural remedy like Liv-52 during hepatotoxic steroid administration, they do not provide complete assurance that this remedy can prevent liver damage.

History:

Liv-52 is an herbal product that has its roots in ayurvedic medicine, an age old form of Hindu science and medicine that centers on the use of natural remedies. Liv-52 is manufactured by the Himalaya Drug Co. in Bombay, India, and was first introduced to the global market in 1955. Over the years it came to be a widely distributed and popular natural product. In 2002, the Swiss government actually classified Liv-52 as a pharmaceutical product, which is believed to be the first time an herbal remedy was adopted as a prescription drug in Western Europe.[905] Liv-52 had already been popular with steroid using bodybuilders and athletes for many years by this point, and further clinical support only cemented this position. Liv-52 presently remains the most commonly used form of natural liver support among the steroid-using community today.

How Supplied:

Liv-52 is supplied in capsules containing a 450 mg of a blend of caper bush (capparis spinosa), arjuna (terminalia arjuna), wild chicory (cichorium intybus), yarrow (achillea millefolium), black nightshade (solanum nigrum), tamarisk (tamarix gallica), and negro coffee (cassia occidentalis).

Side Effects:

Liv-52 is a natural herbal supplement medication and is not expected to have notable side effects.

Administration:

For general liver support or as an adjunct to hepatotoxic pharmaceuticals, Liv-52 is generally taken at a dosage of 1-2 capsules 2 times per day.

Availability:

Liv-52 is produced exclusively by the Himalaya Drug Company, and is distributed widely in many areas of the world. In some regions, including the United States, the product is marketed under the LiverCare® trade name.

Liver Stabil™

Description:

Liver Stabil is a liver support supplement. It contains more than a dozen natural ingredients designed to help protect and detoxify the liver, and may be specifically useful during exposure to hepatotoxic substances such as oral anabolic/androgenic steroids. At the foundation of this formula are several clinically studied ingredients similar to those found in Liv-52 and Essentiale forte. For example, cichorium intybus, which was originally an old Turkish folk medicine, has been the subject of modern studies showing it can protect the liver from toxic substance damage. It has specifically been shown to lower liver enzymes (aspartate aminotransferase and alanine aminotransferase) and bilirubin levels after toxic exposure.[906] Arjuna is also used, and again has been shown to lower liver enzyme levels and stress markers following hepatotoxic substance administration.[907] Yarrow (achillea millefolium) was also included, and may help reduce hepatic inflammation and regulate bile secretion.[908] Phosphatidylcholine (a key constituent of cellular membranes including liver cells) and a combination of key vitamins round out the Liv-52/Essential forte-like base of the Liver Stabil formula.

Lipid Stapil expands on its foundation with four additional well-studied liver health ingredients. The most prevalent of these are N-acetyl cysteine and L-glutathione. Both nutrients are important to maintaining ongoing liver health, and may be especially useful in countering hepatic glutathione depletion,[909] an effect common with oral AAS toxicity.[910] Next, milk thistle extract standardized for silymarin content is included. Silymarin contains several key flavonolignans that protect and detoxify the liver. In fact, this natural remedy is one of the most extensively studied and proven liver detoxification supplements, and in some regions is widely prescribed by physicians to treat numerous liver diseases including alcohol cirrhosis. An extensive review of more than a dozen placebo-controlled studies with the use of silymarin on patients with cirrhosis have shown it to consistently reduce aspartate aminotransferase levels and even liver-related mortality.[911] Regardless of the chosen liver support regimen, milk thistle should be included. Lastly, wasabi japonica is a rich source of 6-methylsulfinylhexyl isothiocyanate (6-HITC). The nutrient 6-HITC is an inhibitor of glutathione S-transferase, an enzyme that breaks down hepatic glutathione.[912]

History:

Liver Stabil was developed in 2008 by Molecular Nutrition (United States). The focus was specifically on designing a supplement that can help support liver health in users of hepatotoxic substances such as oral anabolic/androgenic steroids. The formula was intended to target several key areas of steroid-induced liver toxicity including general liver strain and hepatic enzyme elevations, glutathione depletion, inflammation, and bile secretion and transport. Liver Stabil can be found through international distribution, most notably in Canada, Australia, and certain parts of Europe. Note that in some regions with strict controls over nutritional supplements Liver Stabil may be considered a natural drug product, and may be subject to certain rules and regulations concerning its importation and sale.

How Supplied:

Liver Stabil is supplied in capsules containing a blend of N-acetyl cysteine, milk thistle extract, wild chicory (cichorium intybus), L-glutathione, wasabi japonica, arjuna (terminalia arjuna), phosphatidylcholine, yarrow (achillea millefolium), vitamin B1, vitamin B2, vitamin B6, vitamin B12, vitamin E, and niacin.

Side Effects:

Liver Stabil is a natural dietary supplement and is not expected to have notable side effects.

Administration:

For general liver support or as an adjunct to hepatotoxic pharmaceuticals, Liver Stabil is taken at a dosage of 3 capsules per day. A dosage of up to 6 capsules per day may be taken during periods of heightened hepatic strain. Note that a natural product such as Liver Stabil may help reduce the level of liver toxicity, but cannot be relied upon to completely eliminate potential damage from the abuse of hepatotoxic drugs. Care should always be taken to monitor liver health when taking liver toxic substances.

Availability:

Liver Stabil is produced in the U.S. by Molecular Nutrition. It is available for export, and may be found in Canada, Europe, Australia, and some other international markets.

REDUCTASE INHIBITORS Drug Profiles

Avodart® (dutasteride)

Description:

Dutasteride is an inhibitor of the 5-alpha reductase enzyme. Reductase inhibitors are designed to prevent the conversion of testosterone to its more androgenic counterpart DHT (dihydrotestosterone). DHT is implicated in a number of disorders in men including male pattern hair loss and benign prostate enlargement. Dutasteride is specifically approved for the treatment of symptomatic benign prostate hyperplasia (BPH). While dutasteride is similar in structure and action to finasteride, it differs from the first generation reductase inhibitor in its tissue selectivity. Finasteride inhibits the type-2 isozyme of the 5-alpha reductase enzyme, found prominently in the scalp and prostate. Dutasteride is non-specific for isotype, and inhibits both type-1 and type-2 reductase. As such, it inhibits DHT conversion in all tissues including the scalp, liver, prostate, and skin. Because of this it also lowers systemic levels of DHT much more effectively than finasteride.

The DHT inhibiting effects of dutasteride make this drug of some interest to bodybuilders and athletes, particularly those concerned with the androgenic component of testosterone-based steroids. Dutasteride is capable of reducing the androgenic side effects produced by DHT conversion, changing the profile of testosterone drugs measurably. Provided moderate doses of testosterone are being used, the result can be a substantial reduction in the occurrence of oily skin and acne. For those prone to male pattern hair loss, dutasteride may also reduce the harsh impact of testosterone on the hairline. Note that as a selective type-2 inhibitor, finasteride is also effective at lowering DHT levels in the scalp (and reducing hairline impact of testosterone use), but does not work as well for reducing oily skin and acne.

In terms of overall potency, a study published in the *Journal of Clinical Endocrinology and Metabolism* (May 2004) directly compared dutasteride to its closest pharmaceutical counterpart, finasteride.[913] In this investigation 399 males suffering from benign prostatic hypertrophy were assembled and separated into three general groups, each receiving dutasteride (subdivided by doses of .01, .05, .5, 2.5, or 5.0 mg daily), finasteride (.5 mg daily) or placebo, for a period of 24 weeks. Over the 24-week period, the dutasteride group noted the strongest level of DHT inhibition. The beneficial effects of this drug also occurred over a wide range of dosages. For example, a 5 mg daily amount caused 98.4% inhibition in DHT levels, while 1/10th of this amount (.5 mg daily, the adopted therapeutic dose) lowered levels by an average of 94.7%. This was in great contrast to the 5 mg finasteride group, which noticed only 70.8% inhibition. Researchers also noted that there was significantly more of a variation in the results of the finasteride group, with some patients noting DHT suppression in the range of only 50-55%.

Just as there can be benefits to lowering 5-alpha reductase activity by way of less androgenic side effects, there can also be some drawbacks. For one, a strong androgen like DHT helps with neuromuscular interaction, fostering strength and muscle gain. Users of reductase inhibitors often report a drop in their maximum lifts soon after the drug is initiated. Libido may also decline as DHT concentrations are lowered. A small percentage of men even find the need to keep Viagra on hand, as dutasteride renders them otherwise impotent. Dihydrotestosterone also serves as a potent endogenous anti-estrogen, as this non-aromatizable steroid competes with other substrates (like testosterone, which aromatizes) to bind with the aromatase enzyme. Gynecomastia or other estrogenic side effects may occur when this competition is absent. Gynecomastia is listed in the warnings for this product, although the frequency of this in testing was very low (1.1% of users).

History:

Dutasteride was first described in 1997.[914] It was developed by the U.S. based pharmaceutical company GlaxoSmithKline. It was approved by the FDA in November 2001, and introduced to market the following year by Glaxo under the Avodart trade name. GlaxoSmithKline also markets the drug in a number of other countries in Europe and South America under the same trade name.

How Supplied:

Dutasteride is supplied in soft gelatin capsules containing .5 mg each.

Structural Characteristics:

Dutasteride is a synthetic 4-azasteroid. It has the chemical designation (5·,17,)-N-{2,5 bis(trifluoromethyl)phenyl}-3-

oxo-4-azaandrost-1-ene-17-carboxamide.

Warnings (Pregnancy):

This drug must never be taken during pregnancy. Be aware that dutasteride can be absorbed through the skin. Women who are, or might become pregnant, should never handle dutasteride capsules. The DHT blocking action of dutasteride can cause severe developmental problems to an unborn male fetus, even in very small amounts. Unaltered dutasteride can also be recovered in the semen. It is unknown if the drug can be absorbed during sexual intercourse enough to harm a developing male fetus. The use of condoms or abstinence is recommended during therapy.

Side Effects:

The most common adverse reactions to dutasteride therapy are impotence, reduced libido, and difficulty ejaculating. Gynecomastia was also noted during clinical trials, but occurred in less than 1% of patients. Some patients have also developed allergic reactions to the drug, including rash, itching, edema, and hives.

Administration (General Considerations):

Reductase inhibitors cannot completely protect against androgenic side effects such as steroid-induced hair loss, oily skin, and acne. Reductase inhibitors lessen these side effects by reducing, not eliminating, the level of androgenic activity in the skin and scalp. Androgenic and anabolic effects are both mediated by the same receptor, and there is presently no way known to completely separate these two properties. Dihydrotestosterone is also not unique in its ability to facilitate androgenetic alopecia (male pattern hair loss). DHT inhibition, therefore, does not offer complete protection against this side effect.

Reductase inhibitors are only applicable with testosterone, methyltestosterone, and fluoxymesterone. These three drugs are converted to stronger "dihydro" derivatives by the reductase enzyme. Nandrolone and some of its derivatives become weaker upon interaction with this enzyme, as their "dihydro" metabolites bind the androgen receptor very poorly. Reductase inhibition may intensify their androgenic side effects. Methandrostenolone and boldenone undergo conversion to stronger 5-alpha reduced metabolites, but at such small levels that reductase inhibitors have little effect on their androgenicity. Most other synthetic anabolic steroids are unaffected by the reductase enzyme and reductase inhibitors.

Administration:

When used medically for the treatment of symptomatic benign prostatic hyperplasia (BPH), dutasteride is taken in a dosage of .5 mg (1 capsule) per day. When used by bodybuilders and athletes to reduce the androgenicity of testosterone, methyltestosterone, or fluoxymesterone, dutasteride is commonly taken in a dosage of .5 mg (1 capsule) once every 1-2 days. The drug is typically administered for as long as the offending steroids are also taken.

Availability:

GlaxoSmithKline distributes this drug in the U.S., Europe, and South America under the Avodart trade name. Additionally, a number of other brands can be found in different markets including Austria (Avolve, Zyfetor), Greece (Duagen), India (Duprost), Netherlands (Duagen), Portugal (Duagen), and Spain (Duagen).

Proscar® (finasteride)

Description:

Finasteride is an inhibitor of 5a-reductase, which is the enzyme responsible for converting testosterone into DHT (dihydrotestosterone). This drug can efficiently reduce the serum concentration of DHT, thereby minimizing the unwanted androgenic effects that result from its presence. The effect of this drug is quite rapid, suppressing serum DHT concentrations as much as 65% within 24 hours after taking a single 1mg tablet. Medically, this drug is used to treat benign prostate hyperplasia (prostate enlargement) and androgenetic alopecia (male pattern hair loss). It is also being investigated as a potential treatment for hirsutism, which describes male patterned hair growth on the face or body of a woman. Male athletes and bodybuilders are interested in finasteride for its ability to reduce the androgenic side effects associated with the use of testosterone and certain derivatives.

Finasteride is a specific inhibitor of the Type-II 5a reductase enzyme. There are actually two isozymes of reductase in the human body, labeled as Type-I and Type-II. Type-I 5a-reductase is predominantly found in the liver and sebaceous glands of the skin. Type-II 5a-reductase is primarily found in the prostate and hair follicles. The Type-II enzyme is responsible for about 2/3rd of the circulating DHT, while the Type-I enzyme produces the remaining 1/3rd. As an inhibitor of Type-II reductase only, finasteride has a more pronounced effect with regard to preventing hair loss, but is somewhat less effective at mitigating oily skin and acne. Since hair loss is the primary worry among most male steroid users who use reductase inhibitors, finasteride remains a popular ancillary drug in spite of its inability to block DHT conversion in all tissues.

Finasteride is considered a highly specific drug, as it has little spillover effect on the other hormones in the body. It has no affinity for the androgen or estrogen receptors, and therefore does not exhibit any androgenic, anti-androgenic, estrogenic, or anti-estrogenic properties. It has no appreciable impact on circulating levels of cortisol, thyroid-stimulating hormone, or thyroxine, nor does it appear to alter HDL/LDL cholesterol levels. Changes in luteinizing hormone (LH) or follicle-stimulating hormone (FSH) are also not notable, and it is not shown to have a significant effect on the hypothalamic-pituitary-testicular axis. Finasteride has been shown to increase the circulating levels of testosterone by roughly 15%, however, since a greater amount of the androgen is being left unaltered by the reductase enzyme.

History:

The first release of finasteride in the U.S. was under the brand name of Proscar® (Merck), which was approved by the FDA in 1992. It was specifically given approval for use by patients with benign prostate hyperplasia (prostate enlargement). In December 1997, the Food and Drug Administration again approved finasteride, this time for a different purpose, namely the treatment of male pattern hair loss. Merck released the drug under a different brand name for this purpose, Propecia®, which contained only 1/5th of the Proscar® dosage. Today, both Proscar® and Propecia® remain the dominant brands of finasteride on the global market.

How Supplied:

Finasteride is most commonly supplied in tablets of 1 mg and 5 mg.

Structural Characteristics:

Finasteride is a synthetic 4-azasteroid. It has the chemical designation 4-azaandrost-1-ene-17-carboxamide,N-(1,1-dimethylethyl)-3-oxo-,(5·,17,)-.

Warnings (Pregnancy):

This drug must never be taken during pregnancy. Finasteride can be absorbed through the skin. Women who are, or might become pregnant, should never handle broken or uncoated finasteride tablets. The DHT blocking action of finasteride can cause severe developmental problems to an unborn male fetus, even in very small amounts. Unaltered finasteride can also be recovered in the semen. It is unknown if enough drug can be absorbed during sexual intercourse to harm a developing male fetus. The use of condoms or abstinence is recommended during therapy.

Side Effects:

Adverse reactions commonly associated with the short-term (1 year) use of finasteride include impotence (8.1%), decreased libido (6.4%), decreased ejaculate volume (3.7%), ejaculation disorder (.8%), gynecomastia (.5%), breast tenderness (.4%), and rash (.5%).

Administration (General Considerations):

Reductase inhibitors cannot completely protect against androgenic side effects such as steroid-induced hair loss, oily skin, and acne. Reductase inhibitors lessen these side effects by reducing, not eliminating, the level of androgenic activity in the skin and scalp. Androgenic and anabolic effects are both mediated by the same receptor, and there is no way presently known to completely separate these two properties. Dihydrotestosterone is also not unique in its ability to facilitate androgenetic alopecia (male pattern hair loss). DHT inhibition, therefore, does not offer complete protection against this side effect.

Reductase inhibitors are only applicable with testosterone, methyltestosterone, and fluoxymesterone. These three drugs are converted to stronger "dihydro" derivatives by the reductase enzyme. Nandrolone and some of its derivatives become weaker upon interaction with this enzyme, as their "dihydro" metabolites bind the androgen receptor very poorly. Reductase inhibition may intensify their androgenic side effects. Methandrostenolone and boldenone undergo conversion to stronger 5-alpha reduced metabolites, but at such small levels that reductase inhibitors have little effect on their androgenicity. Most other synthetic anabolic steroids are unaffected by the reductase enzyme and reductase inhibitors.

Administration:

When used medically for the treatment of male pattern hair loss (androgenetic alopecia) in men, the recommended dosage is 1mg per day. When used for the treatment of benign prostatic hyperplasia (BPH), 5 mg per day is usually administered. When used by bodybuilders and athletes to reduce the androgenicity of testosterone, methyltestosterone, or fluoxymesterone, finasteride is commonly taken in a dosage of 1mg per day. The drug is typically administered for as long as the offending steroids are also taken. Since DHT inhibition can lessen strength and possibly muscle gains during testosterone, methyltestosterone, or fluoxymesterone therapy (given the positive actions of androgens on the neuromuscular system), a "use only when necessary" approach is usually taken with regard to this drug.

Availability:

Finasteride is widely available in most regions of the world. The most prominent brand names in commerce are Proscar® (5 mg) and Propecia® (1mg), although a number of other brand and generic forms of the drug can also be located.

TANNING AGENTS Drug Profiles

Oxsoralen (methoxsalen)

Description:

Methoxsalen is a repigmenting agent that is similar in structure and action to Trisoralen (trioxsalen). These drugs belong to a class of medicines known as psoralens, which are used along with ultra violet (UV) light exposure to treat certain disorders of the skin such as vitiligo (where skin pigment is lost) and psoriasis (a skin condition characterized by red and scaly blotches). Although the exact underlying mechanism behind these agents is unknown, they ultimately work to increase the output of melanin in response to stimulation by sunlight or artificial UV exposure. This enhances the rate of pigmentation, which in many cases will allow the lighter areas of the skin to become more evenly colored.

Bodybuilders are attracted to psoralens because they may be used to help them develop that deep tan that is so favored in the world of competition and modeling. A good tan helps bring out muscle separation and definition, to the point that it is just about considered a necessity (most bodybuilders who won't tan on their own will apply an artificial brush-on tan). A natural tan usually looks much better (at least in an immediate sense), especially when you are going to be seeing people face to face. This drives many fairer skinned people to look for drugs that can help them achieve a deep bronze look that is otherwise difficult or impossible to achieve on their own. In this regard, methoxsalen seems to deliver for many people who carefully and correctly use the drug.

History:

The first successful treatment with methoxsalen was documented in 1948.[915] By the 1950s this agent was an established medicine in many markets. It has been sold in the United States for decades under the brand name Oxsoralen, manufactured by Valeant Pharmaceuticals (formerly known as ICN Pharmaceuticals). The drug is FDA approved for the symptomatic control of severe, recalcitrant, disabling psoriasis not adequately responsive to other forms of therapy and when the diagnosis has been supported by biopsy.

How Supplied:

Methoxsalen is most commonly supplied in regular or rapid-release capsules of 10 mg. It is also commonly supplied as a cream for topical application.

Structural Characteristics:

Methoxsalen is a photoactive substance belonging to a class of compounds known as psoralens. It has the chemical designation 9-methoxy-7H-furo [3,2-g] [1] benzopyran-7-one.

Warnings (Heightened sensitivity to light):

Psoralen drugs do not protect the skin from sun damage. These drugs increase the skin's sensitivity to sunlight, and can increase the likelihood of skin damage, skin aging, and skin cancer. Medical professionals do not prescribe psoralens for cosmetic purposes (tanning) due to these potential risks.

Warnings (Ocular damage):

Psoralen drugs can increase susceptibility to ocular damage and cataracts. Goggles with complete UVA blocking properties must be worn at all times during light exposure therapy, and for 24 hours following exposure. The medical use of psoralens drugs does not appear to increase the rate of cataract formation when proper eye protection is used.

Side Effects:

The most common adverse reactions to methoxsalen therapy include nausea and severe itching, which occur in approximately 10% of patients. Reddening of the skin (erythema) is also common, and is an inflammatory reaction distinct from normal sunburn. Other adverse reactions include nausea, nervousness, insomnia, depression, edema, dizziness, headache, malaise, pigmentation irregularities, cyst, blister, rash, herpes simplex, prickly heat, inflammation of the hair follicles, gastrointestinal disturbances, skin touch sensitivity, leg cramps, low blood pressure, and exacerbated psoriasis.

Administration:

When used medically to control severe psoriasis, methoxsalen is administered in conjunction with scheduled and controlled doses of long wave ultraviolet radiation. The dosage of methoxsalen is determined by bodyweight, and will range from 10 mg to 70 mg per application. UV exposure levels are determined after consideration of skin type and individual responsiveness to sun exposure. Therapy is usually initiated with drug and UV exposure commencing 2-3 times per week (clearing phase), followed by a schedule of once every 1 to 3 weeks (maintenance phase).

Methoxsalen is taken with a low fat meal or milk prior to UV exposure. Exposure is scheduled around the time of peak photosensitivity. Time of peak photosensitivity following administration is 1.5 to 2.1 hours with rapid-release capsules (Oxsoralen-Ultra), and 3.9 to 4.25 hours for regular methoxsalen capsules. The patient is instructed not to sunbathe 24 hours before and 48 hours after each dose of methoxsalen, and to avoid all sun exposure (even through clouds or glass) for 8 hours after each dose. The patient also must wear eyewear with full UVA protection for 24 hours following each application to protect the eyes from cataracts.

Dosage (by weight)

(kg)	(lbs)	(mg)
<30	<66	10
30-50	66-110	20
51-65	112-143	30
66-80	146-176	40
81-90	179-198	50
91-115	201-254	60
>115	>254	70

When used (off-label) for cosmetic (tanning) purposes, the drug is usually initiated at a low dosage (10 mg), which will be slowly worked upwards by no more than 10 mg each application. The maximum dose will never exceed the recommended medical dose for a given bodyweight. As with medical use, UV light exposure is scheduled approximately 2 to 4 hours after administration of regular capsules, or 1.5 to 2 hours for rapid release capsules. The amount of time spent exposed to UV light (usually a normal tanning bed) is also increased slowly, starting with very brief intervals, as the user becomes accustomed to the drug. In an effort to have better control over skin tone and reduce the likelihood of burns or injury, each application period is typically separated by several days or more of drug abstinence.

Availability:

Methoxsalen is available in more than 30 countries. The most common brand name is Oxsoralen from Valeant, although a number of other trade and generic forms can be located. This drug is not a common target of drug counterfeiting operations.

Trisoralen® (trioxsalen)

Description

Trioxsalen is a melanizing agent of the psoralen family. The normal pigmentation of the skin is due to melanin, a chemical produced in melanocytes located in the base layers of the epidermis (skin). Melanin is formed by an enzyme reaction, which involves the conversion of tyrosine to DOPA via the enzyme tyrosinase. Radiant energy in the form of ultraviolet light is needed to complete this process. The exact mechanism that trioxsalen uses to exert its action on melanin is not clear. Some investigators feel that this drug has a direct impact on the epidermis, or more specifically the melanocytes. Others feel its action is an inflammatory one, and that the process of increased melanogenesis is only a secondary effect. Regardless of the exact mechanism, trioxsalen is widely regarded as an effective mediator of skin pigmentation.

Trioxsalen is used medically to treat conditions associated with pigmentation dysfunction. The most known of these disorders is vitiligo, a condition that involves a marked loss of skin pigmentation (often in a very blotchy and uneven appearance). Treatment usually involves several consecutive months of regular trioxsalen use combined with UV light exposure. This is undertaken in an effort to slowly and safely rebuild the skin's appearance. In many instances periodic treatment (maintenance) will be required indefinitely to control the disease. Trioxsalen has also been used to increase a patient's tolerance to sunlight, which is accomplished by the increased retention of melanin in the skin. At one time this drug was regularly prescribed to fair skinned people to reduce the likelihood of sunburn, however, due to the potential for adverse reactions the drug is no longer widely used for this purpose.

Competitive bodybuilders often regard trioxsalen as an extremely useful finishing tool when readying for a stage appearance. It is no secret that a dark tan is considered important to the bodybuilding physique. Muscle features seem to be markedly improved with tanning, resulting in a more "ripped" and impressive look on stage. Many bodybuilders, especially fair skinned individuals, have trouble developing a very dark skin base. Although the use of various skin dyes (sun-less tanning products) may be popular, a tanning agent like trioxsalen is also a very common choice. While both may be valid methods for completing a competition physique, many individuals regard the process of using trioxsalen, which produces actual pigmentation changes in the skin, as being more desirable.

History:

Trioxsalen was developed after methoxsalen, and first became an established a medicine in the U.S. during the 1960s. It has been most notably associated with ICN Pharmaceuticals, who sold the drug under the Trisoralen brand name for many years (the company has since changed its name to Valeant Pharmaceuticals). Trisoralen was FDA approved for the repigmentation of idiopathic vitiligo, for increasing tolerance to sunlight, and for enhancing pigmentation. In some instances the drug would be prescribed to fair skin people before sun exposure (such as a tropical vacation or summer beach excursions). This was done in an effort to increase sun tolerance and the likelihood of tanning instead of burning. Later studies demonstrated the potential for psoralens to increase skin cancer risk and cataracts, however, eventually eliminating the use of Trisoralen for this purpose. Prescriptions for this drug have since been largely focused on the treatment of vitiligo.

While trioxsalen remained for sale in many nations over the years, it was never able to supplant methoxsalen in the pharmaceutical market. To the contrary, trioxsalen came to be regardless as a secondary medication to the much more readily prescribed methoxsalen capsules. By 2000, Valeant Pharmaceuticals began discontinuing its Trisoralen products in almost all of its remaining markets worldwide. U.S. brand Trisoralen tablets were included in the discontinuations, and have been unavailable for many years now. Trioxsalen tablets are still sold today, but only in a select few markets. This drug has for all intents and purposes been disregarded by Western medicine.

How Supplied:

Trioxsalen is most commonly supplied in tablets of 5 mg.

Structural Characteristics:

Trioxsalen is a photoactive substance belonging to a class of compounds known as psoralens. It has the chemical designation 2,5,9-trimethyl-7H-furo [3,2-g] [1] benzopyran-

7-one.

Warnings (Heightened sensitivity to light):

Psoralen drugs do not protect the skin from sun damage. These drugs increase the skin's sensitivity to sunlight, and can increase the likelihood of skin damage, skin aging, and skin cancer. Medical professionals do not prescribe psoralens for cosmetic purposes (tanning) due to these potential risks.

Warnings (Ocular damage):

Psoralen drugs can increase susceptibility to ocular damage and cataracts. Goggles with complete UVA blocking properties must be worn at all times during light exposure therapy, and for 24 hours following exposure. The medical use of psoralens drugs does not appear to increase the rate of cataract formation when proper eye protection is used.

Side Effects:

The most common adverse reactions to trioxsalen therapy include nausea, itching, and reddening of the skin (erythema). Other adverse reactions include nausea, nervousness, insomnia, depression, edema, dizziness, headache, malaise, pigmentation irregularities, cyst, blister, rash, herpes simplex, prickly heat, inflammation of the hair follicles, gastrointestinal disturbances, skin touch sensitivity, leg cramps, low blood pressure, and exacerbated psoriasis.

Administration:

When used medically to increase tolerance to sunlight, a dose of 10 mg is usually given 2 to 4 hours prior to UV light exposure. Treatment may be given once daily, but continued for no longer than 14 consecutive days. This medication is normally taken with food or milk.

When used (off-label) for cosmetic ("tanning") purposes, a dosage of 10 mg per application is typically used. As with medical use, UV light exposure is scheduled approximately 2 to 4 hours after administration. The amount of time spent exposed to UV light is also increased slowly, starting with very brief intervals as the user becomes accustomed to the drug. In an effort to minimize the potential for unwanted side effects, most users will limit the intake of trioxsalen to no more than two weeks of regular use. Cautious individuals usually opt to wait 48 hours between applications.

Availability:

Trixosalen is produced for sale in select markets including Finland (Tripsor), Greece (Trisoralen), and Malaysia (Puvadin). This medication is not readily available, nor a popular target for drug counterfeit operations.

TESTOSTERONE STIMULATING AGENTS Drug Profiles

hCG (human chorionic gonadotropin)

Description:

Human Chorionic Gonadotropin (hCG) is a prescription medication containing chorionic gonadotropin obtained from a natural (human) origin. Chorionic gonadotropin is a polypeptide hormone normally found in the female body during the early months of pregnancy. It is synthesized in syncytiotrophoblast cells of the placenta, and is responsible for increasing the production of progesterone, a pregnancy-sustaining hormone. Chorionic gonadotropin is present in significant amounts only during pregnancy, and is used as an indicator of pregnancy by standard over-the-counter pregnancy test kits. Blood levels of chorionic gonadotropin become noticeable as early as seven days after ovulation, and rise evenly to a peak at approximately two to three months into gestation. After this point, the hormone level will drop gradually until the point of birth.

Although it possesses minor FSH-like (Follicle Stimulating Hormone) activity, the physiological actions of chorionic gonadotropin mainly mimic those of the gonadotropin luteinizing hormone (LH). As a clinical drug, hCG is used as an exogenous form of LH. It is typically applied to support ovulation and pregnancy in women, most specifically those suffering from infertility due to low concentrations of gonadotropins and an inability to ovulate. Due to the ability of LH to stimulate the Leydig's cells in the testes to manufacture testosterone, hCG is also used with men to treat hypogonadotropic hypogonadism, a disorder characterized by low testosterone levels and insufficient LH output. The drug is also used in the treatment of prepubertal cryptochidism, a condition in which one or both of the testicles have failed to descend into the scrotum. HCG is used by male athletes for its ability to increase endogenous testosterone production, generally during, or at the conclusion of, a steroid cycle, when natural hormone production has been interrupted.

History:

Chorionic gonadotropin was first discovered in 1920,[916] and was identified as a pregnancy hormone approximately 8 years later.[917] The first drug preparation containing chorionic gonadotropin came in the form of an animal pituitary extract, which was developed as a commercial product by Organon. Organon introduced the extract in 1931, under the trade name Pregnon. A trademark dispute forced the company to change the name Pregnyl, however, which reached market in 1932. Pregnyl is still sold by Organon to this day, although it no longer comes in the form of a pituitary extract. Manufacturing techniques were introduced in 1940 that allowed the hormone to be obtained by filtering and purifying the urine of pregnant women, and by the late 1960's were adopted by all manufacturers formerly using animal extracts. Over the years the process and manufacturing protocols have been refined, but hCG is made in essentially the same way today as it was decades ago. While modern preparations are of biological origin, the risks of biological contaminants are said to be low (although cannot be completely excluded).

Early on, the indicated uses for chorionic gonadotropin preparations were much broader than they are presently. Product literature from the 1950's and '60's recommended the use of these drugs for, among other things, the treatment of uterine bleeding and amenorrhea, Froehlich's syndrome, cryptochidism, female sterility, obesity, depression, and male impotence. A good example of the wide uses of chorionic gonadotropin are illustrated in the preparation Glukor, which was described in 1958 as being, "Three times more effective than testosterone. For tired young men in male climacteric. For tired old men in male senility. Beneficial in impotence, angina and coronary heart disease, neuropsychosis, prostatitis, [and] myocarditis." Such recommendations, however, reflect an era less tightly regulated by government agency and less reliant on proven clinical trials. Today, FDA-approved indications for hCG are limited to the treatment of hypogonadotropic hypogonadism and cryptocridism in men, and anovulatory infertility in women.

HCG has no significant thyroid-stimulating activity, and is not an effective fat loss agent. This is specifically pointed out because hCG was once widely used for the treatment of obesity. The trend seemed to have become popular in 1954, after a paper was published by Dr. A.T.W. Simeons claiming that chorionic gonadotropin was an effective adjunct to dieting. According to the study, patients were able to effectively stave off hunger with severely low-calorie diets provided they took the hormone injections. Dubbed the Simeons diet, people everywhere were soon subjecting themselves to severe calorie restriction (500 calories per day) and taking hCG injections. Soon after, the hormone itself became the main focus for fat loss. In fact, by 1957 it was said that hCG was the most commonly prescribed medication for weight loss. More recent and comprehensive investigations, however, refute that there is any anorexic or metabolic advantage to the use of hCG, and the drug has been summarily abandoned for this purpose.[918]

Back in 1962, the Journal of the American Medical Association had already been warning consumers about the hCG-inclusive Simeons diet, stating the more basic fact that severe calorie restriction, which causes the body to sacrifice muscle and organ tissue to obtain necessary protein, was more hazardous than obesity itself. By 1974, the FDA had had enough of the hCG fat loss claims, and mandated the following statement to be included with all prescribing literature. "HCG HAS NOT BEEN DEMONSTRATED TO BE EFFECTIVE ADJUNCTIVE THERAPY IN THE TREATMENT OF OBESITY. THERE IS NO SUBSTANTIAL EVIDENCE THAT IT INCREASES WEIGHT LOSS BEYOND THAT RESULTING FROM CALORIC RESTRICTION, THAT IT CAUSES A MORE ATTRACTIVE OR 'NORMAL' DISTRIBUTION OF FAT, OR THAT IT DECREASES THE HUNGER AND DISCOMFORT ASSOCIATED WITH CALORIE-RESTRICTED DIETS." This warning persists on all product sold in the U.S. today.

Human Chorionic Gonadotropin is a widely popular drug preparation today, owing to the fact that it remains an indispensable part of ovulation therapy for many cases of female infertility. Popular preparations in the U.S. presently include Pregnyl (Organon), Profasi (Serono), and Novarel (Ferring), although many other trade names have been popular for chorionic gonadotropin preparations over the years. This drug is also sold widely outside of the United States, and can be found under many additional trade names, too numerous to list here. Owing to the fact that this drug is not controlled on a federal level, U.S. athletes and bodybuilders unable to find a local physician willing to prescribe the drug to treat steroid-induced hypogonadism often order the product from international pharmacy sources. Given that this drug is cheap and rarely counterfeited, most international sources are trusted. Although recombinant forms of chorionic gonadotropin have been introduced to market in recent years, the vast supply and low cost of biological hCG continues to make it a staple product for both labeled and off-label uses.

Structural Characteristics:

Chorionic gonadotropin is an oligosaccharide glycoprotein composed of 244 amino acids. It has an alpha subunit that is 92 amino acids long and identical to that of luteinizing hormone (LH), follicle-stimulating hormone (FSH), and thyroid-stimulating hormone (TSH). It has a beta subunit that is unique to hCG.

How Supplied:

Human Chorionic Gonadotropin is widely available in various human and veterinary drug markets. Composition and dosage may vary by country and manufacturer, but typically contain 1,000, 1,500, 2,500, 5,000, or 10,000 international units (IU) per dose. All forms are supplied as a lyophilized powder, requiring reconstitution with sterile diluent (water) before use.

Administration (General):

Human Chorionic Gonadotropin is generally given by intramuscular (IM) injection. The subcutaneous route is also used, and has been deemed to be roughly equivalent therapeutically to IM injections.[919] Peak concentrations of chorionic gonadotropin occur approximately 6 hours after intramuscular injection, and 16 to 20 hours after subcutaneous injection.

Administration (Men):

When used to treat hypogonadotropin hypogonadism, current FDA-approved protocols recommend either a short 6-week program, or a long-term program lasting up to 1 year, depending on the individual needs of the patient. Prescribing guidelines for short-term use recommend that 500 to 1,000 units to be given 3 times a week for 3 weeks, followed by the same dose twice a week for 3 weeks. The long-term recommendations call for 4,000 units to be administered 3 times weekly for 6 to 9 months, after which point the dosage is reduced to 2,000 USP units 3 times weekly for an additional 3 months. Bodybuilders and athletes use hCG either on cycle, in an effort to maintain testicular integrity during steroid administration, or after a cycle, to help restore hormonal homeostasis more quickly. Both types of use are deemed effective when properly applied.

Post-Cycle:

Human Chorionic gonadotropin is often used with other medications as part of an in-depth Post Cycle Therapy (PCT) program focused on restoring endogenous testosterone production more rapidly at the end of a steroid cycle. Restoring endogenous testosterone production is a special concern at the conclusion of each cycle, a time when subnormal androgen levels (due to steroid induced suppression) could be very costly to the physique. The main concern is the action of cortisol, which in many ways is balanced out by the effect of androgens. Cortisol sends the opposite message to the muscles than testosterone, or to breakdown protein in the cell. Left unchecked by a low level of testosterone, cortisol can quickly strip much of your new muscle mass away. Protocols for the post-cycle use of hCG generally call for the administration of 1500-4000 Units every 4th or 5th day, taken for no longer than 2 or 3 weeks. If used for too long or at too high a dose, the drug may actually function to desensitize the Leydig's cells to luteinizing hormone, further hindering a return to homeostasis. For a more comprehensive view of hCG's role in a proper hormonal-recovery program, please refer to the Post Cycle Therapy section of this book.

On-Cycle:

Bodybuilders and athletes may also administer Human Chorionic Gonadotropin throughout a steroid cycle, in an effort to avoid testicular atrophy and the resulting reduced ability to respond to LH stimulus. In effect, this practice is used to avoid the problem of testicular atrophy, instead of trying to correct it later on when the cycle is over. It is important to remember that the dosage needs to be carefully monitored with this type of use, as high levels of hCG may cause increased testicular aromatase expression (raising estrogen levels),[920] and also desensitize the testes to LH.[921] As such, the drug may actually induce primary hypogonadism when misused, greatly prolonging, not improving, the recovery window. Current protocols for the use of hCG in this manner involve administering 250IU subcutaneously twice per week (every 3rd or 4th day) throughout the length of the steroid cycle. Higher doses may be necessary for some individuals, but at no point should exceed 500IU per injection.

These on-cycle hCG protocols were developed by Dr. John Crisler, a well-known figure in the anti-aging and hormone-replacement field, for use with his testosterone replacement therapy (TRT) patients. Although TRT is often administered on a long-term basis, testicular atrophy is a common cosmetic complaint of patients irrespective of the maintenance of normal androgen levels. Dr. Crisler's hCG program is designed to alleviate this concern in a manner that is acceptable for longer-term use. For those interested in precisely timing their hCG shots in relation to a prescribed testosterone replacement program, Dr. Crisler recommends the following in his paper, "An Update to the Crisler hCG Protocol," "…my test cyp TRT patients now take their hCG at 250IU two days before, as well as the day immediately previous to, their IM shot. All administer their hCG subcutaneously, and dosage may be adjusted as necessary (I have yet to see more than 350IU per dose required)… Those TRT patients who prefer a transdermal testosterone, or even testosterone pellets (although I am not in favor of same), take their hCG every third day."

Administration (Women):

When used to induce ovulation and pregnancy in anovulatory infertile woman, a dose of 5,000 to 10,000 units is administered one day following the last dose of menotropins. The timing is specific so that the hormone is given precisely at the right moment in the ovulation cycle. Human Chorionic Gonadotropin is not used by women for physique- or performance-enhancing purposes.

Availability:

When we find hCG, we see it is always packaged in 2 different vials/ampules (one with a powder and the other with a sterile solvent). These need to be mixed before injecting, and any leftover drug should be refrigerated for later use. Make sure your product matches this description. Human Chorionic Gonadotropin is widely manufactured, and easily obtained on the black market. To date, counterfeits have not been much of a concern, although a couple of oddities have popped up (all in multi-dose vials).

Endnotes

BIBLIOGRAPHY

1. Role of androgens in growth and development of the fetus, child, and adolescent. Rosenfeld R.L. Adv Pediatr. 19 (1972) 172-213
2. Metabolism of Anabolic Androgenic Steroids, Victor A. Rogozkin, CRC Press 1991
3. Androgens and Erythropoeisis. J Clin Pharmacol. Feb-Mar 1974 p94-101
4. Effects of various modes of androgen substitution therapy on erythropoiesis. Jockenhovel F, Vogel E, Reinhardt W, Reinwein D. Eur J Med Res 1997 Jul 28;2(7):293-8
5. Testosterone increases lipolysis and the number of beta-adrenoceptors in male rat adipocytes. Xu XF, De Pergola G, Bjorntorp P. Endocrinology 1991 Jan;128(1):379-82
6. The effects of androgens on the regulation of lipolysis in adipose precursor cells. Endocrinol 126 (1990) 1229-34
7. Visceral fat accumulation in men is positively associated with insulin, glucose, and C-peptide levels, but negatively with testosterone levels. Seidell JC, Bjorntorp L, Sjostrom L, et al.Metabolism 39 (1990) 897-901
8. Effects of testosterone and estrogens on deltoid and trochanter adipocytes in two cases of transsexualism. Vague J, Meignen J.M. and Negrin J.F. Horm. Metabol. Res. 16 (1984) 380-381
9. Testosterone injection stimulates net protein synthesis but not tissue amino acid transport. Fernando A, Tipton K, Doyle D et al. Am J. Physiol (Endocrinology and Metabolism) 38:E864-71,1998.
10. Glucorticoid antagonism by exercise and androgenic-anabolic steroids. Hickson RC, Czerwinski SM, Falduto MT, Young AP. Med Sci Sports Exerc 22 (1990) 331-40
11. Binding of glucorticoid antagonists to androgen and glucorticoid hormone receptors in rat skeletal muscle. Danhaive PA, Rousseau GG. J Steroid Biochem Mol Biol 24 (1986) 481-71
12. Evidence for a sex-dependent anabolic response to androgenic steroids mediated by muscle glucorticoid receptors in the rat. Danhaive PA, Rousseau GG. J. Steroid Biochem Mol Biol. 29 (1988) 575-81
13. Glucorticoid antagonism by exercise and androgenic-anabolic steroids. Hickson RC, Czerwinski SM, Falduto MT, Young AP. Med Sci Sports Exerc 22 (1990) 331-40
14. The source of excess creatine following methyl testosterone. Samuels L.T., Sellers D.M., McCaulay C.J. J. Clin. Endocrinol. Metab. 6 (1946) 655-63
15. Ontogeny of growth hormone, insulin-like growth factor, estradiol and cortisol in the growing lamb: effect of testosterone. Arnold AM, Peralta JM,Tonney MI. J Endocrinol 150 (1996) 391-9 12.Jun;130(6):3677-83. 81, 2001.
16. Testosterone administration to elderly men increases skeletal muscle strength and protein synthesis. Am J Physiol 269 (1995) E820-6
17. Testosterone deficiency in young men: marked alterations in whole body protein kinetics, strength, and adiposity. Mausas N, Hayes V, Welch S et al. J Clin Endocrin Metab 83 (1998) 1886-92
18. Endocrinology 114(6):2100-06 1984 June, "Relative Binding Affinity of Anabolic-Androgenic Steroids...", Saartok T; Dahlberg E; Gustafsson JA
19. Endocrinology 114(6):2100-06 1984 June, "Relative Binding Affinity of Anabolic-Androgenic Steroids...", Saartok T; Dahlberg E; Gustafsson JA
20. Sex Hormone-Binding Globulin Response to the Anabolic Steroid Stanozolol: Evidence for Its Suitability as a Biological Androgen Sensitivity Test. J Clin Endocrinol Metab 68:1195,1989
21. Twenty two weeks of transdermal estradiol increases sex hormone-binding globulin in surgical menopausal women. Eur J Obstet Gynecol Reprod Biol 73: 149-52,1997
22. Aromatization of androgens by muscle and adipose tissue in vivo. Longcope C, Pratt JH, Schneider SH, Fineberg SE. J Clin Endocrinol Metab 1978 Jan;46(1):146-52
23. The aromatization of androstenedione by human adipose and liver tissue. J Steroid Biochem. 1980 Dec;13(12):1427-31.
24. Aromatase expression in the human male. Brodie A, Inkster S, Yue W. Mol Cell Endocrinol 2001 Jun 10;178(1-2):23-8
25. A review of brain aromatase cytochrome P450. Lephart ED. Brain Res Brain Res Rev 1996 Jun;22(1):1-26
26. Aromatization by skeletal muscle. Matsumine H, Hirato K, Yanaihara T, Tamada T, Yoshida M. J Clin Endocrinol Metab 1986 Sep;63(3):717-20
27. Pentose Cycle Activity in Muscle from Fetal, Neonatal and Infant Rhesus Monkeys. Arch Biochem Biophys 117:275-81 1966
28. The pentose phosphate pathway in regenerating skeletal muscle. Biochem J 170: 17 1978
29. Aromatization of androgens to estrogens mediates increased activity of glucose 6-phosphate dehydrogenase in rat levator ani muscle. Endocrinol 106(2):440-43 1980
30. Influence of tamoxifen, aminoglutethimide and goserelin on human plasma IGF-1 levels in breast cancer patients. J steroid Biochem Mol Bio 41:541-3,1992
31. Activation of the somatotropic axis by testosterone in adult males: Evidence for the role of aromatization. J Clin. Endocrinol Metab 76:1407-12 1993
32. Testosterone administration increases insulin-like growth factor-I levels in normal men. J Clin Endocrinol Metab 77(3):776-9 1993
33. Androgen-stimulated pubertal growth:the effects of testosterone and dihydrotestosterone on growth hormone and insulin-like growth factor-I in the treatment of short stature and delayed puberty. J Clin Endocrinol Metab 76(4)996-1001 1993
34. Modulation of the cytosolic androgen receptor in striated muscle by sex steroids. Endocrinology. 1984 Sep;115(3):862-6.
35. Effect of estrogen-serotonin interactions on mood and cognition. Zenab Amin et al. Behav Cogn Neurosci Reviews 4(1) 2005:43-58
36. Serotonin and the sleep/wake cycle: special emphasis on miscodialysis studies. Chiara M Portas et al. Progress in Neurology 60(200) 13-35.
37. Reduction of serotonin transporters of patients with chronic fatigue syndrome. Neuroreport 2004 Dec 3;15(17):2571-4
38. Association between serotonin transporter gene polymorphism and chronic fatigue syndrome. Narita M et al. Biochem Biophys Res Commun 2003 Nov 14;311(2)264-6
39. Premenstrual Syndrome. Dickerson LM et al. Am Fam Physician 2003 Apr 15;67(8):1743-52
40. Phase II trial of anastrozole in women with asymptomatic mullerian cancer. Gynecol Oncol. 2003 Dec;91(3):596-602.

41. Letrozole. A review of its use in postmenopausal women with advanced breast cancer. Drugs. 1998 Dec;56(6):1125-40. Review.
42. Exemestane: a review of its clinical efficacy and safety. Breast. 2001 Jun;10(3):198-208.
43. A study of fadrozole, a new aromatase inhibitor, in postmenopausal women with advanced metastatic breast cancer. J Clin Oncol. 1992 Jan;10(1):111-6.
44. Neural androgen receptor regulation: effects of androgen and antiandrogen. Lu S, Simon NG, Wang Y, Hu S. J Neurobiol 1999 Dec;41(4):505-12
45. A comparative study of the metabolic fate of testosterone, 17alpha-methyltestosterone, 19-nor-testosterone, 17alpha-methyl-19-nor-testosterone and 17alpha-methyl-estr-5(10)-ene-17beta-ol-3-one in normal males. Dimick D, Heron M, et al. Clin Chim Acta 6(1961) 63-71.
46. Unique steroid congeners for receptor studies. Ojasoo T, Raynaud J. Cancer Research 38 (1978) 4186-98
47. Cytosolic androgen receptor in regenerating rat levator ani muscle. Max S.R. Mufti S, Carlson B.M. J Biochem 200 (1981) 77
48. In vitro binding and metabolism of androgens in various organs: a comparative study. Kreig M., Voigt K.D. J Steroid Biochem 7 (1976) 1005
49. Androgen concentrations in sexual and non-sexual skin as well as striated muscle in man. Deslypere J.P., Sayed A., Verdonck L., Vermeulen A. J Steroid Biochem 13 (1980) 1455-8
50. Age related testosterone level changes and male andropause syndrome. Wu CY, Yu TJ, Chen MJ. Chang Gung Med J. 2000 Jun;23(6):348-53.
51. Osteoporosis in male hypogonadism: responses to androgen substitution differ among men with primary and secondary hypogonadism. Schubert M, Bullmann C et al. Horm Res. 2003;60(1):21-8.
52. Effect of testosterone replacement therapy on lipids and lipoproteins in hypogonadal and elderly men. Zgliczynski S, Ossowski M et al. Atherosclerosis. 1996 Mar;121(1):35-43.
53. Testosterone and other anabolic steroids as cardiovascular drugs. Shaprio J, Christiana J et al. Am J Ther 1999 May;6(3):167-74
54. Androgen deficiency as a predictor of metabolic syndrome in aging men: an opportunity for intervention? Kapoor D, Jones TH. Drugs Aging. 2008;25(5):357-69.
55. The effect of testosterone replacement on endogenous inflammatory cytokines and lipid profiles in hypogonadal men. Malkin CJ, Pugh PJ et al. J Clin Endocrinol Metab. 2004 Jul;89(7):3313-8.
56. Testosterone treatment in hypogonadal men: prostate-specific antigen level and risk of prostate cancer. Guay AT, Perez JB, Fitaihi WA, Vereb M. Endocr Pract. 2000 Mar-Apr;6(2):132-8.
57. Prostate volume and growth in testosterone-substituted hypogonadal men are dependent on the CAG repeat polymorphism of the androgen receptor gene: a longitudinal pharmacogenetic study. Zitzmann M, Depenbusch M, Gromoll J, Nieschlag E. J Clin Endocrinol Metab. 2003 May;88(5):2049-54.
58. Obstructive sleep apnea syndrome induced by testosterone administration. Sandblom RE, Matsumoto AM, Schoene RB, Lee KA, Giblin EC, Bremner WJ, Pierson DJ. N Engl J Med. 1983 Mar 3;308(9):508-10.
59. Testosterone therapy and obstructive sleep apnea: is there a real connection? Hanafy HM. J Sex Med. 2007 Sep;4(5):1241-6. Epub 2007 Jul 21.
60. Intramuscular testosterone treatment in elderly men: evidence of memory decline and altered brain function. Maki PM, Ernst M et al. J Clin Endocrinol Metab. 2007 Nov;92(11):4107-14. Epub 2007 Aug 28.
61. Exogenous testosterone alone or with finasteride does not improve measurements of cognition in healthy older men with low serum testosterone. Vaughan C, Goldstein FC, Tenover JL. J Androl. 2007 Nov-Dec;28(6):875-82. Epub 2007 Jul 3.
62. Testosterone improves spatial memory in men with Alzheimer disease and mild cognitive impairment. Cherrier MM, Matsumoto AM et al. Neurology. 2005 Jun 28;64(12):2063-8.
63. Characterization of Verbal and Spatial Memory Changes from Moderate to Supraphysiological increases in Serum Testosterone in Healthy Older Men. M Cherrier et al. Psychoneuroendocrinology 2007 Jan 32(1): 72-79.
64. Danazol and stanozolol in long-term prophylactic treatment of hereditary angioedema. Agostoni A, Cicardi M. J Allergy Clin Immunol. 1980 Jan;65(1):75-9.
65. Endocrine and intracrine sources of androgens in women: inhibition of breast cancer and other roles of androgens and their precursor
66. Effects of androgens on haemostasis. Winkler UH. Maturitas. 1996 Jul;24(3):147-55.
67. Anabolic steroids and fibrinolysis. Lowe GD. Wien Med Wochenschr. 1993;143(14-15):383-5.
68. Plasma fibrinolytic activity following oral anabolic steroid therapy. Walker ID, Davidson JF. Thromb Diath Haemorrh. 1975 Sep 30;34(1):236-45.
69. The effect of mesterolone on sperm count, on serum follicle stimulating hormone, luteinizing hormone, plasma testosterone and outcome in idiopathic oligospermic men. Varma TR, Patel RH. Int J Gynaecol Obstet. 1988 Feb;26(1):121-8.
70. Mesterolone treatment of patients with pathospermia. Szöllösi J, Falkay GY, Sas M. Int Urol Nephrol. 1978;10(3):251-6.
71. Oxandrolone therapy in constitutionally delayed growth and puberty. Bio-Technology General Corporation Cooperative Study Group. Wilson DM, McCauley E, Brown DR, Dudley R. Pediatrics. 1995 Dec;96(6):1095-100.
72. Growth and growth hormone responses to oxandrolone in boys with constitutional delay of growth and puberty (CDGP). Clayton PE, Shalet SM, Price DA, Addison GM. Clin Endocrinol (Oxf). 1988 Aug;29(2):123-30.
73. Oxandrolone in constitutional delay of growth: analysis of the growth patterns up to final stature. Bassi F, Neri AS, Gheri RG, Cheli D, Serio M. J Endocrinol Invest. 1993 Feb;16(2):133-7.
74. Oxandrolone treatment of constitutional short stature in boys during adolescence: effect on linear growth, bone age, pubic hair, and testicular development. Marti-Henneberg C, Niirianen AK, Rappaport R. J Pediatr. 1975 May;86(5):783-8.
75. Anabolic steroids in postmenopausal osteoporosis. Need AG et al. Wien Med Wochenschr. 1993;143(14-15):392-5.
76. Nandrolone decanoate: pharmacological properties and therapeutic use in osteoporosis. Geusens P. Clin Rheumatol. 1995 Sep;14 Suppl 3:32-9.
77. Nandrolone decanoate: pharmacological properties and therapeutic use in osteoporosis. Geusens P. Clin Rheumatol. 1995 Sep;14 Suppl 3:32-9.
78. Nandrolone decanoate for men with osteoporosis. Hamdy RC, Moore SW, Whalen KE, Landy C. Am J Ther. 1998 Mar;5(2):89-95.
79. Effects of nandrolone decanoate on bone mass in established osteoporosis. Passeri M, Pedrazzoni M, Pioli G, Butturini L, Ruys AH, Cortenraad MG. Maturitas. 1993 Nov;17(3):211-9.
80. Nandrolone decanoate: pharmacological properties and therapeutic use in osteoporosis. Geusens P. Clin Rheumatol. 1995 Sep;14 Suppl 3:32-9.
81. Effects of nandrolone decanoate (Decadurabolin) on serum Lp(a), lipids and lipoproteins in women with postmenopausal osteoporosis. Lippi G, Guidi

G, Ruzzenente O, Braga V, Adami S. Scand J Clin Lab Invest. 1997 Oct;57(6):507-11.
82. Turner's syndrome. Guarneri MP, Abusrewil SA et al. J Pediatr Endocrinol Metab. 2001 Jul;14 Suppl 2:959-65.
83. Underweight, overweight and obesity as risk factors for mortality and hospitalization. Gunilla Ringbäck Weitoft. Scandinavian Journal of Public Health, Vol. 36, No. 2, 169-176 (2008)
84. Catabolic illness. Strategies for enhancing recovery. Wilmore DW. N Engl J Med. 1991 Sep 5;325(10):695-702.
85. A randomized, placebo-controlled trial of nandrolone decanoate in human immunodeficiency virus-infected men with mild to moderate weight loss with recombinant human growth hormone as active reference treatment. Storer TW, Woodhouse LJ et al. J Clin Endocrinol Metab. 2005 Aug;90(8):4474-82. Epub 2005 May 24.
86. Double-blind, randomized, placebo-controlled phase III trial of oxymetholone for the treatment of HIV wasting. Hengge UR, Stocks K et al. AIDS. 2003 Mar 28;17(5):699-710.
87. Oxandrolone in the treatment of HIV-associated weight loss in men: a randomized, double-blind, placebo-controlled study. Grunfeld C, Kotler DP et al. J Acquir Immune Defic Syndr. 2006 Mar;41(3):304-14.
88. Use of anabolic steroids and associated health risks among gay men attending London gyms. Bolding G, Sherr L, Elford J. Addiction. 2002 Feb;97(2):195-203.
89. Hepatic lipase activity influences high density lipoprotein subclass distribution in normotriglyceridemic men: genetic and pharmacological evidence. Grundy S et al. J Lipid Res 1999 40: 229-34.
90. Changes in lipoprotein-lipid levels in normal men following administration of increasing doses of testosterone cypionate. Kouri EM et al. Clin J Sport Med 1996 Jul;6(3):152-7.
91. Contrasting effects of testosterone and stanozolol on serum lipoprotein levels. JAMA 261:1165-8,1989
92. High-Density Lipoprotein Cholesterol Is Not Decreased if an Aromatizable Androgen Is Administered. Metabolism, 39:69-74,1990
93. Relationship of cardiac size to maximal oxygen uptake and body size in men and women. Hutchinson PL, Cureton KJ, Outz H, Wilson G. Int J Sports Med. 1991 Aug;12(4):369-73.
94. Androgenic anabolic steroids also impair right ventricular function. Kasikcioglu E et al. Int J Cardiol 2008 Feb 11 E Pub.
95. Cardiac effects of anabolic steroids. Payne J. et al. Heart 2004; 90:473-75.
96. Adverse effects of anabolic androgenic steroids on the cardiovascular, metabolic and reproductive systems of anabolic substance abusers. Tuomo Karila. Publications of the National Public Health Institute ISBN 951-740-388-2
97. Absense of left ventricular wall thickening in athletes engaged in intense power training. Pelliccia A et al. Am J Cardiol 1993; 72: 1048-54.
98. Left ventricular hypertrophy by Sokolow-Lyon voltage criterion predicts mortality in overweight hypertensive subjects. Antikainen RL, Grodzicki T. J Hum Hypertens. 2008 Aug 28. [Epub]
99. Hypertensive heart disease. A complex syndrome or a hypertensive cardiomyopathy? Lip GYH et al. Eur Heart J 2000; 21: 1653-65.
100. Adverse effects of anabolic androgenic steroids on the cardiovascular, metabolic and reproductive systems of anabolic substance abusers. Tuomo Karila. Publications of the National Public Health Institute ISBN 951-740-388-2
101. Left ventricular hypertrophy and QT dispersion in hypertension. Mayet J et al. Hypertension 1996; 28: 791-96.
102. Cardiac arrest following anaesthetic induction in a world-class bodybuilder. Angelilli A, Katz ES, Goldenberg RM. Acta Cardiol. 2005 Aug;60(4):443-4.
103. Effects of training on left ventricular structure and function. An echocardiographic study. Shapiro CM et al. Br. Heart J 1983; 50: 534-39.
104. Are the cardiac effects of anabolic steroid abuse in strength athletes reversible? Urhausen A, Albers T, Kindermann W. Heart. 2004 May;90(5):496-501.
105. The effects of anabolic-androgenic steroids on primary myocardial cell cultures. Melchert RB et al. Med Sci Sports Exerc 1992; 24:266-12
106. Cardiovascular effects of anabolic-androgenic steroids. Melchert RB et al. Med Sci Sports Exerc 1995;27: 1252-62
107. Cause and manner of death among users of anabolic androgenic steroids. Thiblin I et al. J Forensic Sci 2000;45:16-23
108. Anabolic steroid abuse and cardiac death. Kennedy MC et al. Med J Aust 1993; 158:346-48.
109. Serious cardiovascular side effects of large doses of anabolic steroids in weight lifters. Nieminen MS et al. Eur Heart J 1996; 17:1576-83.
110. Sudden cardiac death during anabolic steroid abuse: morphologic and toxicologic findings in two fatal cases of bodybuilders. Fineschi V et al. Int J Legal Med 2007 Jan;121(1):48-53. Epub 2005 Nov 15. Review.
111. Blood pressure and rate pressure product response in males using high-dose anabolic androgenic steroids (AAS). Grace F, Sculthorpe N, Baker J, Davies B. J Sci Med Sport. 2003 Sep;6(3):307-12.
112. Are the cardiac effects of anabolic steroid abuse in strength athletes reversible? A Urhausen et al. Heart 2004;90:496-501.
113. Cardiovascular side effects of anabolic-androgenic steroids. Herz. 2006 Sep;31(6):566-73.
114. Anabolic steroids and fibrinolysis. Lowe GD. Wien Med Wochenschr. 1993;143(14-15):383-5.
115. Effect of anabolic steroids on plasma antithrombin III. alpha2 macroglobulin and alpha1 antitrypsin levels. Walker ID, Davidson JF, Young P, Conkie JA. Thromb Diath Haemorrh. 1975 Sep 30;34(1):106-14.
116. Depo-Testosterone. Pharmacia. U.S. Prescribing Information. Revised August 2002.
117. Anabolic-androgenic steroid abuse in weight lifters: evidence for activation of the hemostatic system. Am J Hematol. Ferenchick GS, Hirokawa S, Mammen EF, Schwartz KA. 1995 Aug;49(4):282-8.
118. Raised concentrations of C reactive protein in anabolic steroid using bodybuilders. F M Grace, B Davies et al. Br J Sports Med 2004;38:97-98.
119. Testosterone increases human platelet thromboxane A2 receptor density and aggregation responses. Ajayi AA, Mathur R, Halushka PV. Circulation. 1995 Jun 1;91(11):2742-7.
120. Androgenic-anabolic steroid abuse and platelet aggregation: a pilot study in weight lifters. Ferenchick G, Schwartz D, Ball M, Schwartz K. Am J Med Sci. 1992 Feb;303(2):78-82.
121. Pulmonary embolism associated with the use of anabolic steroids. Liljeqvist S, Helldén A, Bergman U, Söderberg M. Eur J Intern Med. 2008 May;19(3):214-5. Epub 2007 Sep 19.
122. Coronary thrombosis and ectasia of coronary arteries after long-term use of anabolic steroids. Tischer KH, Heyny-von Haussen R, Mall G, Doenecke P. Z Kardiol. 2003 Apr;92(4):326-31.
123. Massive pulmonary embolus and anabolic steroid abuse. Gaede JT, Montine TJ. JAMA. 1992 May 6;267(17):2328-9.

124. Steroid anabolic drugs and arterial complications in an athlete--a case history. Laroche GP. Angiology. 1990 Nov;41(11):964-9.
125. Death caused by pulmonary embolism in a body builder taking anabolic steroids (metanabol). Siekierzyƒska-Czarnecka A, Polowiec Z, Kulawiƒska M, Rowinska-Zakrzewska E. Wiad Lek. 1990 Oct 1-15;43(19-20):972-5.
126. Coagulation abnormalities associated with the use of anabolic steroids. Ansell JE, Tiarks C, Fairchild VK. Am Heart J. 1993 Feb;125(2 Pt 1):367-71.
127. Hematocrit and the risk of cardiovascular disease--the Framingham study: a 34-year follow-up. Gagnon DR, Zhang TJ, Brand FN, Kannel WB. Am Heart J. 1994 Mar;127(3):674-82.
128. Homocysteine induced cardiovascular events: a consequence of long term anabolic-androgenic steroid (AAS) abuse. M R Graham, F M Grace et al. Br. J Sports Med. 2006;40:544-48.
129. Homocysteine and cardiovascular disease: time to routinely screen and treat? P. O'Callaghan et al. Br J Cario 2003; 10(2) 115-7.
130. Promotion of vascular smooth muscle cell growth by homocysteine: a link to atherosclerosis. Proc Natl Acad Sci 1994;91:6369-73.
131. Homocystinuria: metabolic studies on three patients. Brenton D et al. J Pediatr 1966;67-58-68.
132. Homocysteine, and atherogenic stimulus, reduces protein C activation by arterial and venous endothelial cell. Rogers G et al. Blood 1990;75:895-901.
133. Homocysteinethiolactone disposal by human arterial endothelial cells and serum in vitro. Dudman N et al. Atherioscler Thromb 1991;11:663-70.
134. Plasma homocysteine levels and mortality in patients with coronary artery disease. Nygard O et al. N Engl J Med 1997;337:230-6.
135. Effects of sex steroids on plasma total homocysteine levels: a study in transsexual males and females. Giltay EJ, Hoogeveen EK et al. J Clin Endocrinol Metab. 1998 Feb;83(2):550-3.
136. Homocysteine levels in men and women of different ethnic and cultural background living in England. Cappuccio FP, Bell R. et al. Atherosclerosis. 2002 Sep;164(1):95-102.
137. Hyperhomocysteinemia in bodybuilders taking anabolic steroids. Ebenbichler CF, Kaser S et al. Eur J Intern Med. 2001 Feb;12(1):43-47.
138. Homocysteine induced cardiovascular events: a consequence of long term anabolic-androgenic steroid (AAS) abuse. M R Graham, F M Grace et al. Br. J Sports Med. 2006;40:544-48.
139. The effect of supraphysiologic doses of testosterone on fasting total homocysteine levels in normal men. Zmuda JM, Bausserman LL, Maceroni D, Thompson PD. Atherosclerosis. 1997 Apr;130(1-2):199-202.
140. Hypertension, stroke, and endothelium. F. Consentino, M. Volpe. Cur Hypertension Rep. January 2005: 7(1); 68-71
141. Differences in Vascular Reactivity Between Men and Women. Bob J. Schank, MS et al. Angiology, Vol. 57, No. 6, 702-708 (2007)
142. Flow-mediated, endothelium-dependent vasodilatation is impaired in male body builders taking anabolic-androgenic steroids. Ebenbichler CF, Sturm W et al. Atherosclerosis. 2001 Oct;158(2):483-90.
143. Impaired vasoreactivity in bodybuilders using androgenic anabolic steroids. Lane HA et al. Eur J Clin Invest 2006 Jul; 36(7): 483-8.
144. The more effective immune system of women against infectious agents. Müller HE. Wien Med Wochenschr. 1992;142(17):389-95
145. Sex hormones, immune responses, and autoimmune diseases. Mechanisms of sex hormone action. Ansar AS et al. Human Repr Upd. 11(4) 411-23. 2005.
146. Sex hormones and the immune response in humans. A Bouman et al. Human Reprod Update 11(4) pp.411-23, 2005.
147. Effect of a single administration of testosterone on the immune response and lymphoid tissue in mice. Fuji H et al. Immunology 20:315-26. 1975.
148. Estrogens and health in males. Lombardi G, Zarrilli S et al. Mol Cell Endocrinol. 2001 Jun 10;178(1-2):51-5.
149. Dichotomy of glucocorticoid action in the immune system. Asadullah K, Schäcke H, Cato AC. Trends Immunol. 2002 Mar;23(3):120-2
150. Anabolic steroid effects on immune function: differences between analogues. Mendenhall CL, Grossman CJ, et al. J Steroid Biochem Mol Biol. 1990 Sep;37(1):71-6.
151. A trial of testosterone therapy for HIV-associated weight loss. Coodley GO, Coodley MK. AIDS. 1997 Sep;11(11):1347-52.
152. Effects of nandrolone decanoate compared with placebo or testosterone on HIV-associated wasting. J Gold,1 MJ Batterham et al. HIV Medicine (2006), 7, 146–155
153. The effect of anabolic steroids and strength training on the immune response. L Calabrese et al. Med and Sci in Sports and Exer. 21(4) pp. 386-92, 1983.
154. Androgens potentiate the effects of erythropoietin in the treatment of anemia of end-stage renal disease. Ballal SH, Domoto DT, Polack DC, Marciulonis P, Martin KJ. Am J Kidney Dis. 1991 Jan;17(1):29-33.
155. Use of androgens in patients with renal failure. Johnson CA. Semin Dial. 2000 Jan-Feb;13(1):36-9.
156. Anabolic effects of nandrolone decanoate in patients receiving dialysis: a randomized controlled trial. Johansen KL, Mulligan K, Schambelan M. JAMA. 1999 Apr 14;281(14):1275-81.
157. Testosterone metabolism and replacement therapy in patients with end-stage renal disease. Johansen KL. Semin Dial. 2004 May-Jun;17(3):202-8.
158. The effect of anabolic steroids on the gastrointestinal system, kidneys, and adrenal glands. Modlinski R, Fields KB. Curr Sports Med Rep. 2006 Apr;5(2):104-9.
159. Wilms tumor in an adult associated with androgen abuse. Prat J, Gray GF, Stolley PD, Coleman JW. JAMA. 1977 May 23;237(21):2322-3
160. Anabolic steroid abuse and renal cell carcinoma. Martorana G, Concetti S, Manferrari F, Creti S. J Urol. 1999 Dec;162(6):2089
161. Anabolic steroid abuse and renal-cell carcinoma. Bryden AA, Rothwell PJ, O'Reilly PH. Lancet. 1995 Nov 11;346(8985):1306-7
162. At what price, glory? Severe cholestasis and acute renal failure in an athlete abusing stanozolol. Yoshida EM, Karim MA, Shaikh JF, Soos JG, Erb SR. CMAJ. 1994 Sep 15;151(6):791-3
163. Severe cholestasis with kidney failure from anabolic steroids in a body builder. Habscheid W, Abele U, Dahm HH. Dtsch Med Wochenschr. 1999 Sep
164. The incidence of post-operative renal failure in obstructive jaundice. Dawson JL. Br J Surg 1965; 52: 663-665.
165. Acute renal failure complicating muscle crush injury. Abassi ZA, Hoffman A, Better OS. Semin Nephrol. 1998 Sep;18(5):558-65
166. Rhabdomyolysis in a bodybuilder using anabolic steroids. Hageloch W, Appell HJ, Weicker H. Sportverletz Sportschaden. 1988 Sep;2(3):122-5.
167. Atraumatic rhabdomyolysis in a 20-year-old bodybuilder. Morocco PA. J Emerg Nurs. 1991 Dec;17(6):370-2.
168. Continuous veno-venous hemofiltration for the immediate management of massive rhabdomyolysis after fulminant malignant hyperthermia in a

bodybuilder. Schenk MR, Beck DH, Nolte M, Kox WJ. Anesthesiology. 2001 Jun;94(6):1139-41.

169. Rhabdomyolysis in a bodybuilder using steroids. Daniels JM, van Westerloo DJ, de Hon OM, Frissen PH. Ned Tijdschr Geneeskd. 2006 May 13;150(19):1077-80.

170. Hypertension and the kidney. Hohenstein K, Watschinger B. Wien Med Wochenschr. 2008;158(13-14):359-64.

171. Hepatic effects of 17 alpha-alkylated anaboli-androgenic steroids. HIV Hotline. 1998 Dec;8(5-6):2-5.

172. Methyltestosterone, related steroids, and liver function. A deLorimier et al. Arch Inter Med Vol. 116 Aug 1965 p 289-94

173. Jaundice associated with norbolethone (Nilevar) therapy. Shaw R K et al. Ann Intern Med 52:428-34 1960.

174. Androgenic/Anabolic steroid-induced toxic hepatitis. Stimac D, Milič S, Dintinjana RD, Kovac D, Ristič S. J Clin Gastroenterol. 2002 Oct;35(4):350-2.

175. Review of oxymetholone: a 17alpha-alkylated anabolic-androgenic steroid. Pavlatos AM, Fultz O, Monberg MJ, Vootkur A, Pharmd. Clin Ther. 2001 Jun;23(6):789-801; discussion 771

176. A pilot study of anabolic steroids in elderly patients with hip fractures. Sloan JP, Wing P, Dian L, Meneilly GS. J Am Geriatr Soc. 1992 Nov;40(11):1105-11.

177. Effects of long-term use of testosterone enanthate. II. Effects on lipids, high and low density lipoprotein cholesterol and liver function parameters. Tyagi A, Rajalakshmi M. et al. Int J Androl. 1999 Dec;22(6):347-55.

178. Cellular distribution of androgen receptors in the liver. Hinchliffe SA, Woods S, Gray S, Burt AD. J Clin Pathol. 1996 May;49(5):418-20.

179. Liver toxicity of a new anabolic agent: methyltrienolone (17-alpha-methyl-4,9,11-estratriene-17 beta-ol-3-one). Kruskemper, Noell. Steroids. 1966 Jul;8(1):13-24

180. T. Feyel-Cabanes, Compt. Rend. Soc. Biol. 157, 1428 (1963)

181. Anabolic-androgenic steroids and liver injury. M Sanchez-Osorio et al. Liver International ISSN 1478-3223 p. 278-82.

182. Androgenic/Anabolic steroid-induced toxic hepatitis. Stimac D et al. J Clin Gastroenterol. 2002 Oct;35(4):350-2.

183. Mechanisms and sites of action of ursodeoxycholic acid in cholestasis. Beuers U. Nat Clin Pract Gastroenterol Hepatol 2006; 3:318-28.

184. Peliosis hepatis in a young adult bodybuilder. Cabasso A. Med Sci Sports Exerc. 1994 Jan;26(1):2-4.

185. Bleeding esophageal varices associated with anabolic steroid use in an athlete. Winwood PJ et al. Post-Grad Med J 1990; 66:864-65.

186. Benign liver-cell adenoma associated with long-term administration of an androgenic-anabolic steroid (methandienone). Hernandez-Nieto L, Bruguera M, Bombi J, Camacho L, Rozman C. Cancer. 1977 Oct;40(4):1761-4

187. Hepatocellular carcinoma in the non-cirrhotic liver. Evert M, Dombrowski F. Pathologe. 2008 Feb;29(1):47-52

188. Intratesticular leiomyosarcoma in a young man after high dose doping with Oral-Turinabol: a case report. Cancer. Froehner M, Fischer R, Leike S, Hakenberg OW, Noack B, Wirth MP. 1999 Oct 15;86(8):1571-5.

189. Hepatocellular carcinoma associated with recreational anabolic steroid use. Gorayski P, Thompson CH, Subhash HS, Thomas AC. Br J Sports Med. 2008 Jan;42(1):74-5; discussion 75.

190. Bodybuilder death steroids warning. Express and Star 2008 09/04. Epub. www.expressandstar.com

191. Effect of testosterone and anabolic steroids on the size of sebaceous glands in power athletes. Kiraly CL et al. Am J Dermatopathol, 1987 Dec, 9:6, 515-9.

192. RU 58841, a new specific topical antiandrogen: a candidate of choice for the treatment of acne, androgenetic alopecia, and hirsutism. Battmann T. et al. J Steroid Biochem Mol Biol. 1994 Jan;48(1):55-60.

193. Androgenetic alopecia and current methods of treatment. Bienová M, Kucerová R. et al. Acta Dermatovenerol Alp Panonica Adriat. 2005 Mar;14(1):5-8.

194. Molecular mechanisms of androgenetic alopecia. Trüeb RM. Exp Gerontol. 2002 Aug-Sep;37(8-9):981-90.

195. The inheritance of common baldness: two B or not two B? Kuster W, Happle R. J Am Acad Dermatol 1984; 11: 921-26.

196. Polymorphism of the Androgen Receptor Gene is Associated with Male Pattern Baldness. Justine A Ellis, Margaret Stebbing and Stephen B Harrap. Journal of Investigative Dermatology (2001) 116, 452–455.

197. EDA2R is associated with androgenetic alopecia. Prodi DA, Pirastu N, et al. J Invest Dermatol. 2008 Sep;128(9):2268-70. Epub 2008 Apr 3.

198. Current understanding of androgenetic alopecia. Part I: Etiopathogenesis. Hoffmann R, Happle R. European Journal of Dermatology. Volume 10, Number 4, 319-27, June 2000

199. Estrogen and progesterone receptors in androgenic alopecia versus alopecia areata. Wallace ML, Smoller BR. Am J Dermatopathol. 1998 Apr;20(2):160-3.

200. Hormonal doping and androgenization of athletes: a secret program of the German Democratic Republic government. Franke WW, Berendonk B. Clin Chem. 1997 Jul;43(7):1262-79.

201. Role of estrogen on bone in the human male: insights from the natural models of congenital estrogen deficiency. Faustini-Fustini, M. et al. Mol Cell Endocrinol. 2001 Jun 10;178(1-2):215-20.

202. Effects of estrogen on growth plate senescence and epiphyseal function. M Weise, S De-Levi et al. Proc Natl Acad Sci June 5, 2001 pp. 6871-6876.

203. The results of short-term (6 months) high-dose testosterone treatment on bone age and adult height in boys of excessively tall stature. Brämswig JH, von Lengerke HJ et al. Eur J Pediatr. 1988 Nov;148(2):104-6.

204. Oxandrolone in constitutional delay of growth: analysis of the growth patterns up to final stature. Bassi F, Neri AS, Gheri RG, Cheli D, Serio M. J Endocrinol Invest. 1993 Feb;16(2):133-7.

205. Salt, hypertension, and edema. Rössler R. Internist (Berl). 1976 Oct;17(10):489-93. Review.

206. Sex hormone effects on body fluid regulation. Stachenfeld NS. Exerc Sport Sci Rev. 2008 Jul;36(3):152-9.

207. Effect of ovarian steroids on vasopressin secretion. Forsling, M. L., P. Stromberg, and M. Akerlund. J. Endocrinol. 95: 147-151, 1982

208. Estrogen influences osmotic secretion of AVP and body water balance in postmenopausal women. Nina S. Stachenfeld, Loretta Dipietro, Steven F. Palter, and Ethan R. Nadel Am J Physiol Regul Integr Comp Physiol 274: R187-R195, 1998.

209. Independent and combined effects of testosterone and growth hormone on extracellular water in hypopituitary men. Johannsson G, Gibney J, et al.

J Clin Endocrinol Metab. 2005 Jul;90(7):3989-94. Epub 2005 Apr 12.

210. Casner, S. W., Early, R. G., and Carlson, B.R. Journal of Sports Med and Phys Fitness, 1971 11,98.

211. The effects of anabolic steroids on growth, body composition, and metabolism in boys with chronic renal failure on regular hemodialysis. Jones RW, El Bishti MM et al. J Pediatr. 1980 Oct;97(4):559-66.

212. A randomized, placebo-controlled trial of nandrolone decanoate in human immunodeficiency virus-infected men with mild to moderate weight loss with recombinant human growth hormone as active reference treatment. Storer TW, Woodhouse LJ, J Clin Endocrinol Metab. 2005 Aug;90(8):4474-82. Epub 2005 May 24.

213. Bodybuilders' Body Composition: Effect of Nandrolone Decanoate. VAN MARKEN LICHTENBELT, W. D., F. HARTGENS, N. B. J. VOLLAARD, S. EBBING, and H. KUIPERS. Med. Sci. Sports Exerc., Vol. 36, No. 3, pp. 484-489, 2004.

214. Severe laryngitis following chronic anabolic steroid abuse. Ray S, Masood A, Pickles J, Moumoulidis I. J Laryngol Otol. 2008 Mar;122(3):230-2. Epub 2007 May 14

215. Estrogen regulation of mammary gland development and breast cancer: amphiregulin takes center stage
Heather L LaMarca1 and Jeffrey M Rosen. Breast Cancer Res. 2007; 9(4): 304.

216. Androgens and mammary growth and neoplasia. Dimitrakakis C, Zhou J, Bondy CA. Fertil Steril. 2002 Apr;77 Suppl 4:S26-33.

217. Surgical treatment of gynecomastia in the body builder. Aiache AE. Plast Reconstr Surg. 1989 Jan;83(1):61-6.

218. Roles of estrogen and progesterone in normal mammary gland development insights from progesterone receptor null mutant mice and in situ localization of receptor. Shyamala G. Trends Endocrinol Metab. 1997 Jan-Feb;8(1):34-9.

219. A report on alterations to the speaking and singing voices of four women following hormonal therapy with virilizing agents. Baker J. J Voice 1999 Dec;13(4):496-507.

220. Fundamental voice frequence during normal and abnormal growth, and after androgen treatment. Vuorenkoski V, Lenko HL, Tjernlund P, Vuorenkoski L, Perheentupa J. Arch Dis Child. 1978 Mar;53(3):201-9.

221. Fluoxymesterone therapy in anemia of patients on maintenance hemodialysis: comparison between patients with kidneys and anephric patients. Acchiardo SR, Black WD. J Dial. 1977;1(4):357-66.

222. Testosterone therapy in women: its role in the management of hypoactive sexual desire disorder. Abdallah RT, Simon JA. Int J Impot Res. 2007 Sep-Oct;19(5):458-63. Epub 2007 Jun 21.

223. Virilization caused by methandrostenolone-containing cream in 2 prepubertal girls. Sorgo W, Zachmann M. Helv Paediatr Acta. 1982 Sep;37(4):401-6.

224. Change in speaking fundamental frequency in hormone-treated patients with Turner's syndrome--a longitudinal study of four cases. Andersson-Wallgren G, Albertsson-Wikland K. Acta Paediatr. 1994 Apr;83(4):452-5.

225. Virilization of the voice in post-menopausal women due to the anabolic steroid nandrolone decanoate (Decadurabolin). The effects of medication for one year. Gerritsma EJ, Brocaar MP, Hakkesteegt MM, Birkenhäger JC. Clin Otolaryngol Allied Sci. 1994 Feb;19(1):79-84.

226. Idiopathic isolated clitoromegaly: A report of two cases. Eray Copcu1, Alper Aktas et al. Reproductive Health 2004, 1:4.

227. Two Cases of Clitoromegaly. Clitoral Reduction Preserving Sensation of Clitoris. NODA KOJIRO (Chiba-ken Kodomo Byoin), UDAGAWA AKIKAZU (Chiba-ken Kodomo Byoin) et al. Journal of Japan Society of Aesthetic Plastic Surgery VOL.22;NO.3;PAGE.90-95(2000).

228. Evaluation and Treatment of Women with Hirsutism. MELISSA H. HUNTER, M.D., and PETER J. CAREK, M.D. Am Fam Physician 2003;67:2565-72.

229. Effects of long-term androgen administration on breast tissue of female-to-male transsexuals. M Slagter, L Gooren et al. J Histochem Cytochem. 54(8): 905-910, 2006.

230. Behavioural effects of androgen in men and women. Christiansen K. J Endocrinol. 2001 Jul;170(1):39-48.

231. Exogenous testosterone enhances responsiveness to social threat in the neural circuitry of social aggression in humans. Hermans EJ, Ramsey NF, van Honk J. Biol Psychiatry. 2008 Feb 1;63(3):263-70. Epub 2007 Aug 28.

232. Underground Steroid Handbook II. Daniel Duchaine. 1989. HLR technical books. Venice, CA.

233. Metabolic and behavioral effects of high-dose, exogenous testosterone in healthy men. Bagatell CJ, Heiman JR, Matsumoto AM, Rivier JE, Bremner WJ. J Clin Endocrinol Metab. 1994 Aug;79(2):561-7.

234. The effects of exogenous testosterone on sexuality and mood of normal men. Anderson RA, Bancroft J, Wu FC. J Clin Endocrinol Metab. 1992 Dec;75(6):1503-7.

235. Psychological and serum homovanillic acid changes in men administered androgenic steroids. Hannan CJ Jr, Friedl KE, Zold A, Kettler TM, Plymate SR. Psychoneuroendocrinology. 1991;16(4):335-43.

236. Psychosexual effects of three doses of testosterone cycling in normal men. Yates WR et al. Biol Psychiatry. 1999;45:254-60.

237. Effects of supraphysiological doses of testosterone on mood and aggression in normal men. H Pope, E Kouri et al. Arch Gen Psychiatry. 2000;57:133-140.

238. Psychiatric side effects induced by supraphysiological doses of combinations of anabolic steroids correlate to the severity of abuse. T Pagonis et al. Eur Psych 21 (2006) 551-62.

239. Violence toward women and illicit androgenic-anabolic steroid use. Choi PY, Pope HG Jr. Ann Clin Psychiatry. 1994 Mar;6(1):21-5.

240. Criminality among individuals testing positive for the presence of anabolic androgenic steroids. Klötz F, Garle M, Granath F, Thiblin I. Arch Gen Psychiatry. 2006 Nov;63(11):1274-9.

241. Homicide and near-homicide by anabolic steroid users. Pope HG Jr, Katz DL. J Clin Psychiatry. 1990 Jan;51(1):28-31.

242. Evidence for physical and psychological dependence on anabolic androgenic steroids in eight weight lifters. K Bower, G Eliopulos et al. Am J Psychiatry 1990; 147:510-12.

243. Muscle dysmorphia. An underrecognized form of body dysmorphic disorder. Pope HG Jr, Gruber AJ, Choi P, Olivardia R, Phillips KA. Psychosomatics. 1997 Nov-Dec;38(6):548-57.

244. "Chocolate addiction": a preliminary study of its description and its relationship to problem eating. Hetherington MM, MacDiarmid JI. Appetite. 1993 Dec;21(3):233-46.

245. Reinforcing aspects of androgens. Wood RI. Physiol Behav. 2004 Nov 15;83(2):279-89.
246. Expression of testosterone conditioned place preference is blocked by peripheral or intra-accumbens injection of alpha-flupenthixol. Packard MG, Schroeder JP, Alexander GM. Horm Behav. 1998 Aug;34(1):39-47.
247. Role of dopamine receptor subtypes in the acquisition of a testosterone conditioned place preference in rats. Schroeder JP, Packard MG. Neurosci Lett. 2000 Mar 17;282(1-2):17-20.
248. Increased dopamine transporter density in the male rat brain following chronic nandrolone decanoate administration. Kindlundh AM, Rahman S, Lindblom J, Nyberg F. Neurosci Lett. 2004 Feb 12;356(2):131-4.
249. Abuse liability of testosterone. Fingerhood MI, Sullivan JT et al. J Psychopharmacol 1997; 11(1):59-63.
250. Anabolic steroid withdrawal depression: a case report. Allnutt S, Chaimowitz G. Can J Psychiatry. 1994 Jun;39(5):317-8.
251. The use of fluoxetine in depression associated with anabolic steroid withdrawal: a case series. Malone DA Jr, Dimeff RJ. J Clin Psychiatry. 1992 Apr;53(4):130-2.
252. New-generation antidepressants, suicide and depressed adolescents: how should clinicians respond to changing evidence? Dudley M, Hadzi-Pavlovic D, Andrews D, Perich T. Aust N Z J Psychiatry. 2008 Jun;42(6):456-66.
253. Anabolic androgenic steroids and suicide. Thiblin I, Runeson B, Rajs J. Ann Clin Psychiatry. 1999 Dec;11(4):223-31.
254. Testosterone deficiency and mood in aging men: pathogenic and therapeutic interactions. Seidman SN. World J Biol Psychiatry. 2003 Jan;4(1):14-20.
255. Treatment strategies of withdrawal from long-term use of anabolic-androgenic steroids. MedraÊ M, Tworowska U. Pol Merkur Lekarski. 2001 Dec;11(66):535-8. Review
256. Psychological moods and subjectively perceived behavioral and somatic changes accompanying anabolic-androgenic steroid use. Bahrke MS, Wright JE, Strauss RH, Catlin DH. Am J Sports Med. 1992 Nov-Dec;20(6):717-24.
257. Insomnia: pathophysiology and implications for treatment. Roth T, Roehrs T, Pies R. Sleep Med Rev. 2007 Feb;11(1):71-9. Epub 2006 Dec 18.
258. When does estrogen replacement therapy improve sleep quality? Polo-Kantola P, Erkkola R, Helenius H, Irjala K, Polo O. Am J Obstet Gynecol. 1998 May;178(5):1002-9.
259. Adverse effects of anabolic androgenic steroids on the cardiovascular, metabolic and reproductive systems of anabolic substance abusers. Tuomo Karila. Publications of the National Public Health Institute ISBN 951-740-388-2
260. Reversible hypogonadism and azoospermia as a result of anabolic-androgenic steroid use in a bodybuilder with personality disorder. A case report. Boyadjiev NP, Georgieva KN, Massaldjieva RI, Gueorguiev SI. J Sports Med Phys Fitness. 2000 Sep;40(3):271-4.
261. Conservative management of azoospermia following steroid abuse. M.R. Gazvani et al. Human Reprod 12(8) (1997) pp. 1706-08.
262. Contraceptive efficacy of testosterone-induced azoospermia in normal men. Lancet, 1990 20;336(8721):955-9.
263. Effects of chronic testosterone administraton in normal men: safety and efficacy of high dose testosterone and parallel dose-dependent suppression of luteinizing hormone, follicle-stimulating hormone, and sperm production. Matsumoto AM. J Clin Endocrinol Metab 1990; 70:282-87.
264. Restorative increases in serum testosterone levels are significantly correlate to improvements in sexual functioning. A Seftel, R Mack et al. J Androl 25(6) 2004 pp. 963-72.
265. Sexual functioning of male anabolic steroid abusers. Moss HB, Panzak GL, Tarter RE. Arch Sex Behav. 1993 Feb;22(1):1-12.
266. Human male sexual functions do not require aromatization of testosterone: a study using tamoxifen, testolactone, and dihydrotestosterone. Gooren
267. Low sex hormone-binding globulin and testosterone levels in association with erectile dysfunction among human immunodeficiency virus-infected men receiving testosterone and oxandrolone. Wasserman P, Segal-Maurer S, Rubin D. J Sex Med. 2008 Jan;5(1):241-7. Epub 2007 Oct 24.
268. Sex steroids and sexual desire mechanism. Rochira V, Zirilli L, Madeo B, Balestrieri A, Granata AR, Carani C. J Endocrinol Invest. 2003;26(3 Suppl):29-36.
269. Testosterone-induced priapism in Klinefelter syndrome. Ichioka K, Utsunomiya N, Kohei N, Ueda N, Inoue K, Terai A. Urology. 2006 Mar;67(3):622.e17-8. Epub 2006 Feb 28.
270. Severe priapism as a complication of testosterone substitution therapy. Zelissen PM, Stricker BH. Am J Med. 1988 Aug;85(2):273-4
271. Testosterone induced priapism in two adolescents with sickle cell disease. Slayton W, Kedar A, Schatz D. J Pediatr Endocrinol Metab. 1995 Jul-Sep;8(3):199-203.
272. Benign hypertrophy and carcinoma of the prostate. Moore RA. Surgery 1944;16:152-67.
273. Guilt by association: a historical perspective on Huggins, testosterone therapy, and prostate cancer. Morgentaler A. J Sex Med. 2008 Aug;5(8):1834-40. Epub 2008 Jun 10.
274. Testosterone therapy in hypogonadal men and potential prostate cancer risk: a systematic review. Shabsigh R, Crawford ED, Nehra A, Slawin KM. Int J Impot Res. 2008 Jul 17. [Epub ahead of print]
275. Long-term psychiatric and medical consequences of anabolic-androgenic steroid abuse: A looming public health concern? Kanayama G, Hudson JI, Pope HG Jr. Drug Alcohol Depend. 2008 Nov 1;98(1-2):1-12. Epub 2008 Jul 2.
276. The many faces of testosterone. Bain J. Clin Interv Aging. 2007;2(4):567-76.
277. Testosterone treatment in hypogonadal men: prostate-specific antigen level and risk of prostate cancer. Guay AT, Perez JB, Fitaihi WA, Vereb M. Endocr Pract. 2000 Mar-Apr;6(2):132-8.
278. Adenocarcinoma of prostate in 40 year old body-builder. Roberts TJ, Essenhigh DM. Lancet 1986;2:742.
279. Testosterone therapy for men at risk for or with history of prostate cancer. Morgentaler A. Curr Treat Options Oncol. 2006 Sep;7(5):363-9.
280. Testosterone replacement therapy and the risk of prostate cancer. Is there a link? Barqawi A, Crawford ED. Int J Impot Res. 2006 Jul-Aug;18(4):323-8. Epub 2005 Nov 10.
281. Volume change of the prostate and seminal vesicles in male hypogonadism after androgen replacement therapy. Sasagawa I, Nakada T, Kazama T, Satomi S, Terada T, Katayama T. Int Urol Nephrol. 1990;22(3):279-84.
282. A four-year efficacy and safety study of the long-acting parenteral testosterone undecanoate. Minnemann T, Schubert M, Hübler D, Gouni-Berthold I, Freude S, Schumann C, Oettel M, Ernst M, Mellinger U, Sommer F, Krone W, Jockenhövel F. Aging Male. 2007 Sep;10(3):155-8.
283. Effect of Testosterone Replacement Therapy on Prostate Tissue in Men With Late-Onset Hypogonadism

A Randomized Controlled Trial Leonard S. Marks, MD; Norman A. Mazer, MD, et al. JAMA. 2006;296:2351-2361.

284. Prognostic value of serum markers for prostate cancer. Stenman UH, Abrahamsson PA, Aus G, Lilja H, Bangma C, Hamdy FC, Boccon-Gibod L, Ekman P. Scand J Urol Nephrol Suppl. 2005 May;(216):64-81.

285. Relationship between prostate specific antigen, prostate volume and age in the benign prostate. Collins GN, Lee RJ, McKelvie GB, Rogers AC, Hehir M. Br J Urol. 1993 Apr;71(4):445-50.

286. Long-term treatment with finasteride results in a clinically significant reduction in total prostate volume compared to placebo over the full range of baseline prostate sizes in men enrolled in the MTOPS trial. Kaplan SA, Roehrborn CG, McConnell JD et al. J Urol. 2008 Sep;180(3):1030-2; discussion 1032-3. Epub 2008 Jul 17.

287. Winning is the Only Thing. Randy Roberts, James S. Olson. JHU Press, 1991. ISBN 0801842409

288. Androgen or Estrogen Effects on Human Prostate. B. Jin, L Turner et al. J Clin Endocrinol Metab. 1996;81(12):4290-95.

289. Fingerprinting the diseased prostate: associations between BPH and prostate cancer. Shah US, Getzenberg RH. J Cell Biochem. 2004 Jan 1;91(1):161-9.

290. Estrogen-regulated development and differentiation of the prostate. McPherson SJ, Ellem SJ, Risbridger GP. Differentiation. 2008 Jul;76(6):660-70. Epub 2008 Jun 28.

291. Estrogen action on the prostate gland: a critical mix of endocrine and paracrine signaling. G Risbridger, S Ellem et al. J Mol Endocrinol (2007) 39, 183-88.

292. Effects of androgen therapy on prostatic markers in hemodialyzed patients. Teruel JL, Aguilera A, Avila C, Ortuño J. Scand J Urol Nephrol. 1996 Apr;30(2):129-31.

293. The role of aromatization in testosterone supplementation. Effects on cognition in older men. M.M. Cherrier, A.M. Matsumoto et al. Neurology 2005;64:290-96.

294. Use of anabolic steroids and associated health risks among gay men attending London gyms. Bolding G, Sherr L, Elford J. Addiction. 2002 Feb;97(2):195-203.

295. Indications of prevalence, practice and effects of anabolic steroid use in Great Britain. Korkia P, Stimson GV. Int J Sports Med. 1997 Oct;18(7):557-62.

296. A combined regimen of cyproterone acetate and testosterone enanthate as a potentially highly effective male contraceptive. C Meriggola et al. J Clin Endocrinol Metab 81(8) 3018-23, 1996.

297. HPGA normalization protocol after androgen treatment. N Vergel, AL Hodge, MC Scally. Program for Wellness Restoration.

298. An update to the Crisler HCG Protocol. John Crisler, DO. 2004.

299. Testicular responsiveness following chronic administration of hCG (1500 IU every six days) in untreated hypogonadotropic hypogonadism. Balducci R, Toscano V, Casilli D, Maroder M, Sciarra F, Boscherini B. Horm Metab Res. 1987 May;19(5):216-21.

300. Estrogen suppression in males: metabolic effects. Mauras N, O'Brien KO, Klein KO, Hayes V. J Clin Endocrinol Metab. 2000 Jul;85(7):2370-7.

301. Progesterone and testosterone in combination act in the hypothalamus of castrated rams to regulate the secretion of LH. Turner AI, Tilbrook AJ, Clarke IJ, Scott CJ. J Endocrinol. 2001 May;169(2):291-8.

302. Football; Alzado Tumor is Rare and Deadly. Elisabeth Rosenthal. NY Times. July 4, 1991.

303. Primary central nervous system lymphoma. O'Neill BP, Illig JJ. Mayo Clin Proc. 1989 Aug;64(8):1005-20.

304. Sports People: Football; Alzado Talks. NY Times. Associated Press Report. June 28, 1991.

305. Alzado believed drug killed him – Ex-Raider star dead from brain cancer. Associated Press. May 15, 1992.

306. 54-year-old man with breast cancer after prolonged testosterone therapy. Sorscher S, Krause W. Clin Adv Hematol Oncol. 2005 Jun;3(6):475; discussion 476.

307. Androgen therapy. Longson D. Practitioner. 1972 Mar;208(245):338-48.

308. Androgen treatment of middle-aged, obese men: effects on metabolism, muscle and adipose tissues. Mårin P, Krotkiewski M, Björntorp P. Eur J Med. 1992 Oct;1(6):329-36.

309. Effects of androgen therapy on adipose tissue and metabolism in older men. Schroeder ET, Zheng L, Ong MD, Martinez C, Flores C, Stewart Y, Azen C, Sattler FR. J Clin Endocrinol Metab. 2004 Oct;89(10):4863-72.

310. Insulin sensitivity, insulin secretion, and abdominal fat: the insulin resistance atherosclerosis study (IRAS) family study. Wagenknecht LE, Langerfeld CD et al. Diabetes 52:2490-2494.

311. Recent developments in the toxicology of anabolic steroids. Graham S, Kennedy M. Drug Saf. 1990 Nov-Dec;5(6):458-76.

312. Insulin resistance and diminished glucose tolerance in powerlifters ingesting anabolic steroids. Cohen JC, Hickman R. J Clin Endocrinol Metab. 1987 May;64(5):960-3.

313. Insulin action and dynamics modelled in patients taking the anabolic steroid methandienone (Dianabol). Godsland IF, Shennan NM, Wynn V. Clin Sci (Lond). 1986 Dec;71(6):665-73

314. The effects of varying doses of T on insulin sensitivity, plasma lipids, apolipoproteins, and C-reactive protein in healthy young men. Singh AB, Hsia S. et al. J Clin Endocrinol Metab. 2002 Jan;87(1):136-43.

315. Nandrolone, a 19-nortestosterone, enhances insulin-independent glucose uptake in normal men. Hobbs CJ, Jones RE, Plymate SR. et al. J Clin Endocrinol Metab. 1996 Apr;81(4):1582-5.

316. Indications of prevalence, practice and effects of anabolic steroid use in Great Britain. Korkia P, Stimson GV. Int J Sports Med. 1997 Oct;18(7):557-62.

317. Cardiovascular complications of respiratory diseases. Chowdhuri S, Crook ED, Taylor HA Jr, Badr MS. Am J Med Sci. 2007 Nov;334(5):361-80.

318. Obesity and hormonal factors in sleep and sleep apnea. Wittels EH. Med Clin North Am. 1985 Nov;69(6):1265-80.

319. Metabolic aspects of sleep apnea. Grunstein RR. Sleep. 1996 Dec;19(10 Suppl):S218-20.

320. Testosterone replacement therapy for older men. Borst SE, Mulligan T. Clin Interv Aging. 2007;2(4):561-6.

321. The Short-Term Effects of High-Dose Testosterone on Sleep, Breathing, and Function in Older Men Peter Y. Liu, Brendon Yee et al. The Journal of Clinical Endocrinology & Metabolism Vol. 88, No. 8 3605-3613

322. Induction of the obstructive sleep apnea syndrome in a woman by exogenous androgen administration. Johnson MW, Anch AM, Remmers JE. Am

Rev Respir Dis. 1984 Jun;129(6):1023-5.

323. Testosterone dose-response relationships in healthy young men. Shalender A, Woodhouse L et al. Am J Physiol Endocrinol Metab 281: e1172-81 2001

324. Metabolic effects of nandrolone decanoate and resistance training in men with HIV. Sattler et al. Am J Physiol Endocrinol Metab 283: e1214-22

325. Effects of an oral androgen on muscle and metabolism in older, community-dwelling men. Schroeder et al. Am J Physiol Endocrinol Metab 284: E120-28

326. Behind the Scenes: Hypertrophy. Gene. Mind and Muscle Magazine 5/2005

327. Regulation of skeletal muscle fiber size, shape and function. J Biomech. 24(suppl1):123-33 (1991)

328. Initial events in exercise-induced muscular injury. Med Sci Sports Exerc 22(4):429-35 (1990)

329. Myostatin negatively regulates satellite cell activation and self-renewal. J Cell Biol. 162:1135-47 (2003)

330. Signaling satellite-cell activation in skeletal muscle: markers, models, stretch, and potential alternative pathways. A Wozniak, J Kong et al. Muscle Nerve 31: 283-300 (2005)

331. Effects of physical exercise on phospholipid fatty acid composition in skeletal muscle. Agneta Andersson et al. Am J Physiol. 274 (Endocrinol. Metab. 37): E432-8 (1998)

332. Effects of Exercise on parameters of blood coagulation, platelet function and the prostaglandin system. H Sinzinger, I Virgolini. Sports Medicine 6: 238-45 (1988)

333. Mechanical stretch induces activation of skeletal muscle satellite cells in vitro. Tatsumi R, Sheehan SM et al. Exp Cell Res 267(1) 107-14 (2001)

334. Release of hepatocyte growth factor from mechanically stretched skeletal muscle satellite cells and role of pH and Nitric Oxide. Ryuichi Tatsumi et al. Mol Biol of the Cell 13 p 2909-18 (2002)

335. Hepatocyte growth factor as a key to modulate anti-ulcer action of prostaglandins in stomach. J Clin Inv 98:2604-11

336. The role of prostaglandins in bone formation. Harada SI, Balena R et al. Connect Tissue Res. 1995;31(4)279-82

337. Prostaglandin F2a stimulates proliferation of clonal osteoblastic MC3T3-E1 cells by up-regulation of Insulin-like Growth Factor 1 receptors. Yoshiyuky Hakeda et al. J Biol Chem 266(31): 21044-50 (1991)

338. Prostaglandin E2 stimulates insulin-like growth factor I synthesis in osteoblast-enriched cultures from fetal bone. McCarthy TL, Centrella M et al. Endocrinology 128(6):2895-900 (1991)

339. Sequence of IGF-I, IGF-II, and HGF expression in regenerating skeletal muscle. Hayashi S et al. Histochem Cell Biol. 122(5):427-34 (2004)

340. Expression of insulin like growth factor-1 splice variants and structural genes in rabbit skeletal muscle induced by stretch and stimulation. G McKoy, W Ashley et al. J Physiol 516(2) 583-92 (1999)

341. Expression of fibroblast growth factor family during postnatal skeletal muscle hypertrophy. P Mitchell, T Steenstrup, K Hannon. J Applied Physiol 86:313-19 (1999)

342. Fibroblast growth factor is stored in fiber extracellular matrix and plays a role in regulating muscle hypertrophy. Medicine and Science in Sports and Exercise 21(5) S173-80 (1989)

343. The insulin-like effect of muscle contraction. Ivy JL. Exerc Sport Sci Rev. 1987;15:29-51.

344. The role of prostaglandins as modulators of insulin-stimulated glucose metabolism in skeletal muscle. Leighton B et al. Horm Metab Res Suppl. 22:89-95 (1990)

345. Differential effects of prostaglandins derived from n-6 and n-3 polyunsaturated fatty acids on COX-2 expression and IL-6 secretion. Dilprit Bagga et al. PNAS 100(4) 1751-56 (2003)

346. The role of arachidonic acid metabolism in the activities of Interleukin 1 and 2. W Farrar, J Humes. J of Immunol 135(2) 1153-9 (1985)

347. Regulation of protein synthesis associated with skeletal muscle hypertrophy by insulin-, amino acid and exercise-induced signaling. D Bolster, L Jefferson, S Kimball. Proc of the Nutrition Society 63: 351-56 (2004).

348. Effect of long-term testosterone oenanthate administration on male reproductive function: Clinical evaluation, serum FSH, LH, Testosterone and seminal fluid analysis in normal men. J. Mauss, G. Borsch et al. Acta Endocrinol 78 (1975) 373-84

349. Desensitization to gonadotropins in cultured Leydig tumor cells involves loss of gonadotropin receptors and decreased capacity for steroidogenesis. Freeman DA, Ascoli M Proc Natl Acad Sci U S A 1981 Oct;78(10):6309-13

350. Acute stimulation of aromatization in Leydig Cells by Human Chorionic Gonadotropin In-vitro. Proc Natl Acad Sci USA 76:4460-3,1079

351. Anabolic Steroids Withdrawal in Strength Trained Athletes: How Does It Affect Skeletal Muscles?," Anders Eriksson and Lars-Eric Thornell. American Physiological Society. The Integrative Biology of Exercise V, Sep 24-27, 2008 Hilton Head, SC.

352. Increased premature mortality of competitive powerlifters suspected to have used anabolic agents. Pärssinen M, Kujala U, Vartiainen E, Sarna S, Seppälä T. Int J Sports Med. 2000 Apr;21(3):225-7.

353. Detection of nandrolone metabolites in urine after a football game in professional and amateur players: a Bayesian comparison. Robinson N, Taroni F, Saugy M, Ayotte C, Mangin P, Dvorak J. Forensic Sci Int 2001 Nov 1;122(2-3):130-5

354. Detection of norbolethone, an anabolic steroid never marketed, in athletes' urine. Catlin D, Ahrens B, Kucherova Y. Rapid Commun. Mass Spectrom. 2002; 16: 1273-75

355. Schanzer W, Donike M. Anal Chim. Acta. 1993; 275: 23

356. Androgens and Anabolic Agents: Chemistry and Pharmacology, Julius A. Vida, Academic Press 1969.

357. Suchowsky GK et al. Exc. Med. (Amsterd.) Congr. Ser. No. 51 (1962):68.

358. K. J. Ryan. Acta Endocrinol. 35, Suppl. 51, 697 (1960).

359. C. Gual, T. Morato, M. Gut, R.I. Dorfman, Endocrinology 71, 920 (1962).

360. 17beta-hydroxy-5alpha-androst-1-en-3-one (1-testosterone) is a potent androgen with anabolic properties. Friedel A, Geyer H, Kamber M, Laudenbach-Leschowsky U, Schanzer W, Thevis M, Vollmer G, Zierau O, Diel P. Toxicol Lett. 2006 Aug 20;165(2):149-55. Epub 2006 Apr 18.

361. Testosterone buciclate (20 Aet-1) in hypogonadal men: pharmacokinetics and pharmacodynamics of the new long-acting androgen ester. Behre HM, Nieschlag E. J Clin Endocrinol Metab. 1992 Nov;75(5):1204-10.

362. New injectable testosterone ester maintains serum testosterone of castrated monkeys in the normal range for four months. Weinbauer GF, Marshall GR, Nieschlag E. Acta Endocrinol (1986) 113:128-32.
363. Potential of testosterone buciclate for male contraception: endocrine differences between responders and nonresponders. Behre HM, Baus S, Kliesch S, Keck C, Simoni M, Nieschlag E. J Clin Endocrinol Metab. 1995 Aug;80(8):2394-403.
364. Enzyme induction by oral testosterone. Johnsen SG, Kampmann JP, Bennet EP, Jorgensen F. Clin Pharmacol Ther (1976) 20:233-237.
365. High-density lipoprotein cholesterol is not decreased if an aromatizable androgen is administered. Friedl K, Hannan C et al. Metabolism 39(1) 1990:69-74.
366. Testosterone dose-response relationships in healthy young men. Bhasin S, Woodhouse L et al. Am J Physiol Endocrinol Metab (2001) 281:E1172-81.
367. The effects of varying doses of T on insulin sensitivity, plasma lipids, apolipoproteins, and C-reactive protein in healthy young men. Singh A, Hsia S, et al. J Clin Endocrinol Metab (2002) 87:136-43.
368. Experiences with a new testosterone isobutyrate crystal suspension. Drescher H. Dtsch Med Wochenschr. 1952 Apr 4;77(14):431-2.
369. Enzyme induction by oral testosterone. Johnsen SG, Kampmann JP, Bennet EP, Jorgensen F. Clin Pharmacol Ther (1976) 20:233-237.
370. High-density lipoprotein cholesterol is not decreased if an aromatizable androgen is administered. Friedl K, Hannan C et al. Metabolism 39(1) 1990:69-74.
371. Testosterone dose-response relationships in healthy young men. Bhasin S, Woodhouse L et al. Am J Physiol Endocrinol Metab (2001) 281:E1172-81.
372. The effects of varying doses of T on insulin sensitivity, plasma lipids, apolipoproteins, and C-reactive protein in healthy young men. Singh A, Hsia S, et al. J Clin Endocrinol Metab (2002) 87:136-43.
373. Camerino B, Patelli B. et al. J Amer. Chem. Soc. 78 (1956):3540.
374. Anabolic Steroids and Sports Volume II. James E. Wright. Sports Science Consultants, Natick, MA 1982.
375. A. Ercoli, R. Gardi, R. Vitali. Chem & Ind. (London) 1284 (1962).
376. Research on enol derivatives of steroid hormones. ERCOLI A, KOLLER M. G Ital Chemioter. 1956 Jul-Dec;3(3-4):380-3. Italian.
377. Metabolism of Boldenone in Man: gas Chromatographic/Mass Spectrometric Identification of Urinary Excreted Metabolites and Determination of Excretion Rates. Schanzer, Donike. Bol Mass Spec. 21 (1992) 3-16.
378. 2-Methyl and 2-hydroxymethylene-androstane derivatives. Ringold HJ et al. J Am Chem Soc 1959;81:427-32.
379. Oxymetholone treatment for the anemia of bone marrow failure. Alexanian R, Nadell J, et al. Blood. 1972; 40:353-6.
380. Les hormones anabolisantes du point de vue experimental. P.A. Desaulles. Helv. Med. Acta 1960:479-503.
381. Studies on anabolic steroids-8. GC/MS characterization of unusual seco acidic metabolites of oxymetholone in human urine. J Steroid Biochem Mol Bio 42 (1992):229-42.
382. Effects of various 17 alpha alkyl substitutions and structural modifications oof steroids on sulfobromophthalein (BSP) renention in rabbits. Lennon HD et al. Steroids 7 (1966): 157-70.
383. Long-term oxymetholone use in HIV patients not associated with significant hepatotoxicity. Hengge UR et al. Poster presented at the Third International Conference on Nutrition and HIV Infection; April 22-25, 1999; Cannes, France.
384. Effects of an oral androgen on muscle and metabolism in older, community-dwelling men. Schroeder et al. Am J Physiol Endocrinol. Metab. 284:E120-28.
385. Anabolic Steroids and Sports Volume II. James E. Wright. Sports Science Consultants, Natick, MA 1982.
386. Diezfalusy E. Acta endocrin. (Kbh.) 35 (1960):59.
387. Biosynthesis of Estrogens, Gual C, Morato T, Hayano M, Gut M, and Dorfman R. Endocrinology 71 (1962):920-25.
388. Aromatization of androstenedione and 19-nortestosterone in human placental, liver and adipose tissues (abstract). Nippon Naibunpi Gakkai Zasshi 62 (1986):18-25.
389. Competitive progesterone antagonists: receptor binding and biologic activity of testosterone and 19-nortestosterone derivatives. Reel JR, Humphrey RR, Shih YH, Windsor BL, Sakowski R, Creger PL, Edgren RA. Fertil Steril 1979 May;31(5):552-61.
390. Studies of the biological activity of certain 19-nor steroids in female animals. Pincus G, Chang M, Zarrow M, Hafez E, Merrill A. December 1956.
391. Different Pattern of Metabolism Determine the Relative Anabolic Activity of 19-Norandrogens. J Steroid Biochem Mol Bio 53(1995):255-7.
392. Relative binding affinities of testosterone, 19-nortestosterone and their 5-alpha reduced derivatives to the androgen receptor and to other androgen-bidning proteins: A suggested role of 5alpha-reductive steroid metabolism in the dissociation of "myotropic" and "androgenic" activities of 19-nortestosterone. Toth M, Zakar T. J Steroid Biochem 17 (1982):653-60.
393. Metabolic effects of nandrolone decanoate and resistance training in men with HIV. Sattler FR, Schroeder ET, Dube MP, Jaque SV, Martinez C, Blanche PJ, Azen S, Krauss RM. Am J Physiol Endocrinol Metab. 2002 Dec;283(6):E1214-22. Epub 2002 Aug 27.
394. Lipemic and lipoproteinemic effects of natural and synthetic androgens in humans. Crist DM, Peake GT, Stackpole PJ. Clin Exp Pharmacol Physiol 1986 Jul;13(7):513-8.
395. The administration of pharmacological doses of testosterone or 19-nortestosterone to normal men is not associated with increased insulin secretion or impaired glucose tolerance. Karl E. Friedl et al. J Clin Endocrinol Metab 68: 971, 1989.
396. Influence of nandrolonedecanoate on the pituitary-gonadal axis in males. Bijlsma J, Duursma S, Thijssen J, Huber O. Acta Endocrinol 101 1982:108-12
397. Underground Steroid Handbook II. Daniel Duchaine. HLR Technical Books, Venice CA, 29.
398. Oxandrolone: A Potent Anabolic Steroid of Novel Chemical Composition. Fox M, Minot AS, and Liddle GW. Journal of Clinical Endocrinology and Metabolism. 1962; Volume 22, Pgs. 921-924.
399. M. Fox et al. J. Clin Endocrinol Metab 22 (1962):921.
400. Published reference of personal communication from Saunders F.J. (April 21, 1961) to author of Methyltestosterone, related steroids, and liver function. Arch Int. Med 116 (1965):289-94.
401. Studies on anabolic steroids. II--Gas chromatographic/mass spectrometric characterization of oxandrolone urinary metabolites in man. Masse R, Bi HG, Ayotte C, Dugal R. Biomed Environ Mass Spectrom. 1989 Jun;18(6):429-38.
402. Methyltestosterone, related steroids, and liver function. DeLorimier, Gordan G, Lowe R. et al. Arch Int. Med 116 (1965):289-94.

403. Effects of Oxandrolone on Plasma Lipoproteins and the Intravenous Fat tolerance in Man. Atherosclerosis 19 (1974):337-46.
404. Oxandrolone and Plasma Triglyceride Reduction: Effect of Triglyceride-Rich Diet and High Density Lipoproteins. Artery 9 (1981):328-41.
405. Plasma and Lipoprotein Lipid Responses to Four Hypolipid Drugs. Lipids 19 (1984):73-79.
406. The effects of oxandrolone on the growth hormone and gonadal axis in boys with constitutional delay of growth and puberty. Malhitra A, Poon E. Et al. Clin Endocrinol (Oxf) 1993 Apr;38(4):393-8.
407. Anabolic Steroids and Sports Volume II. James E. Wright. Sports Science Consultants, Natick, MA 1982.
408. Butenandt AK et al. Ber dtsch chem. Ges. 68 (1935):2097.
409. Comparative pharmacokinetics of three doses of percutaneous dihydrotestosterone gel in healthy elderly men--a clinical research center study. Wang C, Iranmanesh A, Berman N et al. J Clin Endocrinol Metab 1998 Aug;83(8):2749-57.
410. Transdermal dihydrotestosterone treatment of 'andropause'. Ann Med. 1993 Jun;25(3):235-41.
411. Studies on the treatment of idiopathic gynaecomastia with percutaneous dihydrotestosterone. Clin Endocrinol (Oxf). 1983 Oct;19(4):513-20.
412. Gynecomastia: effect of prolonged treatment with dihydrotestosterone by the percutaneous route Presse Med. 1983 Jan 8;12(1):21-5.
413. Contribution of lymphatically transported testosterone undecanoate to the systemic exposure of testosterone after oral administration of two andriol formulations in conscious lymph duct-cannulated dogs. Shackleford D, Faassen W Aet al. J of Pharm and Exper Ther. 306 (2003):925–933.
414. Enzyme induction by oral testosterone. Johnsen SG, Kampmann JP, Bennet EP, Jorgensen F. 1976 Clin Pharmacol Ther 20:233-237.
415. A ten-year safety study of the oral androgen testosterone undecanoate. Gooren LJG , J Androl , 1994 , 15 , 212–5.
416. The effects of testosterone treatment on body composition and metabolism in middle-aged obese men. Mårin P, Holmång S, Jöhnsson L, et al. Int J Obes , 1992 , 16 , 991-7.
417. Enzyme induction by oral testosterone. Johnsen SG, Kampmann JP, Bennet EP, Jorgensen F 1976 Clin Pharmacol Ther 20:233-237.
418. Testosterone replacement, cardiovascular system and risk factors in the aging male. Vigna GB, Bergami E. J Endocrinol Invest. 2005;28(11 Suppl Proceedings):69-74.
419. Evaluation of the pharmacokinetic profiles of the new testosterone topical gel formulation, Testim, compared to AndroGel. Marbury T, Hamill E, Bachand R, Sebree T, Smith T. Biopharm Drug Dispos. 2003 Apr;24(3):115-20.
420. Enzyme induction by oral testosterone. Johnsen SG, Kampmann JP, Bennet EP, Jorgensen F. 1976 Clin Pharmacol Ther 20:233-237.
421. Testosterone replacement, cardiovascular system and risk factors in the aging male. Vigna GB, Bergami E. J Endocrinol Invest. 2005;28(11 Suppl Proceedings):69-74.
422. Enzyme induction by oral testosterone. Johnsen SG, Kampmann JP, Bennet EP, Jorgensen F. 1976 Clin Pharmacol Ther 20:233-237.
423. High-density lipoprotein cholesterol is not decreased if an aromatizable androgen is administered. Karl Friedl, Charles Hannan et al. Metabolism 39(1) (1990):69-74.
424. Testosterone dose-response relationships in healthy young men. Bhasin S, Woodhouse L et al. Am J Physiol Endocrinol Metab 281 (2001):E1172-81.
425. The effects of varying doses of T on insulin sensitivity, plasma lipids, apolipoproteins, and C-reactive protein in healthy young men. Atam Singh, Stanley Hsia, et al. J Clin Endocrinol Metab 87 (2002):136-43.
426. Enzyme induction by oral testosterone. Johnsen SG, Kampmann JP, Bennet EP, Jorgensen F. 1976 Clin Pharmacol Ther 20:233-237.
427. High-density lipoprotein cholesterol is not decreased if an aromatizable androgen is administered. Friedl K, Hannan C et al. Metabolism 39(1) (1990):69-74.
428. Testosterone dose-response relationships in healthy young men. Bhasin S, Woodhouse L et al. Am J Physiol Endocrinol Metab 281 (2001):E1172-81.
429. The effects of varying doses of T on insulin sensitivity, plasma lipids, apolipoproteins, and C-reactive protein in healthy young men. Atam Singh, Stanley Hsia, et al. J Clin Endocrinol Metab 87 (2002):136-43.
430. Enzyme induction by oral testosterone. Johnsen SG, Kampmann JP, Bennet EP, Jorgensen F. 1976 Clin Pharmacol Ther 20:233-237.
431. High-density lipoprotein cholesterol is not decreased if an aromatizable androgen is administered. Friedl K, Hannan C et al. Metabolism 39(1) (1990):69-74.
432. Testosterone dose-response relationships in healthy young men. Bhasin S, Woodhouse L et al. Am J Physiol Endocrinol Metab 281 (2001):E1172-81.
433. The effects of varying doses of T on insulin sensitivity, plasma lipids, apolipoproteins, and C-reactive protein in healthy young men. Atam Singh, Stanley Hsia, et al. J Clin Endocrinol Metab 87 (2002):136-43.
434. Lyster SC, et al. Acta Endocrin (Kbh) 43 (1963):399.
435. The biological activity of 7 alpha-methyl-19-nortestosterone is not amplified in male reproductive tract as is that of testosterone. Endocrinology. 1992 Jun; 130(6):3677-83.
436. Anabolic Steroids and Sports Volume II. James E. Wright. Sports Science Consultants, Natick, MA 1982.
437. De Visser, J. et al. Acta Endocrin. (Kbh.) 35 (1960):405.
438. Biosynthesis of Estrogens, Gual C, Morato T, Hayano M, Gut M and Dorfman R. Endocrinology 71 (1962):920-25.
439. Aromatization of androstenedione and 19-nortestosterone in human placental, liver and adipose tissues (abstract). Nippon Naibunpi Gakkai Zasshi 62 (1986):18-25.
440. Competitive progesterone antagonists: receptor binding and biologic activity of testosterone and 19-nortestosterone derivatives. Reel JR, Humphrey RR, Shih YH, Windsor BL, Sakowski R, Creger PL, Edgren RA. Fertil Steril 1979 May;31(5):552-61.
441. Studies of the biological activity of certain 19-nor steroids in female animals. Pincus G, Chang M, Zarrow M, Hafez E, Merrill A. December 1956.
442. Different Pattern of Metabolism Determine the Relative Anabolic Activity of 19-Norandrogens. J Steroid Biochem Mol Bio 53:255-7,1995.
443. Relative binding affinities of testosterone, 19-nortestosterone and their 5-alpha reduced derivatives to the androgen receptor and to other androgen-binding proteins: A suggested role of 5alpha-reductive steroid metabolism in the dissociation of "myotropic" and "androgenic" activities of 19-nortestosterone. Toth M, Zakar T. J Steroid Biochem 17 (1982):653-60.
444. Metabolic effects of nandrolone decanoate and resistance training in men with HIV. Sattler FR, Schroeder ET, Dube MP, Jaque SV, Martinez C, Blanche PJ, Azen S, Krauss RM. Am J Physiol Endocrinol Metab. 2002 Dec;283(6):E1214-22. Epub 2002 Aug 27.

445. Lipemic and lipoproteinemic effects of natural and synthetic androgens in humans. Crist DM, Peake GT, Stackpole PJ. Clin Exp Pharmacol Physiol 1986 Jul;13(7):513-8.
446. The administration of pharmacological doses of testosterone or 19-nortestosterone to normal men is not associated with increased insulin secretion or impaired glucose tolerance. Karl E. Friedl et al. J Clin Endocrinol Metab 68: 971, 1989.
447. Influence of nandrolonedecanoate on the pituitary-gonadal axis in males. Bijlsma J, Duursma S, Thijssen J, Huber O. Acta Endocrinol 101 (1982):108-12.
448. Effect of nandrolone decanoate therapy on weight and lean body mass in HIV-infected women with weight loss. K Mulligan, R Zackin, et al. Arch Intern Med. (2005):165:578-85.
449. Nandrolone decanoate: Pharmacological properties and therapeutic use in osteoporosis. P Geusens. Clinical Rheumatology, 1995, 14, Suppl. 3.
450. Contraceptive efficacy and adverse effects of testosterone enanthate in Thai men. Sukcharoen N, Aribarg A, Kriangsinyos R, Chanprasit Y, Ngeamvijawat J. J Med Assoc Thai 1996 Dec;79(12):767-73.
451. Enzyme induction by oral testosterone. Johnsen SG, Kampmann JP, Bennet EP, Jorgensen F. 1976 Clin Pharmacol Ther 20:233-237.
452. High-density lipoprotein cholesterol is not decreased if an aromatizable androgen is administered. Friedl K, Hannan C et al. Metabolism 39(1) (1990):69-74.
453. Testosterone dose-response relationships in healthy young men. Bhasin S, Woodhouse L et al. Am J Physiol Endocrinol Metab 281 (2001):E1172-81.
454. The effects of varying doses of T on insulin sensitivity, plasma lipids, apolipoproteins, and C-reactive protein in healthy young men. Atam Singh, Stanley Hsia, et al. J Clin Endocrinol Metab 87 (2002):136-43.
455. Enzyme induction by oral testosterone. Johnsen SG, Kampmann JP, Bennet EP, Jorgensen F. 1976 Clin Pharmacol Ther 20:233-237.
456. High-density lipoprotein cholesterol is not decreased if an aromatizable androgen is administered. Friedl K, Hannan C et al. Metabolism 39(1) (1990):69-74.
457. Testosterone dose-response relationships in healthy young men. Bhasin S, Woodhouse L et al. Am J Physiol Endocrinol Metab 281 (2001):E1172-81.
458. The effects of varying doses of T on insulin sensitivity, plasma lipids, apolipoproteins, and C-reactive protein in healthy young men. Singh A, Hsia S, et al. J Clin Endocrinol Metab 87 (2002):136-43.
459. Biological half-lives of [4-14C]testosterone and some of its esters after injection into the rat. James KC, Nicholls PJ, and Roberts M.J, Pharm. Pharmacol 21 (1969):24-27.
460. Enzyme induction by oral testosterone. Johnsen SG, Kampmann JP, Bennet EP, Jorgensen F. 1976 Clin Pharmacol Ther 20:233-237.
461. High-density lipoprotein cholesterol is not decreased if an aromatizable androgen is administered. Friedl K, Hannan C et al. Metabolism 39(1) 1990:69-74.
462. Testosterone dose-response relationships in healthy young men. Bhasin S, Woodhouse L et al. Am J Physiol Endocrinol Metab 281 (2001):E1172-81.
463. The effects of varying doses of T on insulin sensitivity, plasma lipids, apolipoproteins, and C-reactive protein in healthy young men. Singh A, Hsia S, et al. J Clin Endocrinol Metab 87 (2002):136-43.
464. Vischer E, Meystre C, Wettstein A. Helv Chim Acta 38 (1955):1502.
465. Never Enough / Steroids in Sports: Experiment turns epidemic. Robert Dvorchak. Pittsburgh Post-Gazette January 14, 2005.
466. Comments from Dr. John Ziegler. Strength & Heath Magazine, 1967.
467. Officials bungled steroid regulation from the start. Robert Dvorchak, Pittsburgh Post-Gazette October 3, 2005.
468. Anabolic-androgenic steroid interaction with rat androgen receptor in vivo and in vitro: a comparative study. Feldkoren BI, Andersson S. J Steroid Biochem Mol Biol. 2005 Apr;94(5):481-7. Epub 2005 Mar 17.
469. Kruskemper, H L, Anabolic Steroids, Academic Press, New York, 1968.
470. Relative imporance of 5alpha reduction for the androgenic and LH-inhibiting activities of delta-4-3-ketosteroids. Steroids 29 (1997):331-48.
471. Anabolic steroids in clinical medicine. Liddle GW, Burke jr. H A Helvetica Medica Acta, 5/6 1960:504-13.
472. Effect of anabolic steroid (metandienon) on plasma LH-FSH, and testosterone and on the response to intravenous administration of LRH. Holma P, Adlercreutz. Acta Endocrinol (Copenh) 1976 Deca;83(4):856-64.
473. Anabolic Steroids and Sports Volume II. James E. Wright. Sports Science Consultants, Natick, MA 1982.
474. Mathieu J, Proc Intern. Symp. Drug Res. (1967):134. Chem Inst. Can., Montreal, Canada 1967.
475. Anabolic Steroids and Sports Volume II. James E. Wright. Sports Science Consultants, Natick, MA 1982.
476. Biosynthesis of Estrogens, Gual C, Morato T, Hayano M, Gut M and Dorfman R. Endocrinology 71 (1962):920-25.
477. Aromatization of androstenedione and 19-nortestosterone in human placental, liver and adipose tissues (abstract). Nippon Naibunpi Gakkai Zasshi
478. Competitive progesterone antagonists: receptor binding and biologic activity of testosterone and 19-nortestosterone derivatives. Reel JR, Humphrey RR, Shih YH, Windsor BL, Sakowski R, Creger PL, Edgren RA. Fertil Steril May;31(5) (1979):552-61.
479. Studies of the biological activity of certain 19-nor steroids in female animals. Pincus G, Chang M, Zarrow M, Hafez E, Merrill A. December 1956.
480. Different Pattern of Metabolism Determine the Relative Anabolic Activity of 19-Norandrogens. J Steroid Biochem Mol Bio 53 (1995):255-7.
481. Relative binding affinities of testosterone, 19-nortestosterone and their 5-alpha reduced derivatives to the androgen receptor and to other androgen-bidning proteins: A suggested role of 5alpha-reductive steroid metabolism in the dissociation of "myotropic" and "androgenic" activities of 19-nortestosterone. Toth M, Zakar T. J Steroid Biochem 17 (1982):653-60.
482. Metabolic effects of nandrolone decanoate and resistance training in men with HIV. Sattler FR, Schroeder ET, Dube MP, Jaque SV, Martinez C, Blanche PJ, Azen S, Krauss RM. Am J Physiol Endocrinol Metab. 283(6) Dec (2002):E1214-22. Epub 2002 Aug 27.
483. Lipemic and lipoproteinemic effects of natural and synthetic androgens in humans. Crist DM, Peake GT, Stackpole PJ. Clin Exp Pharmacol Physiol 13(7) Jul (1986):513-8.
484. The administration of pharmacological doses of testosterone or 19-nortestosterone to normal men is not associated with increased insulin secretion or impaired glucose tolerance. Karl E. Friedl et al. J Clin Endocrinol Metab 68 (1989):971.
485. Influence of nandrolonedecanoate on the pituitary-gonadal axis in males. Bijlsma J, Duursma S, Thijssen J, Huber O. Acta Endocrinol 101 (1982):108-12.

486. Inhibition of the estrogenic activity of methylandrostenediol following administration of aminopterin. Boll Soc Ital Biol Sper. 31(9-10) Sep-Oct (1955):1280-4.
487. Overbeek G A, J. de Visser: Acta endocrin. (Kbh.) 24 (1957):209.
488. Biosynthesis of Estrogens, Gual C, Morato T, Hayano M, Gut M and Dorfman R. Endocrinology 71 (1962):920-25.
489. Aromatization of androstenedione and 19-nortestosterone in human placental, liver and adipose tissues (abstract). Nippon Naibunpi Gakkai Zasshi 62 (1986):18-25.
490. Competitive progesterone antagonists: receptor binding and biologic activity of testosterone and 19-nortestosterone derivatives. Reel JR, Humphrey RR, Shih YH, Windsor BL, Sakowski R, Creger PL, Edgren RA. Fertil Steril 31(5) May (1979):552-61.
491. Studies of the biological activity of certain 19-nor steroids in female animals. Pincus G, Chang M, Zarrow M, Hafez E, Merrill A. December 1956.
492. Different Pattern of Metabolism Determine the Relative Anabolic Activity of 19-Norandrogens. J Steroid Biochem Mol Bio 53 (1995):255-7.
493. Relative binding affinities of testosterone, 19-nortestosterone and the 5-alpha reduced derivatives to the androgen receptor and to other androgen-bidning proteins: A suggested role of 5alpha-reductive steroid metabolism in the dissociation of "myotropic" and "androgenic" activities of 19-nortestosterone. Toth M, Zakar T. J Steroid Biochem 17 (1982):653-60.
494. Metabolic effects of nandrolone decanoate and resistance training in men with HIV. Sattler FR, Schroeder ET, Dube MP, Jaque SV, Martinez C, Blanche PJ, Azen S, Krauss RM. Am J Physiol Endocrinol Metab. 283(6) Dec (2002):E1214-22. Epub 2002 Aug 27.
495. Lipemic and lipoproteinemic effects of natural and synthetic androgens in humans. Crist DM, Peake GT, Stackpole PJ. Clin Exp Pharmacol Physiol 13(7) Jul (1986):513-8.
496. Influence of nandrolonedecanoate on the pituitary-gonadal axis in males. Bijlsma J, Duursma S, Thijssen J, Huber O. Acta Endocrinol 101 (1982):108-12.
497. Biosynthesis of Estrogens, Gual C, Morato T, Hayano M, Gut M and Dorfman R. Endocrinology 71 (1962):920-25.
498. Aromatization of androstenedione and 19-nortestosterone in human placental, liver and adipose tissues (abstract). Nippon Naibunpi Gakkai Zasshi 62:18-25,1986.
499. Competitive progesterone antagonists: receptor binding and biologic activity of testosterone and 19-nortestosterone derivatives. Reel JR, Humphrey RR, Shih YH, Windsor BL, Sakowski R, Creger PL, Edgren RA. Fertil Steril 1979 May;31(5):552-61.
500. Studies of the biological activity of certain 19-nor steroids in female animals. Pincus G, Chang M, Zarrow M, Hafez E, Merrill A. December 1956.
501. Different Pattern of Metabolism Determine the Relative Anabolic Activity of 19-Norandrogens. J Steroid Biochem Mol Bio 53:255-7,1995.
502. Relative binding affinities of testosterone, 19-nortestosterone and their 5-alpha reduced derivatives to the androgen receptor and to other androgen-bidning proteins: A suggested role of 5alpha-reductive steroid metabolism in the dissociation of "myotropic" and "androgenic" activities of 19-nortestosterone. Toth M, Zakar T. J Steroid Biochem 17 (1982):653-60.
503. Metabolic effects of nandrolone decanoate and resistance training in men with HIV. Sattler FR, Schroeder ET, Dube MP, Jaque SV, Martinez C, Blanche PJ, Azen S, Krauss RM. Am J Physiol Endocrinol Metab. 2002 Dec;283(6):E1214-22. Epub 2002 Aug 27.
504. Lipemic and lipoproteinemic effects of natural and synthetic androgens in humans. Crist DM, Peake GT, Stackpole PJ. Clin Exp Pharmacol Physiol 1986 Jul;13(7):513-8.
505. The administration of pharmacological doses of testosterone or 19-nortestosterone to normal men is not associated with increased insulin secretion or impaired glucose tolerance. Karl E. Friedl et al. J Clin Endocrinol Metab 68: 971, 1989.
506. Influence of nandrolonedecanoate on the pituitary-gonadal axis in males. Bijlsma J., Duursma S, Thijssen J, Huber O. Acta Endocrinol 101 (1982):108-12.
507. Biosynthesis of Estrogens, Gual C, Morato T, Hayano M, Gut M and Dorfman R. Endocrinology 71 (1962):920-25.
508. Aromatization of androstenedione and 19-nortestosterone in human placental, liver and adipose tissues (abstract). Nippon Naibunpi Gakkai Zasshi 62:18-25,1986.
509. Competitive progesterone antagonists: receptor binding and biologic activity of testosterone and 19-nortestosterone derivatives. Reel JR, Humphrey RR, Shih YH, Windsor BL, Sakowski R, Creger PL, Edgren RA. Fertil Steril 1979 May;31(5):552-61.
510. Studies of the biological activity of certain 19-nor steroids in female animals. Pincus G, Chang M, Zarrow M, Hafez E, Merrill A. December 1956.
511. Different Pattern of Metabolism Determine the Relative Anabolic Activity of 19-Norandrogens. J Steroid Biochem Mol Bio 53:255-7,1995.
512. Relative binding affinities of testosterone, 19-nortestosterone and their 5-alpha reduced derivatives to the androgen receptor and to other
513. Metabolic effects of nandrolone decanoate and resistance training in men with HIV. Sattler FR, Schroeder ET, Dube MP, Jaque SV, Martinez C, Blanche PJ, Azen S, Krauss RM. Am J Physiol Endocrinol Metab. 2002 Dec;283(6):E1214-22. Epub 2002 Aug 27.
514. Lipemic and lipoproteinemic effects of natural and synthetic androgens in humans. Crist DM, Peake GT, Stackpole PJ. Clin Exp Pharmacol Physiol 1986 Jul;13(7):513-8.
515. The administration of pharmacological doses of testosterone or 19-nortestosterone to normal men is not associated with increased insulin secretion or impaired glucose tolerance. Karl E. Friedl et al. J Clin Endocrinol Metab 68: 971, 1989.
516. Influence of nandrolonedecanoate on the pituitary-gonadal axis in males. Bijlsma J, Duursma S, Thijssen J, Huber O. Acta Endocrinol 101 (1982):108-12.
517. Anabolic and androgenic efficacy of thio-substituted androstanes. Kraft, Hans Guenther et al. Merck AG, Darmstadt, Germany. Arzneimittel-Forschung (1964), 14:328-30.
518. Conference Reports: Therapy Congress and Pharmaceutical Exhibition. Angew. Chem. Internat. Edit. Vol. 4 (2) 1965.
519. Anticatabolic effect of steroids with anabolic activity. Luecker P.E. Merck AG, Darmstadt, Germany, Androgens Norm Pathol Cond. Proc. Symp. Steroid Horm., 2nd (1966). Meeting date 1965. 164-7.
520. Anabolic Steroids and Sports Volume II. James E. Wright. Sports Science Consultants, Natick, MA 1982.
521. Biosynthesis of Estrogens, Gual C, Morato T, Hayano M, Gut M and Dorfman R. Endocrinology 71 (1962):920-25.
522. Metabolism of boldenone in man: gas chromatographic/mass spectrometric identification of urinary excreted metabolites and determination of excretion rates. Schanzer, Donike. Bol Mass Spec. 21 (1992):3-16.

523. Biosynthesis of Estrogens, Gual C, Morato T, Hayano M, Gut M, and Dorfman R. Endocrinology 71 (1962):920-25.
524. Metabolism of boldenone in man: gas chromatographic/mass spectrometric identification of urinary excreted metabolites and determination of excretion rates. Schanzer, Donike. Bol Mass Spec. 21 (1992):3-16.
525. Enzyme induction by oral testosterone. Johnsen SG, Kampmann JP, Bennet EP, Jorgensen F 1976 Clin Pharmacol Ther 20:233-237.
526. High-density lipoprotein cholesterol is not decreased if an aromatizable androgen is administered. Friedl K, Hannan C et al. Metabolism 39(1) 1990:69-74.
527. Testosterone dose-response relationships in healthy young men. Bhasin S, Woodhouse L et al. Am J Physiol Endocrinol Metab 281: E1172-81, 2001.
528. The effects of varying doses of T on insulin sensitivity, plasma lipids, apolipoproteins, and C-reactive protein in healthy young men. Singh A, Hsia S, et al. J Clin Endocrinol Metab 87: 136-43, 2002.
529. Butenandt A. K. et al. Ber dtsch chem. Ges. 68 (1935):2097.
530. Formyldienolone. Cornet F, Pedrazzini S. Boll Chim Farm 1972 Nov;111(11):645-8.
531. Arzneimittelforsch 23(11):1583, 1973.
532. Curr Med Res Opinion 3(1):43;1975.
533. Study of non-hypophysiary growth retardation treated with formebolone. Cuatrecasas Membrado JM, Bosch Banyeres JM. An Esp Pediatr. 1985 Jan;22(1): 27-32.
534. Anabolic Steroids and Sports Volume II. James E. Wright. Sports Science Consultants, Natick, MA 1982.
535. Biosynthesis of Estrogens, Gual C, Morato T, Hayano M, Gut M and Dorfman R. Endocrinology 71 (1962):920-25.
536. Aromatization of androstenedione and 19-nortestosterone in human placental, liver and adipose tissues (abstract). Nippon Naibunpi Gakkai Zasshi 62:18-25,1986.
537. Competitive progesterone antagonists: receptor binding and biologic activity of testosterone and 19-nortestosterone derivatives. Reel JR, Humphrey RR, Shih YH, Windsor BL, Sakowski R, Creger PL, Edgren RA. Fertil Steril 1979 May;31(5):552-61.
538. Studies of the biological activity of certain 19-nor steroids in female animals. Pincus G, Chang M, Zarrow M, Hafez E, Merrill A. December 1956.
539. Different pattern of metabolism determine the relative anabolic activity of 19-norandrogens. J Steroid Biochem Mol Bio 53:255-7,1995.
540. Relative binding affinities of testosterone, 19-nortestosterone and their 5-alpha reduced derivatives to the androgen receptor and to other androgen-binding proteins: A suggested role of 5alpha-reductive steroid metabolism in the dissociation of "myotropic" and "androgenic" activities of 19-nortestosterone. Toth M, Zakar T. J Steroid Biochem 17 (1982):653-60.
541. A non-C17-alkylated steroid and long-term cholestasis. Gil VG, et al. Ann Intern Med 1986; 104: 135-6.
542. Metabolic effects of nandrolone decanoate and resistance training in men with HIV. Sattler FR, Schroeder ET, Dube MP, Jaque SV, Martinez C, Blanche PJ, Azen S, Krauss RM. Am J Physiol Endocrinol Metab. 2002 Dec;283(6):E1214-22. Epub 2002 Aug 27.
543. Lipemic and lipoproteinemic effects of natural and synthetic androgens in humans. Crist DM, Peake GT, Stackpole PJ. Clin Exp Pharmacol Physiol 1986 Jul;13(7):513-8.
544. The administration of pharmacological doses of testosterone or 19-nortestosterone to normal men is not associated with increased insulin secretion or impaired glucose tolerance. Karl E. Friedl et al. J Clin Endocrinol Metab 68: 971, 1989.
545. Influence of nandrolonedecanoate on the pituitary-gonadal axis in males. Bijlsma J., Duursma S, Thijssen J, Huber O. Acta Endocrinol 101 (1982):108-12.
546. J. Mathieu, Proc. Intern. Symp. Drug Res. 1967, p 134. Chem. Inst. Can., Montreal, Canada.
547. Unique steroid congeners for receptor studies. Ojasoo, Raynaud. Cancer Research 38 (1978):4186-98.
548. Characterisation of the affinity of different anabolics and synthetic hormones to the human androgen receptor, human sex hormone binding globulin and to the bovine progestin receptor. Bauer, Meyer et al. Acta Pathol Microbiol Imunol Scand Suppl 108 (2000):838-46.
549. Unique steroid congeners for receptor studies. Ojasoo, Raynaud. Cancer Research 38 (1978):4186-98.
550. Disposition of 17 beta-trenbolone in humans. Spranger, Metzler. J Chromatogr 564 (1991):485-92.
551. Cholestasis induced by Parabolan successfully treated with the molecular adsorbent recirculating system. Anand JS et al. ASAIO 2006. Jan-Feb;52(1):117-8.
552. Smith H. et al. Experientia 19 (1963) 394.
553. Evaluation of clinical efficacy and safety of norbolethone in the treatment of idiopathic underweight. Gogate AN. Indian J Med Sci. 1969 Dec;23(12):648-53.
554. Efficacy of norbolethone in stimulating linear growth in stunted children. Gogate AN. Curr Ther Res Clin Exp. 1970 Jun;12(6):323-32.
555. Greenblatt RB et al. Am J Med Sci 1964; 248:317.
556. LeVann LJ et al. Int J Clin Pharmacol 1972; 6:54.
557. Nutritional and metabolic effects of some newer steroids. V. Norbolethone. Albanese AA, Lorenze EJ, Orto LA, Wein EH. N Y State J Med. 1968 Sep;68(18):2392-406.
558. Detection of norbolethone, an anabolic steroid never marketed, in athletes' urine. Catlin DH, Ahrens BD, Kucherova Y. Rapid Commun Mass Spectrom. 2002;16(13):1273-5.
559. A Brief History of Drugs in Sport. Charlie Francis. Oct. 26, 2001 Testosterone Magazine.
560. Relative effects of 17a-alkylated anabolic steroids on sulfobromophthalein (BSP) retention in rabbits. Lennon H. J Pharmacol Exper Thera 151(1) 1966:143-50.
561. Anabolic Steroids and Sports Volume II. James E. Wright. Sports Science Consultants, Natick, MA 1982.
562. Steroids detected in dietary tablets: some contents similar to those used by East German athletes. Amy Shipley. Washington Post, Wednesday, November 30, 2005.
563. Anabolic Steroids and Sports Volume II. James E. Wright. Sports Science Consultants, Natick, MA 1982.
564. Herr, M E, Hogg J A, Levin R H, J Am Chem Soc. 78, 500 (1956).

565. Lyster S C, Lund G H, and Stafford R O, Endocrinology 58, 781 (1956).
566. Testing for fluoxymesterone (Halotestin®) administration to man: Identification of urinary metabolites by gas chromatography-mass spectrometry. Kammerer R, Mardink J, Jangels M et al. J Steroid Biochem 36 (1990):659-66.
567. Eisenberg, E. Modern Trends in Endocrinology (H. Gardiner-Hill, ed) p 46. Hoeber, NY (1961)
568. Methyltestosterone, related steroids, and liver function. deLorimier A, Gilbert G. et al. Arch Intern Med v116 (1965):289-94.
569. The effects of fluoxymesterone administration on testicular function. Jones TM, Fang VS et al. J Clin Endocrinol Metab 1977 Jan;44(1):121-9.
570. Anabolic Steroids and Sports Volume II. James E. Wright. Sports Science CEnsultants, Natick, MA 1982.
571. Anabolic agents. 2,3-Epithioandrostane derivatives. Klimstra PD, Nutting EF, Counsell RE J Med Chem. 1966 Sep;9(5):693-7.
572. Anabolic-androgenic activity of A-ring modified androstane derivatives. II. A comparison of oral activity. Nutting EF, Klimstra PD, Counsell RE. Acta Endocrinol (Copenh). 1966 Dec;53(4):635-43.
573. U.S. Patent # 2,762,818.
574. Sala G, Baldratti G. Proc Soc. Exptl. Biol. Med. 95, 22 (1957).
575. F. A. Kincl. Methods Hormone Res. 4, 21 (1965).
576. Synthesis of deuterium- and tritium-labelled 4-hydroxyandrostene-3,17-dione, an aromatase inhibitor, and its metabolism in nitro and in vivo in the rat. Marsh DA, Romanoff L. et al. Biochem Pharmacol Mar 1;31(5):701-5 1982.
577. Biosynthesis of Estrogens, Gual C, Morato T, Hayano M, Gut M and Dorfman R. Endocrinology 71 (1962):920-25.
578. Aromatization of androstenedione and 19-nortestosterone in human placental, liver and adipose tissues (abstract). Nippon Naibunpi Gakkai Zasshi 62:18-25,1986.
579. Competitive progesterone antagonists: receptor binding and biologic activity of testosterone and 19-nortestosterone derivatives. Reel JR, Humphrey RR, Shih YH, Windsor BL, Sakowski R, Creger PL, Edgren RA. Fertil Steril 1979 May;31(5):552-61.
580. Studies of the biological activity of certain 19-nor steroids in female animals. Pincus G, Chang M, Zarrow M, Hafez E, Merrill A. December 1956.
581. Different pattern of metabolism determine the relative anabolic activity of 19-norandrogens. J Steroid Biochem Mol Bio 53:255-7,1995.
582. Relative binding affinities of testosterone, 19-nortestosterone and their 5-alpha reduced derivatives to the androgen receptor and to other androgen-binding proteins: A suggested role of 5alpha-reductive steroid metabolism in the dissociation of "myotropic" and "androgenic" activities of 19-nortestosterone. Toth M, Zakar T. J Steroid Biochem 17 (1982):653-60.
583. Metabolic effects of nandrolone decanoate and resistance training in men with HIV. Sattler FR, Schroeder ET, Dube MP, Jaque SV, Martinez C, Blanche PJ, Azen S, Krauss RM. Am J Physiol Endocrinol Metab. 2002 Dec;283(6):E1214-22. Epub 2002 Aug 27.
584. Lipemic and lipoproteinemic effects of natural and synthetic androgens in humans. Crist DM, Peake GT, Stackpole PJ. Clin Exp Pharmacol Physiol 1986 Jul;13(7):513-8.
585. The administration of pharmacological doses of testosterone or 19-nortestosterone to normal men is not associated with increased insulin secretion or impaired glucose tolerance. Karl E. Friedl et al. J Clin Endocrinol Metab 68: 971, 1989.
586. Influence of nandrolonedecanoate on the pituitary-gonadal axis in males. Bijlsma J, Duursma S, Thijssen J, Huber O. Acta Endocrinol 101 (1982):108-12.
587. Inhibition of the estrogenic activity of methylandrostenediol following administration of aminopterin. Boll Soc Ital Biol Sper. 1955 Sep-Oct;31(9-10):1280-4.
588. Counsell R E, Adelstein G W et al. J. Med. Chem. 9,685 (1966).
589. Kincl FA, Dorfman RI. Acta Endocrinologica, Supplement 1963; 73:3.
590. Anabolic Steroids and Sports Volume II. James E. Wright. Sports Science Consultants, Natick, MA 1982.
591. 2-Methyl and 2-hydroxymethylene-androstane derivatives. Ringold HJ et al. J Am Chem Soc 1959;81:427-32.
592. Ringold H. J. et al. J. org Chem. 21 (1956):1432.
593. Pharmacokinetics of 7a-methylnortestosterone in men and cynomolgus monkeys. Kumar N. et al. J Androl 18:352-58.
594. Al Segaloff. Steroids 1, 299 (1963).
595. J A Campbell, S C Lyster et al. Steroids 1, 317 (1963).
596. Prostate-sparing effects in primates of the potent androgen 7a-methyl-nortestosterone: A potential alternative to testosterone for androgen replacement and male contraception. Cummings D, Kumar N et al. J Clin Endocrinol Metab. 83: 4212-19:(1998).
597. 7alpha-methyl-19-nortestosterone, a synthetic androgen with high potency: structure-activity comparisons with other androgens. Kumar N. et al. L Steroid Biochem Mol Biol. 1999 Dec 31;71(5-6):213-22.
598. Lyster S C, et al. Acta Endocrin (Kbh) 43 (1963):399.
599. Transdermal testosterone improves sexual function, mood, muscle strength, and body composition parameters in hypogonadal men. J. Clin Endocrinol. Metab. 85: 2839-53.
600. 7alpha-methyl-19-nortestosterone: an ideal androgen for replacement therapy. Sundaram K, Kumar N, Bardin CW. Recent Prog Horm Res. 1994;49:373-6.
601. A clinical trial of 7a-methyl-19-nortestosterone implants for possible use as a long-acting contraceptive for men. S. Eckardstein, G Noe et al. J Clin Enocrinol Metab 88: 5232-39:(2003).
602. 7a-methyl-19-nortestosterone maintains sexual behavior and mood in hypogonadal men. R.A. Anderson, C.W. Martin et al. J Clin Endocrinol Metab. 84:3556-62(1999).
603. Structure-activity relationship study of human liver microsomes-ctalized hydrolysis rate of ester prodrugs of MENT by comparative molecular field analysis (CoMFA). Bursi R. Grootenhuis A. et al. Steroids 2003 Mar;68(3):213-20.
604. Aromatization of 7alpha-methyl-19-nortestosterone by human placental microsomes in vitro. Kumar N. LaMorte et al. J Steroid Biochem Mol Biol. 1994 Feb;48(2-3):297-304.
605. Estrogenic and progestational activity of 7-alpha-methyl-19-nortestosterone, a synthetic androgen. Beri R, Kumar N, Savage T. et al. Steroid Biochem Mol Biol. 1998 Nov;67(3):275-83.

606. Different patterns of metabolism determine the relative anabolic activity of 19-norandrogens. Sundaram K, Kumar N. et al. J Steroid Biochem Mol Biol. 1995 Jun;53(1-6):253-7.
607. Herstellung des 17-metyl-testosterons und anderer Androsten- und Androstanderivate. Ruzicka L, Goldberg MW. Et al. Helv Chim Acta 18 (1935):1487-98.
608. Effect of anabolic steroids on liver function tests and creatine excretion. Marquardt G. H. et al. JAMA 175 (Mar 11, 1961):851-3.
609. Methyltestosterone, related steroids, and liver function. deLorimier A, Gilbert G. et al. Arch Intern Med v116 (1965):289-94.
610. High-density lipoprotein cholesterol is not decreased if an aromatizable androgen is administered. Friedl KE, Hannan CJ Jr, Jones RE, Plymate SR. Metabolism. 1990 Jan;39(1):69-74.
611. Anabolic Steroids and Sports Volume II. James E. Wright. Sports Science Consultants, Natick, MA 1982.
612. Rucicka L et al. Helv Chim. Acta 18 (1935) 1487
613. Anabolic Steroids and Sports Volume II. James E. Wright. Sports Science Consultants, Natick, MA 1982
614. The synthesis of some 7alpha and 7beta methyl steroid hormones. Campbell JA, Babcock JC. J Am Chem Soc 81:4069-74 (1959)
615. NDA 017383 Filed Aug 18, 1972. Approved Feb 20, 1973
616. Male breast cancer: two cases with objective regression from calusterone (7 alpha, 17 beta-dimethyltestosterone) after failure of orchiectomy. Horn Y, Roof B. Oncology 1976;33(4):188-91
617. Calusterone. Brodkin RA, Cooper MR. Ann Intern Med. 1978 Dec;89(6) 945-8.
618. Interference of gestagens and androgens with rat uterine oestrogen receptors. Di Carlo F, Conti G, Reboani C. J Endocrinol. 1978 Apr;77(1):49-55
619. Antitumoral activity of calusterone in advanced mammary carcinoma. Rosso R, Brema, F et al. Tumori 1976 Jan-Feb 61(1):79-84
620. Anabolic Steroids and Sports Volume II. James E. Wright. Sports Science Consultants, Natick, MA 1982
621. Counsell R. E., Klimstra P.D. et al. J. Org. Chem. 27, 248 (1962)
622. Anabolic Steroids and Sports Volume II. James E. Wright. Sports Science Consultants, Natick, MA 1982
623. Perelman M. Farkas E., Forenfeld E.J. et al. J Am Chem Soc. 82 (1960), 2402
624. Anabolic Steroids and Sports Volume II. James E. Wright. Sports Science Consultants, Natick, MA 1982
625. Liver toxicity of a new anabolic agent: methyltrienolone (17-alpha-methyl-4,9,11-estratriene-17 beta-ol-3-one). Kruskemper, Noell. Steroids. 1966 Jul;8(1):13-24.
626. T. Feyel-Cabanes, Compt. Rend. Soc. Biol. 157, 1428 (1963)
627. Protein anabolism produced in man by a new steroid: methyltrienolone. Tremolieres J, Pequignot E. Presse Med. 1965 Nov 6;73(47):2655-8.
628. Specific binding of [3H]-methyltrienolone to both progestin and androgen binding components in human benign prostatic hypertrophy (BPH). Asselin J, Melancon R, Gourdeau Y, Labrie F, Bonne C, Raynaud JP. J Steroid Biochem. 1979 May;10(5):483-6
629. Liver toxicity of a new anabolic agent: methyltrienolone (17-alpha-methyl-4,9,11-estratriene-17 beta-ol-3-one). Kruskemper, Noell. Steroids. 1966 Jul;8(1):13-24.
630. Anabolic Steroids and Sports Volume II. James E. Wright. Sports Science Consultants, Natick, MA 1982
631. M. Shimizu, G. Ohta et al. Chem. & Pharm. Bull. (Tokyo) 13, 895 (1965)
632. Pharmacological studies on experimental nephritic rats. (4) Improvement of hyperlipemic models in rats utilizing anti-rat kidney rabbit serum and effects of anti-hyperlipemic agents on serum lipid levels. Suzuki Y, Honda Y, Ito M. Jpn J Pharmacol. 1978 Oct;28(5):729-38.
633. The use of oxandrolone in hyperlipidaemia. Doyle AE, Pinkus NB, Green J. Med J Aust. 1974 Feb 2;1(5):127-9.
634. G. Sala, in "Hormonal Steroids" (L. Martini and A. Pecile eds.) Vol 1, P. 67 Academic Press, NY (1964)
635. Anabolic Steroids and Sports Volume II. James E. Wright. Sports Science Consultants, Natick, MA 1982
636. Clinical evaluation of a new anabolic agent 7a,17a-dimethyltestosterone (bolasterone). Korst, D. R., Bowers, C. Y., Flokstra, J. H., McMahon, F.G. Clin. Pharmacol. Therap. 4:734-9 (1963).
637. The synthesis of some 7alpha and 7beta methyl steroid hormones. Campbell JA, Babcock JC. J Am Chem Soc 81:4069-74 (1959).
638. Anabolic and androgenic activities of 7a,17a-dimethyltestosterone (U-19,763), a new anabolic steroid. Stucki J. C., Duncan G. W., Lyster S.C.
639. Anabolic Steroids and Sports Volume II. James E. Wright. Sports Science Consultants, Natick, MA 1982.
640. NEBIDO Prescribing Information (2004). Schering AG Germany.
641. Enzyme induction by oral testosterone. Johnsen SG, Kampmann JP, Bennet EP, Jorgensen F 1976 Clin Pharmacol Ther 20:233-237.
642. High-density lipoprotein cholesterol is not decreased if an aromatizable androgen is administered. Karl Friedl, Charles Hannan et al. Metabolism 39(1) 1990:69-74.
643. Testosterone dose-response relationships in healthy young men. Bhasin S, Woodhouse L et al. Am J Physiol Endocrinol Metab 281: E1172-81, 2001.
644. The effects of varying doses of T on insulin sensitivity, plasma lipids, apolipoproteins, and C-reactive protein in healthy young men. Atam Singh, Stanley Hsia, et al. J Clin Endocrinol Metab 87: 136-43, 2002.
645. Preliminary results of experience with a new anabolic steroid, "androisoxazole," in the aged. Antonini FM, Verdi G. Minerva Med. 1961 Oct 6;52:3437-41.
646. Preliminary research in the pediatric field with a new protein anabolic agent: androisoxazole. Research on the serum transaminase and aldolase. Cytological examinations of the vaginal mucosa. Bertolotti E, Lojodice G. Minerva Med. 1961 Oct 6;52:3433-7.
647. Androisoxazole in pediatrics. Kofman I, Calvi C, Rey Carregal R. Rass Clin Ter. 1966;65(6):345-9.
648. Anabolic Steroids and Sports Volume II. James E. Wright. Sports Science Consultants, Natick, MA 1982.
649. Butenandt A. K. et al. Ber dtsch chem. Ges. 68 (1935), 2097.
650. Studies on the treatment of idiopathic gynaecomastia with percutaneous dihydrotestosterone. Clin Endocrinol (Oxf). 1983 Oct;19(4):513-20.
651. Gynecomastia: effect of prolonged treatment with dihydrotestosterone by the percutaneous route Presse Med. 1983 Jan 8;12(1):21-5.
652. Enzyme induction by oral testosterone. Johnsen SG, Kampmann JP, Bennet EP, Jorgensen F 1976 Clin Pharmacol Ther 20:233-237.
653. High-density lipoprotein cholesterol is not decreased if an aromatizable androgen is administered. Karl Friedl, Charles Hannan et al. Metabolism 39(1)

1990:69-74.
654. Testosterone dose-response relationships in healthy young men. Bhasin S, Woodhouse L et al. Am J Physiol Endocrinol Metab 281: E1172-81, 2001.
655. The effects of varying doses of T on insulin sensitivity, plasma lipids, apolipoproteins, and C-reactive protein in healthy young men. Atam Singh, Stanley Hsia, et al. J Clin Endocrinol Metab 87: 136-43, 2002.
656. Colton F.B., Nysted L.N., Riegel B., et al. J Am Chem Soc. 79 (1954), 1123.
657. Studies of the biological activity of certain 19-nor steroids in female animals. Pincus G., Chang M., Zarrow M., Hafez E., Merrill A. December 1956.
658. Anabolic Steroids and Sports Volume II. James E. Wright. Sports Science Consultants, Natick, MA 1982.
659. Enzyme induction by oral testosterone. Johnsen SG, Kampmann JP, Bennet EP, Jorgensen F 1976 Clin Pharmacol Ther 20:233-237.
660. High-density lipoprotein cholesterol is not decreased if an aromatizable androgen is administered. Karl Friedl, Charles Hannan et al. Metabolism 39(1) 1990:69-74.
661. Testosterone dose-response relationships in healthy young men. Bhasin S, Woodhouse L et al. Am J Physiol Endocrinol Metab 281: E1172-81, 2001.
662. The effects of varying doses of T on insulin sensitivity, plasma lipids, apolipoproteins, and C-reactive protein in healthy young men. Atam Singh, Stanley Hsia, et al. J Clin Endocrinol Metab 87: 136-43, 2002.
663. Metabolism of anabolic steroid drugs in man and the marmoset monkey (callithrix jacchus)-I. Nilevar and Orabolin. Ward R, Lawson A.M, Shackleton C.L.H. J Steroid Biochem 8 (1977):1057-63.
664. De Winter, M. S. et al. Chem. and Ind. (London) 1959, 905.
665. Overbeek G.A. et al. Acta Endicrin. (Kbh) 40 (1962):133.
666. Anabolic Steroids and Sports Volume II. James E. Wright. Sports Science Consultants, Natick, MA 1982.
667. Doerner G and Schubert A. Proc. Intern. Congr. Hormonal Steroids, Milan 1962, Excerpta Med. Intern. Congr. Ser. No. 51, 210.
668. Anabolic Steroids and Sports Volume II. James E. Wright. Sports Science Consultants, Natick, MA 1982.
669. Camerino B. et al. Farmaco (Pavia) ediz sci. 11 (1956):586.
670. U.S. Patent # 3,060,201. 4-hydroxy-17alpha-methyl-3-keto-delta4-steroids of androstane and 19-nor-androstane series and esters therof. Camerino, Patelli, Sala. Oct 23, 1962.
671. Anabolic steroid abuse and cardiac death. Kennedy MC, Lawrence C. Med J Aust. 1993 Mar 1;158(5):346-8.
672. Anabolic Steroids and Sports Volume II. James E. Wright. Sports Science Consultants, Natick, MA 1982.
673. Miescher, Wettstein & Tschopp (1936) Schweiz. Med. Wschr. 66, 310.
674. Enzyme induction by oral testosterone. Johnsen SG, Kampmann JP, Bennet EP, Jorgensen F 1976 Clin Pharmacol Ther 20:233-237.
675. High-density lipoprotein cholesterol is not decreased if an aromatizable androgen is administered. Friedl K, Hannan C et al. Metabolism 39(1) 1990: 69-74.
676. Testosterone dose-response relationships in healthy young men. Bhasin S, Woodhouse L et al. Am J Physiol Endocrinol Metab 281: E1172-81, 2001.
677. The effects of varying doses of T on insulin sensitivity, plasma lipids, apolipoproteins, and C-reactive protein in healthy young men. Atam Singh, Stanley Hsia, et al. J Clin Endocrinol Metab 87: 136-43, 2002.
678. Arnold A and Potts GO. Acta Endocrinol. 52, 489 (1966).
679. Overbeek GA and J. de Visser, Acta Endocrinol. 22, 318 (1956).
680. Djerassi, C. et al. J. Am. Chem Soc. 76 (1954):4092.
681. Saunders FJ et al. Proc. Soc. Exp. Biol. (N.Y.) 94 (1957):717.
682. Methylestrenolone, a new progestogenic substance more active than progesterone. Mansani FE. Minerva Ginecol. 1957 Move 30;9(22):935-41.
683. Jaundice during administration of methylestrenolone. Peters RH, Randall AH et al. L Clin Endorcinol Metab, 1958 Jan;18(1):114-5.
684. Anabolic Steroids and Sports Volume II. James E. Wright. Sports Science Consultants, Natick, MA 1982.
685. J. Mathieu, Proc. Intern. Symp. Drug Res. 1967, p 134. Chem. Inst. Can., Montreal, Canada.
686. Unique steroid congeners for receptor studies. Ojasoo, Raynaud. Cancer Research 38 (1978):4186-98.
687. Characterisation of the affinity of different anabolics and synthetic hormones to the human androgen receptor, human sex hormone binding globulin and to the bovine progestin receptor. Bauer, Meyer et al. Acta Pathol Microbiol Imunol Scand Suppl 108 (2000):838-46.
688. Unique steroid congeners for receptor studies. Ojasoo, Raynaud. Cancer Research 38 (1978):4186-98.
689. Disposition of 17 beta-trenbolone in humans. Spranger, Metzler. J Chromatogr 564 (1991):485-92.
690. Cholestasis induced by Parabolan successfully treated with the molecular adsorbent recirculating system. Anand JS et al. ASAIO 2006. Jan-Feb;52(1):117-8.
691. Enzyme induction by oral testosterone. Johnsen SG, Kampmann JP, Bennet EP, Jorgensen F 1976 Clin Pharmacol Ther 20:233-237.
692. High-density lipoprotein cholesterol is not decreased if an aromatizable androgen is administered. Karl Friedl, Charles Hannan et al. Metabolism 39(1) 1990:69-74.
693. Testosterone dose-response relationships in healthy young men. Bhasin S, Woodhouse L et al. Am J Physiol Endocrinol Metab 281: E1172-81, 2001.
694. The effects of varying doses of T on insulin sensitivity, plasma lipids, apolipoproteins, and C-reactive protein in healthy young men. Singh A, Hsia S, et al. J Clin Endocrinol Metab 87: 136-43, 2002.
695. Wiechert R. et al. Chem Ber. 93 (1960):1710.
696. Methenolone acetate, Summary of information for clinical investigators, New Brunswick, NJ. The Squibb Institute for Medical Research, May 30, 1962.
697. Anabolic effects of methenolone enanthate and methenolone acetate in underweight premature infants and children. New York State Journal of Medicine March 1, 1965, 645-8.
698. Kruskemper H L et al, Exc Medica (Amsterd.) Congr. Ser. No. 51 (1962), 209.
699. Weller O. Arzneimittelforsch. 12 (1962):234.
700. Proc. Intern. Congr. Hormonal Steroids, Milan, 1962. Excerpta Med. Intern. Congr. Ser No. 51, p. 209. Excerpta. Med. Found., Amsterdam, 1962.
701. Failure of non-17-alkylated anabolic steroids to produce abnormal liver function tests. J Clin Endocrinol Metab. 1964 Dec;24:1334-6.

702. Fatal outcome of a patient with severe aplastic anemia after treatment with metenolone acetate. Ann Hematol. 1993 Jul;67(1):41-3. Tsukamoto N, Uchiyama T, Takeuchi T, Sato S, Naruse T, Nakazato Y.
703. Comparative studies about the influence of metenoloneacetate and mesterolone on hypophysis and male gonads. Trenkner R, Senge T, Hienz H et al. Arzneimittelforschung. 1970 20(4):545-7.
704. Anabolic Steroids and Sports Volume II. James E. Wright. Sports Science Consultants, Natick, MA 1982.
705. Wiechert R. et al. Chem Ber. 93 (1960):1710.
706. Methenolone enanthate, Summary of information for clinical investigators, New Brunswick, NJ. The Squibb Institute for Medical Research, April 15, 1962.
707. Anabolic effects of methenolone enanthate and methenolone acetate in underweight premature infants and children. New York State Journal of Medicine March 1, 1965, 645-8.
708. Proc. Intern. Congr. Hormonal Steroids, Milan, 1962. Excerpta Med. Intern. Congr. Ser No. 51, p. 209. Excerpta. Med. Found., Amsterdam, 1962.
709. Failure of non-17-alkylated anabolic steroids to produce abnormal liver function tests. J Clin Endocrinol Metab. 1964 Dec;24:1334-6.
710. Relative binding affinity of anabolic-androgenic steroids: comparison of the binding to the androgen receptors in skeletal muscle and in prostate, as well as to sex hormone-binding globulin. Saartok T, Dahlberg E, Gustafsson JA. Endocrinology. 1984 Jun;114(6):2100-6.
711. Influence of various modes of androgen substitution on serum lipids and lipoproteins in hypogonadal men. Jockenhovel F, Bullmann C, Schubert M, Vogel E, Reinhardt W, Reinwein D, Muller-Wieland D, Krone W. Metabolism. 1999 May;48(5):590-6.
712. Comparative studies about the influence of metenolonacetate and mesterolone on hypophysis and male gonads. Trenkner R, Senge T, Hienz A, et al. Arzneim-Forsch. (Drug Res) Jahrgang 30, Nr. 4 (1970):545-7.
713. The effects of mesterolone, a male sex hormone in depressed patients (a double blind controlled study). Itil TM, Michael ST, Shapiro DM, Itil KZ. Methods Find Exp Clin Pharmacol. 1984 Jun;6(6):331-7.
714. Clinical evaluation of the proteo-anabolic activity of dimethazine in patients with genital neoplasms during actinotherapy. Fontana Donatelli G, Dambrosio F. Ann Ostet Ginecol. 1962 Sep;84:773-83. Italian.
715. Biological determination of the secondary hormonal activities of dimethazine. Lupo, C, Matscher R, et al. Bolletino – Societa Italiana di Biologia Sperimentale 38 (1962):990-4.
716. Protracted action of protein anabolism in gynecological oncology and its effect on hepatic function. Dambrosio F, Donatelli G, et al. University of Milan (1963).
717. Inhibition of the estrogenic activity of methylandrostenediol following administration of aminopterin . Boll Soc Ital Biol Sper. 1955 Sep-Oct;31(9-10):1280-4.
718. Enzyme induction by oral testosterone. Johnsen SG, Kampmann JP, Bennet EP, Jorgensen F 1976 Clin Pharmacol Ther 20:233-237.
719. High-density lipoprotein cholesterol is not decreased if an aromatizable androgen is administered. Karl Friedl, Charles Hannan et al. Metabolism 39(1) 1990:69-74.
720. Testosterone dose-response relationships in healthy young men. Bhasin S, Woodhouse L et al. Am J Physiol Endocrinol Metab 281: E1172-81, 2001.
721. The effects of varying doses of T on insulin sensitivity, plasma lipids, apolipoproteins, and C-reactive protein in healthy young men. Singh A, Hsia S, et al. J Clin Endocrinol Metab 87:136-43, 2002.
722. McPhail MK, Physiol J. (London) 83 (1934):145
723. Enzyme induction by oral testosterone. Johnsen SG, Kampmann JP, Bennet EP, Jorgensen F. 1976 Clin Pharmacol Ther 20:233-237.
724. High-density lipoprotein cholesterol is not decreased if an aromatizable androgen is administered. Friedl K, Hannan C et al. Metabolism 39(1) 1990: 69-74.
725. Testosterone dose-response relationships in healthy young men. Bhasin S, Woodhouse L et al. Am J Physiol Endocrinol Metab 281: E1172-81, 2001.
726. The effects of varying doses of T on insulin sensitivity, plasma lipids, apolipoproteins, and C-reactive protein in healthy young men. Singh A, Hsia S, et al. J Clin Endocrinol Metab 87: 136-43, 2002.
727. Enzyme induction by oral testosterone. Johnsen SG, Kampmann JP, Bennet EP, Jorgensen F. 1976 Clin Pharmacol Ther 20:233-237.
728. Testosterone replacement, cardiovascular system and risk factors in the aging male. Vigna GB, Bergami E. J Endocrinol Invest. 2005;28(11 Suppl Proceedings):69-74.
729. 2-Methyl and 2-hydroxymethylene-androstane derivatives. Ringold HJ et al. J Am Chem Soc 1959;81:427-32.
730. Enzyme induction by oral testosterone. Johnsen SG, Kampmann JP, Bennet EP, Jorgensen F. 1976 Clin Pharmacol Ther 20:233-237.
731. High-density lipoprotein cholesterol is not decreased if an aromatizable androgen is administered. Karl Friedl, Charles Hannan et al. Metabolism 39(1) 1990: 69-74.
732. Testosterone dose-response relationships in healthy young men. Bhasin S, Woodhouse L et al. Am J Physiol Endocrinol Metab 281: E1172-81, 2001.
733. The effects of varying doses of T on insulin sensitivity, plasma lipids, apolipoproteins, and C-reactive protein in healthy young men. Singh A, Hsia S, et al. J Clin Endocrinol Metab 87: 136-43, 2002.
734. Product Data Sheet: Sustanon 250. August 31, 2001. Pharmaco (N.Z.) LTD Auckland New Zealand.
735. Enzyme induction by oral testosterone. Johnsen SG, Kampmann JP, Bennet EP, Jorgensen F. 1976 Clin Pharmacol Ther 20:233-237.
736. High-density lipoprotein cholesterol is not decreased if an aromatizable androgen is administered. Friedl K, Hannan C et al. Metabolism 39(1) 1990: 69-74.
737. Testosterone dose-response relationships in healthy young men. Bhasin S, Woodhouse L et al. Am J Physiol Endocrinol Metab 281: E1172-81, 2001.
738. The effects of varying doses of T on insulin sensitivity, plasma lipids, apolipoproteins, and C-reactive protein in healthy young men. Singh A, Hsia S, et al. J Clin Endocrinol Metab 87: 136-43, 2002.
739. History of diethylstilbestrol use in cattle. A. P. Raun and R. L. Preston. 2002, American Society of Animal Science.
740. Enzyme induction by oral testosterone. Johnsen SG, Kampmann JP, Bennet EP, Jorgensen F. 1976 Clin Pharmacol Ther 20:233-237.
741. High-density lipoprotein cholesterol is not decreased if an aromatizable androgen is administered. Friedl K, Hannan C et al. Metabolism 39(1) 1990: 69-74.

742. Testosterone dose-response relationships in healthy young men. Bhasin S, Woodhouse L et al. Am J Physiol Endocrinol Metab 281: E1172-81, 2001.
743. The effects of varying doses of T on insulin sensitivity, plasma lipids, apolipoproteins, and C-reactive protein in healthy young men. Singh A, Hsia S, et al. J Clin Endocrinol Metab 87: 136-43, 2002.
744. Long-term experience with testosterone replacement through scrotal skin. In Nieschlag E and Behre HM (eds) Testosterone. Action, Deficiency, Substitution. Atkinson LE, Chang Y-L and Snyder PJ (1998) Springer, Berlin, Germany 365–388.
745. Enzyme induction by oral testosterone. Johnsen SG, Kampmann JP, Bennet EP, Jorgensen F. 1976 Clin Pharmacol Ther 20:233-237.
746. Testosterone replacement, cardiovascular system and risk factors in the aging male. Vigna GB, Bergami E. J Endocrinol Invest. 2005;28(11 Suppl Proceedings):69-74.
747. New androgen for retarded action; testosterone phenylpropionate. Klotz HP, Avril Y. Therapie. 1955;10(4):588-90.
748. Enzyme induction by oral testosterone. Johnsen SG, Kampmann JP, Bennet EP, Jorgensen F. 1976 Clin Pharmacol Ther 20:233-237.
749. High-density lipoprotein cholesterol is not decreased if an aromatizable androgen is administered. Friedl K, Hannan C et al. Metabolism 39(1) 1990:69-74
750. Testosterone dose-response relationships in healthy young men. Bhasin S, Woodhouse L et al. Am J Physiol Endocrinol Metab 281: E1172-81, 2001.
751. The effects of varying doses of T on insulin sensitivity, plasma lipids, apolipoproteins, and C-reactive protein in healthy young men. Singh A, Hsia S, et al. J Clin Endocrinol Metab 87: 136-43, 2002.
752. Enzyme induction by oral testosterone. Johnsen SG, Kampmann JP, Bennet EP, Jorgensen F. 1976 Clin Pharmacol Ther 20:233-237.
753. Testosterone replacement, cardiovascular system and risk factors in the aging male. Vigna GB, Bergami E. J Endocrinol Invest. 2005;28(11 Suppl Proceedings):69-74.
754. The effects of depot testosterone therapy on serum levels of luteinizing hormone and follicle-stimulating hormone in patients with Klinedelter's syndrome and hypogonadotrophic eunuchoidism. Fukutani K, Isurugi K et al. J Clin Endocrinol Metab 39:856-64.
755. Enzyme induction by oral testosterone. Johnsen SG, Kampmann JP, Bennet EP, Jorgensen F. 1976 Clin Pharmacol Ther 20:233-237.
756. High-density lipoprotein cholesterol is not decreased if an aromatizable androgen is administered. Friedl K, Hannan C et al. Metabolism 39(1) 1990:69-74
757. Testosterone dose-response relationships in healthy young men. Bhasin S, Woodhouse L et al. Am J Physiol Endocrinol Metab 281: E1172-81, 2001.
758. The effects of varying doses of T on insulin sensitivity, plasma lipids, apolipoproteins, and C-reactive protein in healthy young men. Singh A, Hsia S, et al. J Clin Endocrinol Metab 87: 136-43, 2002.
759. Hormonal therapy of endometriosis. Metzger DA, Luciano AA. Obstet Gynecol Clin North Am. 1989 Mar;16(1):105-22.
760. Tetrahydrogestrinone: discovery, synthesis, and detection in urine. Catlin et al. Rapid Commun Mass Spectrom. 2004;18(12):1245-049.
761. Tetrahydrogestrinone Is a Potent Androgen and Progestin. Death A, McGrath K et al. J Clin Endocrinol and Metab. 89: 2498-2500, 2004.
762. Anabolic Steroids and Sports Volume II. James E. Wright. Sports Science Consultants, Natick, MA 1982.
763. Edgren, Peterson, Jones, et al. Recent Progr. Hormone Res. 22, 305 (1966).
764. Absorption and disposition of epithipsteroids in rats (1): Route of administration and plasma levels of epitiostane. T Ichihashi, H Kinoshita et al. Xenobiotica (1991) 21: 865-72.
765. Anabolic agents. 2,3-Epithioandrostane derivatives. Klimstra PD, Nutting EF, Counsell RE J Med Chem. 1966 Sep;9(5):693-7.
766. 2alpha,3alpha-epithio-5alpha-androstan-17beta-yl 1-methoxycyclopentyl ether in the treatment of advanced breast cancer. Cancer 1978 Feb; 41(2):758-60
767. Therapeutic value of mepitiostane in the treatment of advanced breast cancer. Inoue K, Okazaki K et al. Cancer Treat Rep. 1978 May;62(5):743-5
768. J. Mathieu, Proc. Intern. Symp. Drug Res. 1967, p 134. Chem. Inst. Can., Montreal, Canada.
769. Unique steroid congeners for receptor studies. Ojasoo, Raynaud. Cancer Research 38 (1978):4186-98.
770. Characterisation of the affinity of different anabolics and synthetic hormones to the human androgen receptor, human sex hormone binding globulin and to the bovine progestin receptor. Bauer, Meyer et al. Acta Pathol Microbiol Imunol Scand Suppl 108 (2000):838-46.
771. Unique steroid congeners for receptor studies. Ojasoo, Raynaud. Cancer Research 38 (1978):4186-98.
772. Disposition of 17 beta-trenbolone in humans. Spranger, Metzler. J Chromatogr 564 (1991):485-92.
773. Cholestasis induced by Parabolan successfully treated with the molecular adsorbent recirculating system. Anand JS et al. ASAIO 2006. Jan-Feb;52(1):117-8.
774. Unique steroid congeners for receptor studies. Ojasoo, Raynaud. Cancer Research 38 (1978):4186-98.
775. Characterisation of the affinity of different anabolics and synthetic hormones to the human androgen receptor, human sex hormone binding globulin and to the bovine progestin receptor. Bauer, Meyer et al. Acta Pathol Microbiol Imunol Scand Suppl 108 (2000):838-46.
776. Unique steroid congeners for receptor studies. Ojasoo, Raynaud. Cancer Research 38 (1978):4186-98.
777. Disposition of 17 beta-trenbolone in humans. Spranger, Metzler. J Chromatogr 564 (1991):485-92.
778. Cholestasis induced by Parabolan successfully treated with the molecular adsorbent recirculating system. Anand JS et al. ASAIO 2006. Jan-Feb;52(1):117-8.
779. Triolandren: a mixture of testosterone esters with a rapid & sustained effect. Tschopp E, Meier R. Rev Med Cubana. 1957 Sep;68(9):373-8.
780. Enzyme induction by oral testosterone. Johnsen SG, Kampmann JP, Bennet EP, Jorgensen F. 1976 Clin Pharmacol Ther 20:233-237
781. High-density lipoprotein cholesterol is not decreased if an aromatizable androgen is administered. Friedl K, Hannan C et al. Metabolism 39(1) 1990:69-74
782. Testosterone dose-response relationships in healthy young men. Bhasin S, Woodhouse L et al. Am J Physiol Endocrinol Metab 281: E1172-81, 2001.
783. The effects of varying doses of T on insulin sensitivity, plasma lipids, apolipoproteins, and C-reactive protein in healthy young men. Singh A, Hsia S, et al. J Clin Endocrinol Metab 87: 136-43, 2002.
784. Clinton R. O. et al. J. Amer chem. Soc. 81 (1959):1513.
785. U.S. Patent # 3,030,358.

786. Anabolic-androgenic steroid interaction with rat androgen receptor in vivo and in vitro: a comparative study. Feldkoren BI, Andersson S. J Steroid Biochem Mol Biol. 2005 Apr;94(5):481-7. Epub 2005 Mar 17.
787. The differential effects of stanozolol on human skin and synovial fibroblasts in vitro: DNA synthesis and receptor binding. Ellis AJ, Cawston TE, Mackie EJ. Agents Actions. 1994 Mar;41(1-2):37-43.
788. Identification of a specific binding site for the anabolic steroid stanozolol in male rat liver microsomes. Boada LD, Fernandez L et al. J Pharmacol Exp Ther 1996 Dec;279(3):1123-9.
789. Stanozolol and danazol, unlike natural androgens, interact with the low affinity glucocorticoid-binding sites from male rat liver microsomes. Fernandez L, Chirino R, Boada LD, Navarro D, Cabrera N, del Rio I, Diaz-Chico BN. Endocrinology. 1994 Mar;134(3):1401-8.
790. Desaulles P. A. et al. Helv. Med Acta 27 (1960), 479.
791. Sex hormone-binding globulin response to the anabolic steroid stanozolol: Evidence for its suitability as a Biological androgen sensitivity test. G Sinnecker, S Kohler. Journal of Clin Endo Metab. 68: 1195,1989.
792. The influence of 6 months of oral anabolic steroids on body mass and respiratory muscles in undernourished COPD patients. Ivone Martins Ferreira, Ieda Verreschi et al. CHEST 114 (1) July 1998 19-28.
793. Androgenic/Anabolic steroid-induced toxic hepatitis. Stimac D, Milic S, Dintinjana RD, Kovac D, Ristic S. J Clin Gastroenterol. 2002 Oct;35(4):350-2.
794. Contrasting effects of testosterone and stanozolol on serum lipoprotein levels. Thompson PD, Cullinane EM, Sady SP, Chenevert C, Saritelli AL, Sady MA, Herbert PN. JAMA. 1989 Feb 24;261(8):1165-8.
795. The effect of intramuscular stanozolol on fibrinolysis and blood lipids. Small M, McArdle BM, Lowe GD, Forbes CD, Prentice CR. Thromb Res. 1982 Oct 1;28(1):27-36.
796. Alteration of hormone levels in normal males given the anabolic steroid stanozolol. Small M, Beastall GH, Semple CG, Cowan RA, Forbes CD. Clin Endocrinol (Oxf). 1984 Jul;21(1):49-55.
797. Anabolic Steroids and Sports Volume II. James E. Wright. Sports Science Consultants, Natick, MA 1982.
798. The effect of stanozolol on 15nitrogen retention in the dog. Olson ME, Morck DW, Quinn KB. Can J Vet Res. 2000 Oct;64(4):246-8.
799. Protein synthesis in isolated forelimb muscles. The possible role of metabolites of arachidonic acid in the response to intermittent stretching. Smith, Palmer et al. Biochem J. 1983 214,153-61.
800. The influence of changes in tension on protein synthesis and prostaglandin release in isolated rabbit muscles. Palemr, Reeds et al. Biochem J. 1983 214,1011-14.
801. Protein synthesis and degradation in isolated muscle. Effect of n3 and n6 fatty acids. Palmer, Wahle. Biochem J. 1987 242, 615-18.
802. Regular exercise modulates muscle membrane phospholipid profile in rats. Helge et al. J. Nutr. 1999 129:1636-42.
803. Exercise training reduces skeletal muscle membrane arachidonate in obese (fa/fa) Zucker rat. Ayre et al. J. Appl. Physiol. 1998 85(5):1898-1902.
804. Effects of physical exercise on phospholipid fatty acid composition in skeletal muscle. Andersson et al. Am. J. Physiol. 274 (Endocrinol. Metab. 37):E432-38 1998.
805. Effects of an omnivorous diet compared with a lactoovovegetarian diet on resistance-training –induced changes in body composition and skeletal muscle in older men. W Campbell, M Barton et al. Am J Clin Nutr 70(1999):1032-9.
806. The effect of dietary arachidonic acid on plasma lipoprotein distribution, apoproteins, blood lipid levels, and tissue fatty acid composition in humans. G.J. Nelson, P.C. Schmidt et al. Lipids 32: 427-33 (1997).
807. The effect of dietary arachidonic acid on platelet function, platelet fatty acid composition, and blood coagulation in humans. Nelson CJ, Schmidt PC et al. Lipids 32(4):421-5 (1997).
808. Effects of dietary arachidonic acid on human immune response. Kelley DS, Taylor PC et al. Lipids 32(4):449-56 (1997).
809. Dietary intake of N-3 and N-6 fatty acids and the risk of prostate cancer. M Leitzmann, M Stampfer et al. Am J Clin Nutr 80:204-16 (2004).
810. Dietary (n-6) PUFA and intestinal tumorigenesis. J Whelan, M McEntee et al. J Nutr 134:3421S-26S (2004).
811. Action of heptaminol hydrochloride on contractile properties in frog isolated twitch muscle fibre. Allard B, Jacquemond V, Lemtiri-Chlieh F, Pourrias B, Rougier O. Br J Pharmacol. 1991 Nov;104(3):714-8.
812. Heptaminol chlorhydrate: new data. Pourrias B. Ann Pharm Fr. 1991;49(3):127-38.
813. On the mode of action of heptaminol (author's transl)] Grobecker H, Grobecker H. Arzneimittelforschung. 1976;26(12):2167-71.
814. Prostaglandins and the control of muscle protein synthesis and degradation. Prostaglandins Leukot Essent Fatty Acids. 1990 Feb;39(2):95-104
815. Prostaglandin F2(alpha)stimulates growth of skeletal muscle cells via an NFATC2-dependent pathway. Horsley V, Pavlath GK. J Cell Biol. 2003 Apr 14; 161(1):111-8.
816. Stretch-induced prostaglandins and protein turnover in cultural skeletal muscle. Vandenburgh HH, Hatfaludy S, Sohar I, Shansky J. Am J Physiol. 1990 Aug;259(2 Pt 1): C232-40.
817. Skeletal muscle PGF(2)(alpha) and PGE(2) in response to eccentric resistance exercise: influence of ibuprofen acetaminophen. Trappe TA, Fluckey JD, White F, Lambert CP, Evans WJ. J Clin Endocrinol Metab. 2001 Oct;86(10):5067-70.
818. Prostaglandins promote and block adipogenesis through opposing effects on peroxisome proliferator-activated receptor gamma. Reginato MJ, Krakow SL, Bailey ST, Lazar MA. J Biol Chem 1998 Jan 23;273(4):1855-8
819. Isotretinoin in acne vulgaris: a proscpective analysis of 160cases from Kuwait. Al-Mutairi N et al. J drug Dermatol. 2005 May-Jun;4(3):369-73
820. Affective psychosis following Accutane treatment. Barak Y et al. Int Clin Psychopharmacol 2005 Jan;20(1):39-41
821. Isotretinoin (13-cis-retinoic acid) associated atrial tachycardia. Husdemir C. et al. Pacing Clin Electrophysiol. 2005 Apr;28(4):348-9.
822. Hoarseness during isotretinoin therapy. Busso CI, Serrano RI. J Am Acad Dermatol. 2005 Jan;52(1) 168
823. Isotretinoin-associated intracranial hypertension. Fraunfelder FW et al. Ophthalmology 2004 Jun;111(6):1248-50.
824. Complications associated with isotretinoin use after rhinoplasty. Allen BC. Rhec JS. Aestheric Plast Surg. 2005 Mar-Apr;29(2):102-6
825. Functional brain imaging alterations in acne patients treated with isotretinoin. Bremner JD et al. Am J Psychiatry. 2005 May;162(5):983-91
826. Preclinical pharmacology of "Arimidex" (anastrozole; ZD1033)--a potent, selective aromatase inhibitor. J Steroid Biochem Mol Biol 1996 Jul;58(4):439-45

827. Anastrozole alone or in combimation with tamoxifen versus tamoxifen alone for adjunctive treatment of postmenopausal women with early breast cancer. Frist results of the ATAC randomized trial. Lancet 2002; 359:2131-39

828. History and Advancement of Anastrozole in the Treatment of Breast Cancer. Edited by Aman Buzdar & Michael Baum. RSM Press, February 2003

829. Inhibition of adrenal corticosteroid synthesis by aminoglutethimide: Studies on the mechanism of action. Dexter RN, FishmanLM, Ney RC et al. J Clin Endocrinol 27 (1967) 473-80

830. First generation aromatase inhibitors –aminoglutethimide and testololactone. Cocconi G. Breast Cancer Res Treat 1994;30(1):57-80

831. Stereoselective inhibition of aromatase by enantiomers of aminoglutethimide. Graves PE, Salhanick HA. Endocrinol 105 (1979) 52-57

832. Beneficial effects of raloxifene and tamoxifen in the treatment of pubertal gynecomastia. Lawrence SE, Faught et al. J. Pediatr. 2004 Jul;145(1):71-6

833. Effects of raloxifene on gonadotropins, sex hormones, bone turnover and lipids in healthy elderly men. Eur J Endocrinol. 2004 Apr;150(4):539-46

834. Raloxifene decreases serum IGF-1 in male patients with active acromegaly. Dimaraki EV, Symons KV, Barkan AL. Eur J Endocrinol. 2004 Apr;150(4):481-7

835. Fulvestrant, Formerly ICI 182,780, Is as Effective as Anastrozole in Postmenopausal Women With Advanced Breast Cancer Progressing After Prior Endocrine Treatment. Howell A, Robertson JFR, Quaresma Albano J, Aschermannova A, et al. J Clin Oncol. 2002; 1:57.

836. Fulvestrant, an estrogen receptor downregulator, reduces cell turnover index more effectively than tamoxifen. Anticancer Res. 2002 Jul-Aug;22(4):2317-9.

837. Fulvestrant. Cheung KL, Robertson JF. Expert Opin Investig Drugs 2002 Feb;11(2):303-308

838. Effects of estrogen on the release of gonadotropins and prolactin in male pseudohermaphrodites. Barbarino A, De Darinis L et al. J endocrinol Invest. 1979 Jan-Mar;2(1):41-4

839. Estrogen-dependent plasma prolactin response to gonadotropin-releasing hormone in intact and castrated men. Barbarino A, De Marinis L. et al. J Clin Endocrinol Metab. 1982 Dec;55(6):1212-6

840. Effects of progesterone administration on follicle-stimulating hormone and prolactin release in estrogen treated eugonadal adult men. Mancini A, De Marinis L. et al. Andrologia 1991 Sep-Oct;23(5):373-9

841. Inhibitory effect of androgen on estrogen-induced prolactin messenger ribonucleic acid accumulation in the male rat anterior pituitary. Tong Y et al. Endocrinology. 1989 Oct;125(4):1821-8

842. Effects of depot testosterone administration on serum levels of testosterone, FSH, LH and prolactin. Ruiz E. et al. J Endocrinol Invest. 1980 Oct-Dec;3(4):385-8.

843. Response of serum hormones to androgen administration in power athletes. Alen M. Reinila M. et al. Med Sci Sports Exerc. 1985 Jun;17(3):354-9.

844. Effect of androgenic anabolic steroids on sperm quality and serum hormone levels in adult male bodybuilders. Torres-Calleja J. et al. Life Sci. 2001 Mar 2;68(15):1769-74.

845. Anabolic steroid-associated hypogonadism in male hemodialysis patients. Maeda Y. et al. Clin Nephrol. 1989 Oct;32(4):198-201.

846. Prescribing Information for Dostinex Tablets. Pharmacia & Upjohn 2003.

847. Enhancement of linear growth and weight gain by cyproheptadine in children with hypopituitarism receiving growth hormone therapy. Kaplowitz PB, Jennings S. Pediatr. 1987 Jan;110(1):140-3.

848. Megestrol acetate vs cyproheptadine in the treatment of weight loss associated with HIV infection. Summerbell CD, Youle M, McDonald V, Catalan J, Gazzard BG. Int J STD AIDS. 1992 Jul-Aug;3(4):278-80.

849. Cyprohepatdine no longer promoted as an appetite stimulant. WHO Drug Info 1994; 8:66

850. Effects of anethum graveolens and garlic on lipid profile in hyperlipidemic patients. Kojuri J, Vosoughi AR, Akrami M. Lipids Health Dis. 2007 Mar 1;6:5.

851. Effects of garlic extract consumption on blood lipid and oxidant/antioxidant parameters in humans with high blood cholesterol. Durak I, Kavutcu M, Aytaç B, Avci A, Devrim E, Ozbek H, Oztürk HS. J Nutr Biochem. 2004 Jun;15(6):373-7.

852. Antioxidative activity of green tea polyphenol in cholesterol-fed rats. Yokozawa T, Nakagawa T, Kitani K. J Agric Food Chem. 2002 Jun 5;50(12):3549-52.

853. Effect of ground green tea drinking for 2 weeks on the susceptibility of plasma and LDL to the oxidation ex vivo in healthy volunteers. Gomikawa S, Ishikawa Y. et al. Kobe J Med Sci. 2008 May 23;54(1):E62-72.

854. Cardiovascular protective effects of resveratrol. Bradamante S, Barenghi L, Villa A. Cardiovasc Drug Rev. 2004 Fall;22(3):169-88.

855. Phytosterols/stanols lower cholesterol concentrations in familial hypercholesterolemic subjects: a systematic review with meta-analysis. Moruisi KG, Oosthuizen W, Opperman AM. J Am Coll Nutr. 2006 Feb;25(1):41-8. Review.

856. Role of policosanols in the prevention and treatment of cardiovascular disease. Varady KA, Wang Y, Jones PJ. Nutr Rev. 2003 Nov;61(11):376-83. Review.

857. Role of selenium in cytoprotection against cholesterol oxide-induced vascular damage in rats. Huang K, Liu H, Chen Z, Xu H. Atherosclerosis. 2002 May;162(1):137-44.

858. Inositol hexaniacinate. Altern Med Rev. 1998 Jun;3(3):222-3.

859. Pownall JH et al , Atherosclerosis. 1999; 143:285-297

860. Harris WS et al, J Cardio Risk 1997; 4:385-391

861. Clinical overview of Omacor: a concentrated formulation of omega-3 polyunsaturated fatty acids. Bays H. Am J Cardiol. 2006 Aug 21;98(4A):71i-76i. Epub 2006 May 30.

862. Gissi P Study, The Lancet 1999; Vol 354:447-55

863. Omega-3 fatty acid supplementation accelerates chylomicron triglyceride clearance. Park Y, Harris WS. J Lipid Res. 2003 Mar;44(3):455-63. Epub 2002 Dec 1.

864. The hypotriglyceridemic effect of eicosapentaenoic acid in rats is reflected in increased mitochondrial fatty acid oxidation followed by diminished lipogenesis. Willumsen N, Skorve J, Hexeberg S, Rustan AC, Berge RK. Lipids. 1993 Aug;28(8):683-90.

865. Docosahexaenoic acid (DHA) and hepatic gene transcription. Jump DB, Botolin D, Wang Y, Xu J, Demeure O, Christian B. Chem Phys Lipids. 2008 May;153(1):3-13. Epub 2008 Feb 23.

866. Why do omega-3 fatty acids lower serum triglycerides? Harris WS, Bulchandani D. Curr Opin Lipidol. 2006 Aug;17(4):387-93.

867. Effects of modafinil ingestion on exercise time to exhaustion. Jacobs I, Bell DG. Med Sci Sports Exerc. 2004 Jun;36(6):1078-82.
868. A double-blind clinical trial in weight control. Use of fenfluramine and phentermine alone and in combination. Weintraub M, Hasday JD, Mushlin AI, Lockwood DH. Arch Intern Med. 1984 Jun;144(6):1143-8
869. Modalities of the food intake-reducing effect of sibutramine in humans. Chapelot D, Marmonier C, Thomas F, Hanotin C. Physiol Behav. 2000 Jan;68(3):299-308.
870. Thermogenic effects of sibutramine and its metabolites. Connoley IP, Liu YL, Frost I, Reckless IP, Heal DJ, Stock MJ. Br J Pharmacol. 1999 Mar;126(6):1487-95.
871. A randomized, double-blind, placebo-controlled, multicenter study on sibutramine in over-weighted and obese subjects. Zhao Y, Wang X, Yan Z. Zhonghua Yu Fang Yi Xue Za Zhi. 2001 Sep;35(5):329-32.
872. Effects of ketotifen and clenbuterol on beta-adrenergic receptor functions of lymphocytes and on plasma TXB-2 levels of asthmatic patients. Huszar E, Herjavecz I et al. Z Erkr Atmungsorgane 1990;175(3):141-6
873. Effect of prednisolone and ketotifen on beta 2-adrenoceptors in asthmatic patients receiving beta 2-bronchodilators. Brodde OE, Howe U et al. Eur J Clin Pharmacol 1988;34(2):145-50
874. Ketotifen alone or as an additional medication for the long-term control of asthma and wheeze in children. Bassler D, et al. The Cochrane Database of Systematic Reviews; Issue 1. Chichester: John Wiley; 2004.
875. The emergence of endocrinology. Welbourn RB. Gesnerus. 1992;49 Pt 2:137-50.
876. Why do we continue to write for Synthroid? Volume XI, Issue 8 Harold J. DeMonaco, M.S., Director of Drug Therapy Management. A publication of the Drug Therapy Committee, Massachusetts General Hospital and the MAssachusets General Physicians Organization.
877. Bioequivalence of generic and brand-name levothyroxine products in the treatment of hypothyroidism. Dong BJ. Hauck WW. Gambertoglio JG. Gee L. White JR. Bubp JL. Greenspan FS. JAMA. 1997; 277: 1205-1213.
878. Detergent effects of sodium deoxycholate are a major feature of an injectable phosphatidylcholine formulation used for localized fat dissolution. Rotunda AM, Suzuki H et al. Dermatol Surg. 2004 Jul;30(7):1001-8
879. Phosphatidylcholine increases the secretion of triacylglycerol-rich lipoproteins by CaCo-2 cells. Mathur SN, Born E et al. Biochem J. 1996 Mar 1;314 (pt 2):569-75
880. Lipolysis injection with phosphatidylcholine (Lipostabil N) examination of blood values after subcutaneous administration. Dr. Franz Hasengschwandtner. Online Article.
881. Clinical experience and safety using phosphatidylcholine injections for the localized reduction of subcutaneous fat: a multicentre, retrospective UK study. Journal of Cosmetic Dermatology. 5(3):218-226, September 2006. Palmer, Mark MD; Curran, John MD; Bowler, Patrick MD
882. Treatment of pituitary dwarf with human growth hormone. Raben MS. J Clin Endocrinol Metab 18:901-903 1958.
883. Long term mortality in the United States cohort of pituitary-derived growth hormone recipients. J Pediat 144:430-436.
884. Pioneering recombinant growth hormone manufacturing: pounds produced per mile of height. J Pediat 131:55-57.
885. Production of Authentic Recombinant Somatropin. Linda Fryklund. Acta Paediatrica Volume 76 Issue s331 Page 5-8, January 1987.
886. Five-year follow-up of growth hormone antibodies in growth hormone deficient children treated with recombinant human growth hormone. G Massa et al. Clin Endocrinol 38(2) 137-42 (Feb 1993).
887. Identification of an insulin-responsive element in the promoter of the human gene for insulin-like growth factor binding protein-1. J Biol Chem 268:17063-68,1995
888. Evidence supporting a direct suppressive effect of growth hormone on serum IGFBP-1 levels. Experimental studies in normal, obese and GH-deficient adults. Growth Hormone and IGF Research 9:52-60,1999
889. Growth hormone induced increase in serum IGFBP-3 level is reversed by anabolic steroids in substance abusing power athletes. Clin Endocrinol (Oxf) 49:459-63,1998
890. United Kingdom multicentre clinical trial of somatrem. Milner RD, Barnes ND, Buckler JM, Carson DJ, Hadden DR, Hughes IA, Johnston DI, Parkin JM,
891. Antigenicity and efficacy of authentic sequence recombinant human growth hormone (somatropin): first-year experience in the United Kingdom. Buzi F, Buchanan CR, Morrell DJ, Preece MA. Clin Endocrinol (Oxf) 1989 May;30(5):531-8
892. Pioneering recombinant growth hormone manufacturing: pounds produced per mile of height. J Pediat 131:55-57.
893. Protein anabolic actions in the human body. W.M. Bennet et al. Diabetic Medicine 1991, 8 199-207
894. Effect of physiologic hyperinsulinemia on skeletal muscle protein synthesis and breakdown in man. R Gelfand et al. J Clin Invest. 80, July 1987 1-6
895. Insulin action on muscle protein kinetics and amino acid transport during recovery after resistance exercise. G Biolo, B Williams et al. Diabetes Vol 48, May 1999 949-957.
896. Insulin signaling and insulin sensitivity after exercise in human skeletal muscle. Jorgen F. P. Wojtaszewski et al. Diabetes Vol 49, March 2000 325-31
897. Intramuscular injection of insulin lispro or soluble human insulin: pharmacokinetics and glucodynamics in Type 2 diabetes. Z. Milicevic et al. Diabetes UK. Diabetic Medicine, 18 562-566
898. Multivitamins and phospholipids complex protects the hepatic cells from androgenic-anabolic-steroids-induced toxicity. Pagonis TA, Koukoulis GN, Hadjichristodoulou CS, Toli PN, Angelopoulos NV. Clinical Toxicol (2008) 46, 57-66.
899. Hepatoprotective effects of Liv-52 on ethanol induced liver damage in rats. Indian J Exp Biol. 1999 Aug;37(8):762-6.
900. The effect of the heptoprotective agent LIV 52 on liver damage. Cas Lek Cesk. 1997 Dec 17;136(24):758-60.
901. Hepatoprotective effect of Liv-52 and kumaryasava on carbon tetrachloride induced hepatic damage in rats. Indian J Exp Biol. 1997 Jun;35(6):655-7.
902. Role of Liv-52 in protection against beryllium intoxication. Biol Trace Elem Res. 1994 Jun;41(3):201-15.
903. Alcohol hangover and Liv.52. Chauhan BL, Kulkarni RD. Eur J Clin Pharmacol. 1991;40(2):187-8.
904. Hepatoprotective effects of Liv-52 on ethanol induced liver damage in rats. Sandhir R, Gill KD. Indian J Exp Biol. 1999 Aug;37(8):762-6.
905. Himalaya's Liv.52/LiverCare Approved as a Herbal Drug in Switzerland. Houstan (BW HealthWire) April 4, 2002.
906. Anti-hepatotoxic effects of root and root callus extracts of Cichorium intybus L. Zafar R, Mujahid Ali S. J Ethnopharmacol. 1998 Dec;63(3):227-31.
907. Aqueous extract of Terminalia arjuna prevents carbon tetrachloride induced hepatic and renal disorders. Manna P, Sinha M, Sil PC. BMC Complement

Altern Med. 2006 Sep 30;6:33.

908. Achillea millefolium L. s.l. revisited: recent findings confirm the traditional use. Benedek B, Kopp B. Wien Med Wochenschr. 2007;157(13-14):312-4.

909. N-acetyl-cysteine protects liver from apoptotic death in an animal model of fulminant hepatic failure. San-Miguel B, Alvarez M, Culebras JM, González-Gallego J, Tuñón MJ. Apoptosis. 2006 Nov;11(11):1945-57.

910. Toxic effects of anabolic-androgenic steroids in primary rat hepatic cell cultures. Welder AA, Robertson JW, Melchert RB. J Pharmacol Toxicol Methods. 1995 Aug;33(4):187-95.

911. An updated systematic review with meta-analysis for the clinical evidence of silymarin. Saller R, Brignoli R, Melzer J, Meier R. Forsch Komplementmed. 2008 Feb;15(1):9-20.

912. A sulforaphane analogue that potently activates the Nrf2-dependent detoxification pathway. Morimitsu Y, Nakagawa Y et al. J Biol Chem. 2002 Feb 1;277(5):3456-63. Epub 2001 Nov 12.

913. Marked suppression of dihydrotestosterone in men with benign prostatic hyperplasia by dutasteride, a dual 5-alpha reductase inhibitor. Clark RV, Hermann DJ, Cunningham GR et al. J Clin Endocrinol Metab 2004 May;89(5):2179-84

914. Unique preclinical characteristics of GG745, a potent dual inhibitor of 5AR. Bramson HN, Hermann D, Batchelor KW, Lee FW, James MK, Frye SV. J Pharmacol Exp Ther. 1997 Sep;282(3):1496-502.

915. A preliminary clinical report on the treatment of leucoderma with ammi majus linn. El Mofty AM. J Egypt Med Ass 31:651-660, 1948

916. Exogenous stimulation of corpus luteum formation in the rabbit; influence of extracts of human placenta, decidua, fetus, hydatid mole and corpus luteum on the rabbit gonad. Hirose T 1920 J Jpn Gynecol Sot 16:1055.

917. Die Schwangerschaftsdiagnose ausdem Ham durch Nachweis des Hypophysenvorderlappen-hormone. II. Pracktishe und theoretische Ergebnisse aus den hamuntersuchungen. Ascheim S, Zondek B 1928 Klin Wochenschr 7:1453-1457.

918. The effect of human chorionic gonadotropin (HCG) in the treatment of obesity by means of the Simeons therapy: a criteria-based meta-analysis. Lijesen GKS, et al. Br J Clin Pharmacol 1995; 40: 237–43.

919. A randomized three-way cross-over study in healthy pituitary-suppressed women to compare the bioavailability of human chorionic gonadotrophin (Pregnyl) after intramuscular and subcutaneous administration. Mannaerts BM, Geurts TB, Odink J. Hum Reprod. 1998 Jun;13(6):1461-4.

920. Acute stimulation of aromatization in Leydig cells by human chorionic gonadotropin in vitro. Proc Natl Acad Sci USA 76:4460-3,1979.

921. The different mechanisms for suppression of pituitary and testicular function. Sandow J, Engelbart K, von Rechenberg W. Med Biol. 1986;63(5-6):192-200.

GLOSSARY

Glossary

AAS – Anabolic/Androgenic Steroid

Acute – Short duration. An acute effect is one that occurs rapidly, not after long-term administration.

Aerobic – Refers to a process where oxygen is used to generate energy in the muscles from carbohydrates, fats, and protein, in the form of ATP (adenosine triphosphate). Long distance running is an example of an aerobic activity.

Adipose – Fat tissue.

Adrenoceptor – A type of receptor in the body involved in the regulation of heart rate, metabolism, and thermogenesis. Stimulated by endogenous catecholamines such as epinephrine (adrenaline), norepinephrine (noradrenaline), and dopamine.

Agonist – A substance that initiates a biological response. An estrogen agonist acts as an estrogen in the body.

Ampule – A glass container that holds a single dosage unit of a liquid drug product. An ampule must be broken open before use.

Anabolic – A process that involves the building of tissues such as muscle and bone. AAS are most valued by bodybuilders and athletes for their anabolic properties.

Anaerobic – Refers to a process where energy is generated in the muscles from carbohydrates in the form of ATP (adenosine triphosphate) without the use of oxygen. Weight lifting is an example of an anaerobic activity.

Androgenic – Refers to the masculinizing properties of a substance. AAS stimulate male libido, secondary hair growth, acne, and male pattern hair loss via their androgenic properties.

Antagonist – A substance that inhibits a biological response. An estrogen antagonist blocks the action of estrogen in the body.

Arrhythmia – An irregular heartbeat. Arrhythmias may be life threatening or benign in nature.

Atherogenic – Promoting the formation of plaque deposits on the walls of arteries.

Atherosclerosis – A progressive cardiovascular disease characterized by the buildup of plaque deposits in the arteries. This may obstruct blood flow, causing heart attack or stroke.

Bacteriostatic – Inhibits the growth of bacteria. Bacteriostatic water contains ingredients that prevent bacteria from contaminating the liquid.

Contraindicated – Not advisable for use. A contraindication is a condition that would prevent someone from using a particular drug product.

Diabetogenic – Increases blood sugar.

Diastolic - The phase of blood circulation where the pumping chambers of the heart (ventricles) are being filled. Pressure is at its lowest during the diastolic phase.

Downregulate – To reduce in number. Some cellular receptors downregulate with high levels of drug stimulation, inducing tolerance. Anabolic/androgenic steroids generally do not cause a reduction in respective androgen receptor concentrations. Classic downregulation does not occur.

Edema – The retention of excess water in the circulatory system and/or body tissues.

Endogenous – Occurring naturally within the body. Testosterone produced by the testes is an endogenous hormone.

Epiphyses – The growth plates at the end of long bones. The epiphyses plates regulate increases in linear height during development, and fuse at maturity preventing further linear growth.

Erythropoiesis – The process in which red blood cells are produced in the body. Anabolic/androgenic steroids can stimulate erythropoiesis.

Esterified – Refers to a steroid compound that has one or more fatty acids attached to the molecule, usually to slow its release from an injection site. Testosterone cypionate is an esterified form of testosterone.

Exogenous – Caused by an agent outside the body.

Glycemic – Relating to blood sugar levels.

Hepatotoxic – Liver toxic. All c-17 alpha alkylated anabolic/androgenic steroids are considered hepatotoxic.

Homeostasis – A state of equilibrium among physiological processes.

Hyperplasia – Growth that occurs via an increase in cell number.

Hypertrophy – Growth that occurs via increases in existing cell size. Anabolic/androgenic steroids produce growth through hypertrophy.

Metabolic Syndrome – A poorly defined common metabolic disorder characterized by abdominal obesity, an atherogenic lipid profile, insulin resistance, elevated blood pressure, a proinflammatory state, and increased risk of cardiovascular disease.

Multi-dose Vial – A vial with a rubber stopper on the top, designed to be pierced repeatedly by a needle (for multiple uses).

Pathological – Involving or caused by physical disease.

Peripheral – Near the surface of the body. Psychoactive drugs are often regarded as centrally acting (brain/central nervous system), while hormones like anabolic steroids affect both central and peripheral tissues (such as muscle and skin).

Prognostic – Serving to predict the likely outcome of a disease.

Pulmonary – Related to the lungs.

Recombinant – Refers to a synthetic manufacturing technology that involves the splicing of genes or DNA segments and inserting them into a cell culture in order to replicate a specific protein. Recombinant DNA technology is used to manufacture many protein-based drug products including human growth hormone, insulin-like growth factors, and human insulin.

Selective – Describes a drug with a very specific effec, and little spillover into other biological systems.

Subcutaneous – Located beneath the skin and above the muscle.

Supraphysiological – In excess of normal biological levels. High doses of testosterone produce supraphysiological levels of hormone in the blood.

Supratherapeutic – In excess of normally defined therapeutic levels.

Systemic – Affecting the entire body through general circulation.

Systolic – The phase of blood circulation where the pumping chambers of the heart (ventricles) are actively pumping. Pressure is at its highest during the systolic phase.

Upregulate – To increase in number. Usually relating to cellular receptor concentrations. Anabolic/androgenic steroids can increase respective androgen receptor concentrations, possibly increasing sensitivity to androgens.

Notes

Notes

Notes

Notes

Appendix A Drug Availability Tables

Drug Availability Tables
Listings by Country

Generic Name	Trade Name	Dose	Packaging	Company	Country	Status	Vet
testosterone undecanoate	Andriol	40 mg capsules	60 capsule bottle	Organon	Algeria		
testosterone enanthate	Androtardyl®	250 mg/ml	1 ml ampule	Schering	Algeria		
mesterolone	Proviron	25 mg tablet	20 tablet box	Schering	Algeria		
testosterone enanthate	Weratestone 250	250 mg/ml	1 ml ampule	Weimer Pharma	Algeria		
boldenone undecylenate	Ana-Bolde	50 mg/ml	10 ml vial	Forti	Argentina		VET
stanozolol (inj)	Anabolico Cimol	60 mg/ml	5 ml vial	Cimol	Argentina		VET
stanozolol (inj)	Anabolico Produvet	10 mg/ml	25 ml vial	Cimol	Argentina		VET
stanozolol (oral)	Apetil	4 mg/ml	10 ml dropper bottle	Holliday	Argentina		VET
Testoviron (testosterone blend)	Bi-Testo	60 mg/ml	10 ml vial	Cimol	Argentina		VET
boldenone undecylenate	Boldenona	50 mg/ml	10, 50 ml vial	Formula Magistral	Argentina		VET
nandrolone decanoate	Deca-Durabolin®	25, 50 mg/ml	1 ml	Organon	Argentina		
nandrolone decanoate	Deca-Durabolin®	50 mg/ml	2 ml	Organon	Argentina		
stanozolol (inj)	Estanozolol	50 mg/ml	5 ml vial	Calastreme	Argentina		VET
stanozolol (inj)	Estanozolol	50 mg/ml	5, 30 ml vial	Formula Magistral	Argentina		VET
stanozolol (oral)	Estanozolol comp	10 mg tablet	100 tablet bottle	Formula Magistral	Argentina		VET
nandrolone phenylpropionate	Estigor	10 mg/ml	250 ml	Burnet	Argentina		VET
stanozolol (inj)	Estrombol	25 mg/ml	10 ml vial	Fundacion	Argentina		VET
boldenone undecylenate	Ex-Pois	50 mg/ml	10 ml vial	Agofarma	Argentina		VET
fluoxymesterone	Ferona	1 mg tablet	30 tablet box	Sidus	Argentina		VET
nandrolone phenylpropionate	Ganekyl	50 mg/ml	10, 100 ml vial	Over Labs	Argentina		VET
oxandrolone	Lonavar	2.5 mg tablet	n/a	Searle	Argentina	[NLM]	
methandrostenolone	Metandrostenolona FM	10 mg tablet	100 tablet bottle	Formula Magistral	Argentina		VET
stanozolol (inj)	Nabolic	2 mg/ml	50 ml vial	Chinfield Ind.	Argentina		VET
stanozolol (inj)	Nabolic Strong	50 mg/ml	30 ml vial	Chinfield Ind.	Argentina		VET
nandrolone decanoate	Nandrex FM	100 mg/ml	10 ml vial	Formula Magistral	Argentina		VET
nandrolone decanoate	Nandro Plus	100 mg/ml	100 ml vial	PharmaVet	Argentina		VET
testosterone undecanoate (inj)	Nebido	250 mg/ml	4 ml ampule	Schering	Argentina		
testosterone propionate	Propionato de Testosterona	25 mg/ml	20 ml vial	Induvet	Argentina		VET
mesterolone	Proviron®	25 mg tablet	n/a	Schering	Argentina		
Sustanon 250 (testosterone blend)	Sustanon "250"	250 mg/ml	1 ml ampule	Organon	Argentina		
stanozolol (inj)	Tanoxol	25 mg/ml	10 ml vial	Burnet	Argentina		VET
testosterone propionate	Testosterona	50 mg/ml	25 ml vial	Calastreme	Argentina		VET
testosterone propionate	Testosterona FM	100 mg/ml	10 ml vial	Formula Magistral	Argentina		VET
Testoviron (testosterone blend)	Testoviron® Depot	135 mg/ml	1 ml ampule	Schering	Argentina	[NLM]	
testosterone enanthate	Testoviron® Depot	250 mg/ml	1 ml ampule	Schering	Argentina		
trenbolone acetate	Trenbolona FM	75 mg/ml	10 ml vial	Formula Magistral	Argentina		VET
testosterone undecanoate	Undestor	40 mg capsules	n/a	Organon	Argentina		
stanozolol (inj)	Vitabolic	20 mg/ml	10, 100 ml vial	Over Labs	Argentina		VET
testosterone undecanoate	Andriol	40 mg capsules	n/a	Organon	Aruba		
boldenone undecylenate	Anabolic BD	50 mg/ml	10 ml vial	SYD Group	Australia		VET
nandrolone cypionate	Anabolic DN	50 mg/ml	10 ml vial	SYD Group	Australia		VET
methylandrostenediol (blend)	Anabolic NA	75 mg/ml	10 ml vial	SYD Group	Australia		VET
stanozolol (inj)	Anabolic ST	50 mg/ml	20 ml vial	SYD Group	Australia		VET
testosterone cypionate	Anabolic TL	100 mg/ml	10 ml vial	SYD Group	Australia		VET
testosterone suspension	Anabolic TS	100 mg/ml	20 ml vial	SYD Group	Australia		VET
methylandrostenediol dipropionate	Anadiol	5 mg tab	10, 100 tablet bottle	Ilium/Troy	Australia		VET

APPENDIX A-1

Errors or Omissions: Info@AnabolicsBook.com

Drug Availability Tables

Listings by Country

Generic Name	Trade Name	Dose	Packaging	Company	Country	Status	Vet
methylandrostenediol dipropionate	Anadiol Depot	75 mg/ml	10 ml vial	Ilium/Troy	Australia		VET
norethandrolone	Anaplex	5 mg tablet	100 tablet bottle	Jurox	Australia		VET
testosterone undecanoate	Andriol	40 mg capsules	60 capsule bottle	Organon	Australia		
testosterone propionate	AVP Supertest	50 mg/ml	10 ml vial	Vetsearch	Australia		VET
boldenone undecylenate	Boldebal-H	50 mg/ml	10 ml vial	Ilium/Troy	Australia		VET
boldenone undecylenate	Boldenone-50	50 mg/ml	10 ml vial	Jurox	Australia	[NLM]	VET
methylandrostenediol (blend)	Drive	55 mg/ml	10 ml vial	RWR	Australia		VET
Sustanon 250 (testosterone blend)	Durateston	250 mg/ml	5 ml vial	Intervet	Australia		VET
nandrolone cypionate	Dynabol	50 mg/ml	10 ml vial	Jurox	Australia	[NLM]	VET
methylandrostenediol (blend)	Filybol	70 mg/ml	10, 20 ml vial	Ranvet	Australia		VET
nandrolone laurate	Laurabolin	25, 50 mg/ml	10 ml vial	Intervet	Australia		VET
methylandrostenediol (blend)	Libriol	75 mg/ml	10, 20 ml vial	RWR	Australia	[NLM]	VET
methylandrostenediol dipropionate	Methasus 50	50 mg/ml	20 ml vial	Jurox	Australia	[NLM]	VET
ethylestrenol	Nandoral	.5 mg tablet	100, 500 tablet bottle	Intervet	Australia		VET
nandrolone phenylpropionate	Nandrolin	50 mg/ml	25 ml vial	Intervet	Australia		VET
nandrolone phenylpropionate	Nandrolin	25 mg/ml	10 ml vial	Intervet	Australia		VET
ethylestrenol	Nitrotain	15 mg/4gram	60, 250, 1000 gram tube	Nature-Vet	Australia		VET
ethylestrenol	Orabol-H	100 mg/5g paste	30 ml plastic tube	Vetsearch	Australia	[NLM]	VET
Testoviron (testosterone blend)	Primoteston Depot 100	135 mg/ml	1 ml ampule	Schering	Australia	[NLM]	
Testoviron (testosterone blend)	Primoteston Depot 50	75 mg/ml	1 ml ampule	Schering	Australia	[NLM]	
testosterone enanthate	Primoteston®-Depot	250 mg/ml	1 ml ampule	Schering	Australia		
testosterone propionate (implant)	Progro-H (plus estradiol)	20 mg/pellet	n/a	Pro Beef	Australia		VET
methylandrostenediol dipropionate	Protabol	75 mg/ml	10 ml vial	RWR	Australia		VET
mesterolone	Proviron®	25 mg tablet	50 tablet bottle	Schering	Australia		
testosterone cypionate	Ridrot Testosterone Inj.	75 mg/ml	250 ml vial	Troy	Australia		VET
testosterone enanthate	Ropel Liquid Testosterone	75 mg/ml	200 ml vial	Jurox	Australia		VET
testosterone (implant)	Ropel Testosterone Pellets	23.5 mg pellet	450, 600 pellet bottle	Jurox	Australia		VET
methylandrostenediol (blend)	RWR 4 Fillies	75 mg/ml	10 ml vial	RWR	Australia		VET
nandrolone decanoate	RWR Deca 50	50 mg/ml	10 ml vial	RWR	Australia		VET
testosterone suspension	RWR Suspension	100 mg/ml	20 ml vial	RWR	Australia		VET
methylandrostenediol (blend)	Spectriol	65 mg/ml	10 ml vial	RWR	Australia		VET
stanozolol (inj)	Stanabolic	50 mg/ml	20 ml vial	Ilium/Troy	Australia		VET
stanozolol (inj)	Stanazol	50 mg/ml	20, 50 ml vial	RWR	Australia	[NLM]	VET
stanozolol (inj)	Stanosus	50 mg/ml	20 ml vial	Jurox	Australia	[NLM]	VET
methylandrostenediol dipropionate	Superbolin	75 mg/ml	10 ml vial	Vetsearch	Australia		VET
boldenone undecylenate	Sybolin	25 mg/ml	10 ml vial	Ranvet	Australia		VET
testosterone propionate (implant)	Synovex®-H (plus estrogen)	20 mg/pellet	n/a	Fort Dodge	Australia		VET
testosterone propionate	Tepro Hormone	100 mg/ml	500 ml vial	Virbac	Australia		VET
testosterone cypionate	Testo LA	100 mg/ml	10 ml vial	Jurox	Australia	[NLM]	VET
testosterone (gel)	Testogel	25, 50 mg	single dose packet	Schering	Australia		
testosterone suspension	Testosus 100	100 mg/ml	20 ml vial	Jurox	Australia	[NLM]	VET
methylandrostenediol (blend)	Tribolin	75 mg/ml	10, 20 ml vial	Ranvet	Australia		VET
testosterone propionate (implant)	Virbac Tepro Pellets	23.5 mg pellet	450 pellets	Virbac	Australia		VET
testosterone propionate	VR Testprop	50 mg/ml	10 ml vial	Jurox	Australia		VET
testosterone undecanoate	Andriol	40 mg capsules	60 capsule bottle	Organon	Austria		
nandrolone laurate	Laurabolin	50 mg/ml	n/a	Werfft-Chemie	Austria		VET

APPENDIX A-2

Errors or Omissions: Info@AnabolicsBook.com

Drug Availability Tables
Listings by Country

Generic Name	Trade Name	Dose	Packaging	Company	Country	Status	Vet
testosterone undecanoate (inj)	Nebido	250 mg/ml	4 ml ampule	Schering	Austria		
mesterolone	Proviron®	25 mg tablet	50 tablet bottle	Schering	Austria		
nandrolone cyclohexylpropionate	Sanabolicum-Vet	50 mg/ml	10 ml vial	Werfft-Chemie	Austria		VET
testosterone (gel)	Testogel	50 mg	single dose packet	Schering	Austria		
testosterone enanthate	Testoviron®-Depot	250 mg/ml	1 ml ampule	Schering	Austria		
testosterone undecanoate	Andriol	40 mg capsules	n/a	Organon	Bahrain		
testosterone enanthate	Testoviron®-Depot	250 mg/ml	1 ml ampule	Schering	Bahrain	[NLM]	
testosterone undecanoate	Andriol	40 mg capsules	n/a	Organon	Bangladesh		
testosterone undecanoate	Andriol	40 mg capsules	n/a	Organon	Belarus		
dihydrotestosterone	Andractim	25 mg/g	80 gram gel	Piette	Belgium		
nandrolone decanoate	Deca-Durabolin®	25, 50 mg/ml	1 ml ampule, syringe	Organon	Belgium		
mesterolone	Proviron®	25 mg tablet	50 tablet bottle	Schering	Belgium		
Sustanon 250 (testosterone blend)	Sustanon 250®	250 mg/ml	1 ml ampule	Organon	Belgium		
testosterone undecanoate	Undestor	40 mg capsules	60 capsule bottle	Organon	Belgium		
boldenone undecylenate	Boldenona 50 Gen-Far	50 mg/ml	10, 50, 100, 250ml vial	Gen-Far	Bolivia		VET
Sustanon 250 (testosterone blend)	Durateston 250®	250 mg/ml	1 ml ampule	Organon	Bolivia		
boldenone undecylenate	Ganabol	50 mg/ml	500 ml vial	Laboratorios VM	Bolivia		VET
boldenone undecylenate	Ganabol	25, 50 mg/ml	10, 50, 100, 250ml vial	Laboratorios VM	Bolivia		VET
methenolone acetate	Primobolan®	5 mg tablet	n/a	Schering	Bolivia	[NLM]	
testosterone undecanoate	Androxon	40 mg capsules	20 capsule box	Organon	Brazil		
nandrolone decanoate	Deca-Durabolin®	25, 50 mg/ml	1 ml ampule	Organon	Brazil		
testosterone cypionate	Deposteron	100 mg/ml	2 ml ampule	Novaquimica/Sigma	Brazil		
Sustanon 250 (testosterone blend)	Durateston 250®	250 mg/ml	1 ml ampule	Organon	Brazil		
boldenone undecylenate	Equifort	50 mg/ml	10, 50 ml vial	Purina	Brazil		VET
oxymetholone	Hemogenin	50 mg tablet	n/a	Aventis	Brazil		
testosterone undecanoate (inj)	Nebido	250 mg/ml	4 ml ampule	Schering	Brazil		
mesterolone	Proviron®	25 mg tablet	20 tablet box	Schering	Brazil		
methandrostenolone	Bionabol	2, 5 mg tab	40 tablet box	Balkanpharma	Bulgaria	[NLM]	
methandrostenolone	Bionabol	2 mg tablet	40 tablet bottle	Pharmacia	Bulgaria	[NLM]	
methandrostenolone	Bionabol	5 mg tab	40 tablet bottle	Pharmacia	Bulgaria	[NLM]	
nandrolone decanoate	Deca-Durabolin®	25, 50 mg/ml	1 ml ampule	Organon	Bulgaria		
methandrostenolone	Nerobol	5 mg tablet	20 tablet box	Gedeon Richter	Bulgaria	[NLM]	
nandrolone phenylpropionate	Nerobolil	25 mg/ml	1 ml ampule	Godeon Richter	Bulgaria	[NLM]	
Omnadren (testosterone blend)	Omnadren 250	250 mg/ml	1 ml ampule	Jelfa	Bulgaria	[NLM]	
Sustanon 250 (testosterone blend)	Omnadren 250	250 mg/ml	1 ml ampule	Jelfa	Bulgaria	[NLM]	
mesterolone	Proviron®	25 mg tablet	20, 50 tablet box	Schering	Bulgaria		
nandrolone decanoate	Retabolil	25, 50 mg/ml	1 ml ampule	Gedeon Richter	Bulgaria	[NLM]	
testosterone propionate	Testosteron	50 mg/ml	1 ml ampule	Sopharma	Bulgaria		
testosterone enanthate	Testosteron-Depot	250 mg/ml	1 ml ampule	Jenapharm	Bulgaria		
testosterone enanthate	Testosteronum Prolongatum	100 mg/ml	1 ml ampule	Jelfa	Bulgaria	[NLM]	
testosterone undecanoate	Undestor	40 mg capsules	60 capsule bottle	Organon	Bulgaria		
testosterone propionate	Anatest	100 mg/ml	10 ml vial	Sterivet	Canada	[NLM]	VET
testosterone propionate	Anatest	100 mg/ml	10 ml vial	Vetoquinol	Canada		VET
testosterone undecanoate	Andriol	40 mg capsules	60 capsule bottle	Organon	Canada		
testosterone (patch)	Androderm®	12.2 mg patch.	30 patches/box	Pharmascience	Canada		
testosterone (gel)	Androgel	25, 50 mg	single dose packet	Solvay	Canada		

APPENDIX A-3

Drug Availability Tables

Listings by Country

Generic Name	Trade Name	Dose	Packaging	Company	Country	Status	Vet
nandrolone decanoate	Deca-Durabolin®	100 mg/ml	2 ml	Organon	Canada		
testosterone enanthate	Delatestryl	200 mg/ml	5 ml vial	Theramed	Canada		
testosterone cypionate	Depo-Testosterone®	100 mg/ml	10 ml vial	Pharmacia	Canada		
boldenone undecylenate	Equipoise®	25, 50 mg/ml	50 ml vial	Squibb	Canada	[NLM]	VET
boldenone undecylenate	Equipoise®	50 mg/ml	50 ml vial	Wyeth	Canada		VET
methyltestosterone	Geri Tabs	2 mg tablet	50, 200 tablet bottle	Vetcom	Canada		VET
fluoxymesterone	Halotestin®	5 mg tablet	50 tablet bottle	Pharmacia	Canada		
testosterone suspension	Malogen Aqueous	100 mg/ml	10 ml vial	Germiphene	Canada	[NLM]	
testosterone propionate	Malogen In Oil	100 mg/ml	10 ml vial	Germiphene	Canada	[NLM]	
testosterone enanthate	PMS-Testosterone Enanthate	200 mg/ml	10 ml via.	Pharmascience	Canada		
trenbolone acetate	Revalor-H (plus estradiol)	20 mg pellet	70 pellet cartridge	Intervet	Canada		VET
trenbolone acetate	Revalor-S (plus estradiol)	20 mg pellet	60 pellet cartridge	Intervet	Canada		VET
testosterone cypionate	Scheinpharma Testone-Cyp	100 mg/ml	10 ml vial	Schein	Canada		
trenbolone acetate	Synovex plus (plus estradiol)	25 mg pellet	80 pellet cartridge	Wyeth	Canada		VET
testosterone propionate (implant)	Synovex®-H (plus estradiol)	20 mg/pellet	n/a	Ayerst	Canada		
testosterone suspension	Testos 100	100 mg/ml	10 ml vial	Vetcom	Canada		VET
testosterone cypionate	Testosterone Cypionate Inj.	100 mg/ml	2 ml vial	Cytex	Canada		VET
testosterone cypionate	Testosterone Cypionate Inj.	200 mg/ml	10 ml vial	Sabex	Canada		
testosterone cypionate	Testosterone Cypionate Inj.	100 mg/ml	10 ml vial	Sandoz	Canada		
testosterone propionate	Testosterone Propionate Inj.	100 mg/ml	10 ml vial	Cytex	Canada		VET
testosterone propionate	Testosterone Propionate Inj.	100 mg/ml	10 ml vial	Dominion	Canada		VET
testosterone propionate	Uni-Test Inj	100 mg/ml	10 ml vial	Univet	Canada		VET
testosterone suspension	Uni-Test Suspension	100 mg/ml	30 ml vial	Univet	Canada		VET
testosterone suspension	Veto-Test Sus	100 mg/ml	30 ml vial	Austin	Canada		VET
stanozolol (inj)	Winstrol® V	50 mg/ml	10, 30ml vial	Pharmacia	Canada	[NLM]	VET
stanozolol (oral)	Winstrol-V®	2 mg tablet	100 tablet bottle	Pharmacia	Canada	[NLM]	VET
nandrolone decanoate	Anaprolina	25, 50 mg/ml	1 ml ampule	Silesia	Chile		
testosterone enanthate	ciclo-6	300 mg/ml	10 ml vial	Drag Pharma	Chile		VET
testosterone enanthate	ciclo-6	300 mg/ml	2 ml ampule	Drag Pharma	Chile		VET
nandrolone decanoate	Deca-Durabolin®	25, 50, 100 mg/ml	1 ml ampule	Organon	Chile		
nandrolone decanoate	Decanoato Nandrolona	25, 50 mg/ml	1 ml ampule	Astorga	Chile		
nandrolone decanoate	Decanoato Nandrolona	50 mg/ml	1 ml ampule	Biosano	Chile		
boldenone undecylenate	Ganabol	50 mg/ml	500 ml vial	Laboratorios VM	Chile		VET
boldenone undecylenate	Ganabol	25, 50 mg/ml	10, 50, 100, 250ml vial	Laboratorios VM	Chile		VET
nandrolone cyclohexylpropionate	Genadrag	50 mg/ml	10 ml vial	Drag Pharma	Chile		VET
nandrolone decanoate	nandrolona decanoato	50 mg/ml	1 ml ampule	Chile	Chile		
nandrolone decanoate	Nandrosande	25, 50, 100 mg/ml	1 ml ampule	Sanderson	Chile		
Sustanon 250 (testosterone blend)	Sustenan 250	250 mg/ml	1 ml ampule	Organon	Chile		
testosterone undecanoate	Testocaps	40 mg capsules	n/a	Organon	Chile		
testosterone enanthate	testosterona enantato	250 mg/ml	1 ml ampule	Biosano	Chile		
testosterone enanthate	testosterona enantato	250 mg/ml	1 ml ampule	Chile	Chile		
methandrostenolone	Anahexia	10 mg tablet	100 tablet box	Jinan Pharm	China		
oxandrolone	Anavar	5 mg tablet	30 tablet strip	Hubei Huangshi	China		
testosterone undecanoate	Andriol	40 mg capsules	16 capsule box	Organon	China		
oxymetholone	Anemoxic	50 mg tablet	100 tablet box	Jinan Pharm	China		
testosterone propionate	Dubol	25 mg/ml	1 ml ampule	n/a	China		

APPENDIX A-4

Errors or Omissions: Info@AnabolicsBook.com

Drug Availability Tables
Listings by Country

Generic Name	Trade Name	Dose	Packaging	Company	Country	Status	Vet
testosterone propionate	Testosterone Propionate Inj	50 mg/ml	1 ml ampule	n/a	China		
boldenone undecylenate	Biometabol	50 mg/ml	10, 50, 100, 250ml vial	Sharper	Colombia		VET
boldenone undecylenate	Boldebig 50	50 mg/ml	10, 50, 100, 250ml vial	Aurofarma	Colombia		VET
boldenone undecylenate	Boldefox	50 mg/ml	10 ml vial	Biochem	Colombia		VET
boldenone undecylenate	Boldegan	50 mg/ml	10, 50, 100, 250ml vial	Gen-Far	Colombia		VET
boldenone undecylenate	Boldemas	50 mg/ml	50, 250 ml vial	Sintefar	Colombia		VET
boldenone undecylenate	Boldenive	50 mg/ml	50 ml vial	Promevet	Colombia		VET
boldenone undecylenate	Boldenol	25 mg/ml	10, 50, 100, 250ml vial	Comandina	Colombia		VET
boldenone undecylenate	Boldenol R-50	50 mg/ml	10, 50, 100, 250ml vial	Comandina	Colombia		VET
boldenone undecylenate	Boldenona	50 mg/ml	10, 20, 100 ml vial	Biogen	Colombia		VET
boldenone undecylenate	Boldenona	50 mg/ml	10, 50, 100, 250ml vial	Farmabiotech	Colombia		VET
boldenone undecylenate	Boldenona	50 mg/ml	50 ml vial	S.F.C.	Colombia		VET
boldenone undecylenate	Boldenona	50 mg/ml	10, 50, 100, 250ml vial	Vecol	Colombia		VET
boldenone undecylenate	Boldenona 25mg/ml	25 mg/ml	10, 50, 100, 250ml vial	Ind. Maravedi	Colombia		VET
boldenone undecylenate	Boldenona 50	50 mg/ml	50 ml vial	Servinsumos	Colombia		VET
boldenone undecylenate	Boldenona 50	50 mg/ml	10, 50, 100, 250ml vial	Servinsumos	Colombia		VET
boldenone undecylenate	Boldenona 50 Gen-Far	50 mg/ml	10, 50, 100, 250ml vial	Gen-Far	Colombia		VET
boldenone undecylenate	Boldenona Undecilato	50 mg/ml	50 ml vial	Mathieson	Colombia		VET
boldenone undecylenate	Boldenona Undecilato	50 mg/ml	50 ml vial	Rowel	Colombia		VET
boldenone undecylenate	Boldenona Undecilato	50 mg/ml	50 ml vial	Vitrofarma	Colombia		VET
boldenone undecylenate	Boldenona Undecilenato	50 mg/ml	10, 50, 100, 250ml vial	Erma	Colombia		VET
boldenone undecylenate	Boldenone 50mg/ml	50 mg/ml	10, 50, 100, 250ml vial	Ind. Maravedi	Colombia		VET
boldenone undecylenate	Boldesyn	50 mg/ml	50 ml vial	Synthesis LTDA	Colombia		VET
boldenone undecylenate	Boldevet	50 mg/ml	50 ml vial	Andean Veterinary	Colombia		VET
boldenone undecylenate	Cebulin 50	50 mg/ml	10, 50, 250 ml vial	Provet	Colombia		VET
nandrolone decanoate	Deca-Durabolin®	25, 50 mg/ml	1 ml ampule	Organon	Colombia		
boldenone undecylenate	Dynabolin 50	50 mg/ml	10, 50, 100, 250ml vial	Kryovet	Colombia		VET
boldenone undecylenate	Ganabol	50 mg/ml	500 ml vial	Laboratorios VM	Colombia		VET
boldenone undecylenate	Ganabol	25, 50 mg/ml	10, 50, 100, 250ml vial	Laboratorios VM	Colombia		VET
boldenone undecylenate	Insubolden	50 mg/ml	10, 50, 100, 250ml vial	Insuvin	Colombia		VET
nandrolone laurate	Laurabolin	50 mg/ml	10, 50 ml	Intervet	Colombia		VET
boldenone undecylenate	Legacy	50 mg/ml	50 ml vial	Technoquimicas	Colombia		VET
boldenone undecylenate	Mitgan 50	50 mg/ml	50 ml vial	California	Colombia		VET
nandrolone laurate	Nandrolona	50 mg/ml	10, 20, 100 ml vial	Laboratorios VM	Colombia		VET
testosterone undecanoate (inj)	Nebido	250 mg/ml	4 ml ampule	Schering	Colombia		
boldenone undecylenate	Porkybol 1%	10 mg/ml	10, 50, 100 ml vial	Compania California	Colombia		VET
mesterolone	Proviron®	25 mg tablet	20 tablet box	Schering	Colombia		
boldenone undecylenate	Strogen	25 mg/ml	10, 50, 100, 250, 500 ml vial	Vicar	Colombia		VET
boldenone undecylenate	Strogen 50	50 mg/ml	50, 100, 250, 500 ml vial	Vicar	Colombia		VET
testosterone enanthate	Testoviron®-Depot	250 mg/ml	1 ml ampule	Schering	Colombia		
boldenone undecylenate	Boldenona 50 Gen-Far	50 mg/ml	10, 50, 100, 250ml vial	Gen-Far	Colombia		VET
methenolone acetate	Primobolan®	5 mg tablet	n/a	Schering	Costa Rica		
mesterolone	Proviron®	25 mg tablet	n/a	Schering	Costa Rica	[NLM]	
testosterone propionate	Testogan	25 mg/ml	50 ml vial	Laguinsa	Costa Rica		VET
Sustanon 250 (testosterone blend)	Testosterona 250	250 mg/ml	10 ml vial	Qualityvet	Costa Rica		VET
mesterolone	Proviron®	25 mg tablet	20 tablet box	Schering	Croatia		

APPENDIX A-5

Errors or Omissions: Info@AnabolicsBook.com

Drug Availability Tables

Listings by Country

Generic Name	Trade Name	Dose	Packaging	Company	Country	Status	Vet
testosterone undecanoate	Andriol	40 mg capsules	n/a	Organon	Cyprus		
testosterone undecanoate (inj)	Nebido	250 mg/ml	4 ml ampule	Schering	Czech Republic		
testosterone suspension (isobutyrate)	Agoviron-Depot	25 mg/ml	2 ml ampule	Biotika	Czech. Rep.		
mesterolone	Proviron®	25 mg tablet	20, 50 tablet box	Schering	Czech. Rep.		
nandrolone phenylpropionate	Superanabolon	25 mg/ml	1 ml ampule	Spofa	Czech. Rep.		
Sustanon 250 (testosterone blend)	Sustanon 250	250 mg/ml	1 ml ampule	Organon	Czech. Rep.		
testosterone undecanoate	Undestor	40 mg capsules	60 capsule bottle	Organon	Czech. Rep.		
nandrolone hexyloxyphenylpropionate	Anadur	25 mg/ml	2 ml ampule	Lundbeck	Denmark	[NLM]	
nandrolone decanoate	Deca-Durabolin®	25, 50 mg/ml	1 ml	Organon	Denmark	[NLM]	
fluoxymesterone	Halotestin®	5 mg tablet	n/a	Upjohn	Denmark	[NLM]	
mesterolone	Mestoranum	25 mg tablet	n/a	Schering	Denmark		
testosterone undecanoate (inj)	Nebido	250 mg/ml	4 ml ampule	Schering	Denmark		
testosterone undecanoate	Restandol	40 mg capsules	60 capsule bottle	Organon	Denmark		
stanozolol (oral)	Stromba	5 mg tablet	n/a	Winthrop	Denmark	[NLM]	
Testoviron (testosterone blend)	Testoviron® Depot 135	135 mg/ml	1 ml ampule	Schering	Denmark		
testosterone enanthate	Testoviron®-Depot	250 mg/ml	1 ml ampule	Schering	Denmark		
methandrostenolone	Anabolex	3 mg tablet	100 tablet box	Ethical	Dom. Rep.		
boldenone undecylenate	Boldenona 50 Gen-Far	50 mg/ml	10, 50, 100, 250ml vial	Gen-Far	Dom. Rep.		VET
boldenone undecylenate	Ganabol	50 mg/ml	500 ml vial	Laboratorios VM	Dom. Rep.		VET
boldenone undecylenate	Ganabol	25, 50 mg/ml	10, 50, 100, 250ml vial	Laboratorios VM	Dom. Rep.		VET
mesterolone	Proviron®	25 mg tablet	20 tablet bottle	Schering	Dom. Rep.		
testosterone propionate	Testogan	25 mg/ml	50 ml vial	Laguinsa	Dom. Rep.		VET
Testoviron (testosterone blend)	Testoviron® Depot 100	135 mg/ml	1 ml ampule	Schering	Dom. Rep.		
testosterone enanthate	Testoviron®-Depot	250 mg/ml	1 ml ampule	Schering	Dom. Rep.		
testosterone undecanoate	Andriol	40 mg capsules	n/a	Organon	Dutch Antilles		
testosterone undecanoate	Andriol	40 mg capsules	n/a	Organon	Ecuador		
boldenone undecylenate	Boldenona 50 Gen-Far	50 mg/ml	10, 50, 100, 250ml vial	Gen-Far	Ecuador		VET
boldenone undecylenate	Ganabol	50 mg/ml	500 ml vial	Laboratorios VM	Ecuador		VET
boldenone undecylenate	Ganabol	25, 50 mg/ml	10, 50, 100, 250ml vial	Laboratorios VM	Ecuador		VET
methenolone acetate	Primobolan®	5 mg tablet	n/a	Schering	Ecuador	[NLM]	
methenolone enanthate	Primobolan® Depot	100 mg/ml	1 ml ampule	Schering	Ecuador		
testosterone enanthate	Primoteston® Depot	250 mg/ml	1 ml ampule	Schering	Ecuador		
testosterone propionate	Testogan	25 mg/ml	50 ml vial	Laguinsa	Ecuador		VET
testosterone undecanoate	Andriol	40 mg capsules	20 capsule box	Organon/Sedico	Egypt		
testosterone undecanoate	Cioteston Depot	250 mg/ml	1 ml ampule	CID	Egypt		
nandrolone decanoate	Deca-Durabolin®	25, 50 mg/ml	1 ml ampule	Organon/Nile	Egypt		
nandrolone decanoate	Gerabolin	25 mg/ml	1 ml ampule	Nile	Egypt		
nandrolone phenylpropionate	Menabolin	25 mg/ml	1 ml ampule	Theramex/Memphis	Egypt		
methyltestosterone	Neo Aphro	5 mg tablet	30 tablet	Misr	Egypt		
methenolone enanthate	Primobolan Depot	100 mg/ml	1 ml ampule	Schering/CID	Egypt	[NLM]	
testosterone enanthate	Primoteston®-Depot	250 mg/ml	1 ml ampule	Schering/CID	Egypt	[NLM]	
Testoviron (testosterone blend)	Primoteston®-Depot 100	135 mg/ml	1 ml ampule	Schering/CID	Egypt	[NLM]	
mesterolone	Proviron®	25 mg tablet	20 tablet box	Schering/CID	Egypt	[NLM]	
nandrolone decanoate	Retabolil	50 mg/ml	1 ml ampule	Medimpex/Alxndria	Egypt		
nandrolone cyclohexylpropionate	Sanabolicum	25, 50 mg/ml	1 ml ampule	Biochemie/Nile	Egypt		
Sustanon 100 (testosterone blend)	Sustanon '100'®	100 mg/ml	1 ml ampule	Organon/Nile	Egypt		

APPENDIX A-6

Errors or Omissions: Info@AnabolicsBook.com

Drug Availability Tables

Listings by Country

Generic Name	Trade Name	Dose	Packaging	Company	Country	Status	Vet
Sustanon 250 (testosterone blend)	Sustanon '250'®	250 mg/ml	1 ml ampule	Organon/Nile	Egypt		
testosterone propionate	Testone-E	25 mg/ml	1 ml ampule	Misr	Egypt		
Sustanon 100 (testosterone blend)	Testonon 100'®	100 mg/ml	1 ml ampule	Nile	Egypt		
Sustanon 250 (testosterone blend)	Testonon '250'®	250 mg/ml	1 ml ampule	Nile	Egypt		
testosterone blend (misc)	Triolandren	250 mg/ml	1 ml ampule	Novartis	Egypt		
boldenone undecylenate	Boldenona 50 Gen-Far	50 mg/ml	10, 50, 100, 250ml vial	Gen-Far	El Salvador		VET
boldenone undecylenate	Ganabol	50 mg/ml	500 ml vial	Laboratorios VM	El Salvador		VET
boldenone undecylenate	Ganabol	25, 50 mg/ml	10, 50, 100, 250ml vial	Laboratorios VM	El Salvador		VET
methenolone acetate	Primobolan®	5 mg tablet	n/a	Schering	El Salvador	[NLM]	
mesterolone	Proviron®	25 mg tablet	n/a	Schering	El Salvador		
testosterone propionate	Testogan	25 mg/ml	50 ml vial	Laguinsa	El Salvador		VET
testosterone undecanoate (inj)	Nebido	250 mg/ml	4 ml ampule	Schering	Estonia		
testosterone undecanoate	Pantestone	40 mg capsules	60 capsule bottle	Organon	Estonia		
mesterolone	Proviron®	25 mg tablet	20 tablet box	Schering	Estonia	[NLM]	
nandrolone decanoate	Retabolil	50 mg/ml	1 ml ampule	Gedeon Richter	Ethiopia		
Sustanon 250 (testosterone blend)	Sustanon 250®	250 mg/ml	1 ml ampule	Organon	Finland		
testosterone enanthate	Testoviron®-Depot	250 mg/ml	1 ml ampule	Schering	Finland		
nandrolone decanoate	Deca-Durabolin®	25, 50 mg/ml	1 ml	Organon	Finland		
nandrolone phenylpropionate	Deca-Durabolin®	100 mg/ml	1,2 ml	Organon	Finland		
fluoxymesterone	Durabolin®	25 mg/ml	n/a	Organon	Finland		
testosterone undecanoate (inj)	Halotestin®	5 mg tablet	n/a	Upjohn	Finland		
testosterone undecanoate	Nebido	250 mg/ml	4 ml ampule	Schering	Finland		
testosterone enanthate	Pantestone	40 mg capsules	60 capsule bottle	Organon	Finland		
Primoteston®-Depot	Primoteston®-Depot	250 mg/ml	1 ml ampule	Leiras	Finland	[NLM]	
mesterolone	Proviron®	25 mg tablet	n/a	Leiras	Finland		
Sustanon 250 (testosterone blend)	Sustanon 250®	250 mg/ml	1 ml ampule	Organon	Finland		
dihydrotestosterone	Andractim	25 mg/g	100 gram gel	Besins-Iscovesco	France		
testosterone enanthate	Androtardyl®	250 mg/ml	1 ml ampule	Schering	France		
testosterone undecanoate (inj)	Nebido	250 mg/ml	4 ml ampule	Schering	France		
norethandrolone	Nilevar	10 mg tablet	30 tablet bottle	Searle	France		
testosterone undecanoate	Pantestone	40 mg capsules	60 capsule bottle	Organon	France		
trenbolone hexahydrobenzylcarbonate	Parabolan	76 mg/1.5 ml	1.5 ml ampule	Negma	France	[NLM]	
testosterone enanthate	Testosterone Heptylate	50, 100, 250 mg/ml	1 ml ampule	Theramex	France		
testosterone undecanoate	Andriol	40 mg capsules	n/a	Organon	Georgia		
nandrolone decanoate	Anabolicum	25 mg/ml	10, 50 ml vial	Bela-Pharm	Germany		VET
testosterone undecanoate	Andriol	40 mg capsules	30, 60 capsule bottle	Organon	Germany		
testosterone (patch)	Androderm®	12.2 mg patch.	10, 30, 60 patches/box	AstraZenica	Germany		
testosterone (gel)	Androtop Gel	50 mg	single dose packet	Kade/Besins	Germany		
nandrolone laurate	Fortadex	25, 50 mg/ml	n/a	Hydro	Germany		VET
nandrolone laurate	Laurabolin	25, 50 mg/ml	5, 10, 50 ml	Vemie	Germany		VET
testosterone undecanoate (inj)	Nebido	250 mg/ml	4 ml ampule	Schering	Germany		
testosterone (gel)	Testogel	25, 50 mg	single dose packet	Jenapharm	Germany		
testosterone enanthate	Testosteron Depot	250 mg/ml	1 ml ampule	Rotex Medica	Germany		
testosterone enanthate	Testosteron-Depot	250 mg/ml	1 ml ampule	Eifelfango	Germany		
testosterone enanthate	Testosteron-Depot	250 mg/ml	1 ml ampule	Jenapharm	Germany		
testosterone propionate	testosteronpropionat	50 mg/ml	1 ml ampule	Eifelfango	Germany		

Errors or Omissions: Info@AnabolicsBook.com

APPENDIX A-7

Drug Availability Tables

Listings by Country

Generic Name	Trade Name	Dose	Packaging	Company	Country	Status	Vet
testosterone enanthate	Testoviron®-Depot	250 mg/ml	1 ml ampule	Schering	Germany		
boldenone undecylenate	Vebonol	25 mg/ml	10 ml vial	Ciba-Geigy	Germany		VET
testosterone undecanoate	Andriol	40 mg capsules	n/a	Organon	Ghana		
nandrolone decanoate	Anaboline Depot	50 mg/ml	1 ml	Adelco	Greece		
oxymetholone	Anasteron	25 mg tablet	60 tablet bottle	Farmaprod	Greece		
testosterone undecanoate	Andriol Testocaps	40 mg capsules	30 tablet box	Organon	Greece		
nandrolone decanoate	Deca-Durabolin®	50 mg/ml	1 ml vial	Organon	Greece		
nandrolone decanoate	Deca-Durabolin®	100 mg/ml	2 ml vial	Organon	Greece		
nandrolone decanoate	Deca-Durabolin®	100 mg/ml	2 ml vial	Organon	Greece		
nandrolone decanoate	Extraboline	50 mg/ml	2 ml vial	Genepharm	Greece		
fluoxymesterone	Halotestin®	5 mg tablet	20 tablet box	Upjohn	Greece		
nandrolone decanoate	nandrolone decanoate	200 mg/2ml	2 ml vial	Norma Hellas	Greece		
nandrolone decanoate	Nurezan	50 mg/ml	1 ml ampule	Rafarm	Greece		
oxymetholone	Oxybolone	50 mg tablet	20 tablet box	Genepharm	Greece		
methenolone enanthate	Primobolan® Depot	100 mg/ml	1 ml ampule	Schering	Greece	[NLM]	
mesterolone	Proviron®	25 mg tablet	20 tablet bottle	Schering	Greece		
testosterone undecanoate	Restandol	40 mg capsules	60 capsule bottle	Organon	Greece	[NLM]	
stanozolol (oral)	stanozolol	5 mg tablet	30 tablet box	Genepharm	Greece		
stanozolol (oral)	Stromba	5 mg tablet	56 tablet box	n/a	Greece		
methyltestosterone	Teston	25 mg tablet	30 tablet box	Remek	Greece		
testosterone enanthate	Testosterone Enanthate	250 mg/ml	1 ml ampule	Norma Hellas	Greece		
testosterone propionate	Testoviron®	50 mg/ml	1 ml ampule	Schering	Greece		
testosterone enanthate	Testoviron®-Depot	250 mg/ml	1 ml ampule	Schering	Greece		
nandrolone decanoate	Ziremilon	50 mg/ml	1 ml ampule	Demo	Greece		
boldenone undecylenate	Boldenona 50 Gen-Far	50 mg/ml	10, 50, 100, 250ml vial	Gen-Far	Guatemala		VET
boldenone undecylenate	Ganabol	50 mg/ml	500 ml vial	Laboratorios VM	Guatemala		VET
boldenone undecylenate	Ganabol	25, 50 mg/ml	10, 50, 100, 250ml vial	Laboratorios VM	Guatemala		VET
methenolone acetate	Primobolan®	5 mg tablet	n/a	Schering	Guatemala	[NLM]	
methenolone enanthate	Primobolan® Depot	100 mg/ml	1 ml ampule	Schering	Guatemala		
testosterone enanthate	Primoteston®-Depot	250 mg/ml	1 ml ampule	Schering	Guatemala		
mesterolone	Proviron®	25 mg tablet	n/a	Schering	Guatemala		
testosterone propionate	Testogan	25 mg/ml	50 ml vial	Laguinsa	Guatemala		VET
boldenone undecylenate	Boldenona 50 Gen-Far	50 mg/ml	10, 50, 100, 250ml vial	Gen-Far	Honduras		VET
boldenone undecylenate	Ganabol	50 mg/ml	500 ml vial	Laboratorios VM	Honduras		VET
boldenone undecylenate	Ganabol	25, 50 mg/ml	10, 50, 100, 250ml vial	Laboratorios VM	Honduras		VET
methenolone acetate	Primobolan®	5 mg tablet	n/a	Schering	Honduras	[NLM]	
mesterolone	Proviron®	25 mg tablet	n/a	Schering	Honduras		
testosterone propionate	Testogan	25 mg/ml	50 ml vial	Laguinsa	Honduras		VET
testosterone cypionate	Depo-Testermon	200 mg/ml	n/a	Kai Yuen	Hong Kong		
testosterone cypionate	Testosterone Cypionate Inj	200 mg/ml	n/a	Charmaine	Hong Kong		
testosterone propionate	Testosterone Propionate Inj	25 mg/ml	n/a	Charmaine	Hong Kong		
testosterone propionate	Testosterone Propionate Inj	50 mg/ml	n/a	Hong Kong Med	Hong Kong		
methyltestosterone	Testosure	5 mg tablet	n/a	Europharm	Hong Kong		
testosterone enanthate	Testoviron®-Depot	250 mg/ml	1 ml ampule	Schering	Hong Kong		
testosterone undecanoate	Andriol	40 mg capsules	n/a	Organon	Hong-Kong		
nandrolone decanoate	Deca-Durabolin®	50 mg/ml	n/a	Organon	Hong-Kong		

APPENDIX A-8

Errors or Omissions: Info@AnabolicsBook.com

Drug Availability Tables

Listings by Country

Generic Name	Trade Name	Dose	Packaging	Company	Country	Status	Vet
testosterone undecanoate (inj)	Nebido	250 mg/ml	4 ml ampule	Schering	Hong-Kong		
testosterone undecanoate	Andriol	40 mg capsules	n/a	Organon	Hungary		
testosterone propionate	Androfort-Richter	10, 25 mg/ml	n/a	Gedeon Richter	Hungary		
methyltestosterone	Androral	10 mg tablet	n/a	Gedeon Richter	Hungary		
testosterone undecanoate (inj)	Nebido	250 mg/ml	4 ml ampule	Schering	Hungary		
methandrostenolone	Nerobol	5 mg tablet	20 tablet box	Gedeon Richter	Hungary	[NLM]	
nandrolone phenylpropionate	Nerobolil	25 mg/ml	n/a	Gedeon Richter	Hungary	[NLM]	
mesterolone	Proviron®	25 mg tablet	10, 15, 20, 50, 100, 150 tab btl	Schering	Hungary		
nandrolone decanoate	Retabolil	25, 50 mg/ml	1 ml ampule	Gedeon Richter	Hungary		
stanozolol (oral)	Stromba	5 mg tablet	n/a	Sterling-Health	Hungary		
testosterone propionate	Testosteron	5, 10, 25, 50 mg/ml	1 ml ampule	Hemofarm	Hungary	[NLM]	
testosterone enanthate	Testoviron® Depot	250 mg/ml	1 ml ampule	Schering	Hungary	[NLM]	
Testoviron (testosterone blend)	Testoviron® Depot	135 mg/ml	1 ml ampule	Schering	Hungary	[NLM]	
testosterone enanthate	Testoviron®-Depot	250 mg/ml	1 ml ampule	Schering	Iceland		
dihydrotestosterone	Andractim	25 mg/g	100 gram gel	Chemec	India		
oxymetholone	Androyd	5 mg tablet	100 tablet	Parke Davis	India		
testosterone suspension	Aquaviron	25 mg/ml	1 ml ampule	Nicholas	India		
testosterone cypionate	Cypobolin	250 mg/ml	1 ml ampule	Alpha-Pharma	India		
nandrolone decanoate	Deca-Durabolin®	25, 50, 100 mg/ml	1 ml ampule	Infar	India		
nandrolone decanoate	Deca-Evabolin	25 mg/ml	1 ml ampule	Concept	India		
nandrolone decanoate	Decaneurabol	25, 50 mg/ml	1 ml ampule	Cadila	India		
nandrolone decanoate	Decaneurophen	25, 50 mg/ml	1 ml ampule	Ind-Swift	India		
nandrolone decanoate	Deca-Pronabol	100 mg/ml	2 ml ampule	P&B Labs	India		
nandrolone phenylpropionate	Durabolin®	25 mg/ml	1 ml ampule	Infar	India		
nandrolone phenylpropionate	Evabolin	25 mg/ml	1 ml ampule	Concept	India		
Sustanon 250 (testosterone blend)	Gonadon-250	250 mg/ml	1 ml ampule	Belco Pharma	India		
Sustanon 250 (testosterone blend)	Induject	250 mg/ml	1 ml ampule	Alpha-Pharma	India		
stanozolol (oral)	Menabol	5 mg tablet	100 tablet box	n/a	India		
nandrolone phenylpropionate	Metabol	25 mg/ml	1 ml ampule	Jagsonpal	India		
nandrolone decanoate	Metadec	25, 50 mg/ml	1 ml ampule	Jagsonpal	India		
methenolone enanthate	Methenolone Enanthate Inj BP	100 mg/ml	1 ml ampule	Belco Pharma	India		
nandrolone decanoate	Myobolin	25 mg/ml	1 ml ampule	Troikaa	India		
nandrolone decanoate	Nandrobolin	100 mg/ml	2 ml vial	Alpha-Pharma	India		
nandrolone decanoate	Nandrolone Decanoate Inj BP	25, 50, 100 mg/ml	1,2 ml ampule	Belco Pharma	India		
nandrolone phenylpropionate	Nandrolone Phenylpropionate BP	25, 50 mg/ml	1,2 ml ampule	Belco Pharma	India		
nandrolone phenylpropionate	NandroRapid	100 mg/ml	1 ml ampule	Alpha-Pharma	India		
stanozolol (oral)	Neurabol	2 mg capsule	10 capsule box	Cadila	India		
nandrolone phenylpropionate	Neurabol Inj	25 mg/ml	1 ml ampule	Cadila	India		
nandrolone phenylpropionate	Neurophen	25 mg/ml	1 ml ampule	Ind-Swift	India		
testosterone undecanoate	Nuvir	40 mg capsules	30 capsule bottle	Organon	India		
ethylestrenol	Orabolin®	2 mg tablet	10 tablet box	Infar	India		
oxandrolone	Oxandrolone Tablets BP	2.5, 5 mg tablet	n/a	Belco Pharma	India		
oxymetholone	Oxymetholone Tablets BP	5 mg tablet	n/a	Alpha-Pharma	India		
trenbolone hexahydrobenzylcarbonate	Parabolin	76.5 mg/1.5ml	1 ml ampule	Alpha-Pharma	India		
methandrostenolone	Pronabol-5	5 mg tablet	100 tablet box	P&B Labs	India	[NLM]	
mesterolone	Proviron®	25 mg tablet	30 tablet box	Schering	India	[NLM]	

APPENDIX A-9

Errors or Omissions: Info@AnabolicsBook.com

Drug Availability Tables
Listings by Country

Generic Name	Trade Name	Dose	Packaging	Company	Country	Status	Vet
mesterolone	Provironum®	25 mg tablet	30 tablet box	Schering	India		
mesterolone	Restore	25 mg tablet	20 tablet box	Brown & Burk	India		
stanozolol (inj)	Rexogin	50 mg/ml	1 ml ampule	Alpha-Pharma	India		
Sustanon 250 (testosterone blend)	Sistanon 250	250 mg/ml	1 ml ampule	Jackson Labs	India		
stanozolol (oral)	Stanozolol Tablets BP	2 mg tablet	n/a	Belco Pharma	India		
Sustanon 100 (testosterone blend)	Sustanon (Cyctahoh)	100 mg/ml	1 ml ampule	Infar	India		
Sustanon 250 (testosterone blend)	Sustanon 250 (Cyctahoh)	250 mg/ml	1 ml ampule	Infar	India		
testosterone enanthate	Sustaverone	250 mg/ml	1 ml ampule	Jackson Labs	India		
testosterone cypionate	Testacyp	100 mg/ml	2 ml vial	BM Pharmaceuticals	India		
testosterone enanthate	Testen-250	250 mg/ml	2 ml vial	BM Pharmaceuticals	India		
Testoviron (testosterone blend)	Testenon	135 mg/ml	2 ml vial	BM Pharmaceuticals	India		
Testoviron (testosterone blend)	Testenon	135 mg/ml	1 ml ampule	Alpha-Pharma	India		
testosterone enanthate	Testobolin	250 mg/ml	1 ml ampule	Alpha-Pharma	India		
testosterone propionate	Testopin-100	100 mg/ml	2 ml vial	BM Pharmaceuticals	India		
testosterone propionate	Testopin-100	100 mg/ml	1 ml ampule	BM Pharmaceuticals	India		
testosterone propionate	TestoRapid	100 mg/ml	1 ml ampule	Alpha-Pharma	India		
testosterone propionate	Testosterone Propionate Inj BP	10, 25, 50 mg/ml	1, 2 ml ampule	Belco Pharma	India		
testosterone enanthate	Testoviron®-Depot	250 mg/ml	1 ml ampule	German Remedies	India		
testosterone enanthate	Testoviron®-Depot	250 mg/ml	1 ml ampule	Schering	India		
testosterone undecanoate	Andriol	40 mg capsules	n/a	Organon	Indonesia		
nandrolone decanoate	Deca-Durabolin®	25, 50 mg/ml	1 ml ampule	Organon	Indonesia		
nandrolone phenylpropionate	Durabolin®	12.5 mg/ml	2 ml ampule	Organon	Indonesia		
methandrostenolone	Neo-Anabolene	5 mg tablet	10 tablet strip	Haurus	Indonesia		
ethylestrenol	Orgabolin	2 mg tablet	n/a	Organon	Indonesia		
mesterolone	Proviron®	25 mg tablet	n/a	Schering	Indonesia		
Sustanon 250 (testosterone blend)	Sustanon "250"	250 mg/ml	1 ml ampule	Organon	Indonesia		
methandrostenolone	Methandrostenolone 5	5 mg tablet	100 tablet box	Ramopharmin	Iran		
nandrolone decanoate	Nandrolone Decanoate IH	25 mg/ml	1 ml ampule	Iran Hormone	Iran		
nandrolone phenylpropionate	nandrolone phenylpropionate	25 mg/ml	1 ml ampule	Iran Hormone	Iran		
oxymetholone	Oxymetholone 50	50 mg tablet	100 tablet bottle	Alhavi	Iran		
oxymetholone	Oxymetholone IH 50	50 mg tablet	100 tablet bottle	Iran Hormone	Iran		
stanozolol (oral)	Stanozolol 5	5 mg tablet	100 tablet box	Ramopharmin	Iran		
testosterone enanthate	Testosterone Enanthate	100 mg/ml	1 ml ampule	Aburaihan	Iran		
testosterone enanthate	Testosterone Enanthate 250	250 mg/ml	1 ml ampule	Aburaihan	Iran		
nandrolone decanoate	Deca-Durabolin®	n/a	n/a	Organon	Ireland		
testosterone undecanoate (inj)	Nebido	250 mg/ml	4 ml ampule	Schering	Ireland		
Sustanon 250 (testosterone blend)	Sustanon	250 mg/ml	1 ml ampule	Schering	Ireland		
testosterone enanthate	Testoviron® Depot	250 mg/ml	1 ml ampule	Schering	Ireland	[NLM]	
testosterone undecanoate	Androxon	40 mg capsules	30 capsule bottle	Organon	Israel		
oxandrolone	Lonavar	2.5 mg tablet	100 tablet bottle	BTG	Israel		
mesterolone	Proviron®	25 mg tablet	20, 50 tablet box	Schering	Israel		
Sustanon 250 (testosterone blend)	Sustanon	250 mg/ml	1 ml ampule	Organon	Israel		
testosterone enanthate	Testoviron®-Depot	250 mg/ml	1 ml ampule	Schering	Israel		
clostebol acetate	Alfa-Trofodermin	.5% gel	n/a	Pharmacia & Upjohn	Italy		
testosterone undecanoate	Andriol	40 mg capsules	60 capsule bottle	Organon	Italy		
testosterone (patch)	Androderm®	12.2 mg patch.	n/a	Schwarz Pharma	Italy		

APPENDIX A-10

Errors or Omissions: Info@AnabolicsBook.com

Drug Availability Tables

Listings by Country

Generic Name	Trade Name	Dose	Packaging	Company	Country	Status	Vet
nandrolone decanoate	Deca-Durabolin®	25, 50 mg/ml	1 ml ampule	Organon	Italy		
nandrolone undecanoate	Dynabolon	80.5 mg/ml	1 ml ampule	Fournier	Italy		
testosterone propionate	Facovit	1 mg/ml	10 ml vial	Teofarma	Italy		
oxandrolone	Oxandrolone SPA	2.5 mg tablet	30 tablet box	SPA	Italy	[NLM]	
oxandrolone	Oxandrolone SPA (Export)	2.5 mg tablet	30 tablet box	SPA	Italy		
mesterolone	Proviron®	50 mg tablet	20 tablet box	Schering	Italy		
stanozolol (oral)	Stanozololo	2 mg tablet	50 tablet bottle	Acme Stargate	Italy		VET
Sustanon 250 (testosterone blend)	Sustanon®	250 mg/ml	1 ml ampule	Organon	Italy		
testosterone enanthate	Testo-Enant	125 mg/ml	2 ml ampule	Geymonat	Italy		
testosterone enanthate	Testo-Enant	250 mg/ml	1 ml ampule	Geymonat	Italy		
testosterone cypionate	Testosterone Depositum	n/a	n/a	SPA	Italy		
testosterone enanthate	Testoviron®-Depot	250 mg/ml	1 ml ampule	Schering	Italy		
methyltestosterone	Testovis	10 mg tablet	n/a	SIT	Italy		
testosterone propionate	Testovis	50 mg/ml	2 ml ampule	SIT	Italy		
clostebol acetate	Trofodermin Crema	cream	30 gram tube	Carlo Erba OTC	Italy		
clostebol acetate	Trofodermin Spray	n/a	30 ml spray	Carlo Erba OTC	Italy		
oxymetholone	Anadrol	5 mg tablet	n/a	n/a	Japan		
methandrostenolone	Andoredan	5 mg tablet	n/a	Takeshima-Kodama	Japan	[NLM]	
testosterone enanthate	Enarmon-Depot	125 mg/ml	n/a	Teskoku Hormone	Japan		
methandrostenolone	Encephan	5 mg tablet	n/a	Sato	Japan	[NLM]	
fluoxymesterone	Halotestin®	2, 5 mg tablet	n/a	n/a	Japan		
oxandrolone	Lonavar	2 mg tablet	n/a	Dainippon	Japan	[NLM]	
drostanolone propionate	Mastisol	5% injection sol.	n/a	Shionogi	Japan	[NLM]	
furazabol	Miotolan	1 mg tablet	n/a	Daiichi Seiyaku	Japan	[NLM]	
methenolone acetate	Primobolan®	5 mg tablet	100, 1000 tablet box	Schering	Japan		
methenolone enanthate	Primobolan® Depot	50 mg/ml	1 ml ampule	Schering	Japan	[NLM]	
methenolone enanthate	Primobolan® Depot	100 mg/ml	1 ml ampule	Schering	Japan		
testosterone enanthate	Testinon-Depot	n/a	n/a	n/a	Japan		
testosterone enanthate	Testoviron®-Depot	250 mg/ml	1 ml ampule	Schering	Japan		
testosterone enanthate	Testron Depot	125, 250 mg/ml	1 ml vial	n/a	Japan		
oxandrolone	Vasorome	0.5 mg tablet	n/a	Kowa	Japan	[NLM]	
oxandrolone	Vasorome	2 mg tablet	n/a	Kowa	Japan	[NLM]	
stanozolol (oral)	Winstrol	2 mg tablet	n/a	n/a	Japan		
testosterone undecanoate	Andriol	40 mg capsules	n/a	Organon	Jordan		
testosterone enanthate	Primoteston®-Depot	250 mg/ml	1 ml ampule	Schering	Jordan		
testosterone undecanoate	Andriol	40 mg capsules	n/a	Organon	Kenya		
dihydrotestosterone	Andractim	25 mg/g	80 gram gel	n/a	Korea		
testosterone undecanoate	Andriol	40 mg capsules	n/a	Organon	Korea		
testosterone (patch)	Androderm®	12.2 mg patch.	n/a	n/a	Korea		
nandrolone decanoate	Canoate Inj	25, 50 mg/ml	n/a	n/a	Korea		
methyltestosterone	Debosteron	n/a	n/a	n/a	Korea		
nandrolone decanoate	Deca-Durabolin®	25, 50 mg/ml	1 ml ampule	Organon	Korea	[NLM]	
testosterone cypionate	Depo-TCP	200mg/ml	n/a	n/a	Korea		
testosterone cypionate	Depovirin Inj	125 mg/ml	2 ml	n/a	Korea		
nandrolone decanoate	Dynabolon Inj	40 mg/.5 ml	1 ml ampule	n/a	Korea		
testosterone enanthate	Jenasteron Inj	250 mg/ml	n/a	n/a	Korea		

Errors or Omissions: Info@AnabolicsBook.com

APPENDIX A-11

Drug Availability Tables

Listings by Country

Generic Name	Trade Name	Dose	Packaging	Company	Country	Status	Vet
methyltestosterone	KangJungBing	n/a	n/a	n/a	Korea		
oxandrolone	Kicker Tab	2.5 mg tablet	n/a	n/a	Korea		
testosterone cypionate	Miro Depo	125 mg/ml	2 ml vial	Hanil Pharm	Korea		
testosterone undecanoate (inj)	Nebido	250 mg/ml	4 ml ampule	Schering	Korea		
oxymetholone	Oxymetholone DongIndang	n/a	n/a	DongIndang	Korea		
oxymetholone	Oxymetholone HanBul	50 mg tablet	n/a	HanBul	Korea		
oxymetholone	Oxymetholone HanSeo	50 mg tablet	100 tablet bottle	HanSeo	Korea		
oxymetholone	Oxymetholone Korea United	50 mg tablet	n/a	Korea United	Korea		
stanozolol (oral)	Seidon	2 mg tablet	100 tablet box	Seoul Pharm	Korea		
stanozolol (oral)	Stabon	2 mg tablet	n/a	n/a	Korea		
stanozolol (oral)	Terabon	2 mg tablet	10 tablet strip	Jin Yang	Korea		
testosterone propionate	Testo	50 mg/ml	10 ml vial	Samil	Korea		
methyltestosterone	Testo Tab	25 mg tablet	n/a	Samil	Korea		
testosterone enanthate	Testosterone Enanthate Dalim	250 mg/ml	n/a	Dalim	Korea		
mesterolone	Vistimon	25 mg tablet	n/a	n/a	Korea		
testosterone undecanoate	Andriol	40 mg capsules	n/a	Organon	Kuwait		
testosterone enanthate	Primoteston®-Depot	250 mg/ml	1 ml ampule	Schering	Kuwait		
testosterone undecanoate (inj)	Nebido	250 mg/ml	4 ml ampule	Schering	Latvia	[NLM]	
testosterone undecanoate	Panteston	40 mg capsules	n/a	Organon	Latvia		
mesterolone	Proviron®	25 mg tablet	20 tablet box	Schering	Latvia	[NLM]	
testosterone undecanoate	Andriol	40 mg capsules	n/a	Organon	Lebanon		
testosterone enanthate	Testoviron®-Depot	250 mg/ml	1 ml ampule	Schering	Lebanon	[NLM]	
testosterone undecanoate (inj)	Nebido	250 mg/ml	4 ml ampule	Schering	Lithuania		
testosterone undecanoate	Panteston	40 mg capsules	n/a	Organon	Lithuania		
testosterone undecanoate	Undestor	40 mg capsules	n/a	Organon	Luxemburg		
testosterone undecanoate	Andriol	40 mg capsules	60 capsule bottle	Organon	Malaysia		
testosterone suspension	Aquabolic	100 mg/ml	10 ml vial	Asia Pharma	Malaysia		
testosterone propionate	Astrapin	50 mg/ml	1 ml ampule	Astrapin	Malaysia		
boldenone undecylenate	Boldabolic	200 mg/ml	10 ml vial	Asia Pharma	Malaysia		
testosterone cypionate	Cypiobolic	200 mg/ml	10 ml vial	Asia Pharma	Malaysia		
nandrolone decanoate	Decabolic	200 mg/ml	10 ml vial	Asia Pharma	Malaysia		
nandrolone decanoate	Deca-Durabolin®	25 mg/ml	1 ml ampule	Organon	Malaysia		
testosterone cypionate	Depo-Testosterone®	100 mg/ml	n/a	Pharmacia	Malaysia		
nandrolone phenylpropionate	Durabolic	100 mg/ml	10 ml vial	Asia Pharma	Malaysia		
nandrolone phenylpropionate	Durabolin®	25 mg/ml	1 ml ampule	Organon	Malaysia		
testosterone enanthate	Enantbolic	250 mg/ml	10 ml vial	Asia Pharma	Malaysia		
fluoxymesterone	Halobolic	10 mg tablet	100 tablet box	Asia Pharma	Malaysia		
testosterone enanthate	Jenasteron Inj	250 mg/ml	1 ml ampule	Jenahexal	Malaysia		
drostanolone propionate	Mastabolic	100 mg/ml	10 ml vial	Asia Pharma	Malaysia		
methandrostenolone	Methanabolic	10 mg tablet	100 tablet box	Asia Pharma	Malaysia		
oxandrolone	Oxanabolic	10 mg tablet	100 tablet box	Asia Pharma	Malaysia		
oxymetholone	Oxyanabolic	50 mg tablet	100 tablet box	Asia Pharma	Malaysia		
oxymetholone	Oxylone	50 mg tablet	100 tablet bottle	Duopharma	Malaysia		
oxymetholone	oxymetholone	50 mg tablet	n/a	Sime Darby	Malaysia		
methenolone enanthate	Primobolic Inj	100 mg/ml	10 ml vial	Asia Pharma	Malaysia		
methenolone acetate	Primobolic Tablets	50 mg tablet	100 tablet box	Asia Pharma	Malaysia		

Errors or Omissions: Info@AnabolicsBook.com

APPENDIX A-12

Drug Availability Tables

Listings by Country

Generic Name	Trade Name	Dose	Packaging	Company	Country	Status	Vet
testosterone propionate	Propiobolic	100 mg/ml	10 ml vial	Asia Pharma	Malaysia		
nandrolone decanoate	Retabolil	25, 50 mg/ml	1 ml ampule	Gedeon Richter	Malaysia		
stanozolol (inj)	Stanobolic Inj	50 mg/ml	10 ml vial	Asia Pharma	Malaysia		
stanozolol (oral)	Stanobolic Tablets	10 mg tablet	100 tablet box	Asia Pharma	Malaysia		
Sustanon 250 (testosterone blend)	Sustainbolic	250 mg/ml	10 ml vial	Asia Pharma	Malaysia		
Sustanon 250 (testosterone blend)	Sustanon '250'®	250 mg/ml	1 ml ampule	Organon	Malaysia		
testosterone (patch)	Testoderm	15 mg patch	n/a	Alza	Malaysia		
methyltestosterone	Testopropon	25 mg tablet	n/a	Scanpharm	Malaysia		
testosterone enanthate	Testoviron®-Depot	250 mg/ml	1 ml ampule	Schering	Malaysia		
trenbolone acetate	Trenabolic	80 mg/ml	10 ml vial	Asia Pharma	Malaysia		
chlorodehydromethyltestosterone	Turanabolic	10 mg tablet	100 tablet box	Asia Pharma	Malaysia		
testosterone undecanoate	Undriol	40 mg capsules	60 capsule box	Asia Pharma	Malaysia		
testosterone enanthate	Testoviron®-Depot	250 mg/ml	1 ml ampule	Schering	Malta		
testosterone undecanoate	Andriol	40 mg capsules	n/a	Organon	Mauritius		
testosterone enanthate	Primoteston®-Depot	250 mg/ml	1 ml ampule	Schering	Mauritius		
Sustanon 250 (testosterone blend)	4 Test	250 mg/ml	5 ml vial	Quality Vet	Mexico	[NLM]	VET
trenbolone acetate	Acetrenbo 50	50 mg tablet	20 tablet bottle	Loeffler	Mexico	[NLM]	VET
boldenone undecylenate	Anabolic BD	100, 200 mg/ml	10 ml vial	SYD Group	Mexico	[NLM]	VET
nandrolone cypionate	Anabolic DN	50, 300 mg/ml	10 ml vial	SYD Group	Mexico	[NLM]	VET
methylandrostenediol (blend)	Anabolic NA	75 mg/ml	10 ml vial	SYD Group	Mexico	[NLM]	VET
stanozolol (inj)	Anabolic ST	50 mg/ml	20 ml vial	SYD Group	Mexico	[NLM]	VET
testosterone cypionate	Anabolic TL	200 mg/ml	10 ml vial	SYD Group	Mexico	[NLM]	VET
testosterone suspension	Anabolic TS	100 mg/ml	20 ml vial	SYD Group	Mexico	[NLM]	VET
boldenone undecylenate	Anabolic-BD	100 mg/ml	10 ml vial	Grupo Tarasco	Mexico	[NLM]	VET
nandrolone cypionate	Anabolic-DN	50 mg/ml	10 ml vial	Grupo Tarasco	Mexico	[NLM]	VET
methylandrostenediol (blend)	Anabolic-NA	75 mg/ml	10 ml vial	Grupo Tarasco	Mexico	[NLM]	VET
stanozolol (inj)	Anabolic-ST	50 mg/ml	20 ml vial	Grupo Tarasco	Mexico	[NLM]	VET
testosterone suspension	Anabolic-TS	100 mg/ml	20 ml vial	Grupo Tarasco	Mexico	[NLM]	VET
methandrostenolone	Anabol-Jet	25 mg/ml	30, 100, 250 ml vial	Norvet	Mexico	[NLM]	VET
methandrostenolone	Anabol-Jet ADE	30 mg/ml	100, 250 ml vial	Norvet	Mexico	[NLM]	VET
methandrostenolone	Anabol-Pet's	10, 25 mg tablet	200 tablet bottle	Norvet	Mexico	[NLM]	VET
oxymetholone	Anabrol 50	50 mg tablet	100 tablet bottle	Brovel	Mexico	[NLM]	VET
testosterone undecanoate	Andriol capsulas	40 mg capsules	30 capsule bottle	Organon	Mexico		
testosterone suspension	AquaTest	100 mg/ml	10 ml vial	Denkall	Mexico	[NLM]	VET
testosterone propionate	Ara-Test	25 mg/ml	10 ml vial	Aranda Laboratories	Mexico	[NLM]	VET
Testoviron (testosterone blend)	Aratest 2500	250 mg/ml	10 ml vial	Aranda	Mexico		VET
boldenone undecylenate	Bold 200	200 mg/ml	10 ml vial	Animal Power	Mexico	[NLM]	VET
boldenone undecylenate	Bold QV 200	200 mg/ml	10 ml vial	Quality Vet	Mexico	[NLM]	VET
boldenone undecylenate	Boldenon	200 mg/ml	10 ml vial	Ttokkyo	Mexico	[NLM]	VET
boldenone undecylenate	Boldenona 200	200 mg/ml	10 ml vial	Pet's Pharma	Mexico	[NLM]	VET
boldenone undecylenate	Crecibol	25 mg/ml	10, 30 ml vial	Unimed	Mexico		VET
testosterone cypionate	Cypiotest 250	250 mg/ml	10 ml vial	Animal Power	Mexico	[NLM]	VET
testosterone cypionate	CypioTest 250	250 mg/ml	10 ml vial	Denkall	Mexico	[NLM]	VET
testosterone cypionate	Cypriotest L/A	250 mg/ml	10 ml vial	Loeffler	Mexico		VET
methandrostenolone	D-Bol	10 mg tablet	100 tablet bottle	Denkall	Mexico	[NLM]	VET
methandrostenolone	D-Bol	10 mg capsule	96 capsule box	Denkall	Mexico	[NLM]	VET

APPENDIX A-13

Errors or Omissions: Info@AnabolicsBook.com

Drug Availability Tables

Listings by Country

Generic Name	Trade Name	Dose	Packaging	Company	Country	Status	Vet
methandrostenolone	D-Bol	10 mg capsule	300 capsule bottle	Denkall	Mexico	[NLM]	VET
methandrostenolone	D-Bol	25 mg/ml	10 ml vial	Denkall	Mexico	[NLM]	VET
nandrolone decanoate	Deca 300	300 mg/ml	10 ml vial	Animal Power	Mexico	[NLM]	VET
nandrolone decanoate	Deca QV 200	200 mg/ml	10, 50 ml vial	Quality Vet	Mexico	[NLM]	VET
nandrolone decanoate	Deca QV 300	300 mg/ml	10 ml vial	Quality Vet	Mexico	[NLM]	VET
nandrolone decanoate	Decanandrolen	200mg/ml	10 ml vial	Denkall	Mexico	[NLM]	VET
nandrolone decanoate	Decandrol 300	300 mg/ml	10 ml vial	Pet's Pharma	Mexico	[NLM]	VET
nandrolone decanoate	Decanoato de Nandrolona	200 mg/ml	10 ml vial	Tornel	Mexico		VET
methylandrostenediol dipropionate	Denkadiol	75 mg/ml	10 ml vial	Denkall	Mexico	[NLM]	VET
testosterone blend (misc)	Deposterona	60 mg/ml	10 ml vial	Fort Dodge	Mexico		VET
methandrostenolone	Dianabol	10 mg tablet	100 tablet bottle	Salud	Mexico		VET
methandrostenolone	Dianabol	25 mg/ml	10, 50, 100 ml vial	Salud	Mexico		VET
nandrolone decanoate	Dimetabol ADE	25 mg/ml	50, 100 ml vial	Lapisa	Mexico	[NLM]	VET
testosterone enanthate	Enantat QV 250	250 mg/ml	10, 50 ml vial	Quality Vet	Mexico	[NLM]	VET
testosterone enanthate	Enantato 350	350 mg/ml	10 ml vial	Pet's Pharma	Mexico	[NLM]	VET
testosterone enanthate	Enantest 250	250 mg/ml	10 ml vial	Animal Power	Mexico	[NLM]	VET
boldenone undecylenate	Equibold	200 mg/ml	10 ml vial	Brovel	Mexico	[NLM]	VET
boldenone undecylenate	Equi-gan	50 mg/ml	10, 50, 100, 250 ml vial	Tornel	Mexico		VET
boldenone undecylenate	Equipoise®	50 mg/ml	10, 50 ml vial	Fort Dodge	Mexico	[NLM]	VET
stanozolol (oral)	Estano-Pet's	10, 25 mg tablet	100 tablet bottle	Norvet	Mexico	[NLM]	VET
trenbolone acetate	Finaplix-H®	20 mg pellet	70, 100 pellet cartridge	Roussel	Mexico	[NLM]	VET
nandrolone laurate	Fortabol	20 mg/ml	10, 50 ml vial	Parfam	Mexico		VET
methandrostenolone	Ganabol	25 mg/ml	50 ml vial	Salud	Mexico	[NLM]	VET
oxymetholone	Kanestron	50 mg tablet	100 tablet bottle	Loeffler	Mexico	[NLM]	VET
nandrolone laurate	Laudrol LA	250 mg/ml	10 ml vial	Loeffler	Mexico	[NLM]	VET
nandrolone laurate	Laurabolin	20, 50 mg/ml	10, 50, 100 ml vial	Intervet	Mexico		VET
Testoviron (testosterone blend)	Macrotest	250 mg/ml	10 ml vial	CPMax	Mexico		VET
testosterone enanthate	Macrotest E	250 mg/ml	10 ml vial	CPMax	Mexico		VET
boldenone undecylenate	Maxigan	50 mg/ml	10, 50 ml vial	Inpel/Denkall	Mexico	[NLM]	VET
oxymetholone	Metalon Tabs	75 mg tablet	100 tablet bottle	Animal Power	Mexico	[NLM]	VET
methandrostenolone	Metandiabol	25 mg/ml	50 ml vial	Quimper	Mexico	[NLM]	VET
methandrostenolone	Metandiol 60	60 mg/ml	10 ml vial	Pet's Pharma	Mexico	[NLM]	VET
methandrostenolone	Metandiol Tab	10 mg tablet	100 tablet bottle	Pet's Pharma	Mexico	[NLM]	VET
methenolone acetate	Metenol QV	50 mg tablet	50 tablet bottle	Quality Vet	Mexico	[NLM]	VET
methandrostenolone	Methan Tabs	10 mg tablet	100 tablet bottle	Animal Power	Mexico	[NLM]	VET
methandrostenolone	Methandienone	5, 10 mg tablet	100, 1000 tablet bottle	Ttokkyo	Mexico	[NLM]	VET
methyltestosterone	Metil-Test	50 mg tablet	100 tablet bottle	Brovel	Mexico	[NLM]	VET
nandrolone decanoate	Nandrolona 300 L.A.	300mg/ml	10 ml vial	Ttokkyo	Mexico	[NLM]	VET
testosterone undecanoate (inj)	Nebido	250 mg/ml	4 ml ampule	Schering	Mexico		
testosterone undecanoate (inj)	Nebido	250 mg/ml	4 ml ampule	Schering	Mexico		
testosterone decanoate	Neotest 250	250 mg/ml	10 ml bottle	Loeffler	Mexico	[NLM]	VET
nandrolone decanoate	Norandren 20	20 mg/ml	10, 50 ml vial	Brovel	Mexico	[NLM]	VET
nandrolone decanoate	Norandren 200	200 mg/ml	50 ml vial	Brovel	Mexico	[NLM]	VET
nandrolone decanoate	Norandren 200	200 mg/ml	10 ml vial	Brovel	Mexico	[NLM]	VET
nandrolone decanoate	Norandren 50	50 mg/ml	10, 50 ml vial	Brovel	Mexico	[NLM]	VET
testosterone propionate	Oreton	25 mg/ml	n/a	Goldline	Mexico	[NLM]	

APPENDIX A-14

Errors or Omissions: Info@AnabolicsBook.com

Drug Availability Tables

Listings by Country

Generic Name	Trade Name	Dose	Packaging	Company	Country	Status	Vet
oxandrolone	Oxafort	5 mg tablet	100 tablet bottle	Loeffler	Mexico	[NLM]	VET
oxandrolone	Oxandro Tabs	5 mg tablet	100 tablet bottle	Animal Power	Mexico	[NLM]	VET
oxandrolone	Oxandrolone	2.5 tablet	100 tablet bottle	Ttokkyo	Mexico	[NLM]	VET
oxandrolone	Oxandrolone	5 mg tablet	100 tablet bottle	Ttokkyo	Mexico	[NLM]	VET
oxandrolone	Oxandrovet	5 mg tablet	100 tablet bottle	Denkall	Mexico	[NLM]	VET
oxandrolone	Oxavet QV	5 mg tablet	100 tablet bottle	Quality Vet	Mexico	[NLM]	VET
oxymetholone	Oximetalon	75 mg tablet	100 tablet bottle	Denkall	Mexico	[NLM]	VET
oxymetholone	Oxivet QV	75 mg tablet	100 tablet bottle	Quality Vet	Mexico	[NLM]	VET
oxymetholone	Oxymetolona 50	50 mg tablet	100 tablet bottle	Ttokkyo	Mexico	[NLM]	VET
methenolone acetate	Primobolan®	5 mg tablet	n/a	Schering	Mexico	[NLM]	
methenolone enanthate	Primobolan® Depot	50 mg/ml	1 ml ampule	Schering	Mexico	[NLM]	
methenolone enanthate	Primo-Plus 100	100 mg/ml	1 ml ampule	Ttokkyo	Mexico	[NLM]	VET
methenolone acetate	Primo-Plus 50	50 mg tablet	100 tablet bottle	Ttokkyo	Mexico	[NLM]	VET
testosterone enanthate	Primoteston®-Depot	250 mg/ml	1 ml ampule	Schering	Mexico	[NLM]	
testosterone propionate	Propionat QV 100	100 mg/ml	10 ml vial	Quality Vet	Mexico	[NLM]	VET
testosterone propionate	Propiotest 100	100 mg/ml	10 ml vial	Animal Power	Mexico	[NLM]	VET
mesterolone	Proviron®	25 mg tablet	10 tablet box	Schering	Mexico		
methandrostenolone	Reforvit Simple	5, 10, 25 mg tab	100, 500, 1000 tablet bottle	Loeffler	Mexico	[NLM]	VET
methandrostenolone	Reforvit-B	25 mg/ml	10, 50 ml	Loeffler	Mexico	[NLM]	VET
methandrostenolone	Restauvit	2 mg tablet	n/a	Ciba, Rugby	Mexico	[NLM]	
Sustanon 250 (testosterone blend)	Sostenon 250®	250 mg/ml	1 ml ampule	Organon	Mexico		
stanozolol (inj)	Stan 50	50 mg/ml	10 ml vial	Animal Power	Mexico	[NLM]	VET
stanozolol (oral)	Stan QV 10	10 mg tablet	100 tablet bottle	Quality Vet	Mexico	[NLM]	VET
stanozolol (inj)	Stan QV 100	100 mg/ml	20 ml vial	Quality Vet	Mexico	[NLM]	VET
stanozolol (inj)	Stan QV 50	50 mg/ml	20 ml vial	Quality Vet	Mexico	[NLM]	VET
stanozolol (oral)	Stan Tabs	10 mg tablet	100 tablet bottle	Animal Power	Mexico	[NLM]	VET
stanozolol (inj)	Stanazolic	50, 100 mg/ml	20 ml, 10ml vial	Denkall	Mexico	[NLM]	VET
stanozolol (oral)	Stanazolic	6 mg cap	300 capsule bottle	Denkall	Mexico	[NLM]	VET
stanozolol (oral)	Stanazolic	10 mg tablet	100 tablet bottle	Denkall	Mexico	[NLM]	VET
stanozolol (inj)	Stanol-V	50, 100 mg/ml	20 ml vial	Ttokkyo	Mexico	[NLM]	VET
stanozolol (oral)	Stanol-V	10 mg tablet	100, 500 tablet bottle	Ttokkyo	Mexico	[NLM]	VET
Sten (testosterone blend)	Sten	50 mg/ml	2 ml ampule	Atlantis	Mexico		
fluoxymesterone	Stenox	2.5 mg tablet	20 tablet box	Atlantis	Mexico		
Sustanon 250 (testosterone blend)	Super Test-250	250 mg/ml	5, 10 ml vial	Tornel	Mexico		VET
methenolone enanthate	Suprimo 100	100 mg/ml	10 ml vial	SYD Group	Mexico	[NLM]	VET
trenbolone acetate	Synovex plus (plus estradiol)	25 mg pellet	80 pellet cartridge	Fort Dodge	Mexico		VET
testosterone propionate (implant)	Synovex®-H (plus estrogen)	25 mg/pellet	80 pellet cartridge	Fort Dodge	Mexico		VET
testosterone propionate (implant)	Synovex®-H (plus estrogen)	20 mg/pellet	n/a	Syntex	Mexico	[NLM]	
Test 400 (testosterone blend)	Test 400	400 mg/ml	10 ml vial	Denkall	Mexico	[NLM]	VET
Sustanon 250 (testosterone blend)	Testenon 250	250 mg/ml	5 ml vial	Ttokkyo	Mexico	[NLM]	VET
testosterone enanthate	Testoenan L/A	250 mg/ml	10 ml vial	Loeffler	Mexico	[NLM]	VET
Sustanon 250 (testosterone blend)	Testo-Jet L.A.	250 mg/ml	10 ml vial	Norvet	Mexico	[NLM]	VET
testosterone cypionate	Teston QV 200	200 mg/ml	10 ml vial	Quality Vet	Mexico	[NLM]	VET
Testoviron (testosterone blend)	Testoprim-D	250 mg/ml	1 ml ampule	Labs. Tocogino	Mexico		
testosterone propionate	Testopro L/A	250 mg/ml	10 ml vial	Loeffler	Mexico	[NLM]	VET
testosterone propionate	Testosterona 100	100 mg/ml	10 ml vial	Brovel	Mexico		VET

APPENDIX A-15

Drug Availability Tables

Listings by Country

Generic Name	Trade Name	Dose	Packaging	Company	Country	Status	Vet
testosterone enanthate	Testosterona 200	200 mg/ml	10 ml vial	Brovel	Mexico	[NLM]	VET
testosterone propionate	Testosterona 25	25 mg/ml	10, 20 ml vial	Brovel	Mexico		VET
testosterone propionate	Testosterona 50	50 mg/ml	10, 20 ml vial	Brovel	Mexico		VET
Sustanon 250 (testosterone blend)	Testosterona IV L/A	250 mg/ml	10 ml vial	Loeffler	Mexico	[NLM]	VET
testosterone enanthate	Testosterone 200 Depot	200 mg/ml	10 ml vial	Tornel	Mexico		VET
testosterone cypionate	Testosterone Cypionate 200	200 mg/ml	10 ml vial	Ttokkyo	Mexico	[NLM]	VET
testosterone cypionate	Testosterone Cypionate L.A.	100 mg/ml	10 ml vial	Ttokkyo	Mexico	[NLM]	VET
trenbolone acetate	Trembolone QV 75	75 mg/ml	10 ml vial	Quality Vet	Mexico	[NLM]	VET
trenbolone acetate	Trenbo 75	75 mg/ml	10 ml vial	Animal Power	Mexico	[NLM]	VET
trenbolone acetate	Trenbol 75	75 mg/ml	20 ml vial	Ttokkyo	Mexico	[NLM]	VET
trenbolone acetate	Trenbolon 75	75 mg/ml	10, 20 ml vial	Pet's Pharma	Mexico	[NLM]	VET
boldenone undecylenate	Ultragan	100 mg/ml	10 ml vial	Denkall	Mexico	[NLM]	VET
boldenone undecylenate	Ultragan	50 mg/ml	50 ml vial	Denkall	Mexico	[NLM]	VET
oxandrolone	Xtendrol	2.5 mg tablet	30 tablet box	Atlantis	Mexico		
methandrostenolone	Danabol	10, 50 mg tablet	60 tablet box	Balkan Pharm	Moldova		
fluoxymesterone	Halotest	2, 5, 10 mg tablet	60 tablet box	Balkan Pharm	Moldova		
nandrolone decanoate	Nandrolona D	50, 100, 200 mg/ml	1 ml ampule	Balkan Pharm	Moldova		
methenolone acetate	Primobol	50 mg tablet	60 tablet box	Balkan Pharm	Moldova		
methenolone enanthate	Primobol	100 mg/ml	1 ml ampule	Balkan Pharm	Moldova		
stanozolol (oral)	Strombafort	10, 50 mg tablet	60 tablet box	Balkan Pharm	Moldova		
Sustanon 250 (testosterone blend)	Sustamed	125, 250 mg/ml	1 ml ampule	Balkan Pharm	Moldova		
testosterone cypionate	Testosterona C	100, 200 mg/ml	1 ml ampule	Balkan Pharm	Moldova		
testosterone enanthate	Testosterona E	100, 200 mg/ml	1 ml ampule	Balkan Pharm	Moldova		
testosterone propionate	Testosterona P	100, 200 mg/ml	1 ml ampule	Balkan Pharm	Moldova		
testosterone undecanoate	Andriol	40 mg capsules	n/a	Organon	Morocco		
testosterone enanthate	Androtardyl®	250 mg/ml	1 ml ampule	Schering	Morocco		
testosterone enanthate	Weratestone 250	250 mg/ml	1 ml ampule	Weimer Pharma	Mozambique		
testosterone undecanoate	Andriol	40 mg capsules	n/a	Organon	Myanmar/Burma		VET
boldenone (blend)	Equilon 100	100 mg/ml	6 ml vial	WDV	Myanmar/Burma		VET
testosterone blend (misc)	Equitest 200	200 mg/ml	6 ml vial	WDV	Myanmar/Burma		VET
oxandrolone	Oxanol	5 mg tablet	60 tablet box	Xenion	Myanmar/Burma		
trenbolone acetate	Trenol 50	50 mg/ml	6 ml vial	WDV	Myanmar/Burma		VET
nandrolone decanoate	Anabolin Forte	50 mg/ml	10, 50 ml vial	Alfasan	Netherlands		VET
testosterone undecanoate	Andriol	40 mg capsules	n/a	Organon	Netherlands		
testosterone (gel)	Androgel	25, 50 mg	single dose packet	Besins	Netherlands		
testosterone (patch)	Andropatch	12.2 mg patch	30, 60 patch box	Schwarz Pharma	Netherlands		
nandrolone decanoate	Deca-Durabolin®	25, 50 mg/ml	1 ml ampule	Organon	Netherlands		
nandrolone decanoate	Deca-Durabolin®	100 mg/ml	2 ml vial	Organon	Netherlands		
nandrolone phenylpropionate	Durabolin®	25 mg/ml	1 ml ampule	Organon	Netherlands		
nandrolone laurate	Laurabolin V	50 mg/ml	10, 50 ml	Intervet	Netherlands		VET
mesterolone	Proviron®	25 mg tablet	50 tablet bottle	Schering	Netherlands		
stanozolol (oral)	Stromba	5 mg tablet	100 tablet box	Sanofi	Netherlands		
Sustanon 100 (testosterone blend)	Sustanon "100"®	100 mg/ml	1 ml ampule	Organon	Netherlands		
Sustanon 250 (testosterone blend)	Sustanon 250®	250 mg/ml	1 ml ampule	Organon	Netherlands		

APPENDIX A-16

Errors or Omissions: Info@AnabolicsBook.com

Drug Availability Tables

Listings by Country

Generic Name	Trade Name	Dose	Packaging	Company	Country	Status	Vet
testosterone (gel)	Testogel	25, 50 mg	single dose packet	Besins	Netherlands		
nandrolone decanoate	Deca-Durabolin®	50 mg/ml	1 ml ampule	Organon	New Zealand		
testosterone cypionate	Depo-Testosterone®	100 mg/ml	10 ml vial	Pharmacia & Upjohn	New Zealand		
testosterone undecanoate	Panteston capsules	40 mg capsules	n/a	Organon	New Zealand		
testosterone enanthate	Primoteston®-Depot	250 mg/ml	1 ml syringe	Schering	New Zealand		
Sustanon 250 (testosterone blend)	Sustanon 250	250 mg/ml	1 ml ampule	Organon	New Zealand		
boldenone undecylenate	Boldenona 50 Gen-Far	50 mg/ml	10, 50, 100, 250ml vial	Gen-Far	Nicaragua		VET
methenolone acetate	Primobolan®	5 mg tablet	n/a	Schering	Nicaragua	[NLM]	
mesterolone	Proviron®	25 mg tablet	n/a	Schering	Nicaragua		
testosterone propionate	Testogan	25 mg/ml	50 ml vial	Laguinsa	Nicaragua		VET
testosterone undecanoate	Andriol	40 mg capsules	n/a	Organon	Nigeria		
testosterone undecanoate	Androxon	40 mg capsules	60 capsule bottle	Organon	Norway		
testosterone (patch)	Atmos	5 mg patch	30 patch box	Astra Zenica	Norway		
nandrolone decanoate	Deca-Durabolin®	50 mg/ml	1 ml ampule	Organon	Norway		
testosterone undecanoate (inj)	Nebido	250 mg/ml	4 ml ampule	Schering	Norway		
testosterone enanthate	Primoteston®-Depot	250 mg/ml	1 ml ampule	Schering	Norway		
testosterone undecanoate	Andriol	40 mg capsules	n/a	Organon	Oman		
testosterone undecanoate	Androxon	40 mg capsules	n/a	Organon	Pakistan		
ethylestrenol	Orabolin®	2 mg tablet	100 tablet box	Organon	Pakistan		
Sustanon 250 (testosterone blend)	Sustanon '250'®	250 mg/ml	1ml ampule	Organon	Pakistan		
testosterone enanthate	Testofort Inj	250 mg/ml	1 ml ampule	Albert David	Pakistan		
Sustanon 250 (testosterone blend)	Testonon 250	250 mg/ml	1 ml ampule	Zafa	Pakistan		
testosterone enanthate	Testosterone Enanthate	250 mg/ml	1 ml ampule	Geofman	Pakistan		
testosterone enanthate	Testoviron®-Depot	250 mg/ml	1 ml ampule	Schering	Pakistan		
boldenone undecylenate	Boldenona 50 Gen-Far	50 mg/ml	10, 50, 100, 250ml vial	Gen-Far	Panama		VET
boldenone undecylenate	Ganabol	50 mg/ml	500 ml vial	Laboratorios VM	Panama		VET
boldenone undecylenate	Ganabol	25, 50 mg/ml	10, 50, 100, 250ml vial	Laboratorios VM	Panama		VET
methenolone acetate	Primobolan®	5 mg tablet	n/a	Schering	Panama	[NLM]	
mesterolone	Proviron®	25 mg tablet	n/a	Schering	Panama		
testosterone propionate	Testogan	25 mg/ml	50 ml vial	Laguinsa	Panama		VET
nandrolone decanoate	Decaland Depot	200 mg/ml	5 ml vial	Landerlan	Paraguay		
Sustanon 250 (testosterone blend)	Duratestoland	250 mg/ml	1 ml ampule	Landerlan	Paraguay		
boldenone undecylenate	Ganabol	50 mg/ml	500 ml vial	Laboratorios VM	Paraguay		VET
boldenone undecylenate	Ganabol	25, 50 mg/ml	10, 50, 100, 250ml vial	Laboratorios VM	Paraguay		VET
methyltestosterone	Metiltestosterona	n/a	n/a	Botica	Paraguay		
oxandrolone	Oxandroland	5 mg tablet	100 tablet bottle	Landerlan	Paraguay		
oxymetholone	Oxitoland	50 mg tablet	20 tablet box	Landerlan	Paraguay		
methenolone enanthate	Primobolan® Depot	100 mg/ml	1 ml ampule	Schering	Paraguay		
mesterolone	Proviron®	25 mg tablet	20 tablet box	Schering	Paraguay		
stanozolol (oral)	Stanozoland	10 mg tablet	100 tablet bottle	Landerlan	Paraguay		
stanozolol (inj)	Stanzoland Depot	50 mg/ml	30 ml vial, 1ml ampule	Landerlan	Paraguay		
stanozolol (inj)	Stanozolol 50mg	50 mg/ml	1 ml ampule	Indufar	Paraguay		
testosterone enanthate	Testenat Depot	250 mg/ml	4 ml vial	Landerlan	Paraguay		
testosterone cypionate	Testoland Depot	200 mg/ml	2 ml ampule	Landerlan	Paraguay		
testosterone propionate	Testosterona Propionato	n/a	n/a	Botica	Paraguay		
testosterone enanthate	Testoviron®-Depot	250 mg/ml	1 ml ampule	Schering	Paraguay		

Drug Availability Tables

Listings by Country

Generic Name	Trade Name	Dose	Packaging	Company	Country	Status	Vet
boldenone undecylenate	Boldemax A.P.	50 mg/ml	10, 50, 100, 250ml vial	Agrovet	Peru		VET
boldenone undecylenate	Boldenona 50 Gen-Far	50 mg/ml	10, 50, 100, 250ml vial	Gen-Far	Peru		VET
nandrolone decanoate	Deca-Durabolin®	50 mg/ml	1 ml ampule	Organon	Peru		
boldenone undecylenate	Ganabol	50 mg/ml	500 ml vial	Laboratorios VM	Peru		VET
boldenone undecylenate	Ganabol	25, 50 mg/ml	10, 50, 100, 250ml vial	Laboratorios VM	Peru		VET
testosterone undecanoate	Panteston	40 mg capsules	30, 60 capsule bottle	Organon	Peru		
testosterone enanthate	Testoviron® Depot	250 mg/ml	1 ml ampule	Schering	Peru		
stanozolol (oral)	Anazol	2 mg tablet	100 tablet box	Xelox (export)	Philippines		
stanozolol (oral)	Anazol	2 mg tablet	100, 1000 tablet bottle	Xelox (export)	Philippines		
testosterone undecanoate	Andriol	40 mg capsules	n/a	Organon	Philippines		
nandrolone (blend)	Dinandrol	100 mg/ml	2 ml vial	Xelox (export)	Philippines		
drostanolone	Dromostan	50 mg/ml	5 ml vial	Xelox (export)	Philippines		
fluoxymesterone	Halotestin®	5 mg tablet	n/a	Pharmacia & Upjohn	Philippines		
mesterolone	Mesterolon	25 mg tablet	n/a	Brown & Burk	Philippines		
testosterone cypionate	Vironate	200 mg/ml	5 ml vial	Xelox (export)	Philippines		
nandrolone decanoate	Deca-Durabolin®	50 mg/ml	1 ml ampule	Organon	Poland		
methandrostenolone	Metanabol	5 mg tablet	20 tablet box	Jelfa	Poland		
methandrostenolone	Metanabol	5 mg tablet	20 tablet box	Polfa	Poland	[NLM]	
methandrostenolone	Metanabol	1 mg tablet	20 tablet box	Polfa	Poland	[NLM]	
methandrostenolone	Metanabol	0.5% cream	n/a	Polfa	Poland	[NLM]	
Omnadren (testosterone blend)	Omnadren	250 mg/ml	1ml ampule	Jelfa	Poland		
Omnadren (testosterone blend)	Omnadren	250 mg/ml	1ml ampule	Polfa	Poland	[NLM]	
mesterolone	Proviron®	25 mg tablet	20 tablet box	Schering	Poland		
testosterone enanthate	Testosteronum Prolongatum	100 mg/ml	1 ml ampule	Jelfa	Poland		
testosterone enanthate	Testosteronum Prolongatum	100 mg/ml	1 ml ampule	Polfa	Poland	[NLM]	
testosterone propionate	Testosteronum Propionicum	25 mg/ml	1 ml ampule	Jelfa	Poland		
testosterone undecanoate	Undestor	40 mg capsules	60 capsule bottle	Organon	Poland		
testosterone undecanoate	Andriol	40 mg capsules	n/a	Organon	Portugal		
nandrolone phenylpropionate	Durabolin®	50 mg/ml	n/a	Organon	Portugal		
testosterone undecanoate (inj)	Nebido	250 mg/ml	4 ml ampule	Schering	Portugal		
mesterolone	Proviron®	25 mg tablet	20 tablet box	Schering	Portugal		
Sustenon 250 (testosterone blend)	Sustenon 250®	250 mg/ml	1 ml ampule	Organon	Portugal		
methyltestosterone	Testormon	10 mg tablet	n/a	Unitas	Portugal		
testosterone enanthate	Testoviron®-Depot	250 mg/ml	1 ml ampule	Schering	Portugal		
testosterone undecanoate	Andriol	40 mg capsules	n/a	Organon	Portugal		
testosterone enanthate	Testoviron®-Depot	250 mg/ml	1 ml ampule	Schering	Qatar	[NLM]	
nandrolone decanoate	Anabolin Forte	50 mg/ml	10 ml vial	Alfasan	Rumania		VET
nandrolone decanoate	Deca-Durabolin®	50 mg/ml	1 ml ampule	Organon	Rumania		
nandrolone decanoate	Decanofort	25 mg/ml	1 ml ampule	Terapia	Rumania		
methyltestosterone	Metil Testosteron	10 mg tablet	50 tablet box	Terapia	Rumania		
methandrostenolone	Naposim	5 mg tablet	20 tablet box	Terapia	Rumania		
testosterone phenylpropionate	Testolent	100 mg/ml	1 ml ampule	Sicomed	Rumania	[NLM]	
testosterone propionate	Testosteron	25 mg/ml	1 ml ampule	Sicomed	Rumania	[NLM]	
testosterone undecanoate	Undestor	40 mg capsules	60 capsule bottle	Organon	Rumania		
testosterone undecanoate	Andriol	40 mg capsules	n/a	Organon	Russia		
methandrostenolone	Metandienon	5 mg tablet	100 tablet box	Bioreaktor	Russia	[NLM]	

APPENDIX A-18

Errors or Omissions: Info@AnabolicsBook.com

Drug Availability Tables

Listings by Country

Generic Name	Trade Name	Dose	Packaging	Company	Country	Status	Vet
methandrostenolone	Metandrostenolon	5 mg tablet	100 tablet box	Akrihin	Russia	[NLM]	
methandrostenolone	Metandrostenolon	5 mg tablet	100 tablet box	Akrihin	Russia		
methandrostenolone	Metandrostenolon	5 mg tablet	100 tablet box	Bioreaktor	Russia	[NLM]	
mesterolone	Proviron®	25 mg tablet	20 tablet bottle	Schering	Russia		
Sustanon 250 (testosterone blend)	Sustanon (Cyctahoh 250)	250 mg/ml	1 ml ampule	Organon	Russia		
Testoviron (testosterone blend)	Testenat	100 mg/ml	1 ml ampule	Farmadon	Russia	[NLM]	
testosterone enanthate	Testenat 10%	100 mg/ml	1 ml ampule	Farmadon	Russia	[NLM]	
testosterone enanthate	Testenat 5%	50 mg/ml	1 ml ampule	Farmadon	Russia		
testosterone propionate	Testosterona Propionat	50, 100 mg/ml	1 ml ampule	Farmadon	Russia	[NLM]	
testosterone undecanoate	Andriol	40 mg capsules	n/a	Organon	Saudi Arabia		
testosterone enanthate	Testoviron®-Depot	250 mg/ml	1 ml ampule	Schering	Saudi Arabia		
testosterone undecanoate	Andriol	40 mg capsules	n/a	Organon	Serbia		
nandrolone phenylpropionate	Durabolin®	50 mg/ml	n/a	Organon	Serbia		
mesterolone	Proviron®	25 mg tablet	n/a	Alkoid	Serbia		
testosterone enanthate	Testosteron-Depo	250 mg/ml	1 ml ampule	Galenika	Serbia		
testosterone undecanoate	Andriol	40 mg capsules	60 capsule bottle	Organon	Singapore		
nandrolone decanoate	Deca-Durabolin®	25 mg/ml	1 ml ampule	Organon	Singapore		
testosterone cypionate	Depo-Testosterone®	100 mg/ml	10 ml vial	Pharmacia & Upjohn	Singapore		
mesterolone	Provironum	25 mg tablet	50 tablet bottle	Organon	Singapore		
Sustanon 250 (testosterone blend)	Sustanon "250"	250 mg/ml	1 ml ampule	Organon	Singapore		
mesterolone	Proviron®	25 mg tablet	20, 50 tablet bottle	Schering	Slovakia		
Sustanon 250 (testosterone blend)	Sustanon	250 mg/ml	1 ml ampule	Organon	Slovakia		
testosterone undecanoate	Undestor	40 mg capsules	n/a	Organon	Slovakia		
testosterone undecanoate	Androxon	40 mg capsules	60 capsule bottle	Donmed/Organon	South Africa		
nandrolone decanoate	Deca-Durabolin®	25, 50 mg/ml	1 ml ampule	Donmed/Organon	South Africa		
testosterone cypionate	Depo-Testosterone	100 mg/ml	10 ml vial	Pharmacia & Upjohn	South Africa		
testosterone cypionate	Depotrone	250 mg/ml	2 ml ampule	Propan-Zurich	South Africa		
testosterone undecanoate (inj)	Nebido	250 mg/ml	4 ml ampule	Schering	South Africa		
methenolone acetate	Primobolan® S	25 mg tablet	50 tablet bottle	Schering/Berlimed	South Africa		
mesterolone	Proviron®	25 mg tablet	20, 100 tablet bottle	Schering/Berlimed	South Africa		
Sustanon 250 (testosterone blend)	Sustanon '250'®	250 mg/ml	1 ml ampule	Donmed/Organon	South Africa		
nandrolone decanoate	Anabolin Forte	50 mg/ml	10, 50 ml vial	Alfasan	Spain		VET
nandrolone hexyloxyphenylpropionate	Anadur	25 mg/ml	2 ml ampule	Leo	Spain	[NLM]	
testosterone (patch)	Androderm®	2.5 mg patch	30, 60 patch box	Schwarz Pharma	Spain		
testosterone (patch)	Androderm®	5 mg patch	30 patch box	Schwarz Pharma	Spain		
nandrolone decanoate	Deca-Durabolin®	25, 50 mg/ml	1 ml ampule	Organon	Spain		
methyltestosterone	Longivol (plus estrogen)	1 mg tablet	n/a	Medical S.A.	Spain		
testosterone undecanoate (inj)	Nebido	250 mg/ml	4 ml ampule	Schering	Spain		
methenolone enanthate	Primobolan® Depot	100 mg/ml	1 ml ampule	Scherimed	Spain	[NLM]	
methenolone enanthate	Primobolan® Depot	100 mg/ml	1 ml ampule	Schering	Spain		
mesterolone	Proviron®	25 mg tablet	20 tablet box	Schering	Spain		
testosterone propionate	Testex Leo	25 mg/ml	1 ml ampule	Altana Pharma	Spain	[NLM]	
testosterone propionate	Testex Leo	25 mg/ml	1 ml ampule	Leo	Spain	[NLM]	
testosterone propionate	Testex Leo	25 mg/ml	1 ml ampule	Q Pharma	Spain		
testosterone cypionate	Testex Leo prolongatum	50, 125 mg/ml	2 ml ampule	Altana Pharma	Spain	[NLM]	
testosterone cypionate	Testex Leo prolongatum	50, 125 mg/ml	2 ml ampule	Leo	Spain		

APPENDIX A-19

Errors or Omissions: Info@AnabolicsBook.com

Drug Availability Tables
Listings by Country

Generic Name	Trade Name	Dose	Packaging	Company	Country	Status	Vet
testosterone cypionate	Testex Leo prolongatum	50, 125 mg/ml	2 ml ampule	Q Pharma	Spain		
testosterone (patch)	Testoderm	6 mg patch	10, 30 patch box	Esteve	Spain		
testosterone (patch)	Testoderm	4 mg patch	10 patch box	Esteve	Spain		
testosterone enanthate	Testoviron®-Depot	250 mg/ml	1 ml ampule	Schering	Spain		
stanozolol (oral)	Winstrol®	2 mg/ml	20 tablet box	Desma	Spain		
stanozolol (oral)	Winstrol®	2 mg tablet	20 tablet box	Zambon	Spain	[NLM]	
stanozolol (inj)	Winstrol® Depot	50 mg/ml	1 ml ampule	Desma	Spain		
stanozolol (inj)	Winstrol® Depot	50 mg/ml	1 ml ampule	Zambon	Spain	[NLM]	
testosterone undecanoate	Andriol	40 mg capsules	n/a	Organon	Sri Lanka		
testosterone enanthate	Testoviron®-Depot	250 mg/ml	1 ml ampule	Schering	Sri Lanka		
testosterone enanthate	Primoteston®-Depot	250 mg/ml	1 ml ampule	Schering	Sudan		
testosterone (gel)	Androgel	25, 50 mg	single dose packet	Besins	Sweden		
testosterone (patch)	Atmos	5 mg patch	n/a	Astra	Sweden		
nandrolone decanoate	Deca-Durabolin®	50 mg/ml	1 ml ampule	Organon	Sweden		
testosterone undecanoate (inj)	Nebido	250 mg/ml	4 ml ampule	Schering	Sweden		
testosterone (gel)	Testogel	25, 50 mg	single dose packet	Besins	Sweden		
testosterone enanthate	Testoviron®-Depot	250 mg/ml	1 ml ampule	Schering	Sweden		
testosterone undecanoate	Undestor	40 mg capsules	n/a	Organon	Switzerland		
testosterone undecanoate	Andriol	40 mg capsules	n/a	Organon	Switzerland		
testosterone (patch)	Androderm®	12.2 mg patch	n/a	Astrazenica	Switzerland		
nandrolone decanoate	Deca-Durabolin®	50 mg/ml	1 ml ampule	Organon	Switzerland		
testosterone enanthate	Testoviron®-Depot	250 mg/ml	1 ml ampule	Schering	Switzerland		
fluoxymesterone	Baojen	5 mg capsule	500 capsule bottle	Ta Fong	Taiwan		
testosterone cypionate	Biselmon Depot	50 mg/ml	n/a	Ta Fong	Taiwan		
fluoxymesterone	Chinglicosan	5 mg capsule	n/a	Ciiphar	Taiwan		
methandrostenolone	Chinlipan Tab	2 mg tablet	n/a	Chin Tien	Taiwan		
testosterone cypionate	Cyclo-Testosterone Depot	130 mg/ml	n/a	Astar	Taiwan		
nandrolone phenylpropionate	Daily Reborn Inj	25 mg/ml	n/a	Shiteh	Taiwan		
nandrolone decanoate	Deca-Durabolin®	50 mg/ml	1 ml ampule	Organon	Taiwan		
testosterone cypionate	Depot-Bifuron	50 mg/ml	n/a	Gentle	Taiwan		
testosterone cypionate	Depo-Testermon	200 mg/ml	n/a	CCPC	Taiwan		
testosterone cypionate	Depo-Testerone	200 mg/ml	n/a	Metro	Taiwan		
testosterone enanthate	DepoTestmon Inj	65 mg/ml	n/a	CCPC	Taiwan		
testosterone cypionate	Depo-Testomon	100 mg/ml	n/a	Li Ta	Taiwan		
testosterone cypionate	Depo-Testosterone CPP	100 mg/ml	n/a	Metro	Taiwan		
testosterone cypionate	Depot-Hormon MF	50 mg/ml	n/a	Sintong	Taiwan		
nandrolone phenylpropionate	Durabolin®	25 mg/ml	2 ml vial	Organon	Taiwan		
fluoxymesterone	Flouoxymesterone cap	5 mg capsule	n/a	Yuan Chou	Taiwan		
fluoxymesterone	Floxymesterone	5 mg capsule	n/a	Chen Ho	Taiwan		
fluoxymesterone	Fosteron	5 mg capsule	n/a	Health Chemical	Taiwan		
fluoxymesterone	Fu Lao Shu	10 mg capsule	n/a	Ming Ta	Taiwan		
fluoxymesterone	Fuloan	10 mg capsule	n/a	New Chem & Pharm	Taiwan		
fluoxymesterone	Lipaw	10 mg capsule	n/a	Long Der	Taiwan		
fluoxymesterone	Long	10 mg capsule	n/a	Century	Taiwan		
nandrolone phenylpropionate	Macrabone	25 mg/ml	n/a	Ta Fong	Taiwan		
nandrolone phenylpropionate	Metrobolin	25 mg/ml	n/a	Metro	Taiwan		

APPENDIX A-20

Errors or Omissions: Info@AnabolicsBook.com

Drug Availability Tables — Listings by Country

Generic Name	Trade Name	Dose	Packaging	Company	Country	Status	Vet
testosterone cypionate	Nannismon Depot	50, 100 mg/ml	n/a	Chi Sheng	Taiwan		
testosterone propionate	Nansmon Depot	25 mg/ml	n/a	Chi Sheng	Taiwan		
fluoxymesterone	ODK	5 mg capsule	n/a	Winston	Taiwan		
fluoxymesterone	Oralsterone	5 mg capsule	n/a	Long Der	Taiwan		
nandrolone phenylpropionate	Protosin Inj	25 mg/ml	n/a	Astar	Taiwan		
mesterolone	Proviron	25 mg tablet	50 tablet box	Schering	Taiwan		
testosterone undecanoate	Restandol	40 mg capsules	n/a	Organon	Taiwan		
nandrolone phenylpropionate	Rubolin	25 mg/ml	n/a	Ying Yuan	Taiwan		
fluoxymesterone	Sidomon	5 mg capsule	n/a	n/a	Taiwan		
nandrolone phenylpropionate	Sinbolin	25 mg/ml	n/a	Sinton	Taiwan		
stanozolol (oral)	Stanol	2 mg tablet	n/a	Hua Shin	Taiwan		
stanozolol (oral)	Stanozolol Tab	2 mg tablet	n/a	Chen Ho	Taiwan		
testosterone enanthate	Sunamon Depot Inj	130 mg/ml	n/a	Astar	Taiwan		
testosterone enanthate	Sunamon Inj	250 mg/ml	n/a	Astar	Taiwan		
Sustanon 250 (testosterone blend)	Sustanon 250	250 mg/ml	1 ml ampule	Organon	Taiwan		
fluoxymesterone	Tealigen	5 mg capsule	n/a	Ming ta	Taiwan		
testosterone enanthate	Testenan Depot	250 mg/ml	n/a	Sinton	Taiwan		
testosterone enanthate	Testermon	25 mg/ml	n/a	CCPC	Taiwan		
testosterone cypionate	Testorone Depot	100 mg/ml	n/a	Gentle	Taiwan		
testosterone propionate	Testosteron Depot	25 mg/ml	n/a	Gentle	Taiwan		
testosterone cypionate	Testosterone Cypionate Inj	200 mg/ml	n/a	Gwo Chyang	Taiwan		
testosterone cypionate	Testosterone Cypionate Inj	200 mg/ml	n/a	Tai Yu	Taiwan		
testosterone propionate	Testosterone Propionate Inj	25 mg/ml	n/a	Tai Yu	Taiwan		
testosterone enanthate	Testoviron Depot	250 mg/ml	1 ml ampule	Schering	Taiwan		
fluoxymesterone	Ton Lin	10 mg capsule	n/a	Chin Teng	Taiwan		
testosterone blend (misc)	Triolandren	250 mg/ml	1 ml ampule	Novartis	Taiwan		
fluoxymesterone	Vewon	5 mg tablet	n/a	Yung Shin	Taiwan		
fluoxymesterone	Vi Jane	10 mg capsule	n/a	Shyh Sar	Taiwan		
mesterolone	Vistimon	25 mg tablet	30 tablet box	Jenapharm	Taiwan		
fluoxymesterone	Waromom	5 mg tablet	n/a	Washington	Taiwan		
methandrostenolone	Ammipire	5 mg tablet	1000 tablet bottle	Ammipire	Thailand		
methandrostenolone	Anabol 10	10 mg tablet	500 tablet bottle	British Dispensary	Thailand		
methandrostenolone	Anabol 15	15 mg tablet	100 tablet bottle	British Dispensary	Thailand		
methandrostenolone	Anabol Tablets	5 mg tablet	1000 tablet bottle	British Dispensary	Thailand		
testosterone undecanoate	Andriol	40 mg capsules	10 capsule strip	Organon	Thailand		
oxymetholone	Androlic	50 mg tablet	100 tablet bottle	British Dispensary	Thailand		
stanozolol	Azolol	2.5, 5 mg tablet	400 tablet bottle	British Dispensary	Thailand		
stanozolol	Azolol Plus	2 mg tablet	n/a	British Dispensary	Thailand		
oxymetholone	Bonalone	50 mg tablet	100 tablet bottle	Body Research	Thailand	[NLM]	
oxandrolone	Bonavar	2.5 mg tablet	10 tablet strip	Body Research	Thailand		
stanozolol (oral)	Cetabon	2 mg tablet	10 tablet strip	Therapharma	Thailand		
testosterone cypionate	Cypionax	100 mg/ml	2 ml ampule	T.P. Drug Laboratories	Thailand		
methandrostenolone	Danabol DS	10 mg tablet	500 tablet bottle	Body Research	Thailand		
trenbolone hexahydrobenzylcarbonate	Danabolan	76 mg/ml	1.5 ml ampule	Body Research	Thailand	[NLM]	
nandrolone decanoate	Deca-Durabolin®	25, 50 mg/ml	1 ml ampule	Organon	Thailand		
methandrostenolone	Diabol-10	10 mg tablet	500 tablet bottle	Bukalo Trading Co.	Thailand		

APPENDIX A-21

Errors or Omissions: Info@AnabolicsBook.com

Drug Availability Tables

Listings by Country

Generic Name	Trade Name	Dose	Packaging	Company	Country	Status	Vet
methandrostenolone	Dronabol	10 mg tablet	500, 1000 tablet bottle	Berich	Thailand		
methandrostenolone	Dronabol	5 mg tablet	500 tablet bottle	Plaza Dispensary	Thailand		
fluoxymesterone	Halotestin®	5 mg tablet	100 tablet bottle	Pharmacia	Thailand		
methandrostenolone	Melic	5 mg tablet	1000 tablet box, bottle	Pharmasant	Thailand		
methyltestosterone	Metesto	25 mg tablet	100 tablet bottle	Acdhon	Thailand		
methandrostenolone	Methandon	5 mg tablet	1000 tablet bottle	Acdhon Co.	Thailand		
nandrolone phenylpropionate	Norabon	25 mg/ml	1 ml ampule	Phihalab	Thailand		
methenolone acetate	Primobolan® S	25 mg tablet	n/a	Schering	Thailand	[NLM]	
mesterolone	Provironum	25 mg tablet	150 tablet box	Schering	Thailand		
stanozolol (inj)	Stanol	50 mg/ml	1 ml ampule	Body Research	Thailand		
stanozolol (oral)	Stanol	5 mg tablet	200 tablet bottle	Body Research	Thailand		
stanozolol (oral)	Stanozodon	2 mg tablet	1000 tablet bottle	Acdhon Co.	Thailand		
Sustanon 250 (testosterone blend)	Sustanon '250'®	250 mg/ml	1 ml ampule	Organon	Thailand		
testosterone propionate	Testolic	50 mg/ml	2 ml ampule	T.P. Drug Laboratories	Thailand		
testosterone enanthate	Testoviron®-Depot	250 mg/ml	1 ml ampule	Schering	Thailand		
methyltestosterone	TP Men Hormone	10 mg dragee	24 tablets	TP Drugs	Thailand		
testosterone propionate	Viromone	50, 100 mg/ml	1 ml ampule	Paines	Thailand		
testosterone undecanoate	Andriol	40 mg capsules	n/a	Organon	Tunisia		
methyltestosterone	Androtardyl®	250 mg/ml	1 ml ampule	Schering	Tunisia		
oxymetholone	Afro	25 mg tablet	40 tablet box	Casel	Turkey		
methyltestosterone	Anapolon	50 mg tablet	20 tablet box	Ibrahim	Turkey		
methenolone enanthate	Hormobin	5 mg tablet	40 tablet box	Munrin Sahin	Turkey		
methenolone enanthate	Primobolan® Depot	100 mg/ml	1 ml ampule	Schering	Turkey		
mesterolone	Proviron	25 mg tablet	20 tablet box	Schering	Turkey		
Sustanon 250 (testosterone blend)	Sustanon 250®	250 mg/ml	1 ml ampule	Organon	Turkey		
testosterone undecanoate	Virigen	40 mg capsules	30 capsule bottle	Organon	Turkey		
oxymetholone	Anadrol 50®	50 mg tablet	100 tablet bottle	Alaven	U.S.		
oxymetholone	Anadrol 50®	50 mg tablet	100 tablet bottle	Unimed	U.S.	[NLM]	
testosterone (patch)	Androderm®	12.2 mg patch	60 patches/box	SmithKline Beecham	U.S.	[NLM]	
testosterone (patch)	Androderm®	12.2, 24.3 mg patch	60 patches/box	Watson Pharma	U.S.		
testosterone (gel)	Androgel	50, 75, 100 mg	single dose packet	Unimed	U.S.		
methyltestosterone	Android	10, 25 mg tablet	100 tablet bottle	Valeant	U.S.		
trenbolone acetate	ComponentTE-G® (+ estradiol)	20 mg pellet	40 pellet cartridge	VetLife	U.S.		VET
trenbolone acetate	ComponentTE-S® (+ estradiol)	20 mg pellet	120 pellet cartridge	VetLife	U.S.		VET
trenbolone acetate	ComponentT-H®	20 mg pellet	200 pellet cartridge	VetLife	U.S.		VET
trenbolone acetate	ComponentT-S®	20 mg pellet	140 pellet cartridge	VetLife	U.S.		VET
nandrolone decanoate	Deca-Durabolin®	100 mg/ml	1, 2 ml vial	Organon	U.S.	[NLM]	
nandrolone decanoate	Deca-Durabolin®	200 mg/ml	1 ml vial	Organon	U.S.	[NLM]	
testosterone enanthate	Delatestryl	200 mg/ml	1 ml syringe	BTG	U.S.	[NLM]	
testosterone enanthate	Delatestryl	200 mg/ml	5 ml vial	BTG	U.S.	[NLM]	
testosterone enanthate	Delatestryl	200 mg/ml	1 ml syringe	Indevus	U.S.		
testosterone enanthate	Delatestryl	200 mg/ml	5 ml vial	Indevus	U.S.		
testosterone cypionate	Depo-Testosterone®	100, 200 mg/ml	10 ml vial	Pharmacia & Upjohn	U.S.		
testosterone cypionate	Depo-Testosterone®	200 mg/ml	1 ml vial	Pharmacia & Upjohn	U.S.		
boldenone undecylenate	Equipoise®	25, 50 mg/ml	50 ml vial	Fort Dodge	U.S.		VET
trenbolone acetate	Finaplix-H®	20 mg pellet	100 pellet cartridge	Intervet	U.S.		VET

Errors or Omissions: Info@AnabolicsBook.com

Drug Availability Tables
Listings by Country

Generic Name	Trade Name	Dose	Packaging	Company	Country	Status	Vet
fluoxymesterone	Fluoxymesterone	10 mg tablet	100 tablet bottle	Rosemont	U.S.		
fluoxymesterone	Fluoxymesterone	10 mg tablet	100 tablet bottle	USL Pharma	U.S.		
fluoxymesterone	Fluoxymesterone	2, 5, 10 mg tablet	100 tablet bottle	USL Pharma	U.S.		
fluoxymesterone	Halotestin®	2, 5, 10 mg tablet	100 tablet bottle	Pharmacia & Upjohn	U.S.		
testosterone propionate (implant)	Implus-H	22 mg/pellet	n/a	Upjohn	U.S.		VET
methyltestosterone	Methyltestosterone	10 mg tablet	n/a	Global	U.S.		
mibolerone	mibolerone drops	100 mcg/ml	55 mg bottle	Wedgewood	U.S.		VET
nandrolone decanoate	nandrolone decanoate	50, 100, 200 mg/ml	1, 2 ml vial	Steris	U.S.	[NLM]	
nandrolone decanoate	Nandrolone Decanoate Inj	100 mg/ml	2 ml vial	Watson Pharma	U.S.	[NLM]	
nandrolone decanoate	Nandrolone Decanoate Inj	200 mg/ml	1 ml vial	Watson Pharma	U.S.	[NLM]	
oxandrolone	Oxandrin®	2.5, 10 mg tablet	100 tablet bottle	BTG	U.S.		
oxandrolone	Oxandrin®	2.5, 10 mg tablet	100 tablet bottle	Savient	U.S.		
oxandrolone	Oxandrolone	2.5, 10 mg tablet	100 tablet bottle	Kali Labs	U.S.		
oxandrolone	Oxandrolone	2.5, 10 mg tablet	100 tablet bottle	Roxane	U.S.		
oxandrolone	Oxandrolone	2.5, 10 mg tablet	100 tablet bottle	Sandoz	U.S.		
oxandrolone	Oxandrolone	2.5, 10 mg tablet	100 tablet bottle	Upsher Smith	U.S.		
trenbolone acetate	Revalor-200 (plus estradiol)	20 mg pellet	100 pellet cartridge	Intervet	U.S.		VET
trenbolone acetate	Revalor-G (plus estradiol)	20 mg pellet	20 pellet cartridge	Intervet	U.S.		VET
trenbolone acetate	Revalor-H (plus estradiol)	20 mg pellet	70 pellet cartridge	Intervet	U.S.		VET
trenbolone acetate	Revalor-IH (plus estradiol)	20 mg pellet	40 pellet cartridge	Intervet	U.S.		VET
trenbolone acetate	Revalor-IS (plus estradiol)	20 mg pellet	40 pellet cartridge	Intervet	U.S.		VET
trenbolone acetate	Revalor-S (plus estradiol)	20 mg pellet	60 pellet cartridge	Intervet	U.S.		VET
trenbolone acetate	Synovex plus (plus estradiol)	25 mg pellet	80 pellet cartridge	Fort Dodge	U.S.		VET
testosterone propionate (implant)	Synovex®-H (plus estrogen)	20 mg/pellet	n/a	Fort Dodge	U.S.		VET
testosterone cypionate	testosterone cypionate	100, 200 mg/ml	10 ml vial	Schein	U.S.	[NLM]	
testosterone cypionate	testosterone cypionate	200 mg/ml	1, 10 ml vial	Sicor	U.S.		
testosterone cypionate	testosterone cypionate	100, 200 mg/ml	10 ml vial	Steris	U.S.	[NLM]	
testosterone cypionate	Testosterone Cypionate Inj	200 mg/ml	1, 10 ml vial	Paddock Laboratories	U.S.		
testosterone cypionate	Testosterone Cypionate Inj	200 mg/ml	10 ml vial	Watson Pharma	U.S.		
testosterone enanthate	testosterone enanthate	100, 200 mg/ml	10 ml vial	Schein	U.S.	[NLM]	
testosterone enanthate	testosterone enanthate	200 mg/ml	5 ml vial	Steris	U.S.	[NLM]	
testosterone enanthate	Testosterone Enanthate Inj	200 mg/ml	5, 10 ml vial	Paddock Laboratories	U.S.		
testosterone enanthate	Testosterone Enanthate Inj	200 mg/ml	10 ml vial	Watson Pharma	U.S.		
testosterone propionate	testosterone propionate	100 mg/ml	10 ml vial	Steris	U.S.	[NLM]	
testosterone suspension	testosterone suspension	50, 100 mg/ml	10, 30 ml vial	Schein	U.S.	[NLM]	
testosterone suspension	testosterone suspension	50, 100 mg/ml	10, 30 ml vial	Steris	U.S.	[NLM]	
methyltestosterone	Testred	10 mg capsule	100 capsule bottle	ICN	U.S.		
methyltestosterone	Virilon (time released)	10 mg capsule	100, 1000 capsule bottle	Star	U.S.		
stanozolol (inj)	Winstrol®-V	50 mg/ml	10, 30ml vial	Pharmacia & Upjohn	U.S.	[NLM]	VET
stanozolol (oral)	Winstrol®-V	2 mg tablet	100 tablet bottle	Pharmacia & Upjohn	U.S.	[NLM]	VET
stanozolol (oral)	Winstrol®-V	2 mg chewable tab	100 tablet bottle	Pharmacia & Upjohn	U.S.	[NLM]	VET
testosterone undecanoate	Andriol	40 mg capsules	n/a	Organon	Ukraine		
testosterone undecanoate (inj)	Nebido	250 mg/ml	4 ml ampule	Schering	Ukraine		
mesterolone	Proviron®	25 mg tablet	20 tablet box	Schering	Ukraine		
testosterone propionate	Testosterony Propionat	50 mg/ml	1 ml ampule	Farmak	Ukraine		
testosterone undecanoate	Andriol	40 mg capsules	n/a	Organon	United Arab E		

APPENDIX A-23

Drug Availability Tables

Listings by Country

Generic Name	Trade Name	Dose	Packaging	Company	Country	Status
testosterone (patch)	Andropatch	2.5 mg patch	60 patches/box	GSK	United Kingdom	
testosterone (patch)	Andropatch	5 mg patch	30 patches/box	GSK	United Kingdom	
nandrolone decanoate	Deca-Durabolin®	50 mg/ml	1 ml ampule	Organon	United Kingdom	
testosterone undecanoate (inj)	Nebido	250 mg/ml	4 ml ampule	Schering	United Kingdom	
testosterone enanthate	Primoteston®-Depot	250 mg/ml	1 ml ampule	Schering	United Kingdom	
mesterolone	Proviron®	25 mg tablet	30 tablet box	Schering	United Kingdom	
testosterone undecanoate	Restandol	40 mg capsules	28, 56 capsule box	Organon	United Kingdom	
Sustanon 100 (testosterone blend)	Sustanon '100'®	100 mg/ml	1 ml ampule	Organon	United Kingdom	
Sustanon 250 (testosterone blend)	Sustanon '250'®	250 mg/ml	1 ml ampule	Organon	United Kingdom	
testosterone enanthate	Testosterone Enanthate	250 mg/ml	1 ml ampule	Cambridge	United Kingdom	
testosterone propionate	Virormone	50 mg/ml	2 ml ampule	Nordic	United Kingdom	
dihydrotestosterone	Andractim	25 mg/g	80 gram gel	Servimedic	Uruguay	
methyltestosterone	Glando Stridox	10 mg tablet	20 tablet box	Ion	Uruguay	
methyltestosterone	Metil Thomsina S	10 mg tablet	20 tablet box	Celsius	Uruguay	
mesterolone	Proviron®	25 mg tablet	n/a	Schering	Uruguay	
testosterone propionate	Testoforte 2.000	20 mg/ml	50 ml vial	Agofarma	Uruguay	VET
testosterone cypionate	Testosterona Ultra Lenta	100 mg/ml	20 ml vial	Dispert Labs.	Uruguay	
testosterone cypionate	Testosterona Ultra Lenta Fuerte	200 mg/ml	5 ml ampule	Dispert Labs.	Uruguay	VET
testosterone cypionate	Testosterona Ultra Lenta Fuerte	200 mg/ml	20 ml vial	Dispert Labs.	Uruguay	VET
testosterone enanthate	Testoviron®-Depot	250 mg/ml	1 ml ampule	Schering	Uruguay	VET
testosterone undecanoate	Andriol capsulas	40 mg capsules	n/a	Organon	Venezuela	
nandrolone decanoate	Deca-Durabolin®	25 mg/ml	1 ml ampule	Organon	Venezuela	
nandrolone decanoate	Deca-Durabolin®	50 mg/ml	1 ml syringe	Organon	Venezuela	
boldenone undecylenate	Ganabol	50 mg/ml	500 ml vial	Laboratorios VM	Venezuela	VET
boldenone undecylenate	Ganabol	25, 50 mg/ml	10, 50, 100, 250ml vial	Laboratorios VM	Venezuela	VET
testosterone undecanoate (inj)	Nebido	250 mg/ml	4 ml ampule	Schering	Venezuela	
methyltestosterone	Oreton	n/a	n/a	n/a	Venezuela	
Sustanon 250 (testosterone blend)	Polysteron 250	250 mg/ml	1 ml ampule	Organon	Venezuela	
mesterolone	Proviron®	25 mg tablet	15 tablet box	Schering	Venezuela	
testosterone enanthate	Proviron®-Depot	250 mg/ml	1 ml ampule	Schering	Venezuela	
testosterone undecanoate	Andriol	40 mg capsules	n/a	Organon	Vietnam	
Sustanon 250 (testosterone blend)	Sustanon "250"	250 mg/ml	1ml ampule	Organon	Vietnam	
testosterone undecanoate	Andriol	40 mg capsules	n/a	Organon	Yemen	
testosterone enanthate	Testoviron®-Depot	250 mg/ml	1 ml ampule	Schering	Yemen	
testosterone enanthate	Weratestone 250	250 mg/ml	1 ml ampule	Weimer Pharma	Zimbabwe	
testosterone enanthate	Weratestone 250	250 mg/ml	1 ml ampule	Weimer Pharma	Zimbabwe	

APPENDIX A-24

Errors or Omissions: Info@AnabolicsBook.com

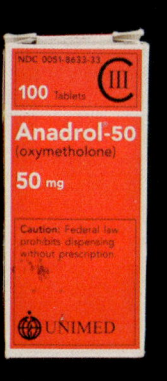

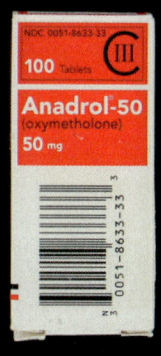

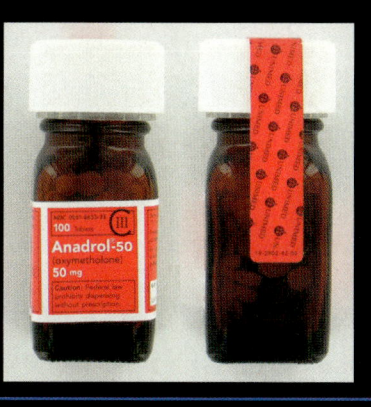

U.S. Anadrol-50 (Unimed, NLM)

Counterfeit U.S. Anadrol (Unimed)

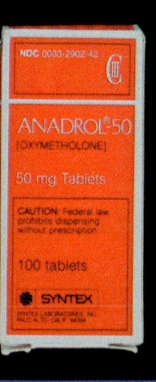

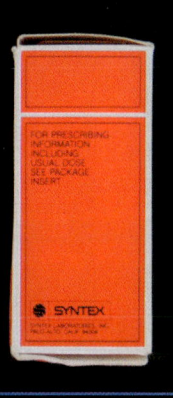

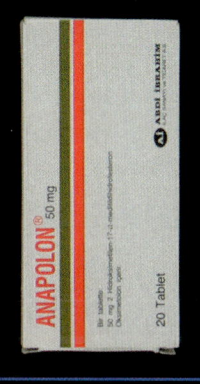

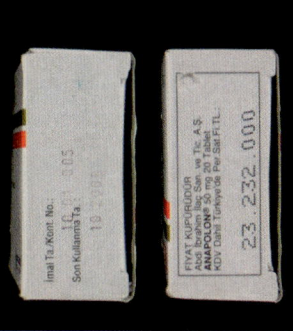

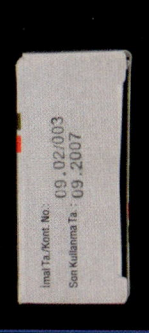

Counterfeit U.S. Anadrol (Syntex)

Anapolon from Turkey (real box)

Counterfeit Anapolon #1

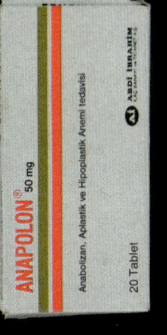

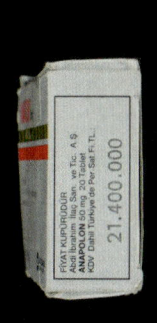

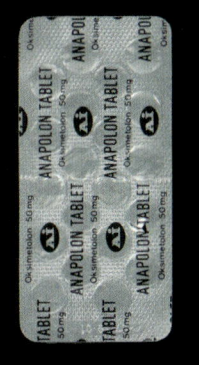

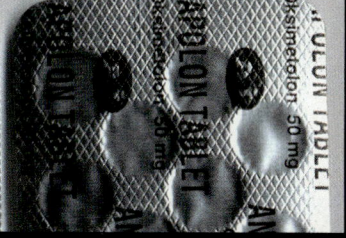

Counterfeit Anapolon #2

Real and Counterfeit Anapolon Strips (Real on Left)

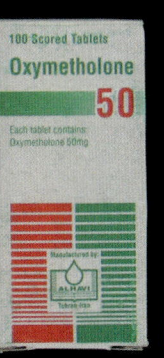

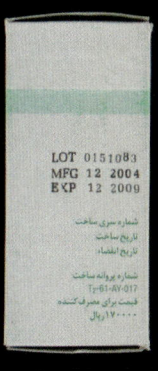

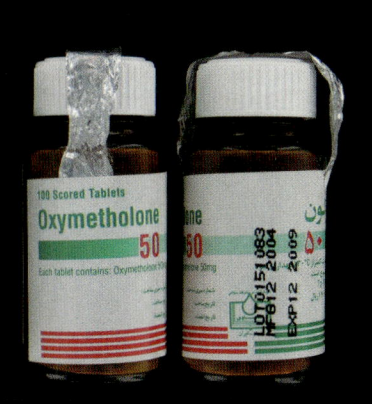

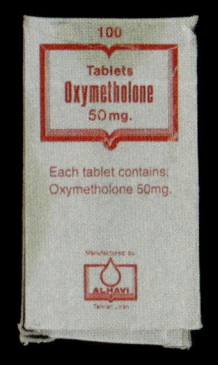

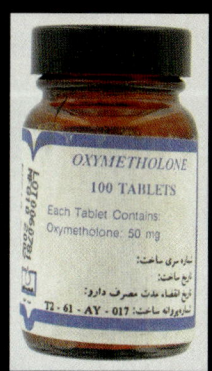

Generic from Alhavi (Iran)

Alhavi - Previous packaging

Appendix B

B-1

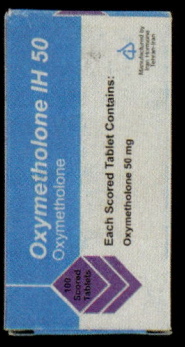

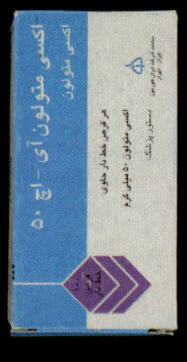

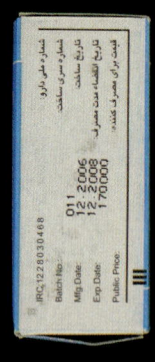

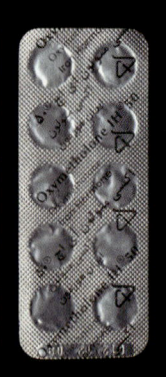

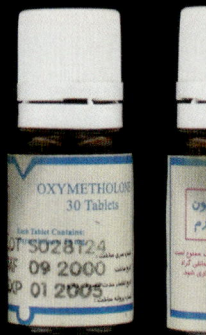

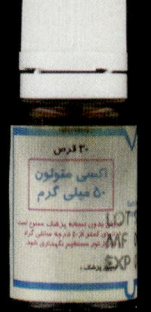

Oxymetholone IH (Iran)

Older bottle from Iran

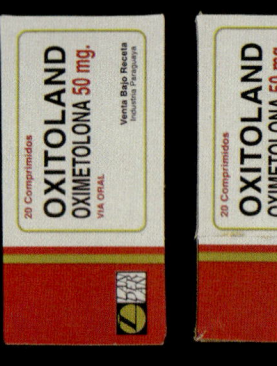

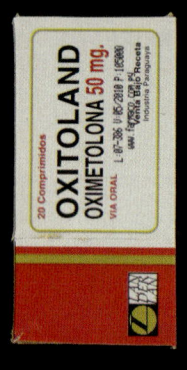

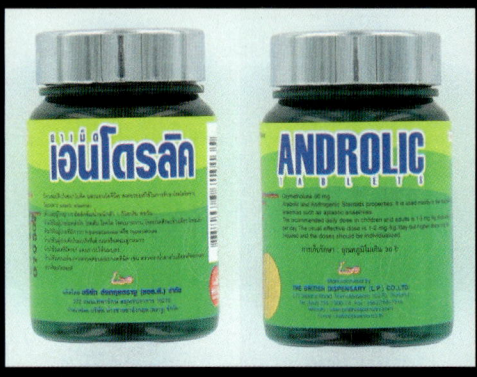

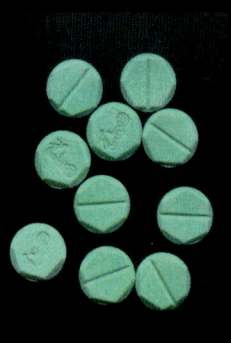

Oxitoland (Paraguay)

Androlic from British Dispensary (Thailand)

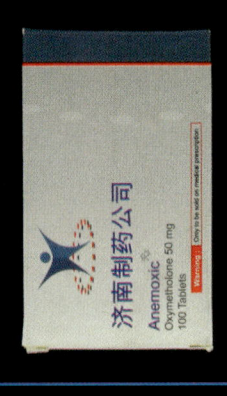

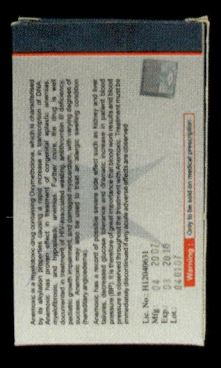

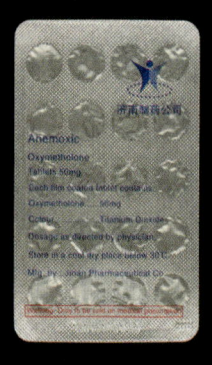

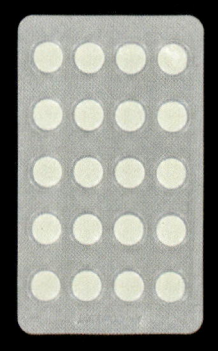

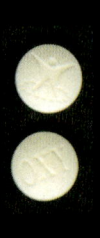

Anemoxic from Jinan Pharmaceuticals (China, Export)

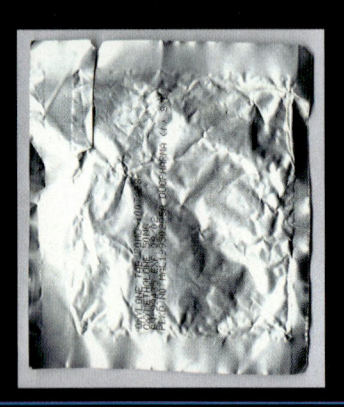

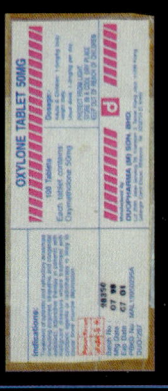

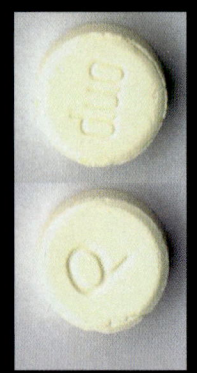

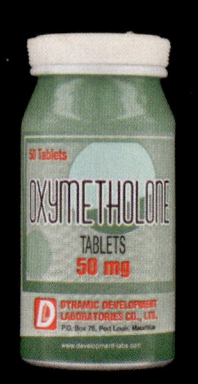

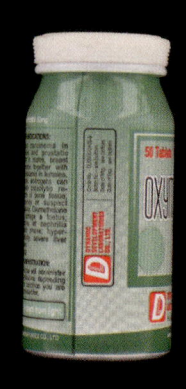

Oxylone from Duopharma (Malaysia)

Generic from Development Labs (Mauritius, Export)

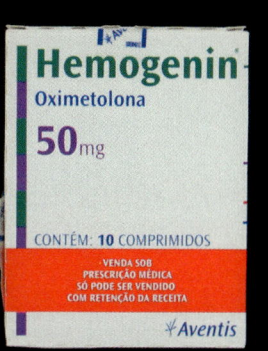

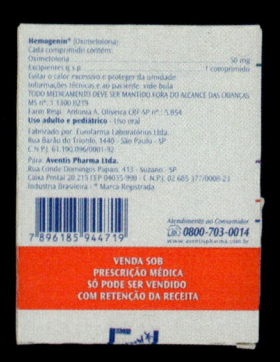

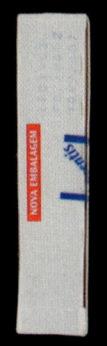

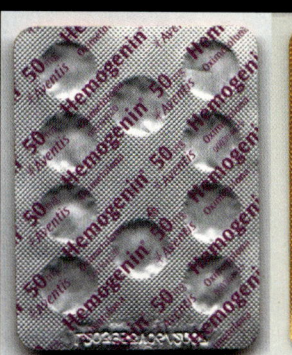

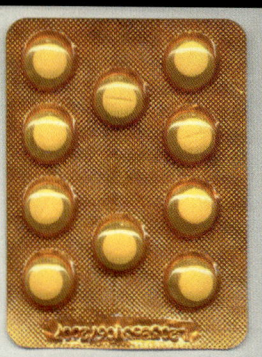

Hemogenin from Aventis Brazil

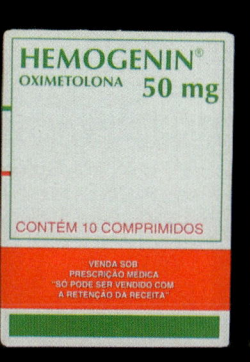

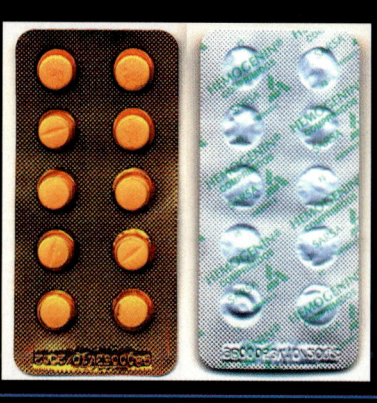

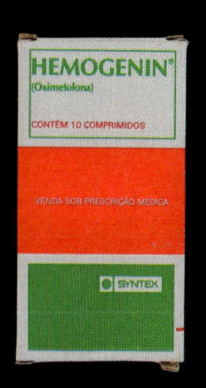

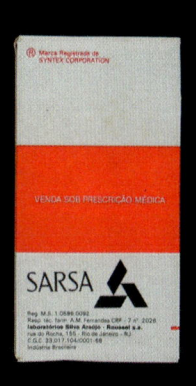

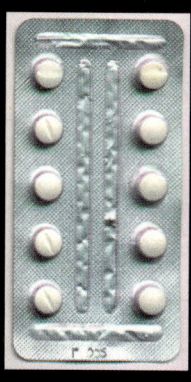

Another Older Hemogenin box and tablet strip

Hemogenin from Syntex/Sarsa Brazil (NLM)

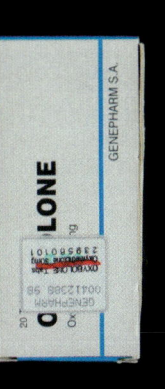

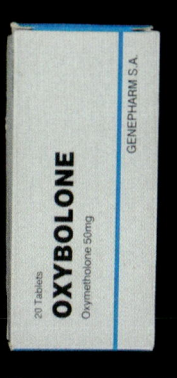

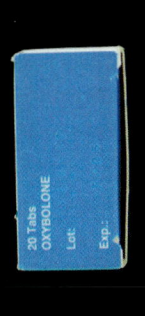

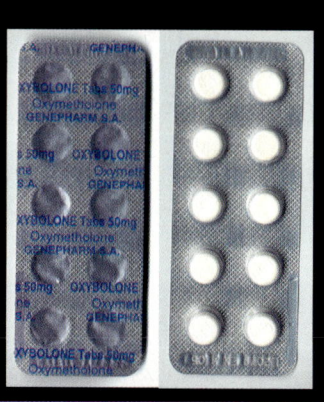

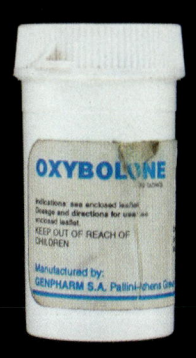

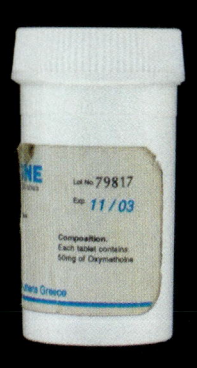

Oxybolone from Genepharm (Greece)

Counterfeit Oxybolone

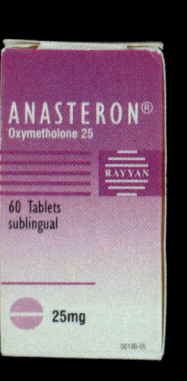

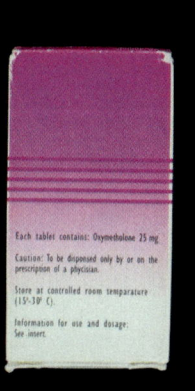

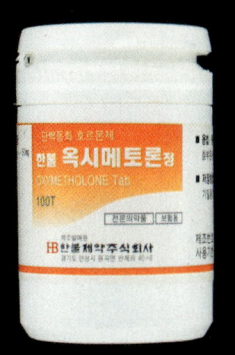

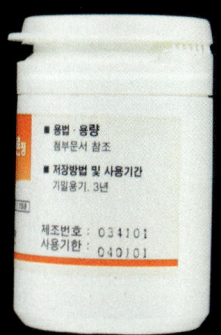

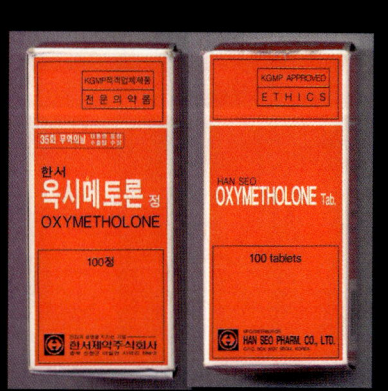

Fake Anasteron (Greece, Export)

Han Bul Generic (Korea)

Han Seo Oxymetholone (Korea)

Appendix B

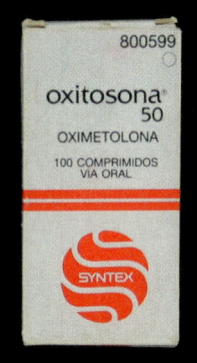

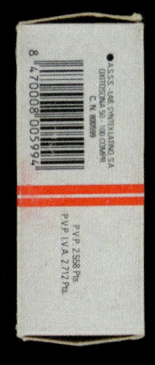

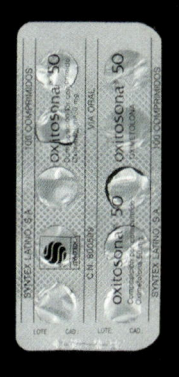

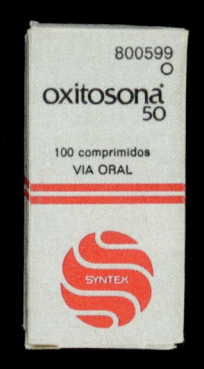

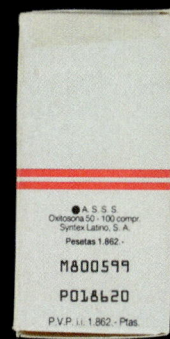

Oxitosona from Spain (NLM)

Counterfeit Oxitosona

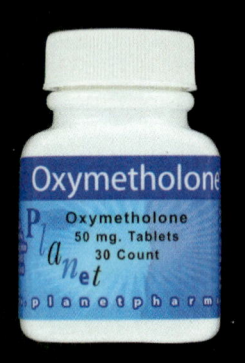

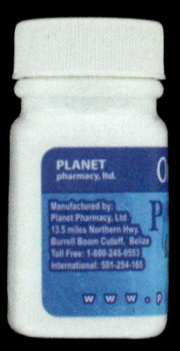

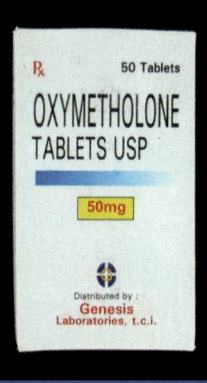

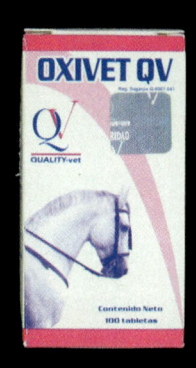

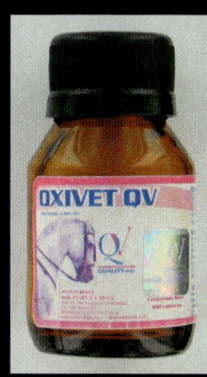

Planet Pharmacy (Belize) NLM

Genesis (Singapore) NLM

Oxivet from Quality Vet (Mexico) NLM

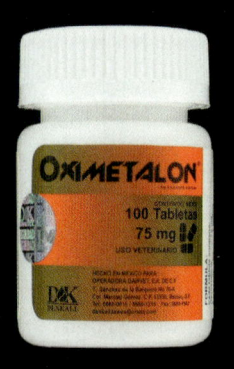

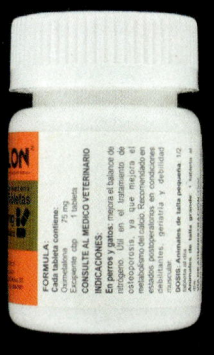

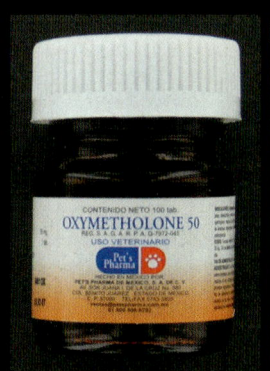

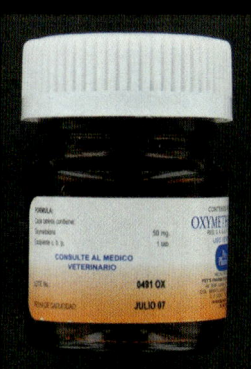

Oximetalon from Denkall (Mexico) NLM

Generic from Pet's Pharma (Mexico) NLM

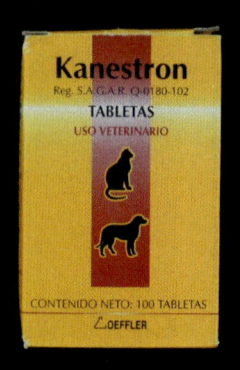

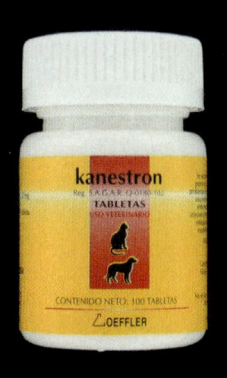

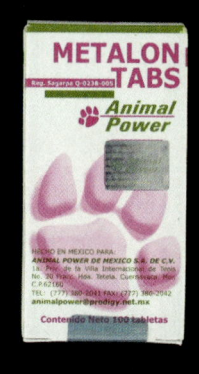

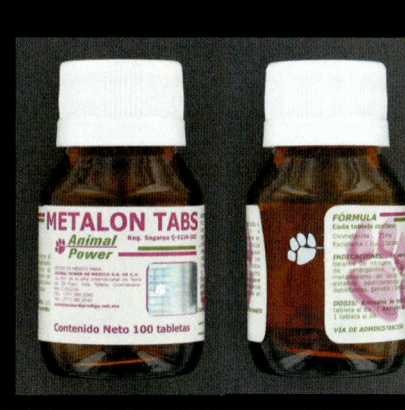

Kanestron from Loeffler (Mexico) NLM

Metalon from Animal Power (Mexico) NLM

B-4

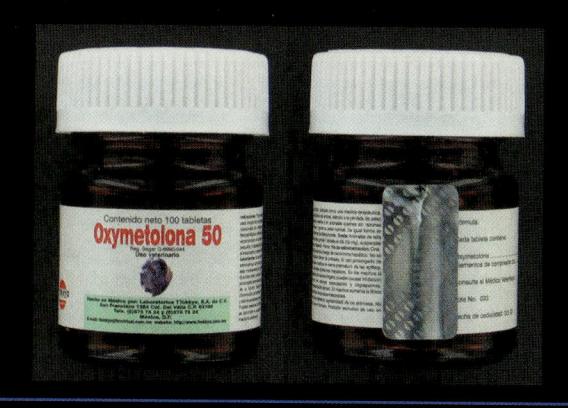

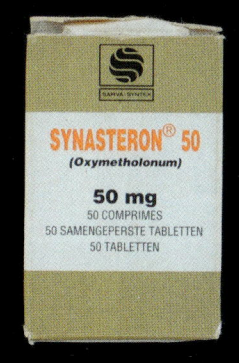

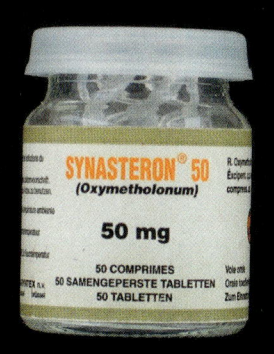

Oxymetolona from Ttokkyo Mexico (NLM)

Counterfeit Synasteron (Belgium)

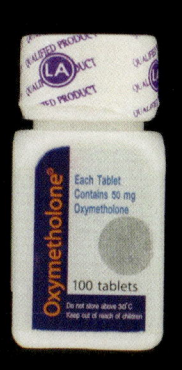

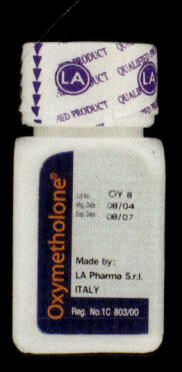

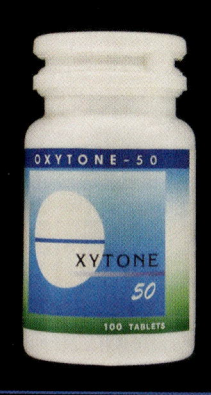

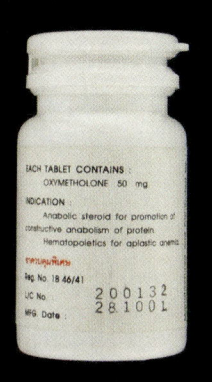

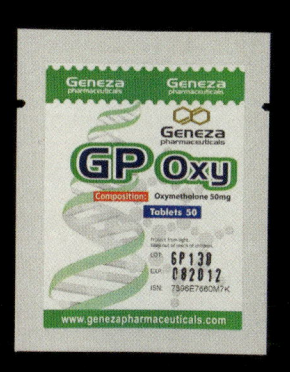

LA Pharma (Thai UG)

Oxytone from SB Laboratories (Thai UG)

Geneza (Underground)

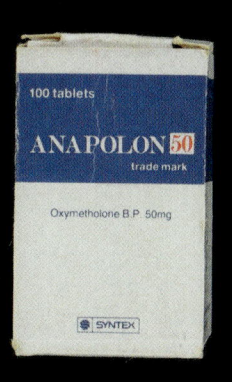

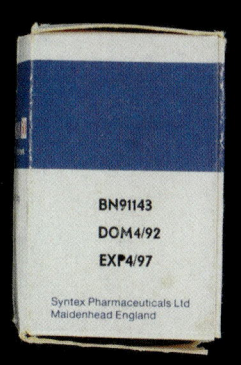

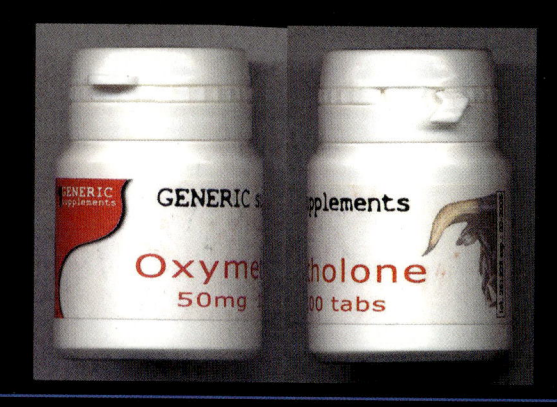

Counterfeit Anapolon from the U.K.

Oxy from Generic Supplements (Underground)

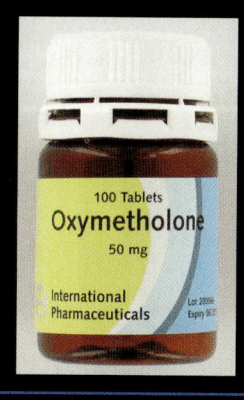

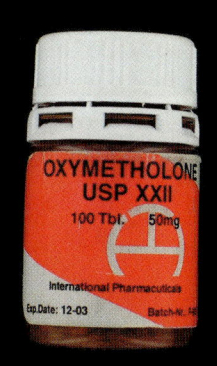

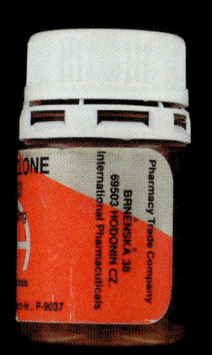

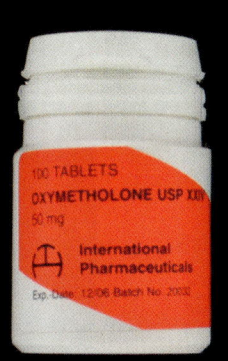

International Pharmaceuticals (UG)

Counterfeit IP bottle

Counterfeit IP bottle

Appendix B

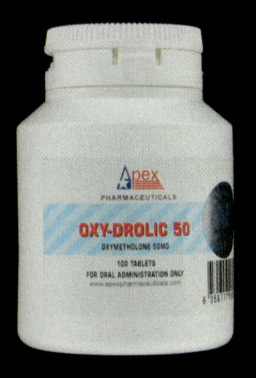

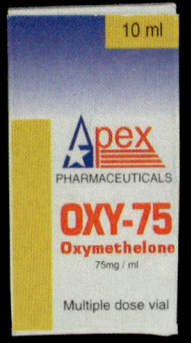

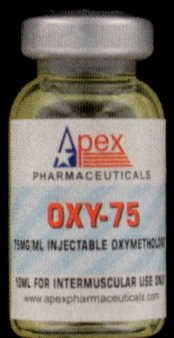

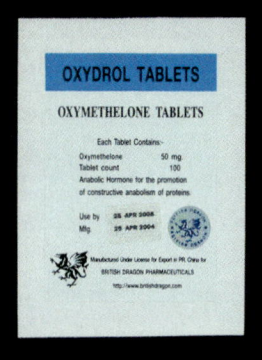

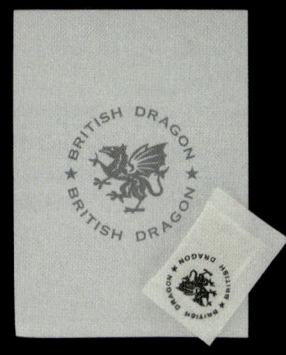

Apex oral and injectable oxymetholone products (Underground)

British Dragon Oxydrol (Underground, NLM)

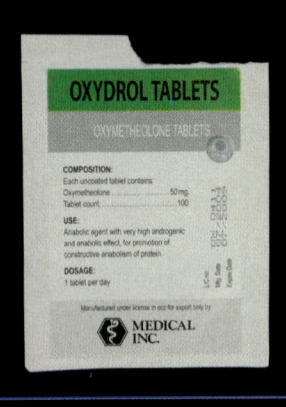

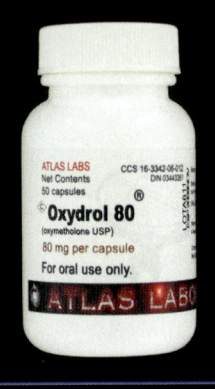

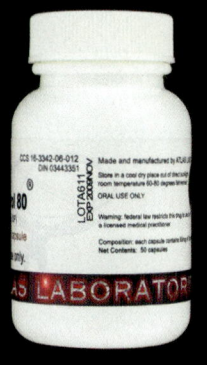

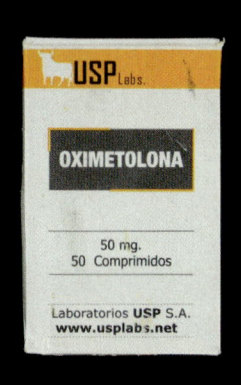

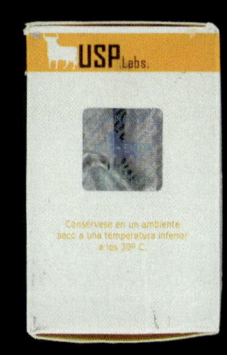

Oxydrol from Medical (UG)

Atlas (UG, NLM)

USP Labs (Underground)

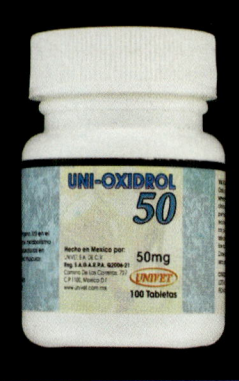

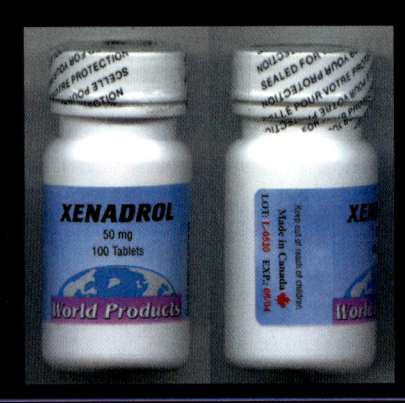

Univet (Mexico, UG)

Xenadrol from World (Underground)

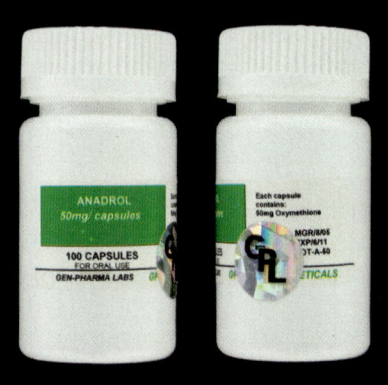

Gen-Pharma (UG, NLM)

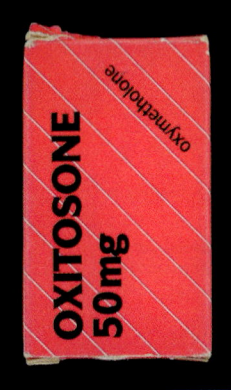

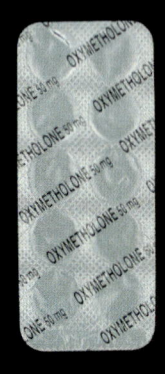

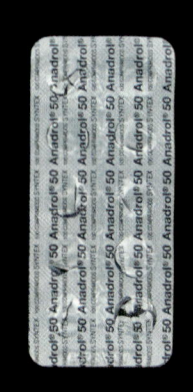

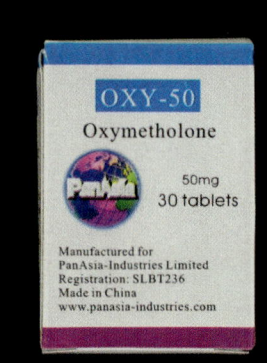

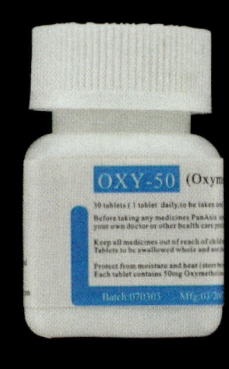

Fake Oxitosone (no such brand exists)

Fake tablet strip

Panasia (Underground)

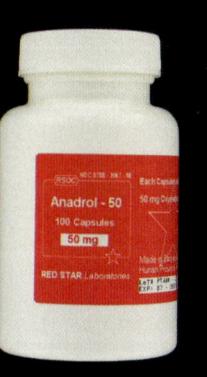

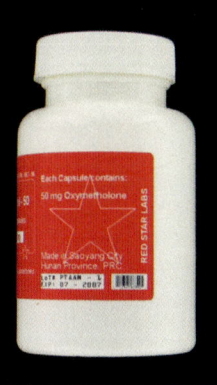

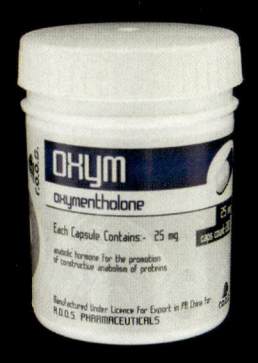

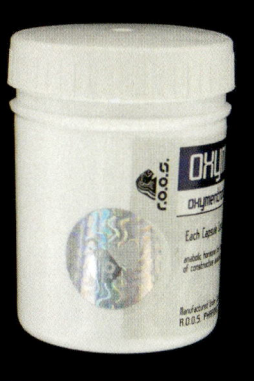

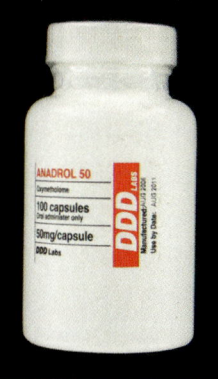

Underground Products from Red Star (NLM), R.O.O.S., and DDD

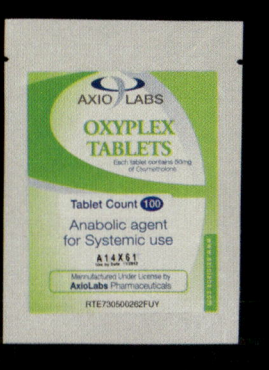

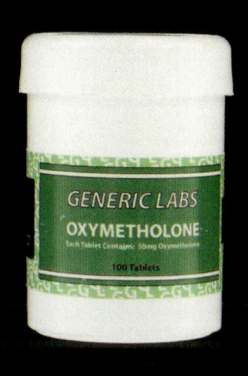

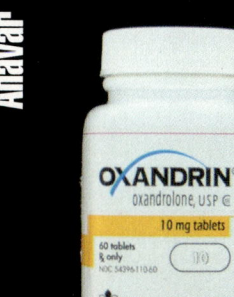

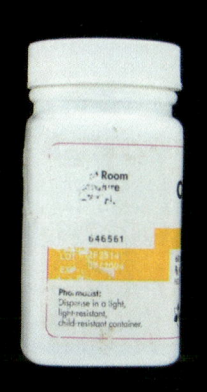

Anavar

Axio Labs (Underground) | Generic Labs (Underground) | U.S. Oxandrin 10mg tablets (BTG, NLM)

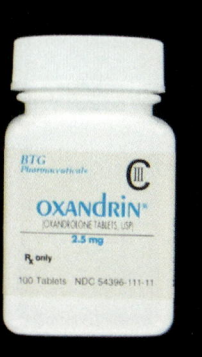

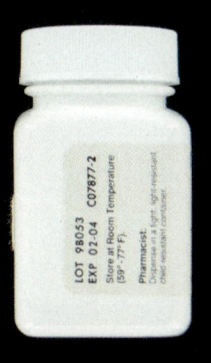

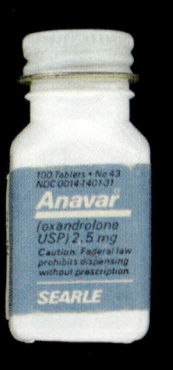

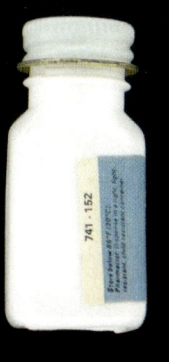

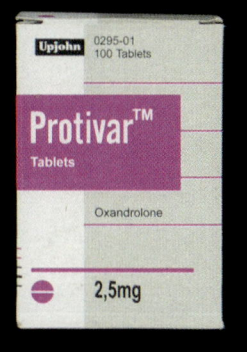

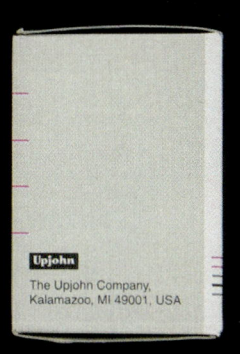

Old bottle of 2.5mg Oxandrin (U.S.) | Fake U.S. Anavar | Fake U.S. Protivar

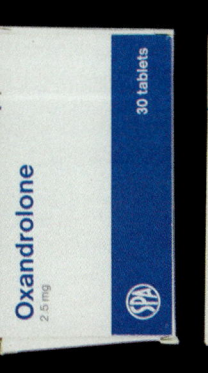

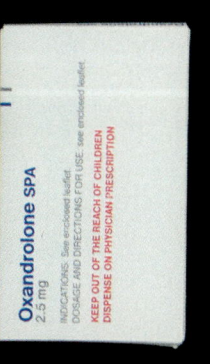

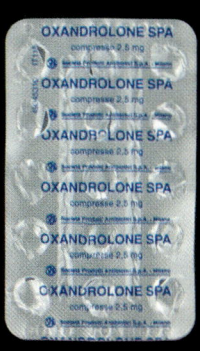

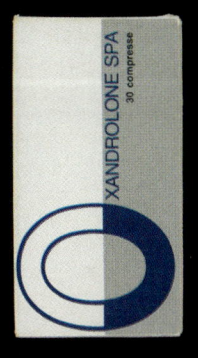

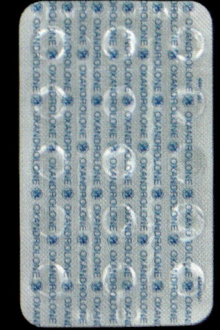

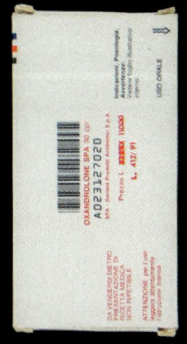

Real Italian Export (from SPA) | Italian domestic from SPA (NLM)

Appendix B

B-7

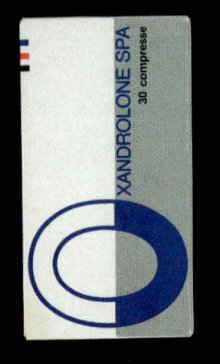

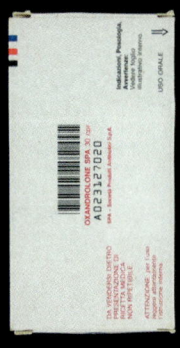

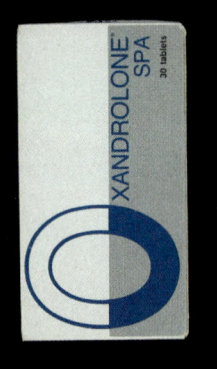

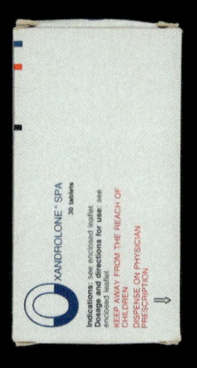

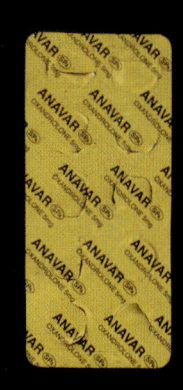

Counterfeit SPA #1

Counterfeit SPA #2

Counterfeit Anavar (Italy)

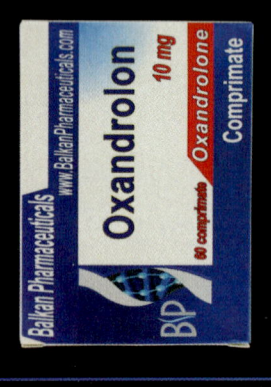

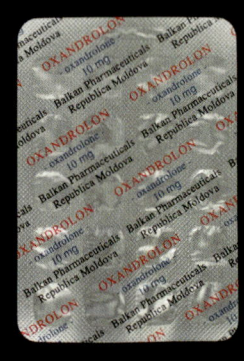

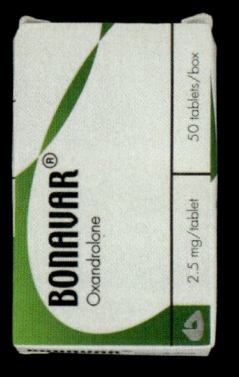

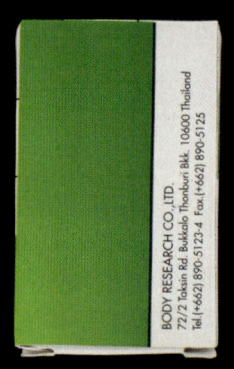

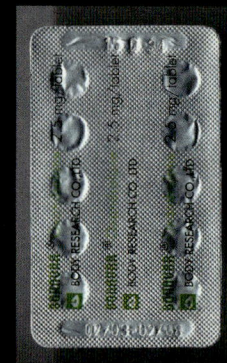

Oxandrolon from Balkan (Moldova)

Bonavar from Body Research (Thailand)

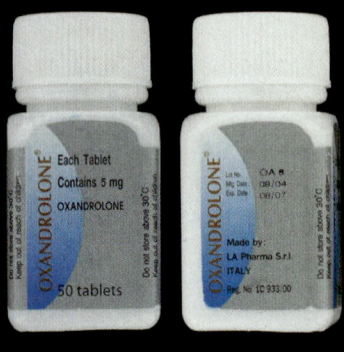

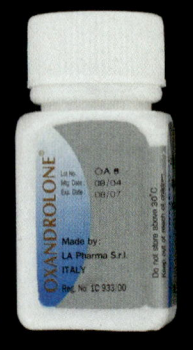

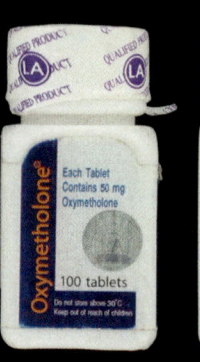

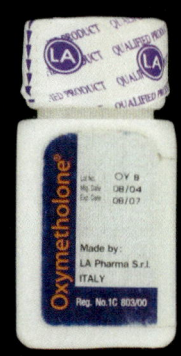

Bogus Italian export (found in Thailand)

Underground common in Thailand

Genesis (Singapore) NLM

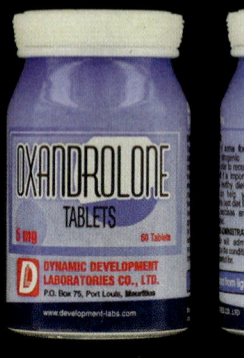

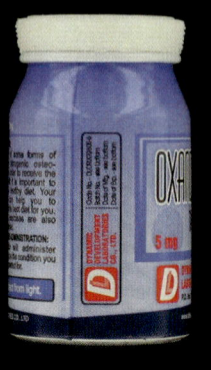

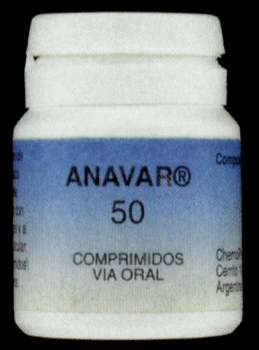

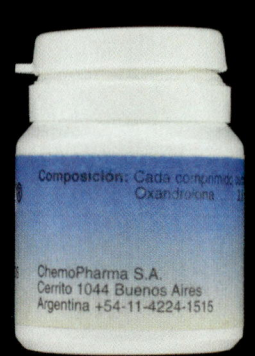

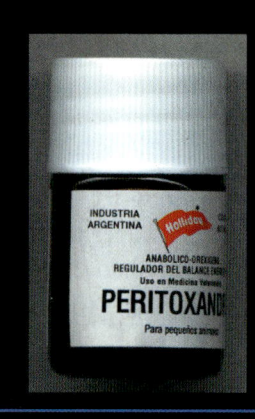

Development Labs generic (Mauritius, Export)

Fake Anavar from Argentina

Another Fake (Argentina)

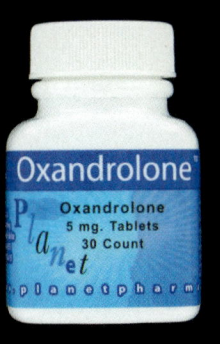

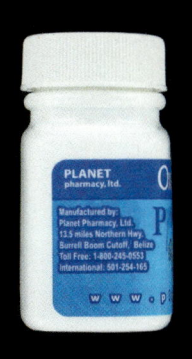

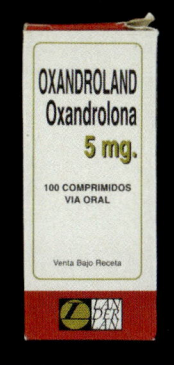

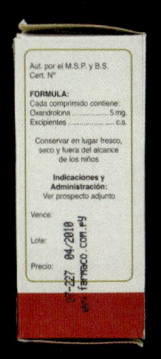

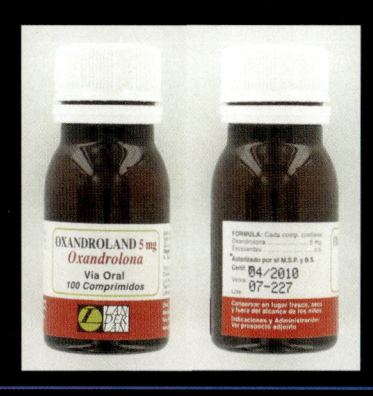

Planet Pharmacy generic (Belize) NLM

Oxandroland from Landerlan (Paraguay)

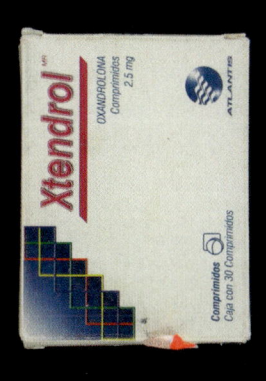

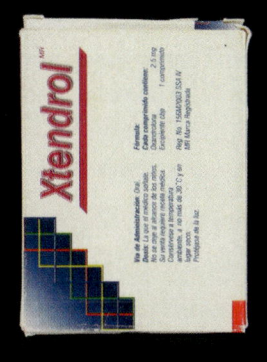

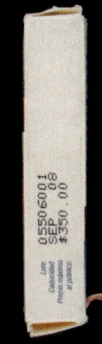

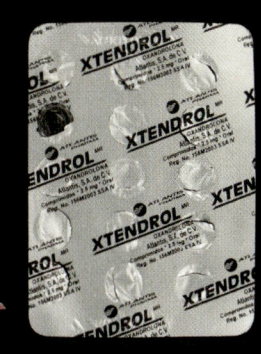

Xtendrol from Atlantis (Mexico)

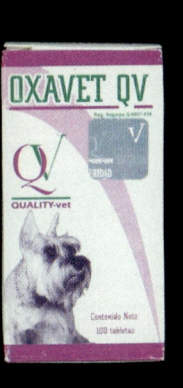

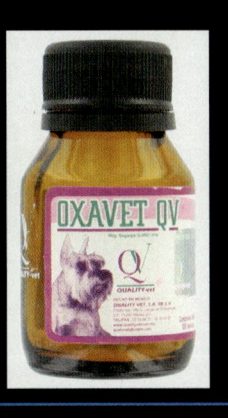

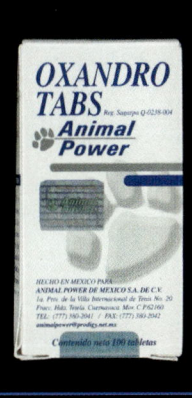

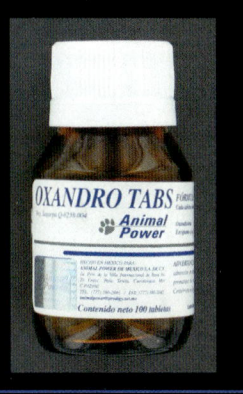

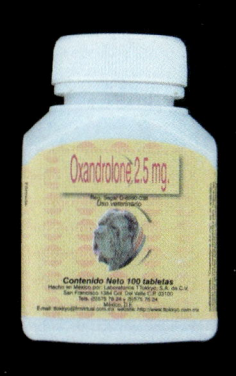

Oxavet from Quality Vet (Mexico) NLM

Oxandro Tabs from Animal Power (Mexico) NLM

Ttokkyo Mexico (NLM)

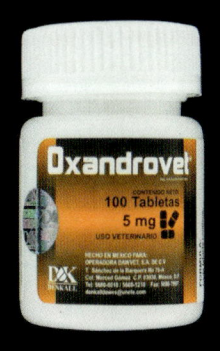

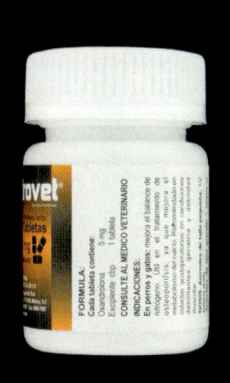

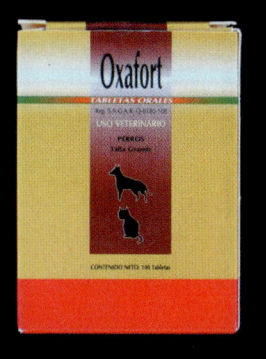

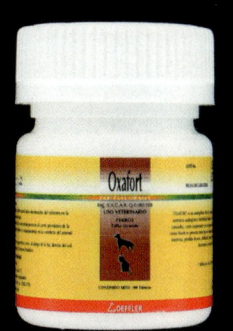

Oxandrovet from Denkall (Mexico) NLM

Loeffler's Oxafort (Mexico) NLM

Appendix B

B-9

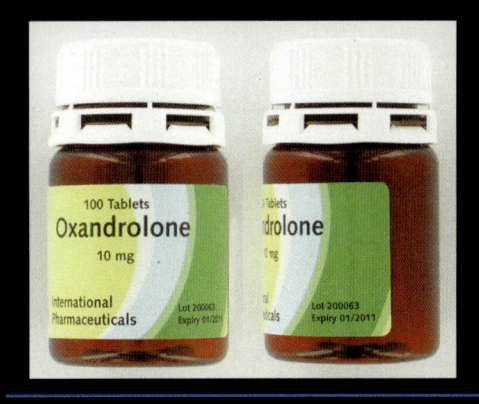

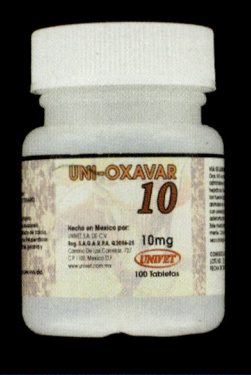

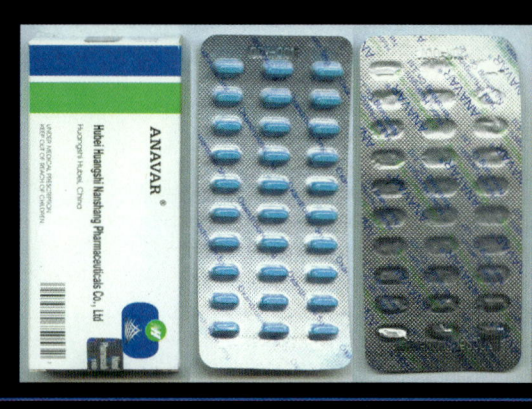

International Pharmaceuticals (UG)   Univet (Mexico, UG)   Fake Hubei product (China)

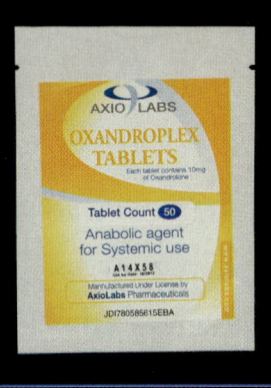

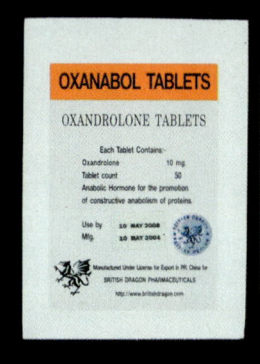

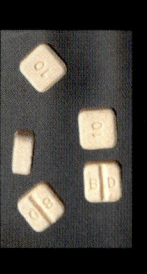

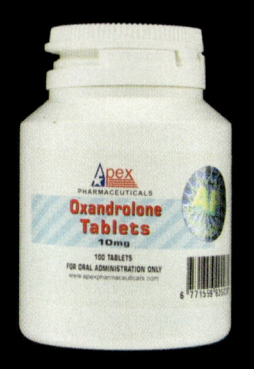

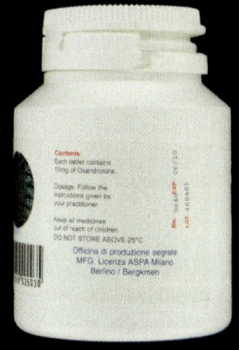

Axio Labs (Underground)   British Dragon (Underground) NLM   Apex (Underground)

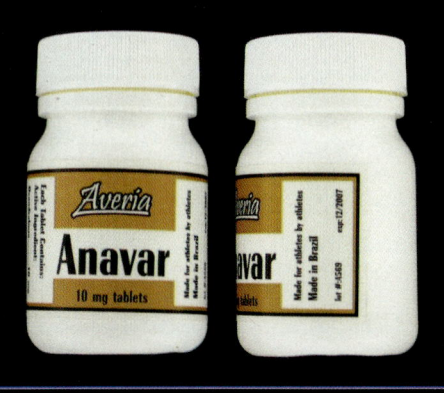

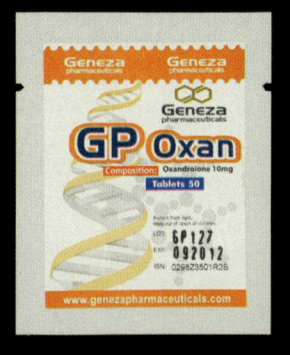

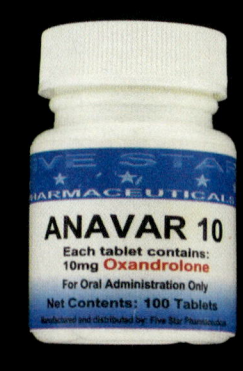

Averia (Underground)   Geneza (Underground)   Five Star Anavar (UG)

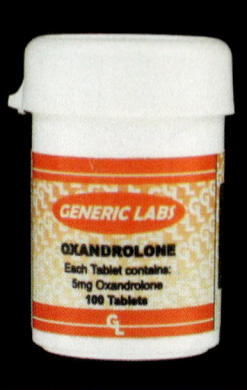

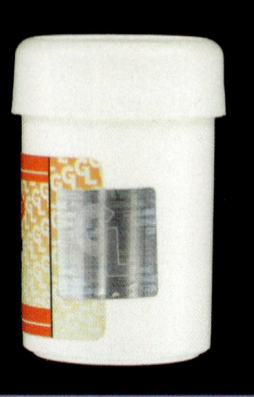

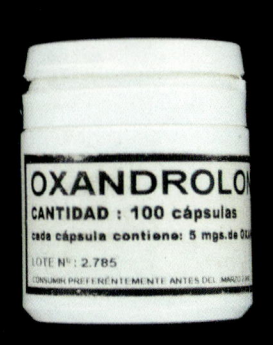

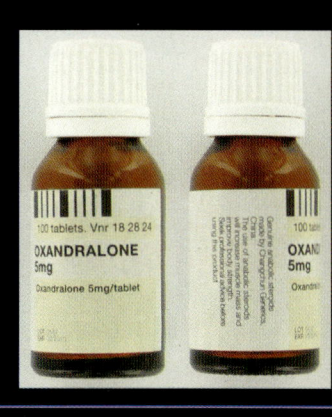

Generic Labs (UG)   Fake generic bottle   Another fake oxandrolone

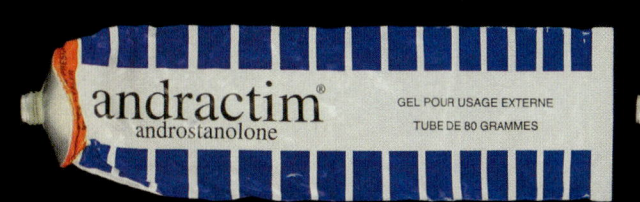

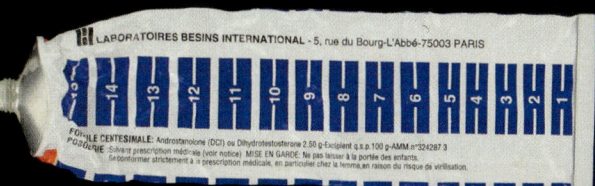

Andractim

Andractim from Besins (France)

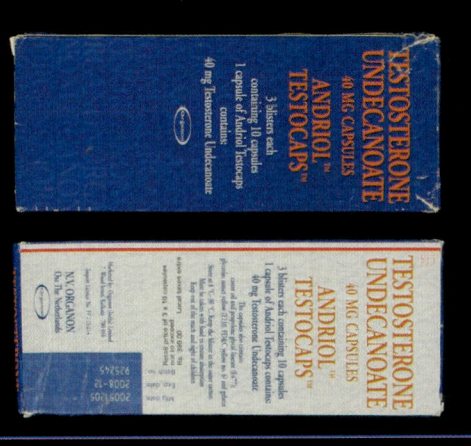

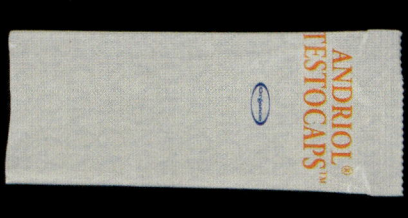

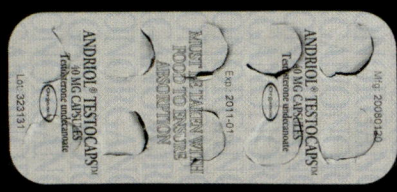

Andriol

Greek Andriol Testocaps

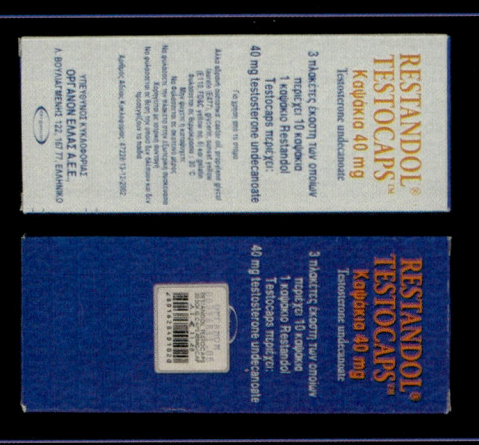

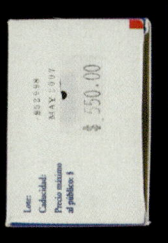

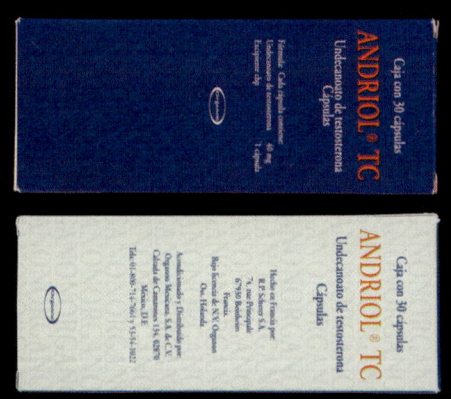

Restandiol from Greece (NLM)

Andriol Testocaps (Mexico)

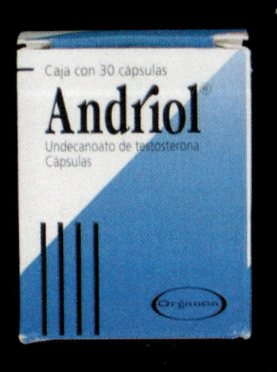

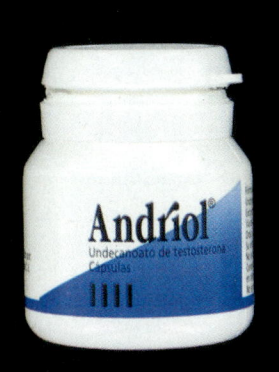

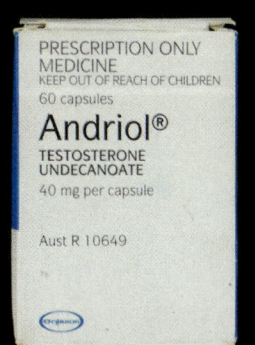

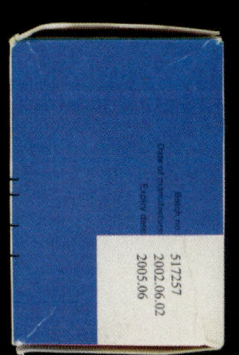

Old Andriol from Mexico

Andriol from Australia

Appendix B

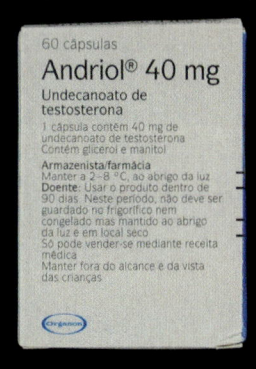

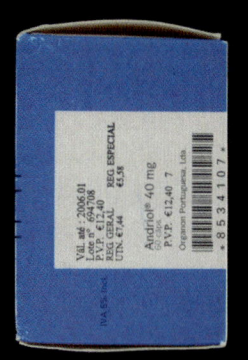

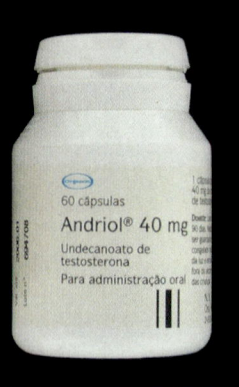

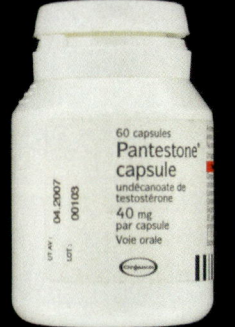

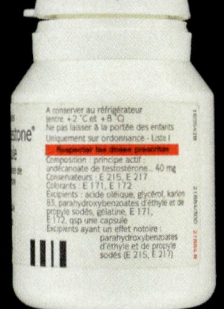

Andriol from Portugal | Pantestone (France)

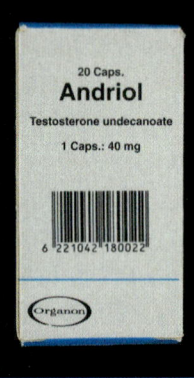

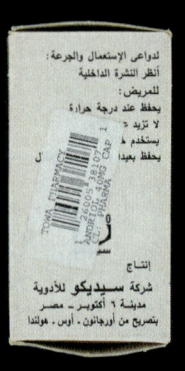

Andriol from Egypt | Andriol Testocaps (India)

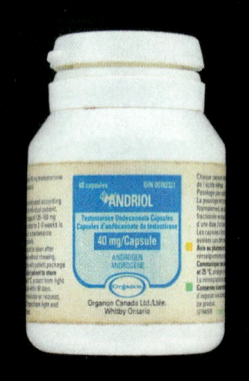

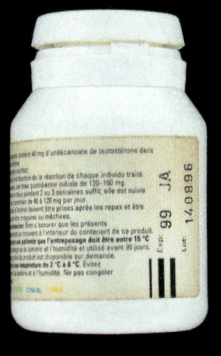

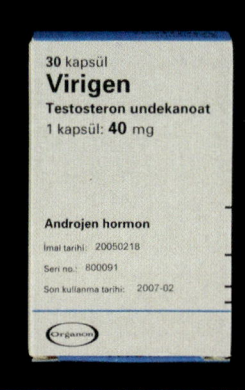

Canadian Andriol | Virigen from Turkey

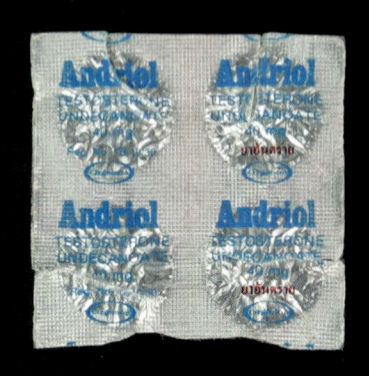

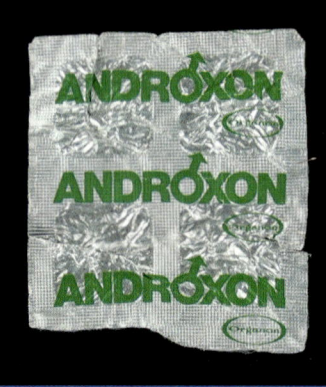

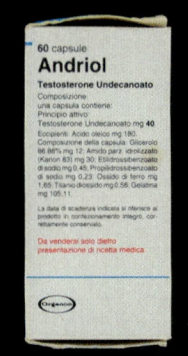

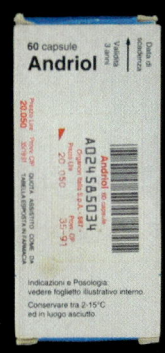

Andriol strip from Thailand | Androxon (Brazil) | Italian Andriol

Androderm

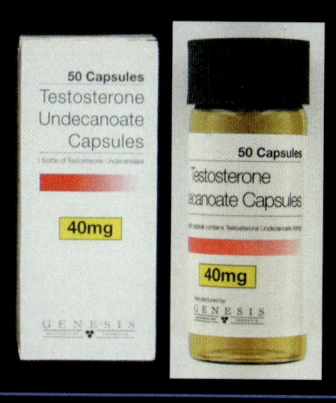

Genesis (Singapore) NLM

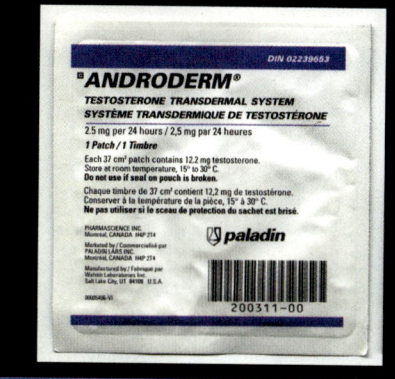

Canadian Androderm

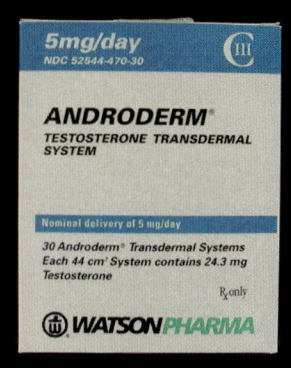

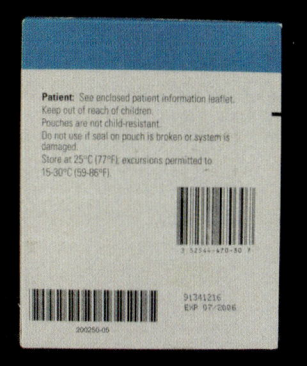

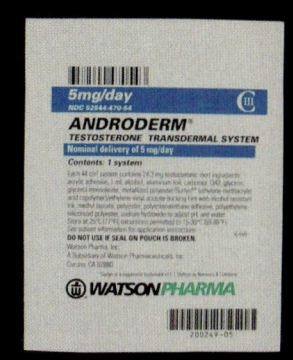

U.S. Androderm from Watson Pharma (5mg)

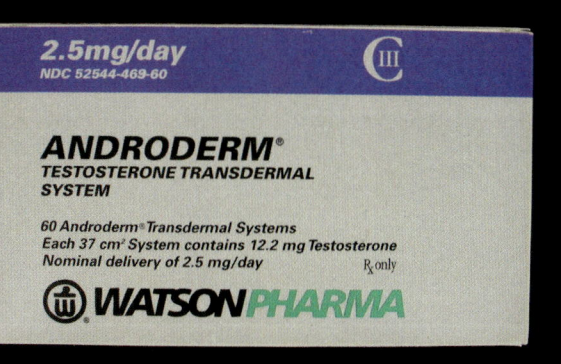

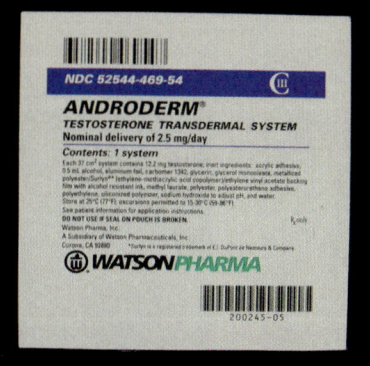

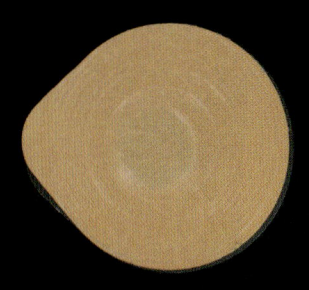

U.S. Androderm (2.5mg)

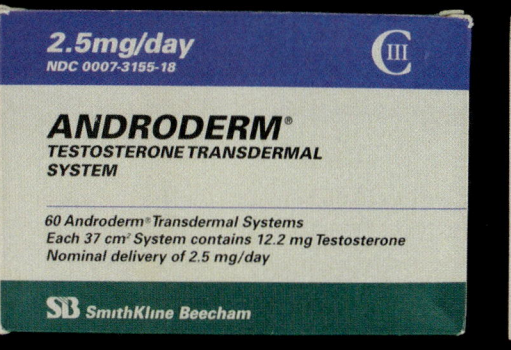

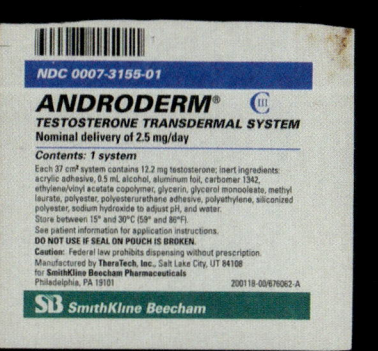

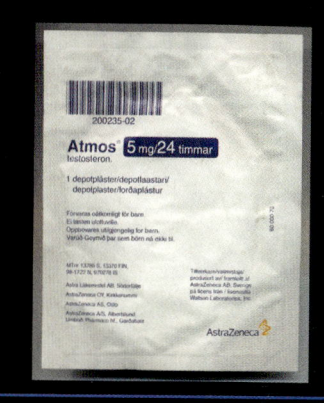

Old U.S. packaging

Atmos from Sweden

Appendix B

Androgel

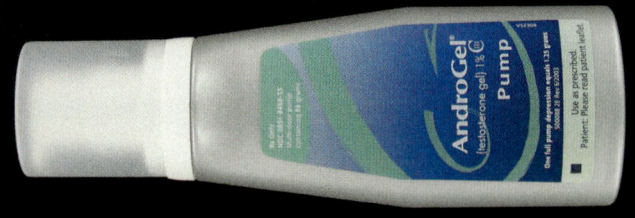

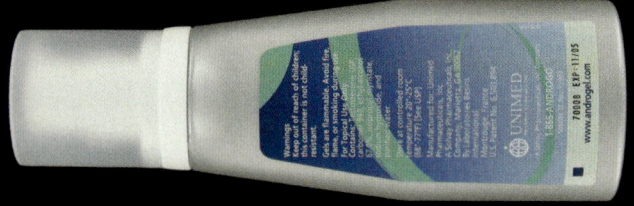

Androgel Pump (U.S.)

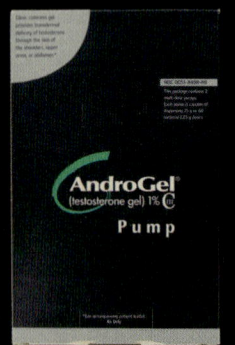

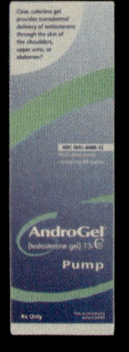

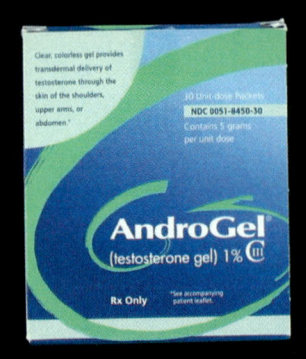

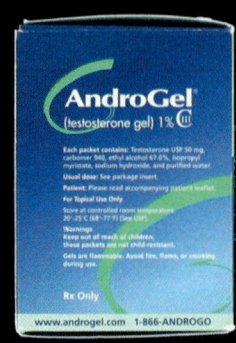

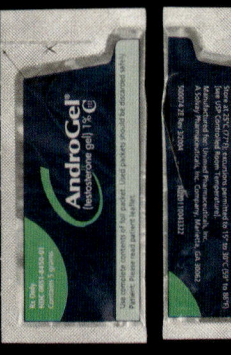

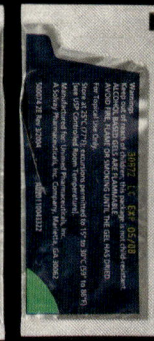

Androgel Pump boxes

U.S. Androgel box and gel packet

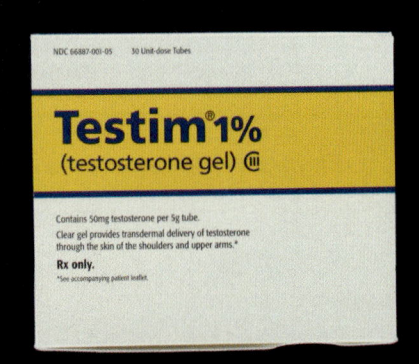

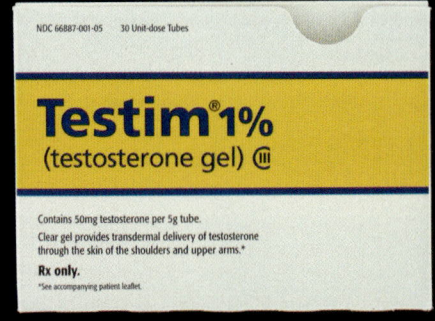

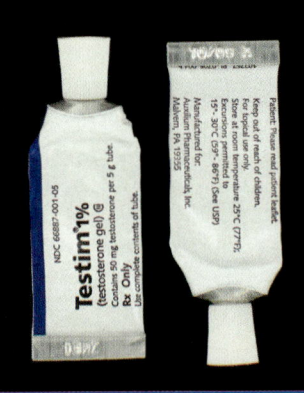

U.S. Testim

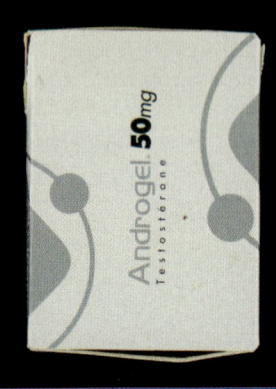

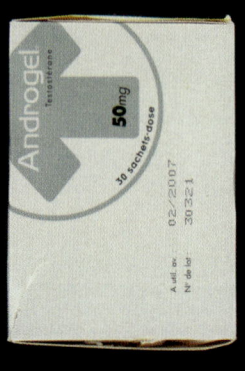

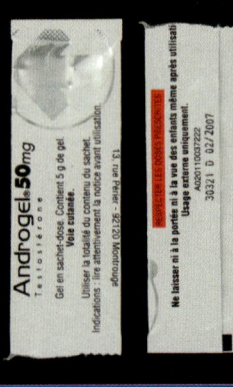

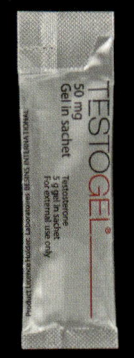

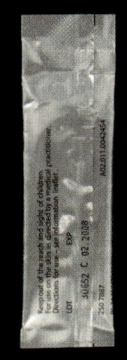

Androgel (France)

Testogel (UK)

B-14

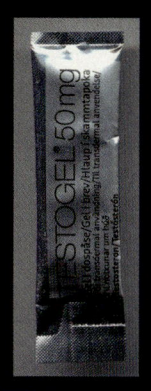

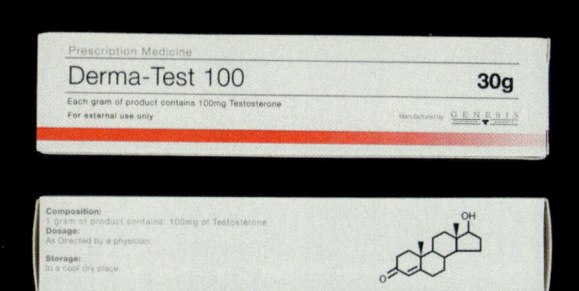

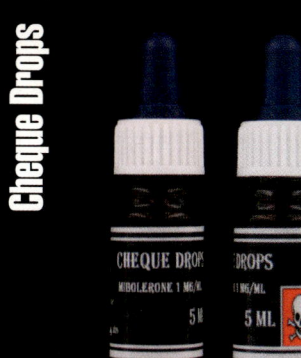

Testogel (Iceland) | Derma-Test 100 from Genesis (Singapore) NLM | Cheque Drops | Hardcore Labs (Underground)

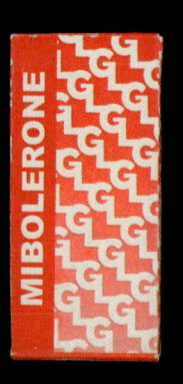

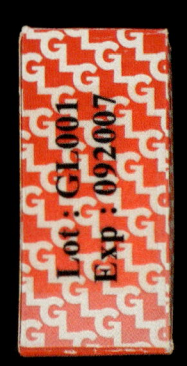

Deca-Durabolin

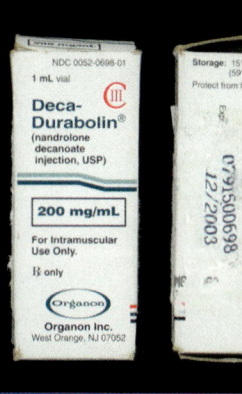

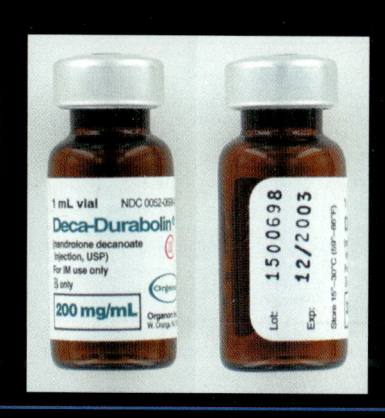

Generic from GL (UG) | U.S. Deca-Durabolin from Organon (NLM)

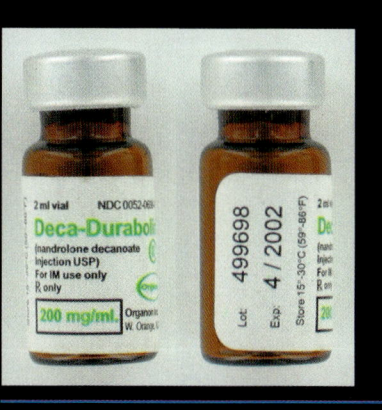

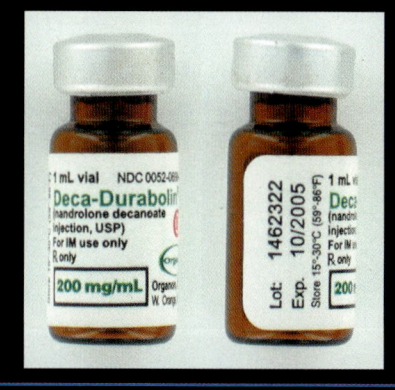

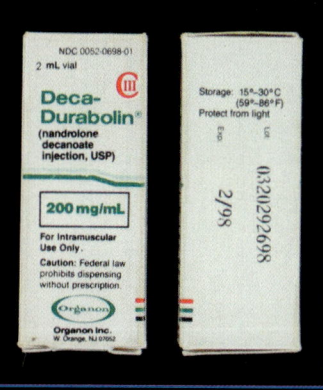

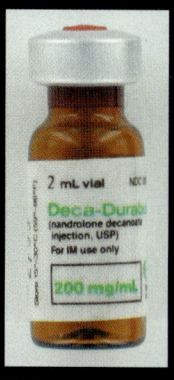

Three different U.S. Organon countefeits

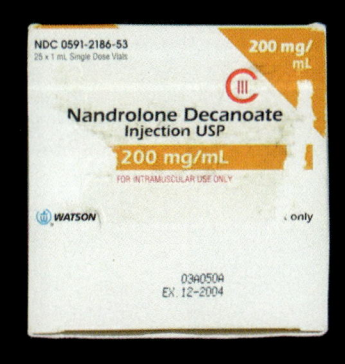

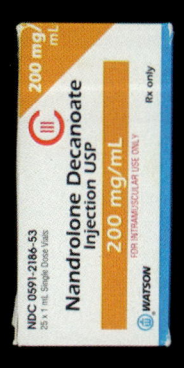

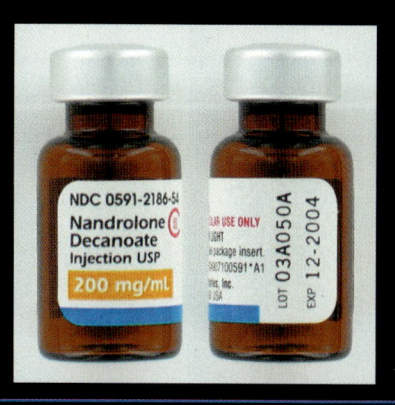

U.S. Watson Generic (NLM)

Appendix B

B-15

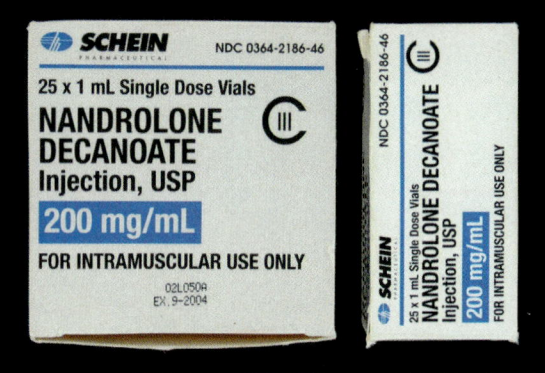

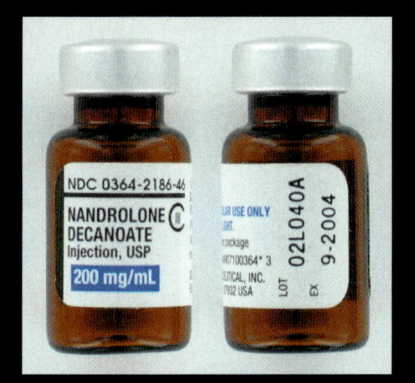

Schein generic box and vial (U.S.)

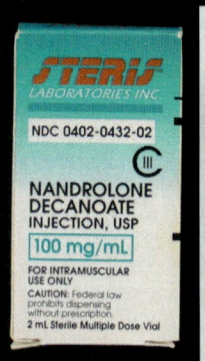

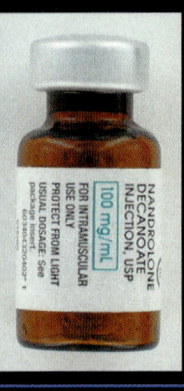

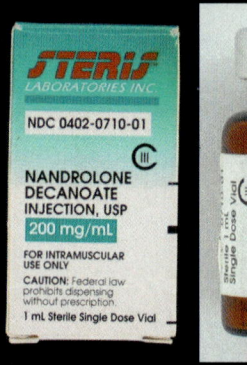

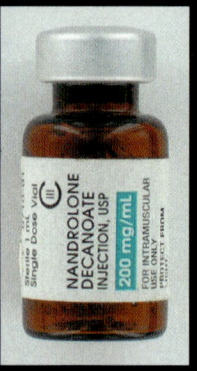

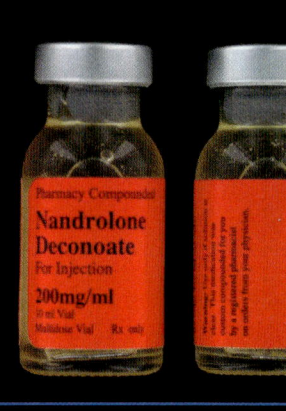

Counterfeit U.S. Steris generics - 100mg/ml and 200mg/ml (NLM)　　　　Signature Pharmacy (U.S.)

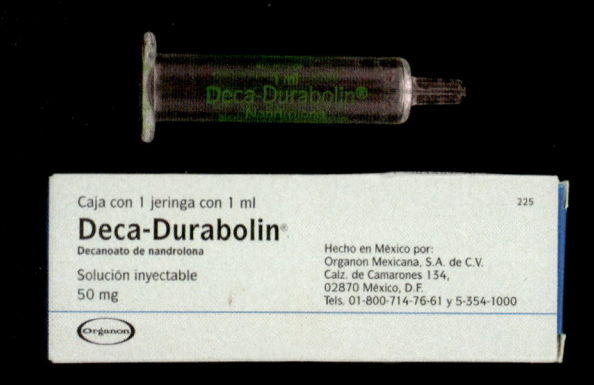

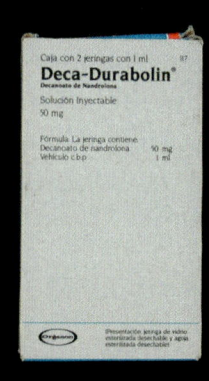

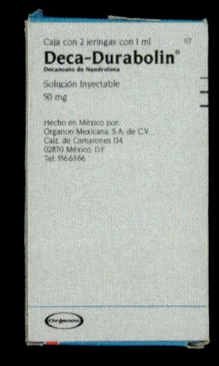

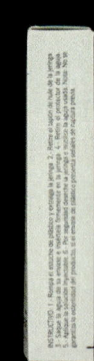

Deca-Durabolin from Organon (Mexico)

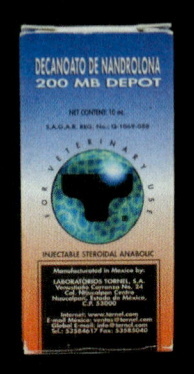

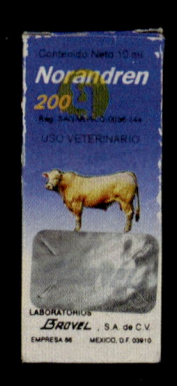

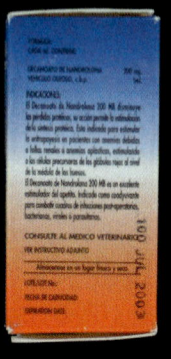

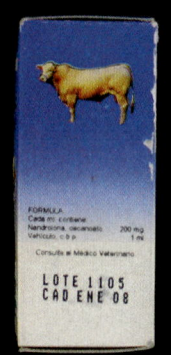

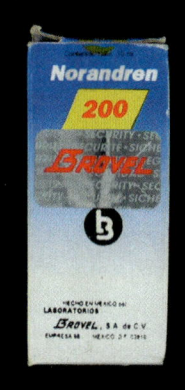

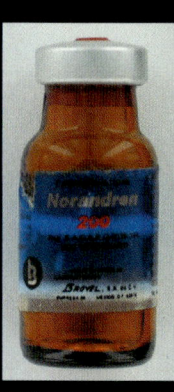

Tornel generic (Mexico)　　　　Brovel Norandren 200 (Mexico) NLM　　　　Older Norandren box and vial (10ml)

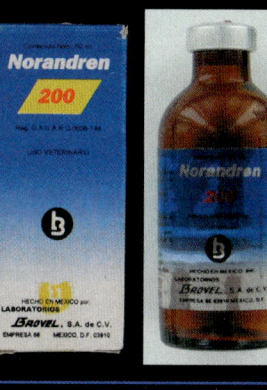

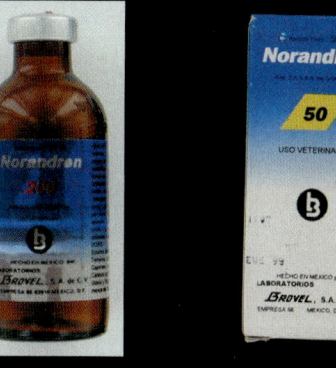

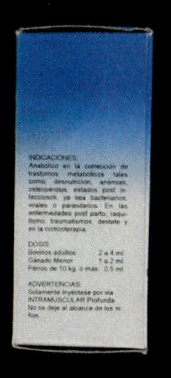

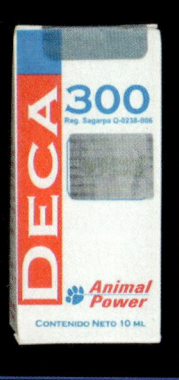

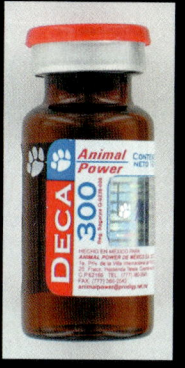

Older 50ml box and vial　　　　Old Norandren 50 (Mexico)　　　　Animal Power Deca 300 (Mexico) NLM

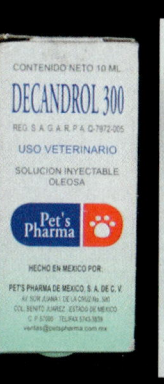

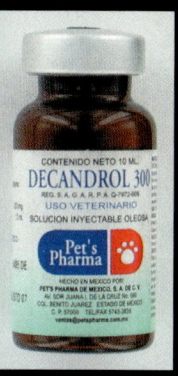

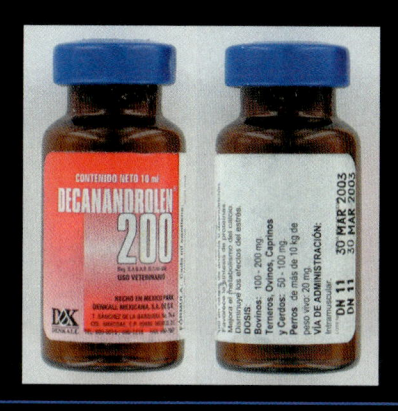

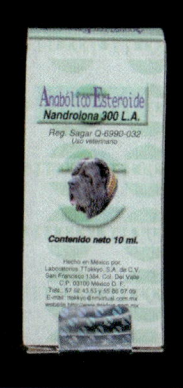

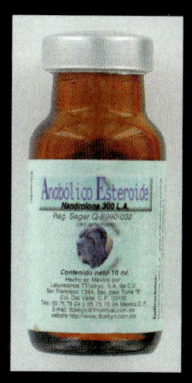

Pet's Pharma (Mexico) NLM　　Denkall Decanandrolen (Mexico) NLM　　Ttokkyo Nandrolona (Mexico, NLM)

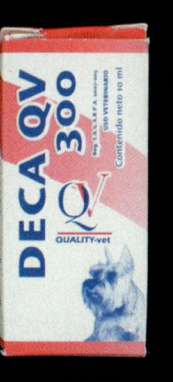

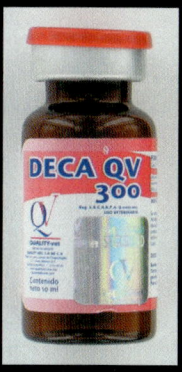

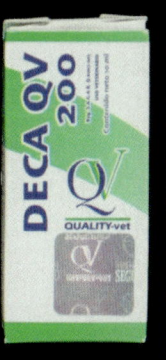

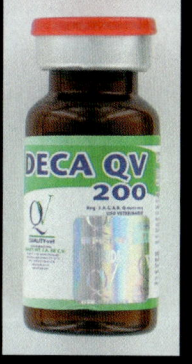

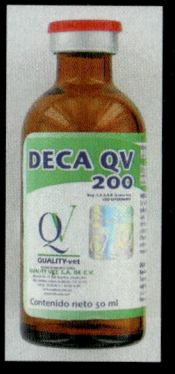

Deca from Quality Vet (Mexico) NLM　　QV Deca 200 (10ml) NLM　　QV Deca 200 (50ml) NLM

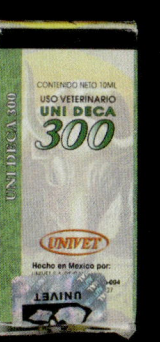

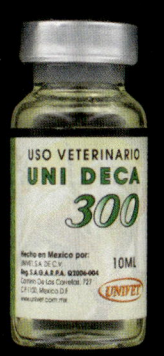

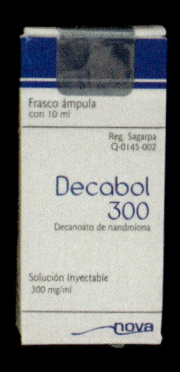

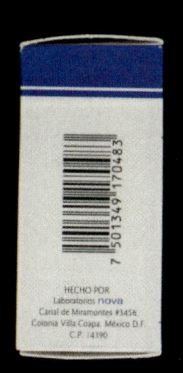

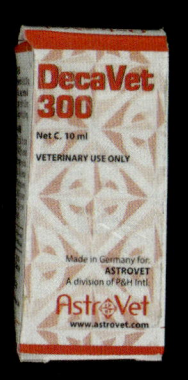

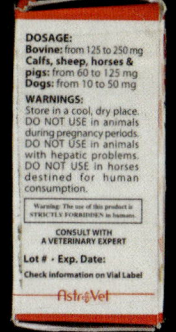

Three different Mexican underground products from Univet, Nova, and Astrovet

Appendix B

B-17

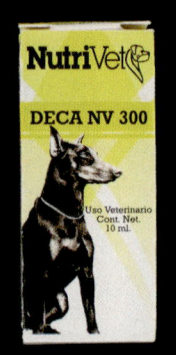

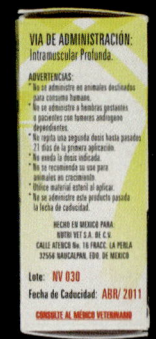

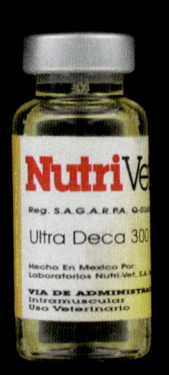

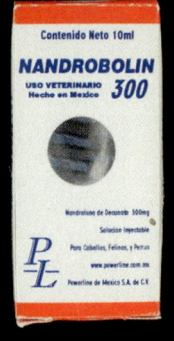

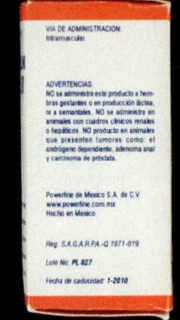

Ultra Deca from Nutri-Vet (Mexico, UG) NLM

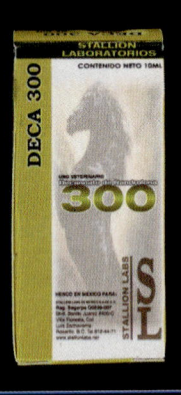

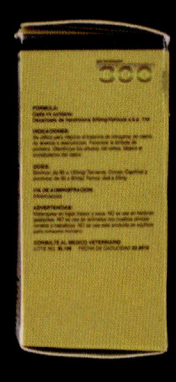

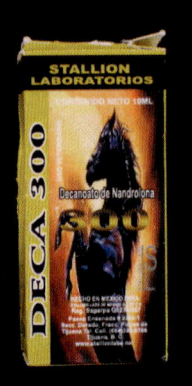

Nandrobolin from Powerline (MX UG) NLM

Deca 300 from Stallion (MX, UG) NLM

Decatron - MX Underground (NLM)

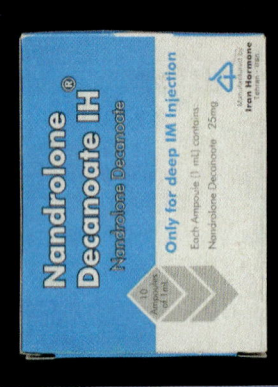

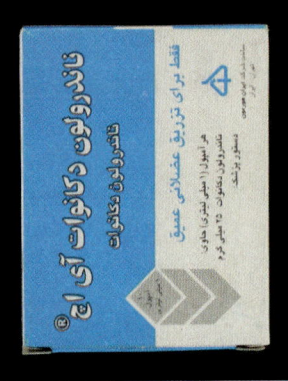

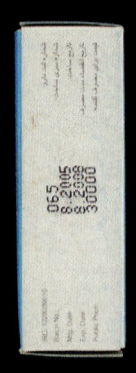

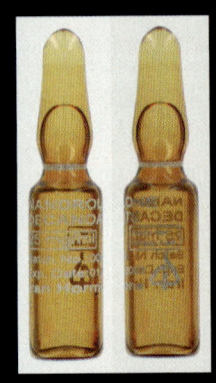

Nandrolone from Iran Hormone (Iran)

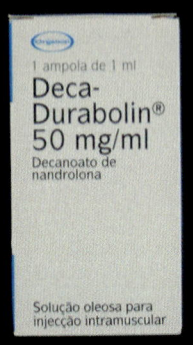

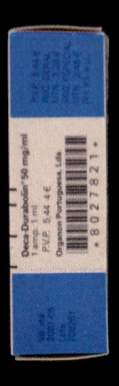

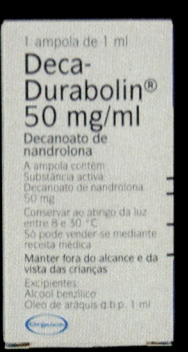

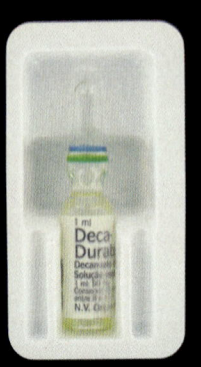

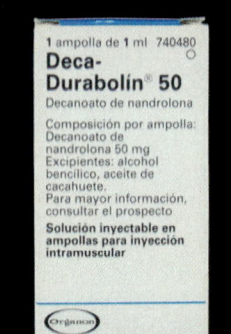

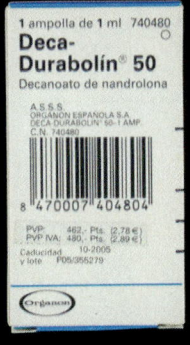

Deca-Durabolin from Portugal

Deca-Durabolin 50mg (Spain)

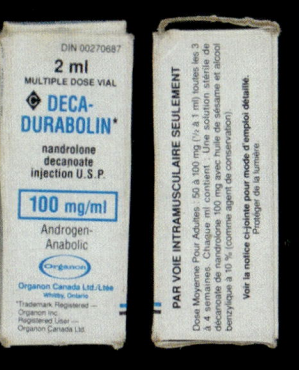

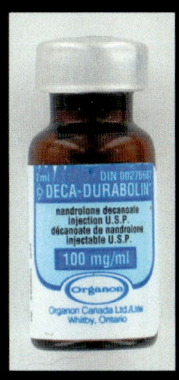

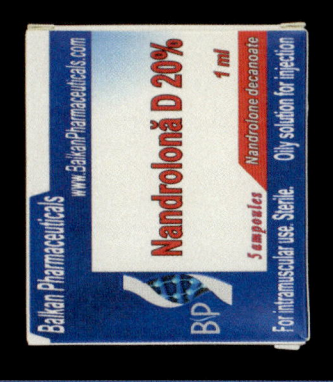

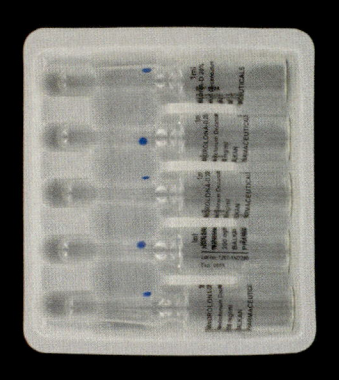

Canadian Deca-Durabolin

Balkan Pharmaceuticals (Moldova)

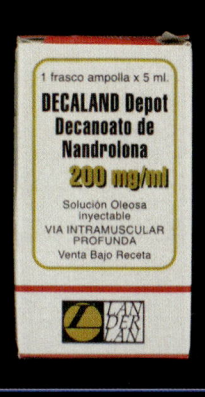

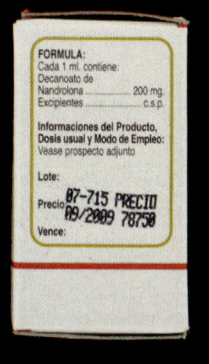

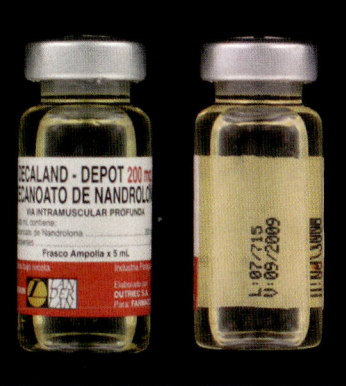

Decaland from Landerlan (Paraguay)

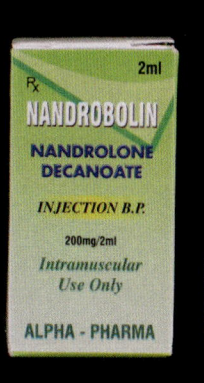

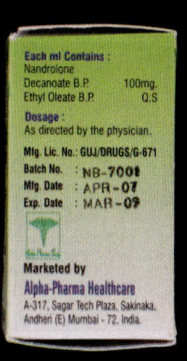

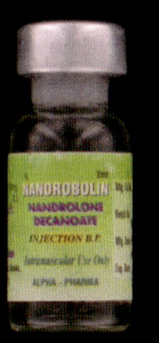

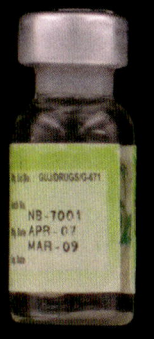

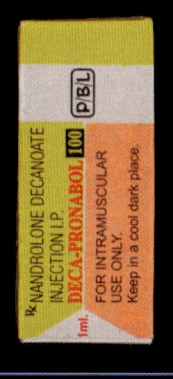

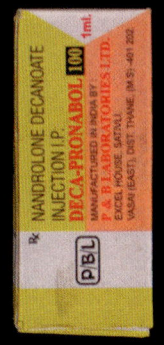

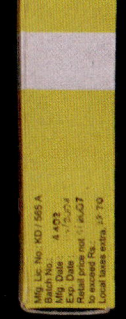

Nandrobolin from Alpha-Pharma (India, export)

Deca-Pronabol from India

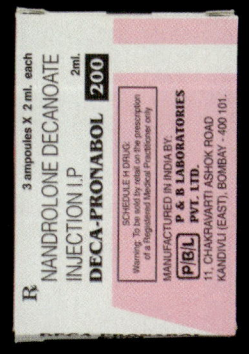

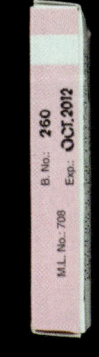

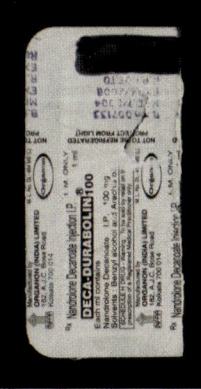

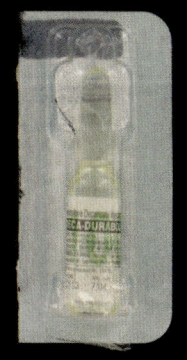

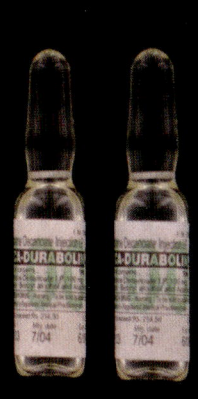

Old Deca-Pronabol box

100mg Deca-Durabolin from Organon/Infar (India)

Appendix B

B-19

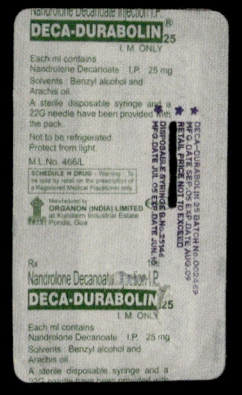

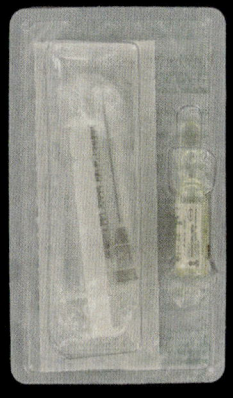

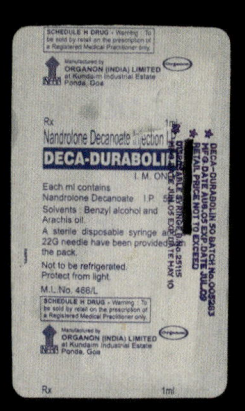

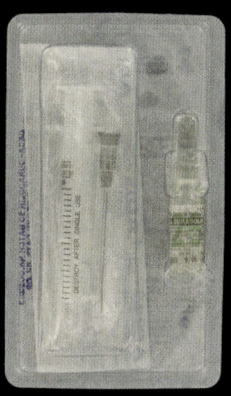

50mg and 25mg Deca-Durabolin from Organon/Infar (India)

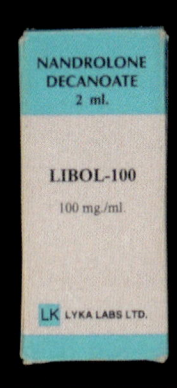

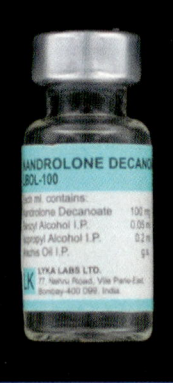

Fake Indian Libol 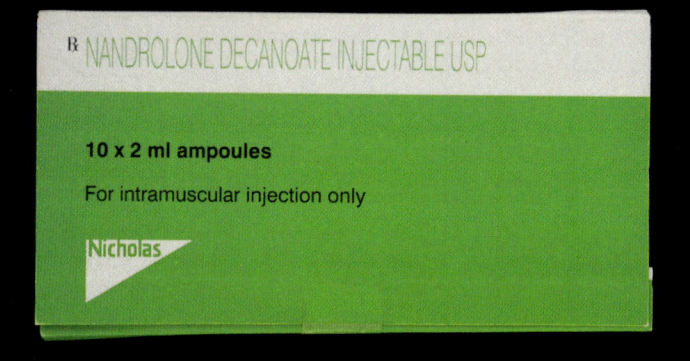   Fake Deca from Nicholas (India) 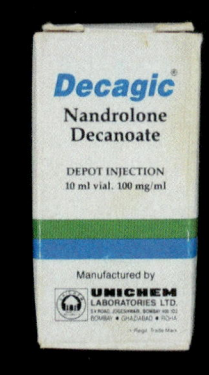   Decagic India (NLM)

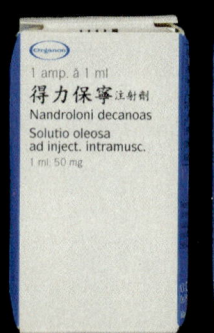

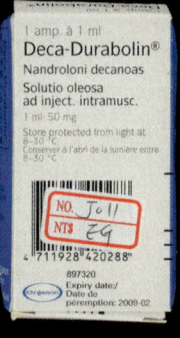

Deca-Durabolin (China) 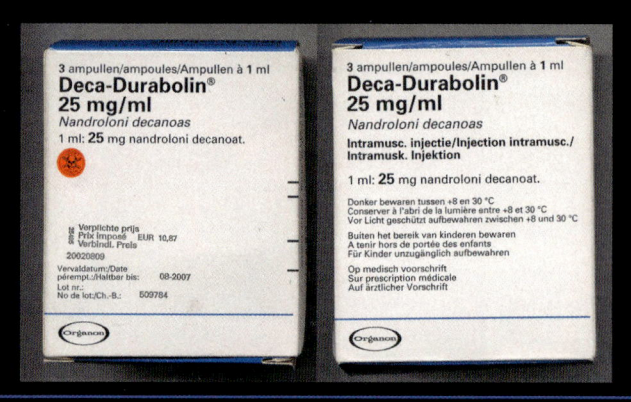   Deca-Durabolin from Organon (Belgium)

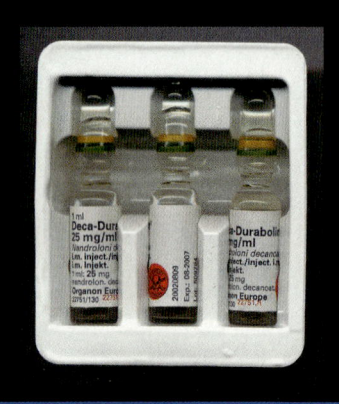

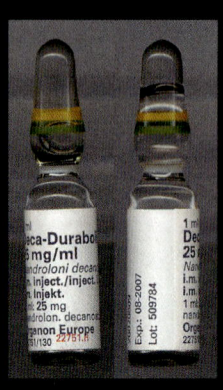

Ampules from Belgium 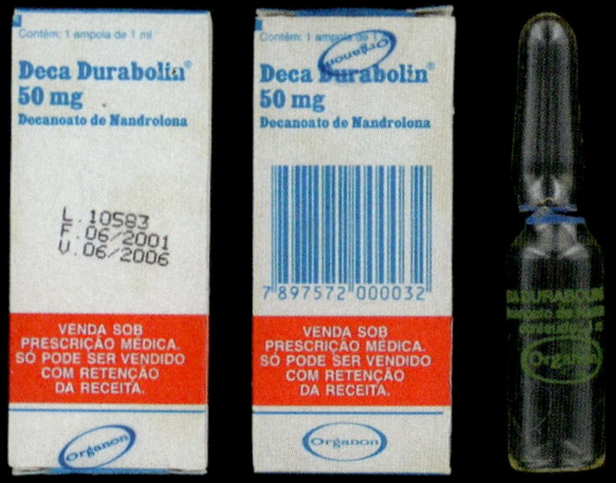   Deca-Durabolin from Brazil

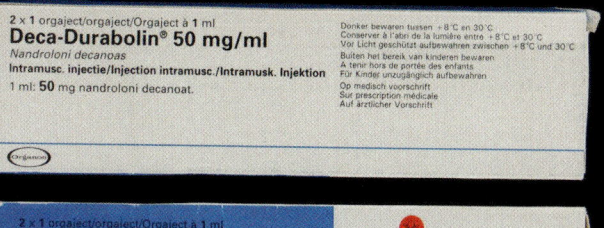

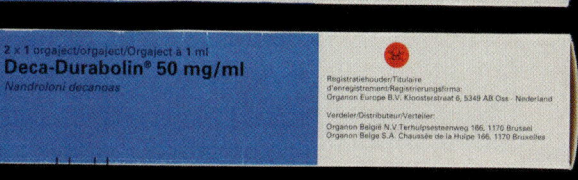

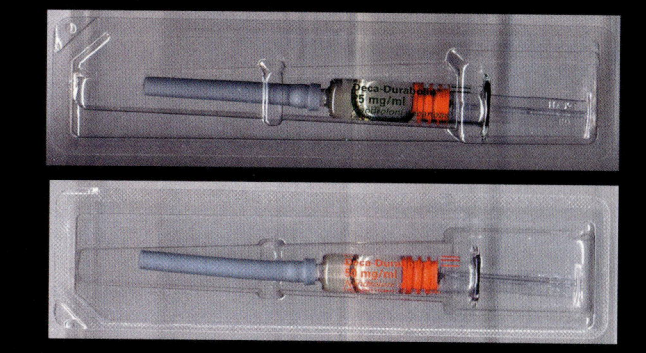

Deca-Durabolin pre-load (Belgium)

Belgian pre-loaded syringes (25 top, 50mg bottom)

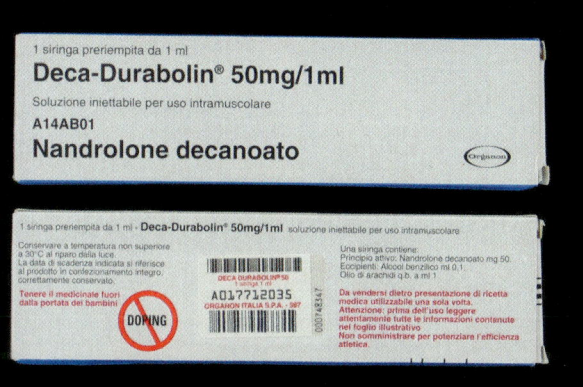

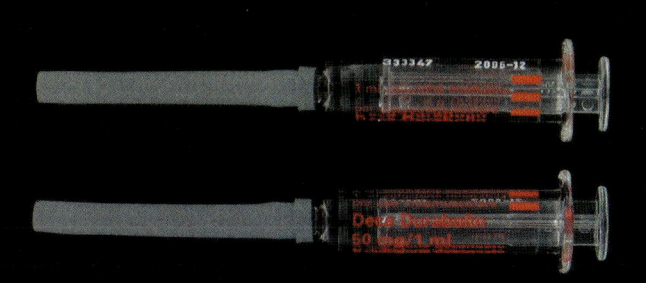

Organon pre-loaded syringes from Italy

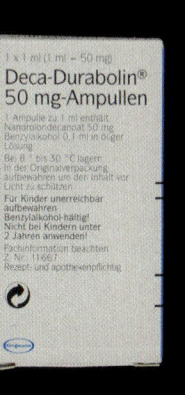

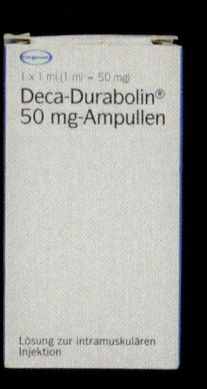

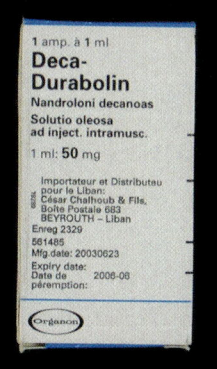

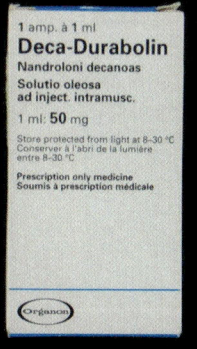

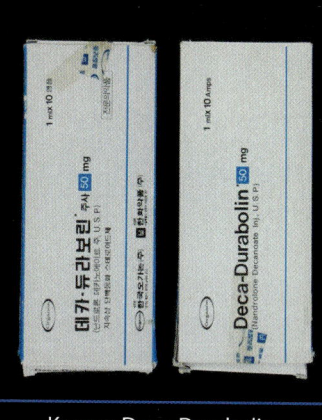

Deca-Durabolin from Austria

Deca-Durabolin from Organon Libya

Korean Deca-Durabolin

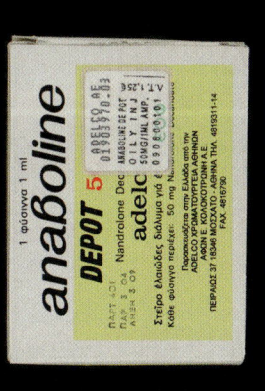

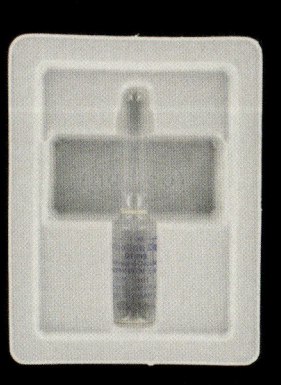

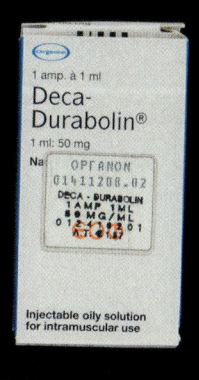

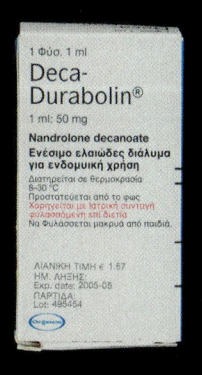

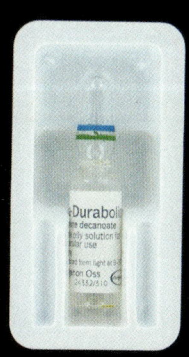

Greek Anaboline Depot

Greek 50mg Deca-Durabolin box and ampule

Appendix B

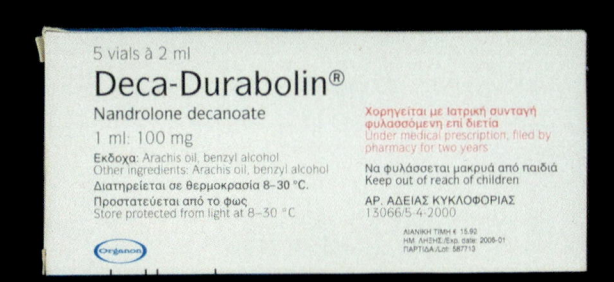

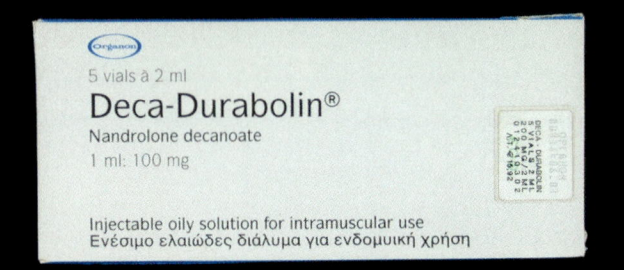

Deca-Durabolin multi-dose vials from Organon Greece

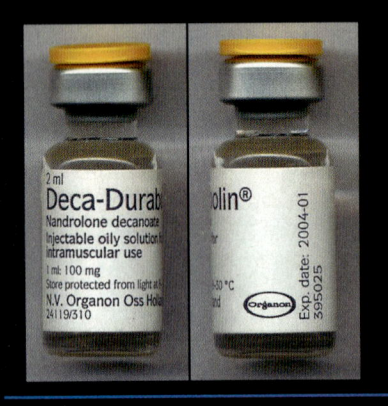

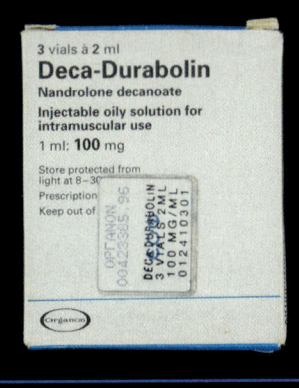

Greek "Yellow Top" vials 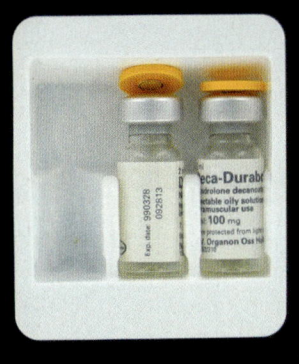 | Previous Greek box and vials 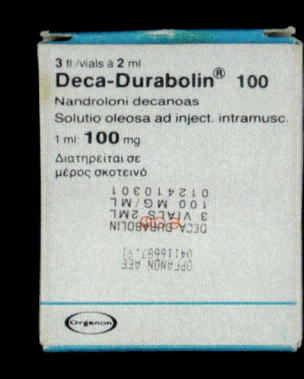 | Greek Deca circa 1991

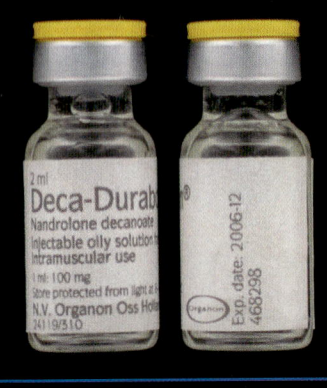

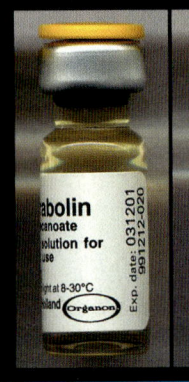

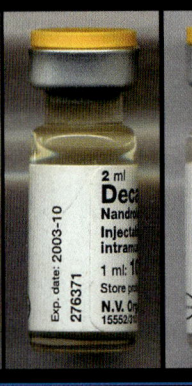

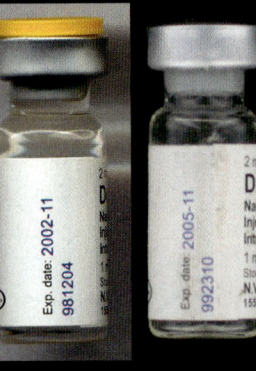

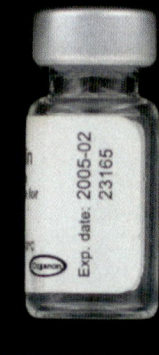

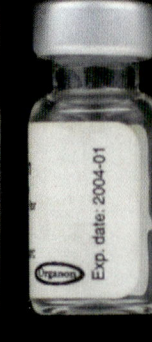

Counterfeit Greek Deca #1 | #2 | #3 | #4 | #5 | #6 | #7

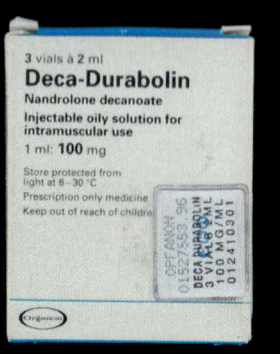

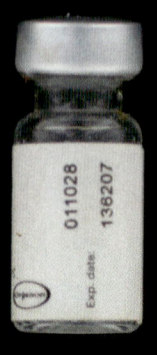

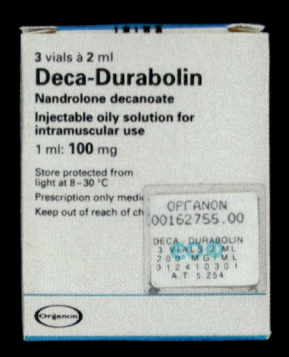

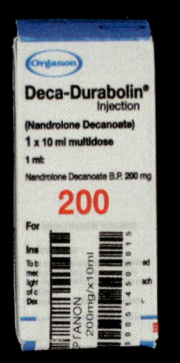

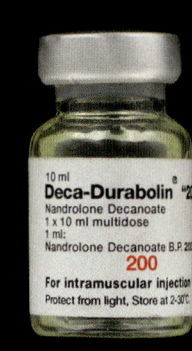

Three more counterfeits with mock pharmacy stickers (#8, #9, #10)

B-22

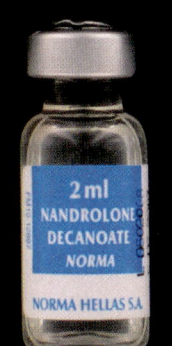

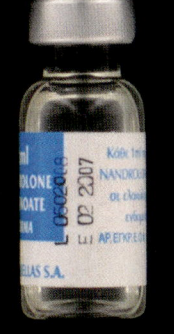

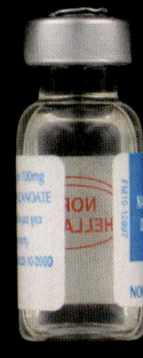

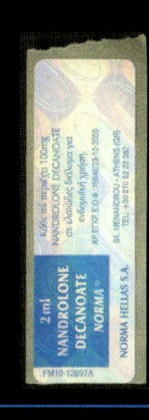

Norma Hellas generic from Greece - Holographic security label on right

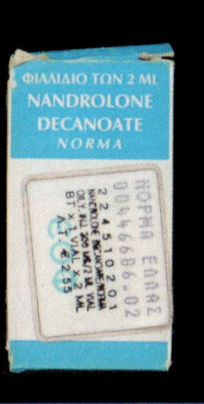

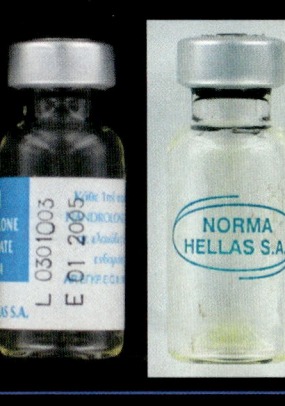

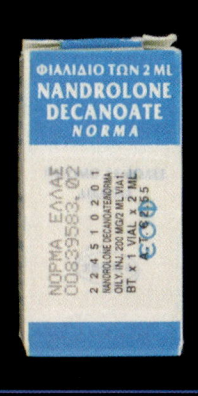

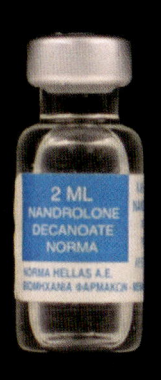

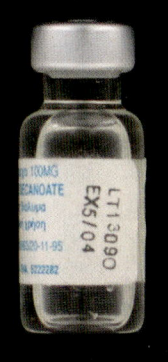

Older Norma with blue etching under label

Counterfeit Norma #1 with bogus pharm sticker

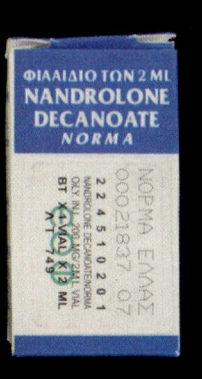

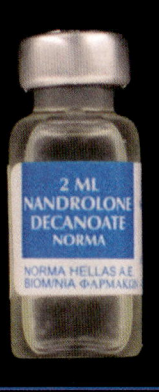

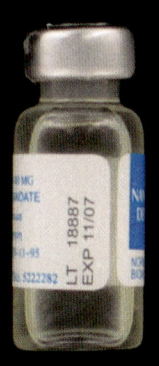

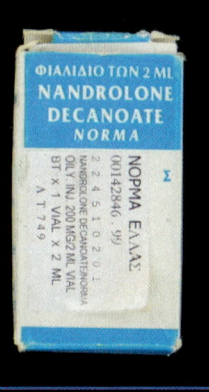

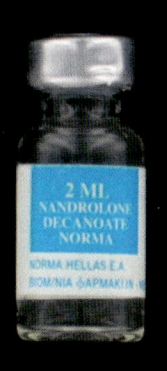

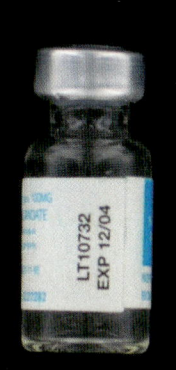

Counterfeit #2, also with mock pharmacy sticker

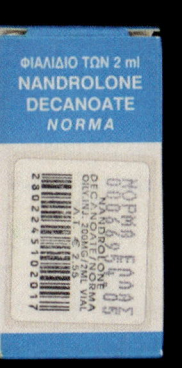

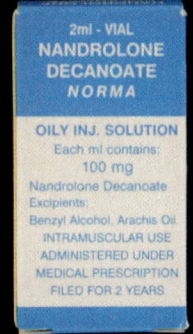

Counterfeit Norma #3

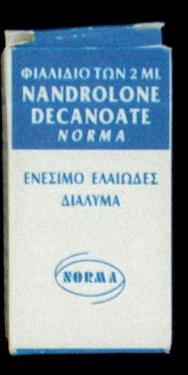

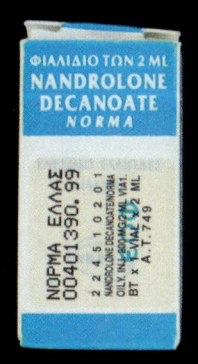

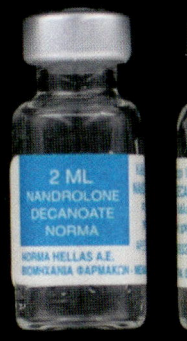

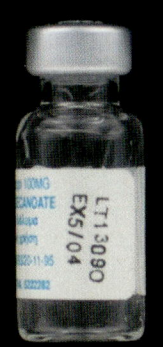

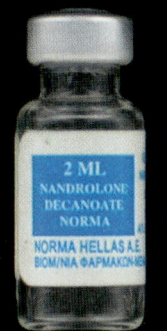

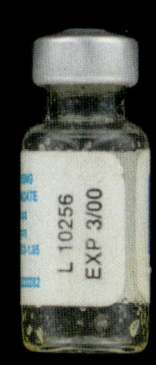

Counterfeit #4

Counterfeit #5

Counterfeit #6

Appendix B

B-23

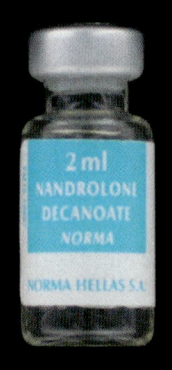

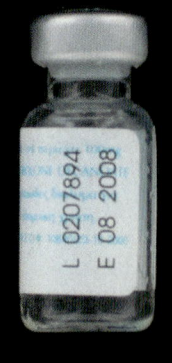

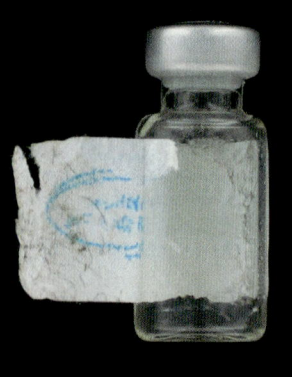

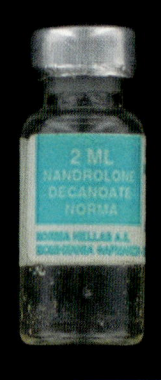

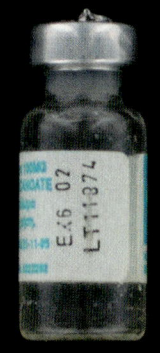

Counterfeit #7 - Logo peels off with label

Counterfeit #8

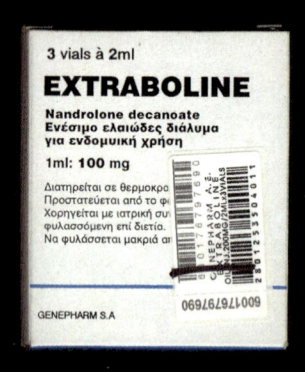

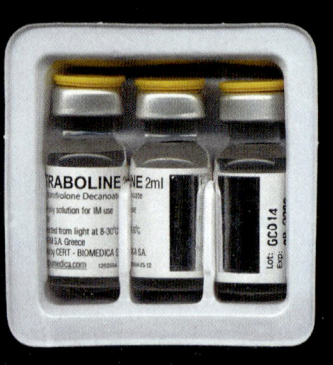

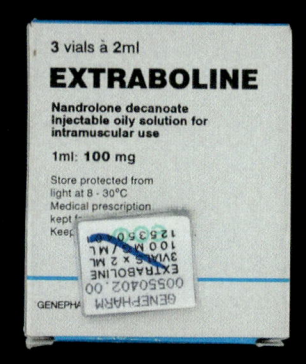

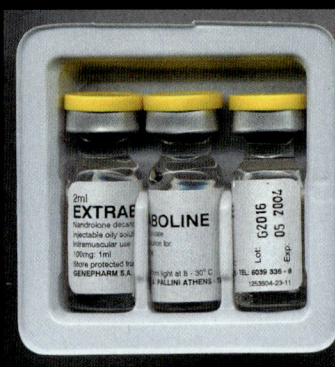

Greek Extraboline (with holograms)

Older Greek Extraboline

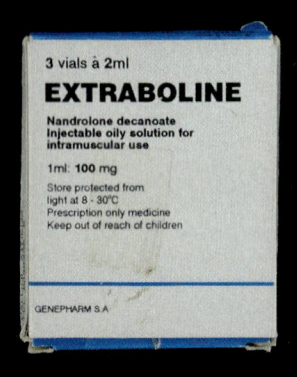

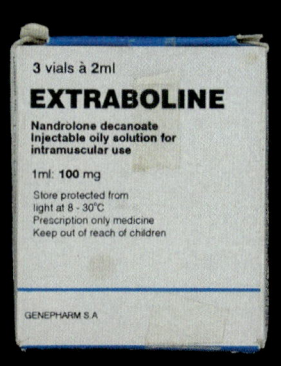

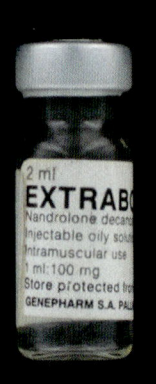

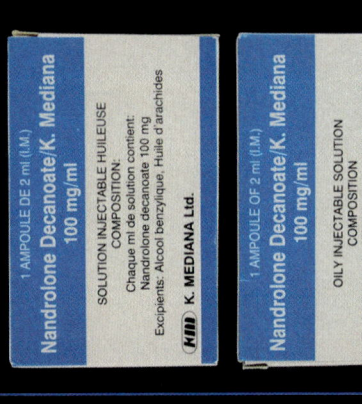

Counterfeit Extraboline box and vial

Fake Mediana Deca (Greece)

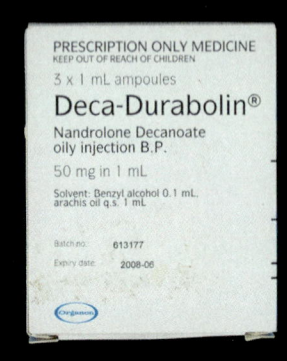

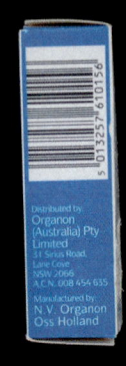

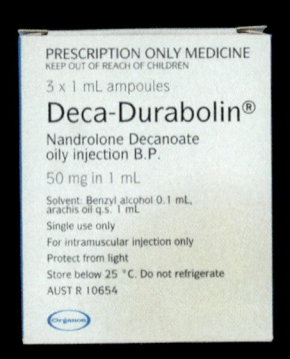

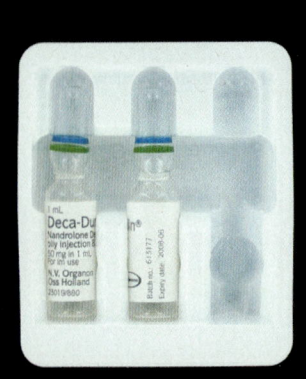

Deca-Durabolin from Organon Australia

B-24

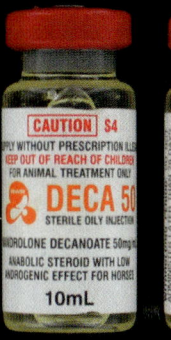

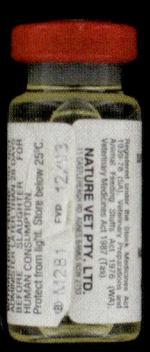

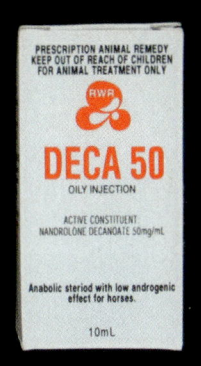

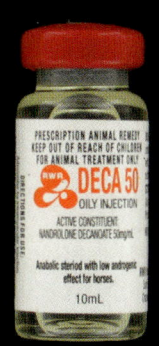

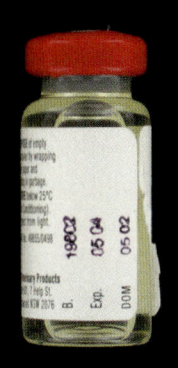

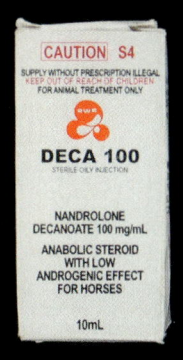

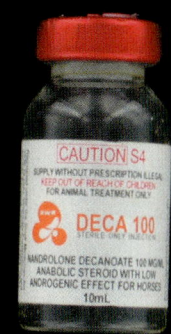

Counterfeit RWR Deca (Australia)   RWR counterfeit box and vial (#2)   Fake RWR Deca 100

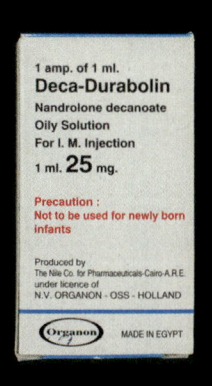

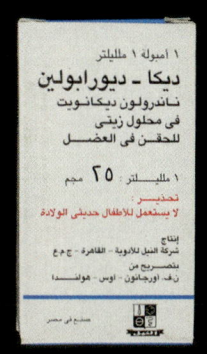

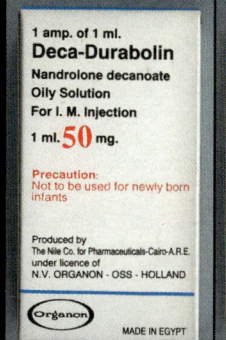

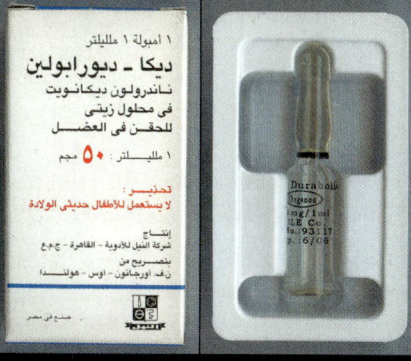

Deca-Durabolin from Nile Co. 25mg and 50mg (Egypt)

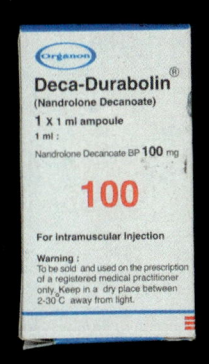

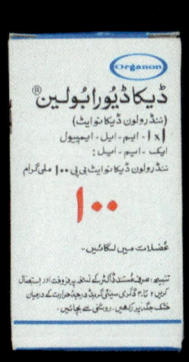

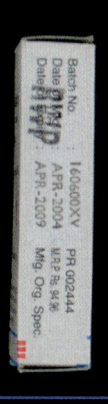

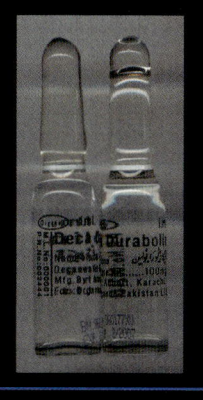

Deca-Durabolin from Pakistan   Counterfeit amps

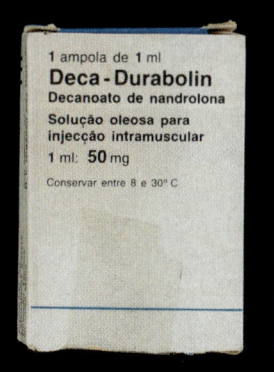

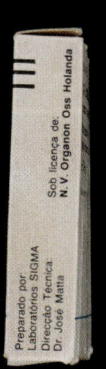

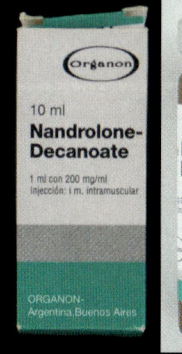

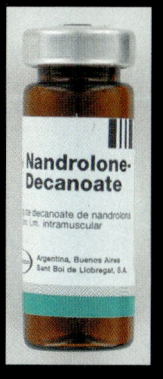

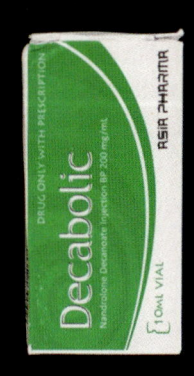

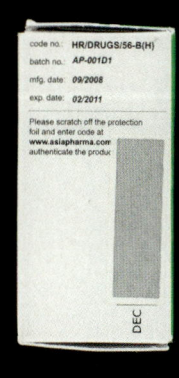

Deca-Durabolin from Argentina   Counterfeit Deca (Argentina)   Decabolic from Asia Pharma (Malaysia)

Appendix B

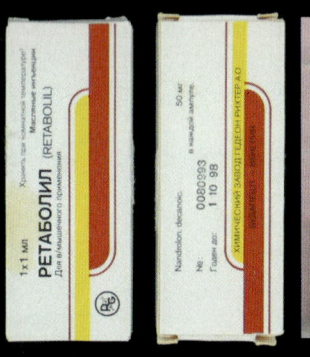

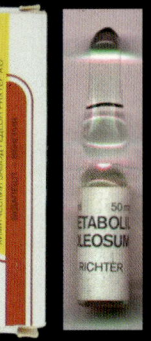

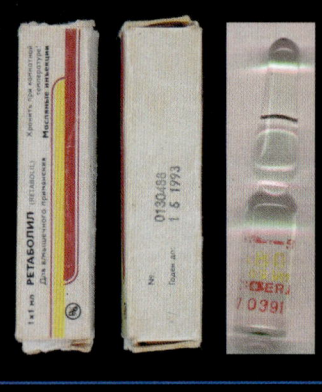

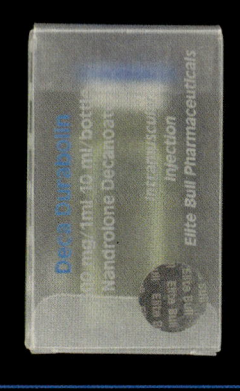

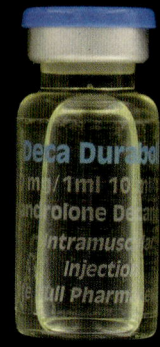

Retabolil from Gedeon Richter (Bulgaria) older style on right

Elite Bull (Hong Kong, Export)

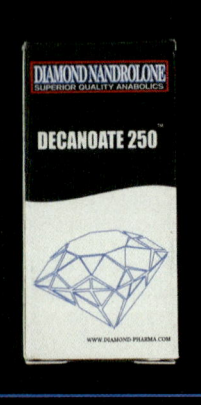

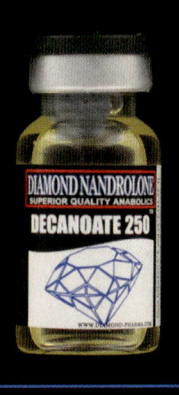

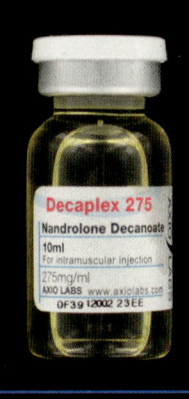

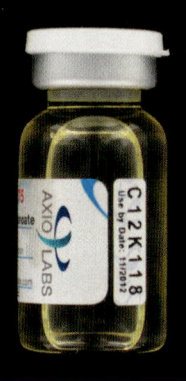

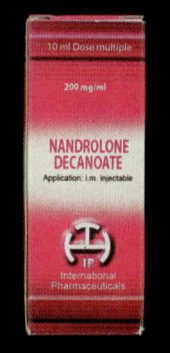

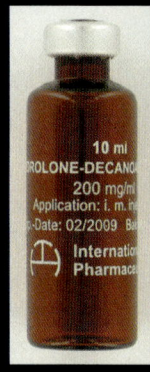

Diamond Decanoate (UG)

Axio Labs (underground)

International Pharmaceuticalss (UG)

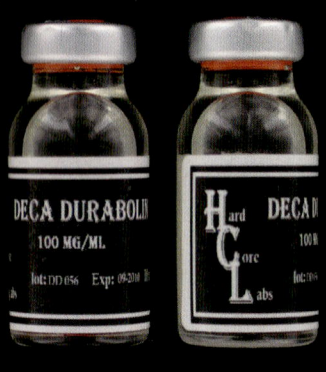

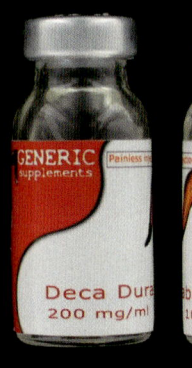

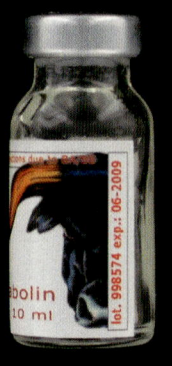

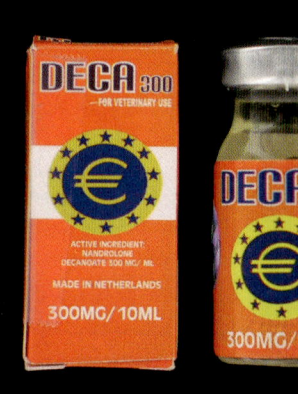

Hardcore Labs (Underground)

Generic Supplements (Underground)

Euro-Vet (Underground)

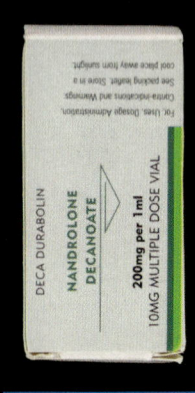

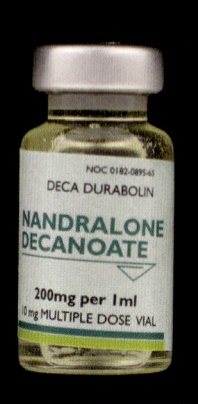

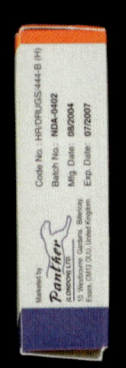

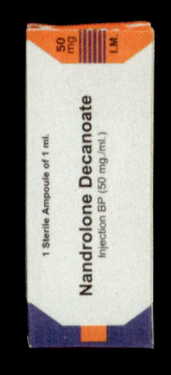

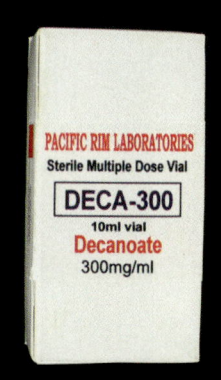

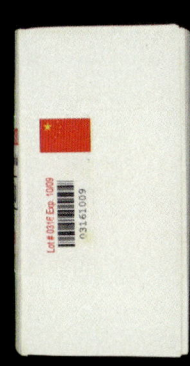

Three more Underground products from Changchun, Panther, and Pacific Rim

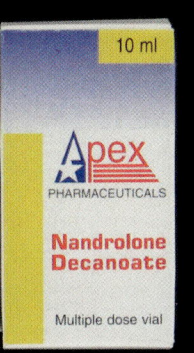

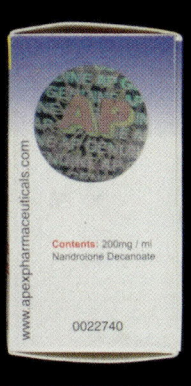

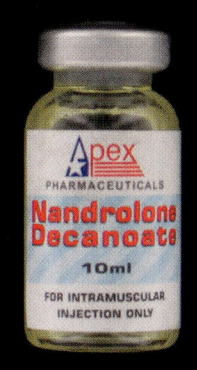

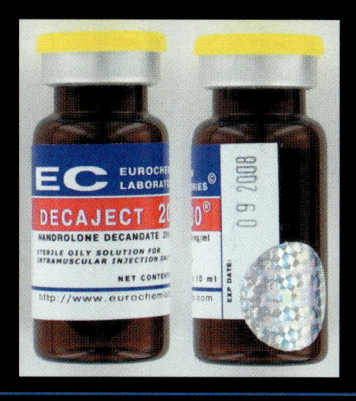

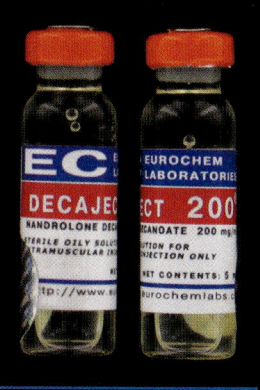

Apex generic (Underground)

Eurochem Decaject (Underground) 10ml and 5ml vials

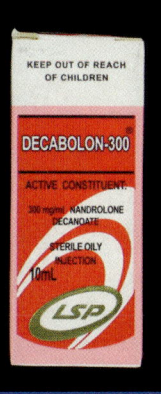

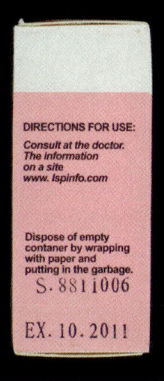

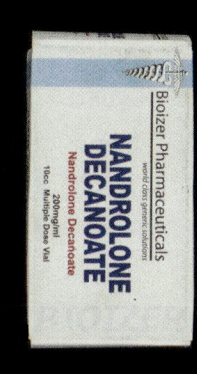

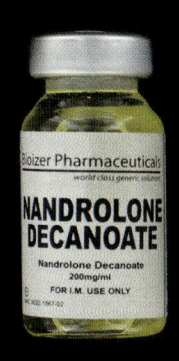

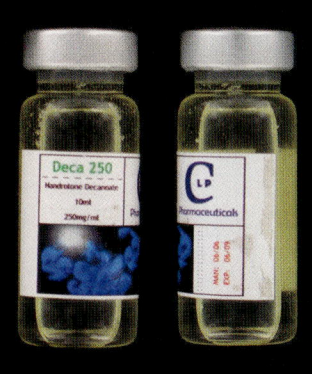

Underground products from LSP, Bioizer Pharmaceuticals, and CLP

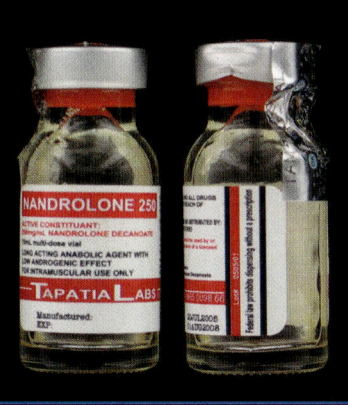

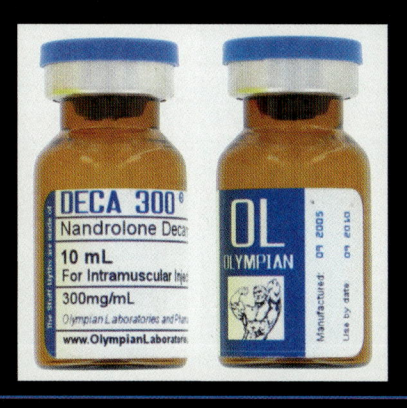

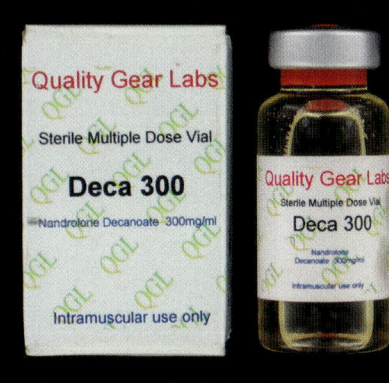

Underground products from Tapatia, Olympian, and Quality Gear Labs

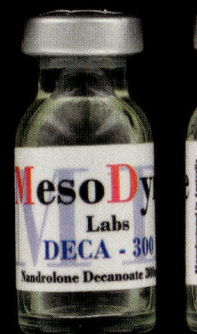

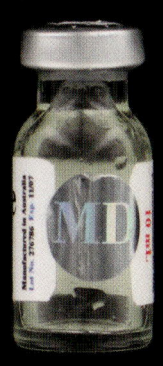

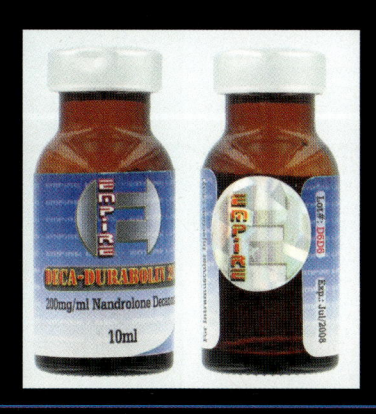

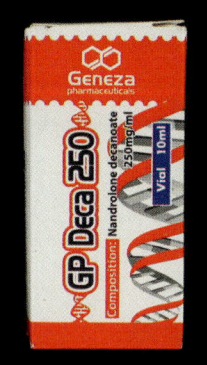

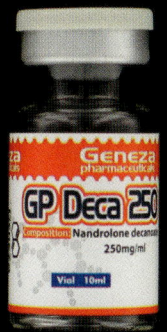

Underground product from MesoDyne, Empire, and Geneza

Appendix B

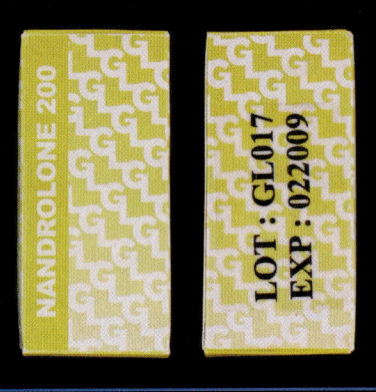

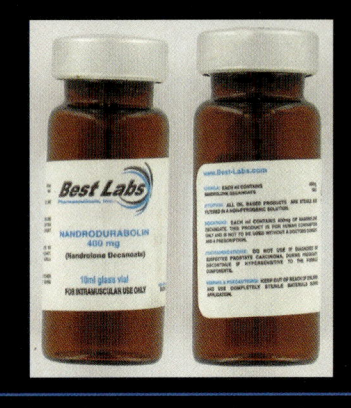

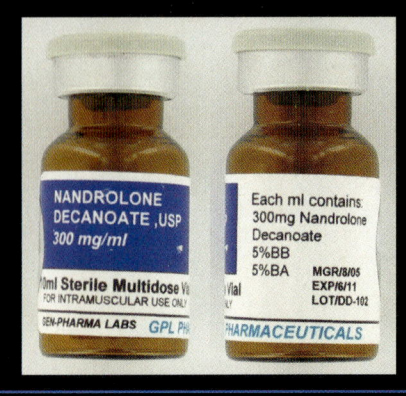

Underground products from GL, Best Labs, and Gen-Pharma (NLM)

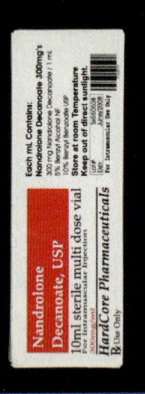

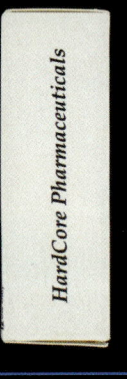

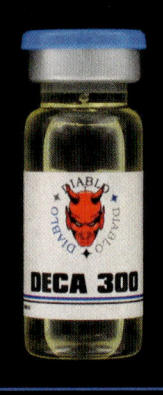

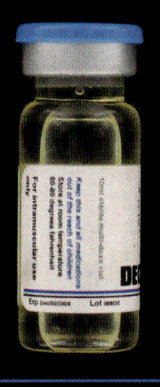

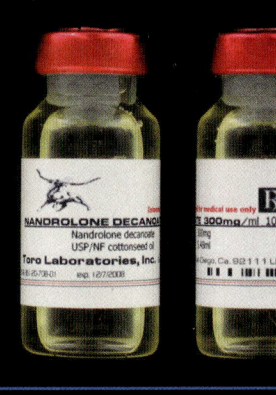

Underground products from HardCore Pharmaceuticals, Diablo, and Toro

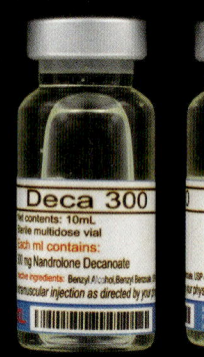

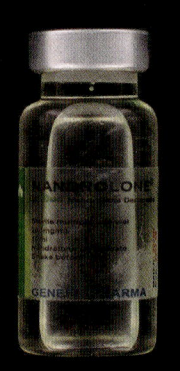

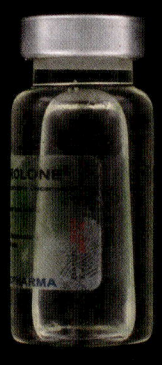

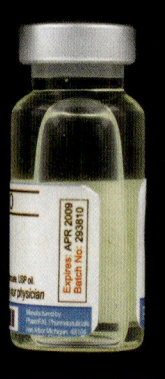

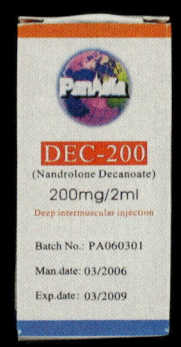

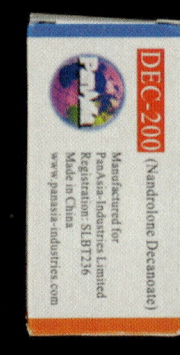

Underground products from PharmRXL,, Generic Pharma, and Panasia

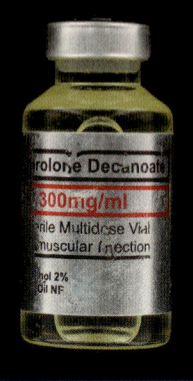

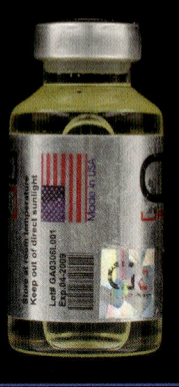

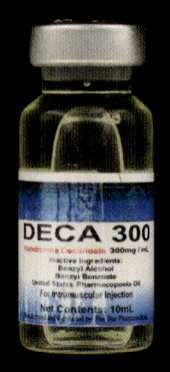

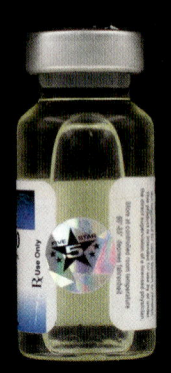

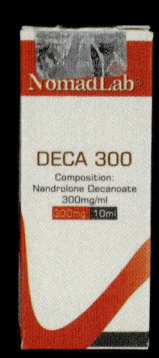

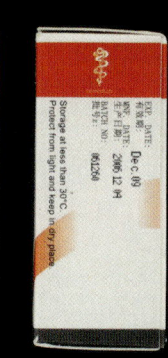

Underground products from GA, 5 Star, and Nomad

B-28

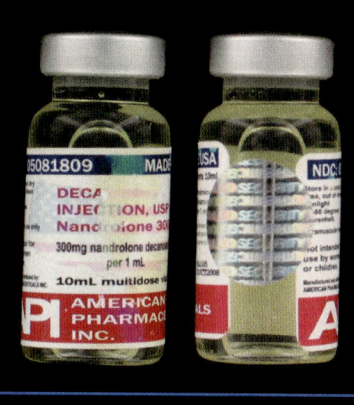

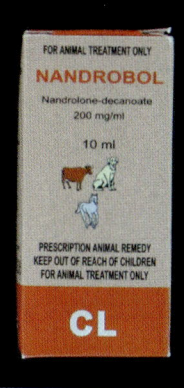

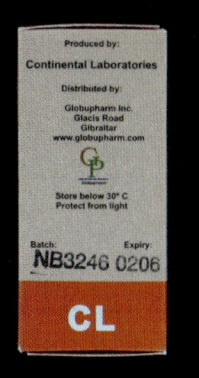

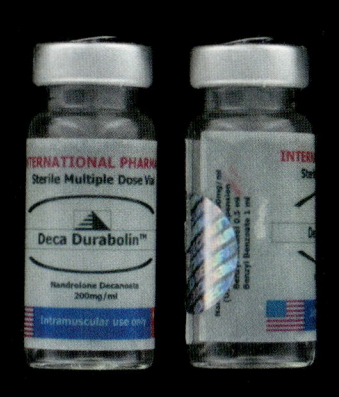

API (UG) | Continental Labs (Underground) | Underground from Int. Pharmacy

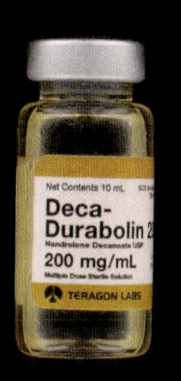

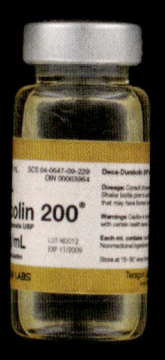

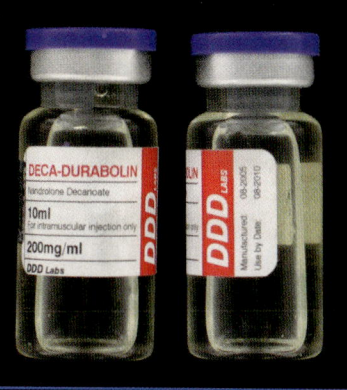

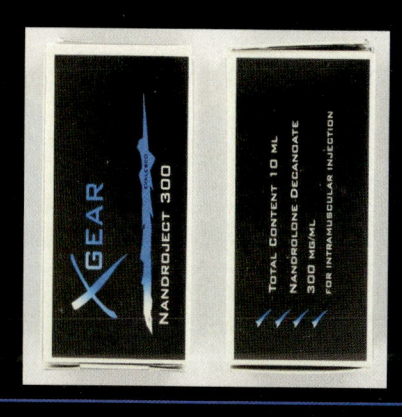

UG from Teragon (NLM) | DDD (Underground) | X Gear (Underground)

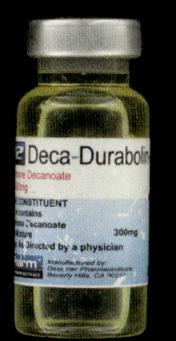

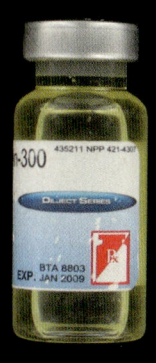

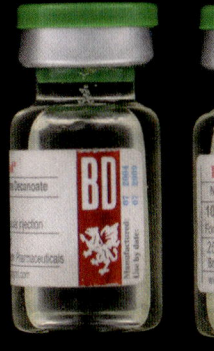

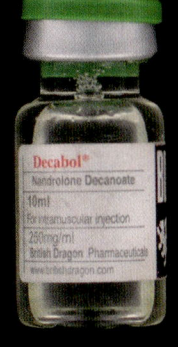

UG from Designer Pharm | British Dragon Underground (NLM) | Fake Deca 300 by Lifetech (U.S.)

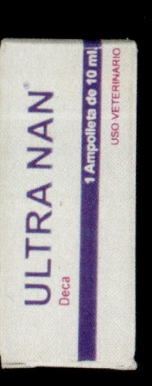

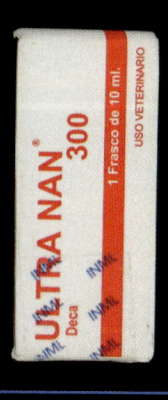

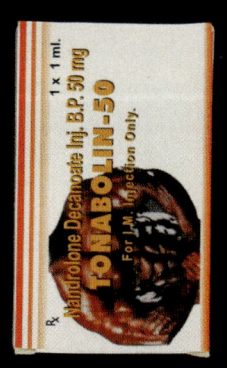

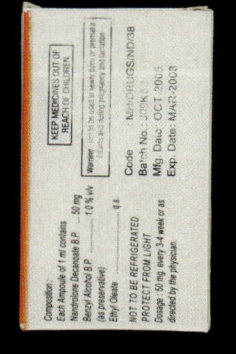

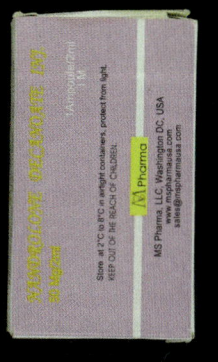

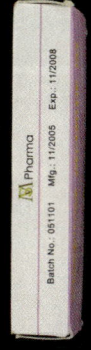

Four different fake nandrolone decanoate products

Appendix B

B-29

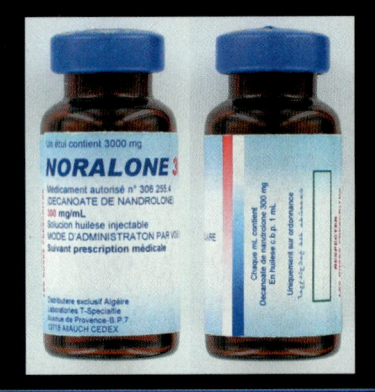

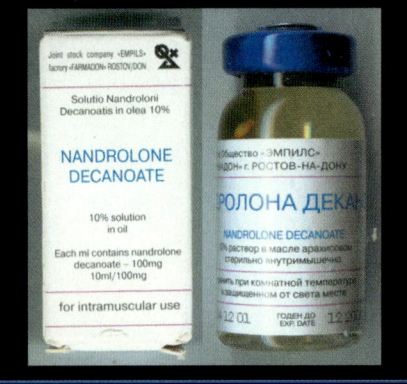

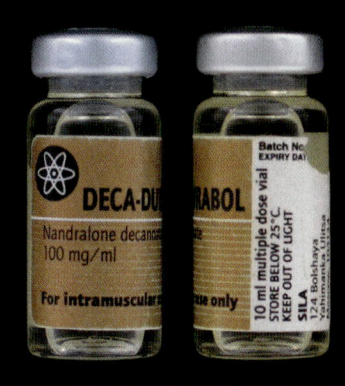

Fake French Noralone — Farmadon counterfeit (Russia) — Fake Sila (Russia)

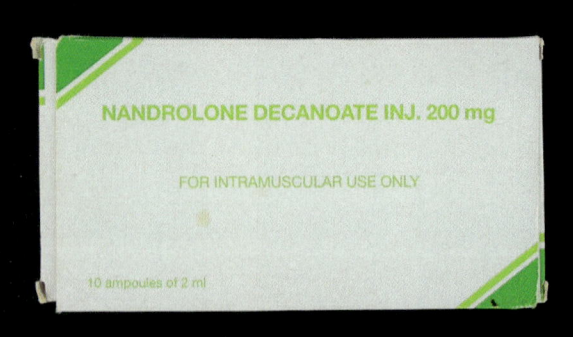

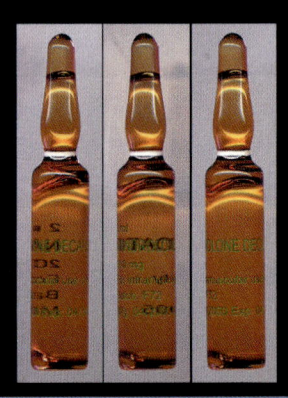

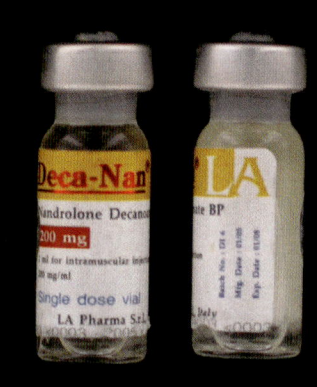

Bogus generic box (with no manufacturer name) and ampules — Deca-Nan (Thai, UG)

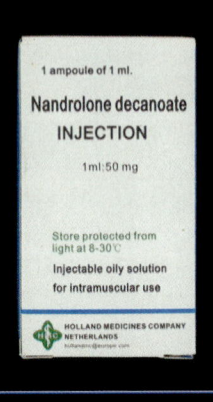

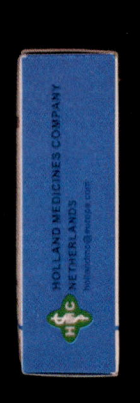

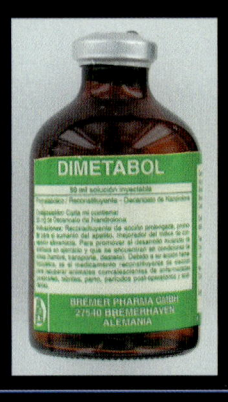

Fake Dutch generic — Counterfeit Dimetabol — Fake Decanoate

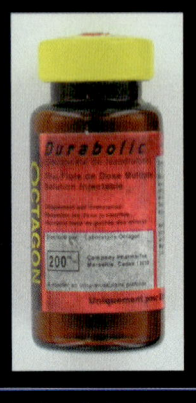

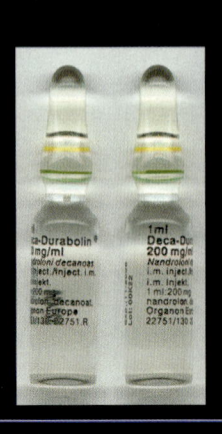

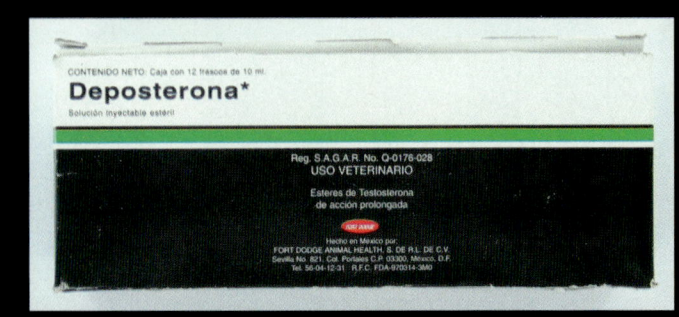

Fake Durabolic (France) — Fake Organon Amps — Deposterona from Fort Dodge (Mexico)

Dianabol

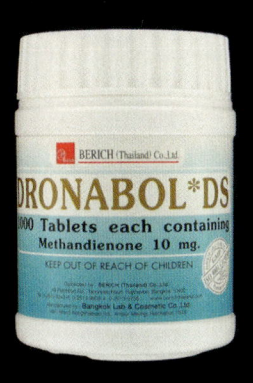

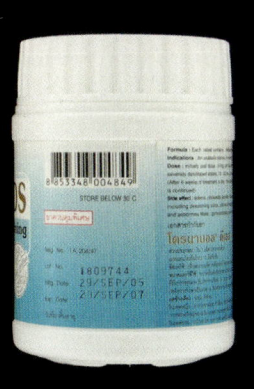

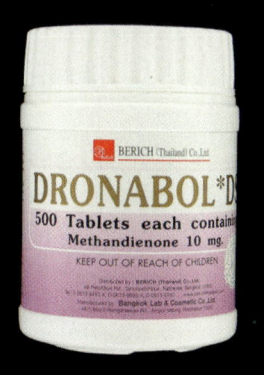

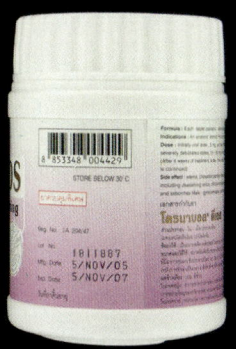

1,000 tablet and 500 tablet bottles of Dronabol DS from Berich (Thailand)

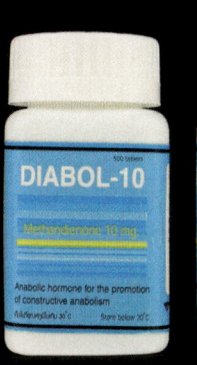

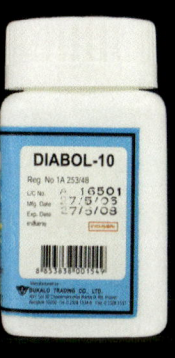

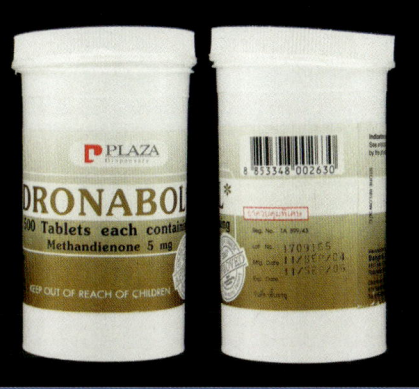

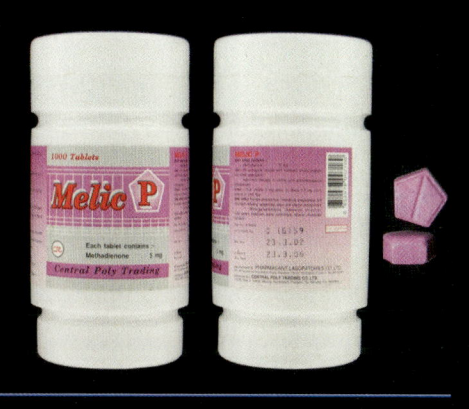

Diabol-10 (Thailand)　　　Dronabol from Plaza (Thailand)　　　Melic from Thailand

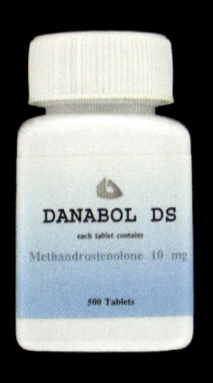

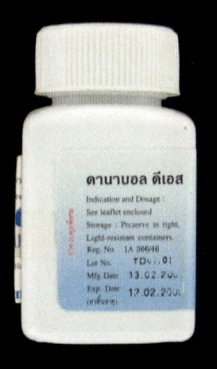

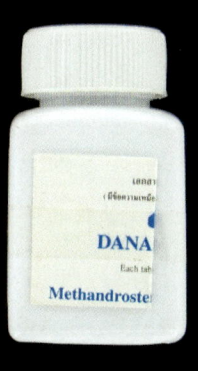

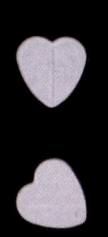

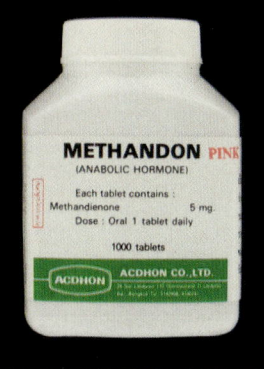

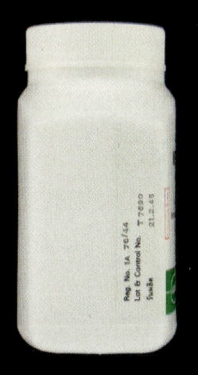

Danabol DS (Thailand)　　　　　　　　　　Methandon (Thailand)

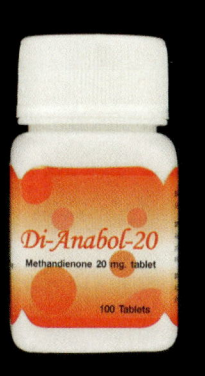

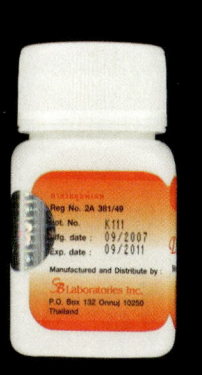

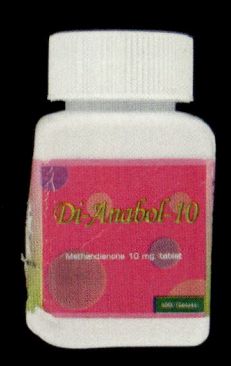

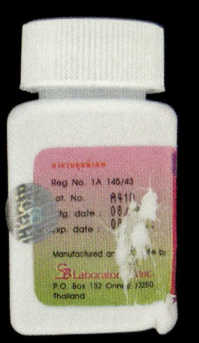

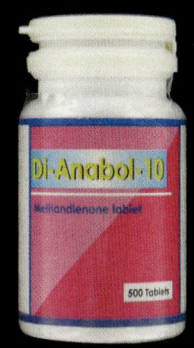

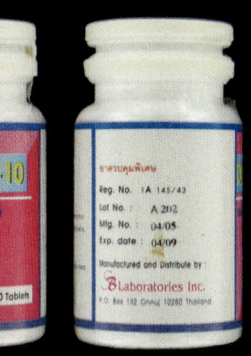

Di-Anabol from SB Labs (Thailand, Underground)

Appendix B

B-31

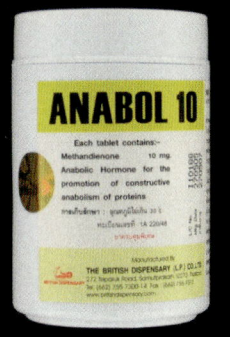

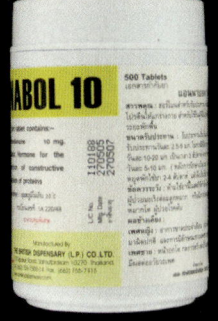

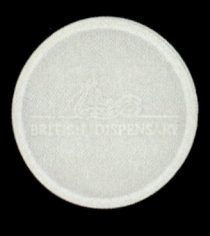

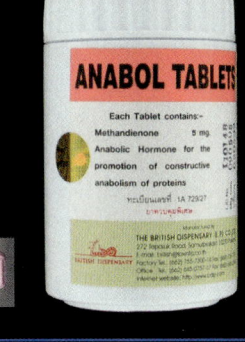

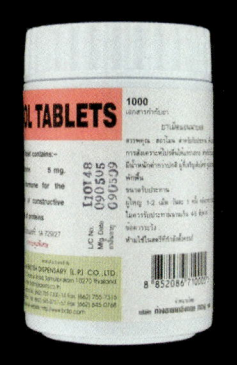

Anabol 10 from British Dispensary (Thailand)

Anabol 5mg tab and bottle from British Dispensary

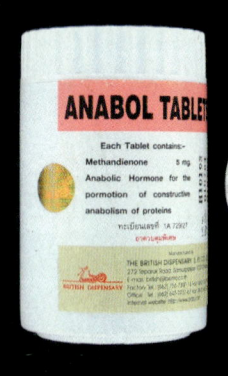

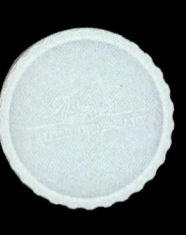

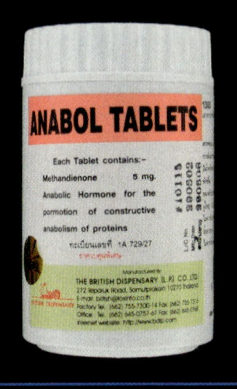

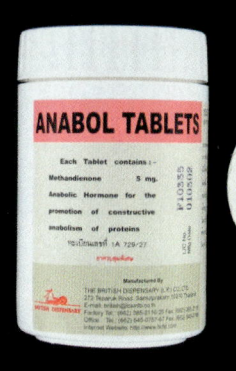

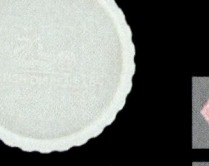

Real bottle with "pormotion" typo

Counterfeit with same typo

Another counterfeit

Counterfeit tabs

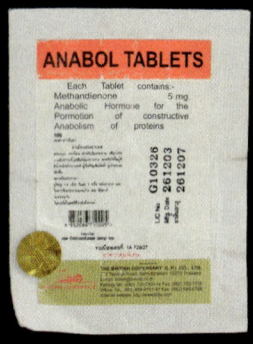

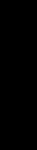

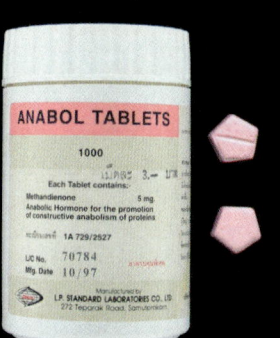

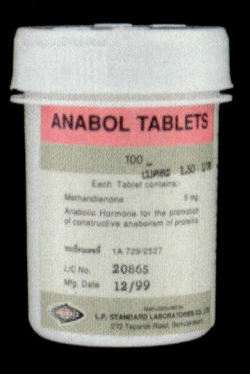

Fake 100 tablet pouch

Old LP Standard Anabol (NLM)

Fake 100 tab LP bottle

LA Generic (Thai, UG)

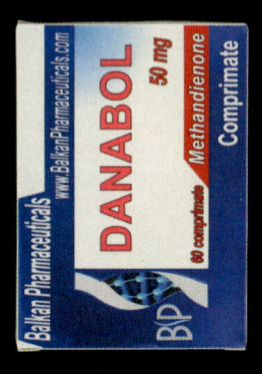

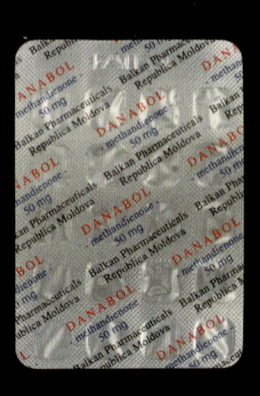

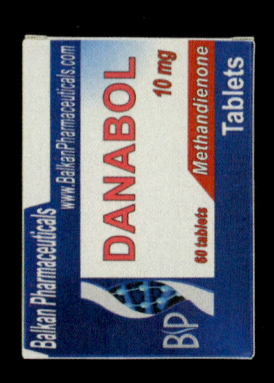

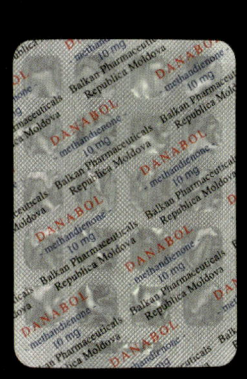

Danabol 50mg and 10mg from Balkan Pharmaceuticals (Moldova)

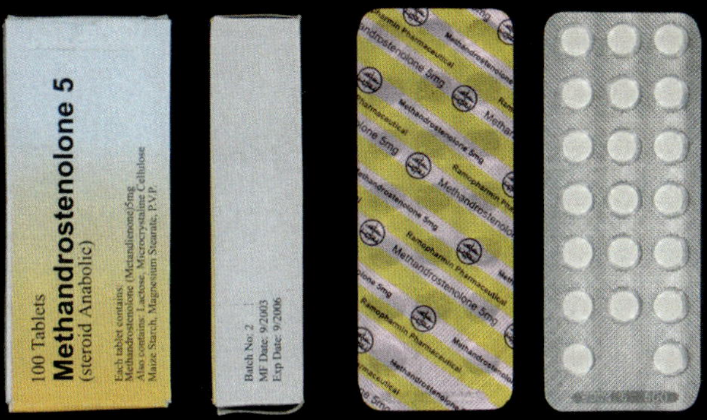

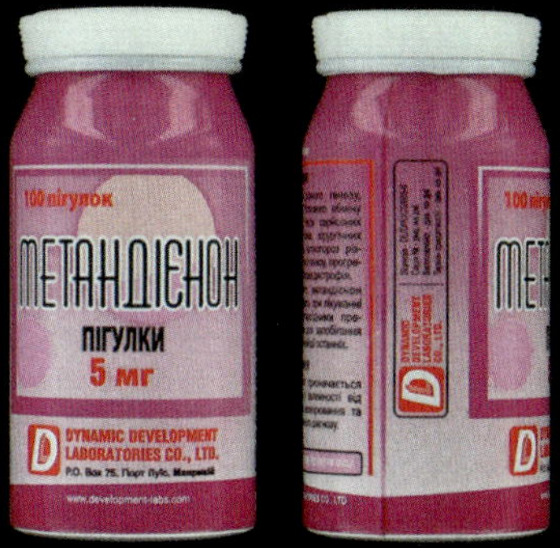

Generic from Ramopharmin (Iran)

Development Labs generic (Mauritius, Export)

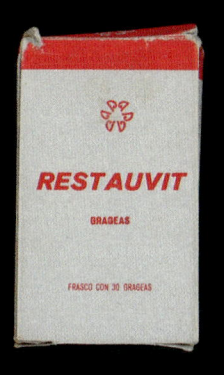

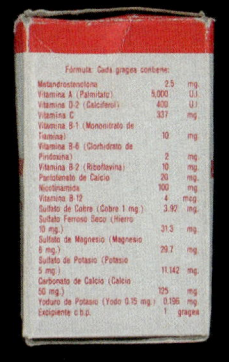

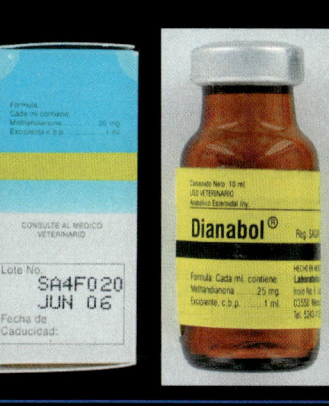

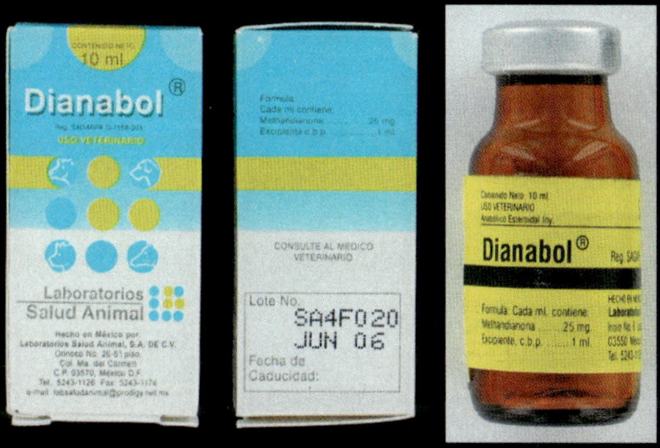

Restauvit Tabs (Mexico)

10ml injectable from Salud

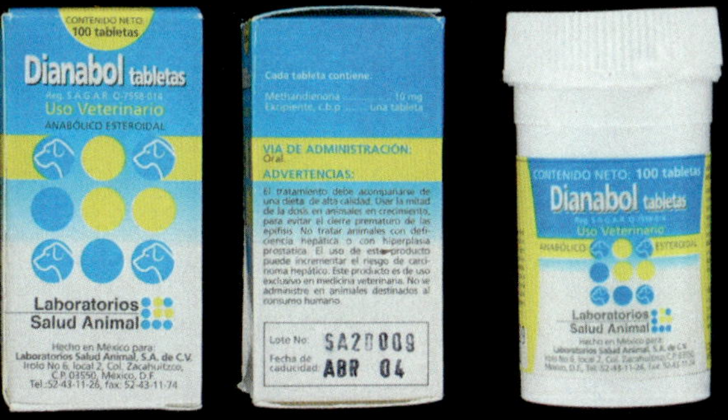

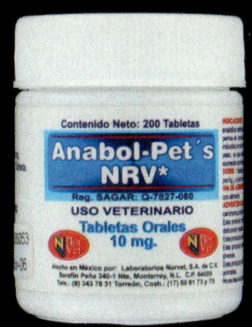

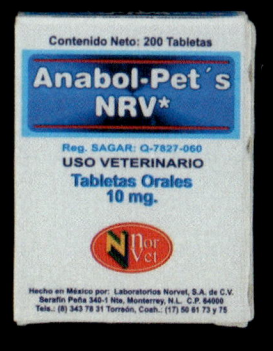

Dianabol tabs from Salud (Mexico)

Anabol-Pet's from Norvet (Mexico) NLM

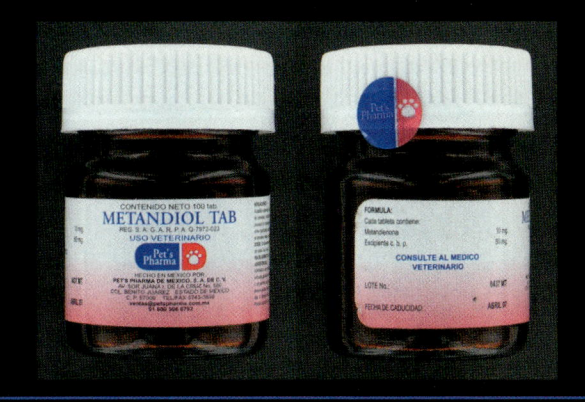

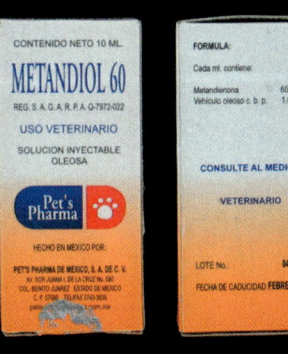

Oral Metandiol from Pet's Pharma (Mexico) NLM

Injectable Metandiol (NLM)

Appendix B

B-33

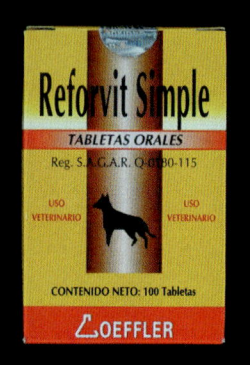

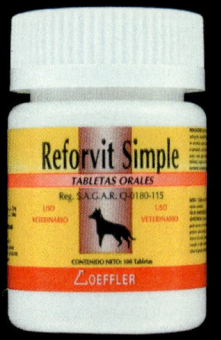

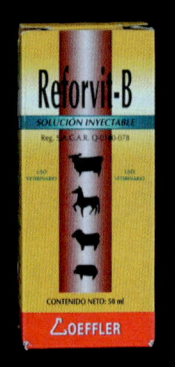

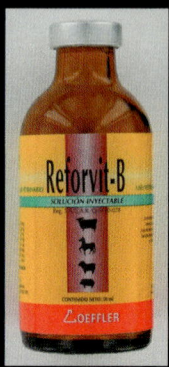

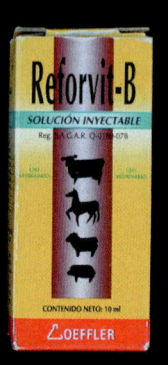

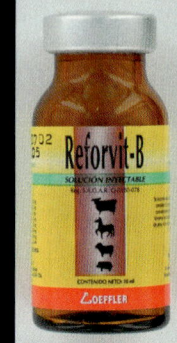

Reforvit tablets and injectables from Loeffler Mexico (NLM)

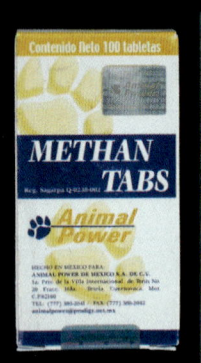

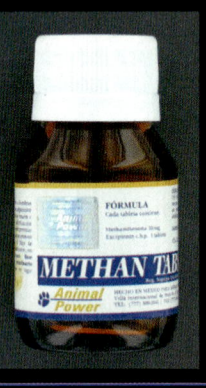

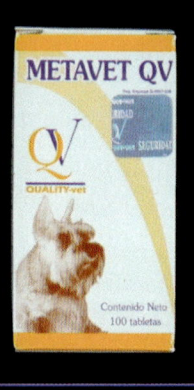

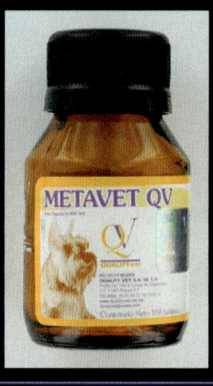

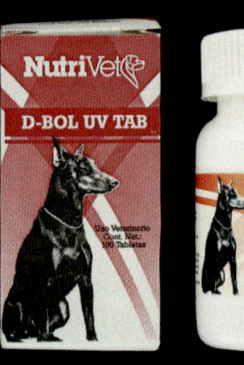

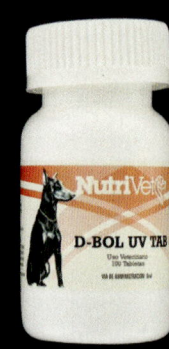

Animal Power (Mexico) NLM — Metavet from Quality Vet (Mexico) NLM — Nutrivet (Mexico, UG) NLM

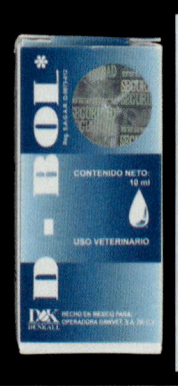

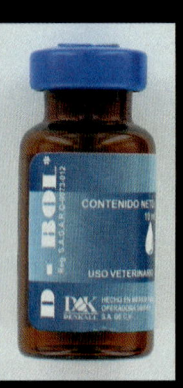

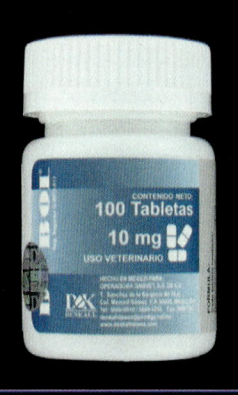

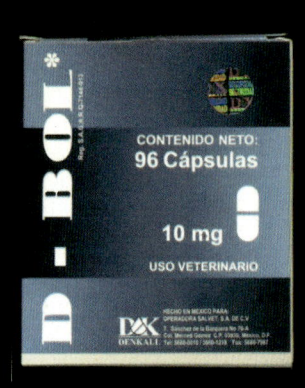

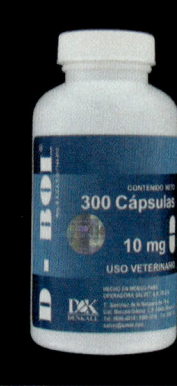

Denkall injectable (Mexico) NLM — Denkall 100 tablet bottle (NLM) — 96 and 300 capsule packaging (NLM)

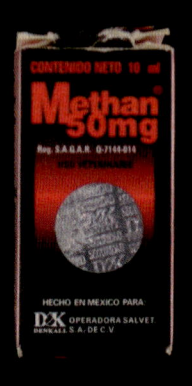

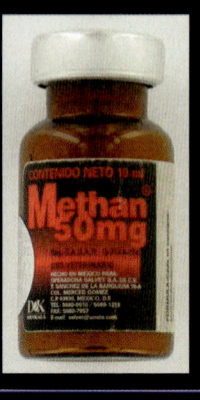

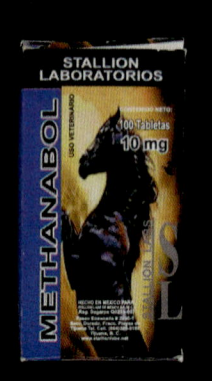

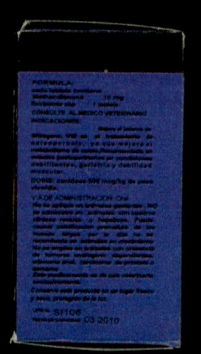

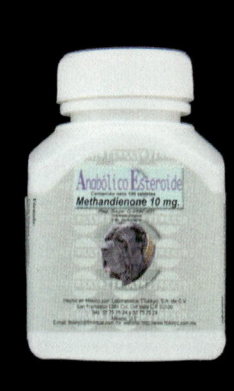

Fake Denkall Methan — Stallion Underground from Mexico (NLM) — Ttokkyo Mexico (NLM)

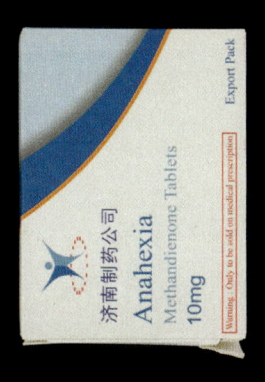

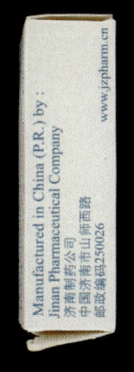

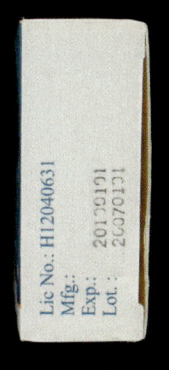

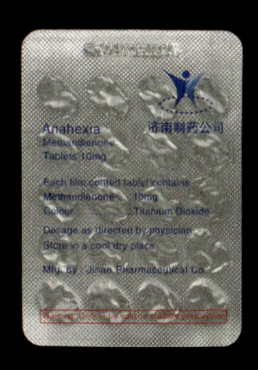

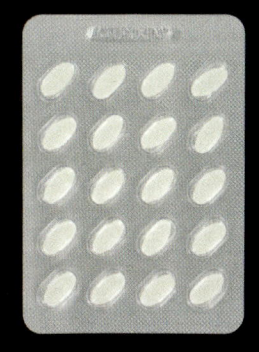

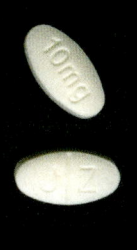

Anahexia from Jinan Pharmaceutical Co. (China)

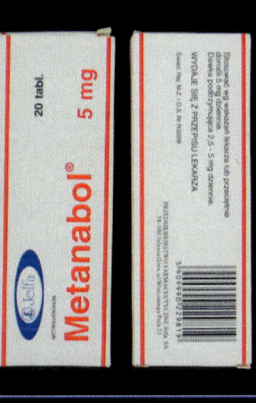

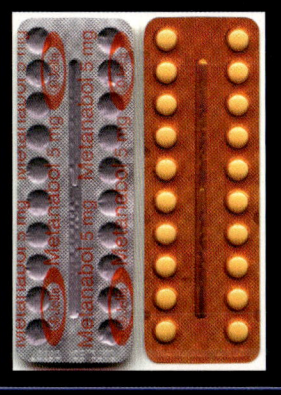

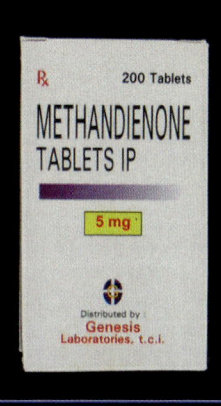

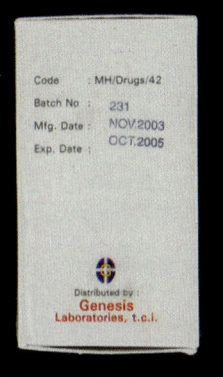

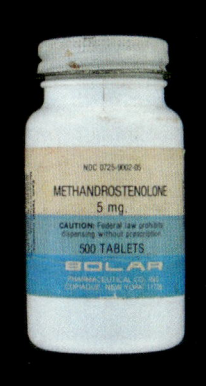

Metanabol from Poland (NLM)　　Genesis (Singapore, export) NLM　　U.S. generic (NLM)

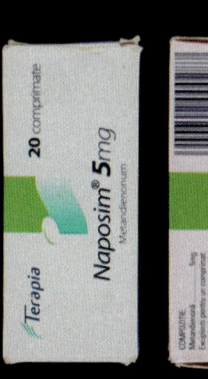

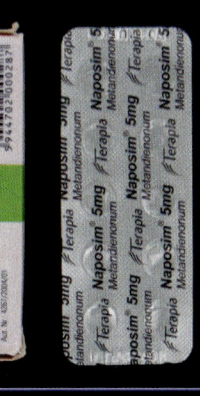

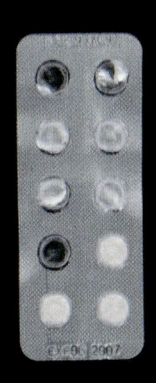

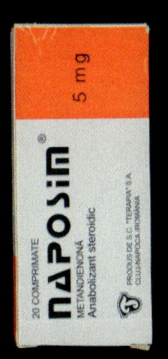

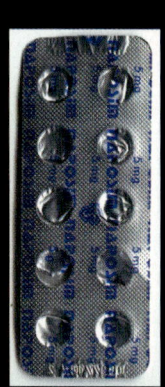

Naposim from Rumania　　Older look to Naposim

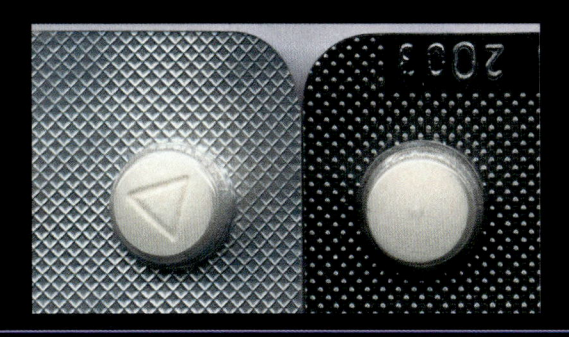

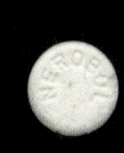

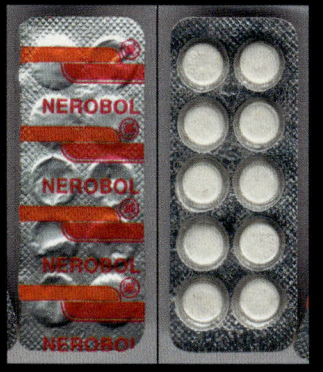

Fake Naposim on left (no nipple on blister, lacks numbers on both ends)　　Nerobol from Hungary (NLM)

Appendix B

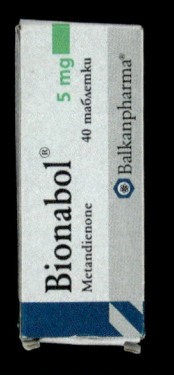

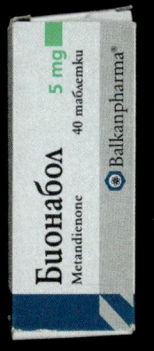

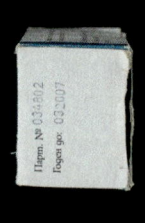

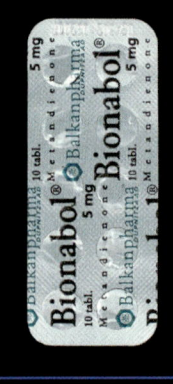

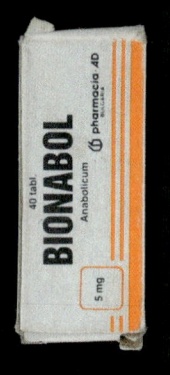

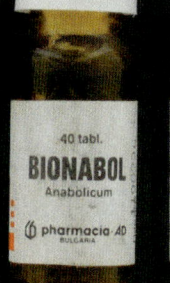

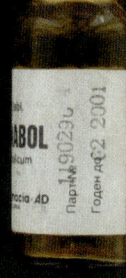

Bionabol from Bulgaria (NLM)

Old Bionabol box and bottle

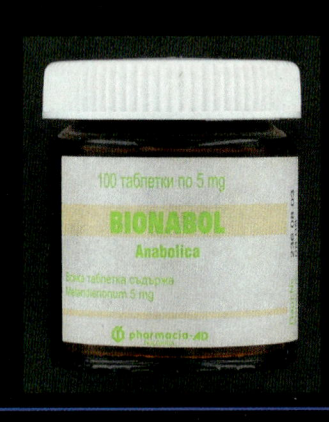

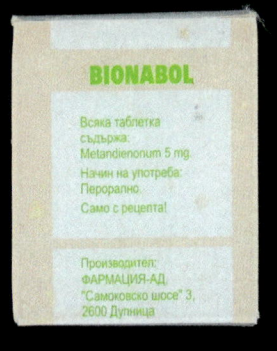

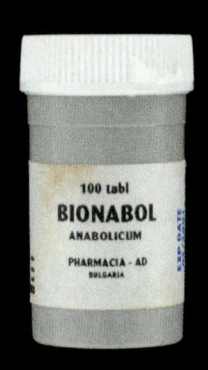

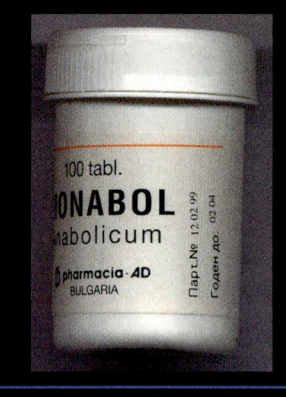

Three different counterfeit Bionabol products

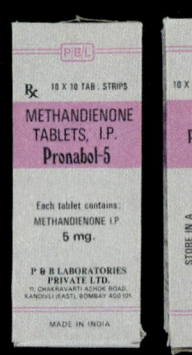

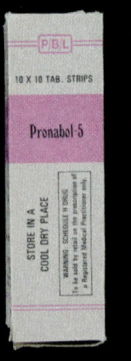

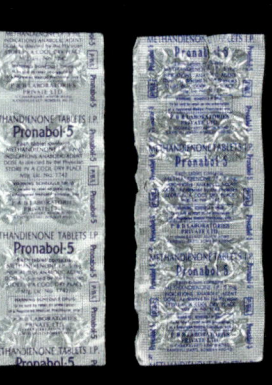

Pronabol from P/B/L India (NLM)

Trinergic from Unichem India (NLM)

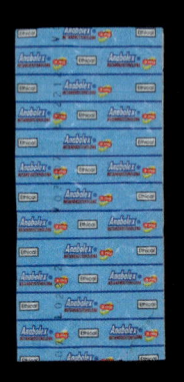

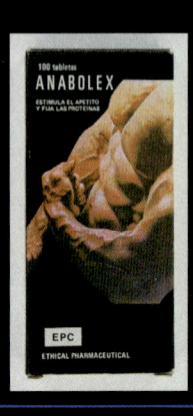

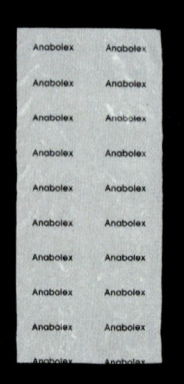

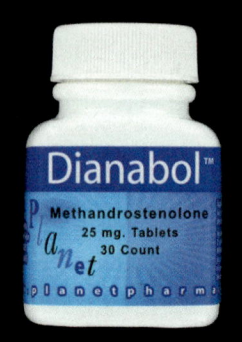

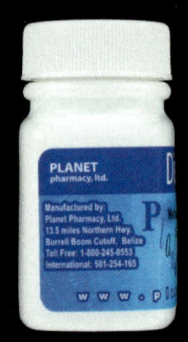

Anabolex from Dominican Republic (old version on right)

Dianabol from Planet Pharmacy (Belize) NLM

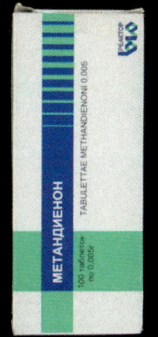

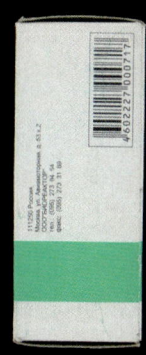

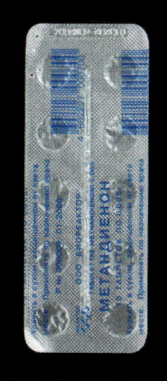

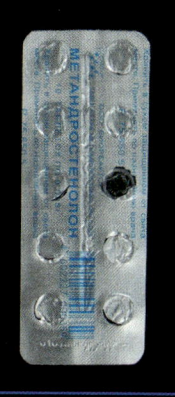

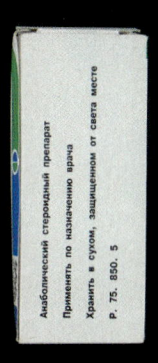

Bioreaktor from Russia (NLM) Counterfeit strip Counterfeit Bioreaktor box

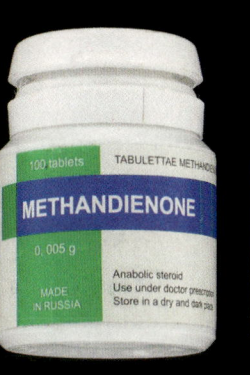

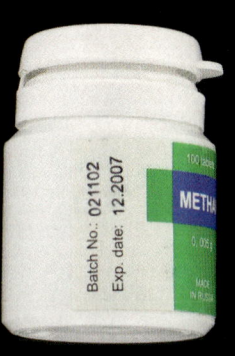

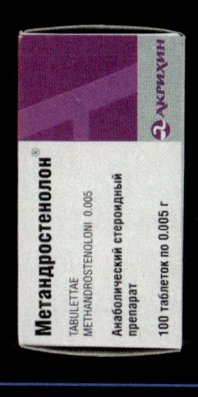

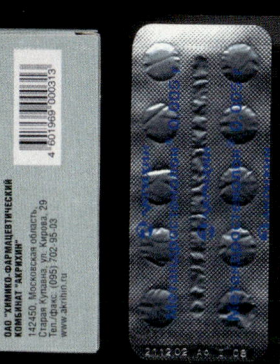

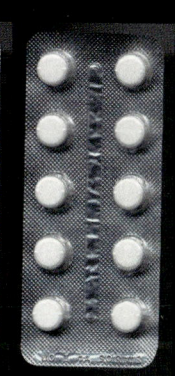

Another counterfeit Bioreaktor Russian Dianabol from Akrikhin

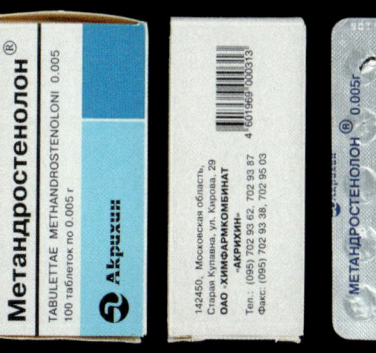

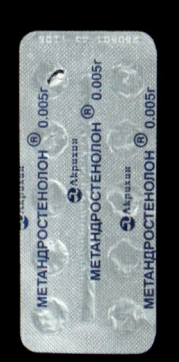

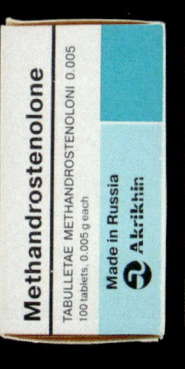

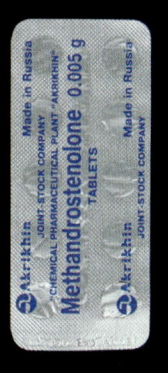

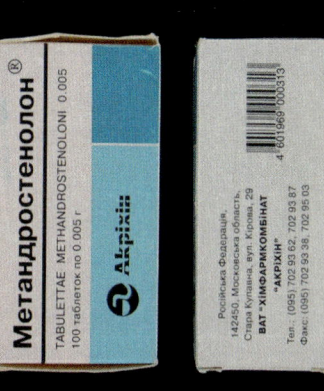

Older packaging Older packaging w/English text Russian Export to Ukraine

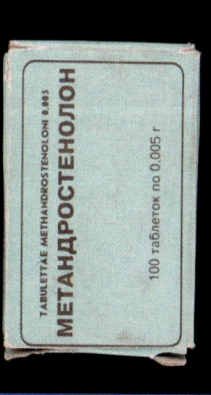

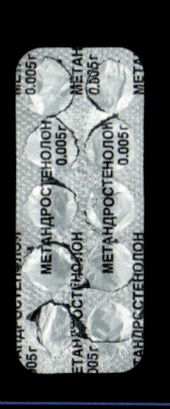

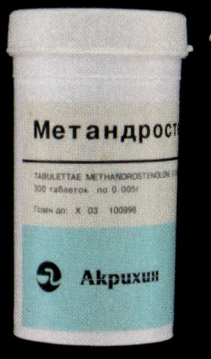

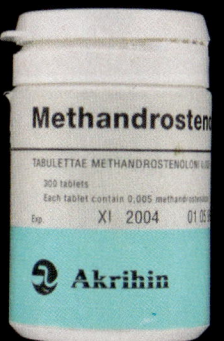

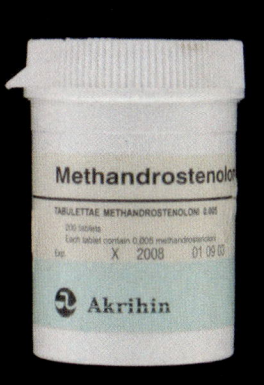

Very old Russian D-Bol Three different counterfeit bottles

Appendix B

B-37

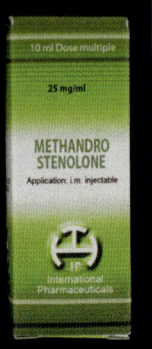

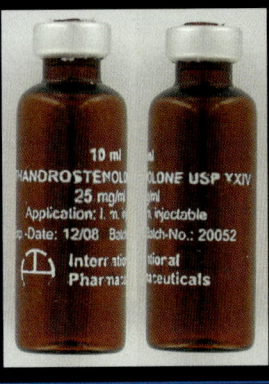

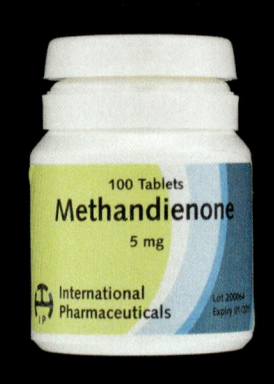

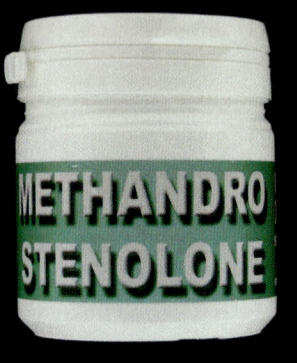

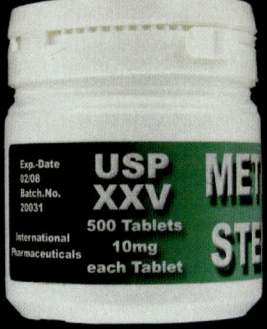

International Pharmaceuticals injectable and and oral products (Underground)

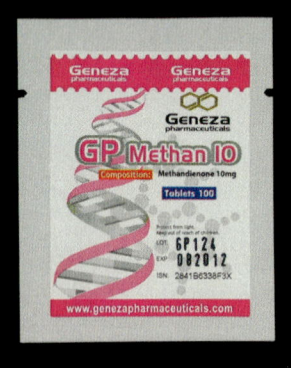

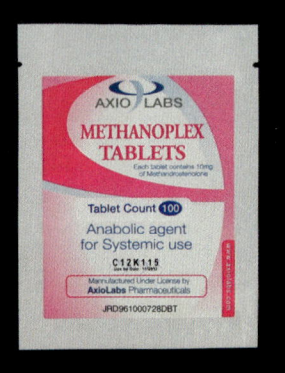

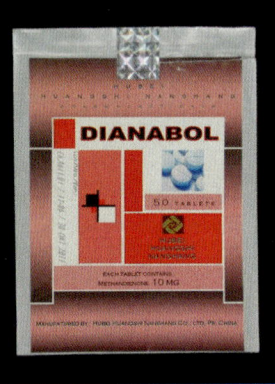

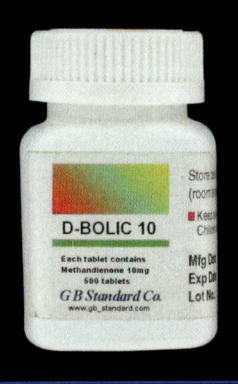

Underground products from Geneza, Hubei, Axio Labs, and G.B. Standard

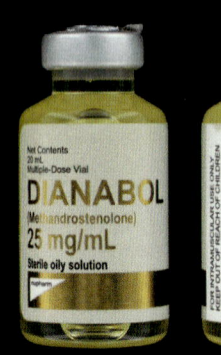

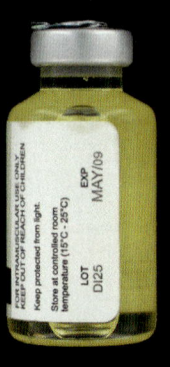

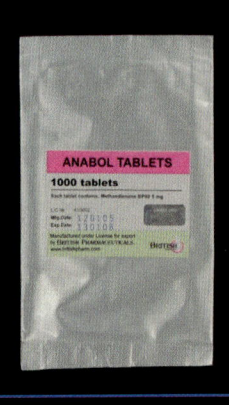

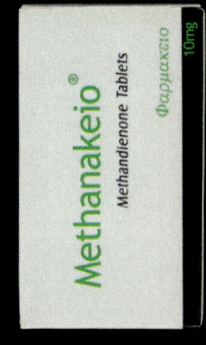

Nupharm (UG)   British Pharm (UG)   Tabs from Farmakeio (UG)

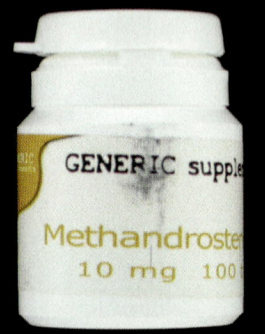

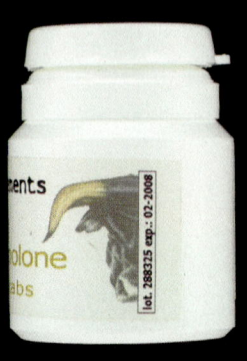

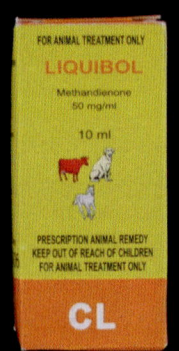

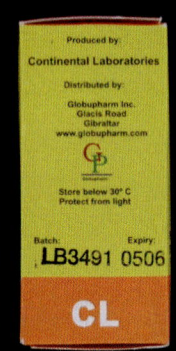

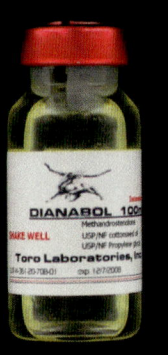

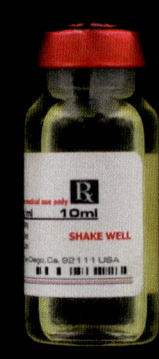

Underground products from Generic Supplements, Continental, and Toro

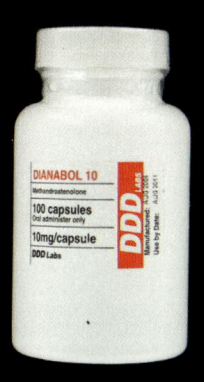

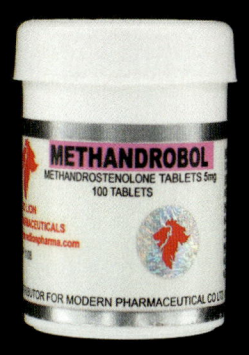

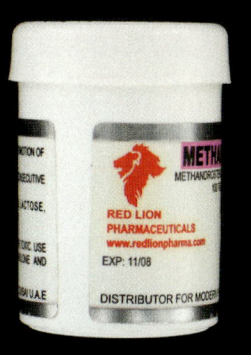

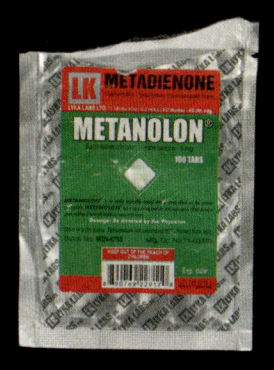

Underground products from DDD, Red Lion, and Lyka

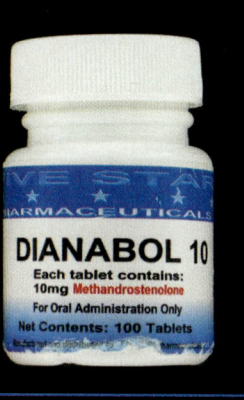

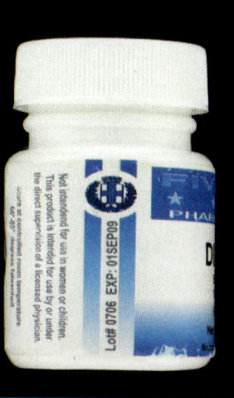

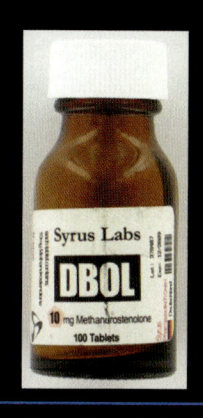

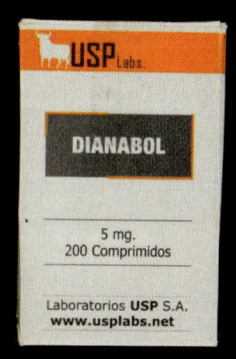

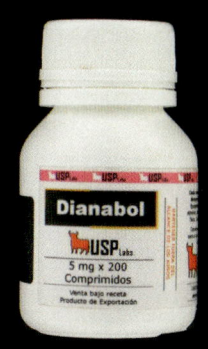

Underground products from 5 Star, Syrus, and USP Labs

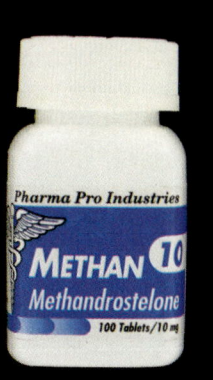

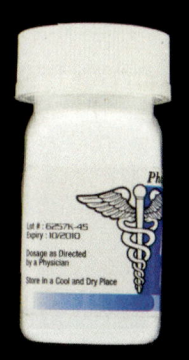

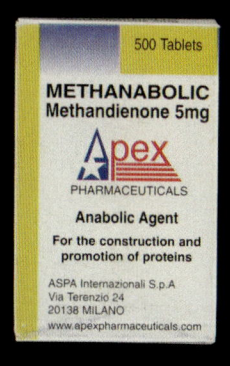

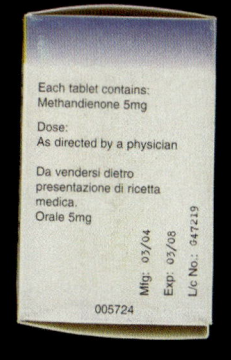

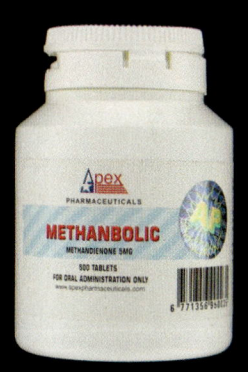

Underground products from Pharma Pro and Apex

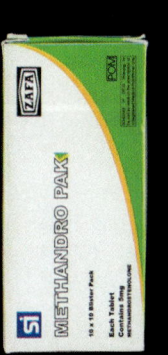

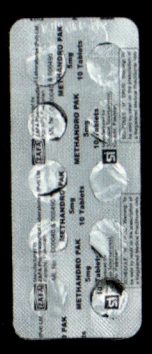

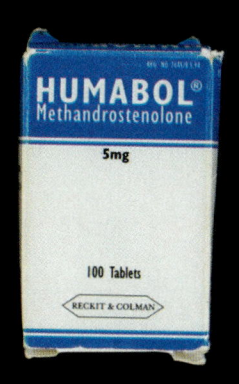

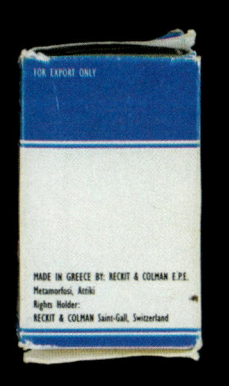

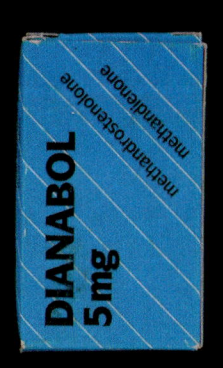

Three fake products with fabricated trade names

Appendix B

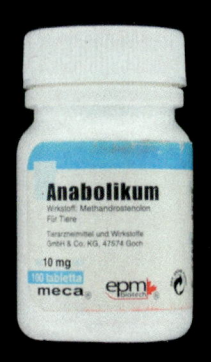

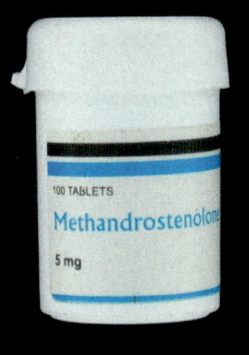

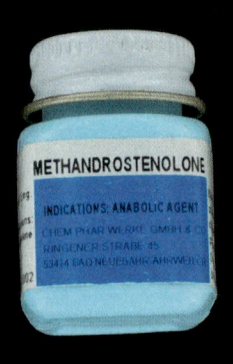

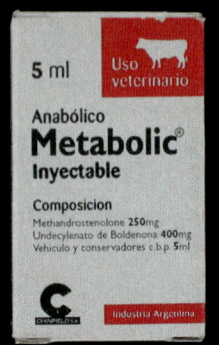

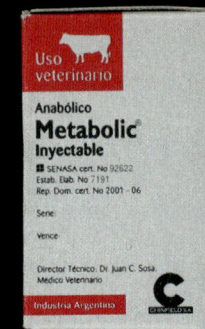

Four more fake methandrostenolone products

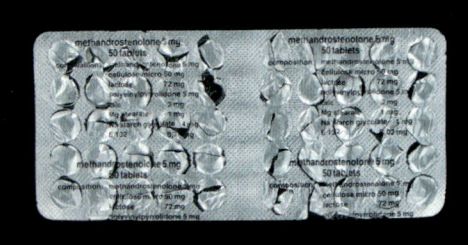

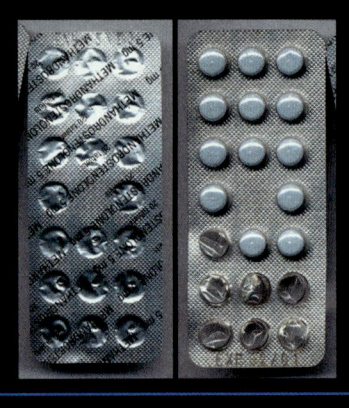

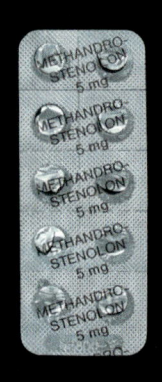

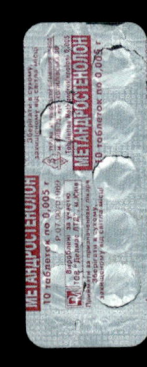

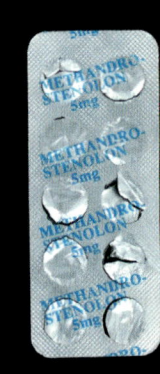

Another five fake Dianabol products

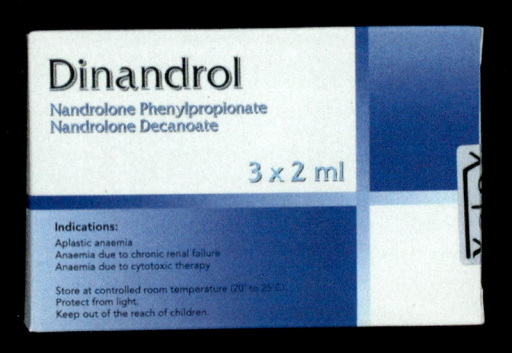

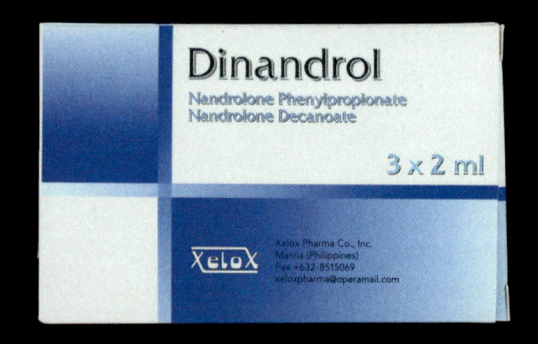

Dinandrol

Dinandrol from Xelox (Philippines)

Drive

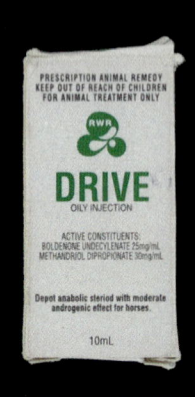

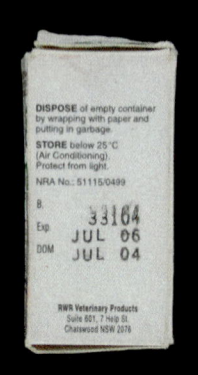

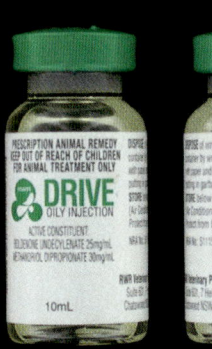

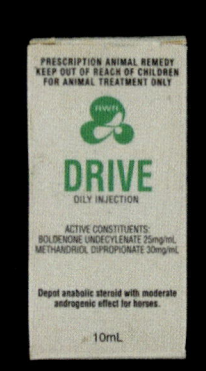

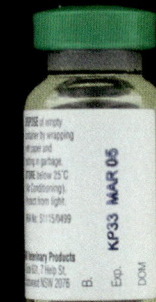

Drive from RWR Australia - older packaging on right

B-40

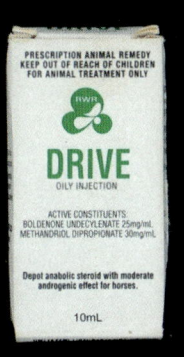

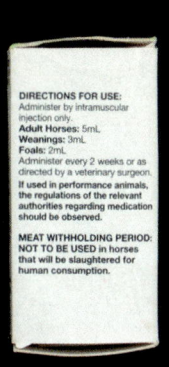

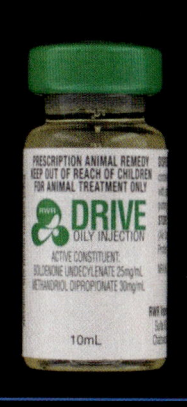

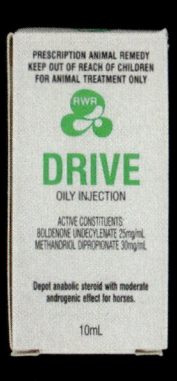

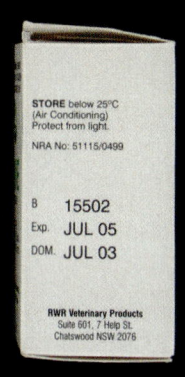

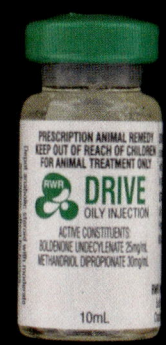

Counterfeit Drive

Another counterfeit box and vial

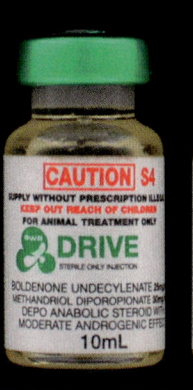

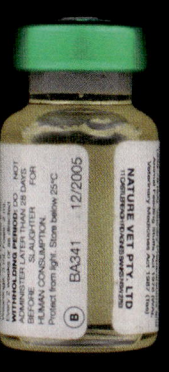

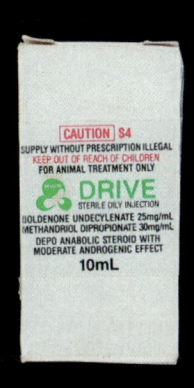

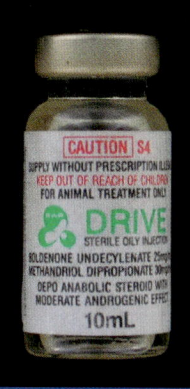

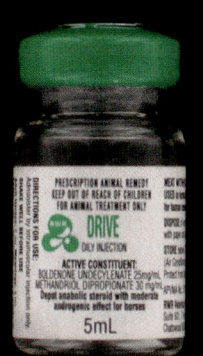

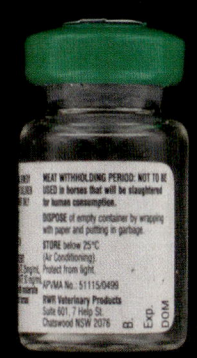

Three additional Drive counterfeits

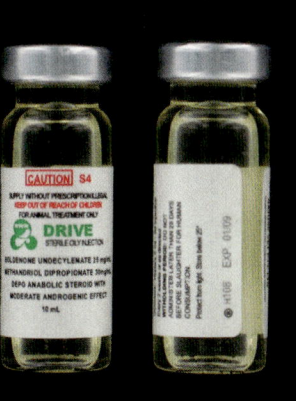

Another counterfeit

Durabolin

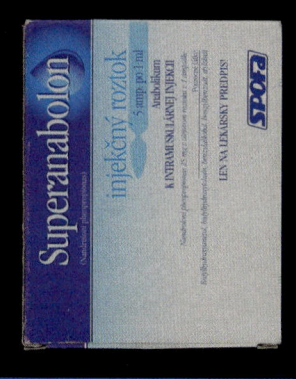

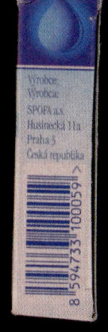

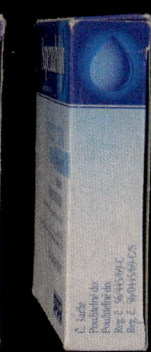

Superanabolan from Spofa (Czech Republic)

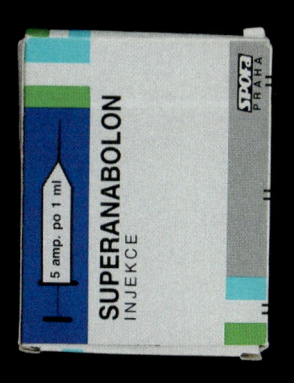

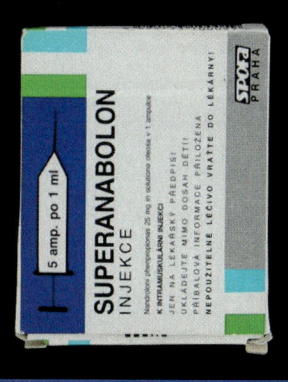

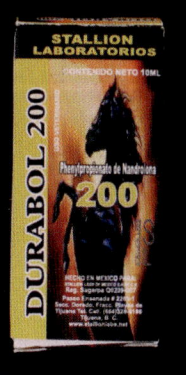

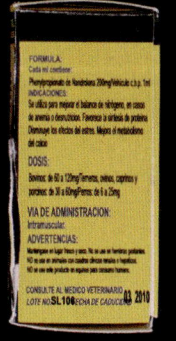

Older Superanabolon box

Stallion Labs (Mexico, UG) NLM

Appendix B

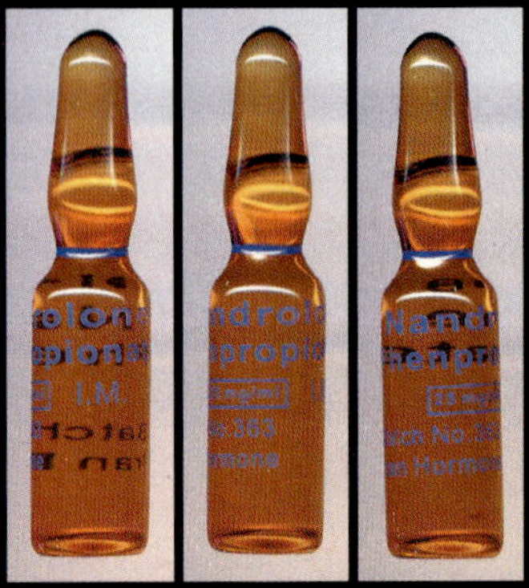

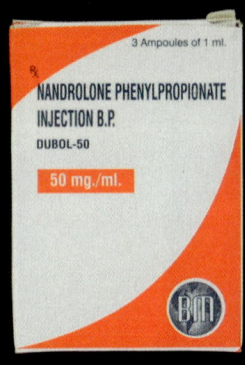

Ampules from Iran Hormone 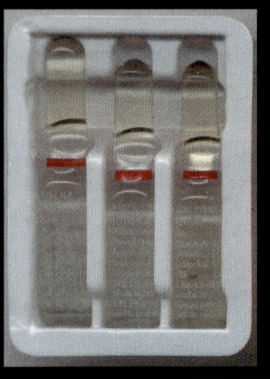   Nandrolone phenylpropionate from BM (India, export) 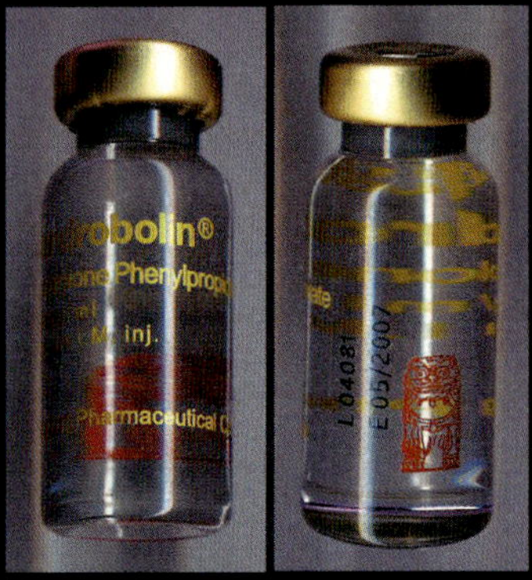   Luoyang (China, export)

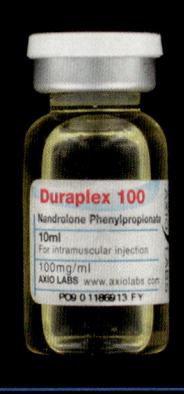

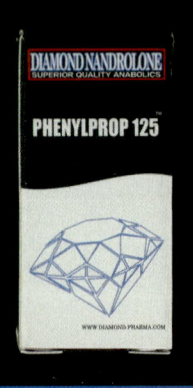

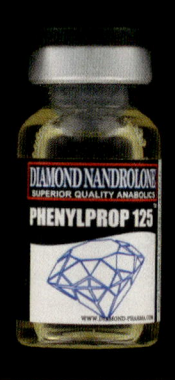

Diamond (Underground) 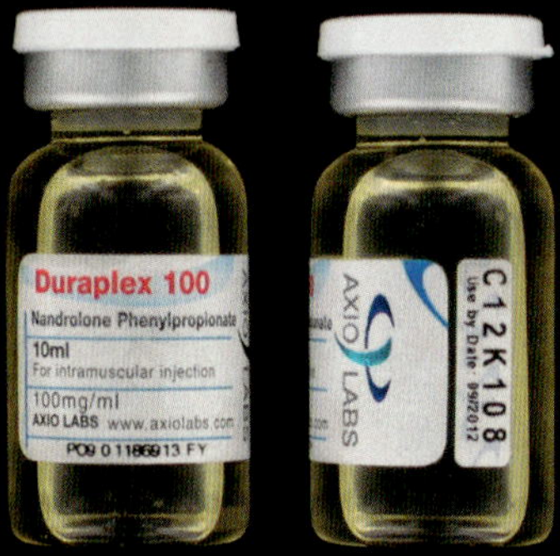   Axio Labs (Underground) 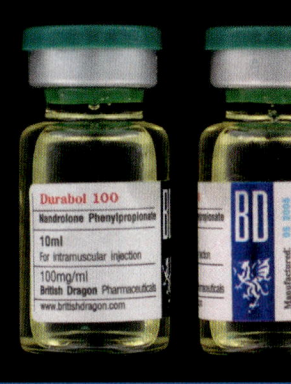   British Dragon Durabol (UG) NLM

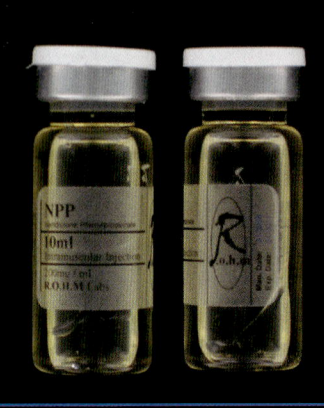

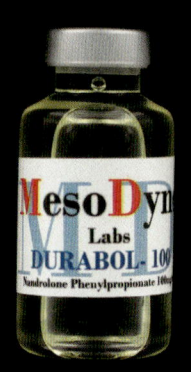

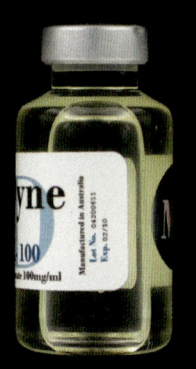

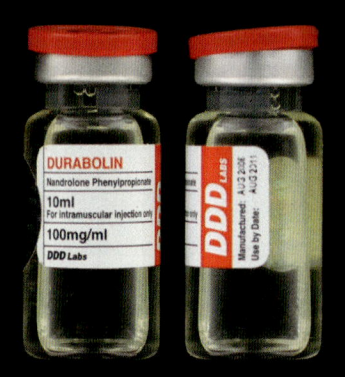

Underground products from R.O.H.M., MesoDyne, and DDD

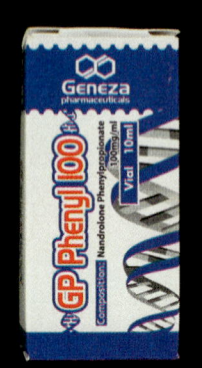

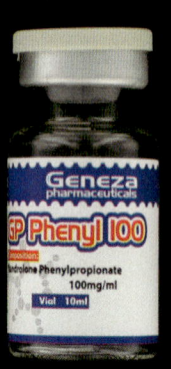

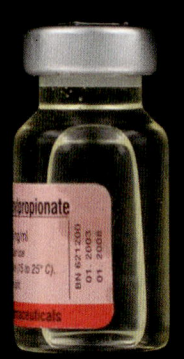

Geneza (Underground) 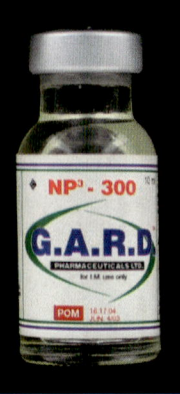   G.A.R.D. (UG) 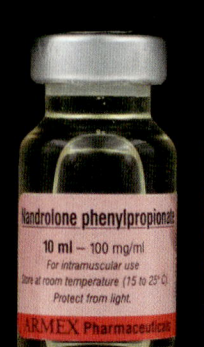   Armex fake 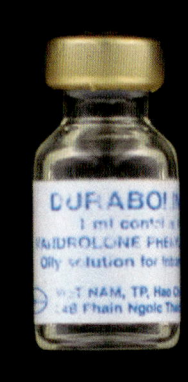   Counterfeit (Vietnam)

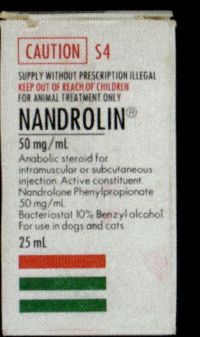

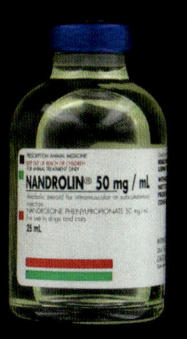

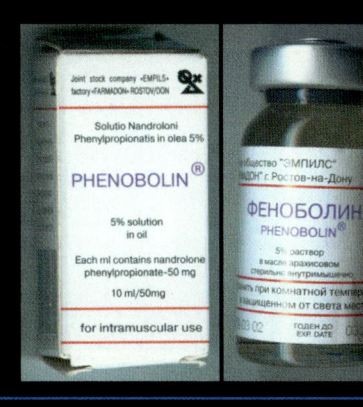

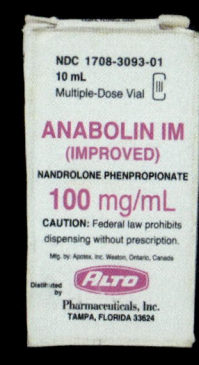

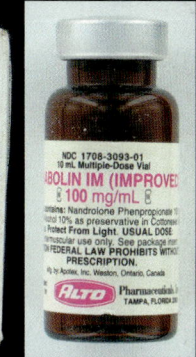

Intervet counterfeit (Australia)　　Farmadon counterfeit (Russia)　　Fake U.S. Anabolin

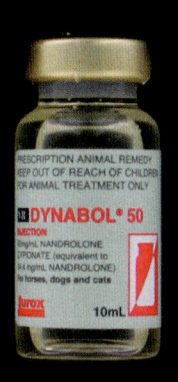

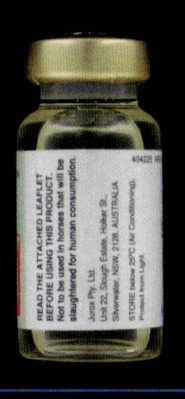

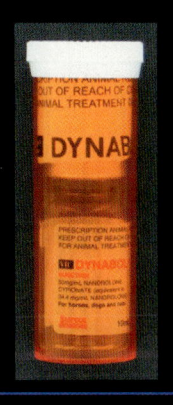

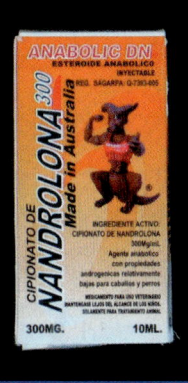

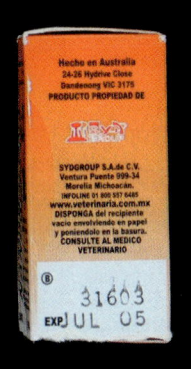

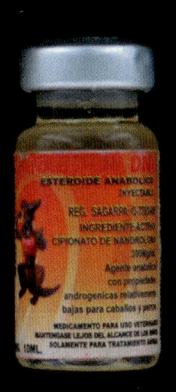

Dynabol

Dynabol 50 from Jurox Australia (NLM)　　Anabolic DN from SYD Group (Mexico) NLM

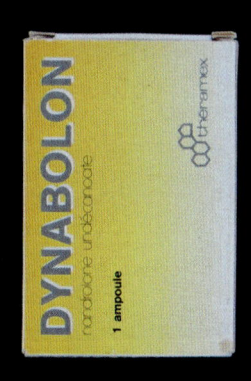

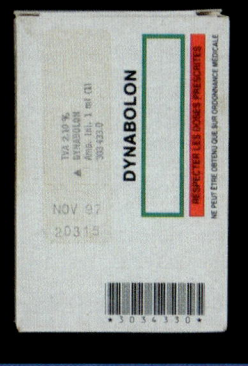

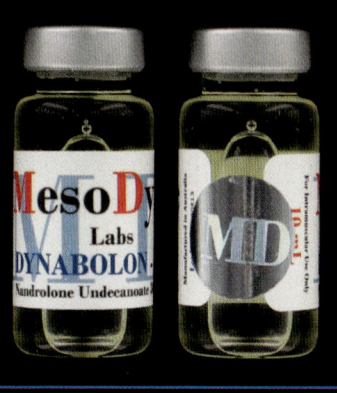

Dynabolon

Dynabolon from France (NLM)　　MesoDyne vial (Underground)

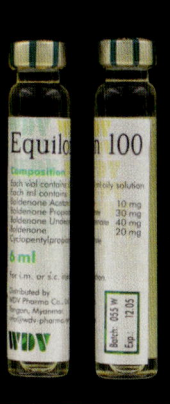

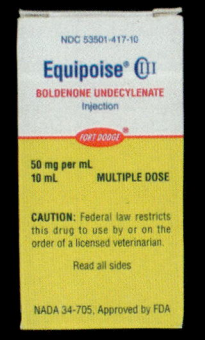

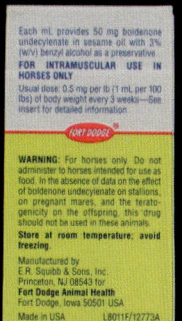

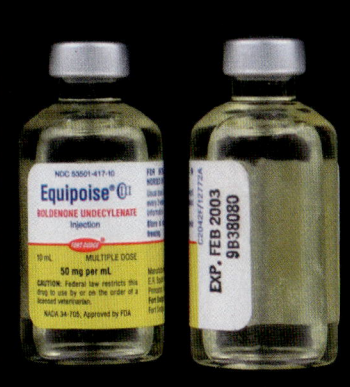

Equilon　　**Equipoise**

Equilon (Myanmar)　　Equipoise from Fort Dodge (U.S.)

Appendix B

B-43

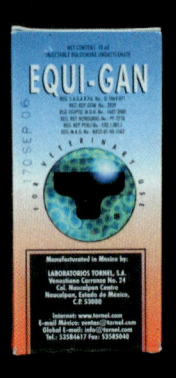

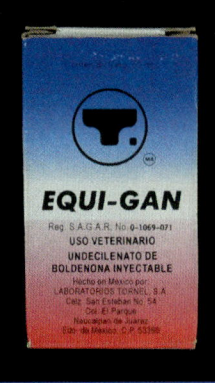

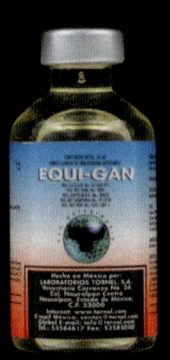

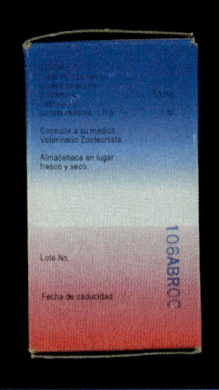

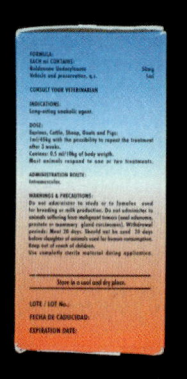

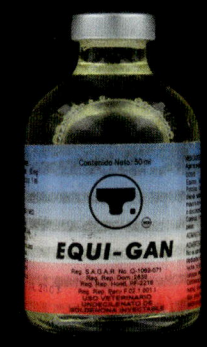

Equi-Gan 10ml from Tornel (Mexico)

Equi-Gan 50ml - older style packaging

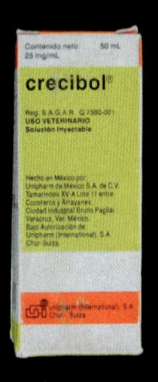

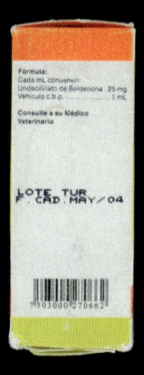

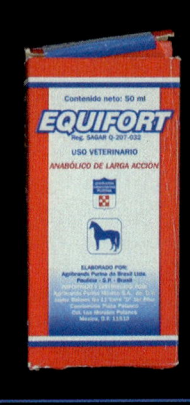

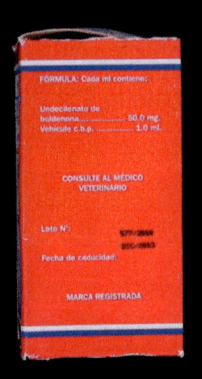

Mexican Crecibol

Equifort from Purina (Mexico)

Gorilla Power (Mexico, UG)

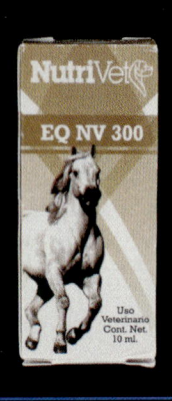

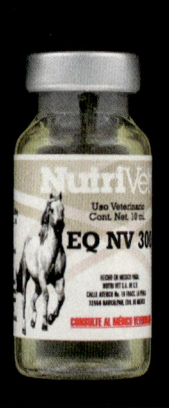

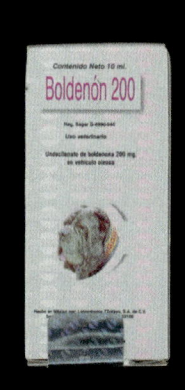

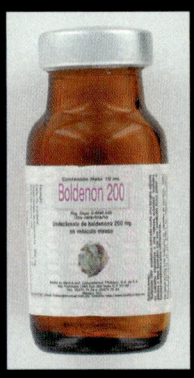

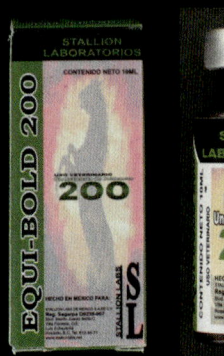

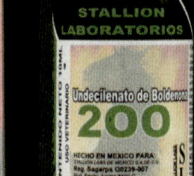

Underground EQ NV (Mexico) NLM

Ttokkyo Mexico (NLM)

Stallion Mexican UG (NLM)

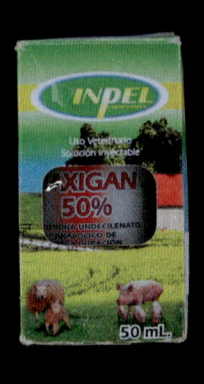

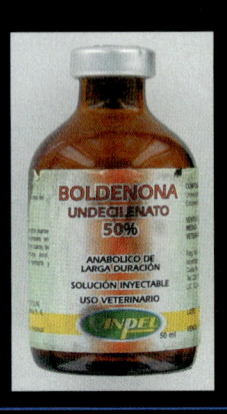

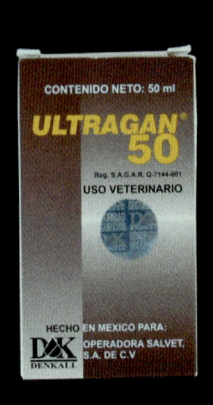

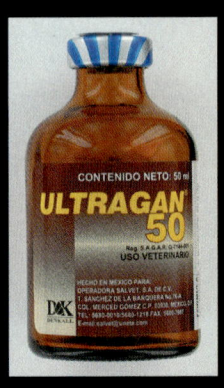

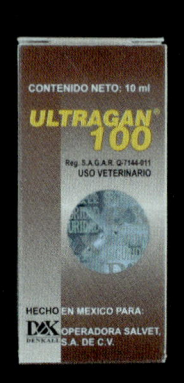

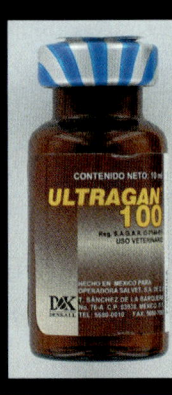

Maxigan from Inpel/Denkall Mexico (NLM)

Ultragan 50ml and 10ml from Denkall Mexico (NLM)

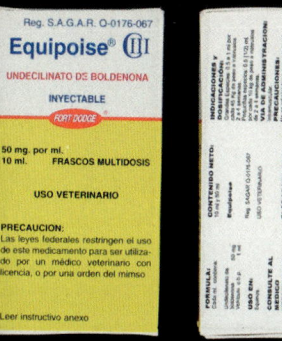

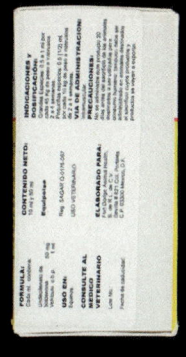

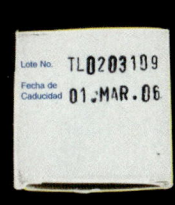

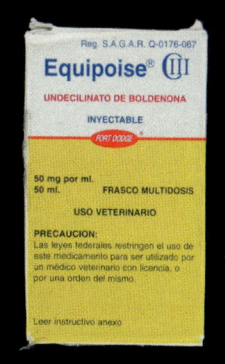

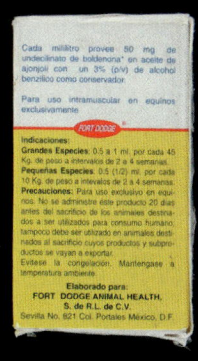

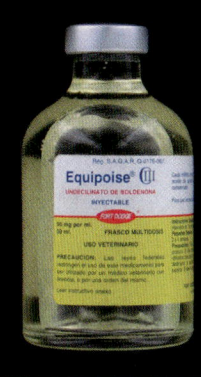

Fort Dodge 10ml from Mexico (NLM)

50ml box and vial from Mexico (NLM)

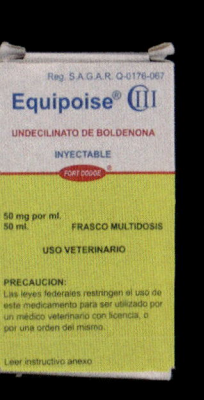

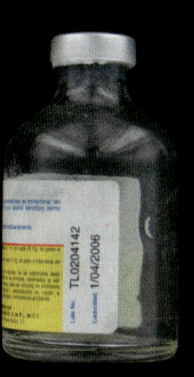

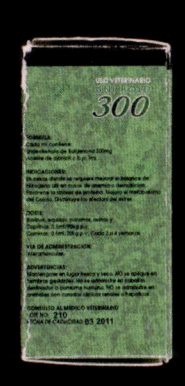

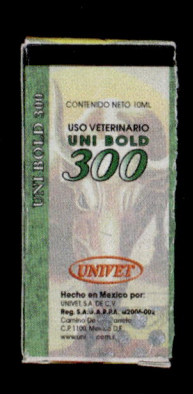

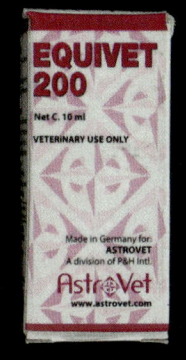

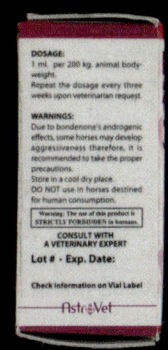

Counterfeit box and vial (Mexico)

Univet (Mexico, underground)

AstroVet (Mexico, UG)

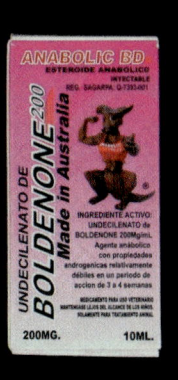

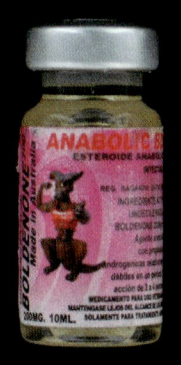

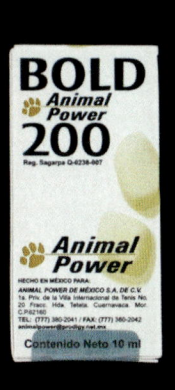

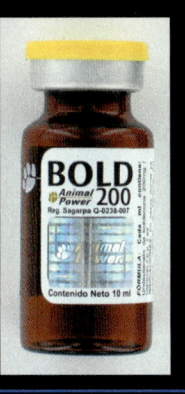

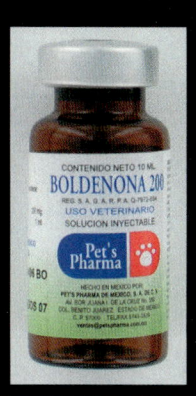

SYD Group Anabolic BD (Mexico) NLM

Animal Power Bold 200 (Mexico) NLM

Pet's Pharma generic (Mexico) NLM

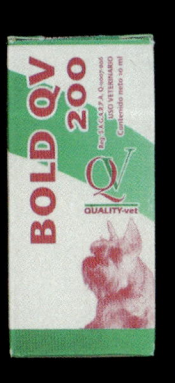

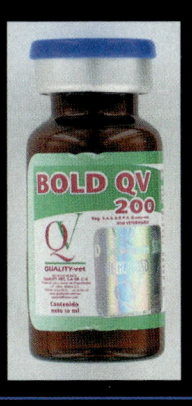

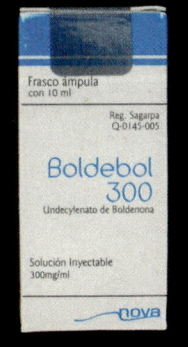

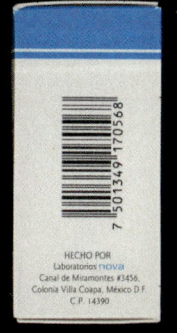

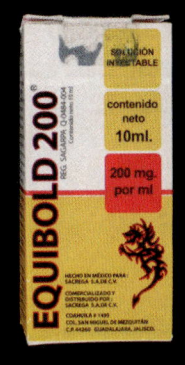

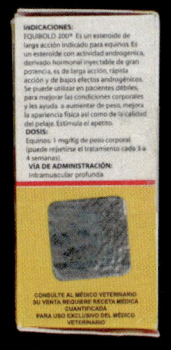

Quality Vet Bold 200 (Mexico) NLM

Nova Underground (Mexico)

Sacrega (Mexico, Underground)

Appendix B

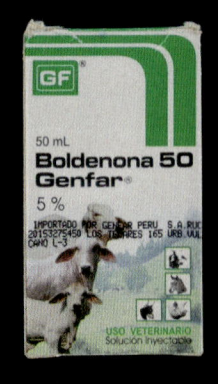

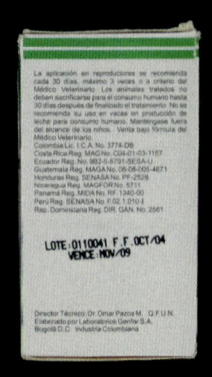

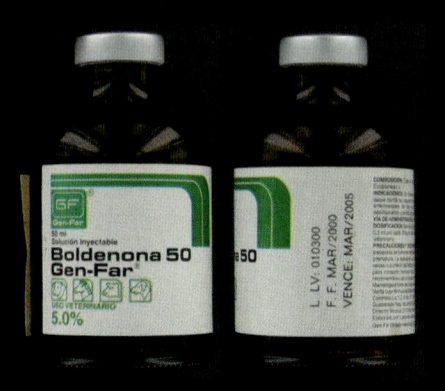

Boldenona 50 from Genfar (Colombia)

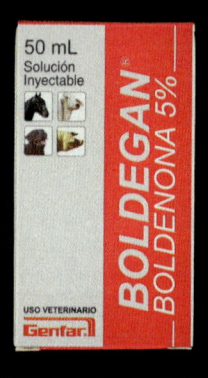

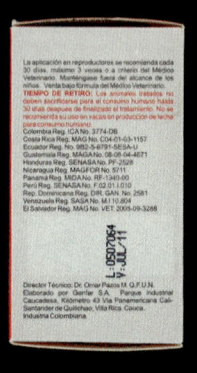

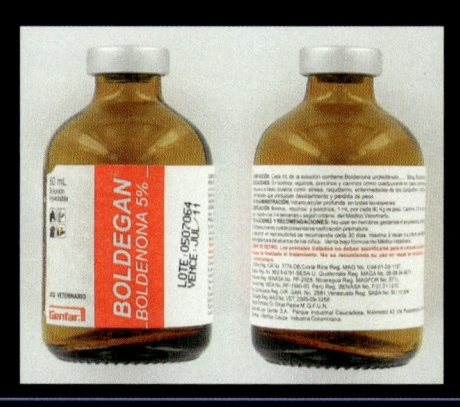

Genfar's Boldegan product (Colombia)

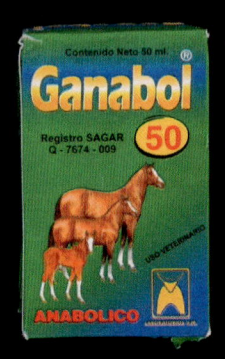

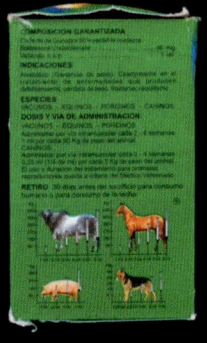

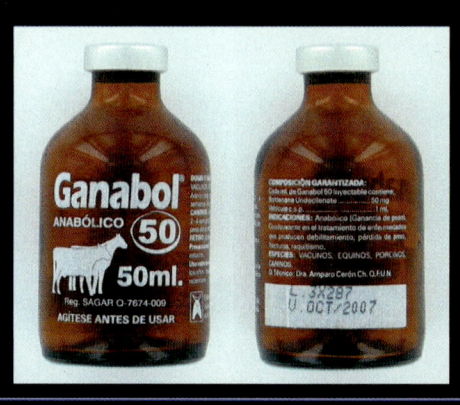

Ganabol from Colombia

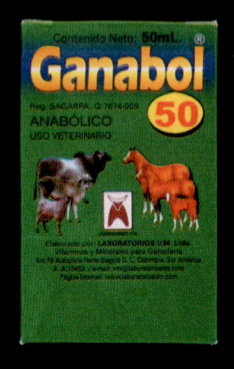

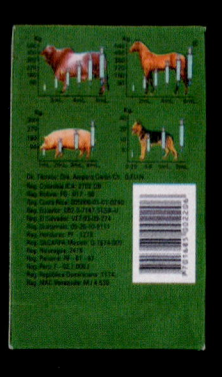

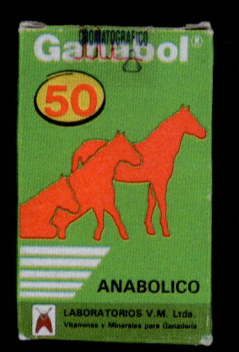

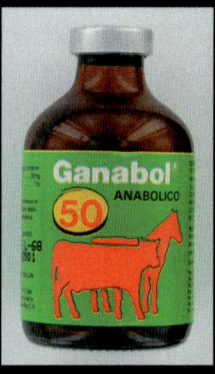

Another South American box   Previous Ganabol packaging (Colombia)

B-46

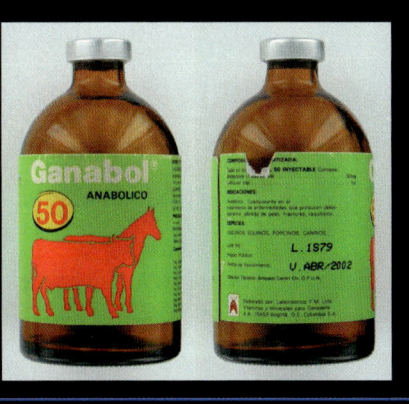

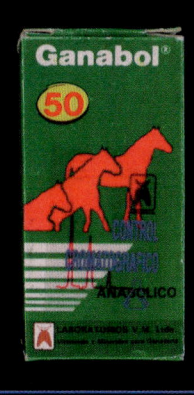

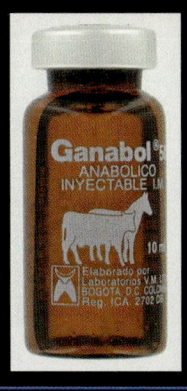

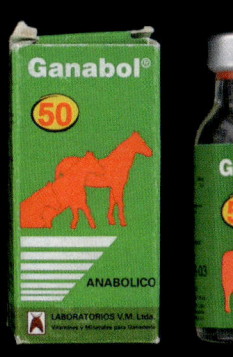

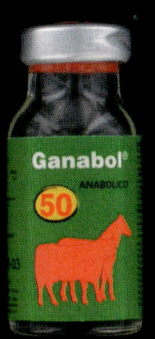

Old 100ml vial

Ganabol counterfeit box and vial

Another counterfeit Ganabol

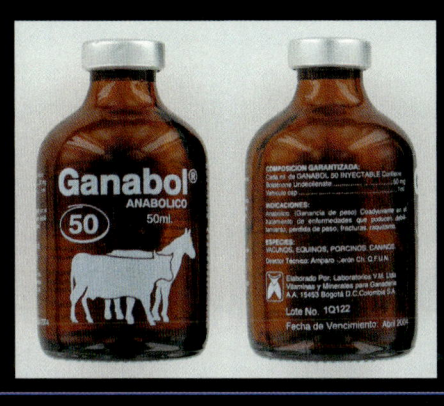

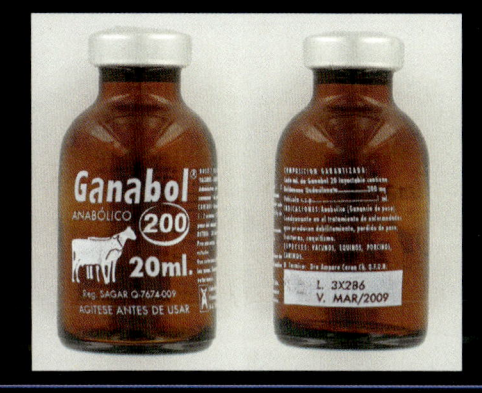

Counterfeit 50ml vial

Fake 200mg/mL version

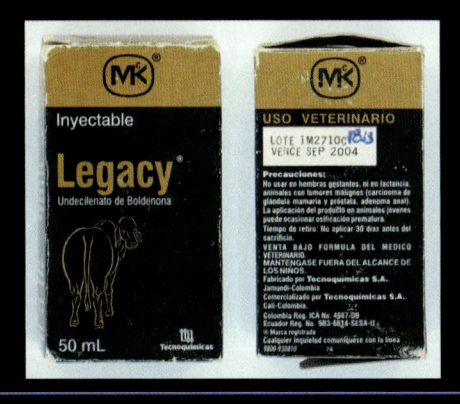

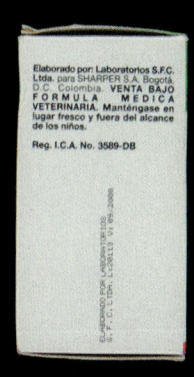

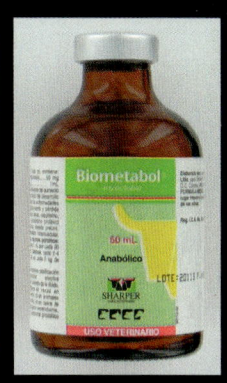

Legacy 50ml product (Colombia)

Biometabol from Colombia

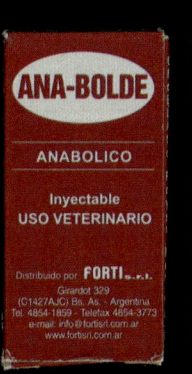

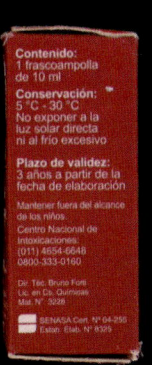

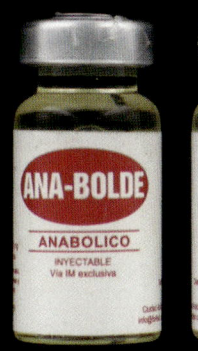

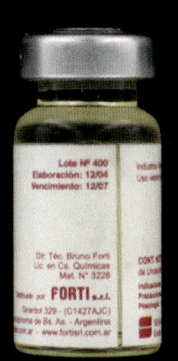

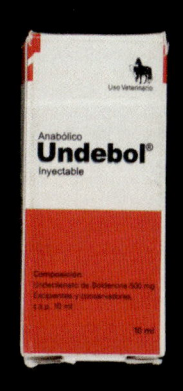

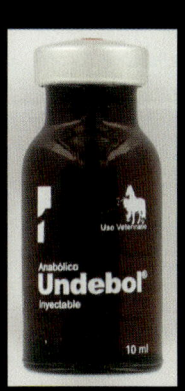

Ana-Bolde from Argentina

Fake Undebol (Argentina)

Appendix B

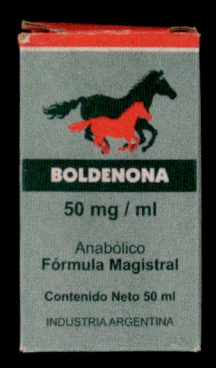

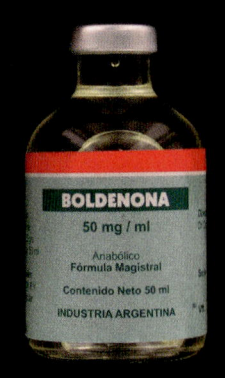

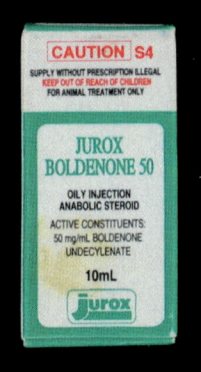

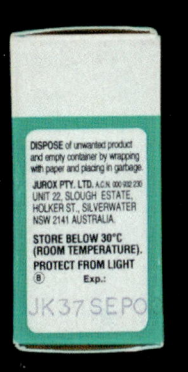

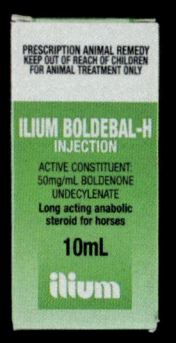

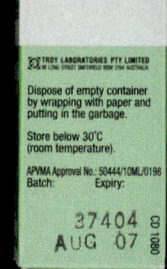

Magistral counterfeit (Argentina)   Australian Jurox Boldenone 50 (NLM)   Ilium Boldebal-H (Australia)

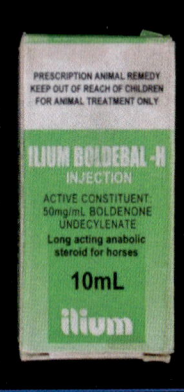

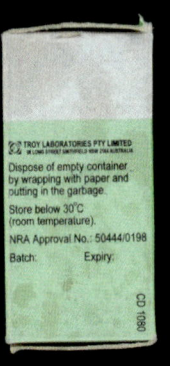

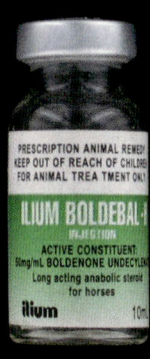

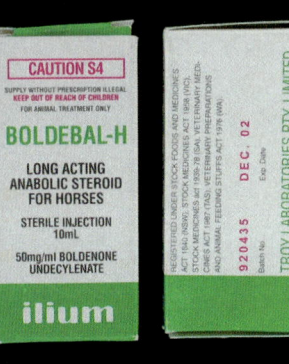

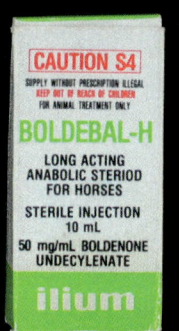

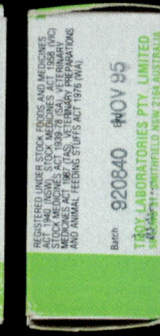

Boldebal-H counterfeit #1   Counterfeit #2   Counterfeit #3

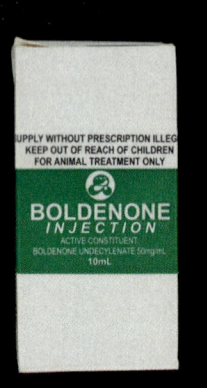

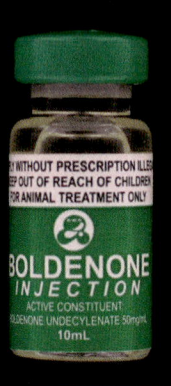

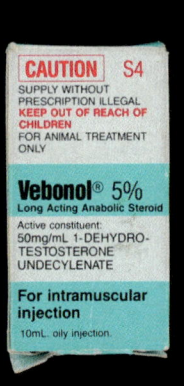

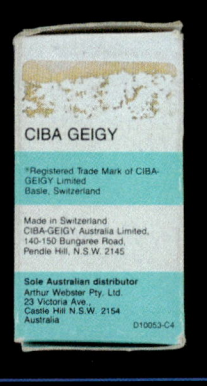

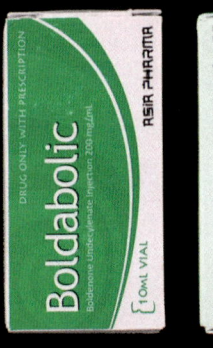

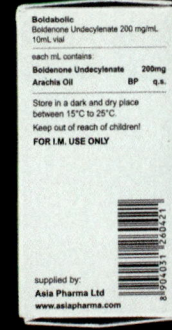

RWR counterfeit (Australia)   Vebonol from Australia (NLM)   Boldabolic (Malaysia)

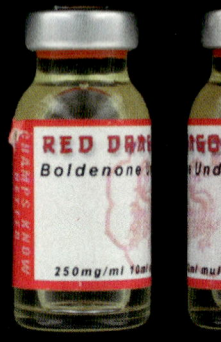

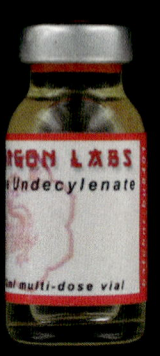

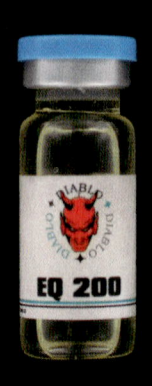

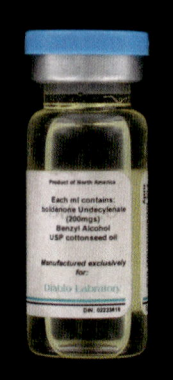

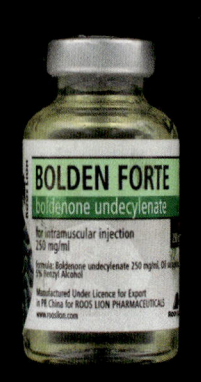

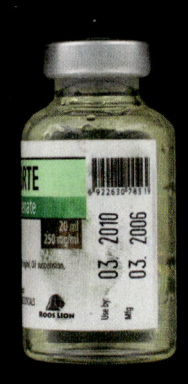

Underground products from Red Dragon, Diablo, and Roos Lion

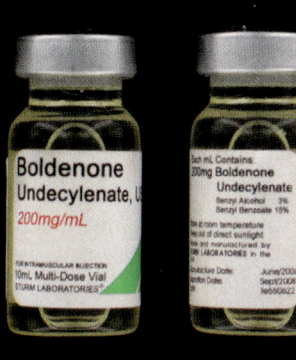

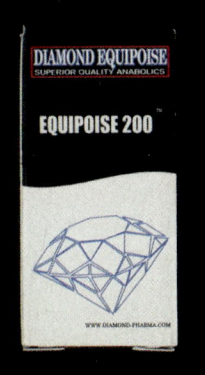

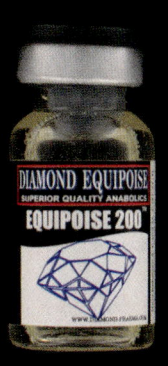

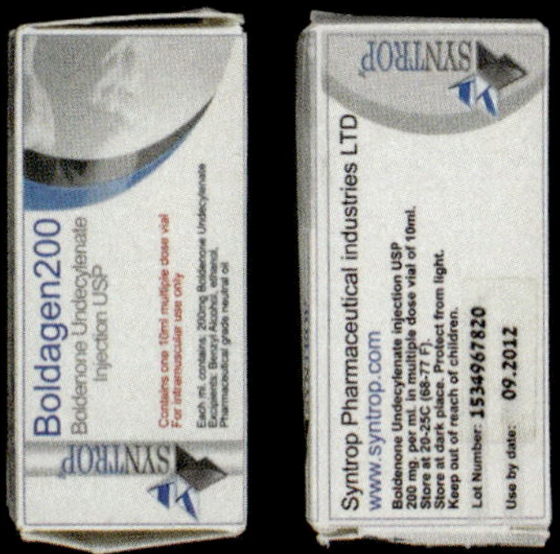

Underground products from Sturm, Diamond, and Syntrop

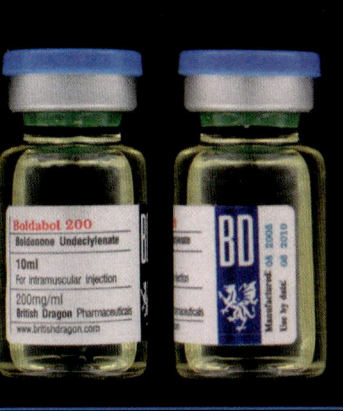

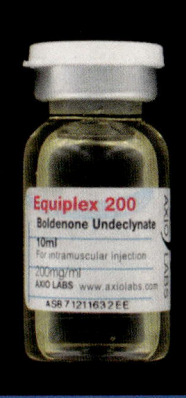

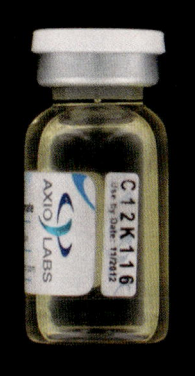

British Dragon (Underground) NLM   Axio Labs (Underground) 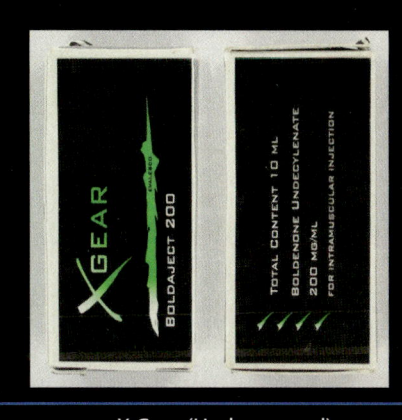   X Gear (Underground)

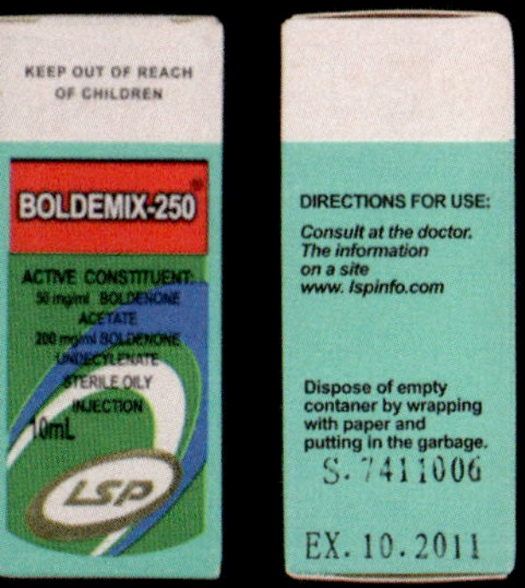

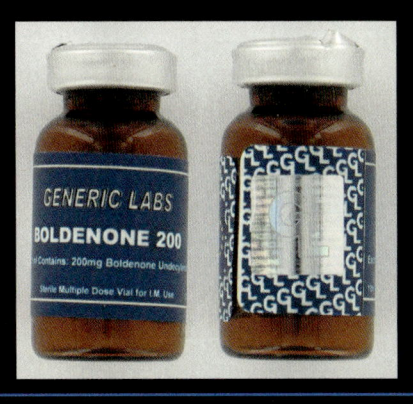

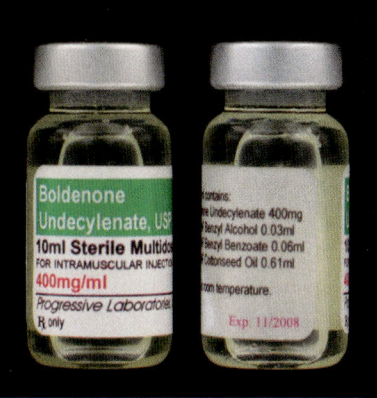

Underground products from LSP, Generic, and Progressive

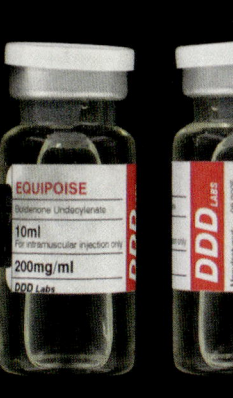

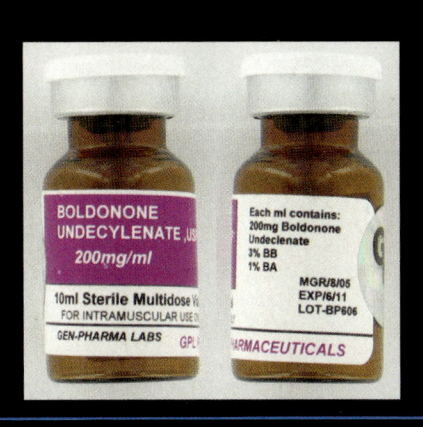

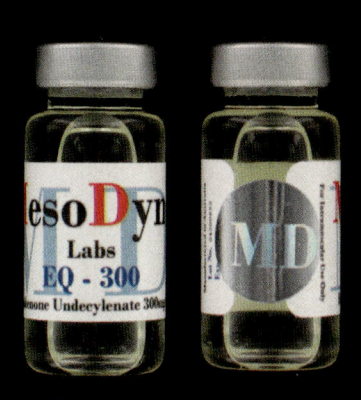

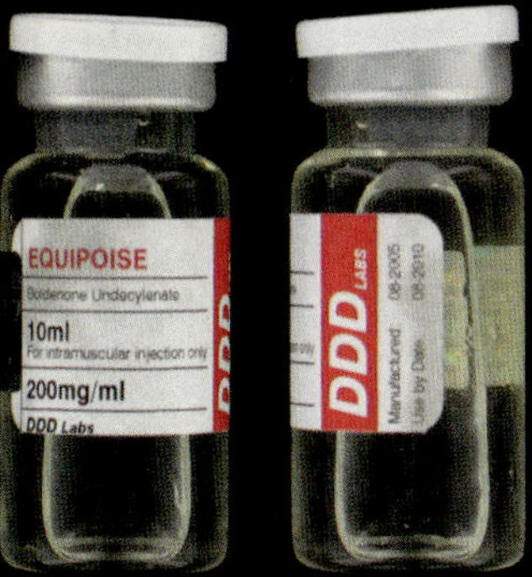

Underground products from DDD, GPL, and MesoDyne

Appendix B

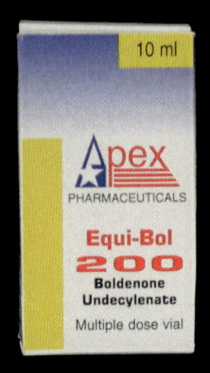

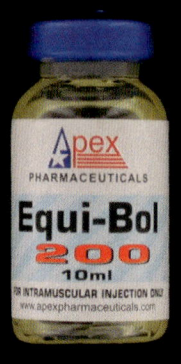

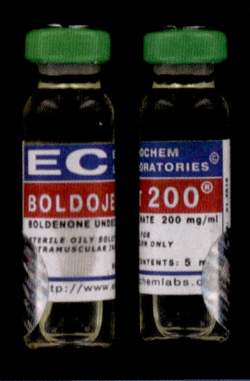

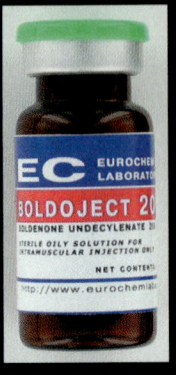

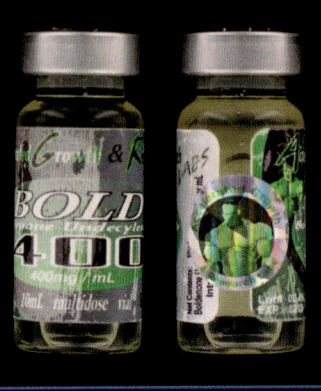

Underground Equi-Bol from Apex

Eurochem 5ml and 10ml vials (Underground)

Accelerated Growth (UG)

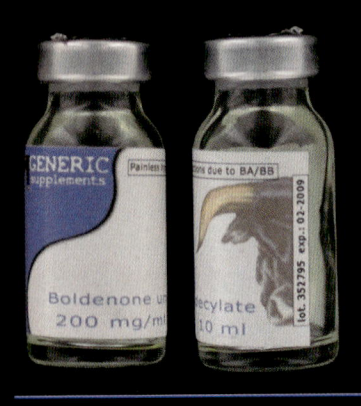

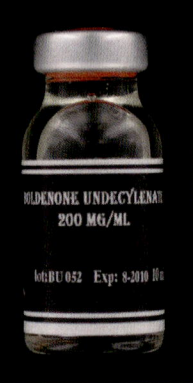

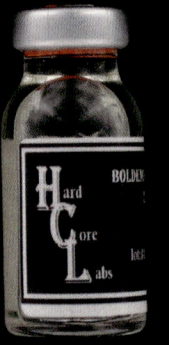

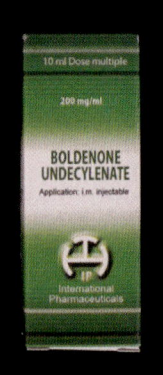

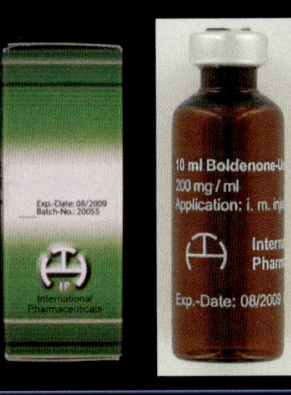

Generic Supplements (UG)

Hardcore Labs (Underground)

International Pharmaceuticals (UG)

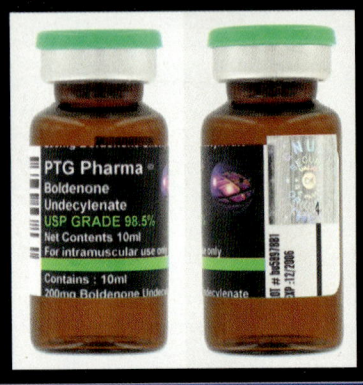

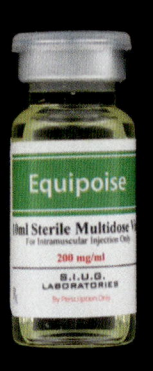

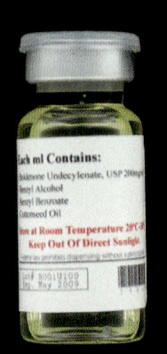

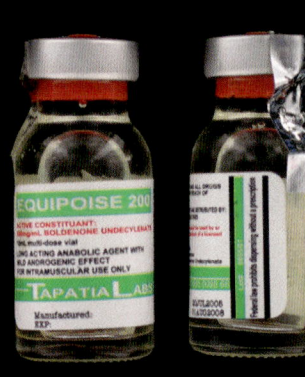

Underground vials from PTG Pharma, SIUG (NLM), and Tapatia Labs

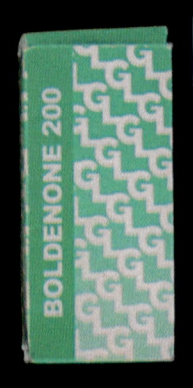

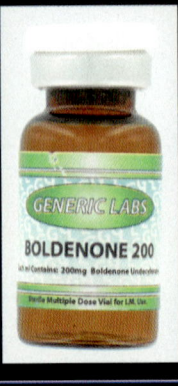

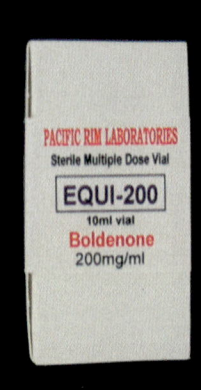

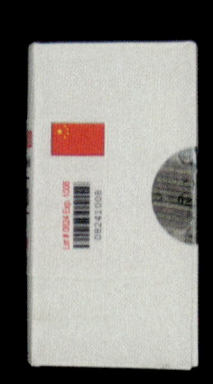

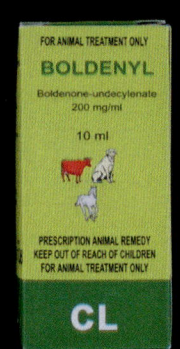

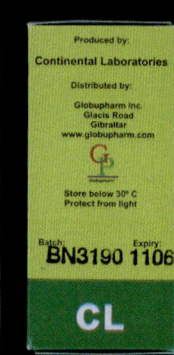

Underground products from Generic Labs, Pacific Rim, and Continental Labs

B-50

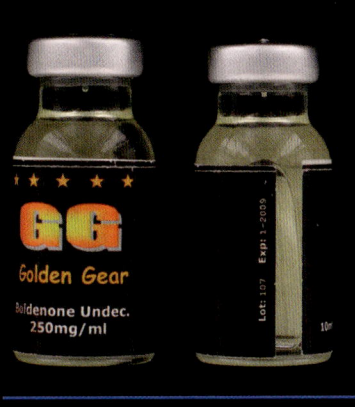

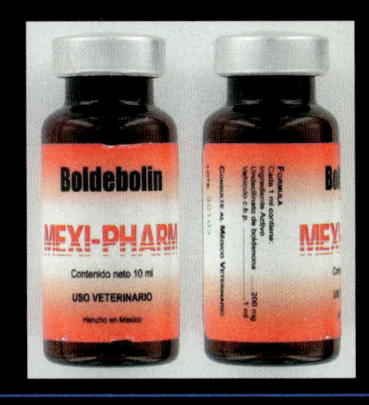

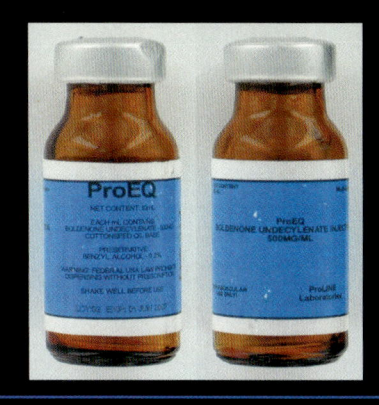

Underground vials from Golden Gear, Mexi-Pharm, and Proline

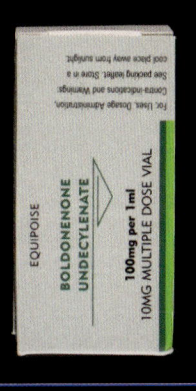

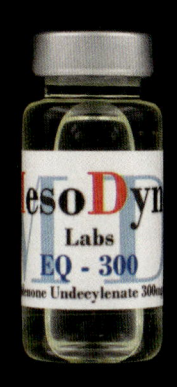

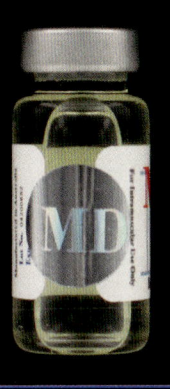

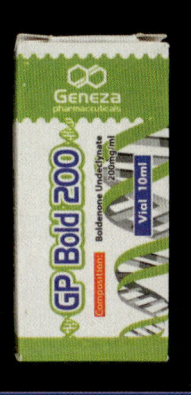

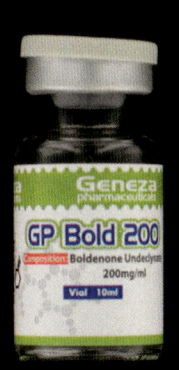

Changchun (UG) MesoDyne (UG) Geneza (Underground)

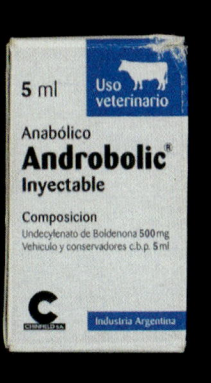

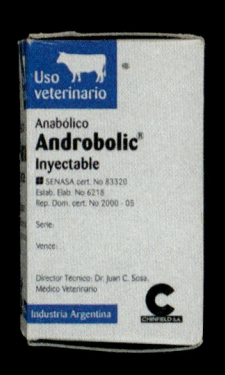

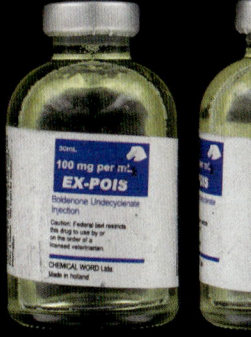

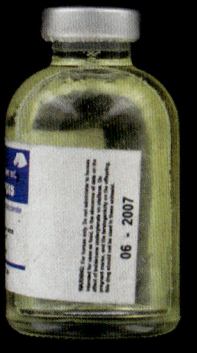

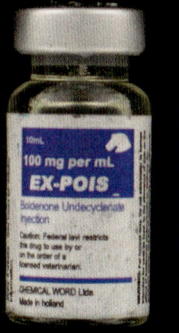

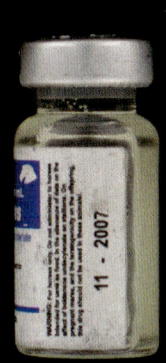

Fake Androbolic (Argentina) Two counterfeit vials of Ex-Pois (Holland)

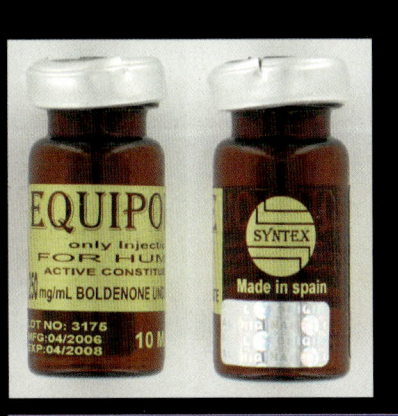

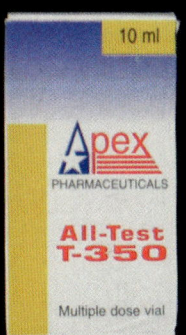

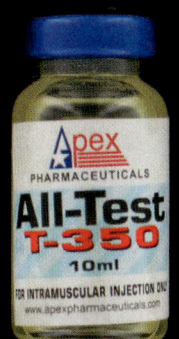

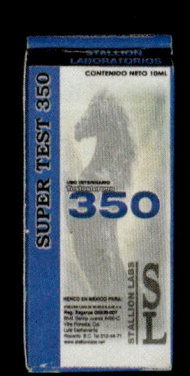

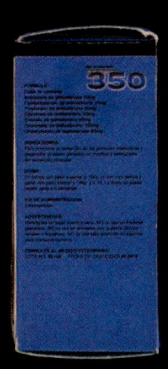

Equitest 200

Fake Spanish Equipoise Similar blends from Apex (UG) and Stallion (MX, UG) NLM

Appendix B

Estandron

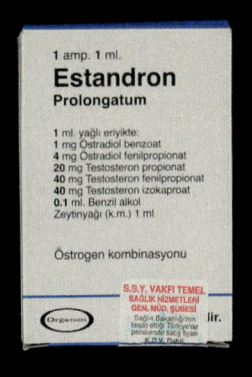

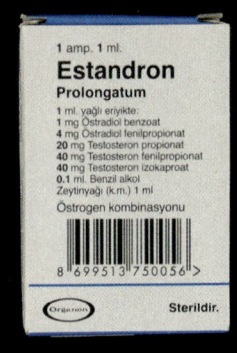

Estandron from Turkey

Halotestin

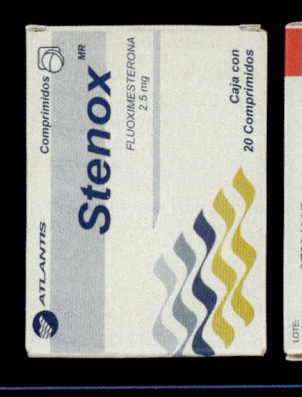

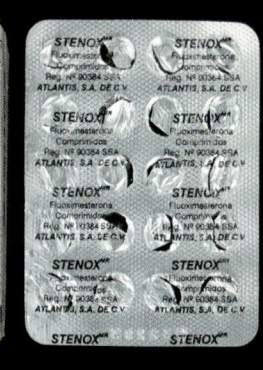

Stenox from Atlantis (Mexico)

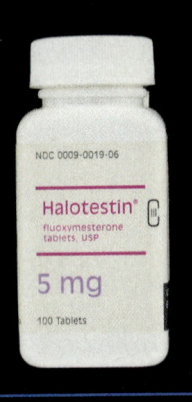

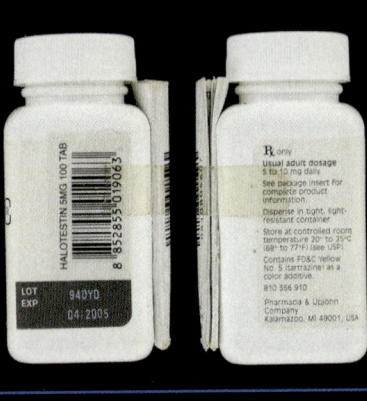

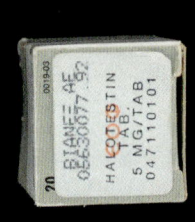

Halotestin from Pharmacia & Upjohn (U.S.) NLM

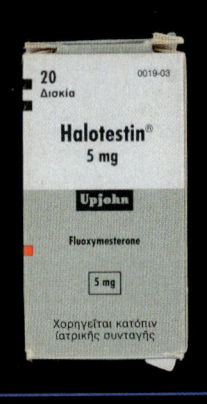

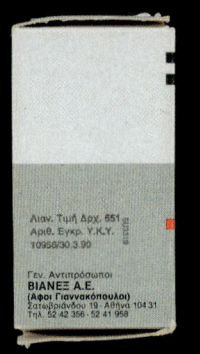

Greek Halotestin (NLM)

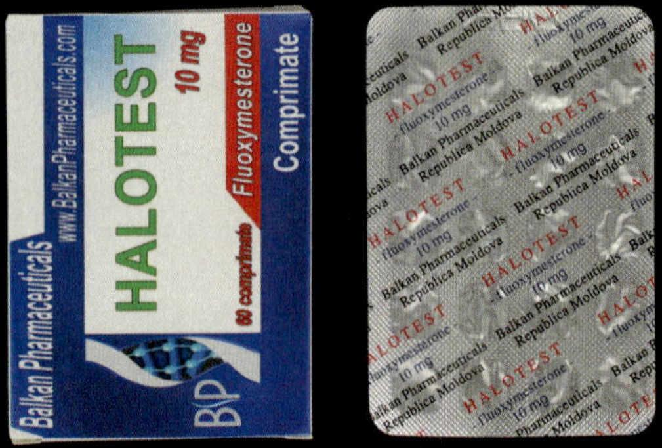

Halotest from Balkan (Moldova)

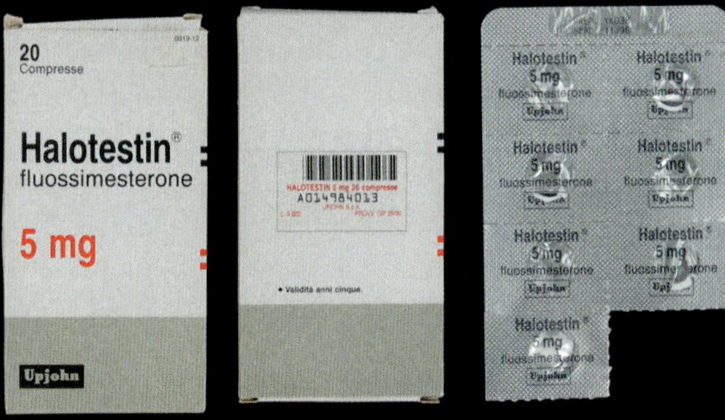

Upjohn Halotestin from Italy (NLM)

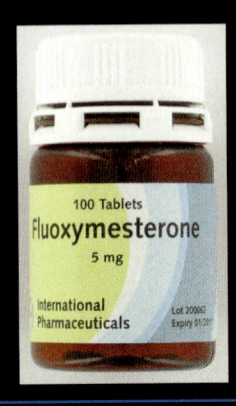

International Pharm (UG)

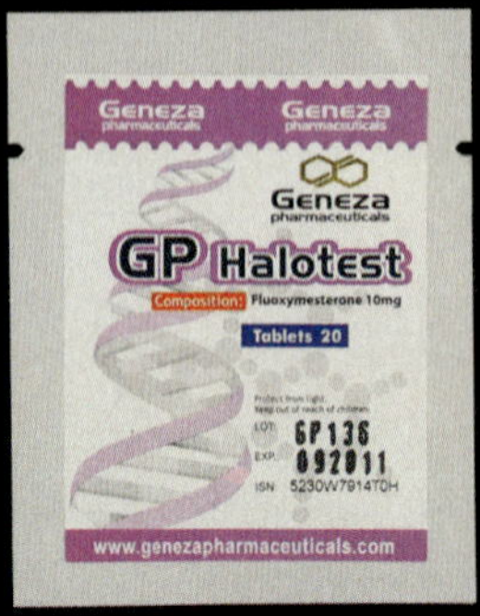

Geneza (Underground)

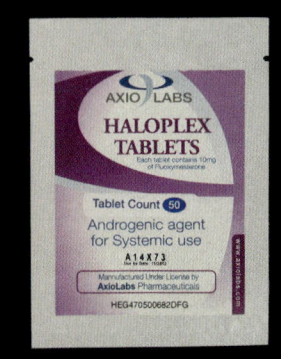

Axio (Underground)

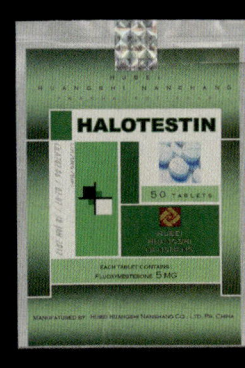

Hubei (Underground)

B-52

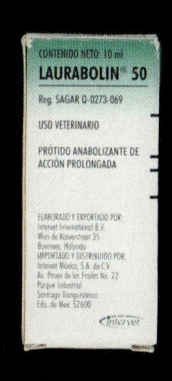

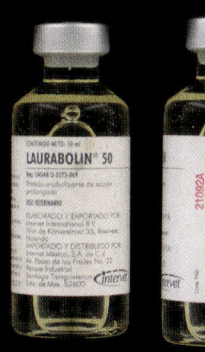

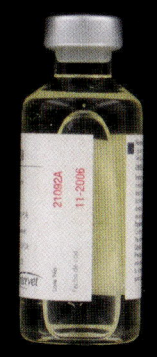

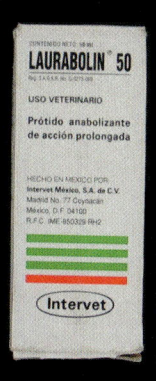

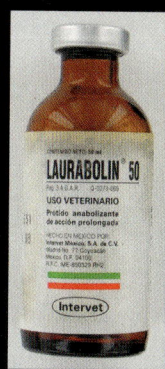

Laurabolin

Laurabolin 10ml box and vial (Mexico)

Old Laurabolin packaging (Mexico)

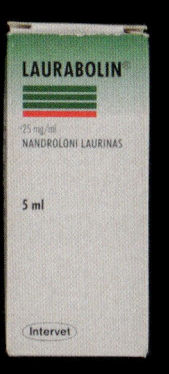

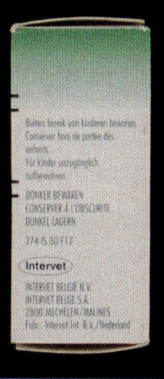

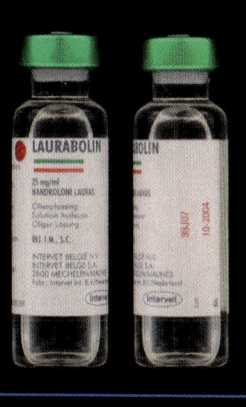

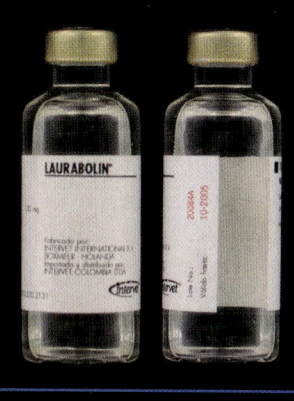

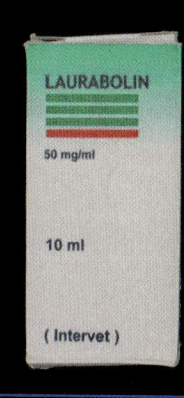

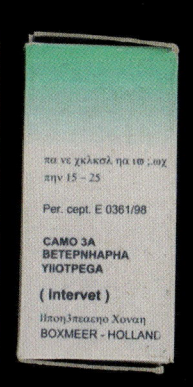

Older packaging from Belgium

Vial from Colombia

Counterfeit from Holland

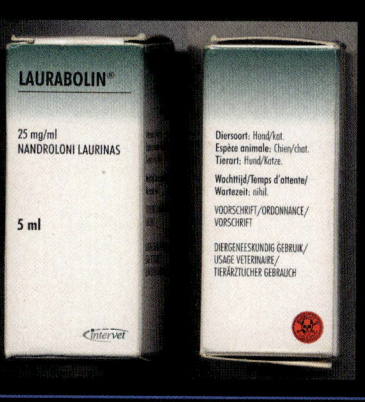

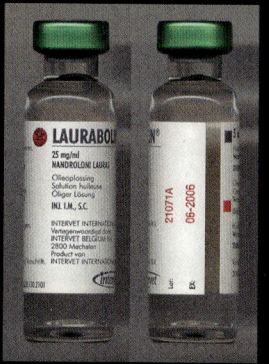

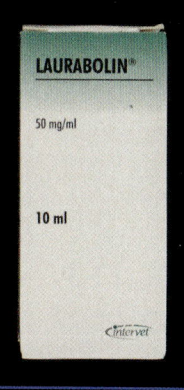

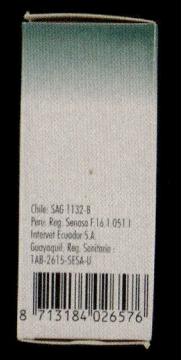

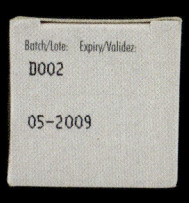

Laurabolin from Belgium

Laurabolin from Ecuador

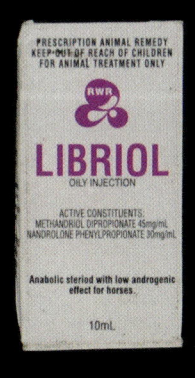

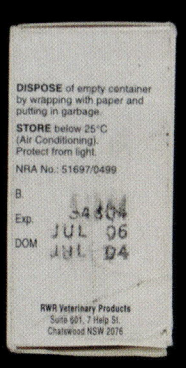

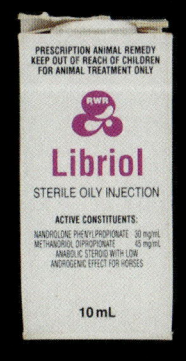

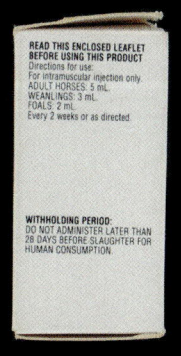

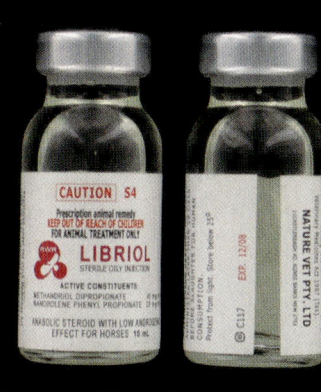

Libriol

Libriol (Australia)

Two different Libriol counterfeits

Appendix B

B-53

Masteron

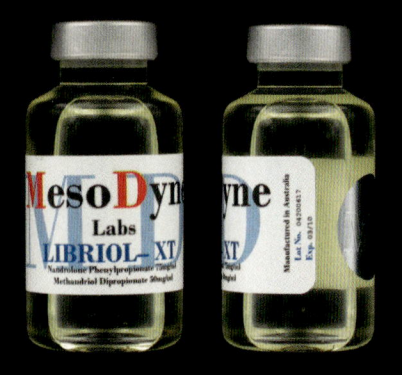

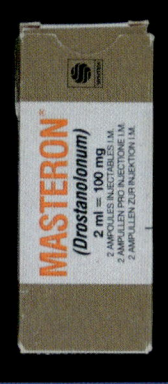

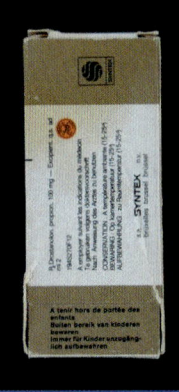

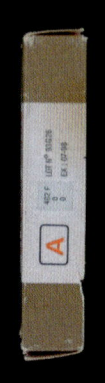

Libriol from MesoDyne (UG)

Masteron from Syntex Belgium (NLM)

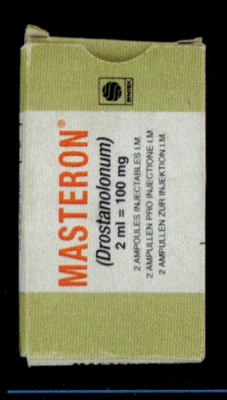

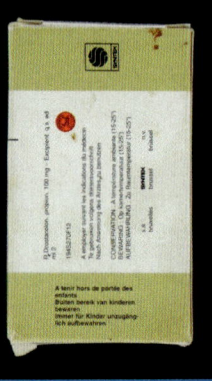

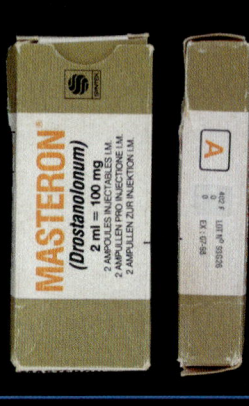

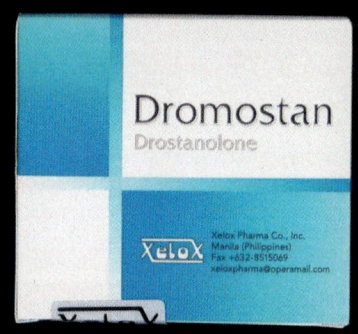

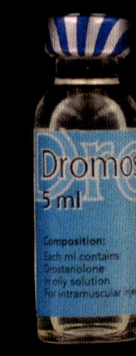

Two Masteron counterfeits

Dromostan from Xelox (Philippines)

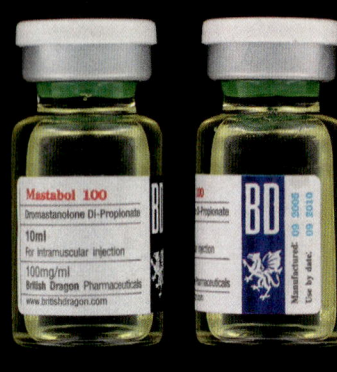

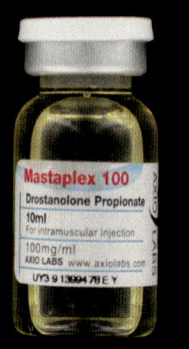

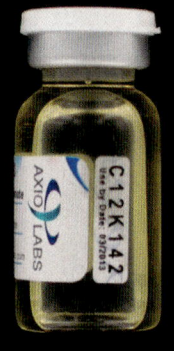

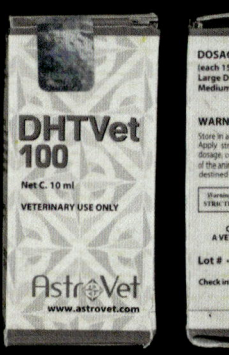

British Dragon (Underground) NLM

Axio Labs (Underground)

AstroVet (Mexico, UG)

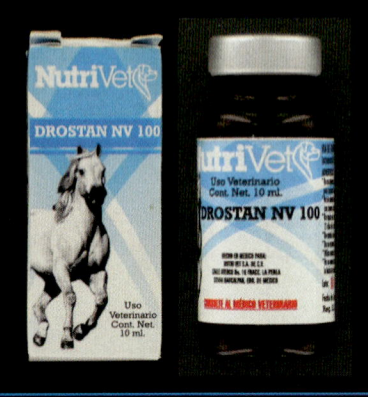

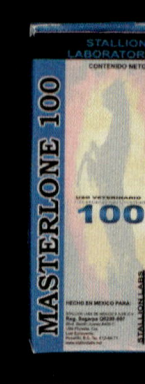

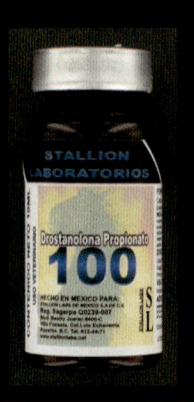

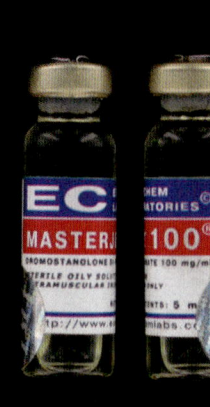

NutriVet (Mexico, UG) NLM

Stallion (Mexico, UG) NLM

Eurochem (UG)

B-54

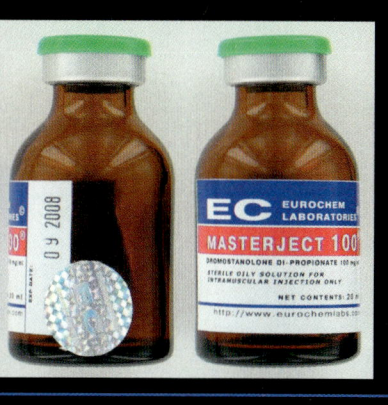

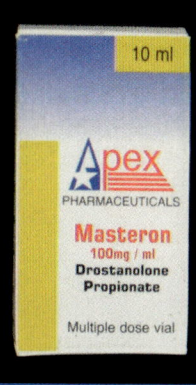

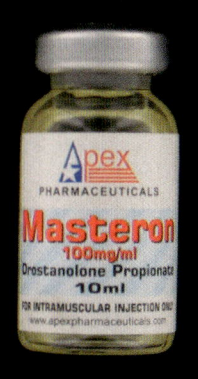

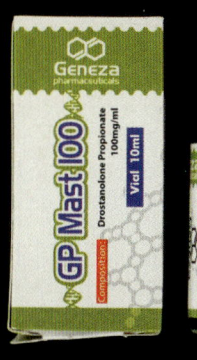

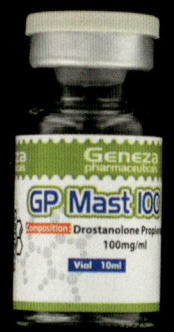

Eurochem 20ml vial

Masteron from Apex (Underground)

Geneza (Underground)

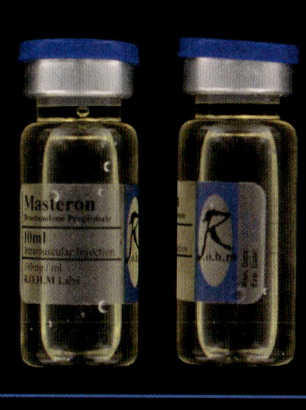

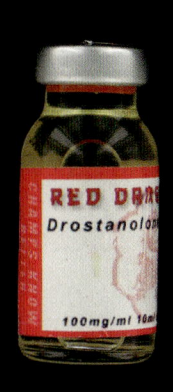

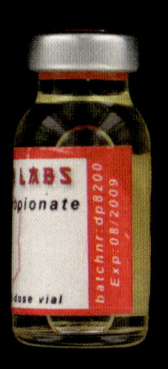

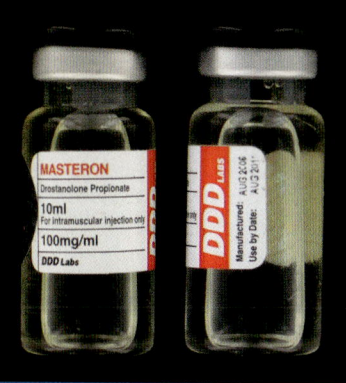

Underground vials from R.O.H.M., Red Dragon, and DDD

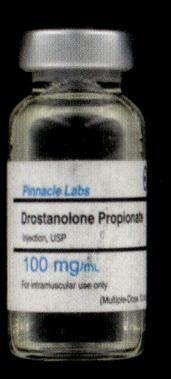

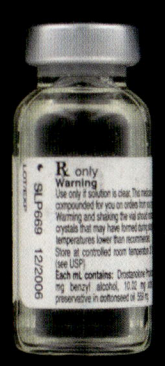

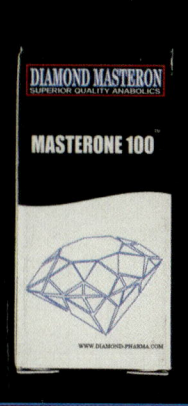

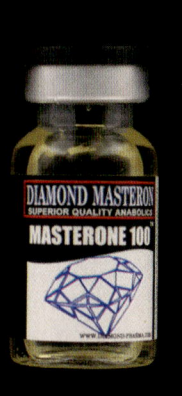

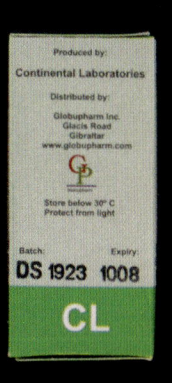

Pinnacle Labs (UG)

Diamond (Underground)

Continental (UG)

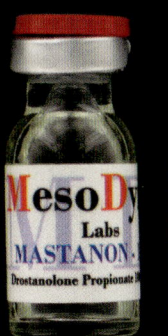

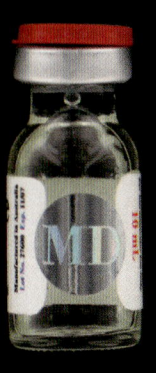

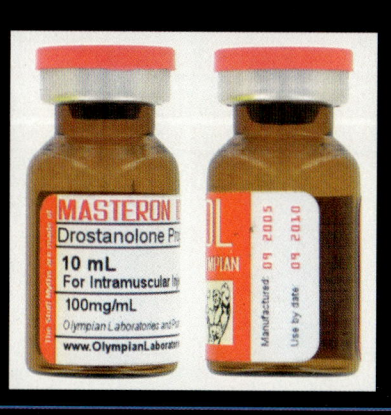

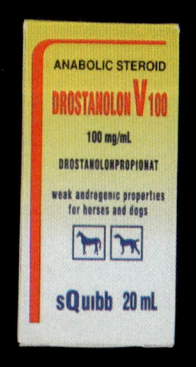

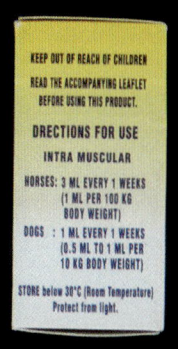

MesoDyne (UG)

Olympian (UG)

Fake Squbb Drostanolon

Appendix B

Methandriol

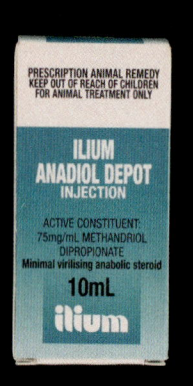

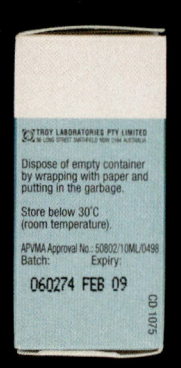

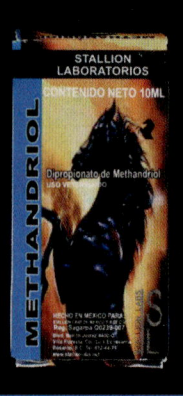

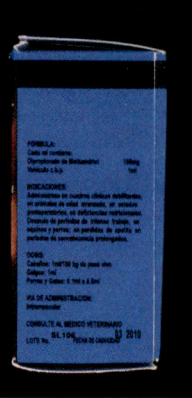

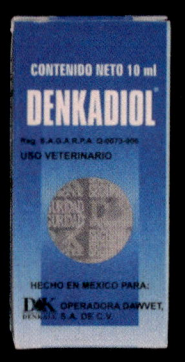

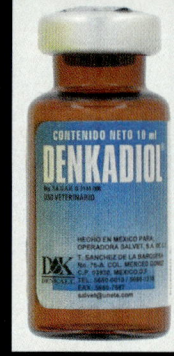

Anadiol Depot (Australia)   Generic from Stallion (MX, UG) NLM   Denkadiol from (Mexico) NLM

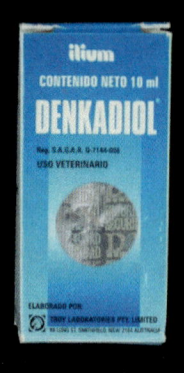

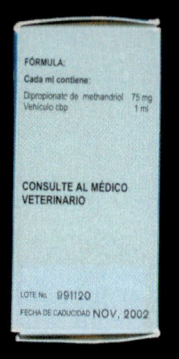

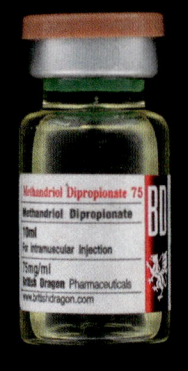

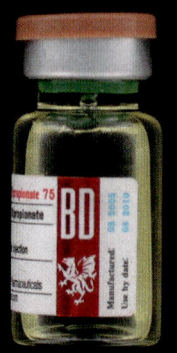

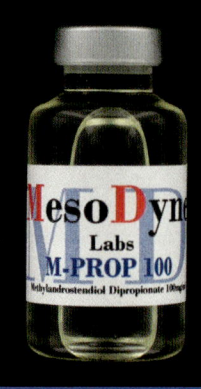

Old box when Ilium made for DK   British Dragon (Underground) NLM   MesoDyne (UG)

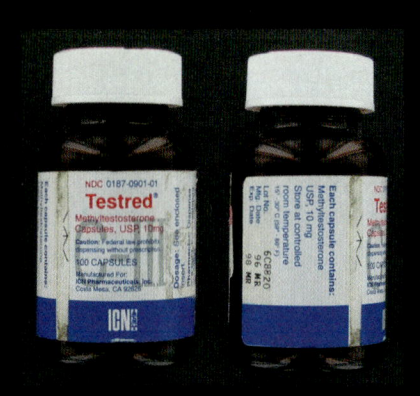

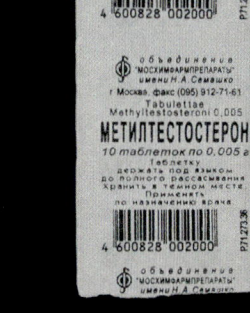

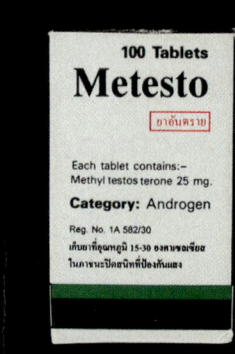

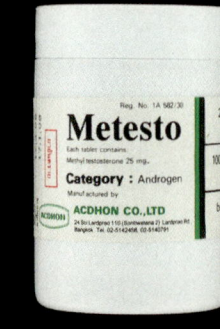

Methyltestosterone

U.S. Testred   Russian generic   Metesto from Acdhon (Thailand)

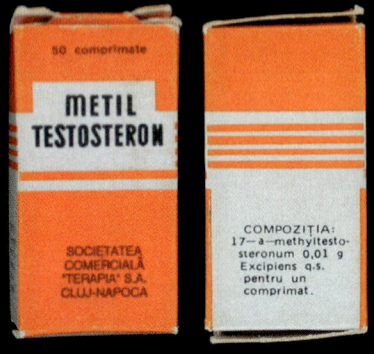

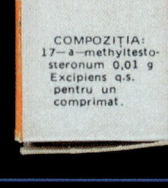

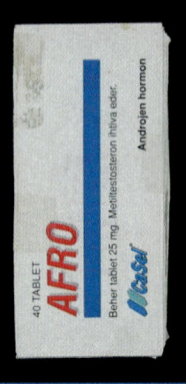

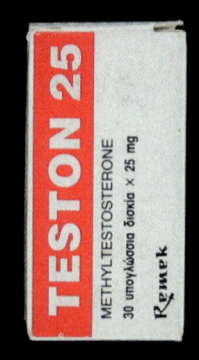

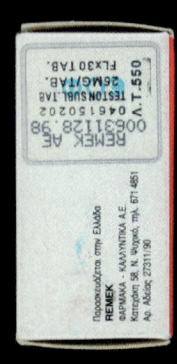

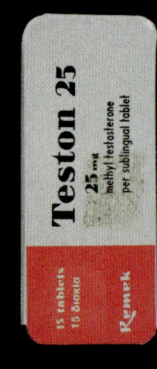

Generic from Rumania   Afro (Turkey)   Greek Teston 25 - Older tin on right

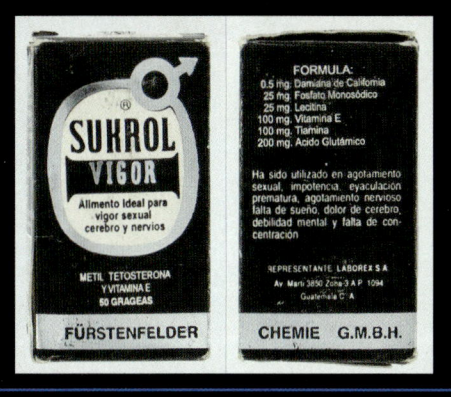

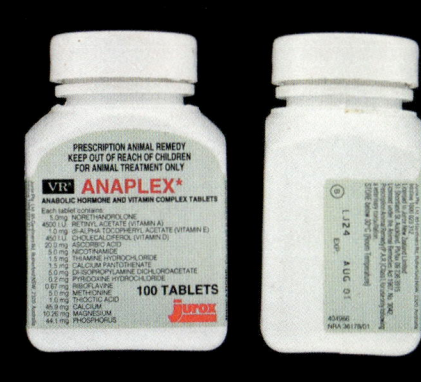

Sukrol Vigor (Guatemala)

Nilevar

Anaplex from Jurox (Australia)

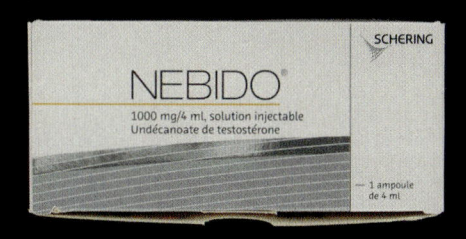

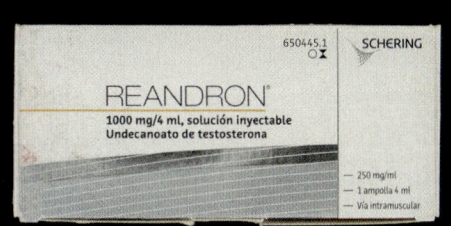

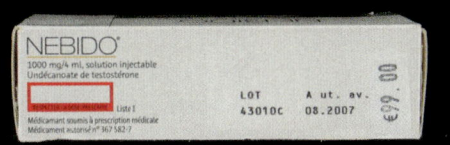

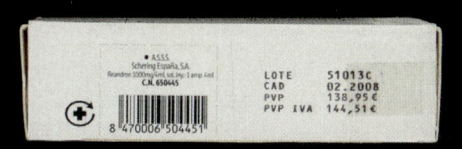

Nebido from France

Reandron from Spain

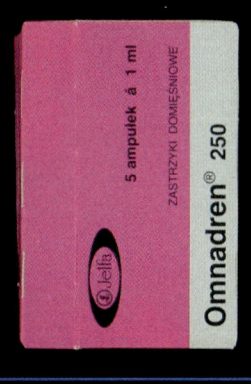

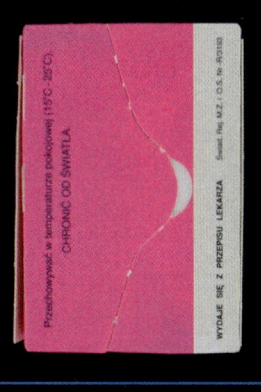

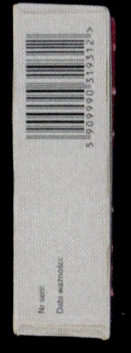

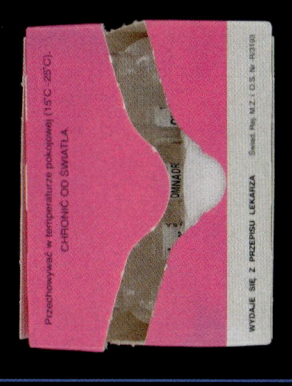

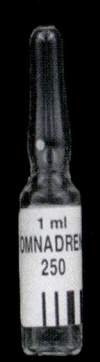

Omnadren from Poland - NLM (in this formula)

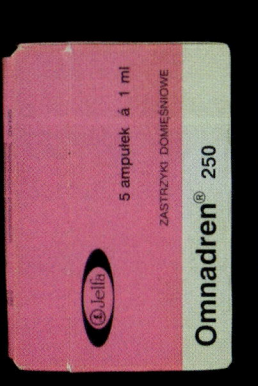

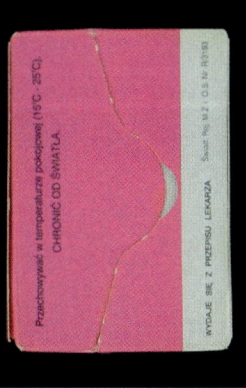

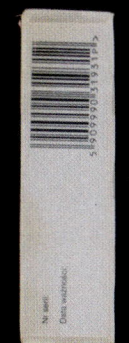

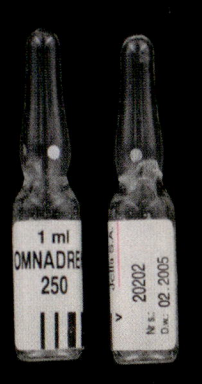

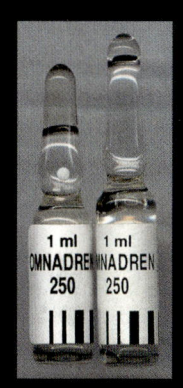

Excellent looking counterfeit box and ampule

Fake ampule is shorter

Appendix B

B-57

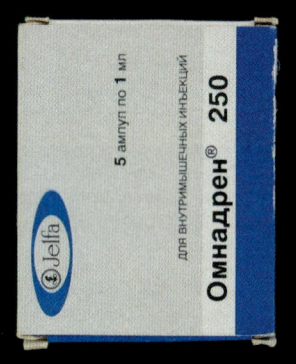

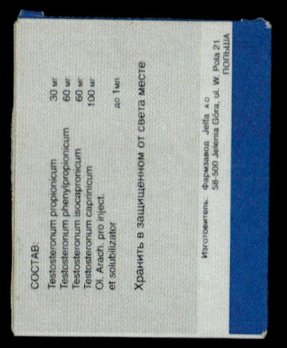

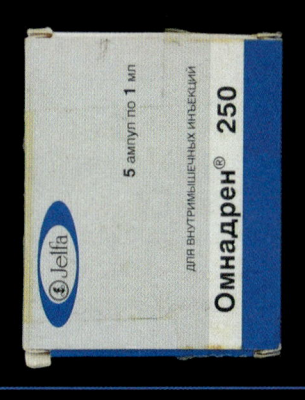

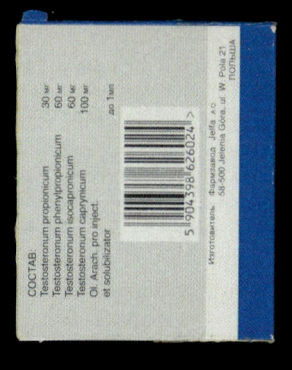

Two different versions of the older packaging

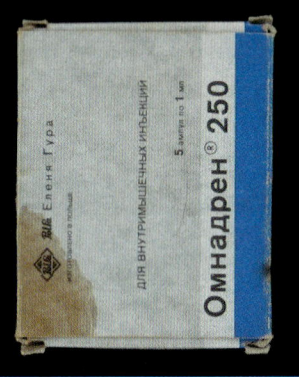

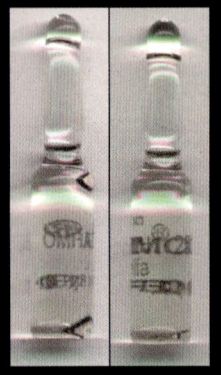

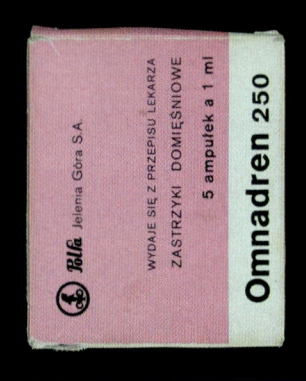

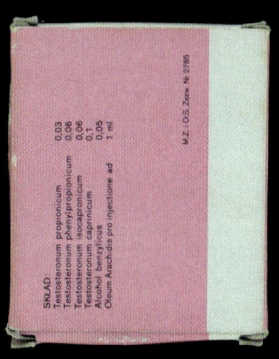

Two different examples of Omnadren when the company was still called Polfa

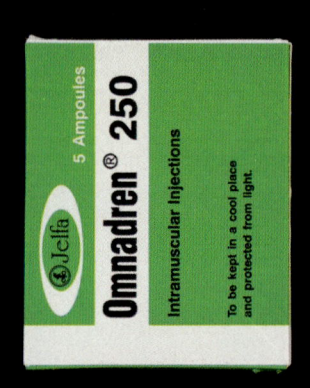

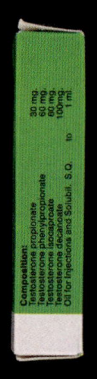

Orabolin

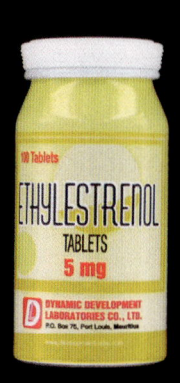

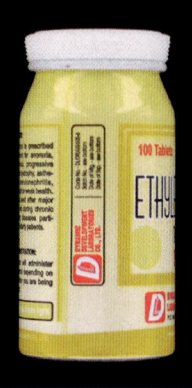

Another counterfeit Omnadren

Generic from Development Labs (Mauritius, export)

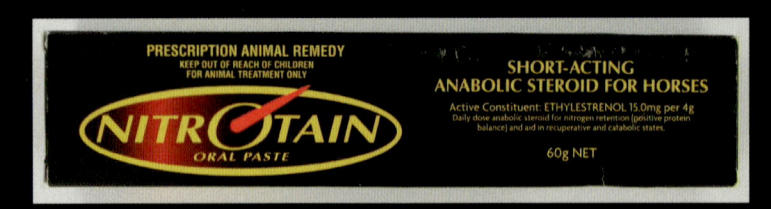

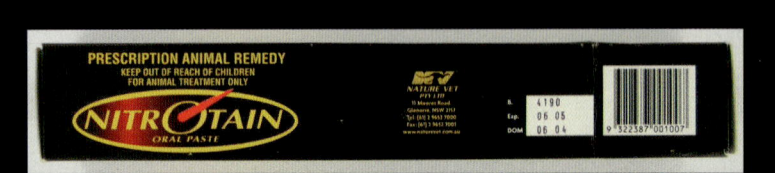

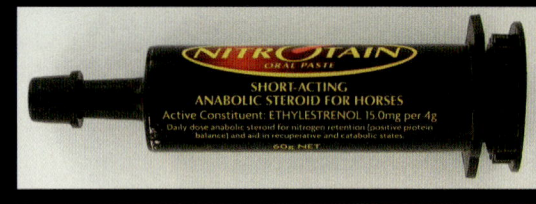

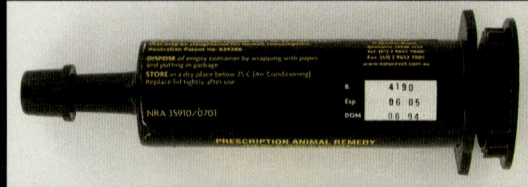

Nitrotain from Australia

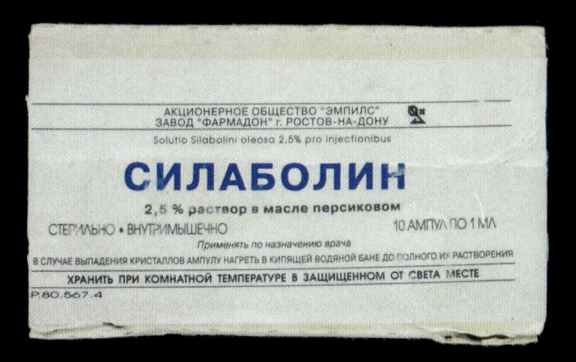

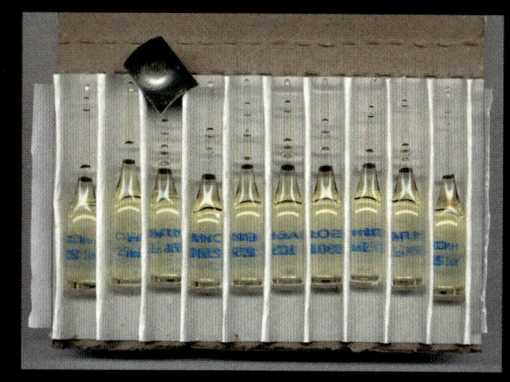

Counterfeit Russian Silabolin

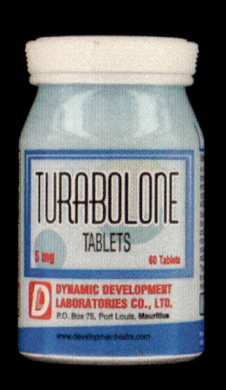

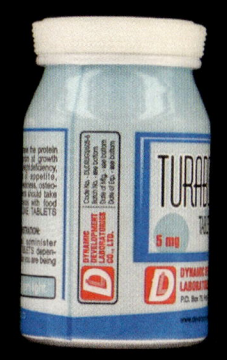

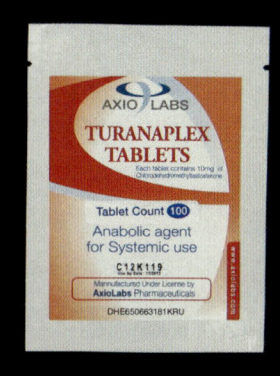

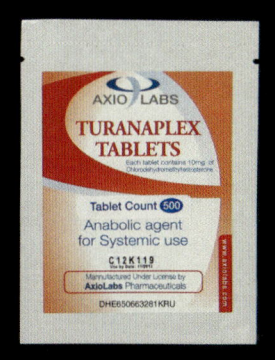

Oral Turinabol

Generic from Development Labs (Mauritius, export)

Axio Labs (Underground)

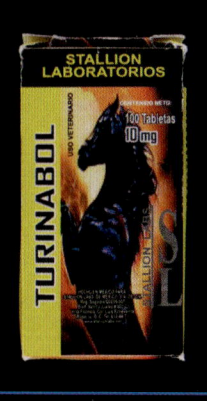

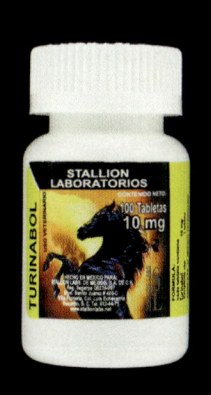

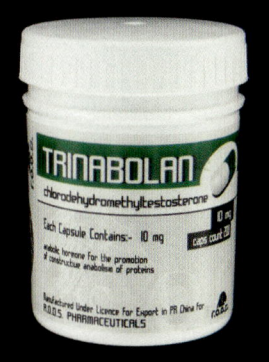

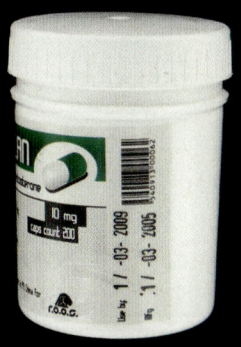

Stallion (Mexico, Underground) NLM

R.O.O.S. (Underground)

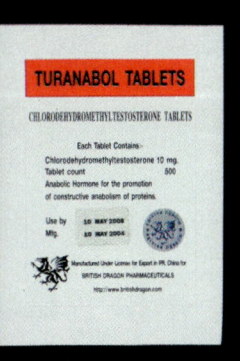

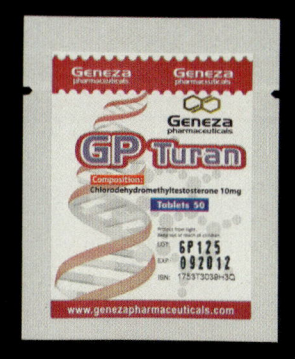

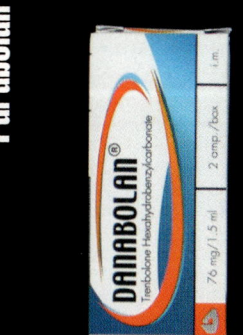

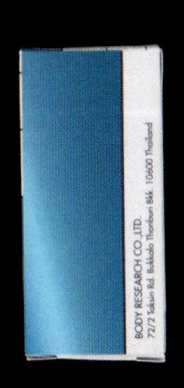

Parabolan

British Dragon (UG) NLM

Geneza (Underground)

Danabolan from Thailand (NLM)

Appendix B

B-59

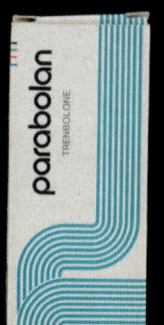

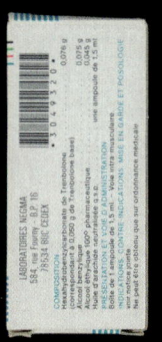

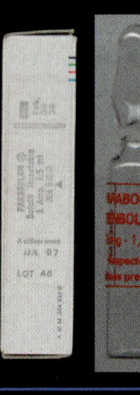

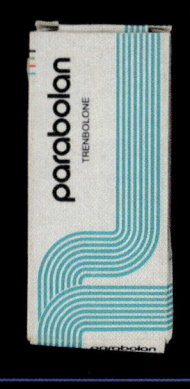

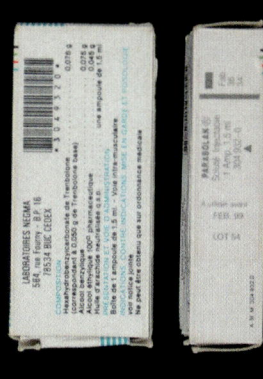

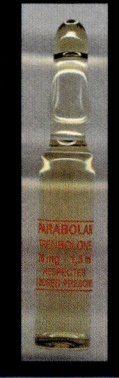

Real French Parabolan (NLM)

Counterfeit Parabolan box and ampule

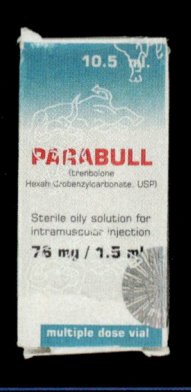

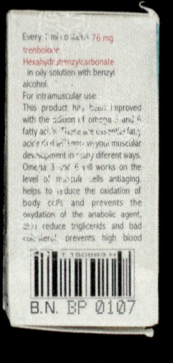

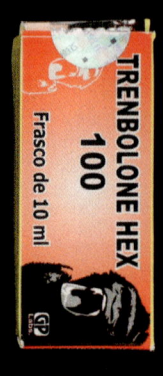

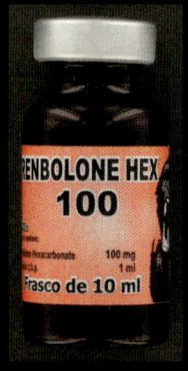

Parabull (Underground)

Gorilla Power (Mexico, UG)

MesoDyne Labs (UG)

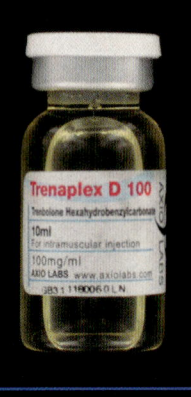

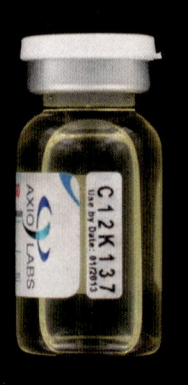

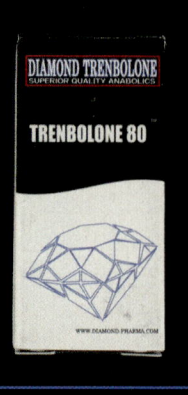

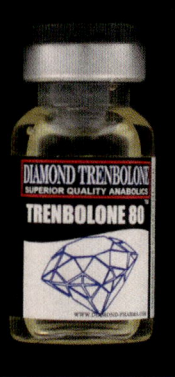

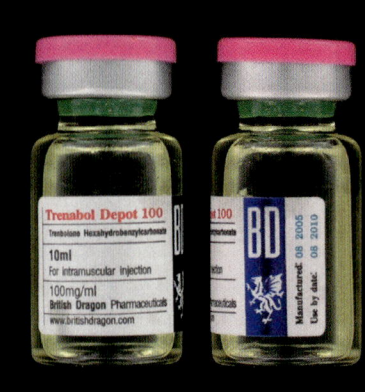

Axio Labs (Underground)

Diamond (Underground)

British Dragon (Underground) NLM

Primobolan Depot

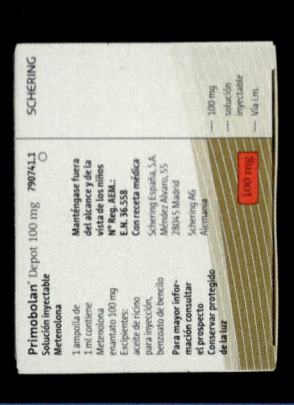

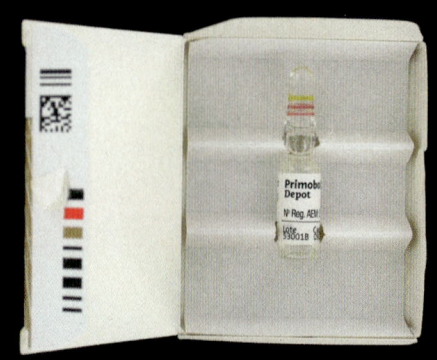

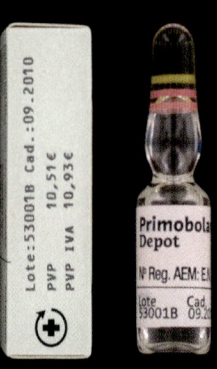

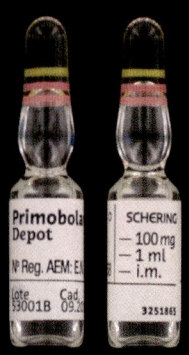

Primobolan Depot from Schering (Spain)

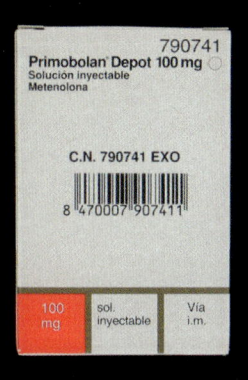

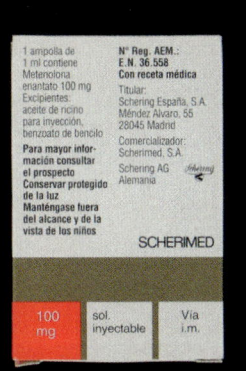

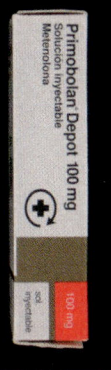

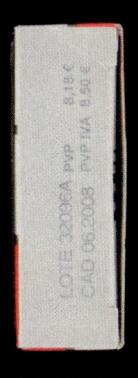

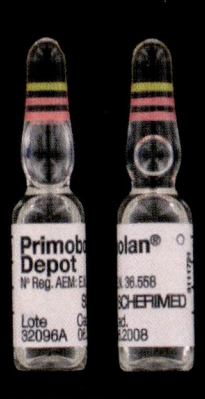

Primobolan Depot from former name Scherimed (Spain) NLM

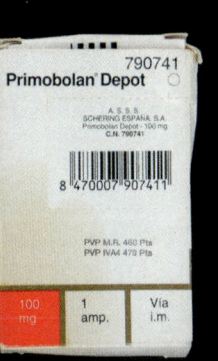

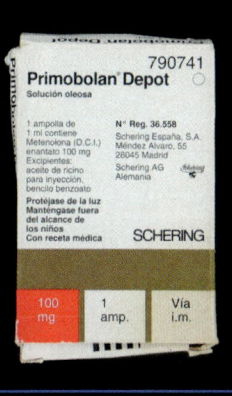

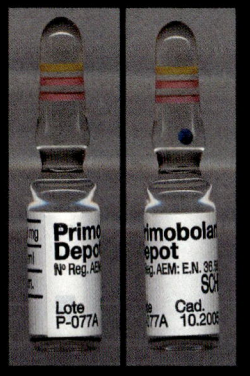

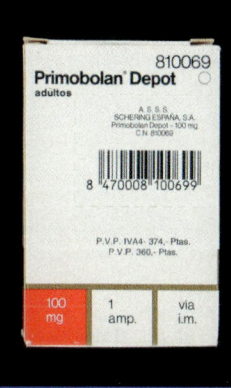

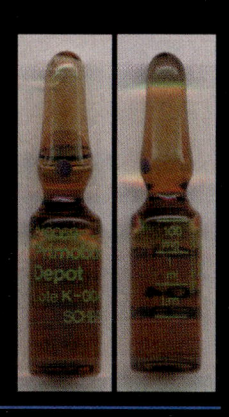

Earlier packaging for Spanish Primobolan

An even earlier box and ampule

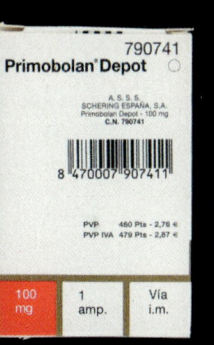

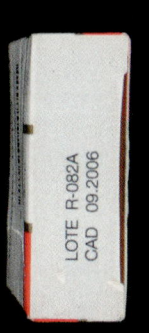

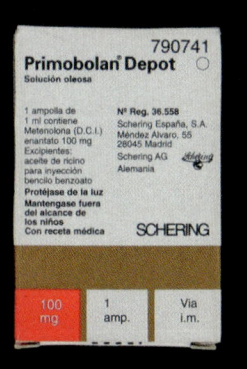

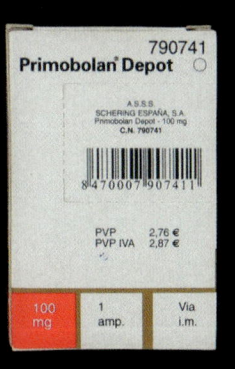

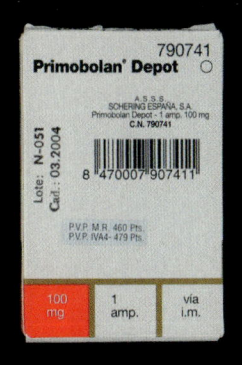

Counterfeit #1

Counterfeit #2

Counterfeit #3

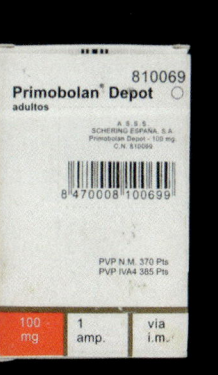

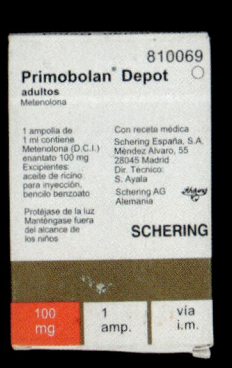

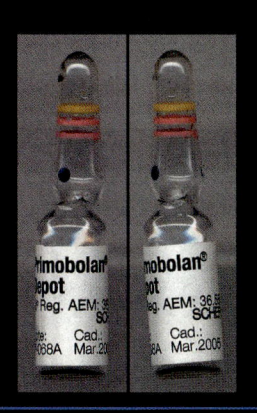

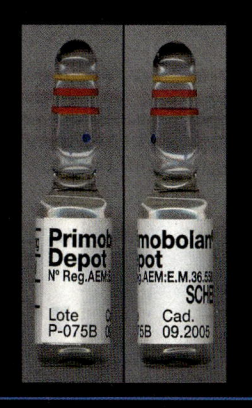

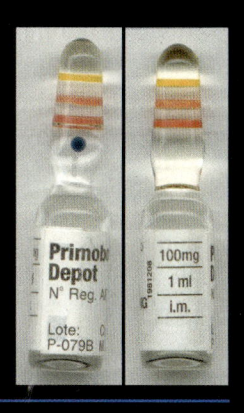

Counterfeit #4

Counterfeit #5

Counterfeit #6

Counterfeit #7

Appendix B

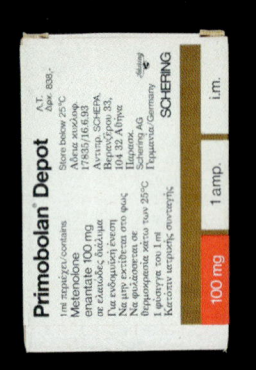

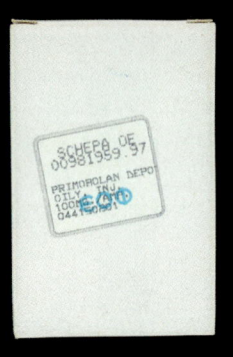

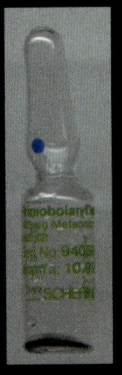

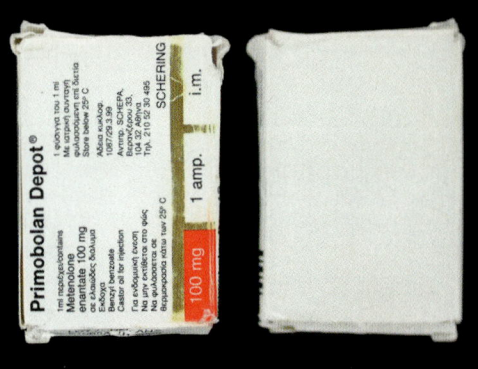

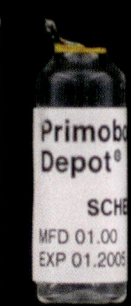

Greek Primobolan (NLM)　　　　　　　　　　Greek counterfeit box and amp

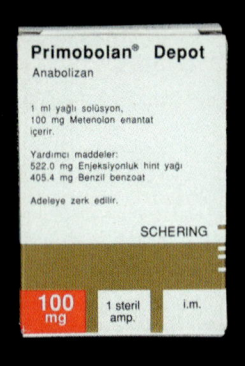

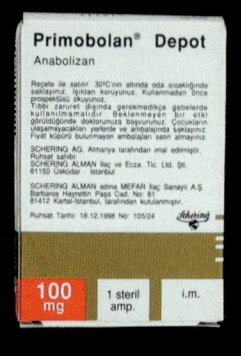

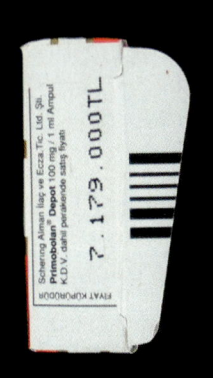

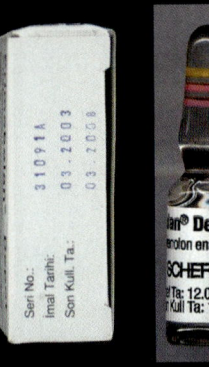

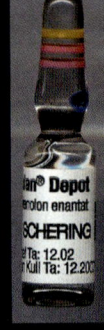

Primobolan Depot from Turkey

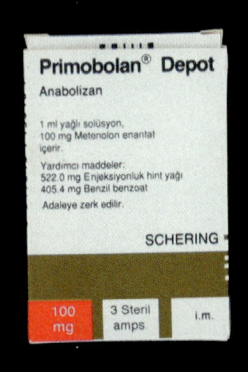

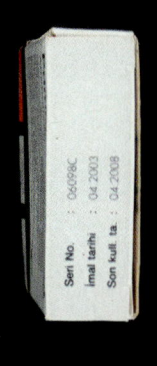

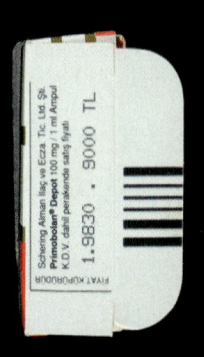

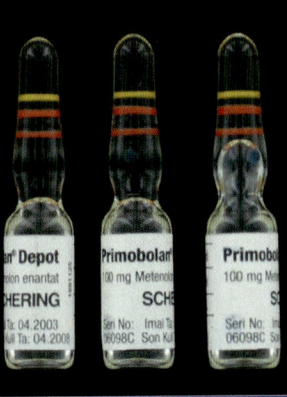

Counterfeit box and ampules (Turkey)

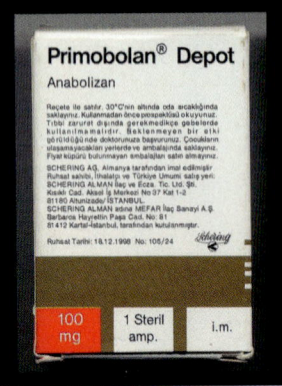

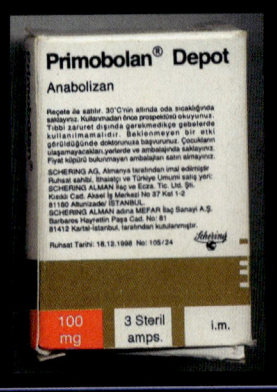

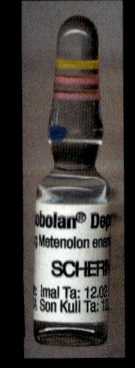

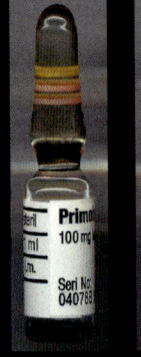

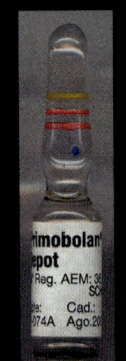

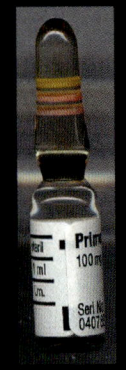

Turkish Counterfeit #2　　　Counterfeit #3　　　#4　　#5　　#6　　#7

B-62

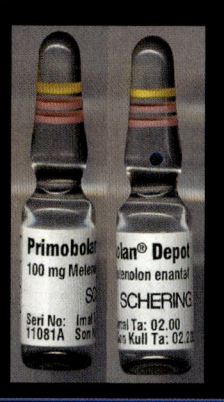

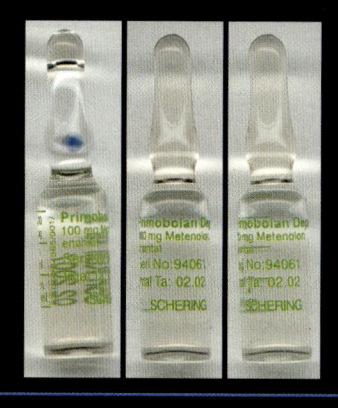

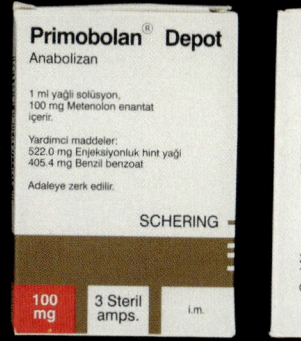

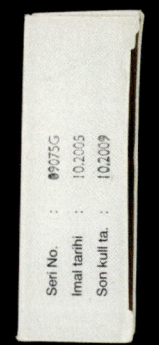

Counterfeit #8 · Turkish counterfeit #9 · Turkish counterfeit #10

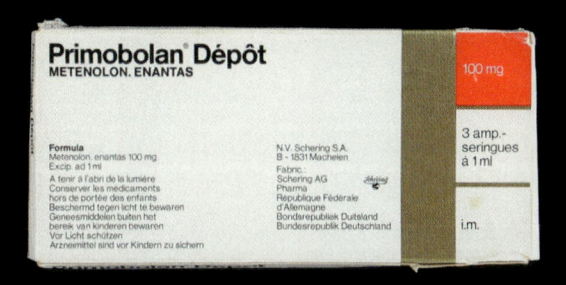

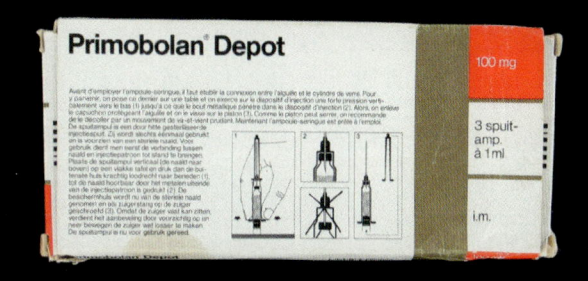

Pre-loaded syringe from Belgium (NLM)

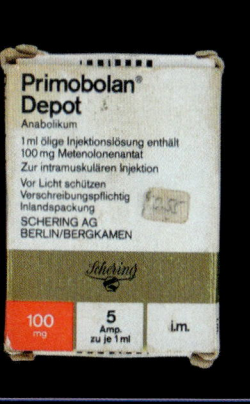

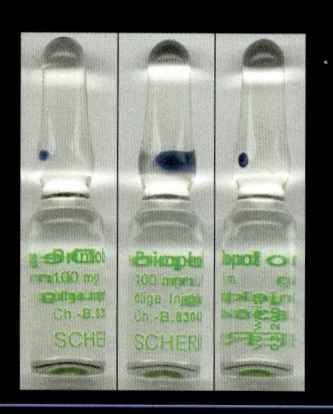

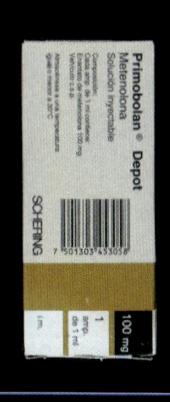

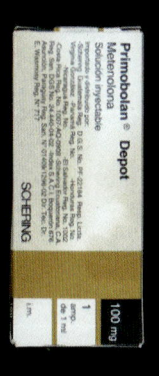

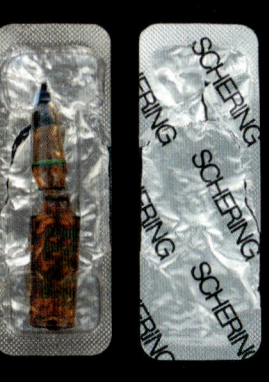

Old German box (NLM) · Counterfeit German amps · Primobolan Depot from Colombia

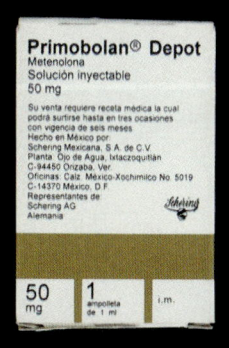

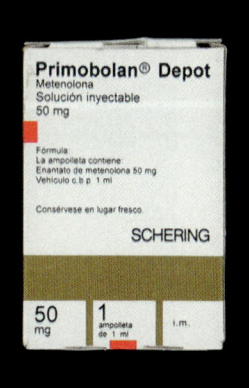

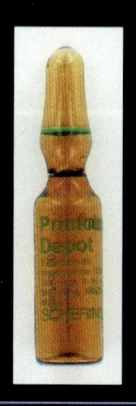

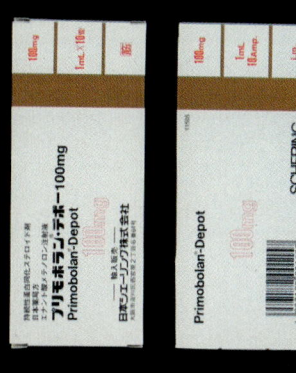

Primobolan from Mexico · Primobolan from Japan

Appendix B

B-63

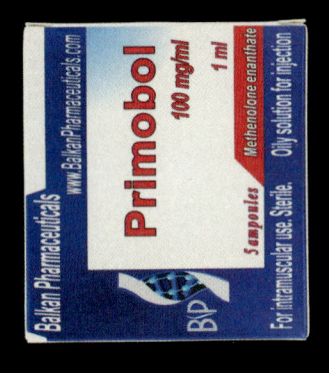

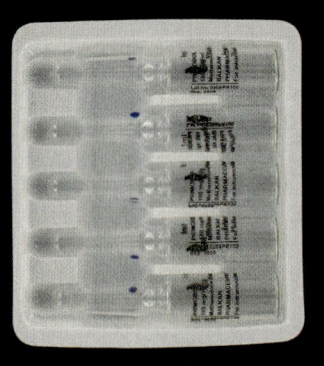

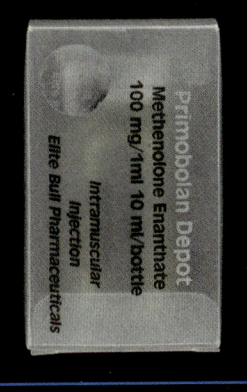

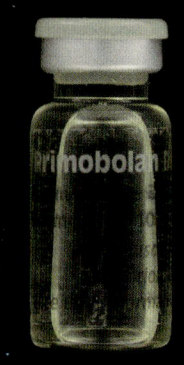

Primobol from Balkan (Moldova)

Elite Bull (Hong Kong, export)

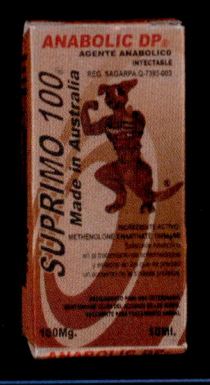

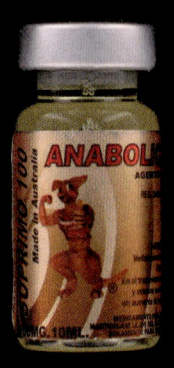

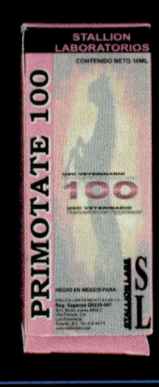

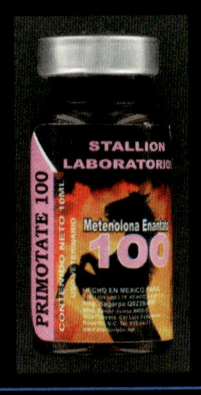

Suprimo 100 (Mexico) NLM

Stallion (Mexico, Underground) NLM

AstroVet (Mexico, Underground)

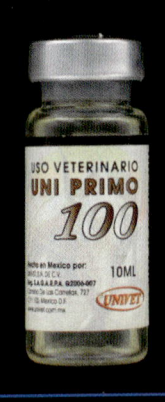

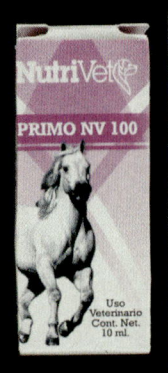

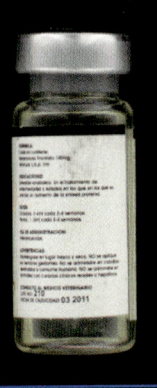

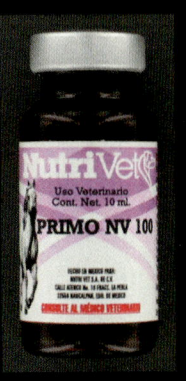

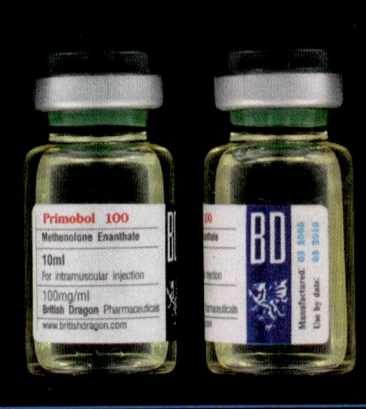

Univet (Mexico, Underground)

NutriVet (Mexico, Underground) NLM

British Dragon (Underground) NLM

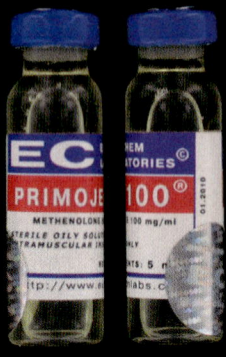

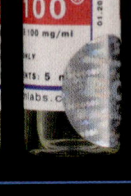

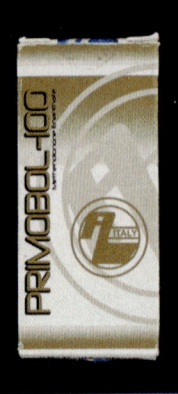

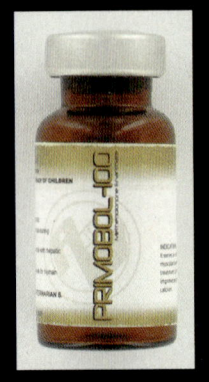

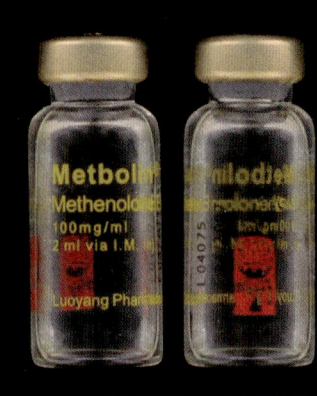

Eurochem vial (UG)

Primobol-100 from AL (UG)

Metbolin from LP (China, export)

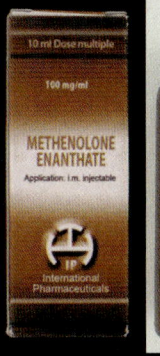

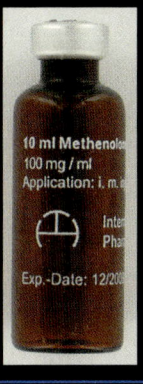

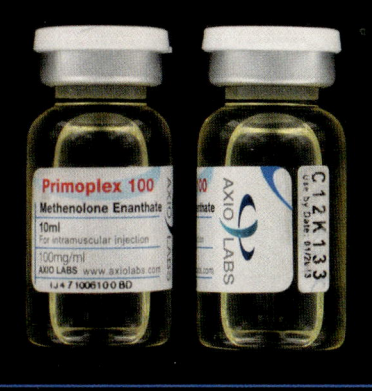

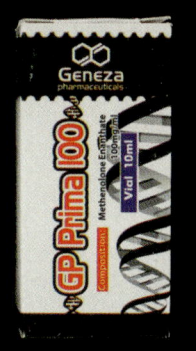

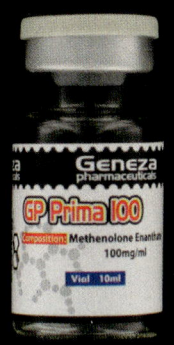

International Pharm (Underground) | Axio Labs (Underground) | Geneza (Underground)

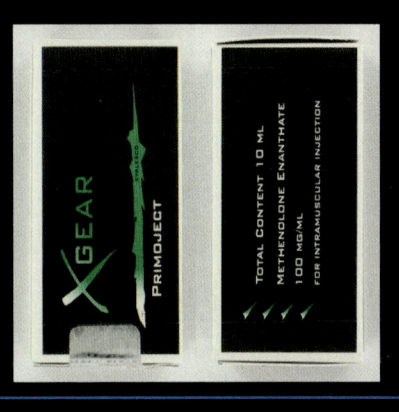

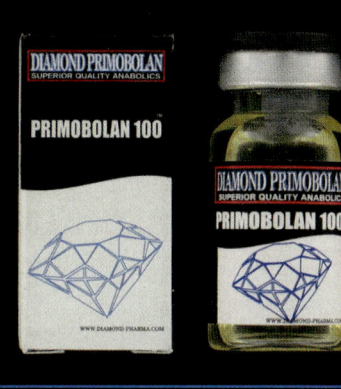

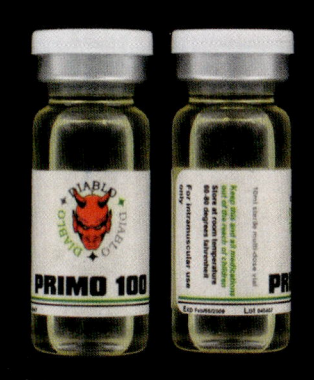

Underground products from X Gear, Diamond, and Diablo

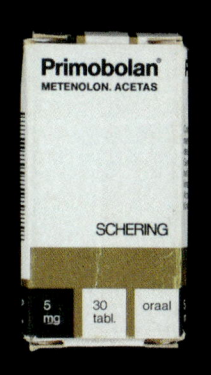

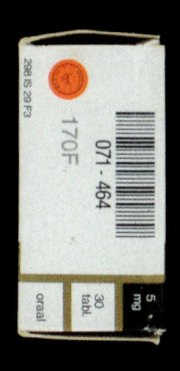

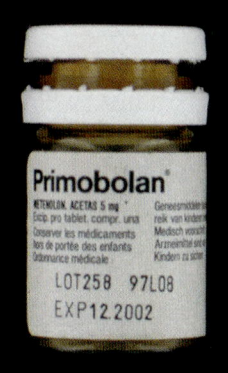

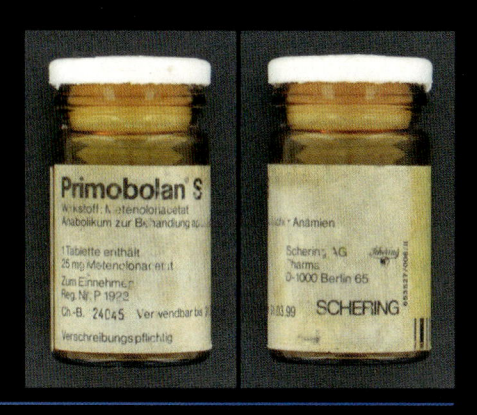

Primobolan Oral

Primobolan tablets from Belgium and Germany (both NLM)

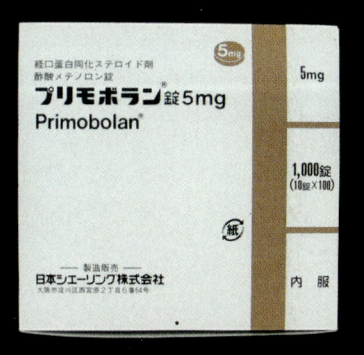

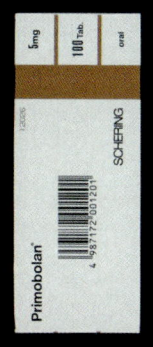

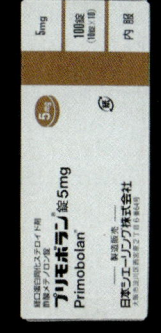

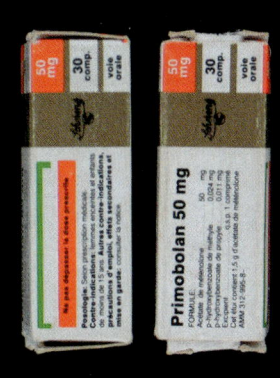

Primobolan from Japan 1,000 and 100 tab box | Counterfeit of French product NLM

Appendix B

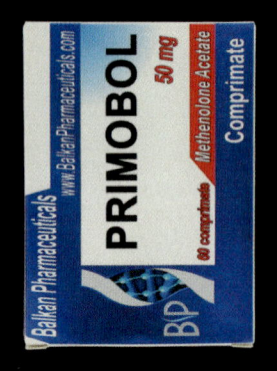

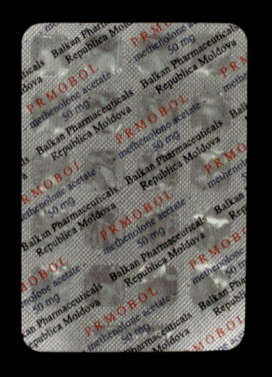

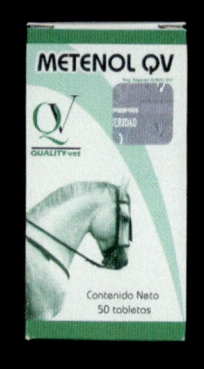

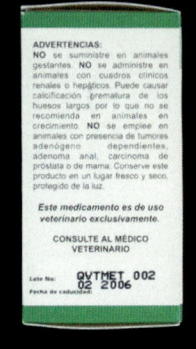

Primobol 50mg from Balkan (Moldova)

Metenol from Quality Vet (Mexico) NLM

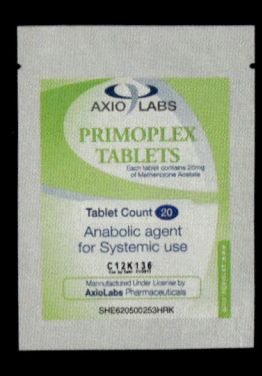

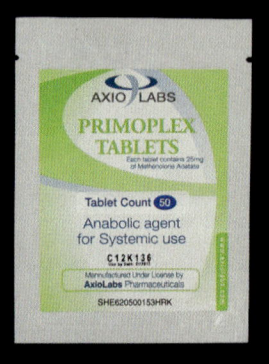

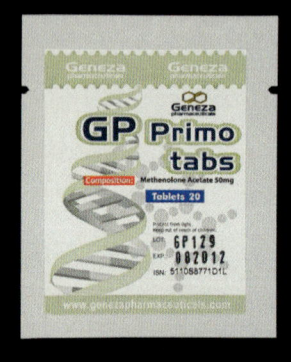

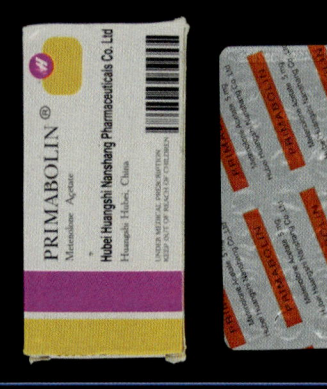

Axio Labs (Underground)

Geneza (Underground)

Fake Primobolan from Hubei China

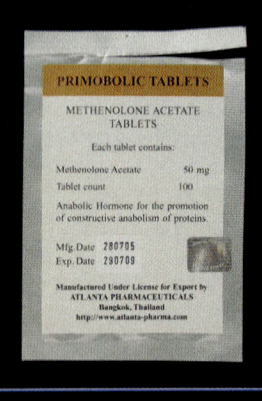

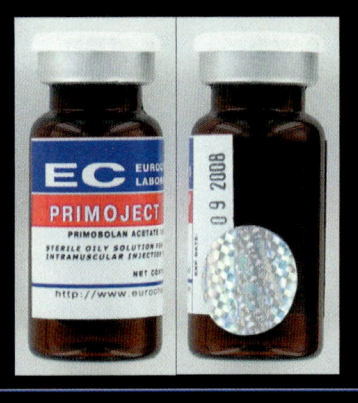

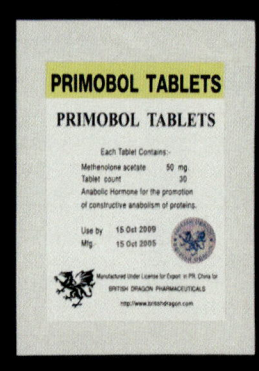

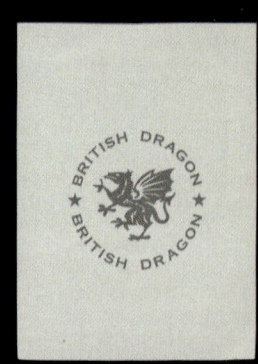

Atlanta (UG) NLM

Eurochem Primo Acetate injectable (UG)

Primobol Tabs from British Dragon (UG) NLM

Proviron

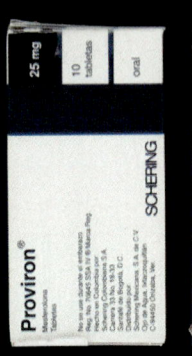

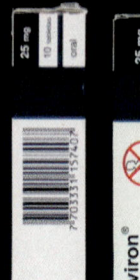

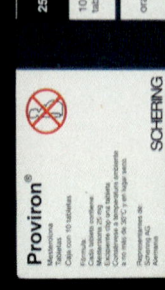

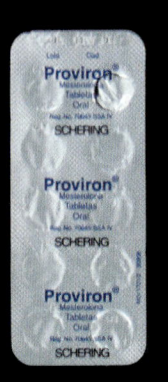

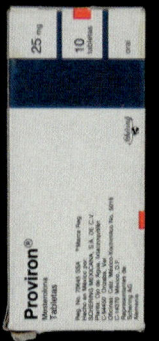

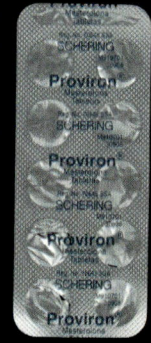

Proviron from Mexico

Older Mexican packaging

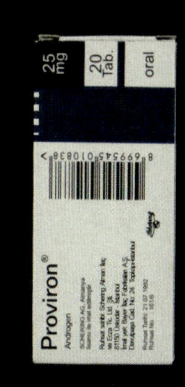

Pro-Viron from the UK

Proviron from Turkey

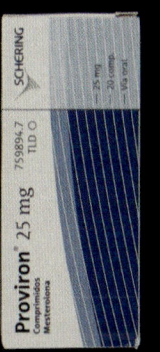

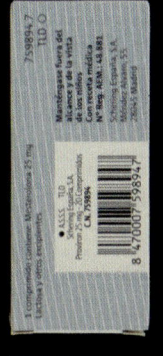

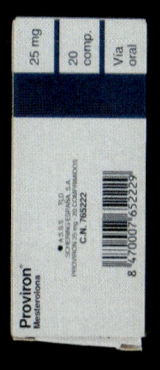

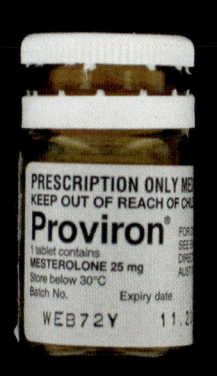

Spanish Proviron

Previous Spanish packaging

Proviron from Australia

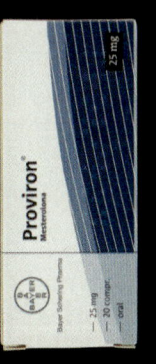

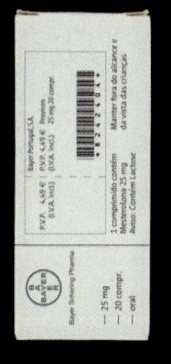

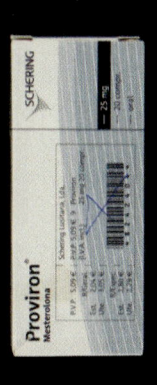

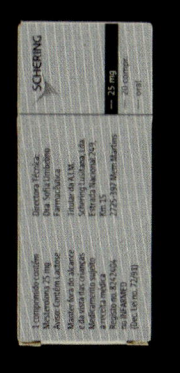

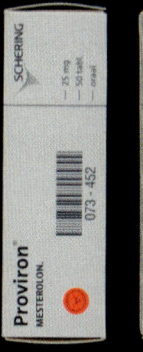

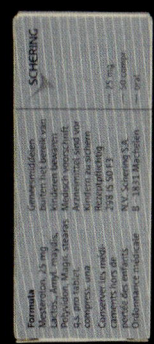

Proviron from Portugal

Previous packaging from Portugal

Belgian Proviron

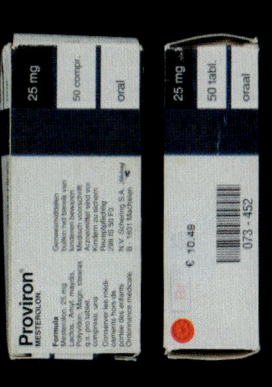

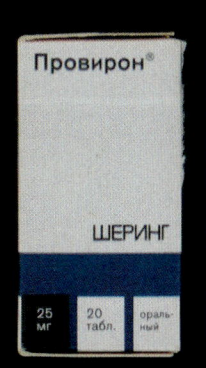

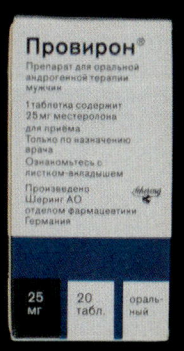

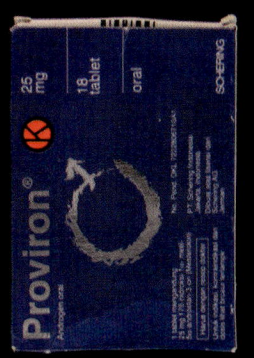

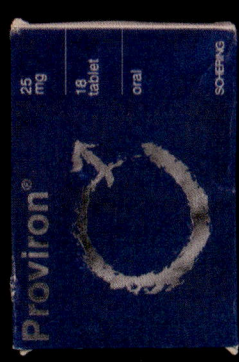

Previous Belgian packaging

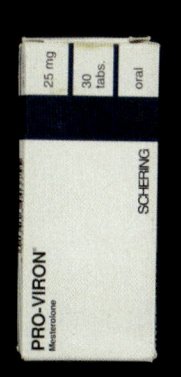

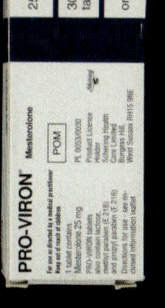

Russian Proviron

Proviron from Indonesia

Appendix B

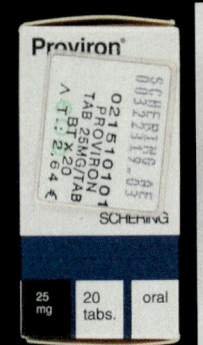

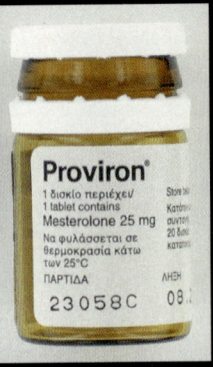

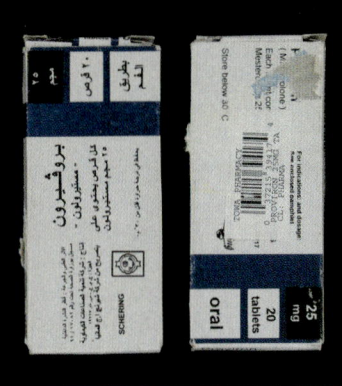

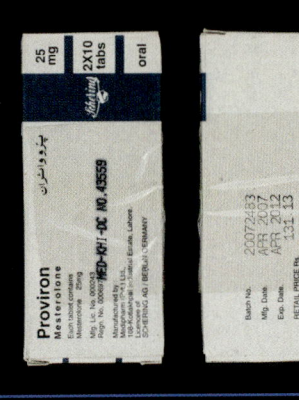

Proviron from Greece

Proviron from Egypt

Proviron from Pakistan

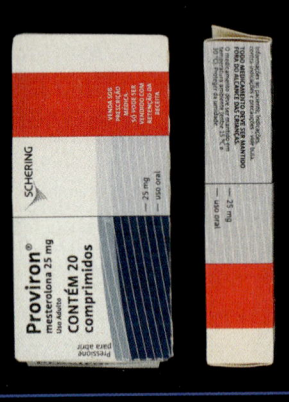

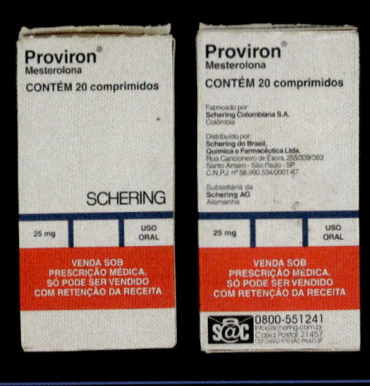

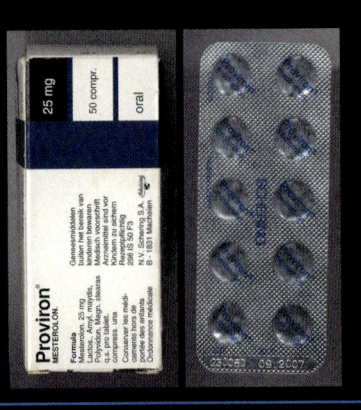

Proviron from Brazil

Older Brazilian Proviron

German Proviron

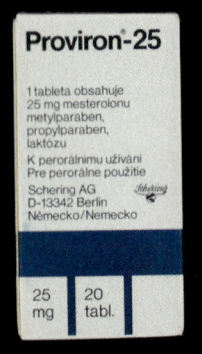

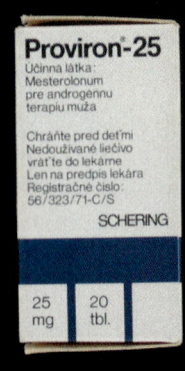

Czech Proviron

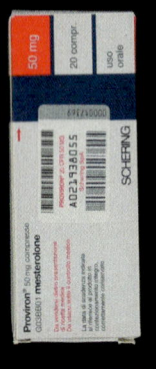

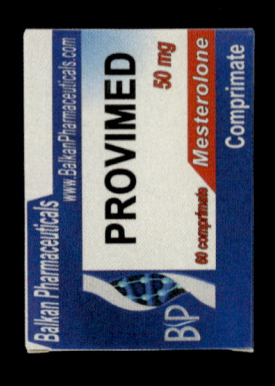

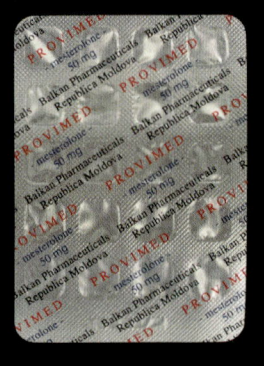

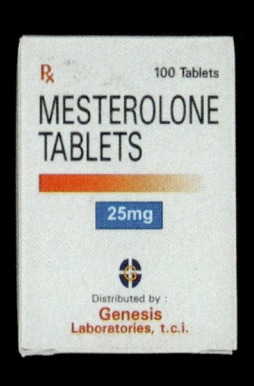

Provironum from India

Older box from India

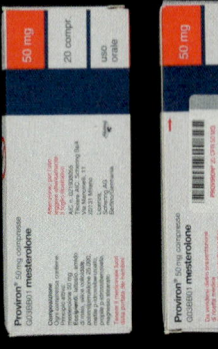

Italian Proviron

Provimed from Balkan (Moldova)

Genesis (Singapore) NLM

Sanabolicum, Fherbolico

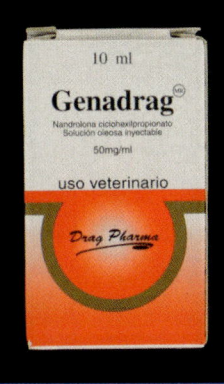

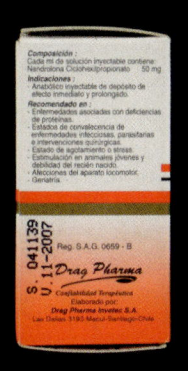

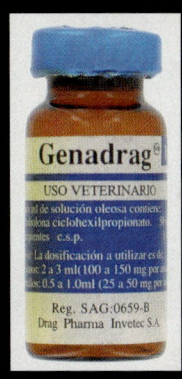

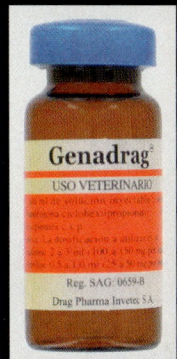

Genadrag from Chile - both vials are legit and from same production run

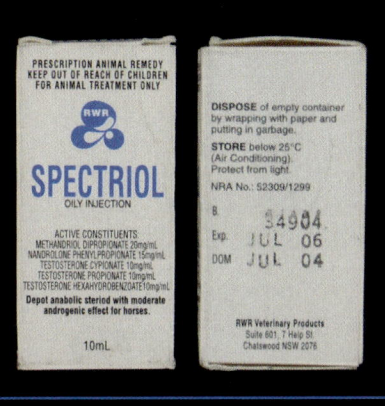

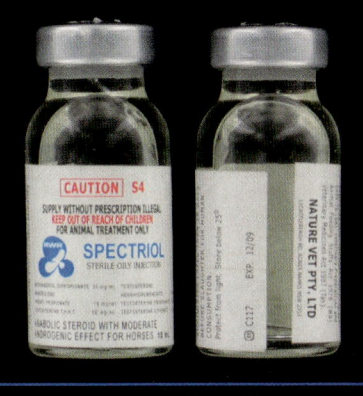

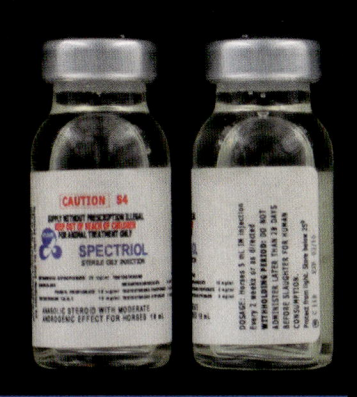

Spectriol

Spectriol (Australia)　　　　　　　　　Two different counterfeits of Australian Spectriol

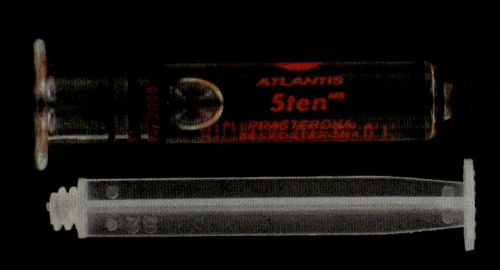

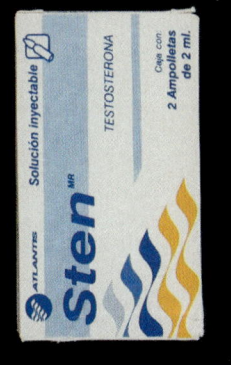

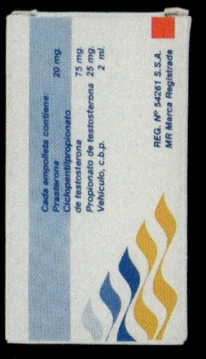

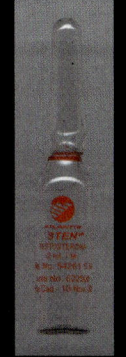

Sten

Sten pre-loaded syringe from Atlantis (Mexico)　　　　　　　　　Older version in ampules

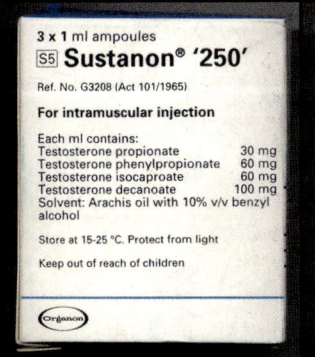

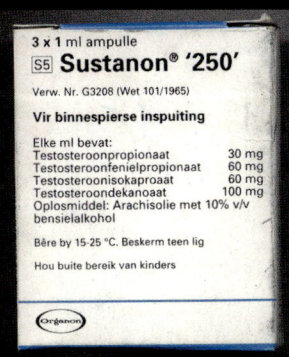

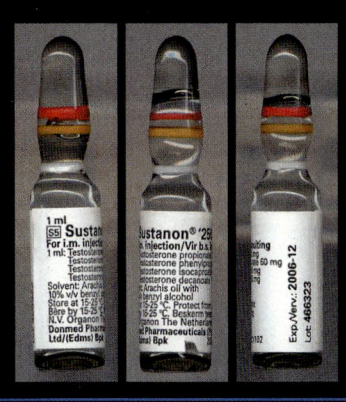

Sustanon

Sustanon '250' from South Africa

Appendix B

B-69

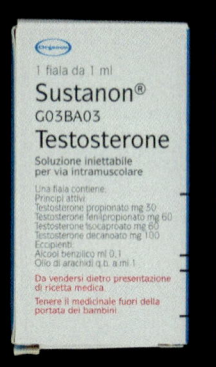

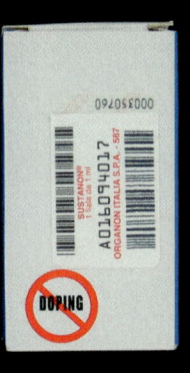

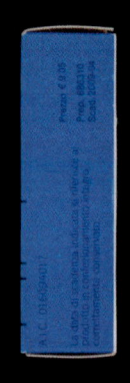

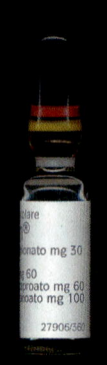

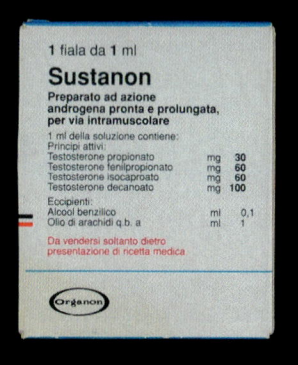

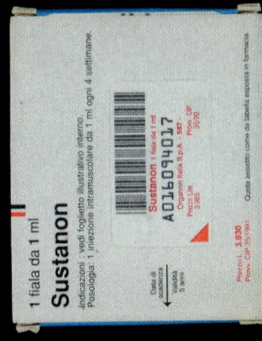

Sustanon from Italy

Old Italian packaging

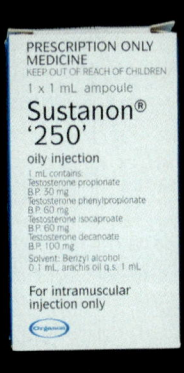

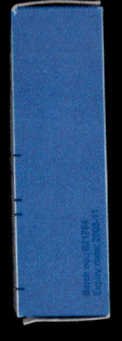

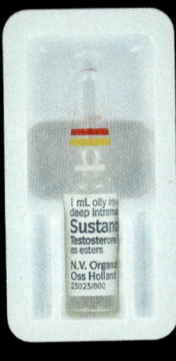

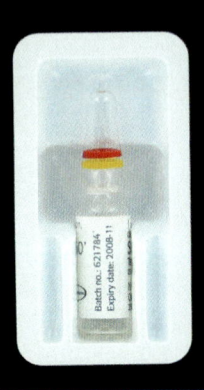

Sustanon '250' from Australia

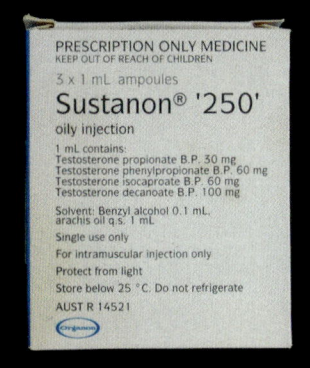

3 ampule box (Australia)

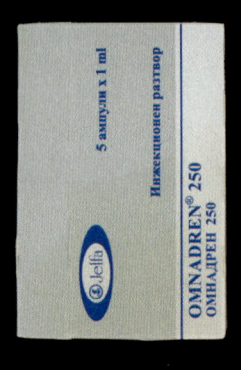

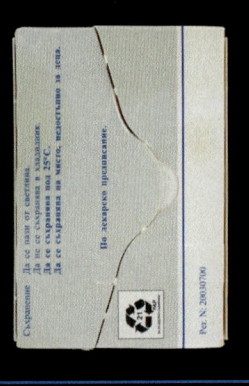

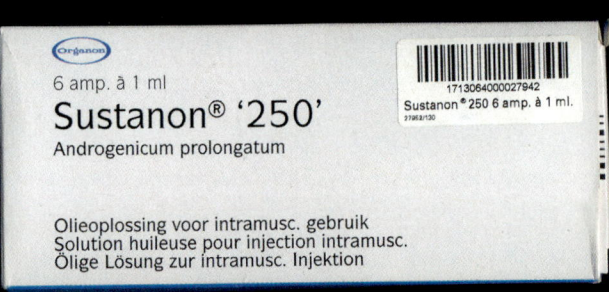

Omnadren 250 (Poland)

Sustanon '250' from Belgium

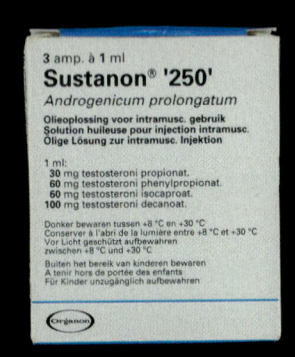

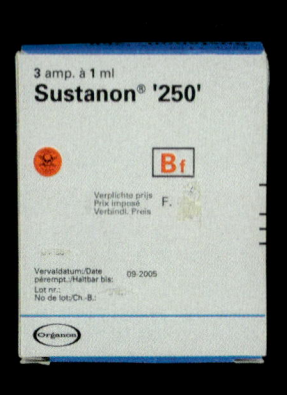

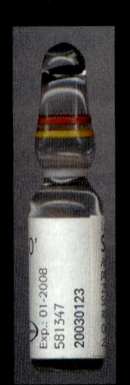

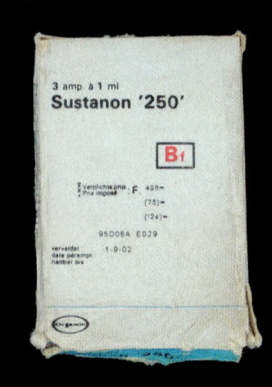

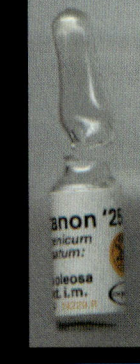

Older Sustanon '250' (Belgium)

Belgian counterfeit

B-70

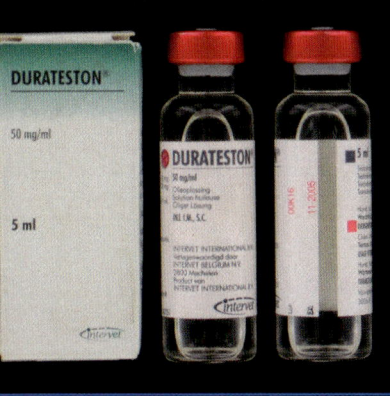

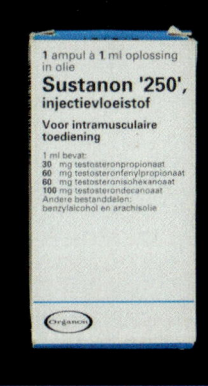

Belgian Durateston (50mg/mL) 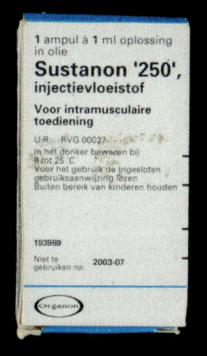 — Sustanon '250' from Holland 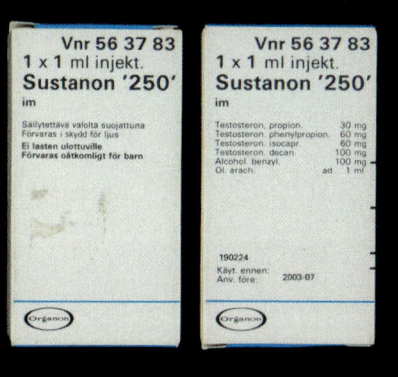 — Sustanon '250' from Estonia

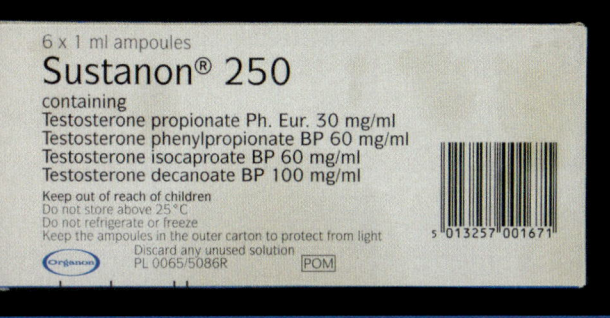

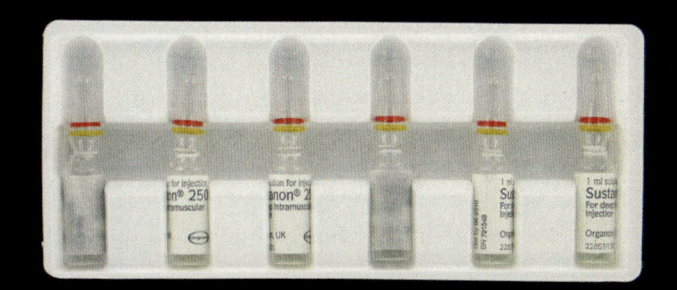

Sustanon 250 (U.K.)

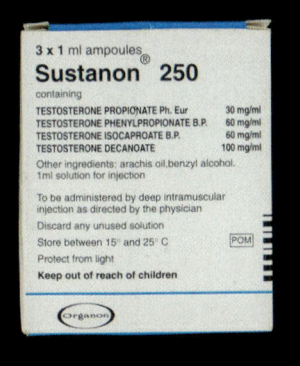

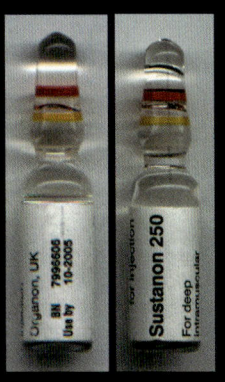

Previous UK packaging 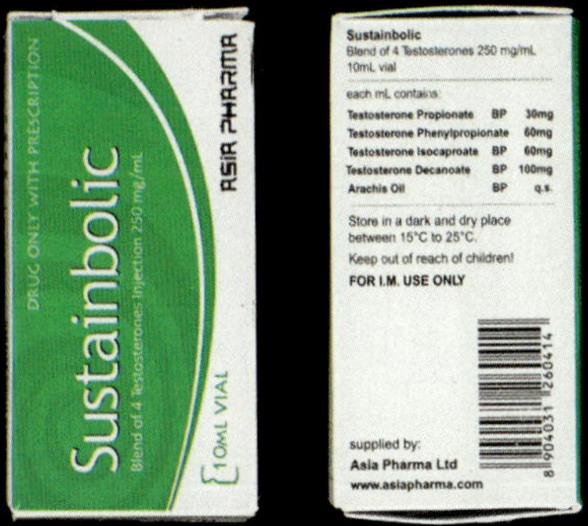 — Sustainbolic (Malaysia)

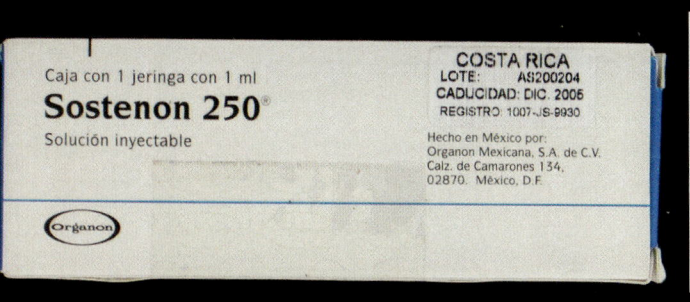

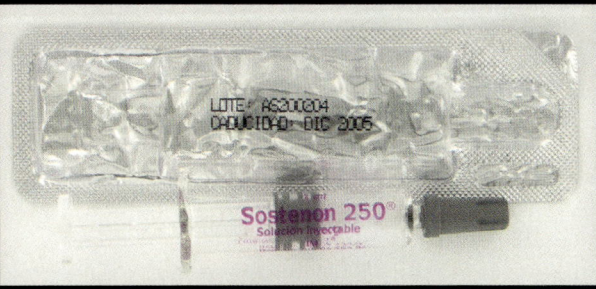

Sustanon 250 (Costa Rica)

Appendix B

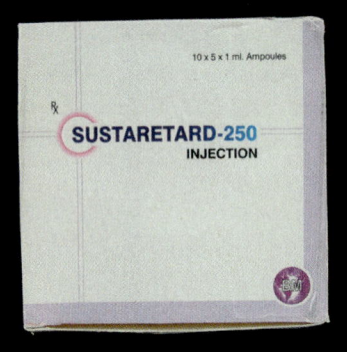

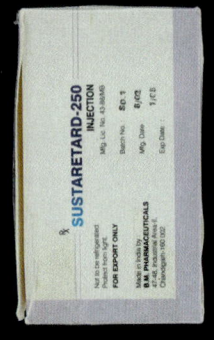

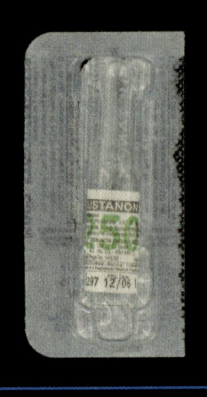

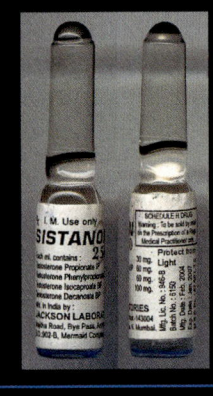

Sustaretard-250 from BM (India, export)   Infar (India)   Sistanon (India)

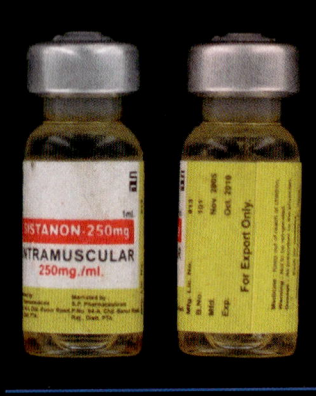

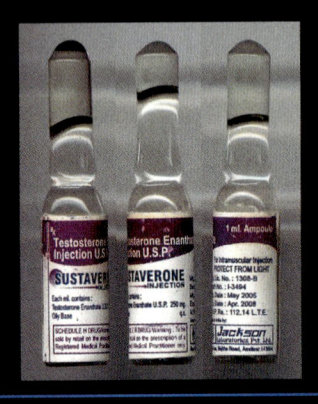

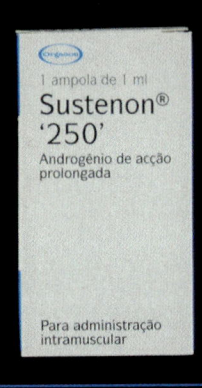

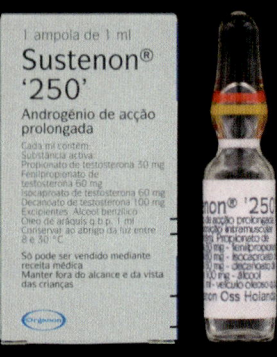

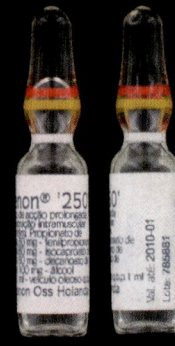

Counterfeit Sistanon and Sustaverone (India)   Sustenon '250' (Portugal)

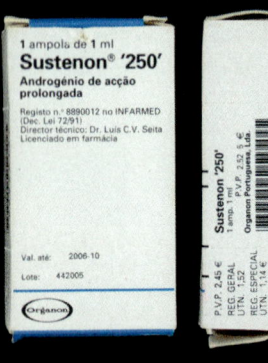

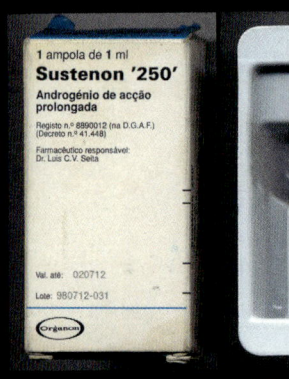

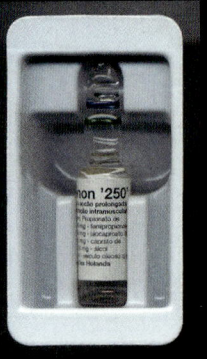

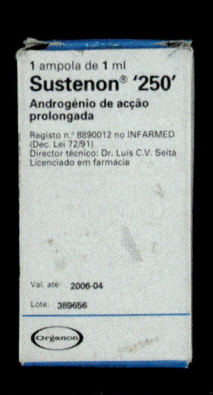

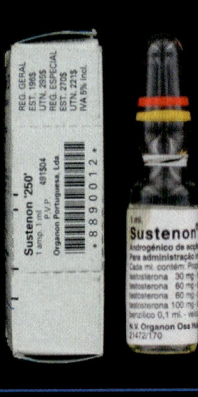

Portuguese counterfet #1   Counterfeit #2   Counterfeit #3

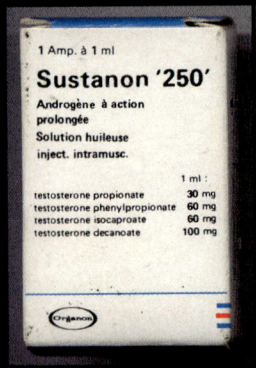

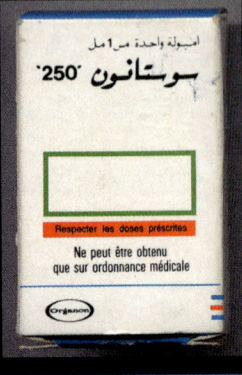

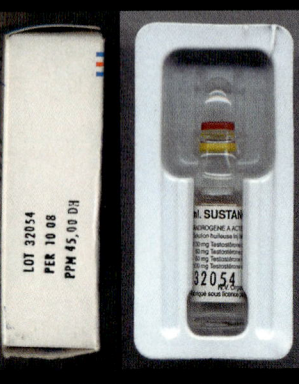

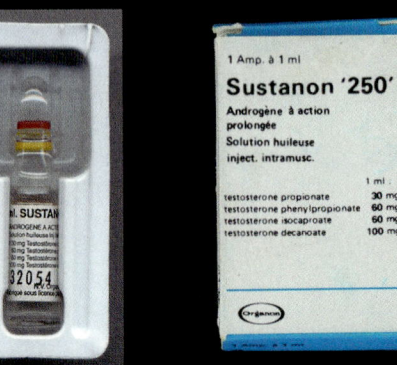

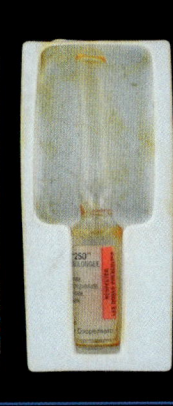

Sustanon '250' from Morocco   Moroccan counterfeit

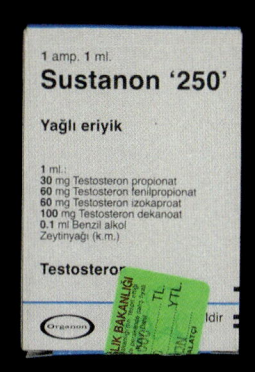

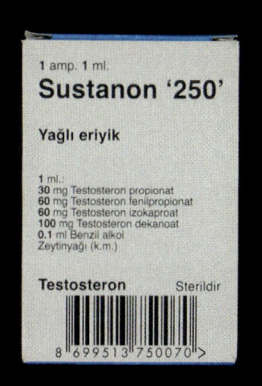

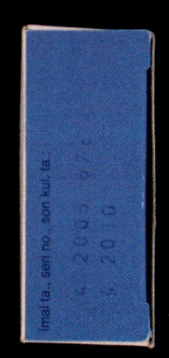

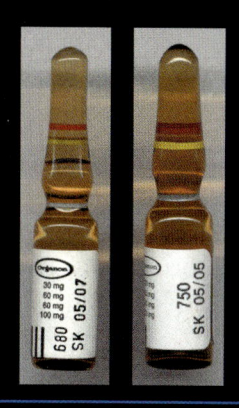

Sustanon '250' from Turkey   Real   Fake

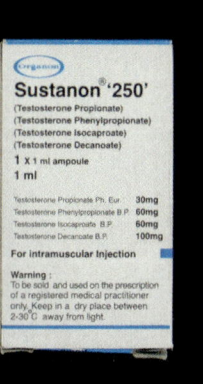

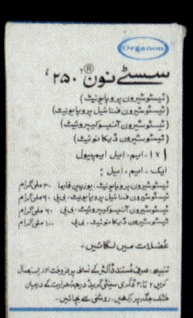

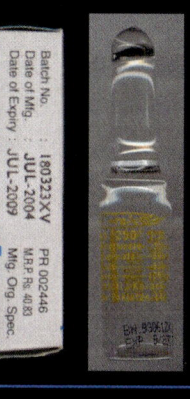

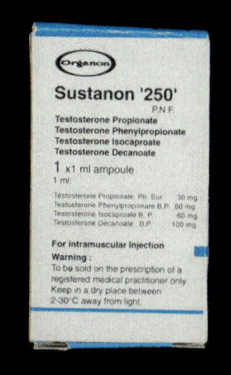

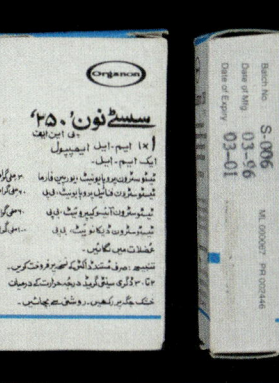

Sustanon '250' from Pakistan   Old box of Pakistani Sustanon '250'

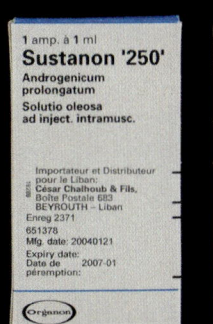

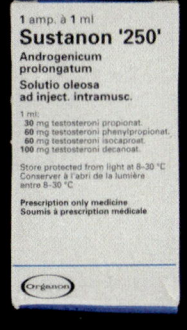

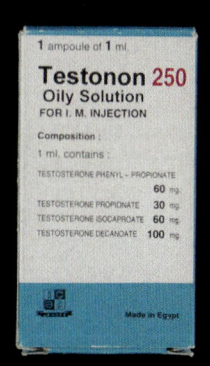

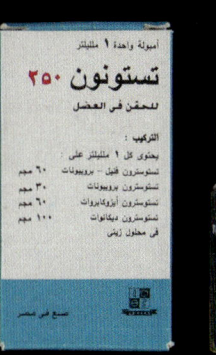

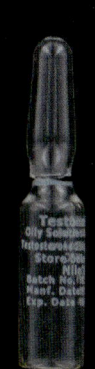

Sustanon '250' from Lebanon   Testonon 250 by The NILE Co. (Egypt)

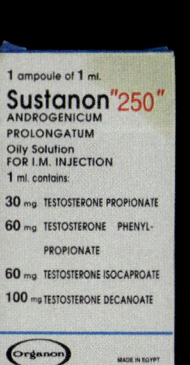

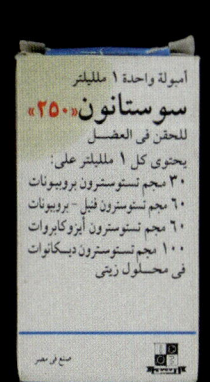

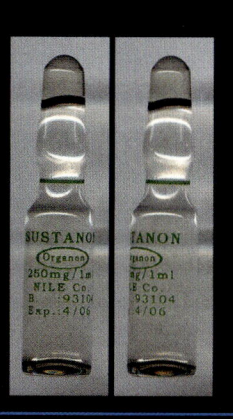

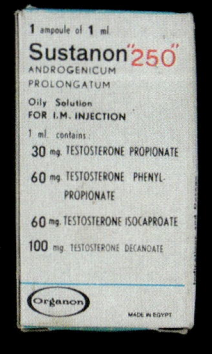

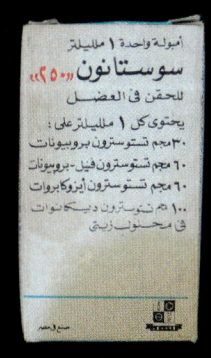

Sustanon "250" by The NILE Co. (Egypt)   Older NILE Sustanon "250" box

Appendix B

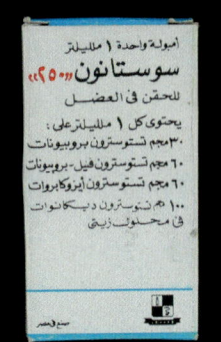

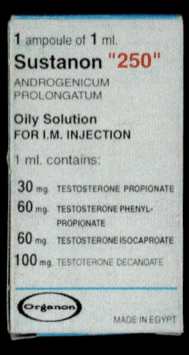

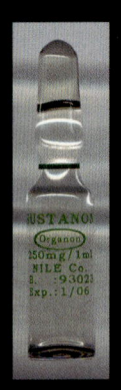

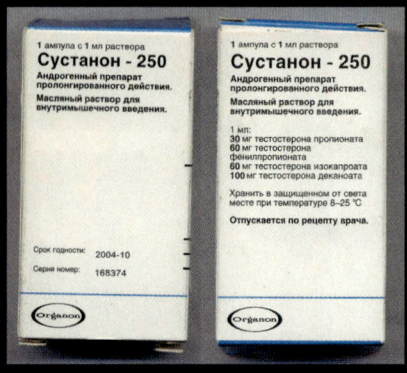

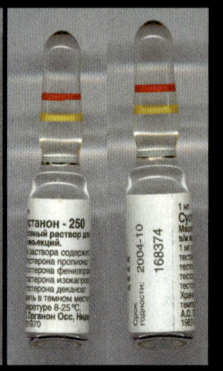

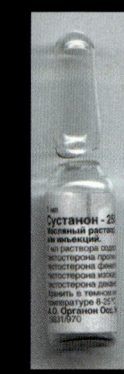

Counterfeit Sustanon "250" by The NILE Co. (Egypt)　　　　Russian Sustanon 250 from Organon　　　　Fake

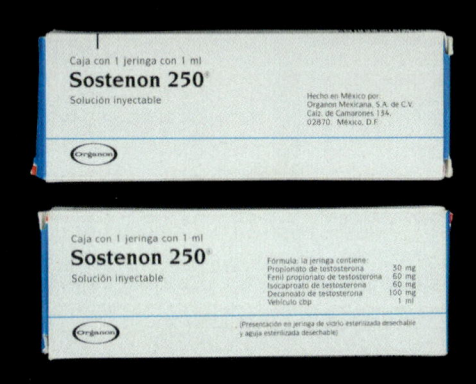

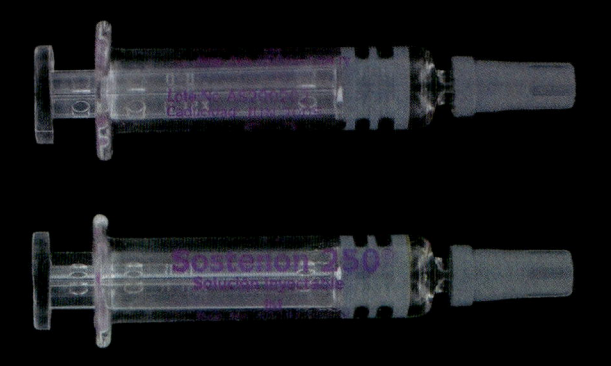

Sostenon 250 pre-loaded synringe from Organon (Mexico)

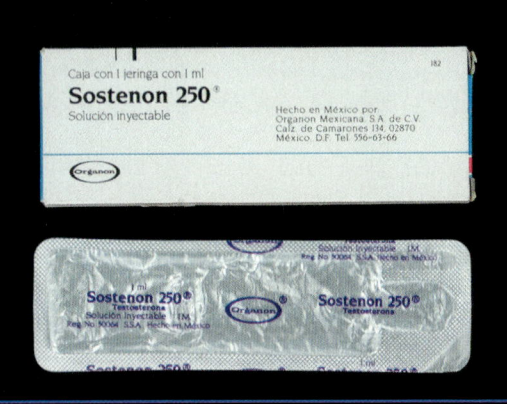

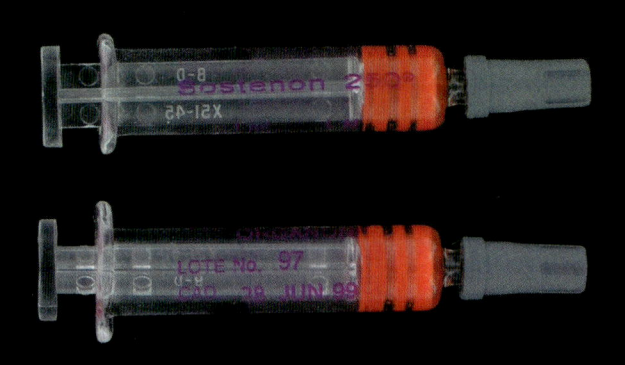

Older packaging for Mexican Sustanon

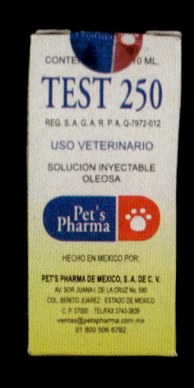

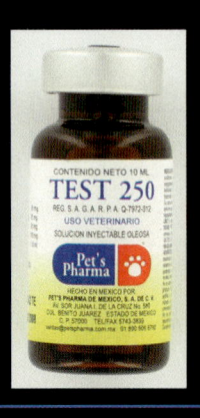

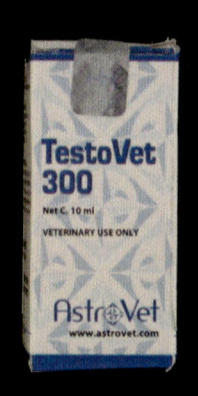

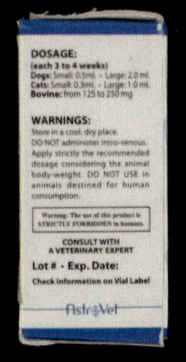

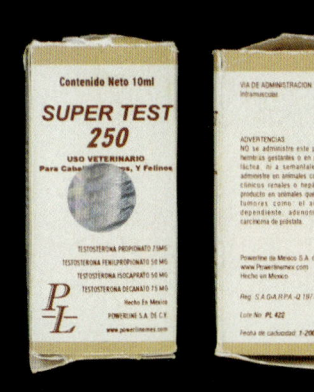

Test 250 from Pet's Pharma (Mexico) NLM　　　　TestoVet from AstroVet (Mexico, UG)　　　　Powerline (Mexico, UG) NLM

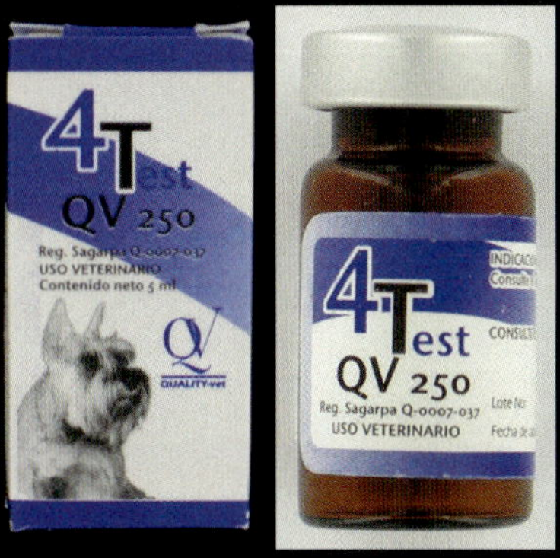

4Test from Quality Vet (Mexico) NLM 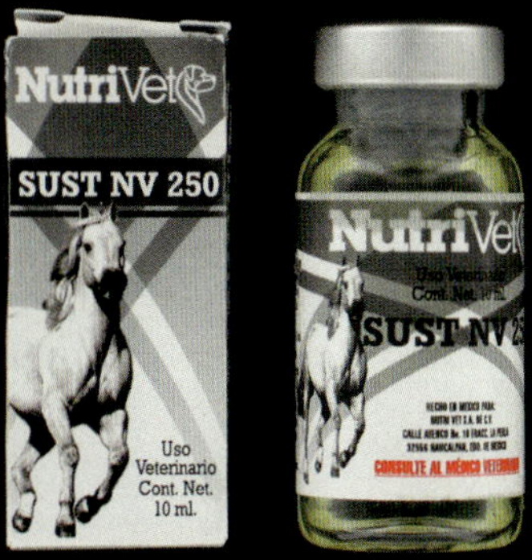 | NutriVet (Mexico, UG) NLM 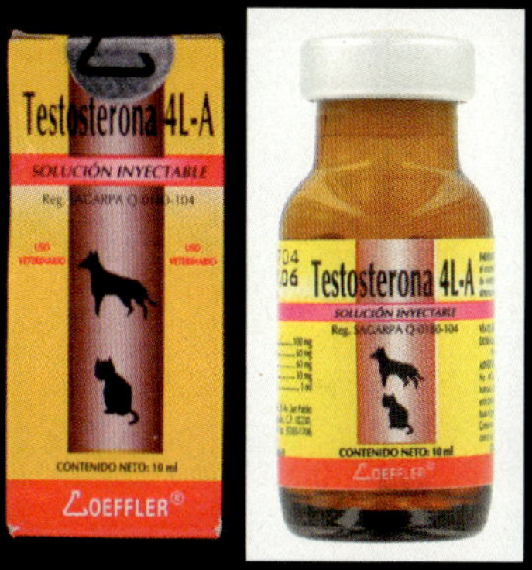 | Loeffler (Mexico) NLM

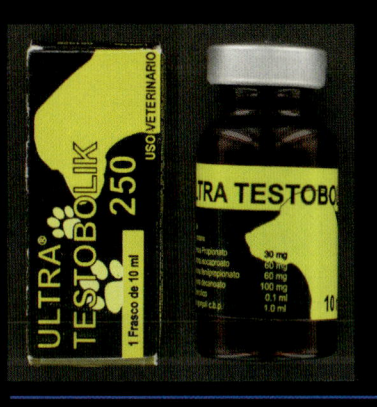

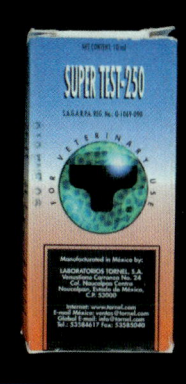

Inmunolab (Mexico, UG) 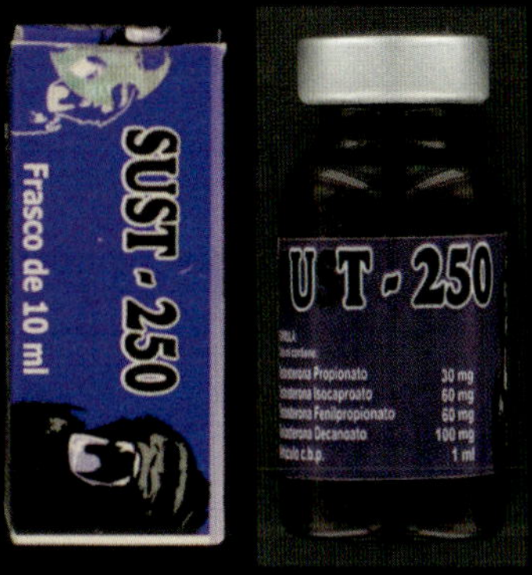 | Gorilla Power (Mexico, UG) 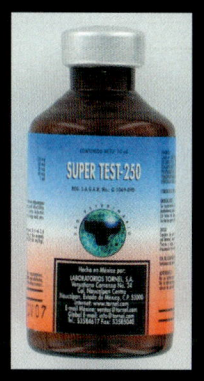 | SuperTest-250 from Tornel (Mexico)

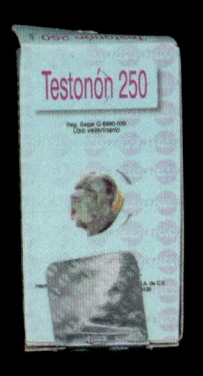

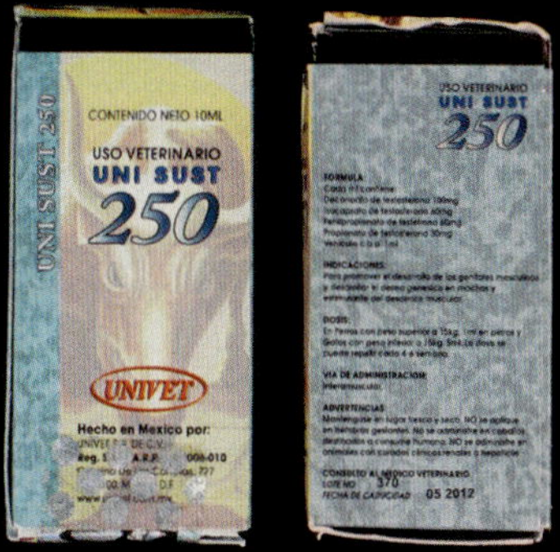

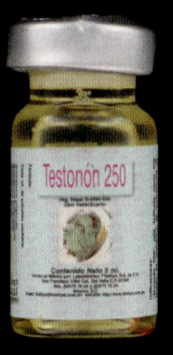

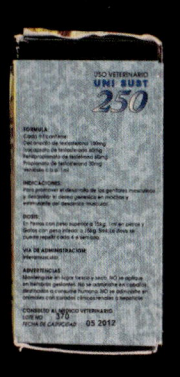

Teston 250 from Ttokkyo Mexico (NLM) 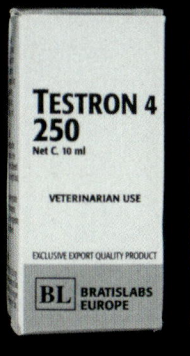 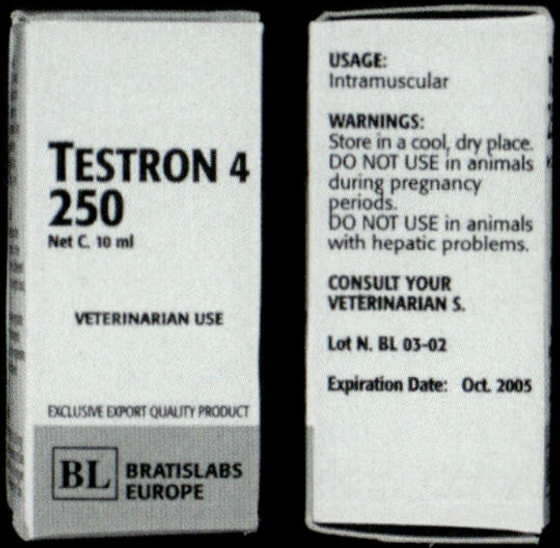 | Mexican UG product from Bratis (NLM) | Univet (Mexico, Underground)

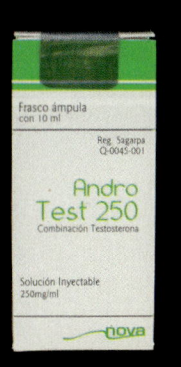

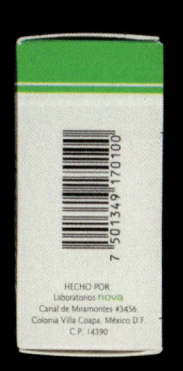

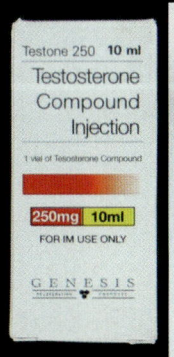

Nova (Mexico, Underground) 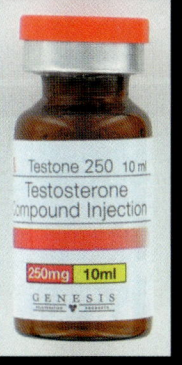 | Testone 250 (Singapore) NLM 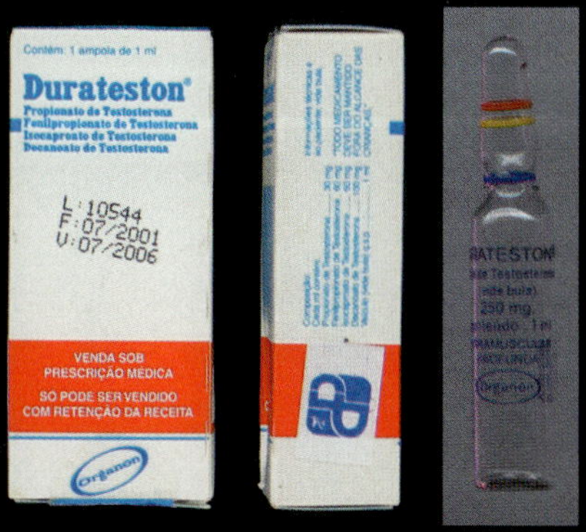 | Durateston (Brazil)

Appendix B

B-75

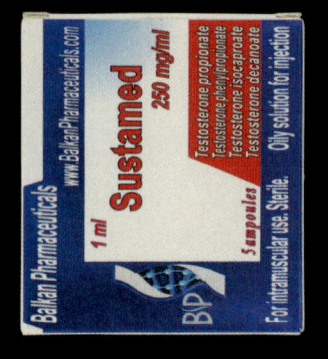

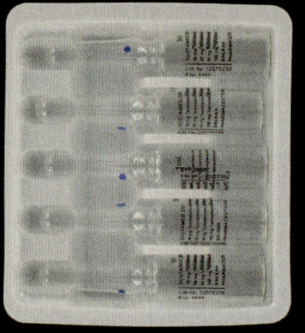

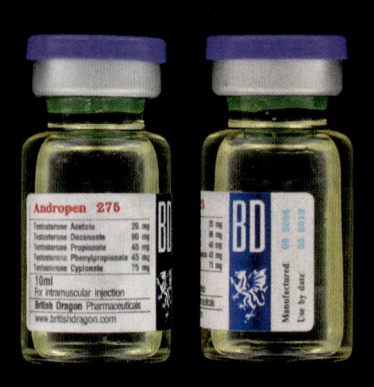

Sustamed from Balkan Pharmaceuticals (Moldova)   British Dragon (Underground) NLM

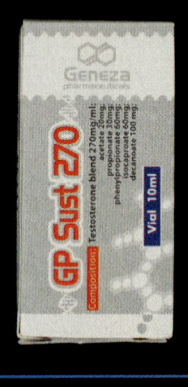

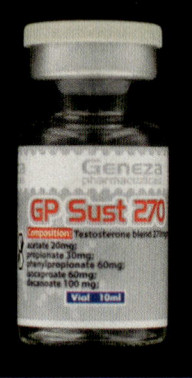

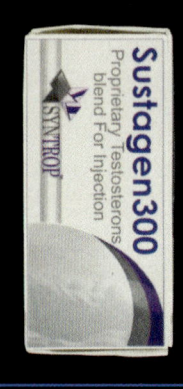

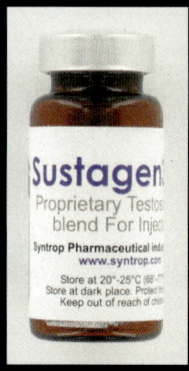

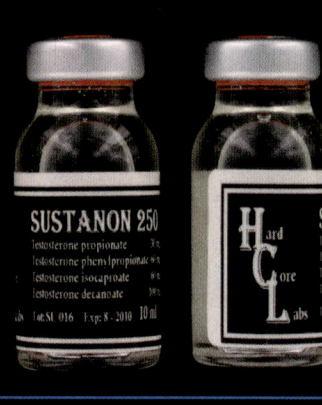

Geneza (Underground)   Syntrop (Underground)   Hardcore Labs (UG)

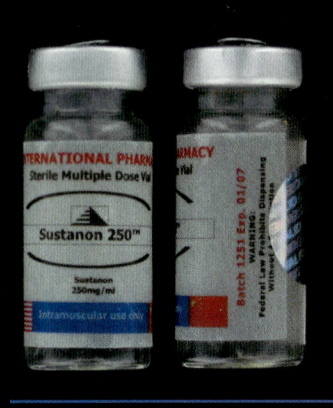

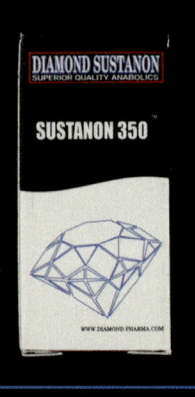

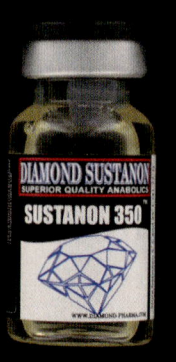

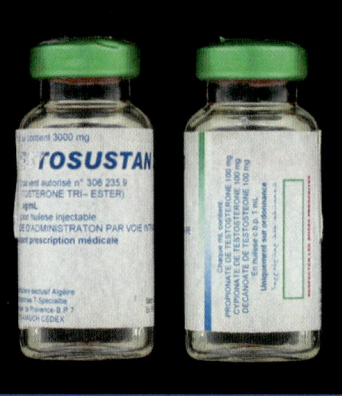

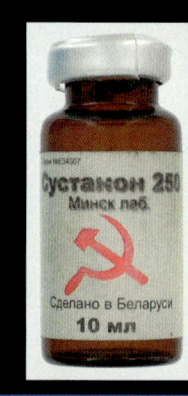

Int Pharmacy (Underground)   Diamond (UG)   Fake French product   Russian fake

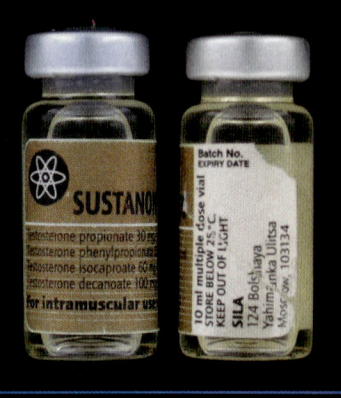

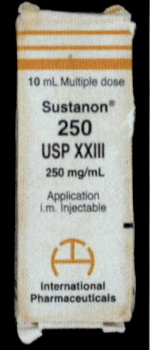

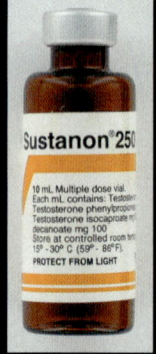

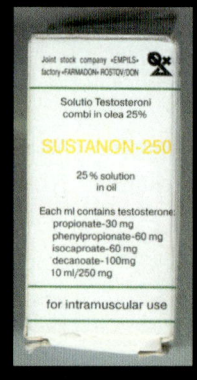

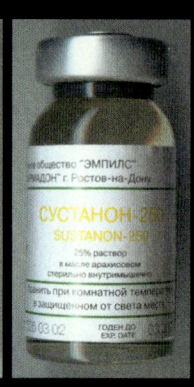

Another fake Russian Sustanon   Fake IP Sustanon   Fake Farmadon box and vial (Russia)

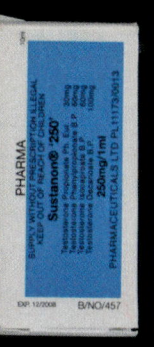

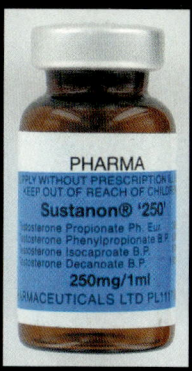

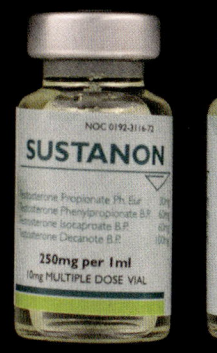

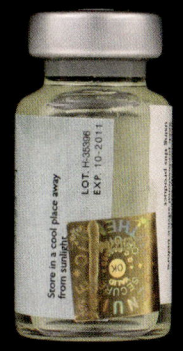

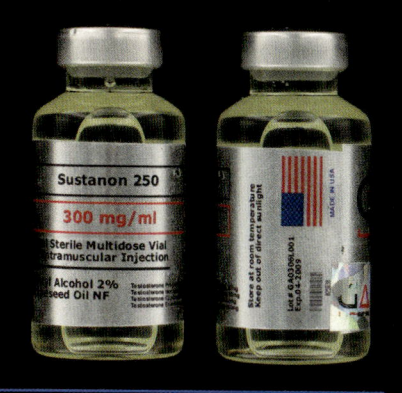

Underground products from Pharma, Changchun, and GA

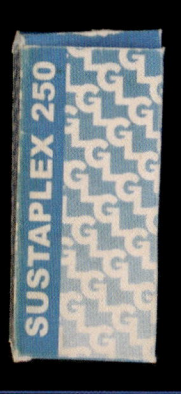

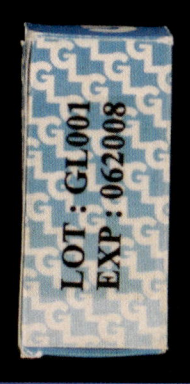

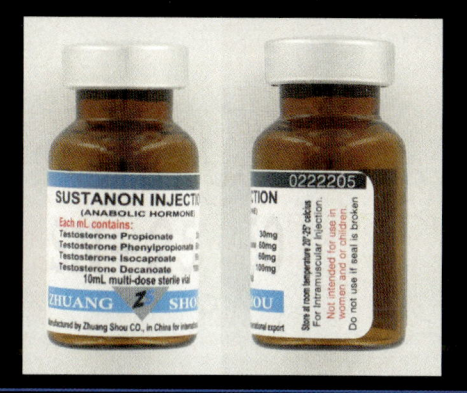

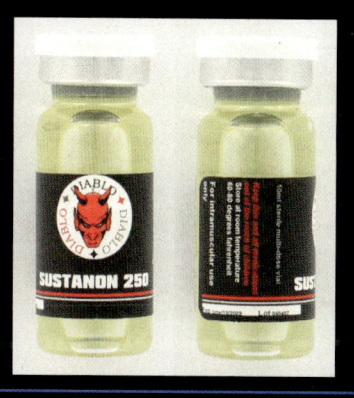

Underground products from Generic Labs, Zhuang, and Diablo

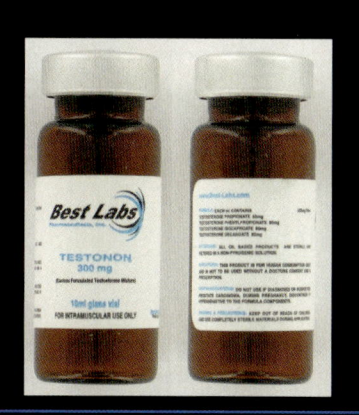

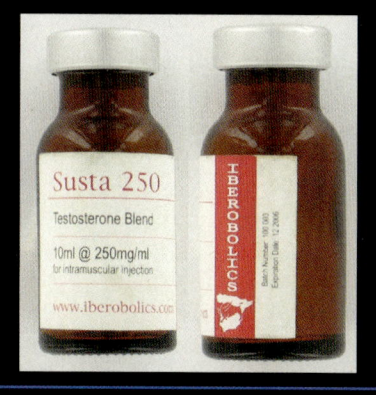

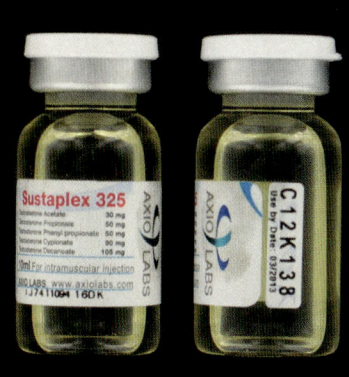

Underground products from Best Labs, Iberobolics, and Axio Labs

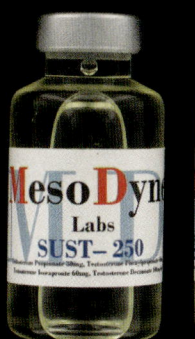

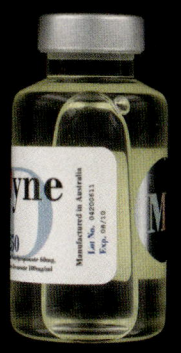

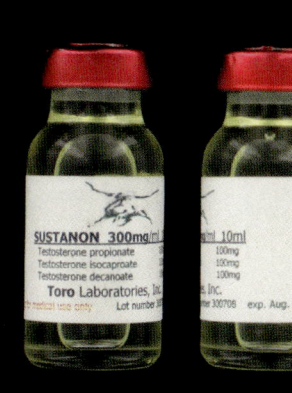

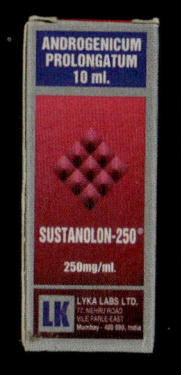

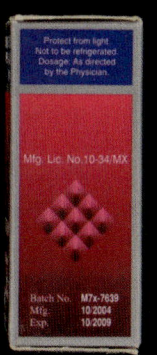

MesoDyne (UG)   Toro (UG)   Lyka (UG)

Appendix B

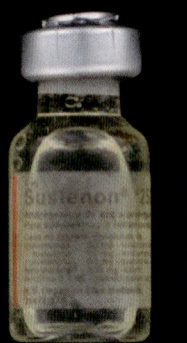

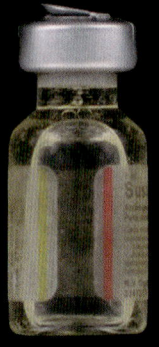

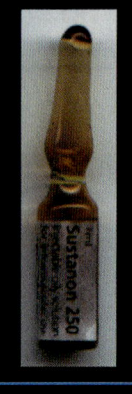

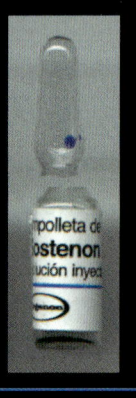

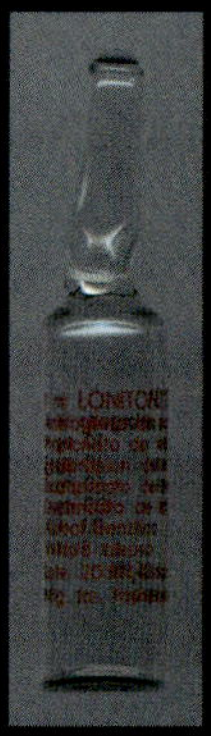

Counterfeit vial (Portugal)   Two counterfeit ampules   Fake Loniton

Synovex

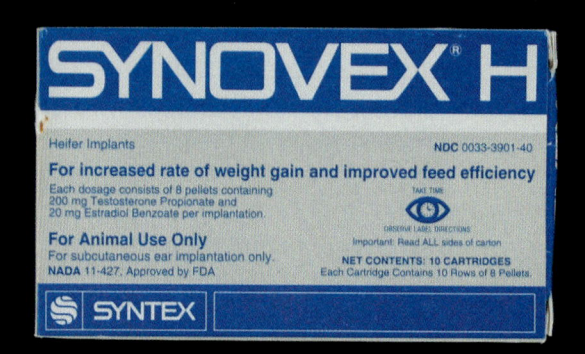

Synovex H (U.S.)

Test400

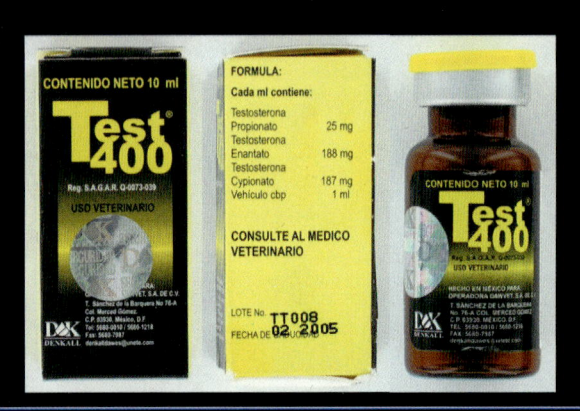

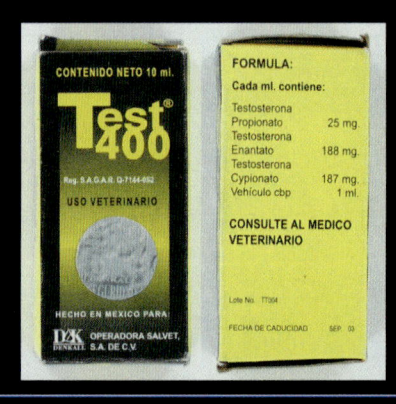

Test 400 from Denkall (Mexico) NLM   Counterfeit Test 400 with fake hologram

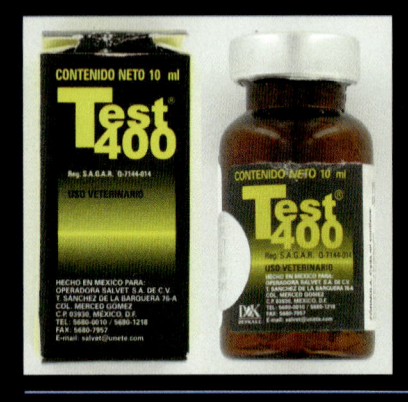

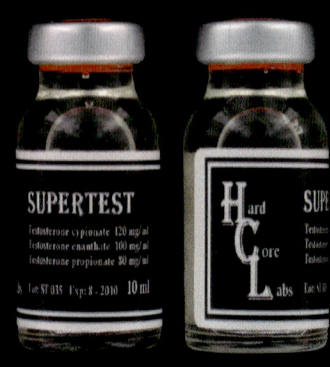

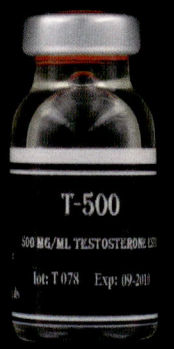

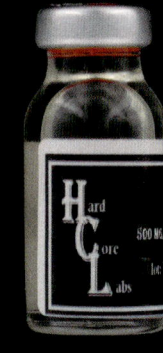

Another counterfeit   300mg/mL clone from Hardcore Labs (UG)   HCL 500mg/mL similar blend

B-78

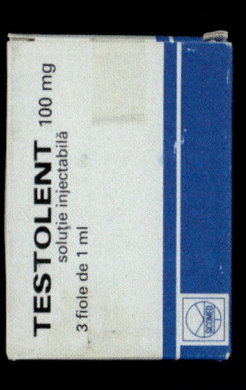

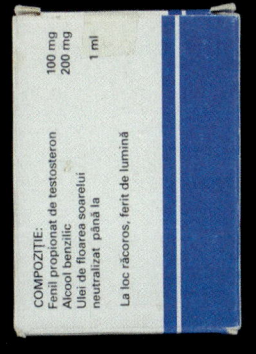

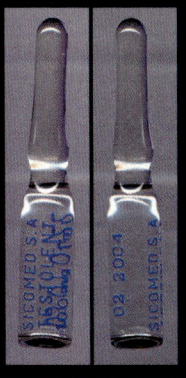

Testolent

Testolent from Romania (NLM)

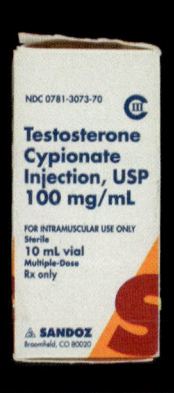

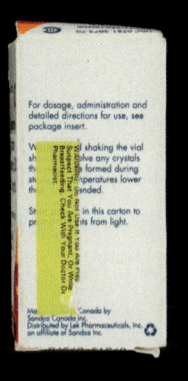

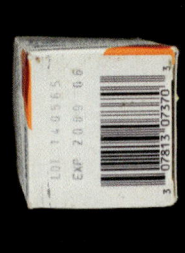

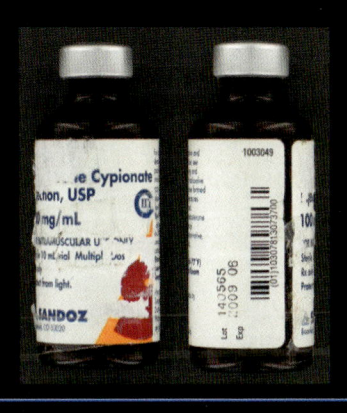

Testosterone Cypionate

U.S. generic from Sandoz

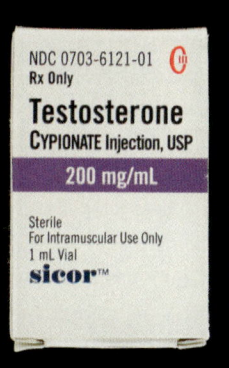

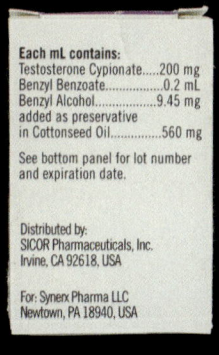

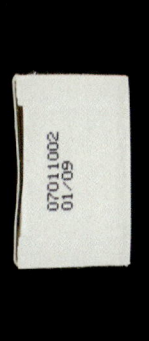

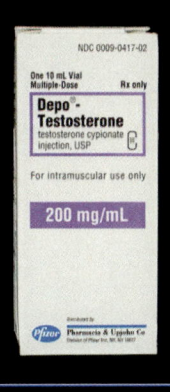

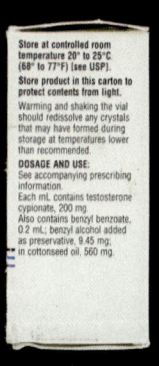

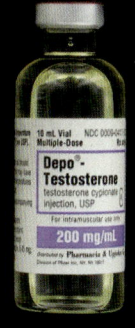

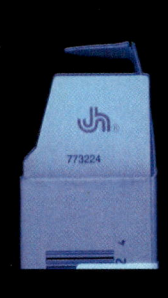

Generic from Sicor (U.S.)

Depo-Testosterone (U.S.) "Jh" appears on flap under UV light

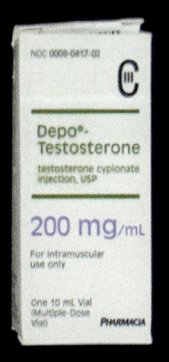

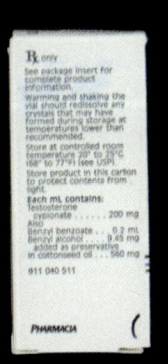

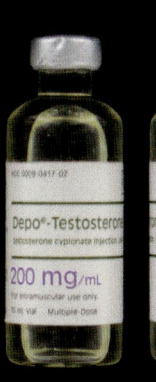

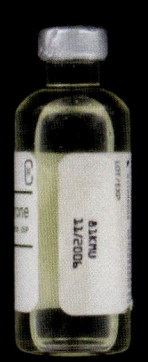

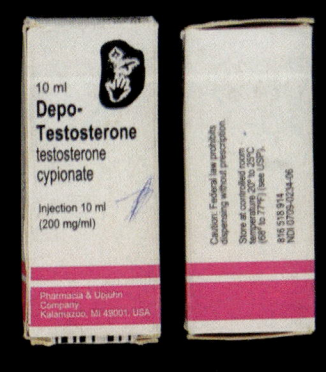

Older packaging for U.S. Depo-Testosterone

Counterfeit Depo Testosterone

Appendix B

B-79

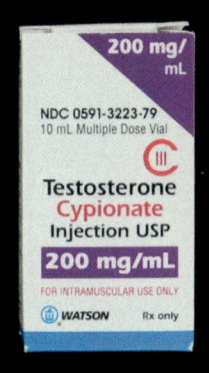

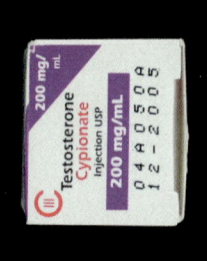

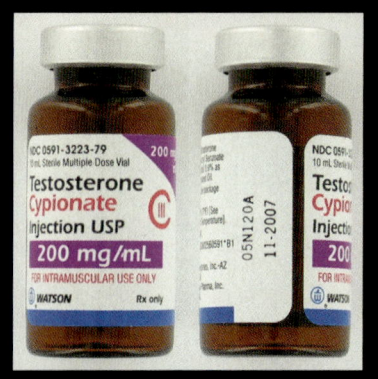

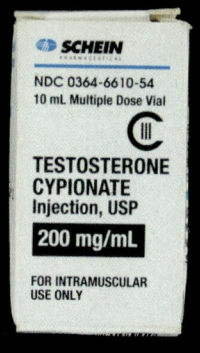

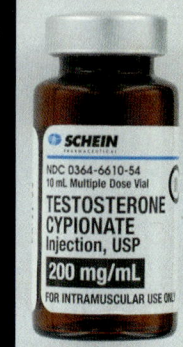

Watson generic (U.S.)

Generic from Schein/Steris (NLM)

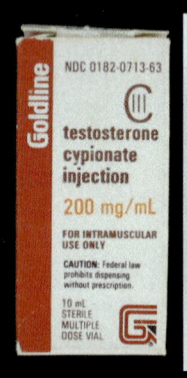

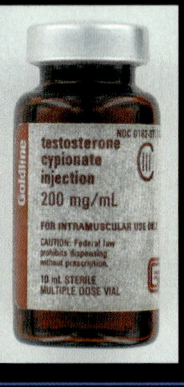

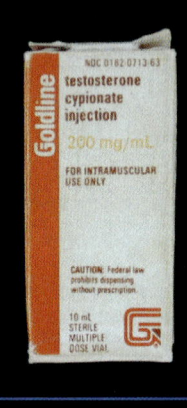

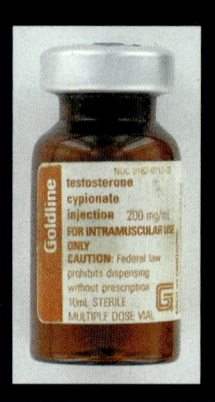

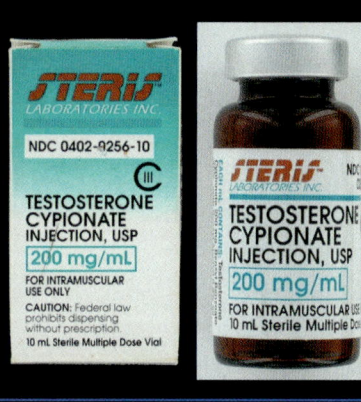

U.S. Goldline generic (NLM)

Goldline Counterfeit

Counterfeit U.S. Steris cypionate

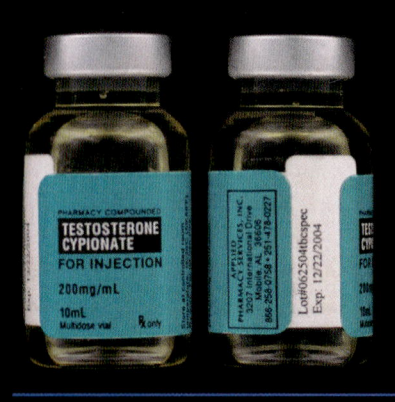

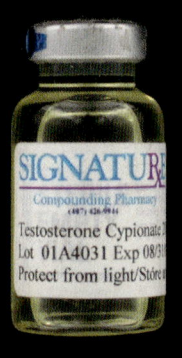

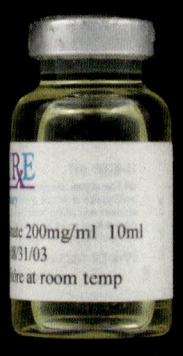

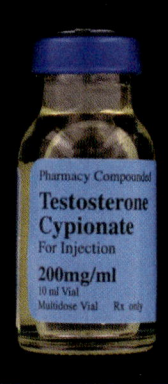

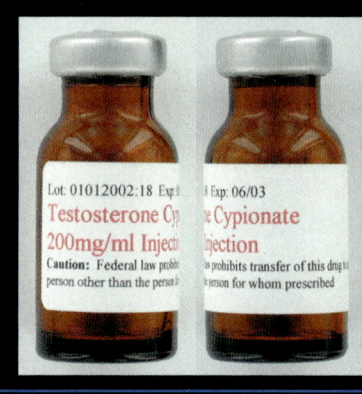

Four different cypionate vials compounded in pharmacies (U.S.)

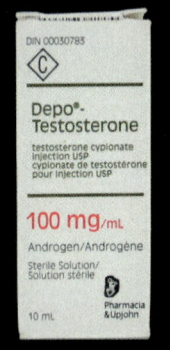

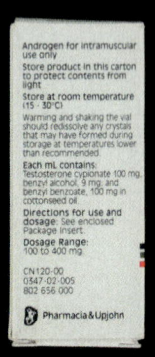

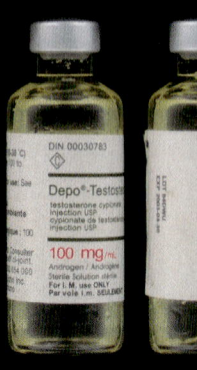

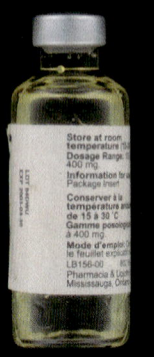

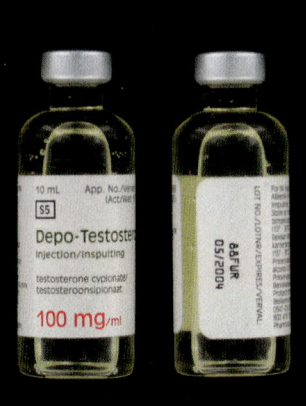

Canadian Depo Testosterone from Pharmacia

Depo Testosterone from Pharmacia S. Africa

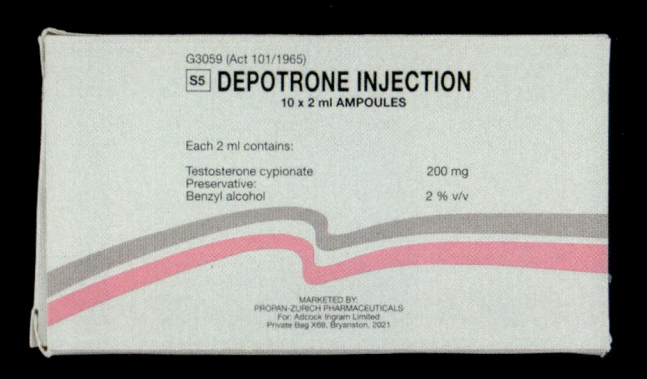

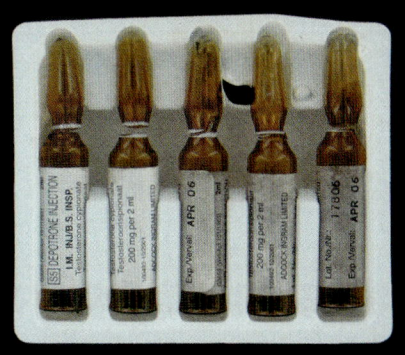

Depotrone from South Africa

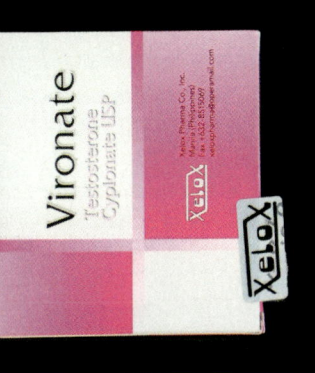

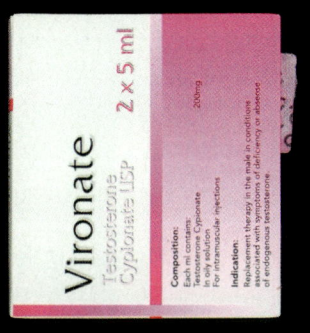

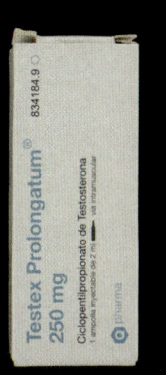

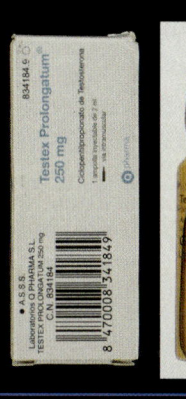

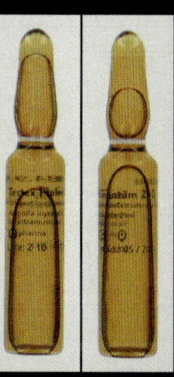

Vironate from WDV (Philippines)

Testex from Q Pharma (Spain)

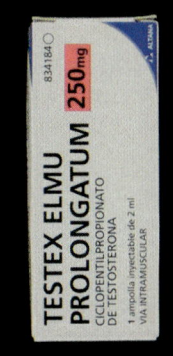

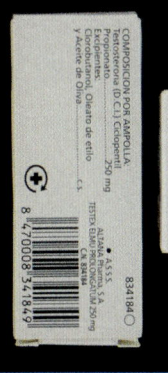

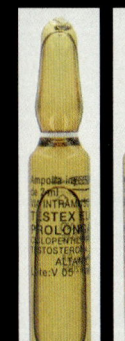

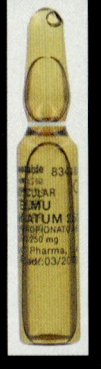

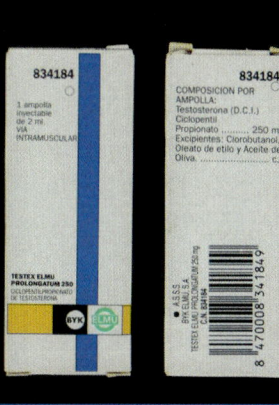

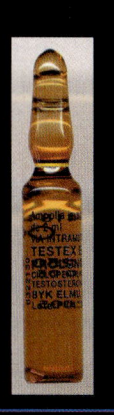

Testex Prolongatum from Altana (Spain) NLM

Old Spanish Testex from BYK/ELMU (NLM)

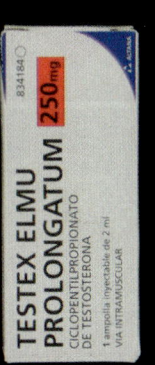

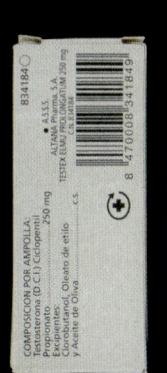

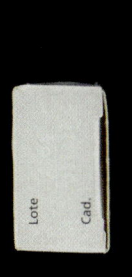

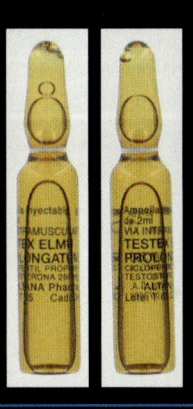

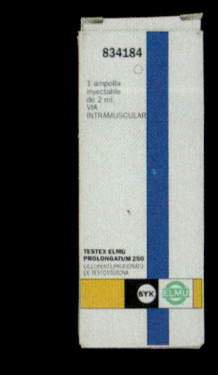

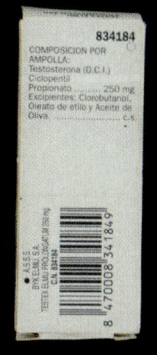

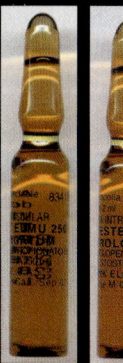

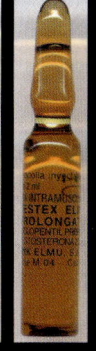

Detailed counterfeit of Altana Testex

Detailed counterfeit of previous Testex brand

Appendix B

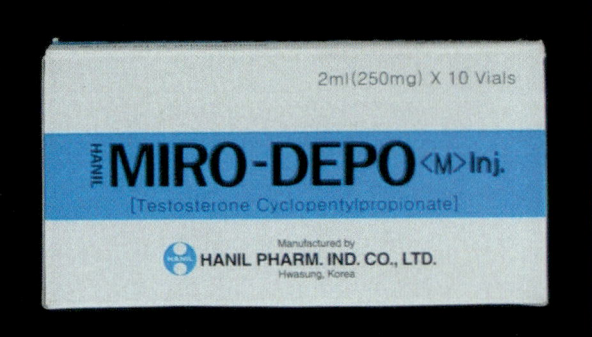

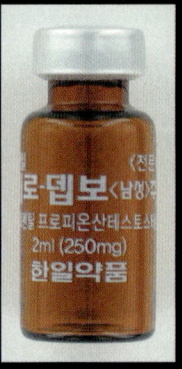

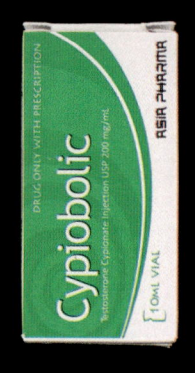

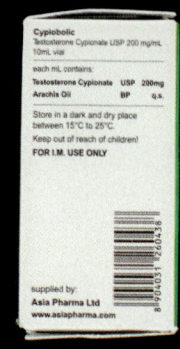

Miro-Depo from Hanil (Korea)

Cypiobolic from Asia Pharma (Malaysia)

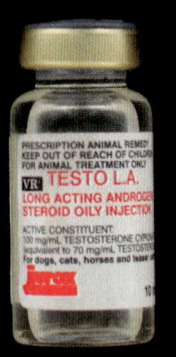

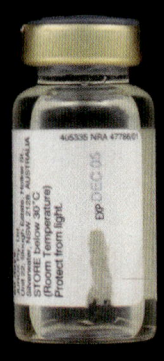

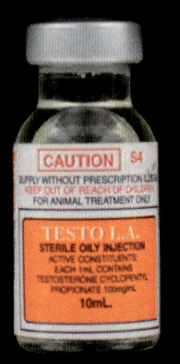

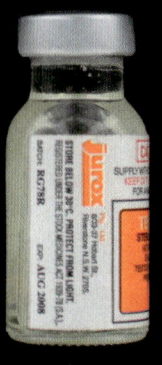

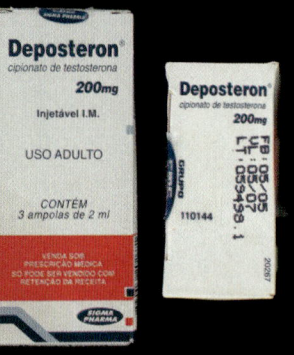

Testo LA from Jurox (Australia)

Counterfeit Jurox Testo LA

Deposteron from Brazil

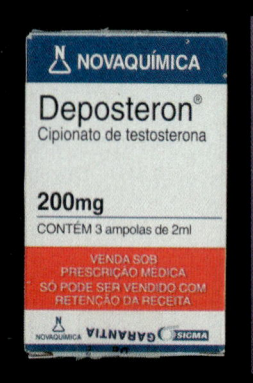

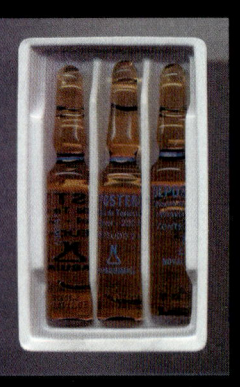

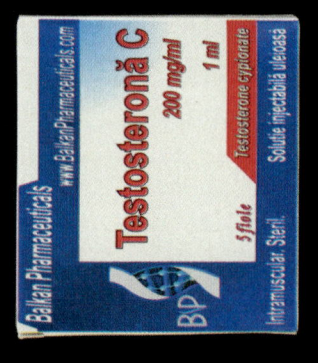

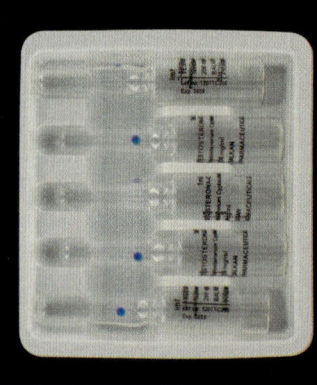

Older Deposteron from Brazil

Testosterona C from Balkan (Moldova)

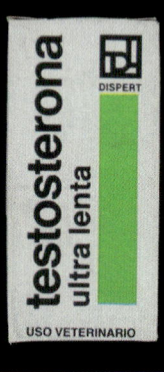

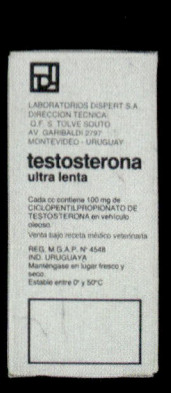

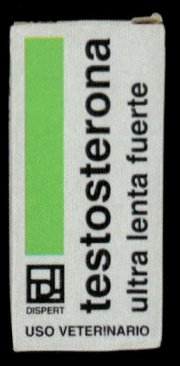

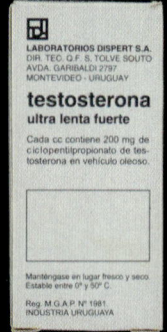

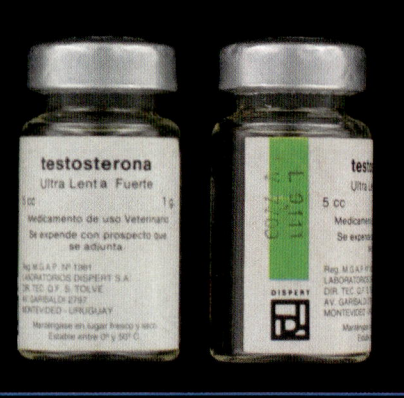

100mg/mL and 200mg/mL products from Dispert Labs (Uruguay)

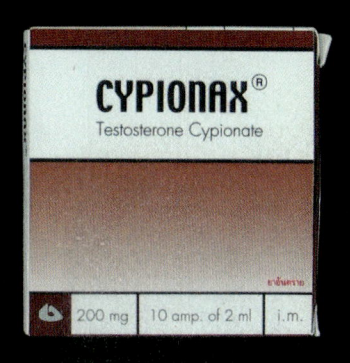

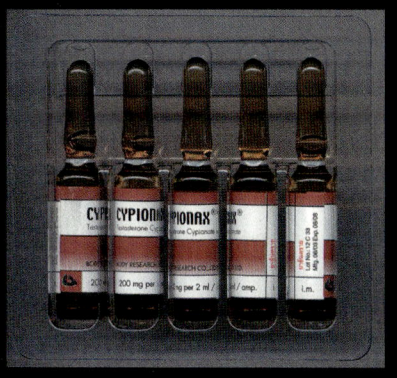

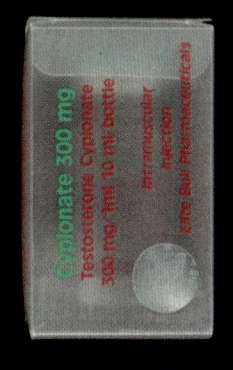

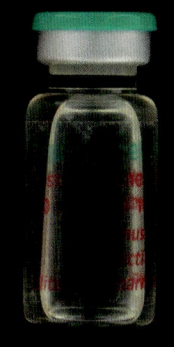

Cypionax (Thailand)

Elite Bull (Hong Kong, export)

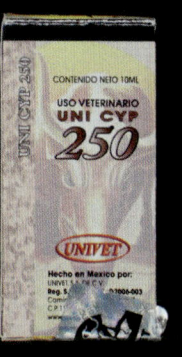

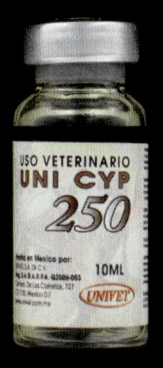

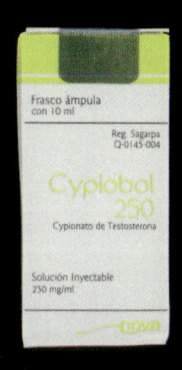

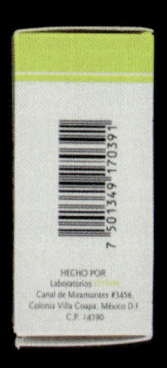

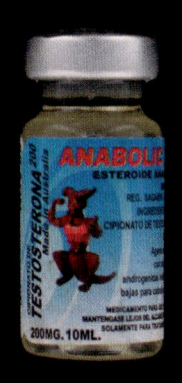

Univet (Mexico, UG)

Nova (Mexico, UG)

SYD Group (Mexico) NLM

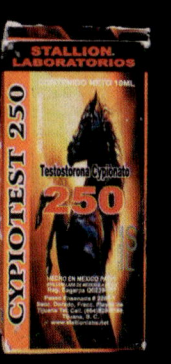

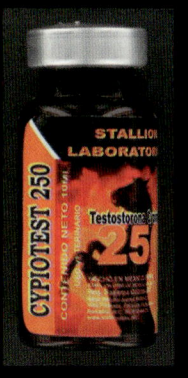

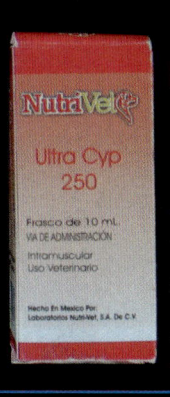

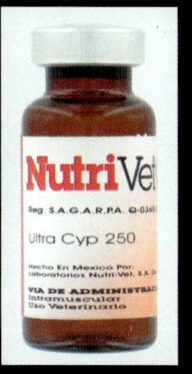

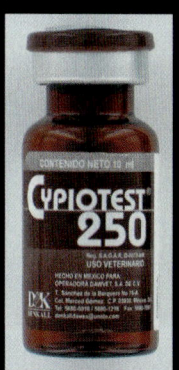

Stallion Labs (Mexico, UG) NLM

Nutri-Vet Ultra Cyp 300 (Mexico, UG)

Denkall (Mexico) NLM

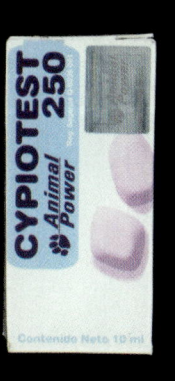

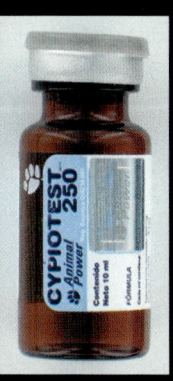

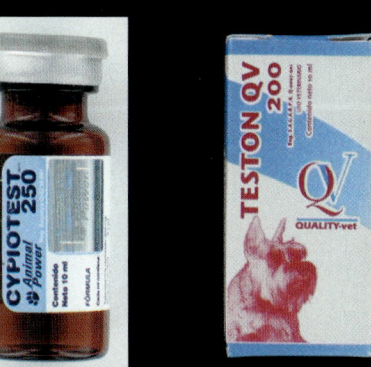

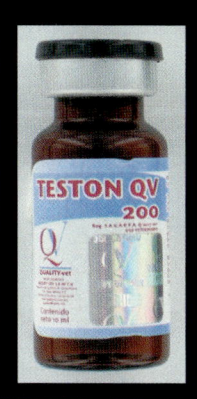

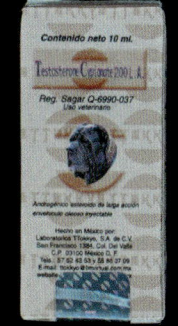

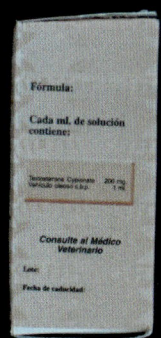

Animal Power (Mexico) NLM

Quality Vet (Mexico) NLM

Ttokkyo (Mexico) NLM

Appendix B

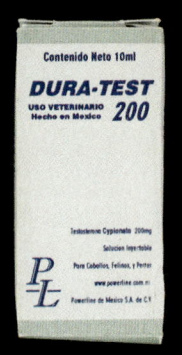

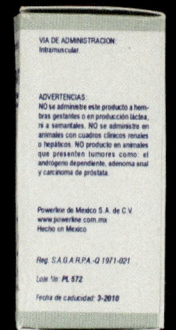

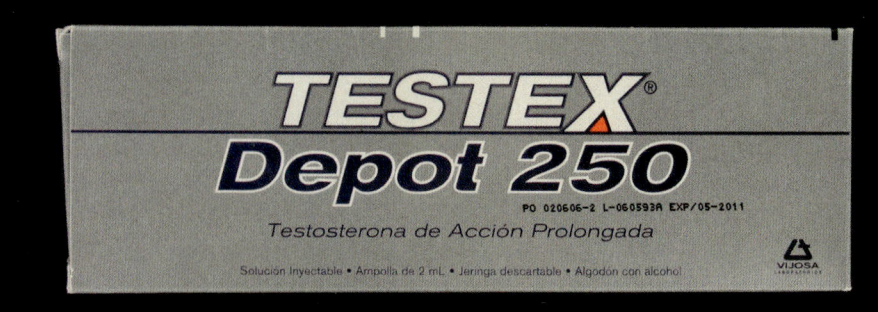

PowerLine (Mexico) NLM · Testex (El Salvador)

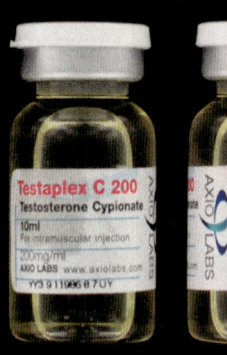

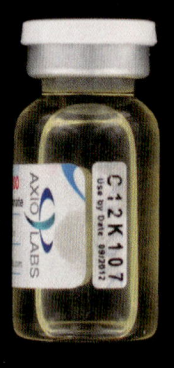

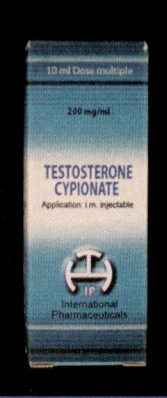

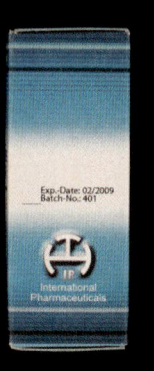

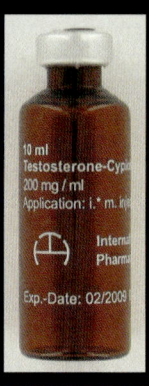

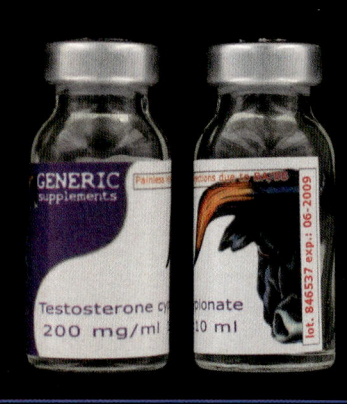

Axio Labs (UG) · International Pharmaceuticals (UG) · Generic Supplements (UG)

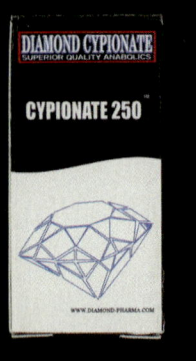

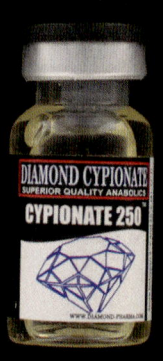

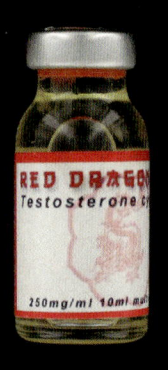

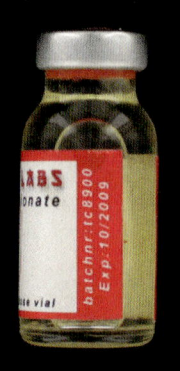

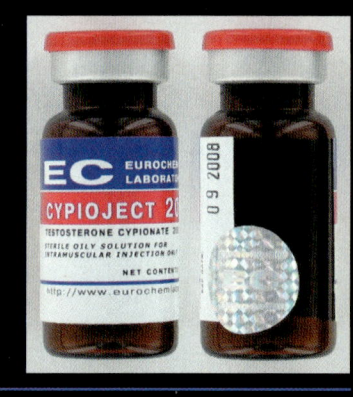

Diamond (Underground) · Red Dragon (Underground) · Eurochem (Underground)

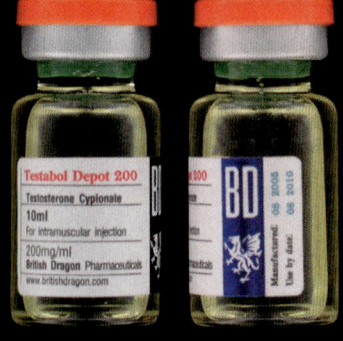

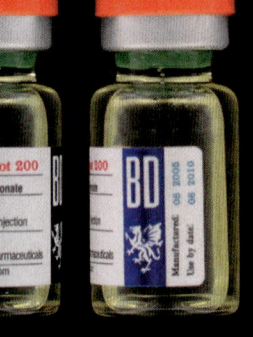

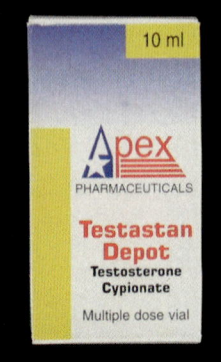

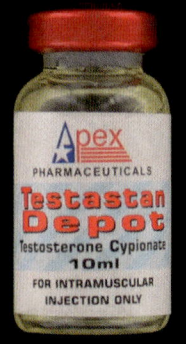

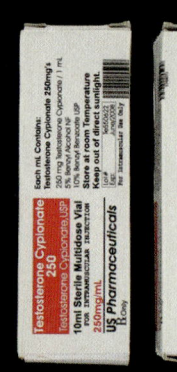

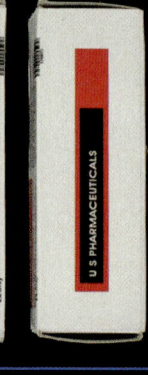

British Dragon (Underground) NLM · Apex (Underground) · U.S. Pharm (Underground)

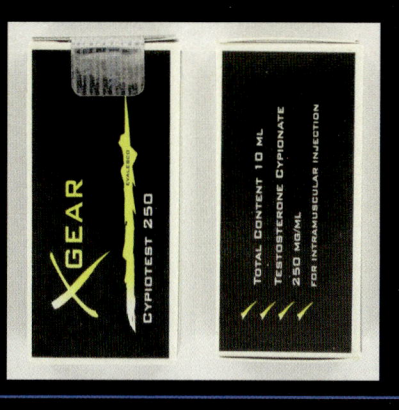

X Gear (Underground) 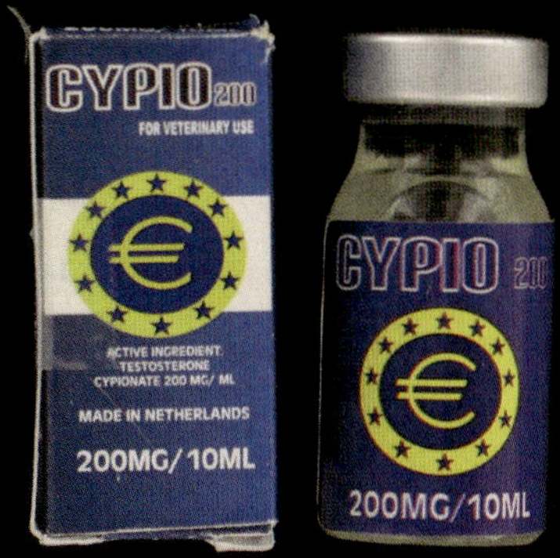 EuroVet (Underground) 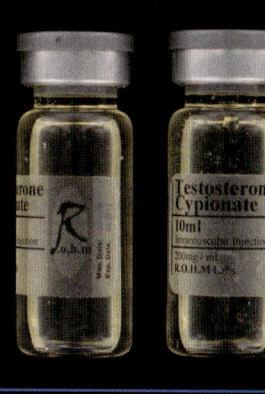 R.O.H.M. (Underground)

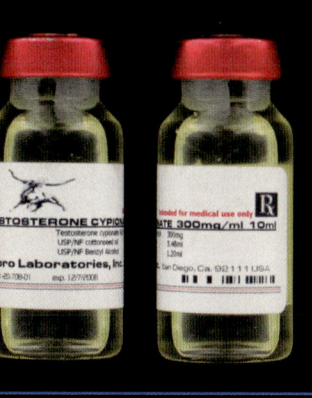

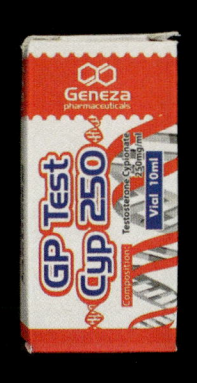

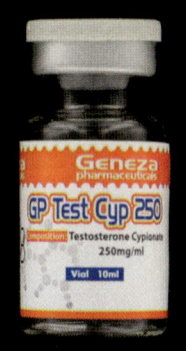

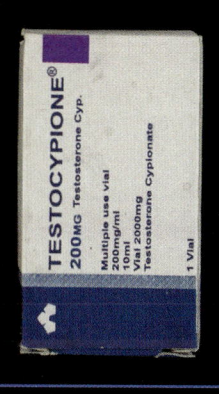

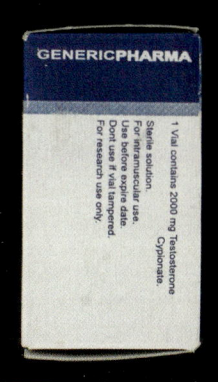

Underground products from Toro, Geneza, and GenericPharma

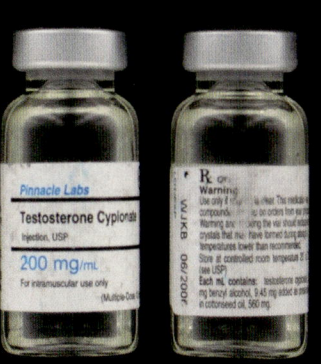

Pinnacle (Underground) 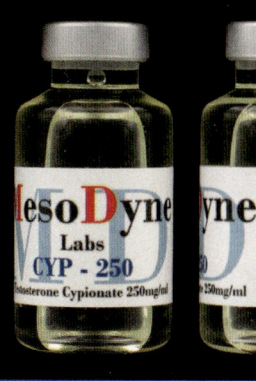 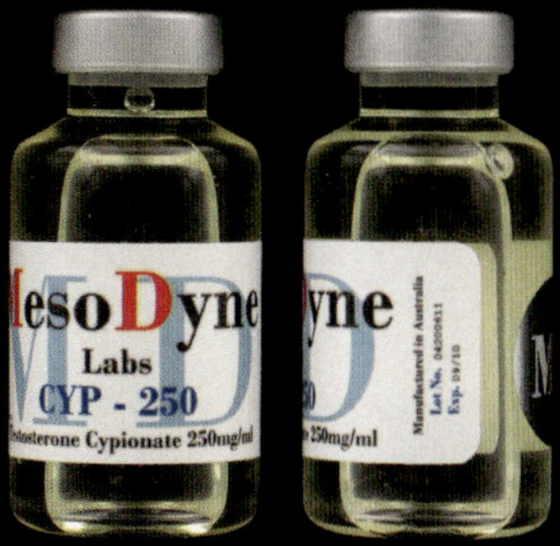 MesoDyne (Underground) 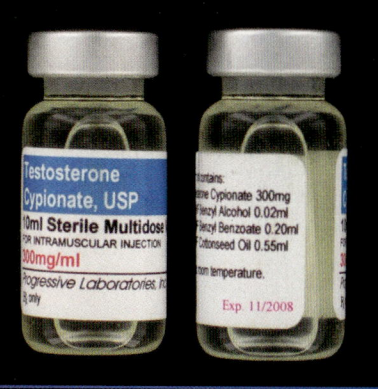 Progressive (Underground)

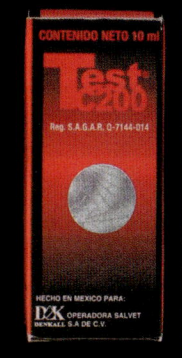

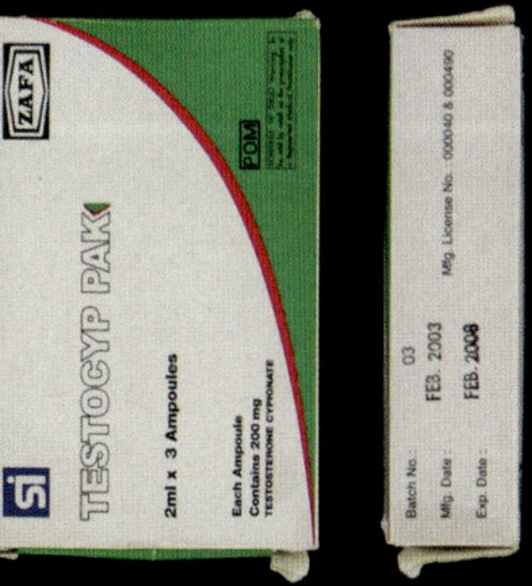

Fake cypionate from India 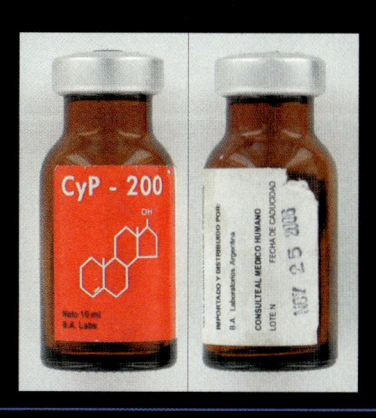 Fake Cyp 200 (Argentina) 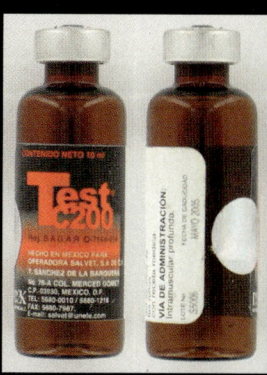 Fake Denkall TestC200

Appendix B

Testosterone Enanthate

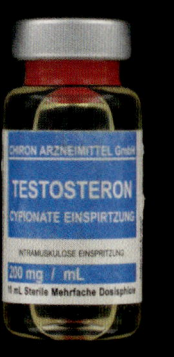

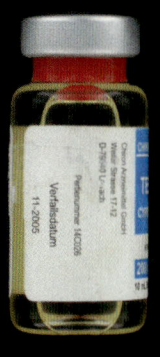

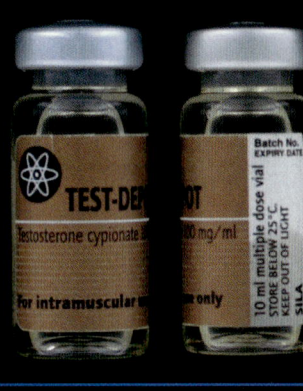

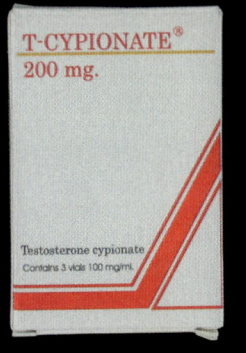

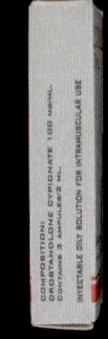

Fake Chiron (Germany)   Fake Test-Depo (Russia)   Fake cypionate from Australia

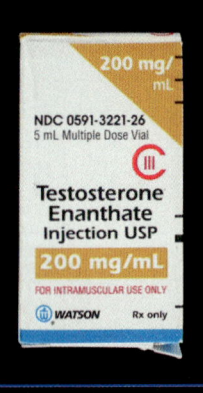

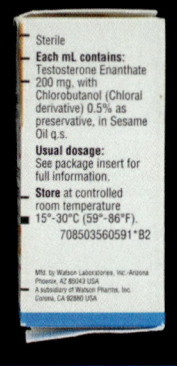

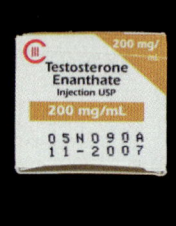

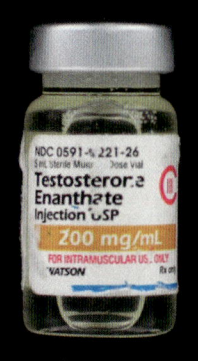

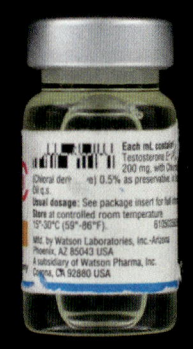

Enanthate generic from Watson (U.S.)

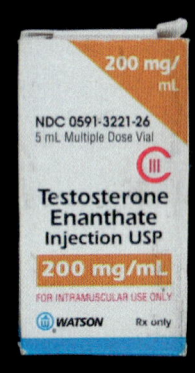

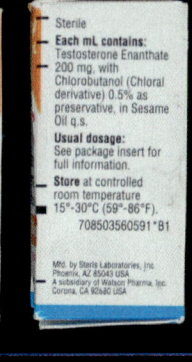

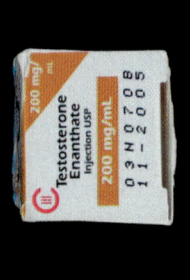

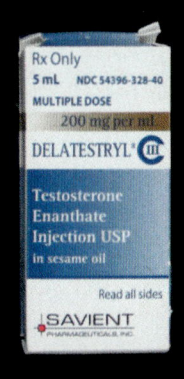

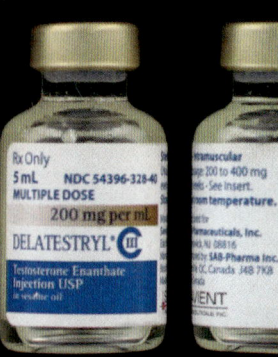

10mL version from Watson (U.S.)   Delatestryl from Savient (U.S.)

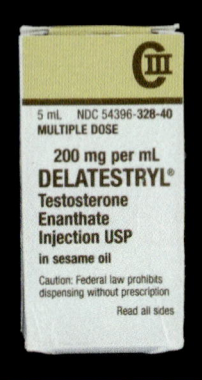

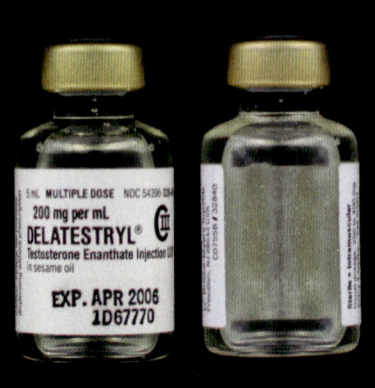

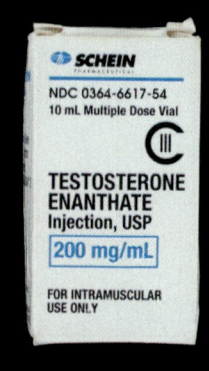

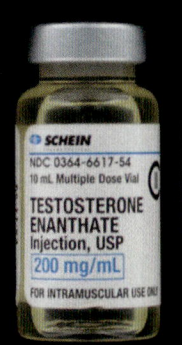

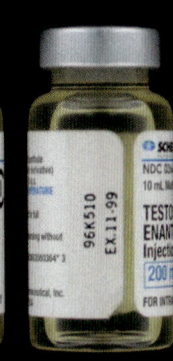

U.S. Delatestryl (older BTG version)   U.S. Schein generic [NLM]

B-86

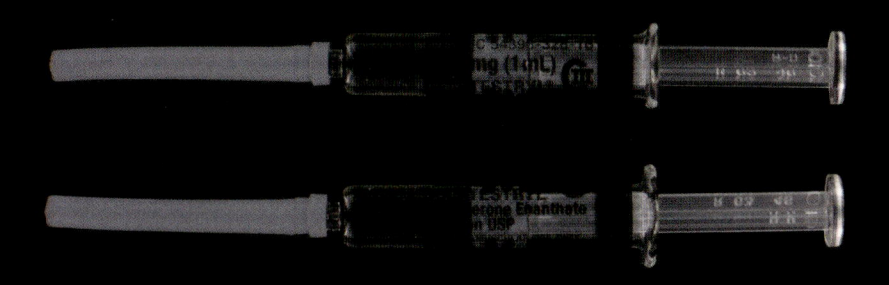

BTG Delatestryl syringes (U.S.)

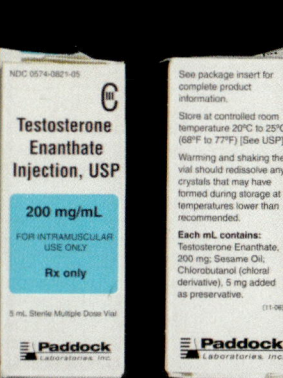

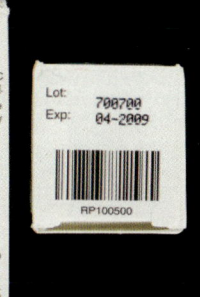

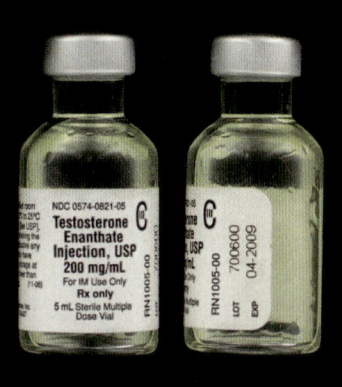

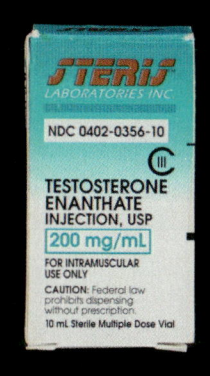

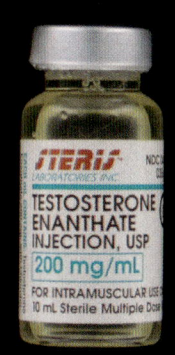

Enanthate generic from Paddock (U.S.)   Counterfeit Steris (U.S.)

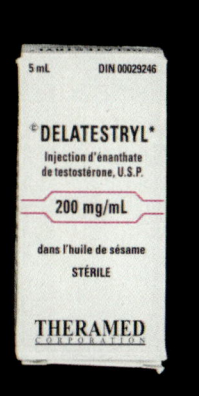

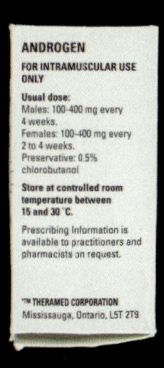

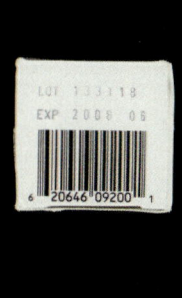

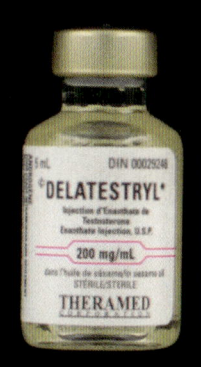

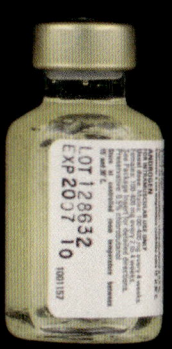

Delatestryl from Theramed Canada

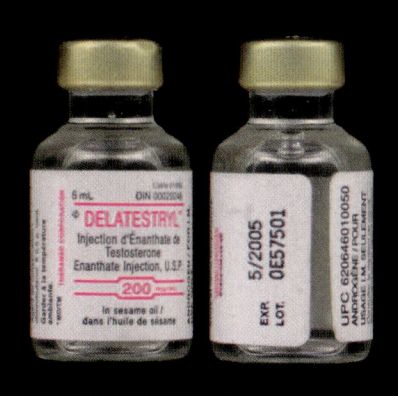

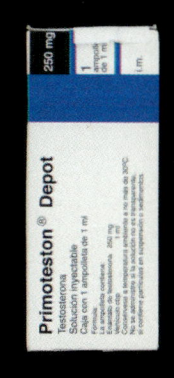

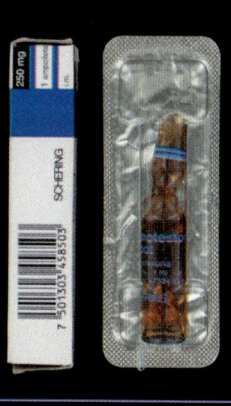

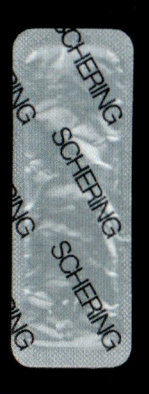

Older Delatestryl (Canada)   Schering Primoteston Depot (Mexico)

Appendix B

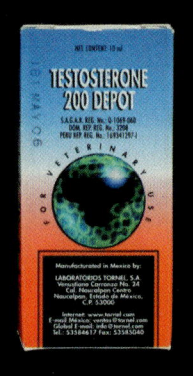

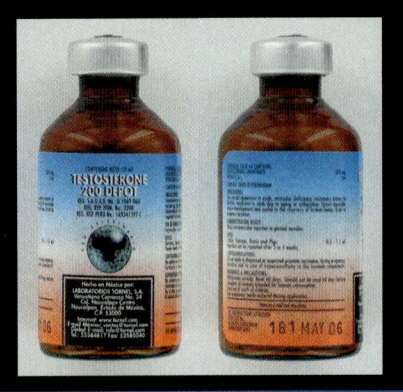

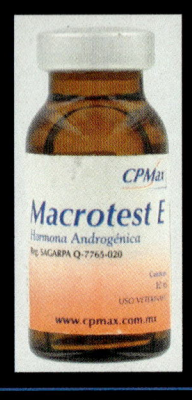

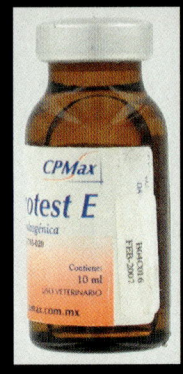

Testosterone 200 Depot from Tornel (Mexico)　　　Macrotest-E from CPMax (Mexico)

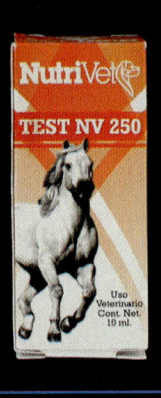

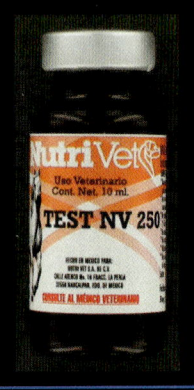

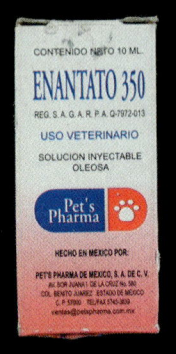

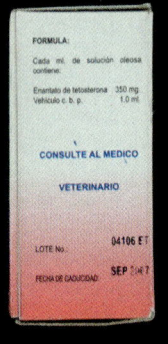

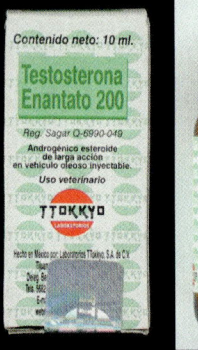

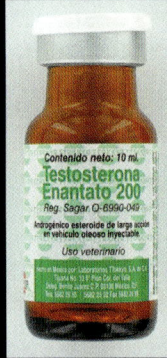

NutriVet (Mexico, UG) NLM　　　Pet's Pharma (Mexico) NLM　　　Ttokkyo generic from Mexico (NLM)

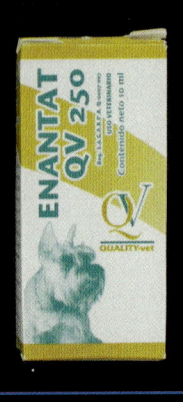

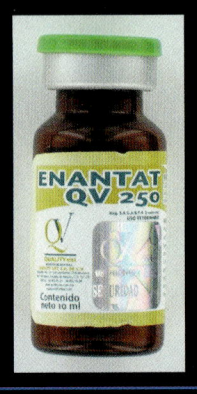

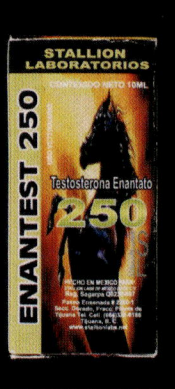

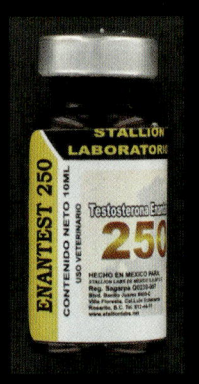

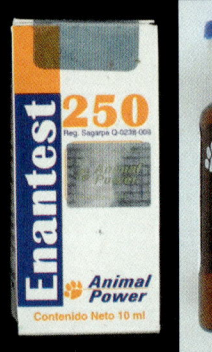

Quality Vet (Mexico) NLM　　　Stallion Labs (Mexico, UG) NLM　　　Animal Power (Mexico) NLM

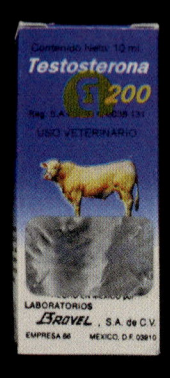

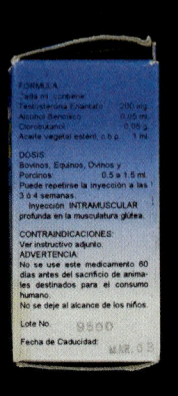

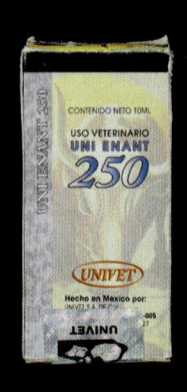

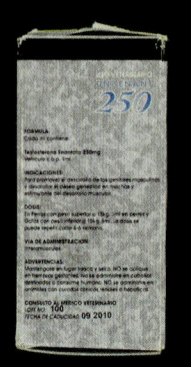

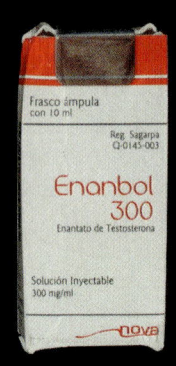

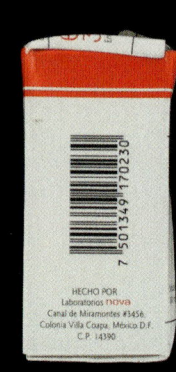

Testosterona 200 from Brovel (Mexico) NLM　　　Univet (Mexico, Underground)　　　Nova (Mexico, Underground)

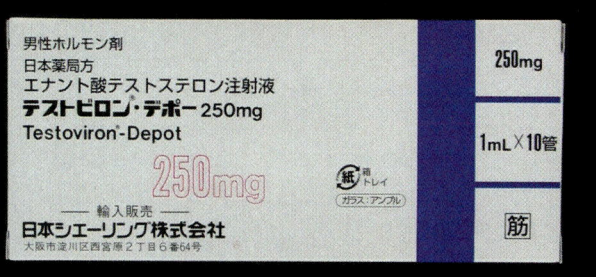

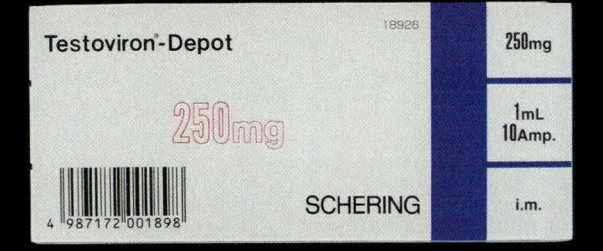

Testoviron from Japan

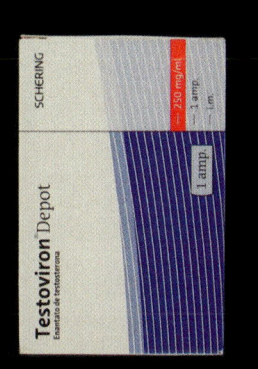

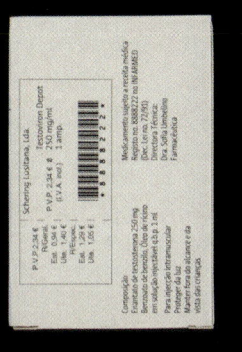

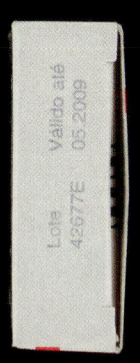

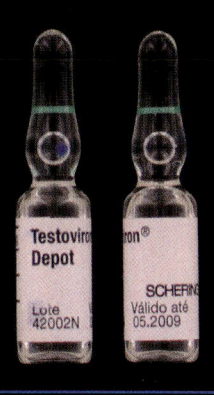

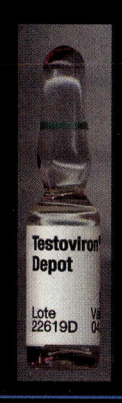

Tesoviron from Portugal (small box)

Counterfeit ampule

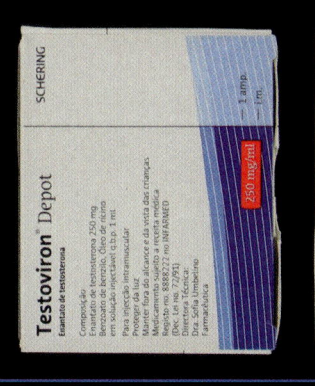

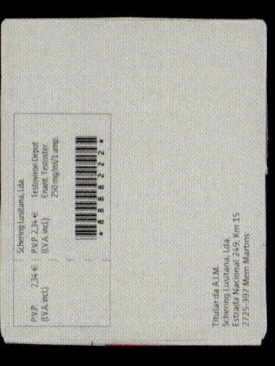

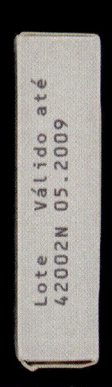

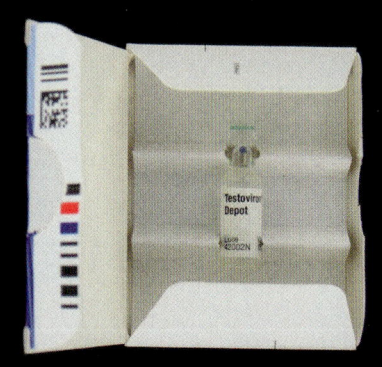

Testoviron from Portugal (slightly larger box)

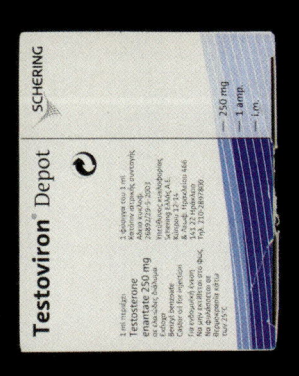

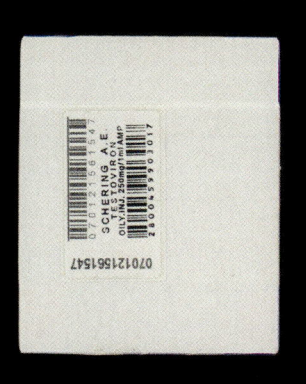

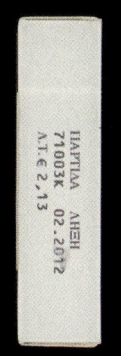

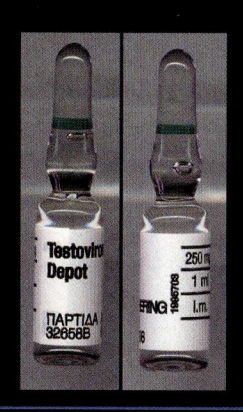

Testoviron from Greece

Appendix B

B-89

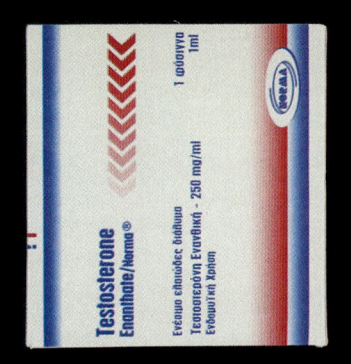

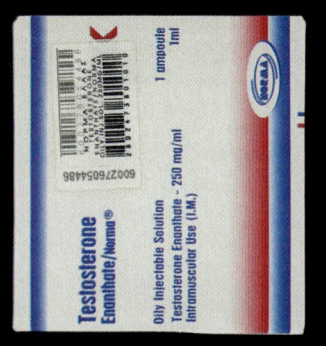

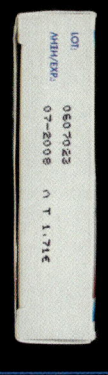

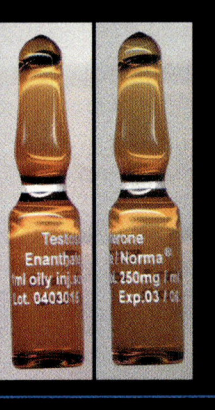

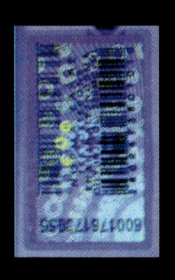

Enanthate from Norma Hellas (Greece)　　　　　　　　　　　　　　　　　　　　　Sticker under UV light

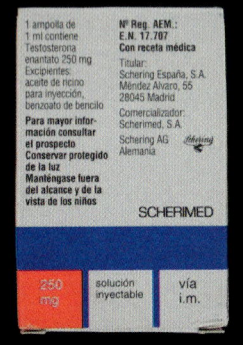

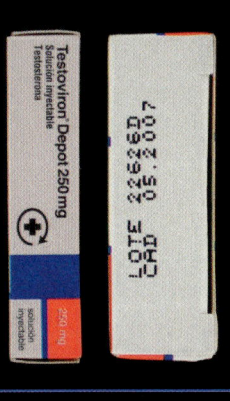

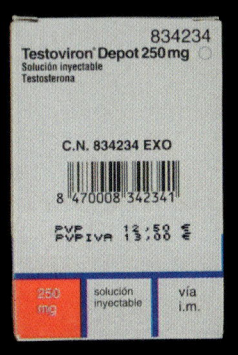

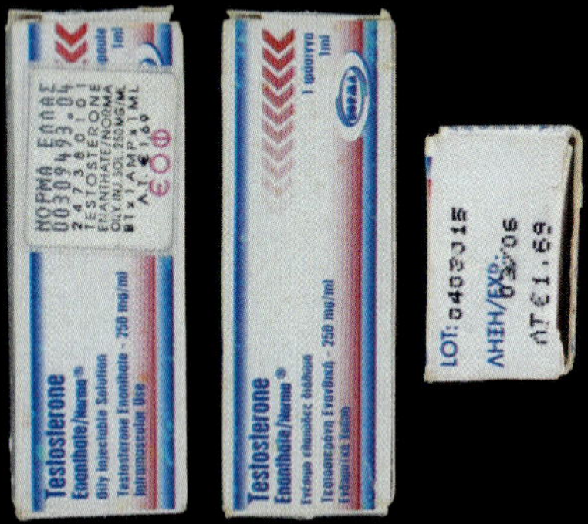

Older Greek box　　　　　　　　　　　　Testoviron from Scherimed (Spain) NLM

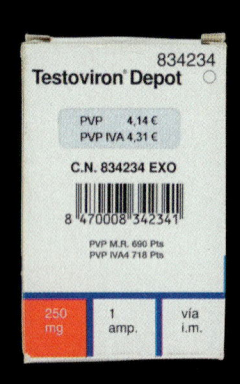

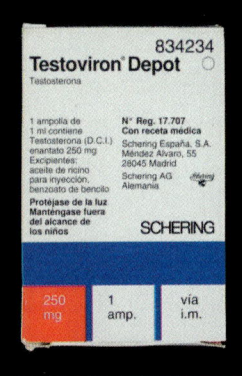

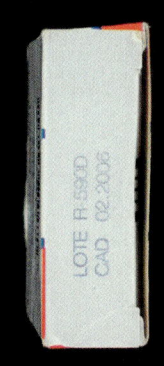

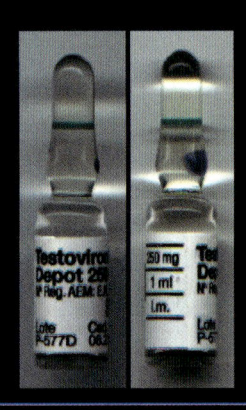

Previous version of Schering Testoviron (Spain)

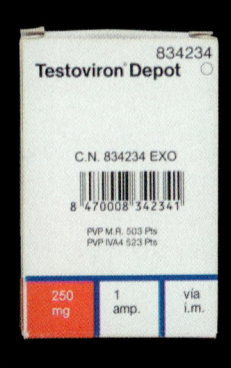

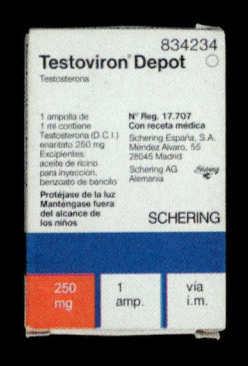

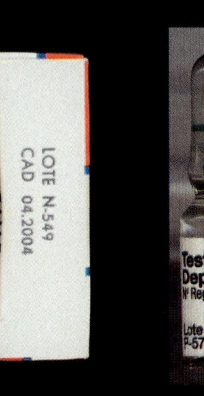

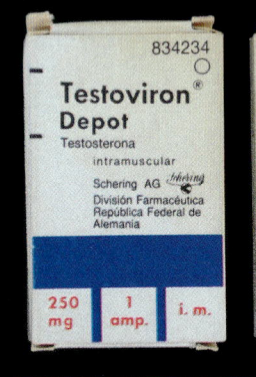

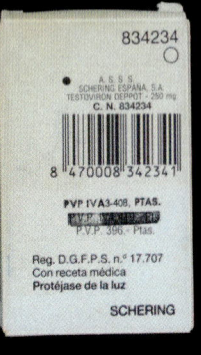

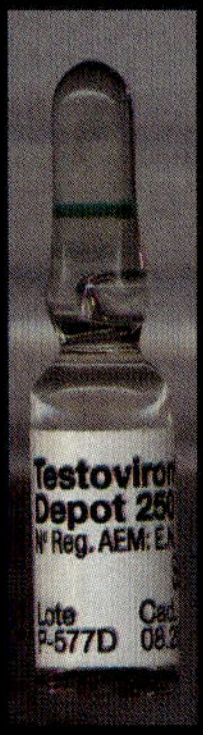

Very old Spanish box　　　　　　　　　Counterfeit Spanish Testoviron　　　　　Fake amp

B-90

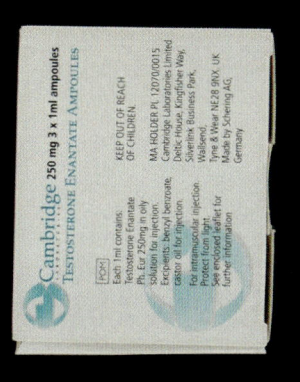

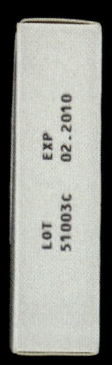

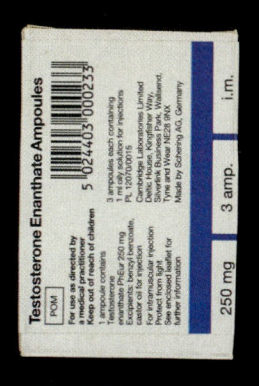

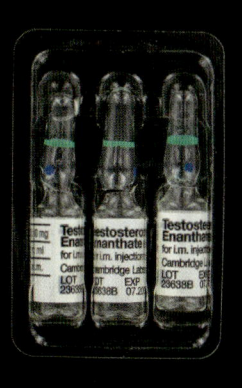

Enanthate from Cambridge (UK)

Older packaging from Cambridge

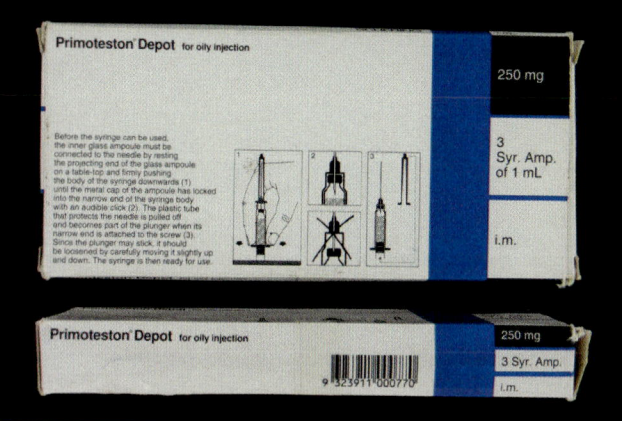

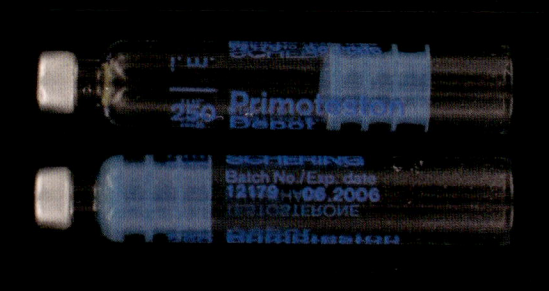

Primoteston Depot redi-ject syringe from Schering (UK)

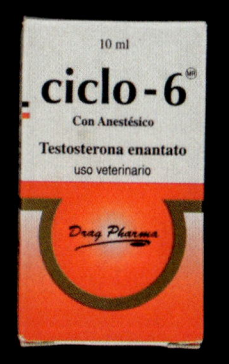

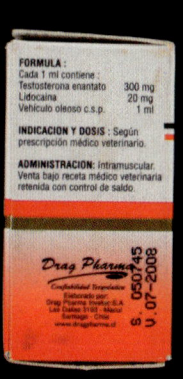

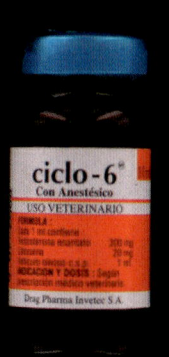

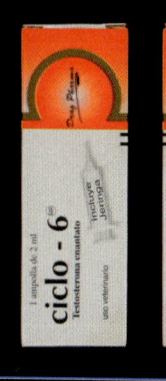

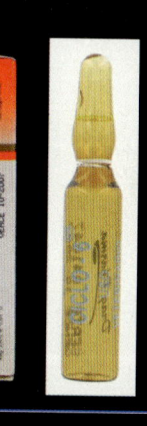

ciclo-6 from Chile - 10mL and 2mL sizes

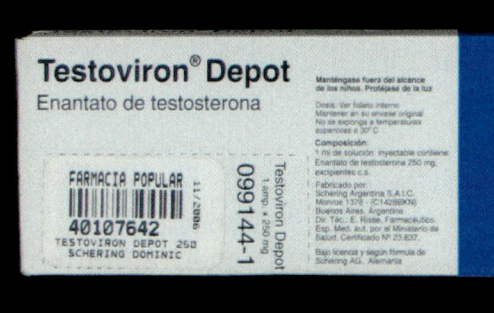

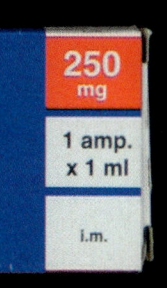

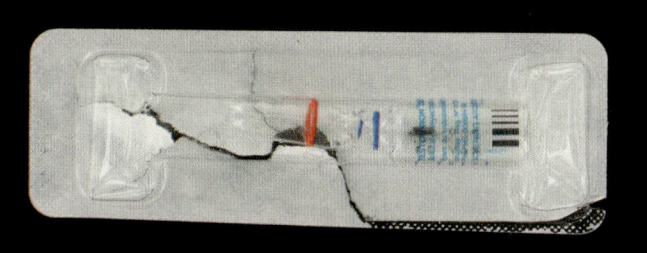

Testoviron Depot from Argentina

Appendix B

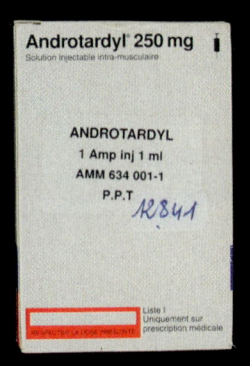

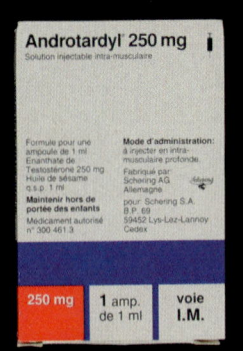

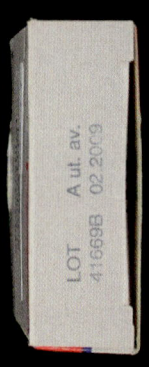

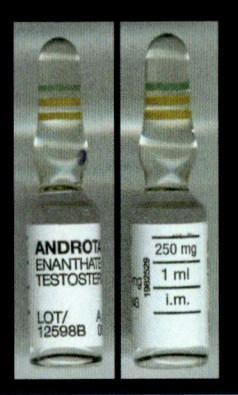

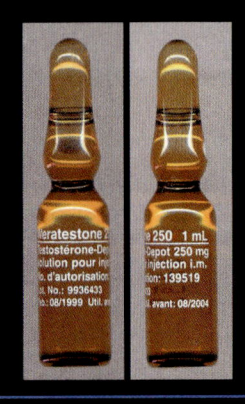

Androtardyl from France

French export Weratestone

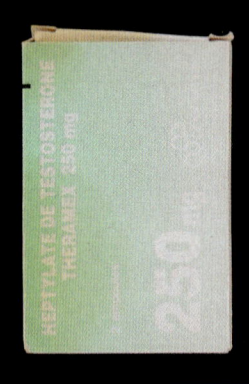

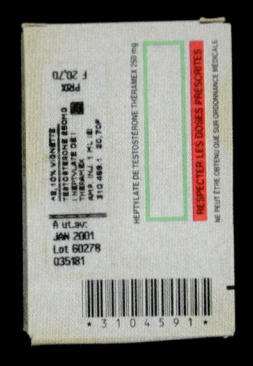

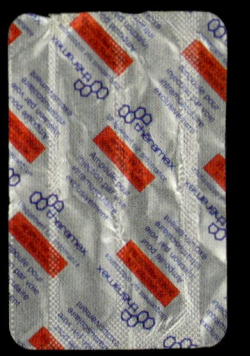

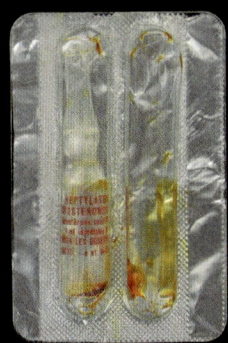

Heptylate de Testosterone from Theramex (France)

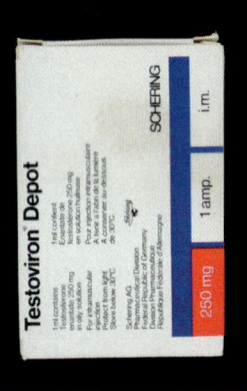

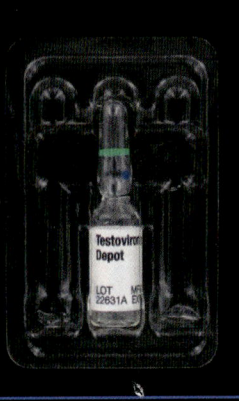

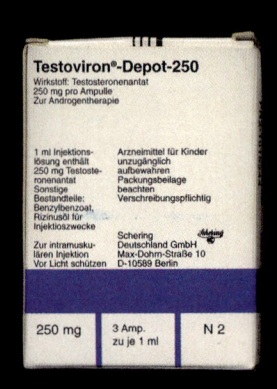

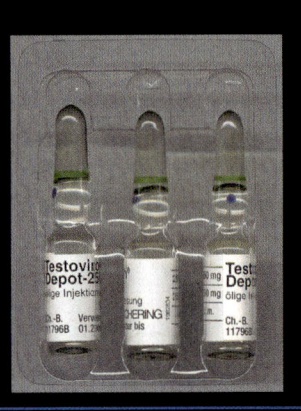

German Testoviron box and (export) amp

Counterfeit German box and ampules

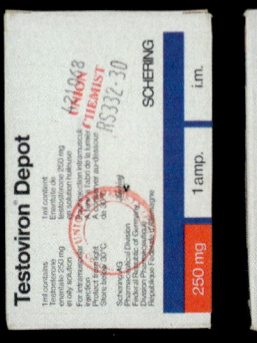

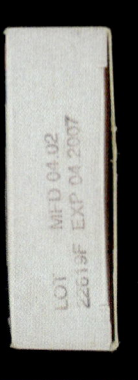

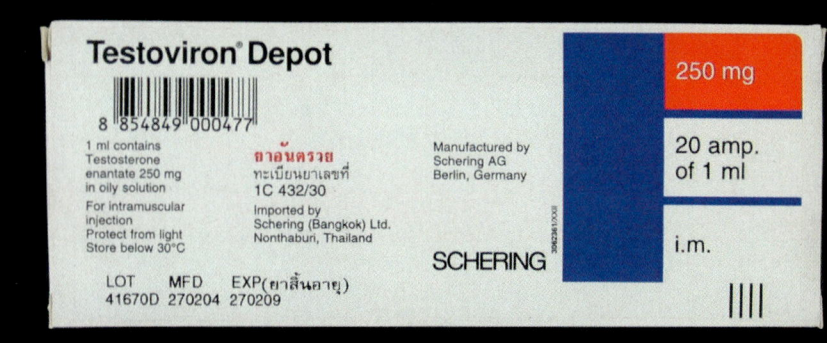

Testoviron from Sri Lanka

Thai Testoviron

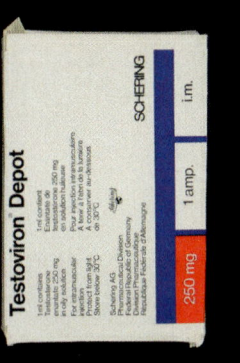

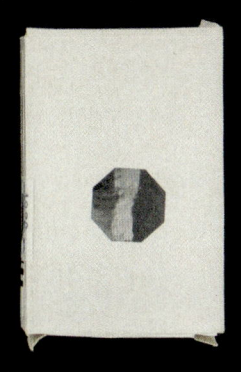

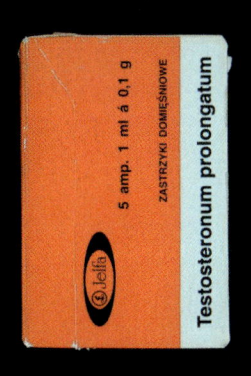

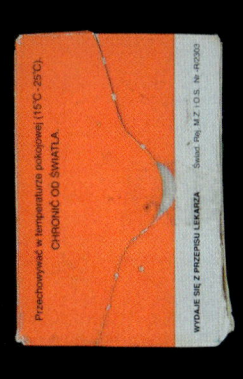

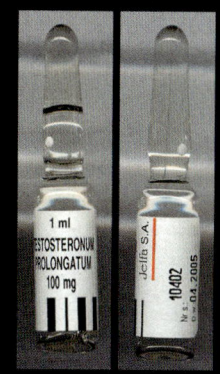

Testoviron Depot from Lebanon

Testosteronum Prolongatum from Jelfa (Poland)

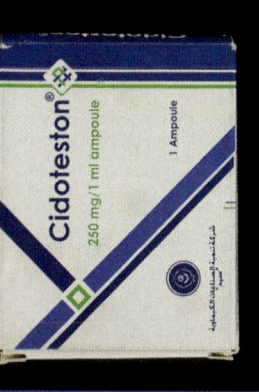

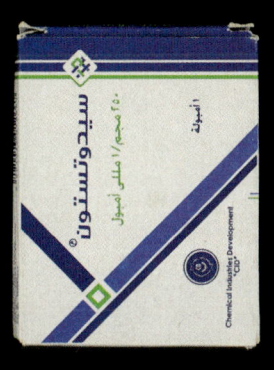

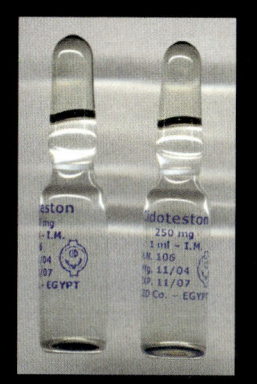

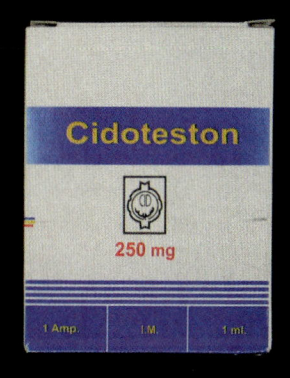

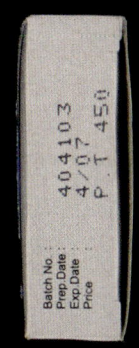

Cidoteston from CID (Egypt)

Older box from CID

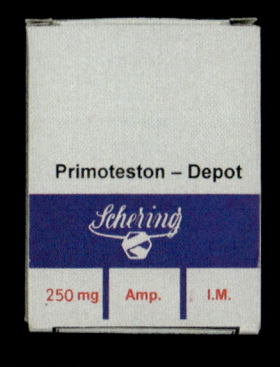

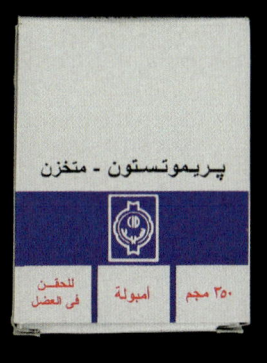

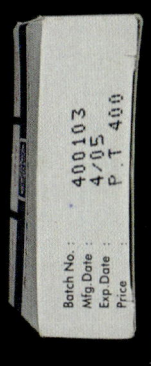

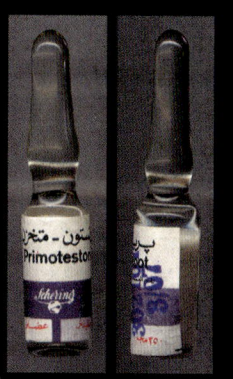

Primoteston-Depot from CID/Schering Egypt (NLM)

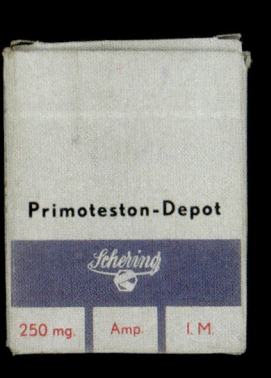

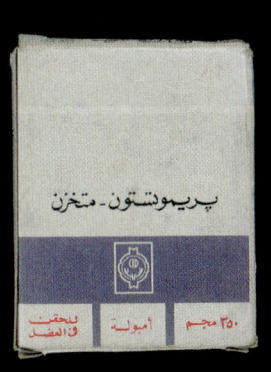

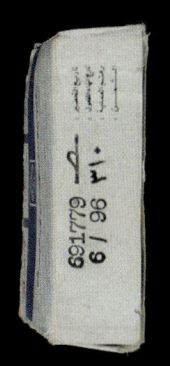

Old Schering/CID packaging

Testoviron from Pakistan

Appendix B

B-93

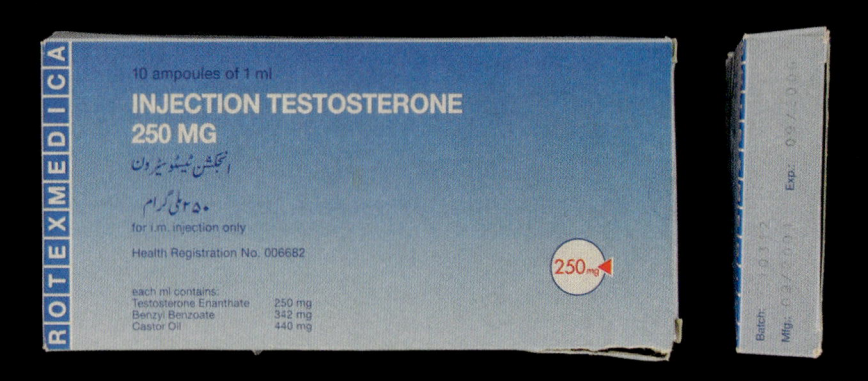

Rotexmedica Testoviron from Pakistan (German export)

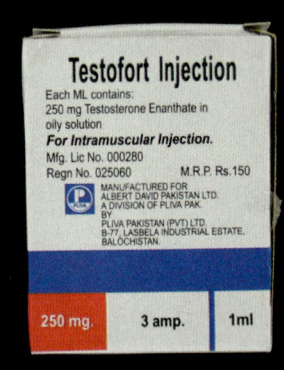

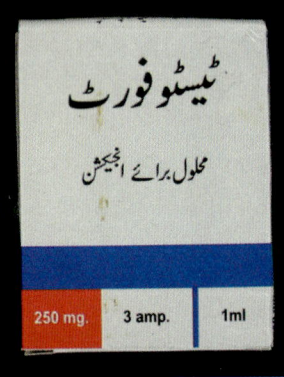

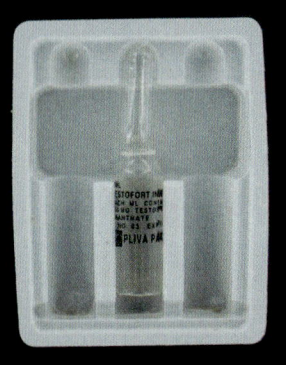

Testofort Injection from Pakistan

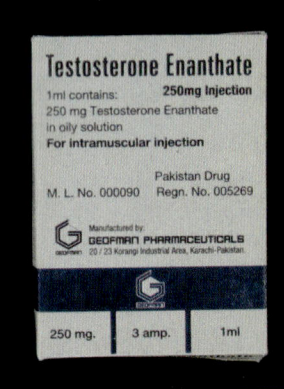

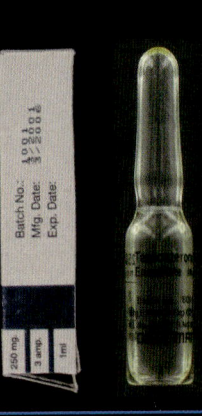

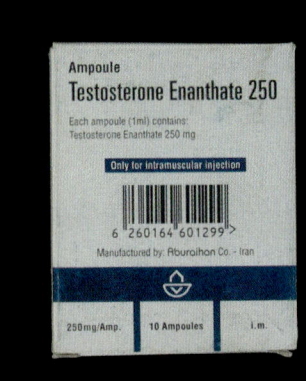

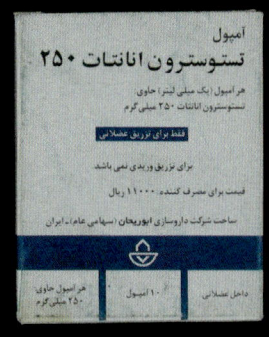

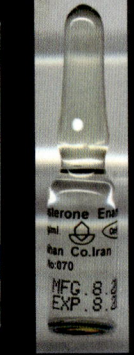

Generic from Geofman (Pakistan)

Generic from Aburihan (Iran)

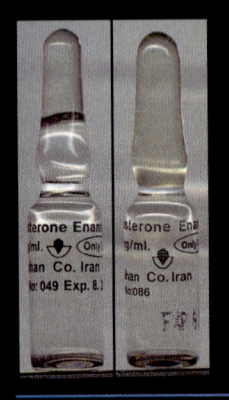

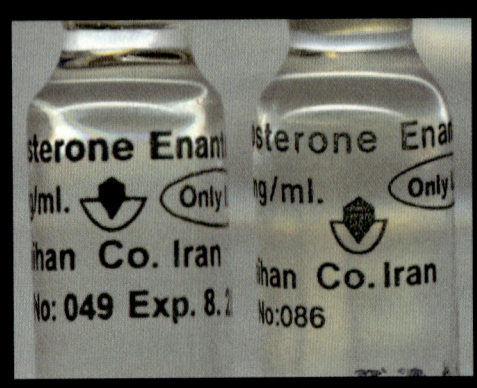

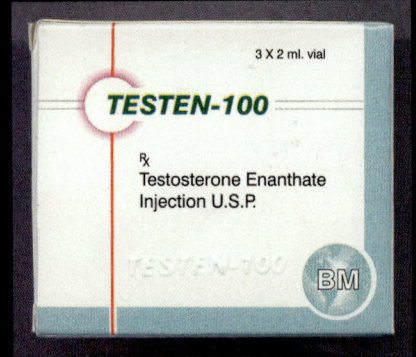

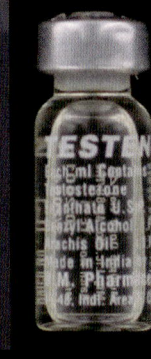

Previous Aburihan ampule - Counterfeit is on left of both picture sets

BM Pharmaceuticals (India, export)

B-94

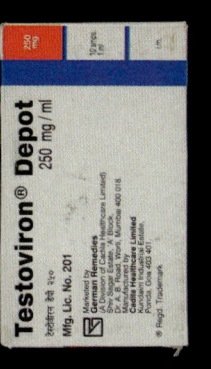

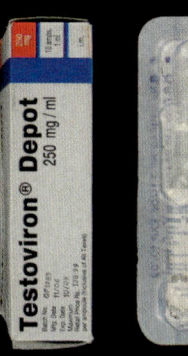

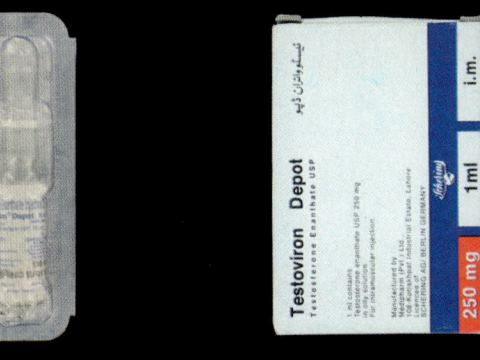

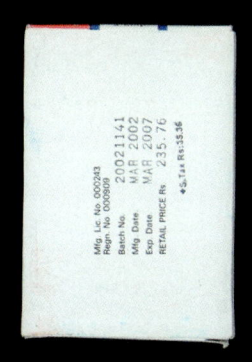

Testoviron Depot from India

Older packaging from India

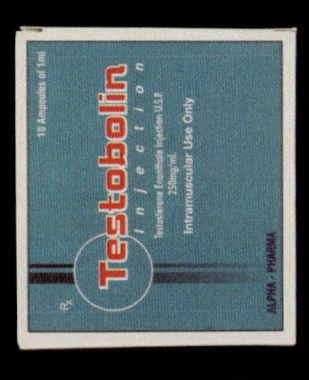

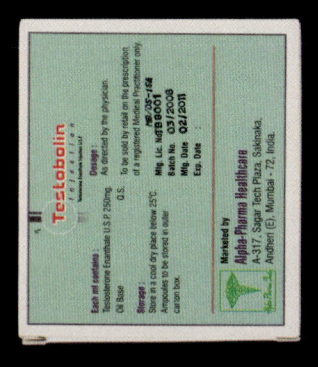

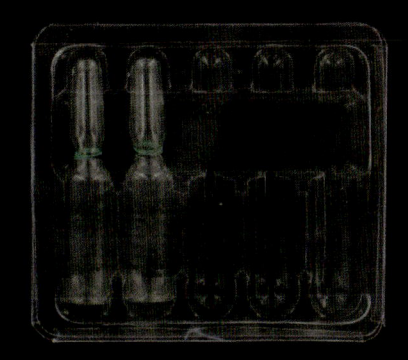

Testobolin from Alpha-Pharma (India, export)

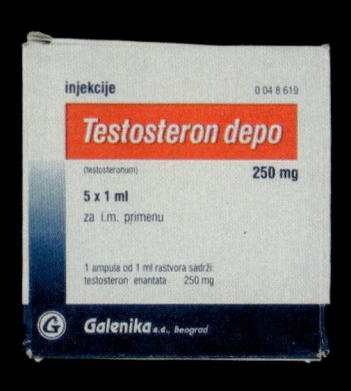

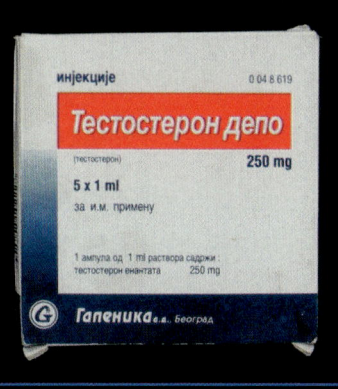

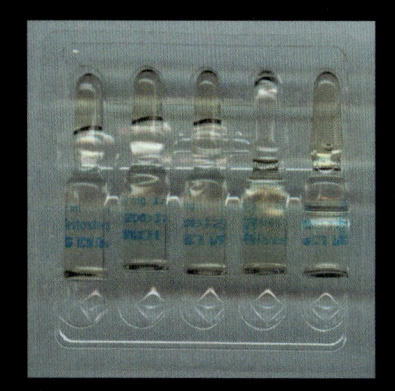

Testosteron Depo from Galenika (Serbia)

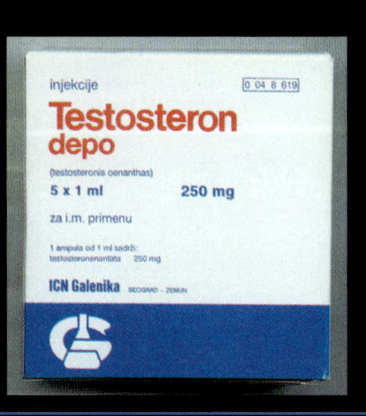

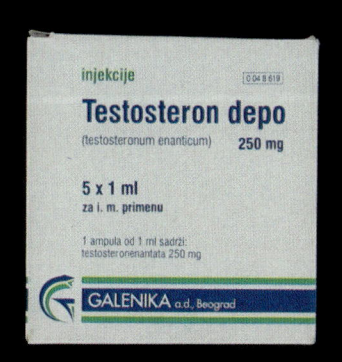

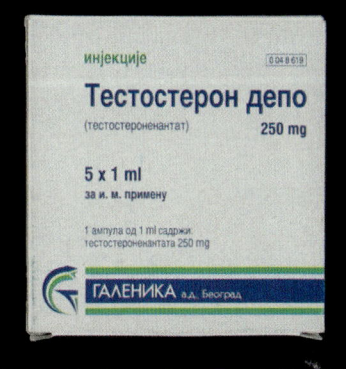

Two different older boxes of Galenika enanthate (Serbia)

Appendix B

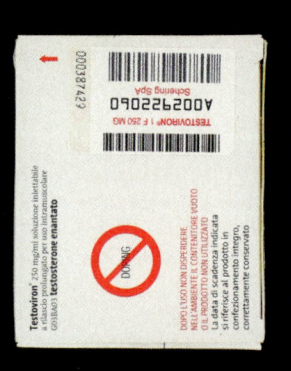

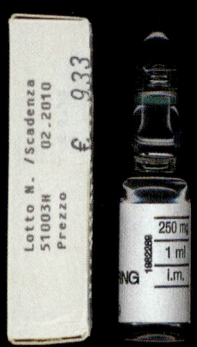

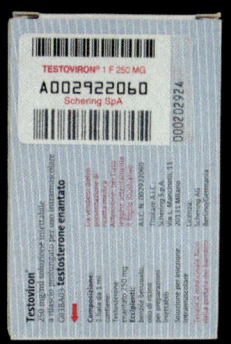

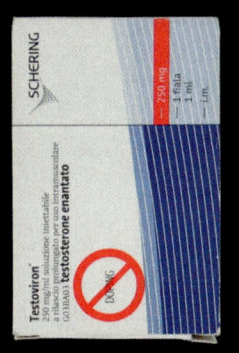

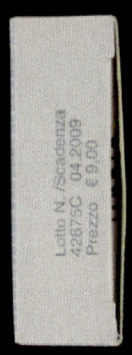

Testoviron from Schering (Italy) older version on right

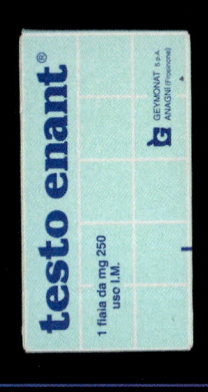

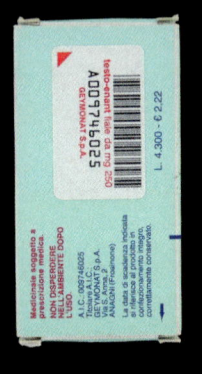

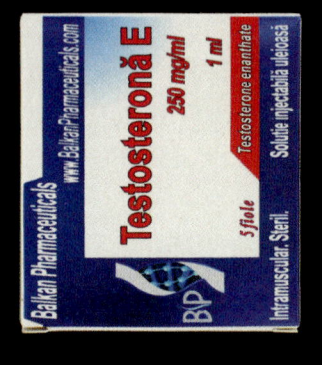

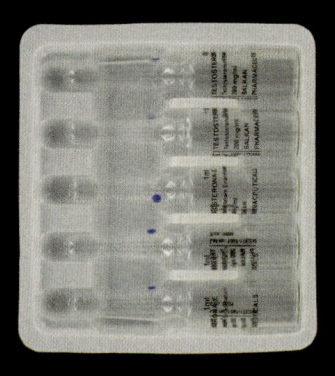

Italian testo enant　　　　　　　　　　Testosterona E from Balkan (Moldova)

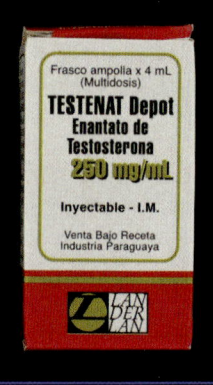

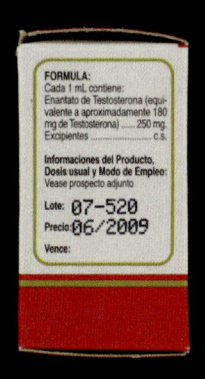

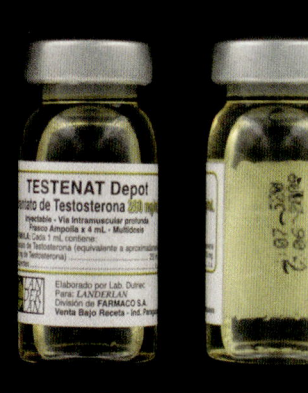

Testenat from Landerlan (Paraguay)

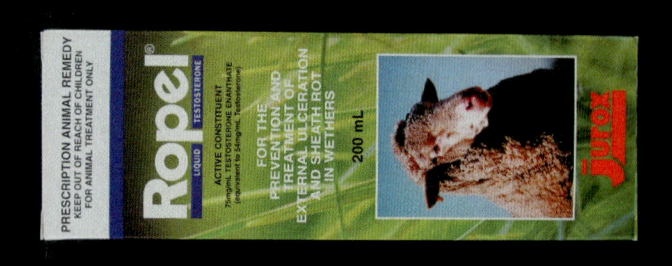

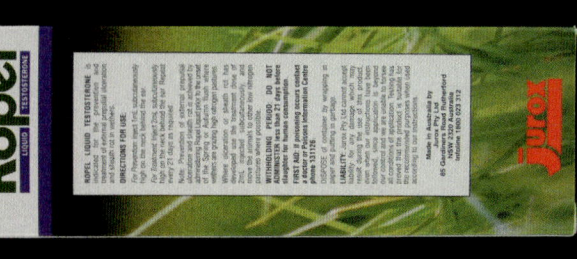

Ropel from Jurox (Australia)

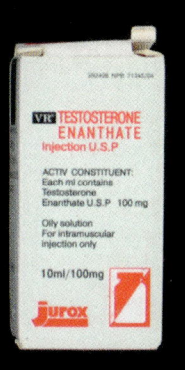

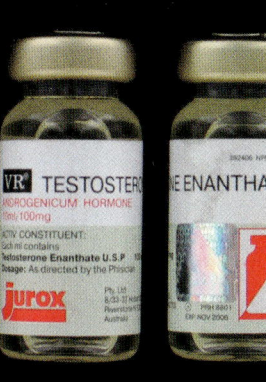

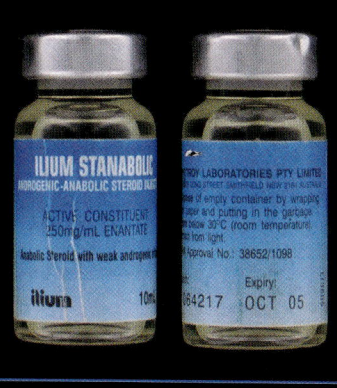

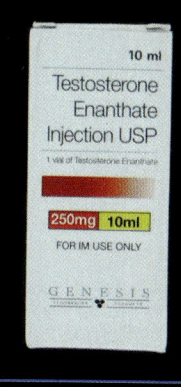

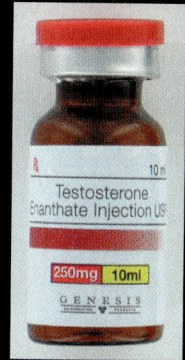

Counterfeit enanthate from Jurox (Australia)   Counterfeit Ilium enanthate (Australia)   Genesis (Singapore) NLM

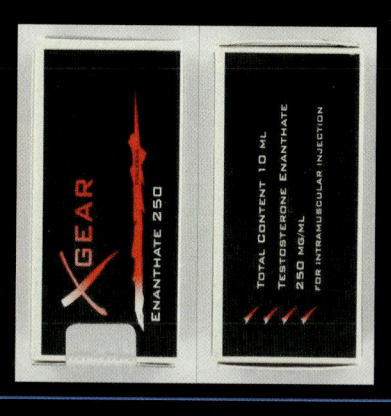

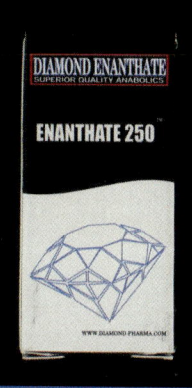

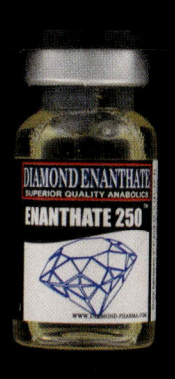

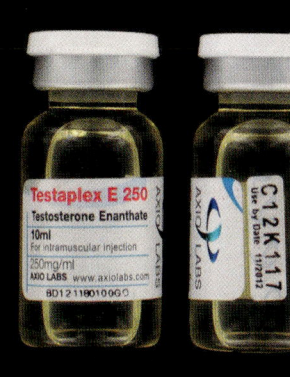

Underground products from X Gear, Diamond, and Axio Labs

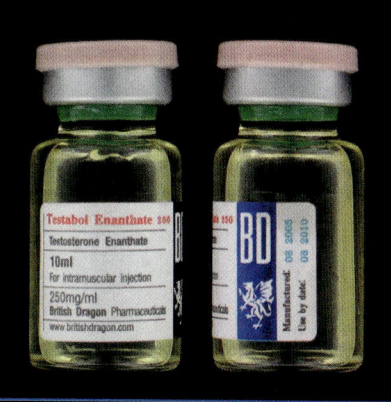

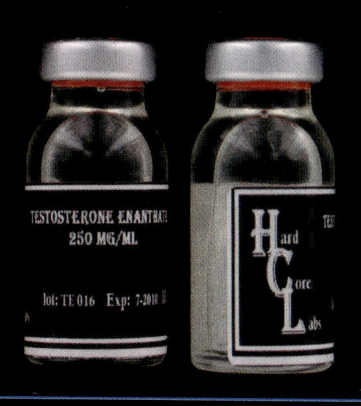

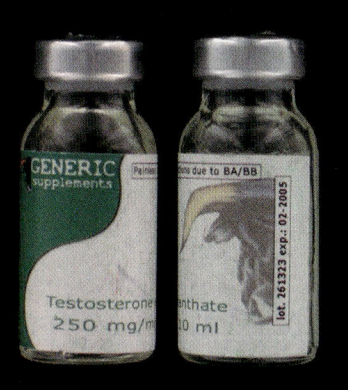

Underground products from British Dragon (NLM), Hardcore Labs, and Generic Supplements

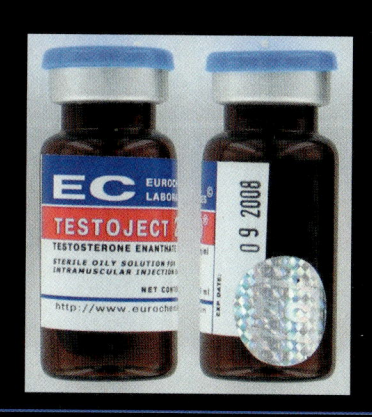

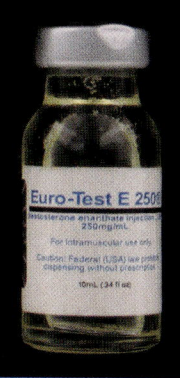

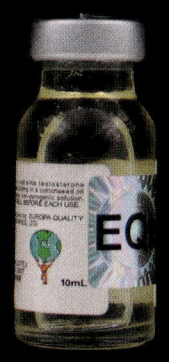

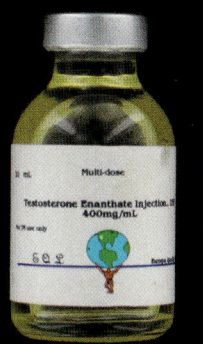

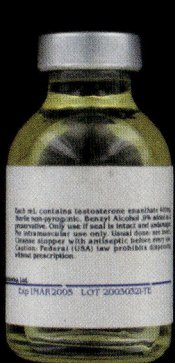

Underground enanthate products from Eurochem and Europa Quality Labs

Appendix B

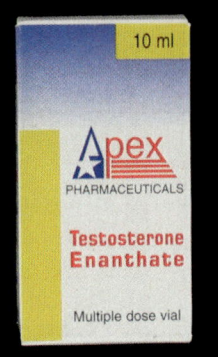

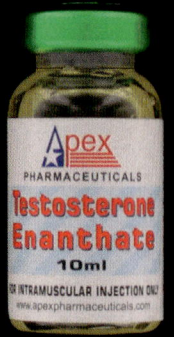

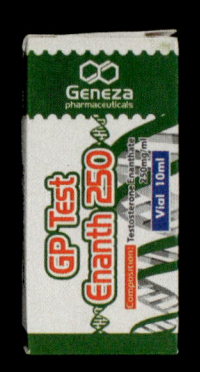

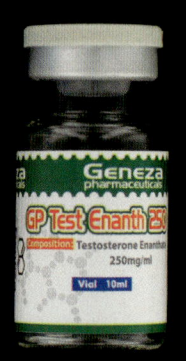

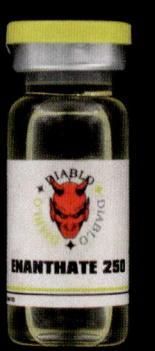

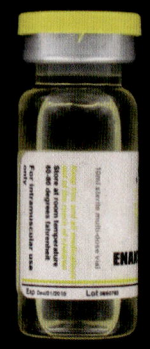

Underground products from Apex, Geneza, and Diablo

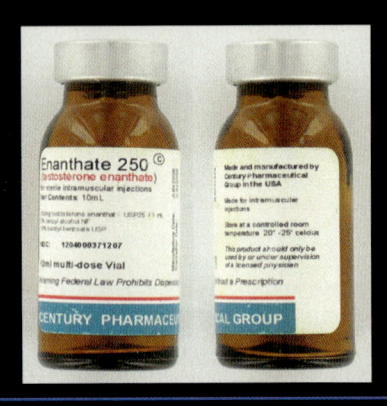

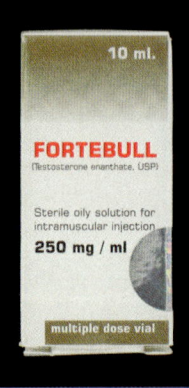

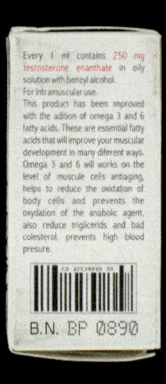

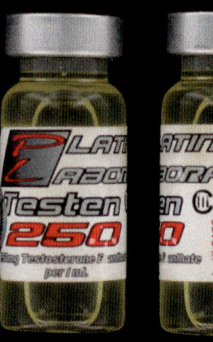

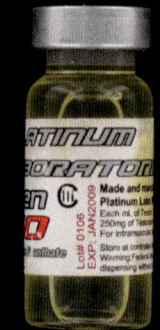

Underground products from Century, Fortebull, and Platinum Labs

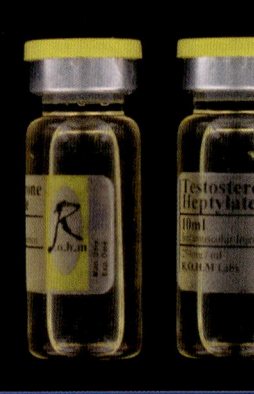

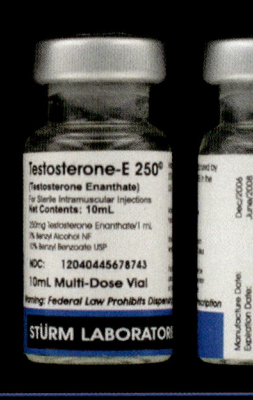

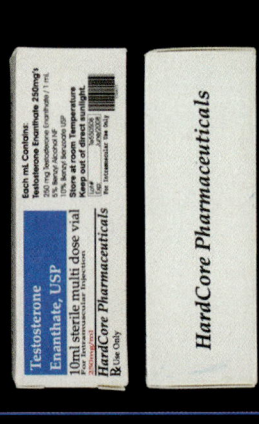

Underground products from R.O.H.M., Sturm, and HardCore

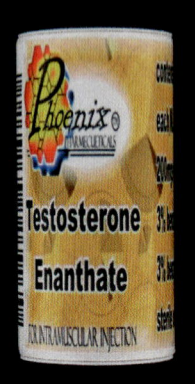

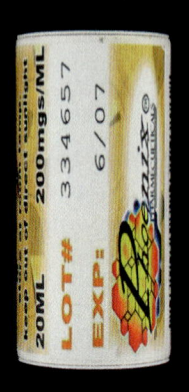

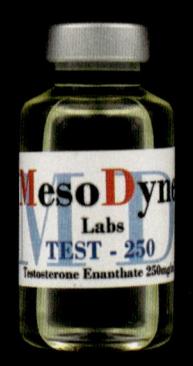

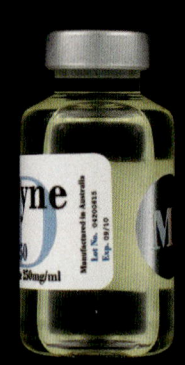

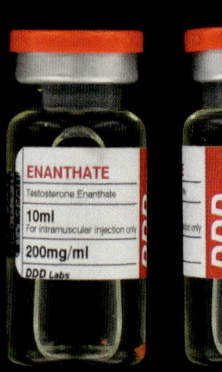

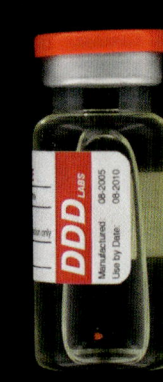

Underground products from Phoenix, MesoDyne, and DDD

B-98

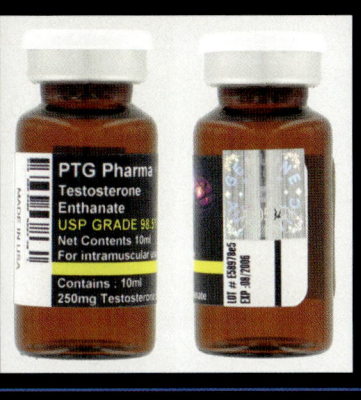

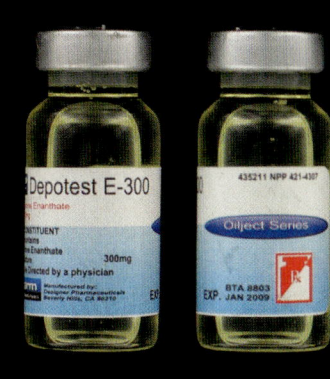

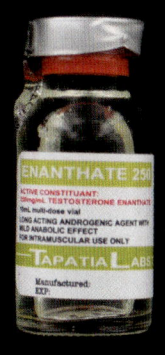

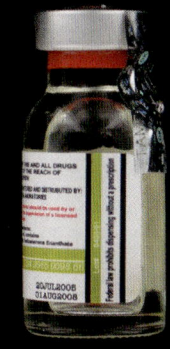

Underground enanthate products from PTG, Designer, and Tapatia

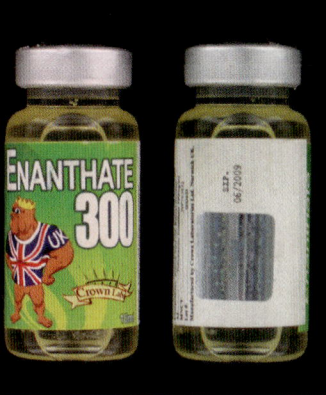

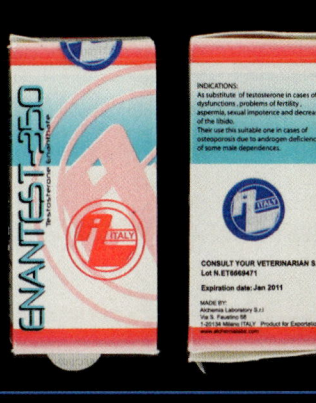

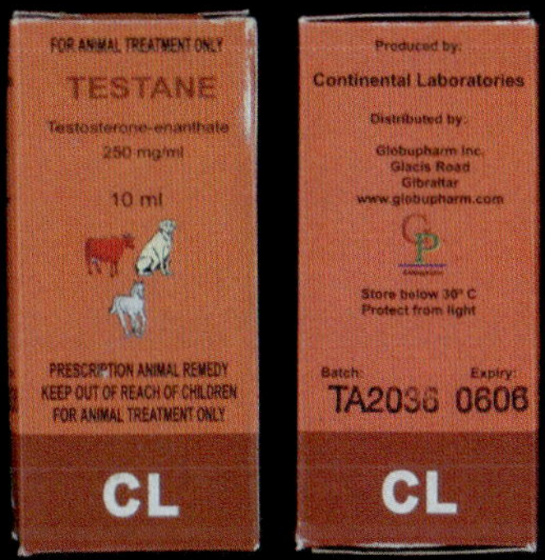

Underground enanthate from Crown Labs, AL Italy, and Continental

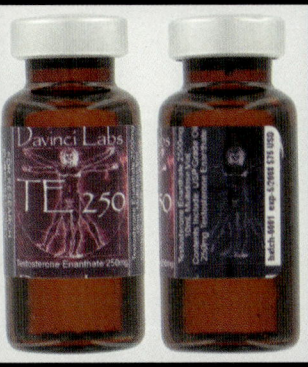

Davinci TE 250 (Underground) 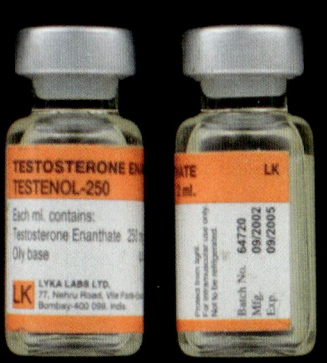   Lyka (Underground) 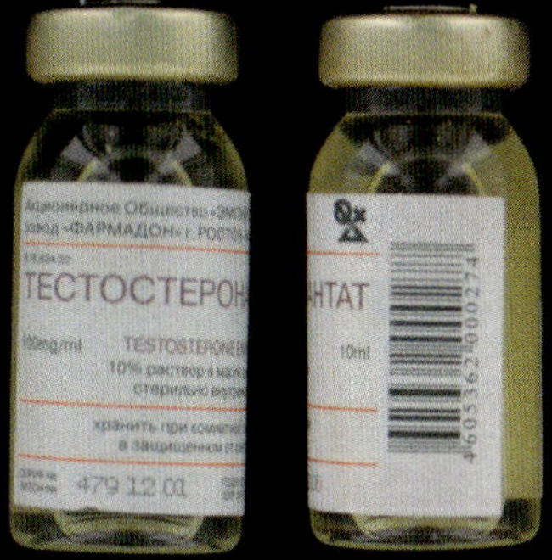   Counterfeit Farmadon vial (Russia)

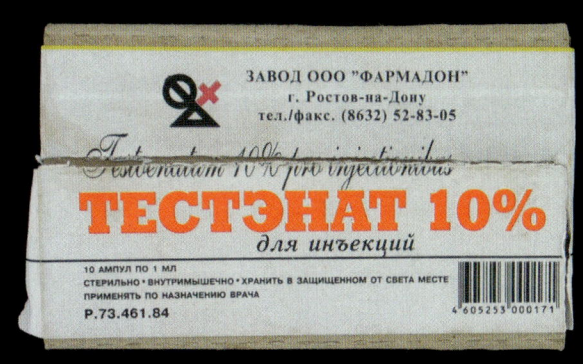

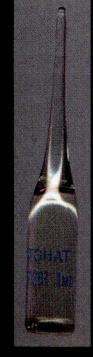

Counterfeit Farmadon box and ampule (Russia)

Appendix B

B-99

Testosterone Propionate

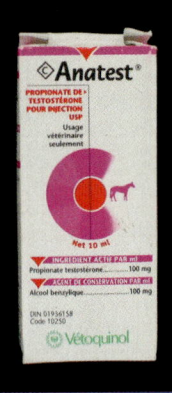

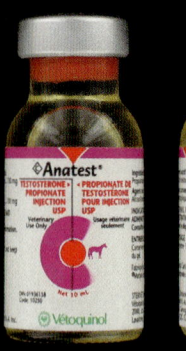

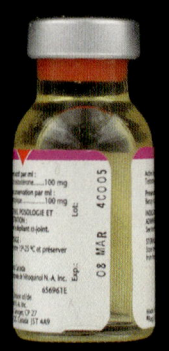

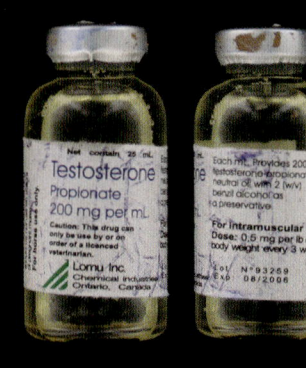

Anatest from Canada — Fake Canadian propionate

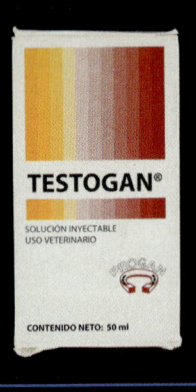

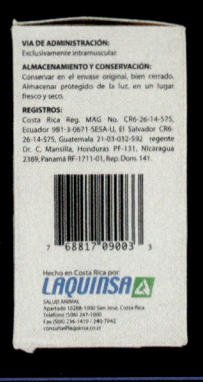

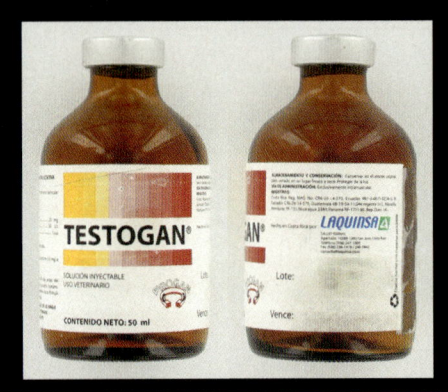

Testogan from Laquinsa (Costa Rica) — Calastreme (Argentina)

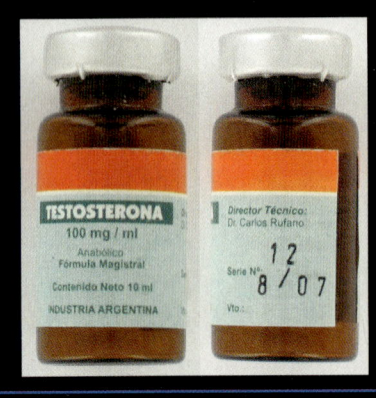

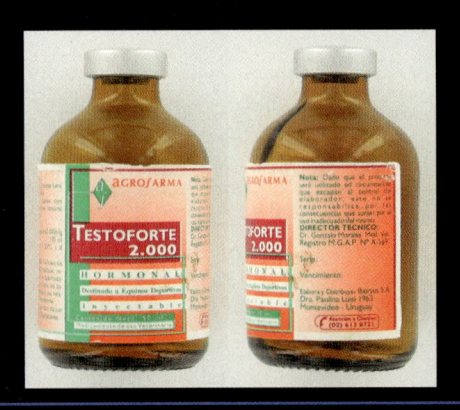

Propionate from Magistral (Argentina) — Testoforte 2.000 (Uruguay) — Quality Vet (Mexico) NLM

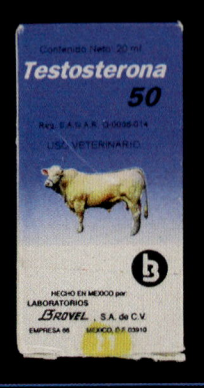

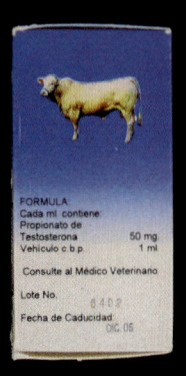

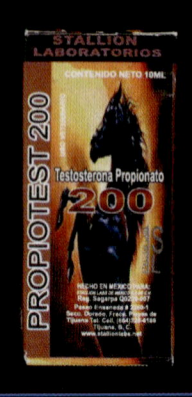

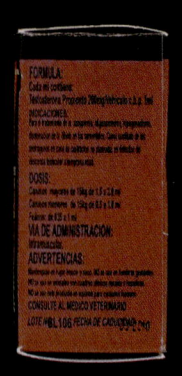

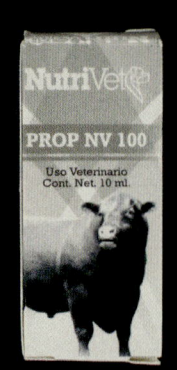

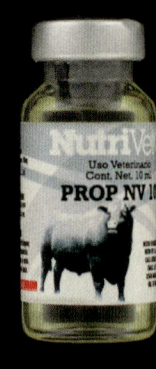

Brovel 50mg/mL propionate (Mexico) — Stallion Labs (Mexico, UG) NLM — NutriVet (Mexico, UG) NLM

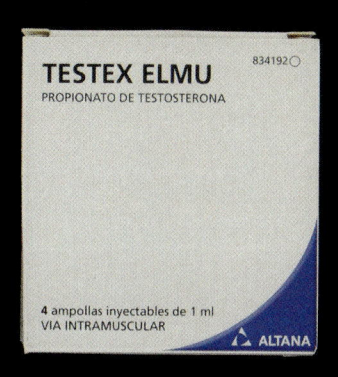

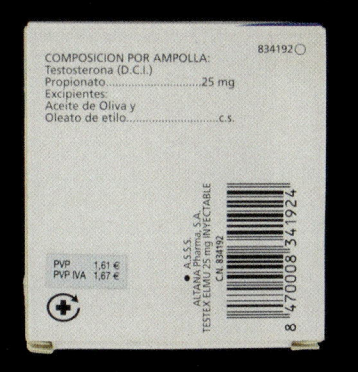

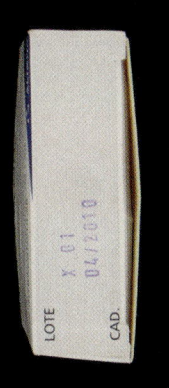

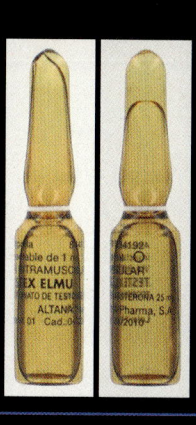

Testex Elmu from Altana (Spain) NLM

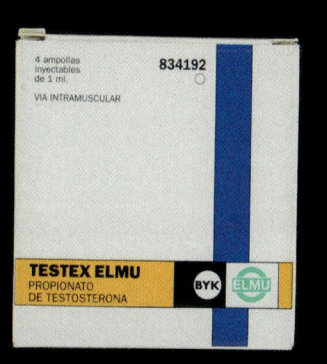

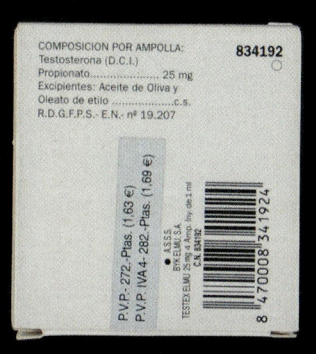

Older packaging of Testex Elmu

German Eifelfango box

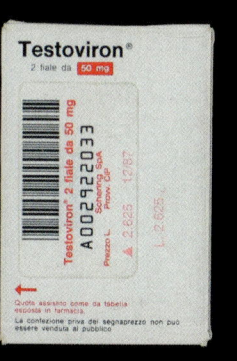

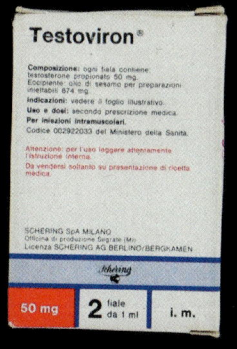

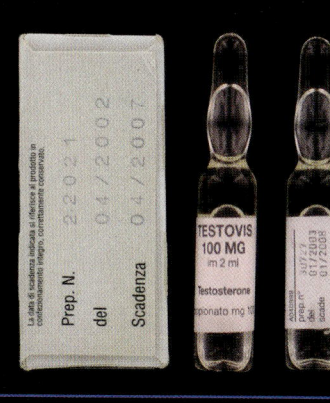

Testoviron from Italy (NLM)

Testovis from Italy

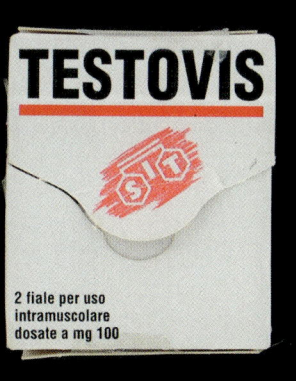

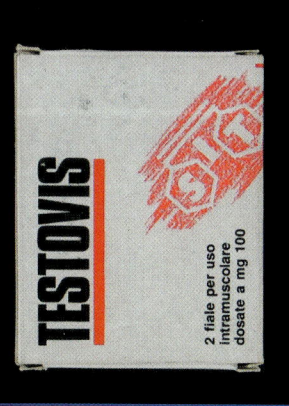

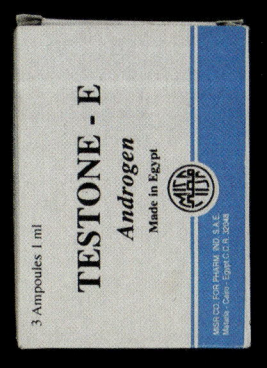

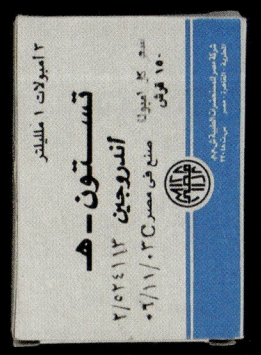

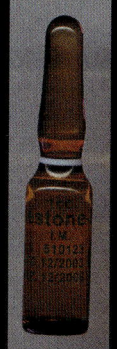

Two older boxes of Italian Testovis

Testone-E from Egypt

Appendix B

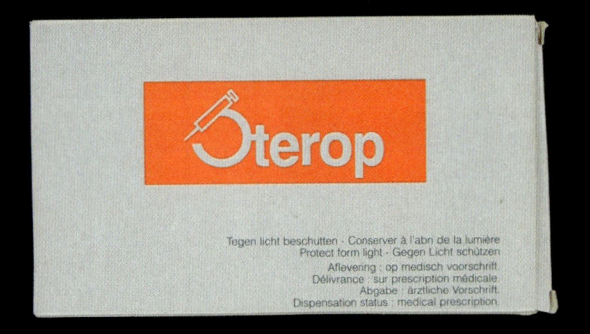

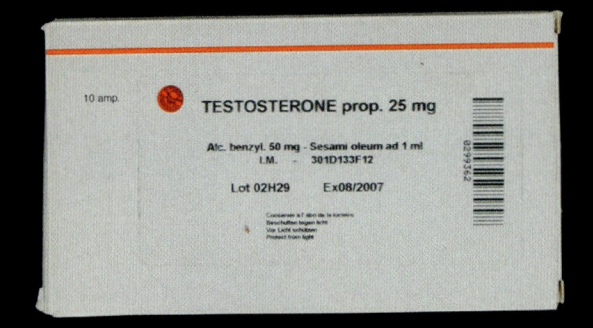

Sterop from Belgium

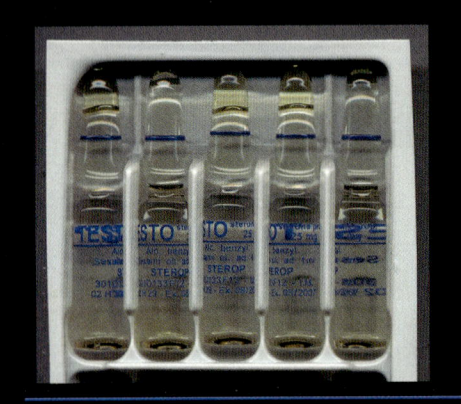

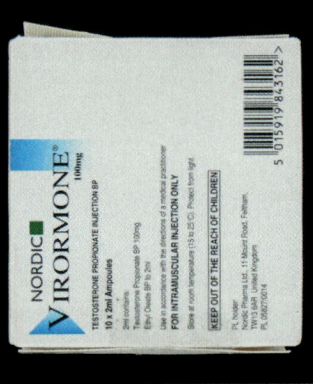

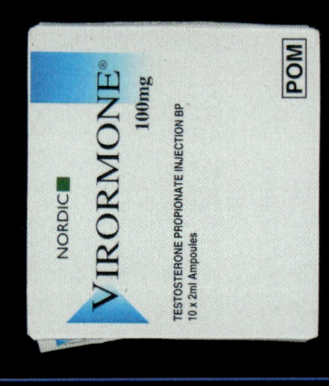

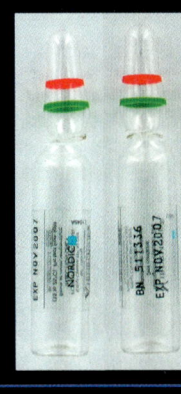

Belgian Sterop ampules

Virormone from the U.K.

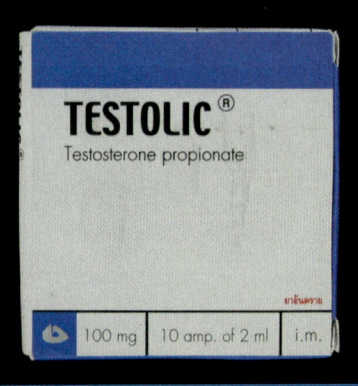

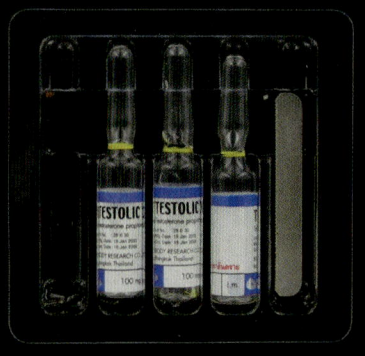

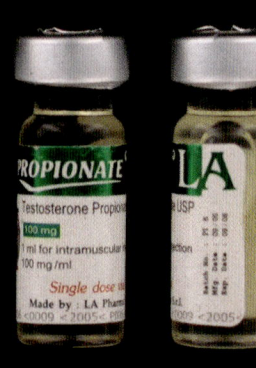

Testolic from Body Research (Thailand)

Generic from LA (Thai, UG)

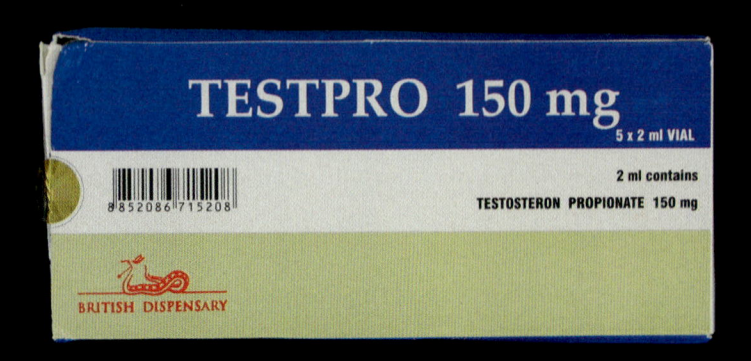

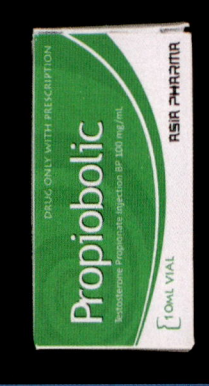

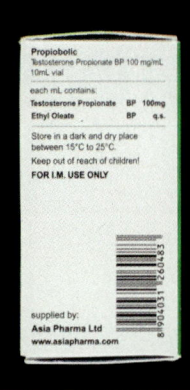

Fake Thai British Dispensary propionate

Propiobolic (Malaysia)

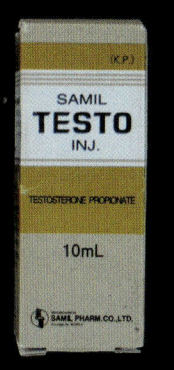

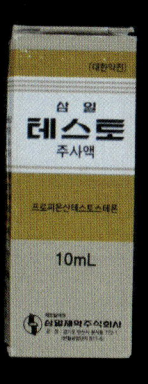

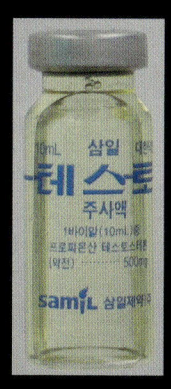

Samil Testo from Korea

Propionate from China

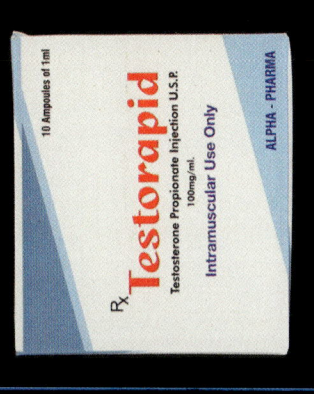

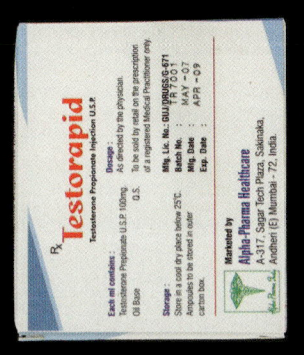

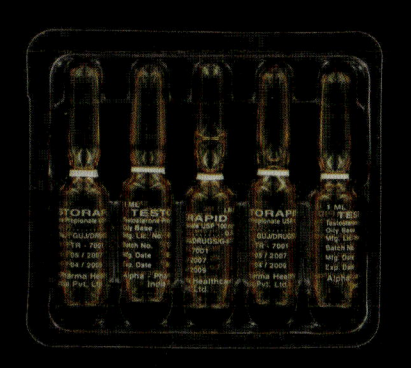

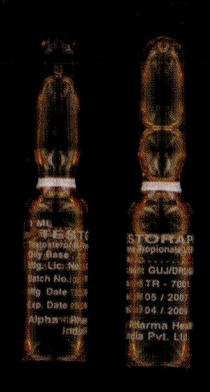

Testorapid from Alpha-Pharma (India, export)

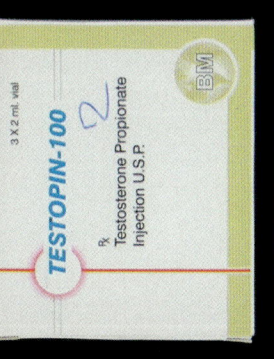

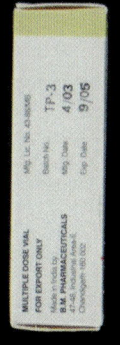

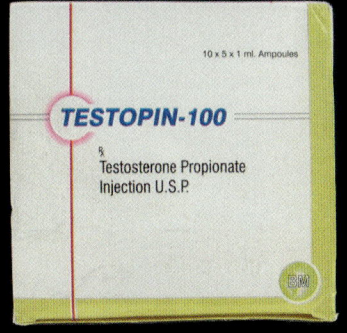

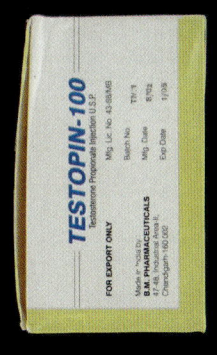

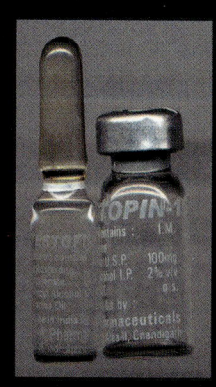

Testopin (vials) box from BM (India, export)

Testopin-100 (ampules)

BM amp and vial

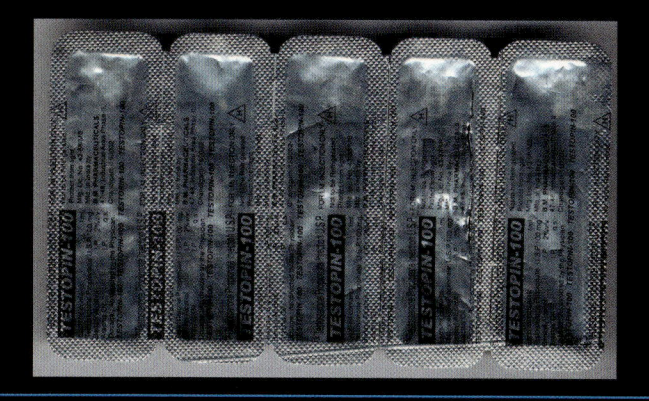

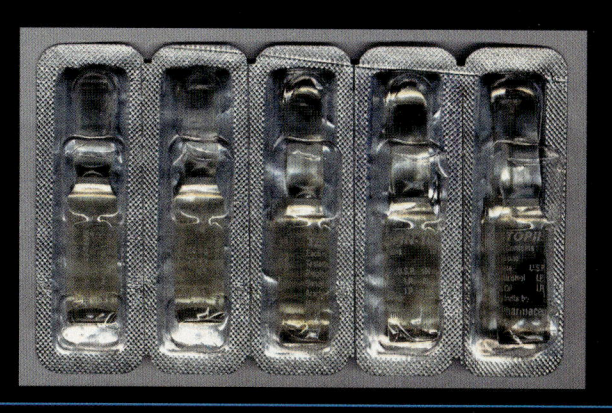

Foil and plastic tray of 5 ampules

Appendix B

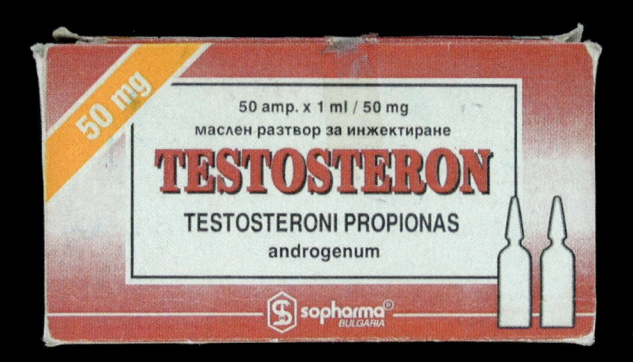

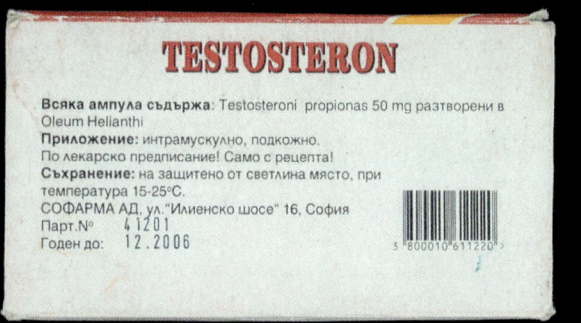

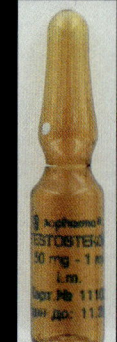

Testosteron from Sopharma (Bulgaria)

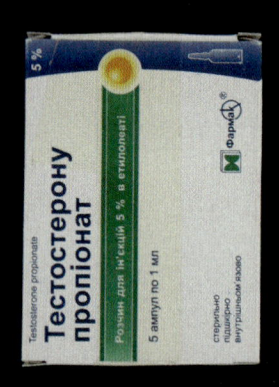

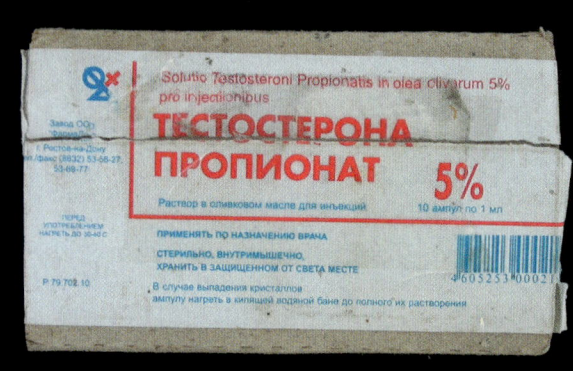

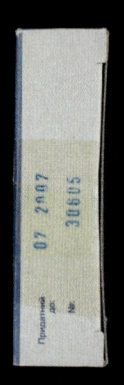

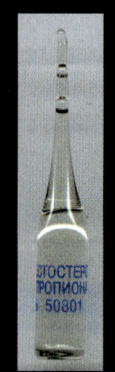

Propionate from Farmak (Ukraine)   Propionate from Farmadon (Russia)

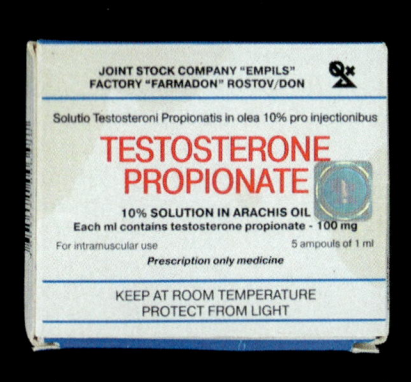

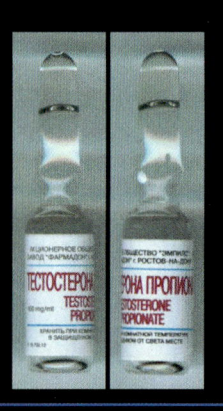

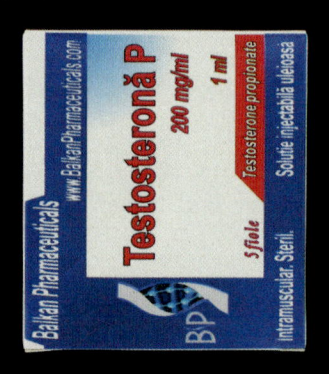

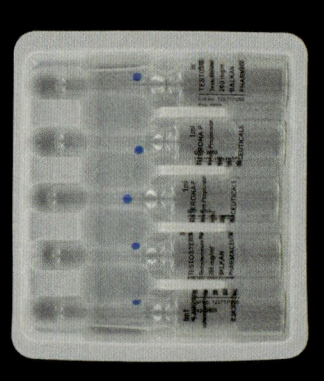

Counterfeit Farmadon box and ampules (Russia)   Testosterona P from Balkan (Moldova)

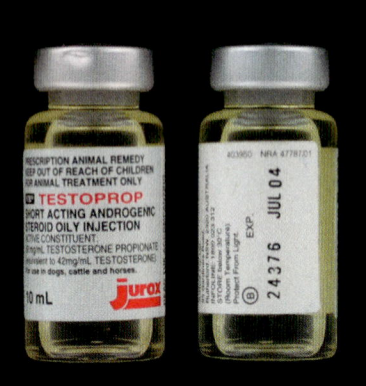

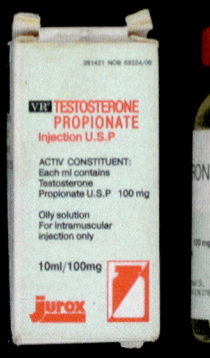

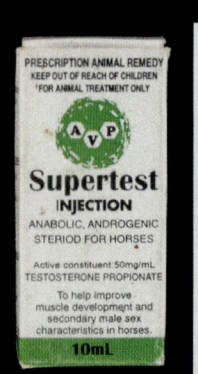

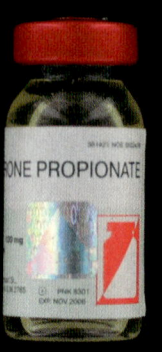

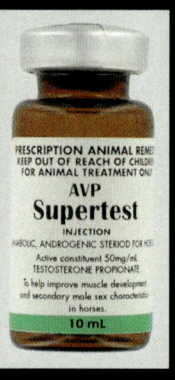

Testoprop from Jurox (Australia)   Counterfeit Jurox   Counterfeit Vetsearch (Australia)

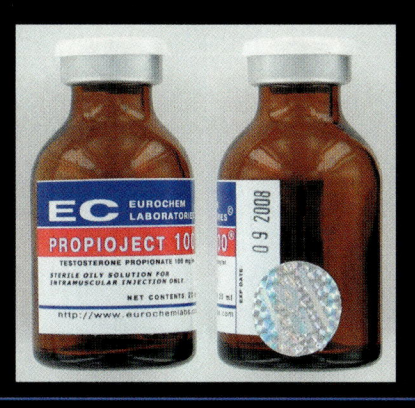

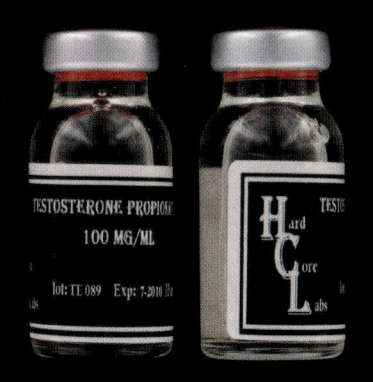

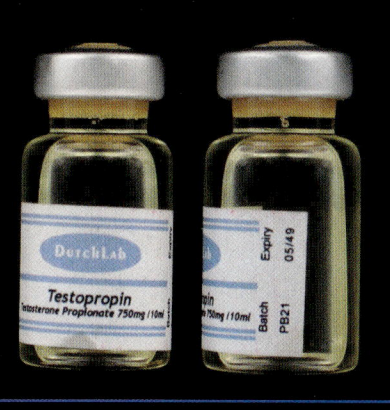

Underground propionate vials from Eurochem, Hardcore Labs, and DutchLab

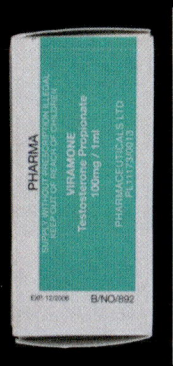

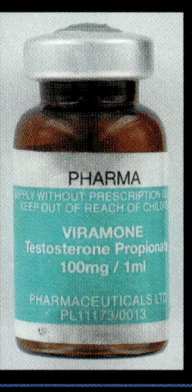

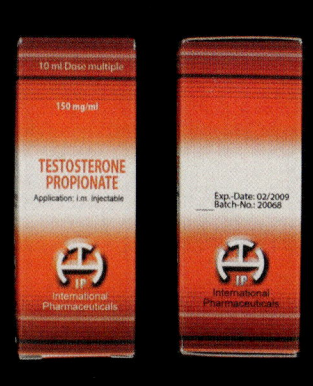

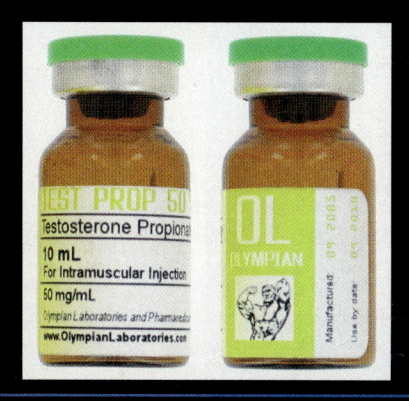

Underground products from Pharma, International Pharmaceuticals, and Olympian

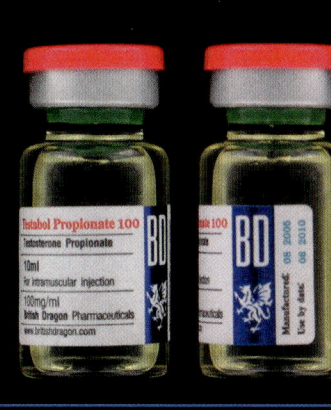

British Dragon (UG) NLM 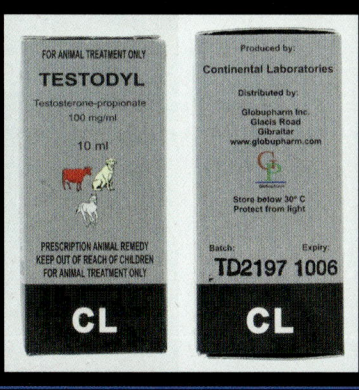   Continental (UG) 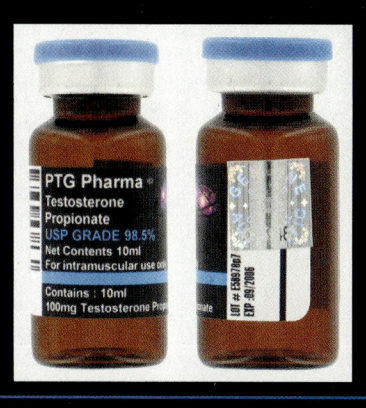   PTG Pharma (UG)

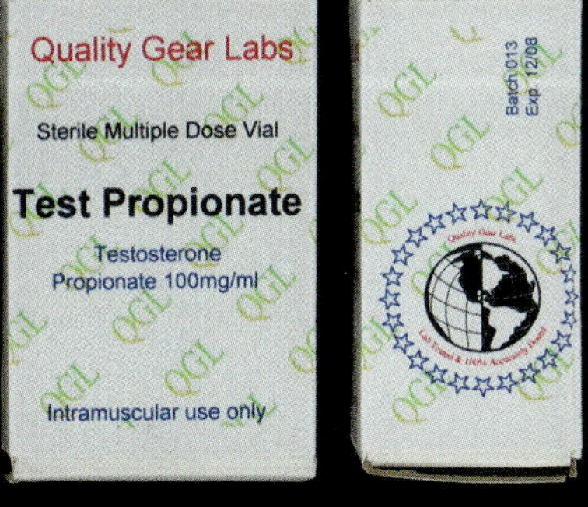

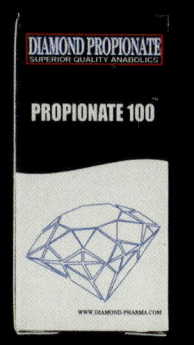

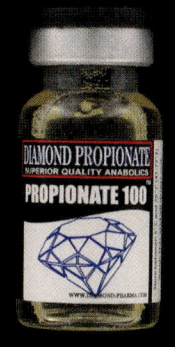

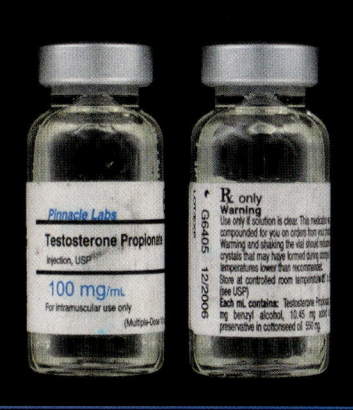

Underground products from Quality Gear Labs, Diamond, and Pinnacle

Appendix B

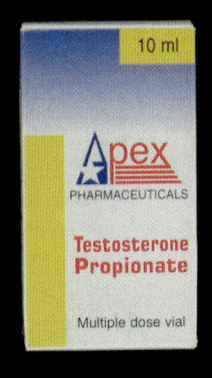

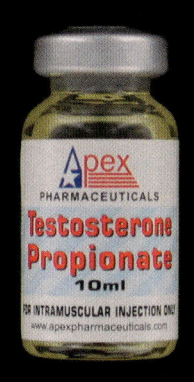

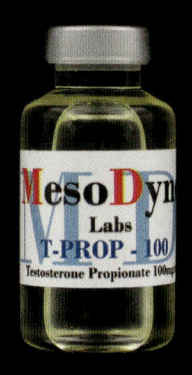

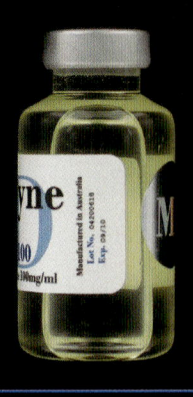

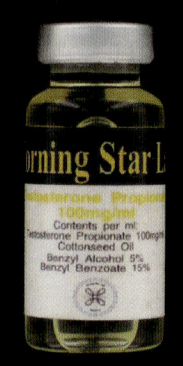

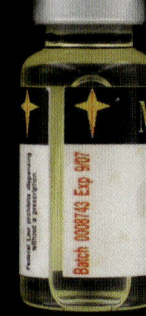

Underground products from Apex, MesoDyne, and Morning Star

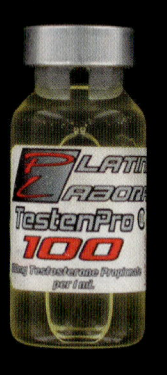

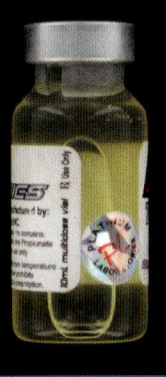

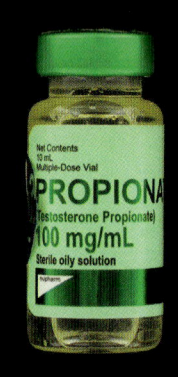

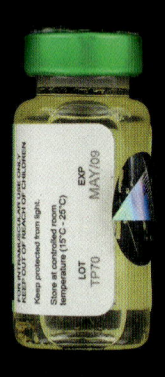

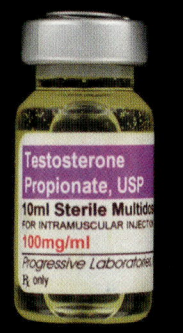

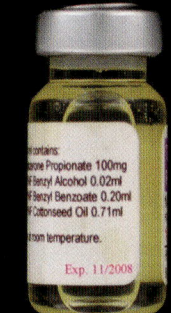

Underground products from Platinum, Nupharm, and Progressive

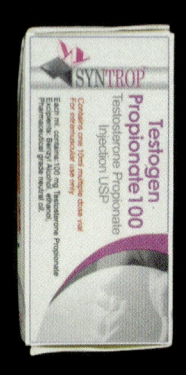

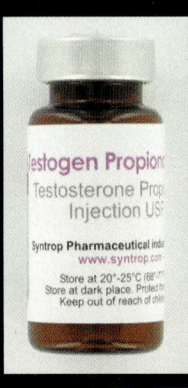

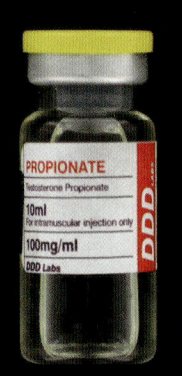

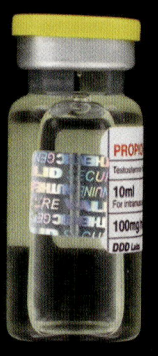

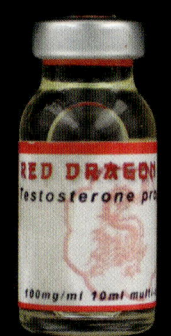

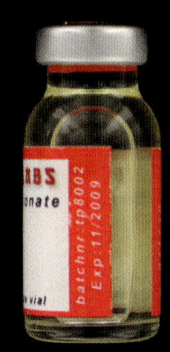

Underground products from Syntrop, DDD, and Red Dragon

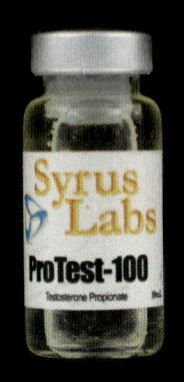

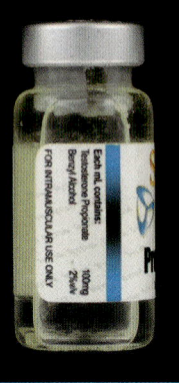

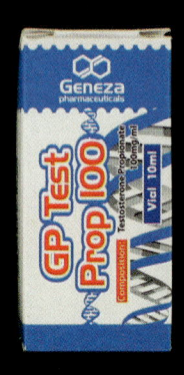

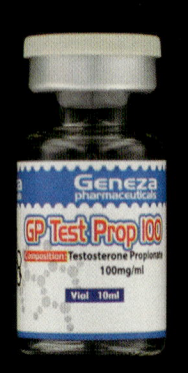

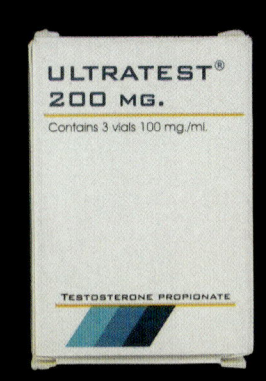

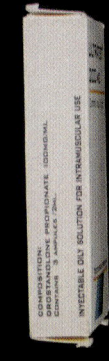

Underground products from Syrus and Geneza Pharm

Fake Australian Ultratest

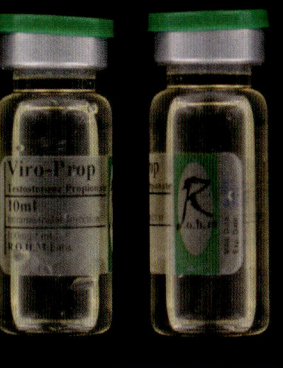

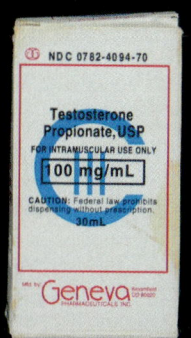

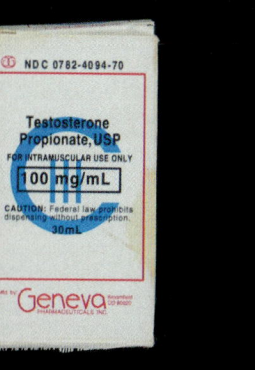

R.O.H.M. (Underground) 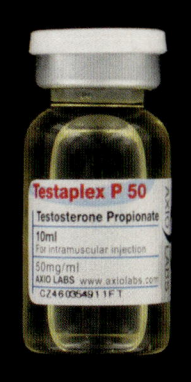 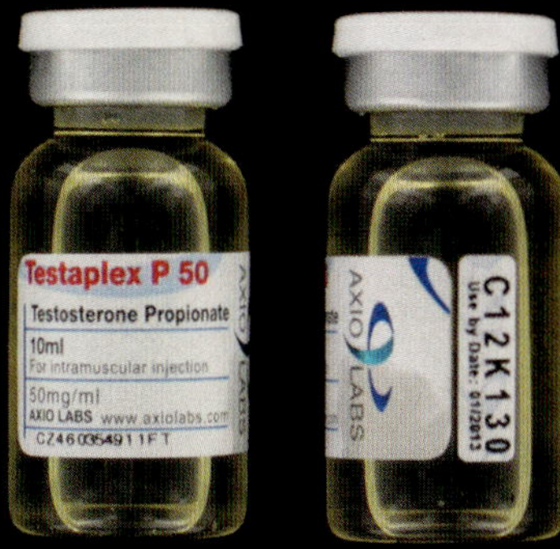   Axio Labs (Underground) 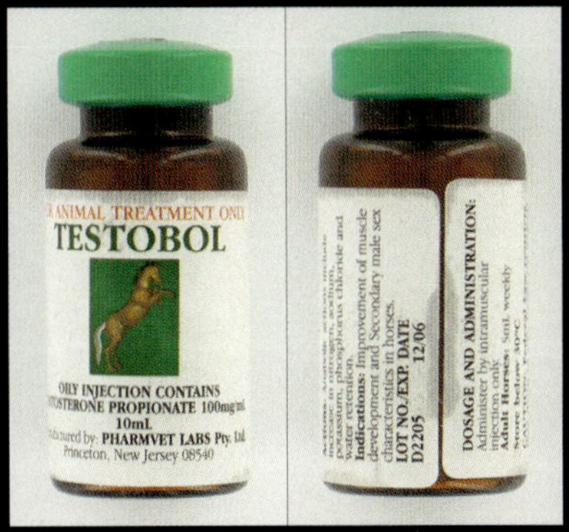   Fake U.S. Pharmvet

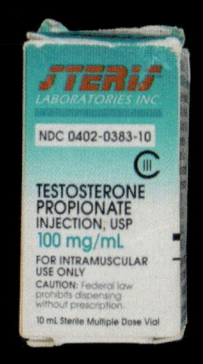

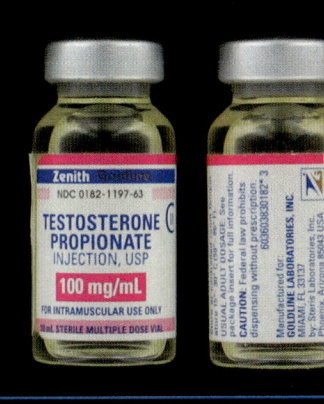

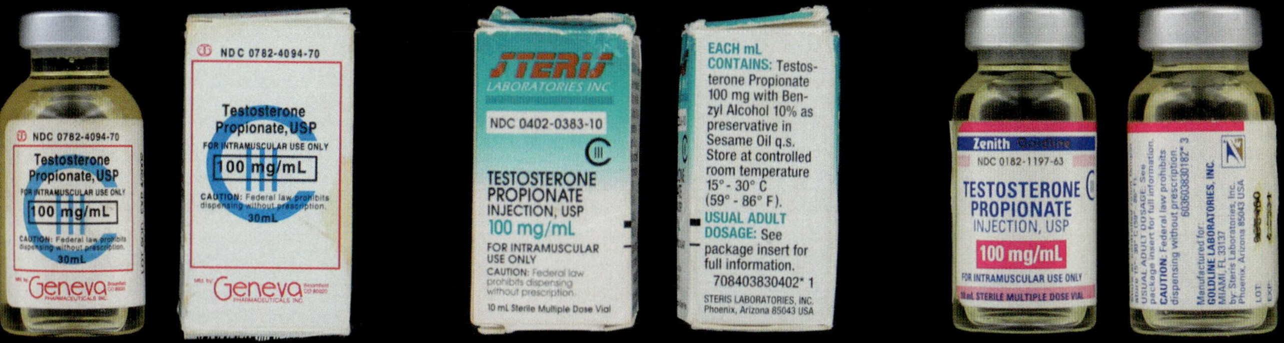

U.S. counterfeits of Geneva, Steris, and Zenith

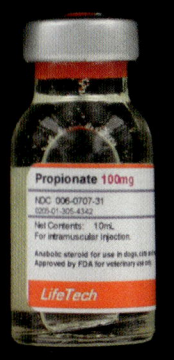

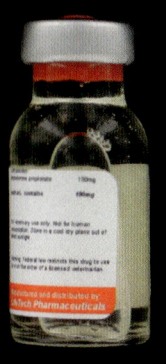

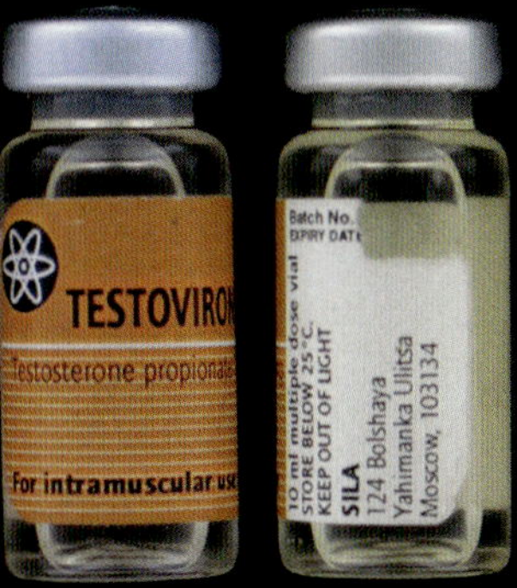

Fake Sila vial from Russia   Fake LifeTech vial 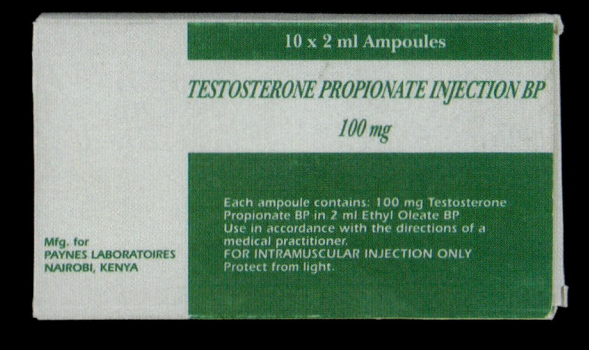   Fake box from Paynes Labs (Kenya)

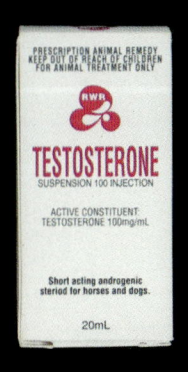

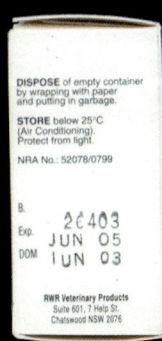

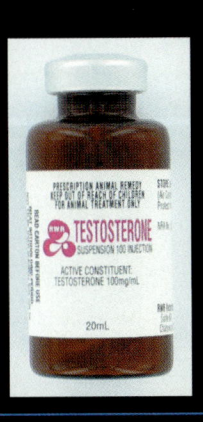

RWR suspension (Australia) 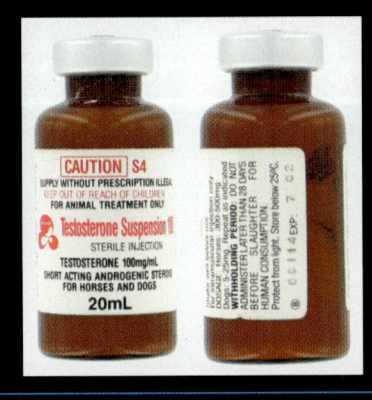   Counterfeit RWR suspension

Testosterone Suspension

Appendix B

B-107

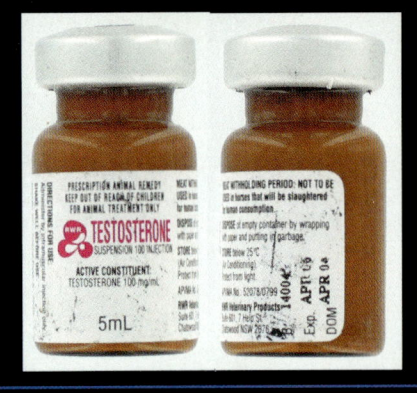

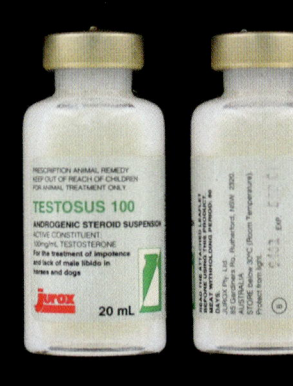

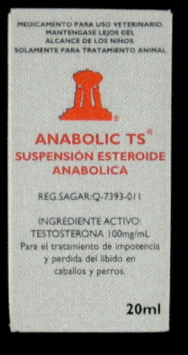

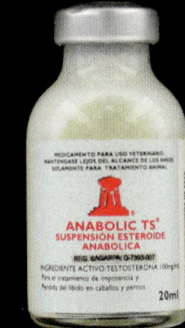

Another counterfeit RWR vial   Jurox suspension (NLM)   Mexican Grupo Tarasco (NLM)

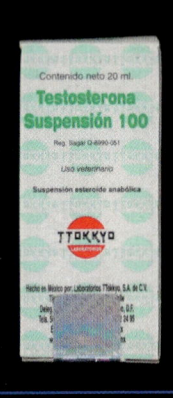

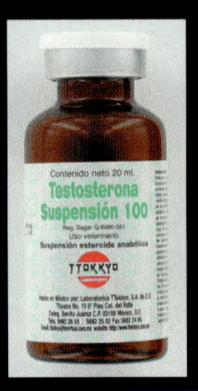

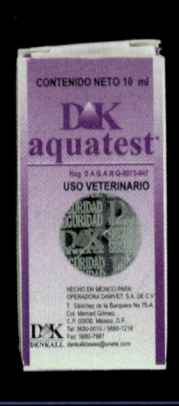

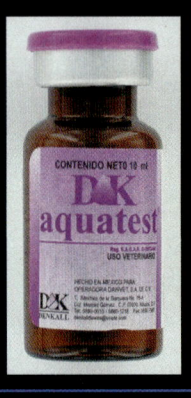

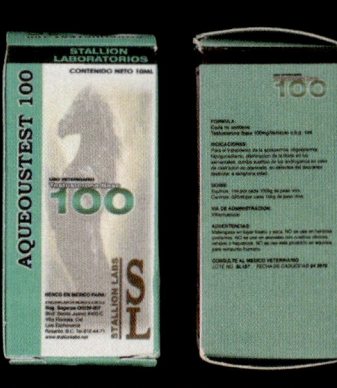

Ttokkyo generic from Mexico (NLM)   Denkall Aquatest (Mexico) NLM   Stallion Labs (Mexico, UG) NLM

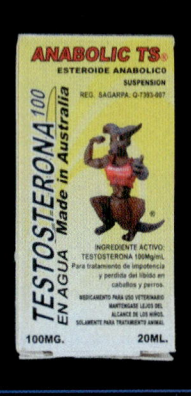

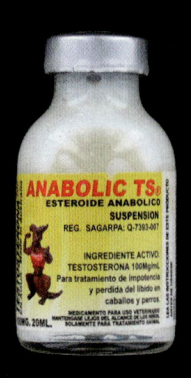

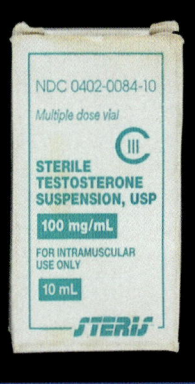

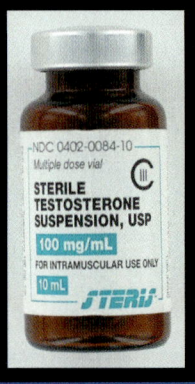

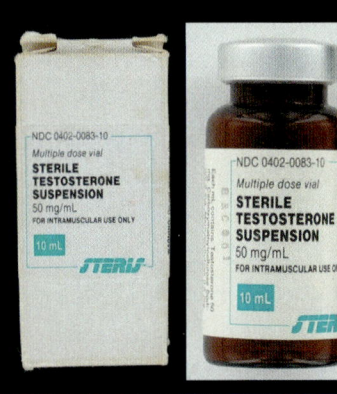

SYD Group (Mexico) NLM   U.S. Steris suspension (NLM)   Steris counterfeit (U.S.)

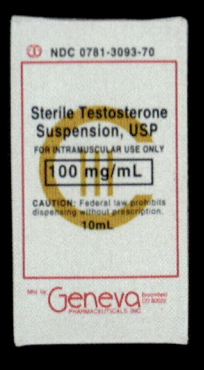

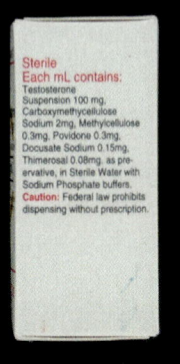

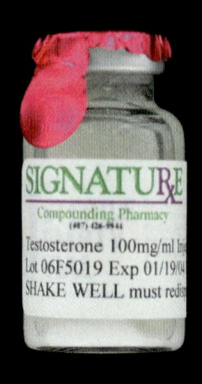

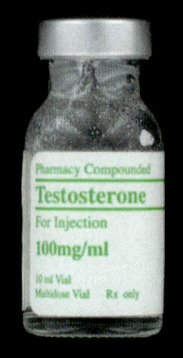

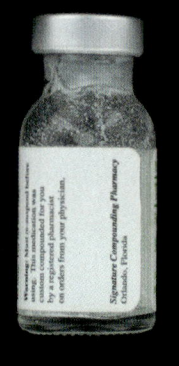

U.S. Geneva counterfeit (NLM)   Signature Pharmacy (U.S.) NLM   Another private label U.S. Product

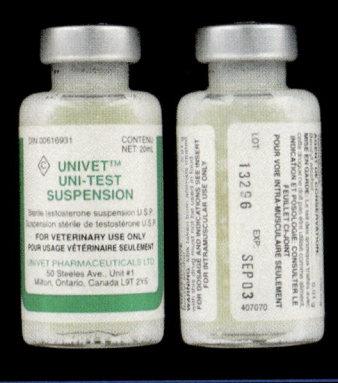

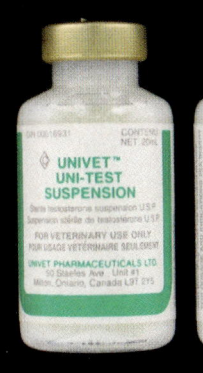

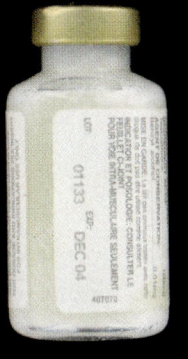

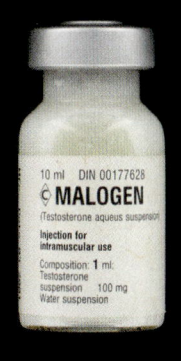

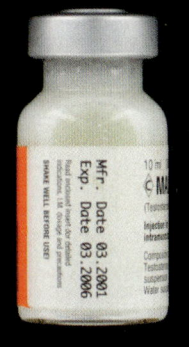

Univet suspension (Canada) | Counterfeit Univet vial | Counterfeit Canadian Malogen

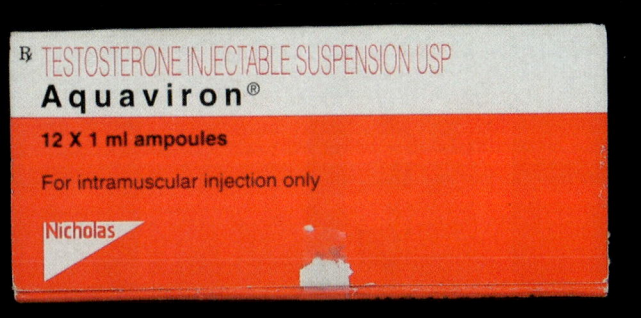

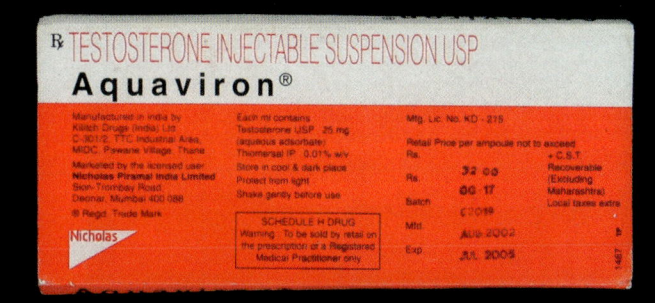

Aquaviron from Nicholas (India)

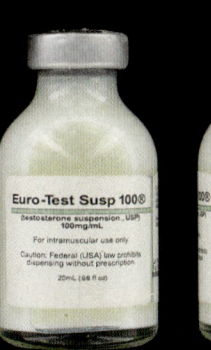

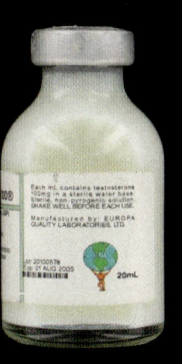

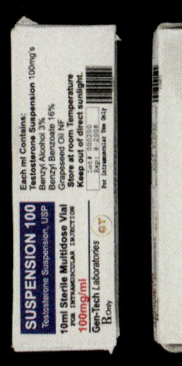

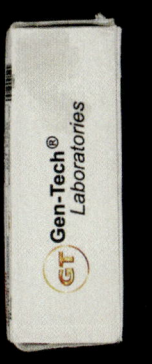

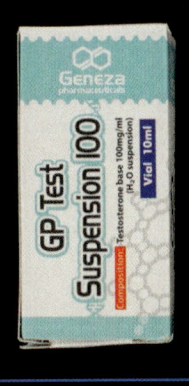

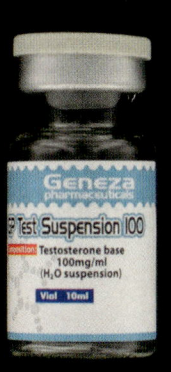

Europa (Underground) | Gen-Tech (Underground) | Geneza (Underground)

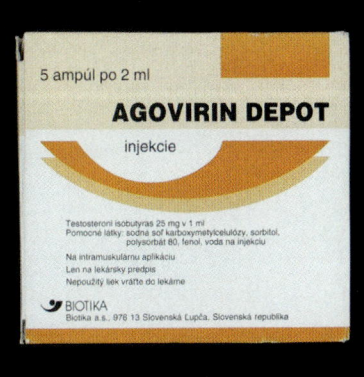

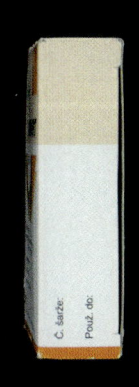

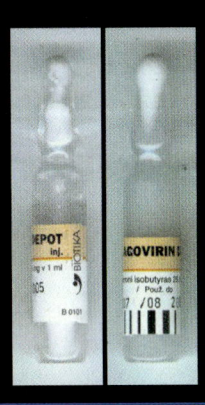

Czech Agovirin Depot from Biotika

Appendix B

Testoviron

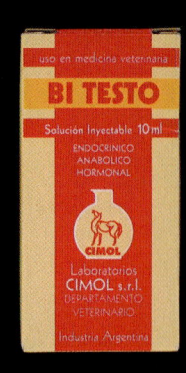

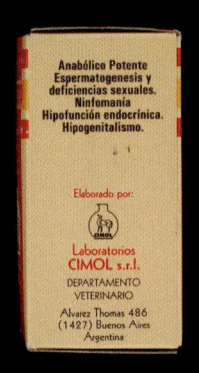

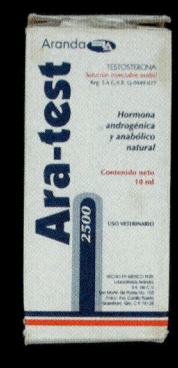

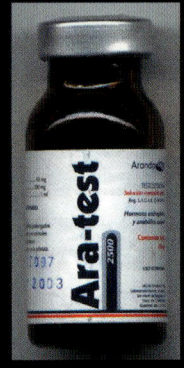

Bi-Testo (Argentina)

Ara-Test (Mexico)

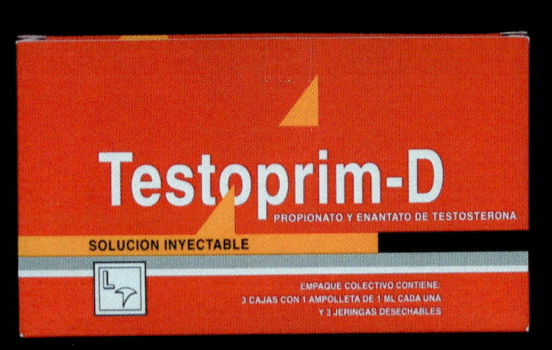

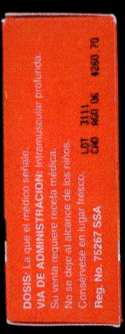

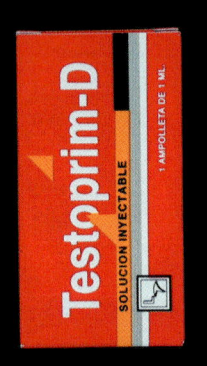

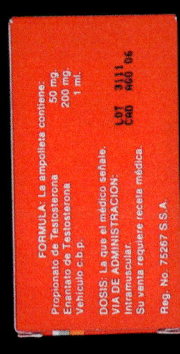

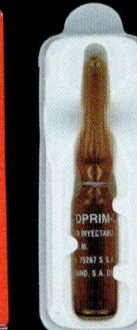

Testoprim-D from Mexico

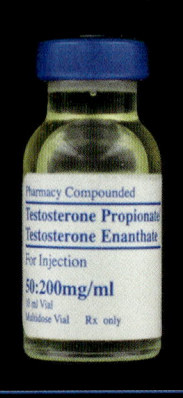

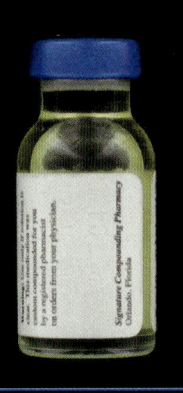

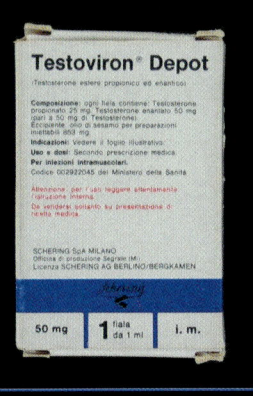

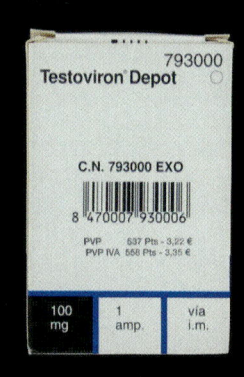

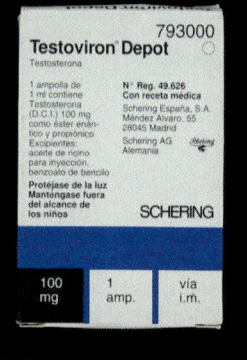

Signature Pharmacy (U.S.) NLM

Italian Testoviron (NLM)

Spanish Testoviron (NLM)

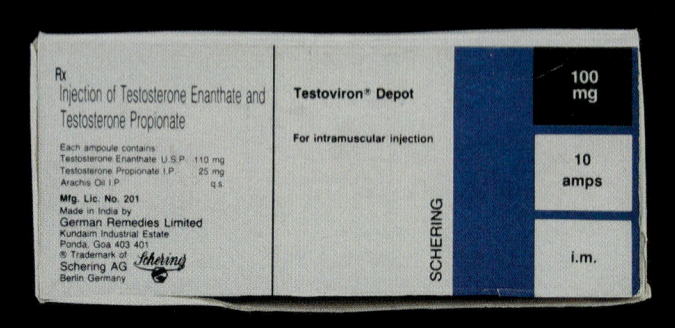

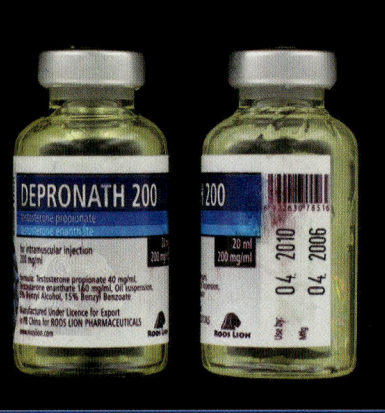

Testoviron Depot from India (NLM)

Roos Lion (Underground)

Trenbolone Acetate

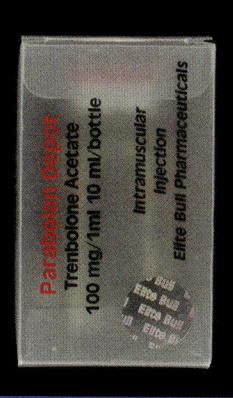

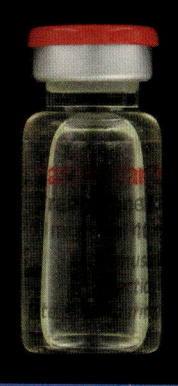

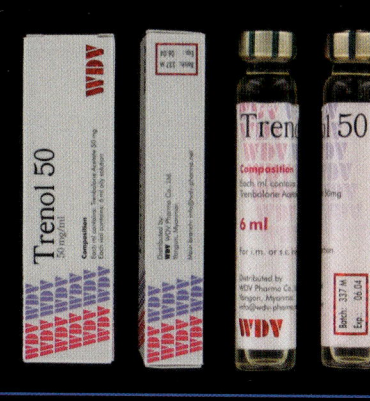

Elite Bull (Hong Kong, export)

Trenol 50 from WDV (Myanmar)

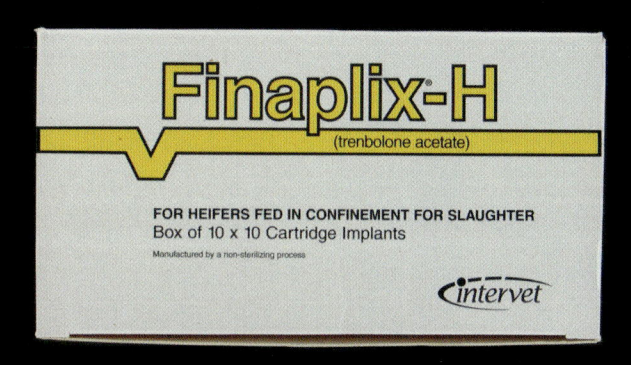

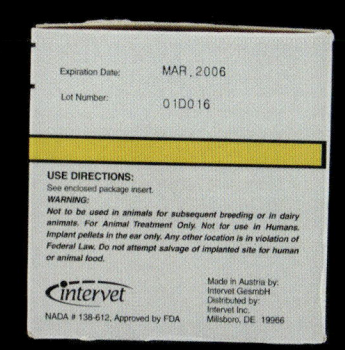

Finaplix-H from Intervet (U.S.)

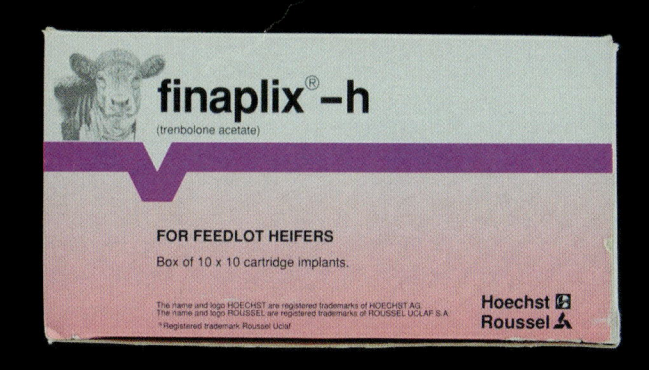

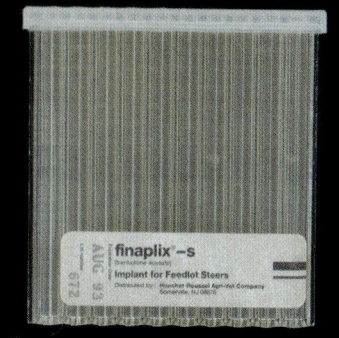

Old U.S. Finaplix-H

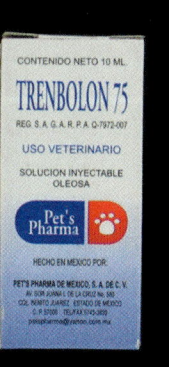

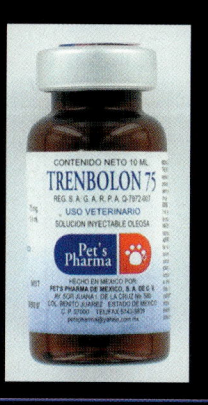

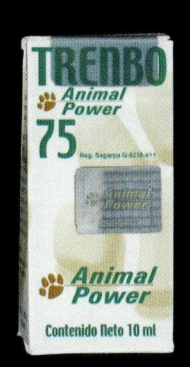

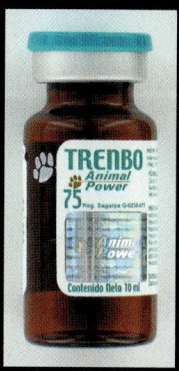

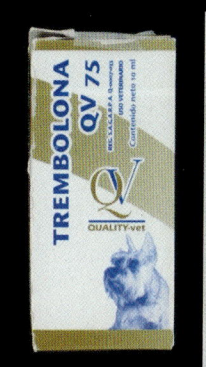

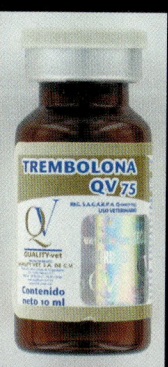

Pet's Pharma (Mexico) NLM

Animal Power (Mexico) NLM

Quality Vet Trembolona (Mexico) NLM

Appendix B

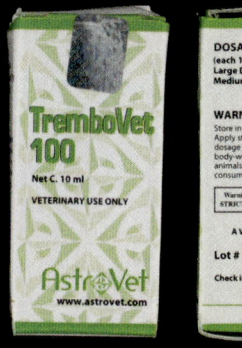

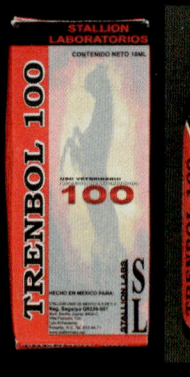

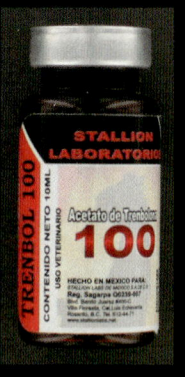

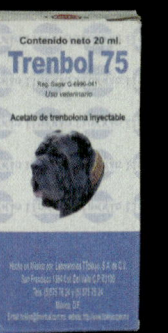

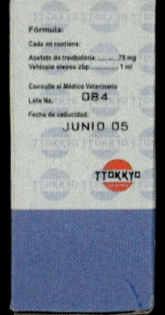

AstroVet (Mexico, Underground) — Stallion Labs (Mexico, UG) NLM — Ttokkyo Trenbol (Mexico) NLM

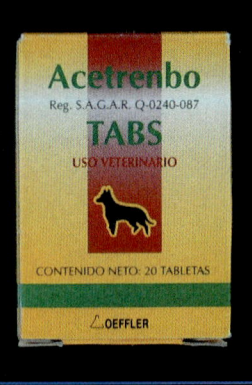

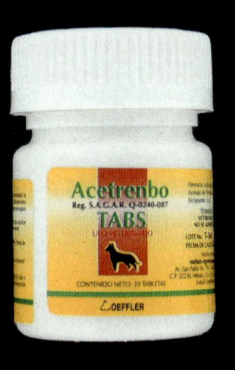

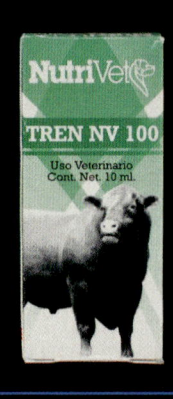

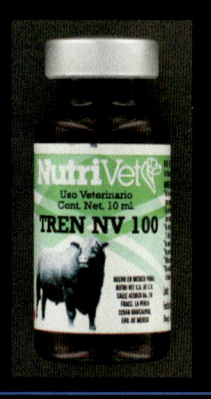

Loeffler Acetrenbo tabs (Mexico) NLM — Nutri-Vet Ultra (Mexico, UG) NLM — Genesis Trenbol (Singapore) NLM

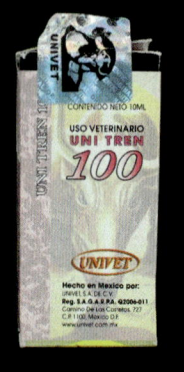

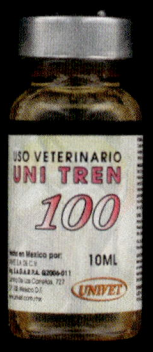

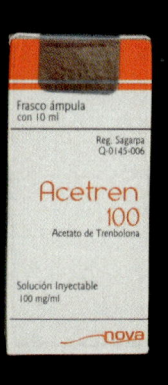

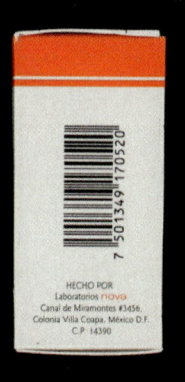

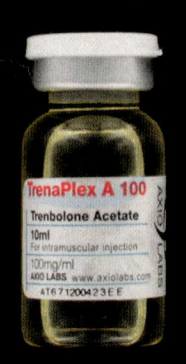

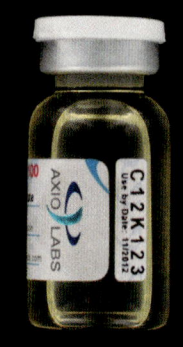

Univet (Mexico, UG) — Nova (Mexico, UG) — Axio Labs (Underground)

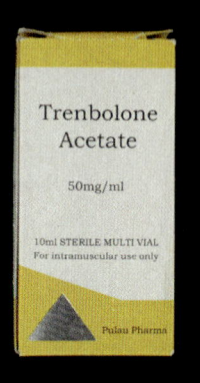

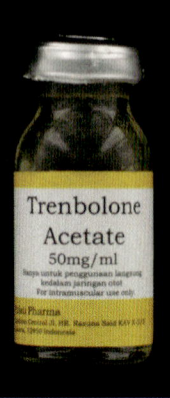

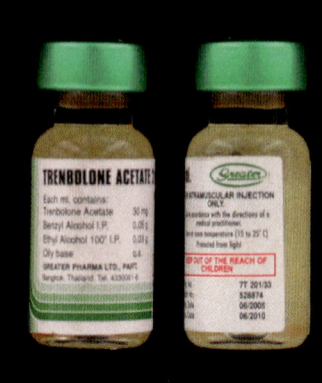

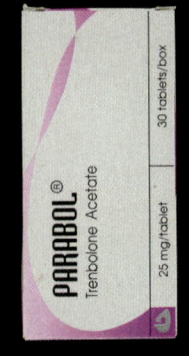

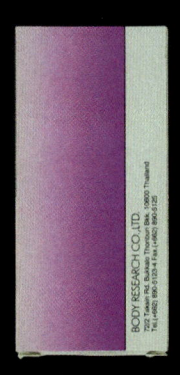

Palau (Underground) — Fake Greater Pharma (Thailand) — Fake Body Research Parabol (Thailand)

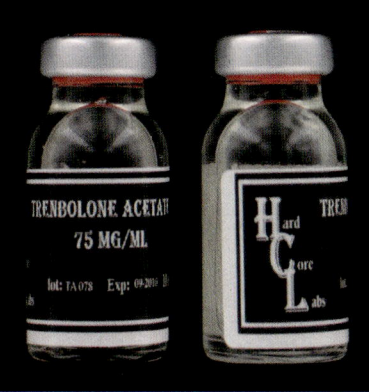

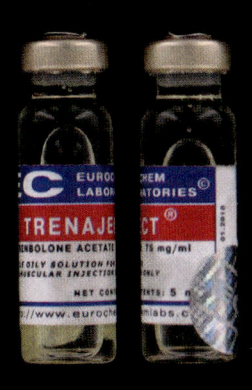

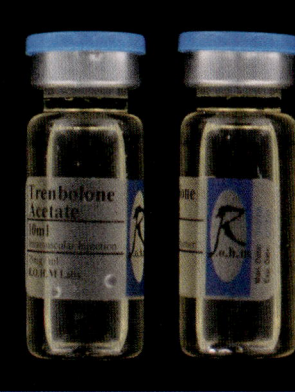

Underground products from Hardcore Labs, Eurochem, and R.O.H.M.

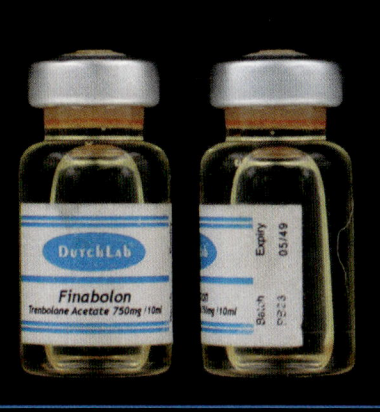

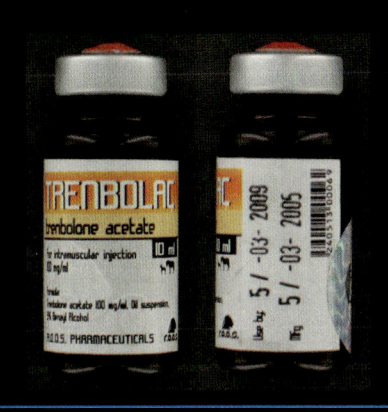

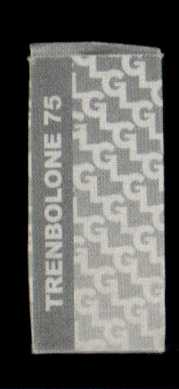

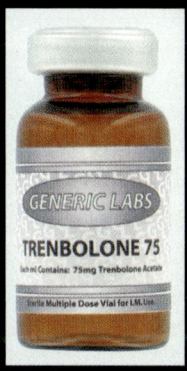

Underground products from Dutchlab, Roos Lion, and Generic Labs

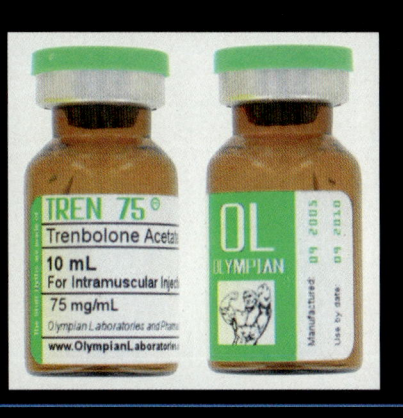

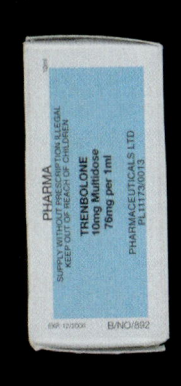

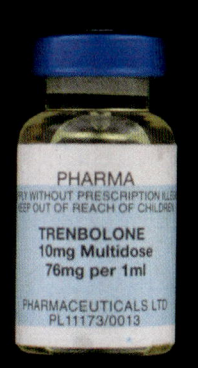

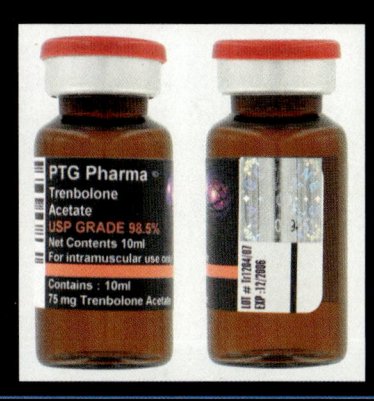

Underground products from Olympian, Pharma, and PTG

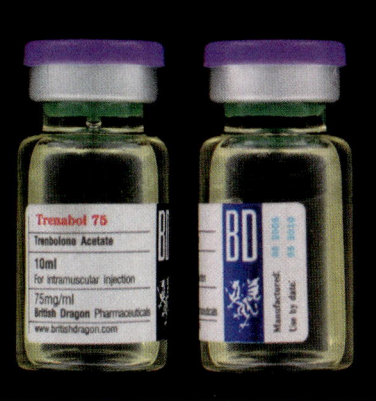

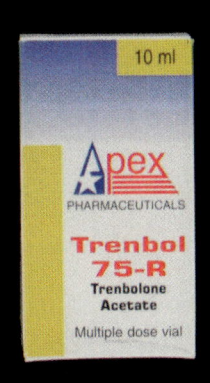

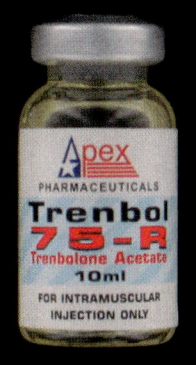

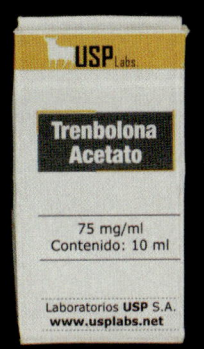

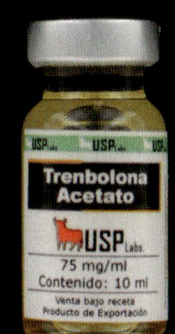

British Dragon (Underground) NLM   Apex (Underground)   USP Labs (Underground)

Appendix B

B-113

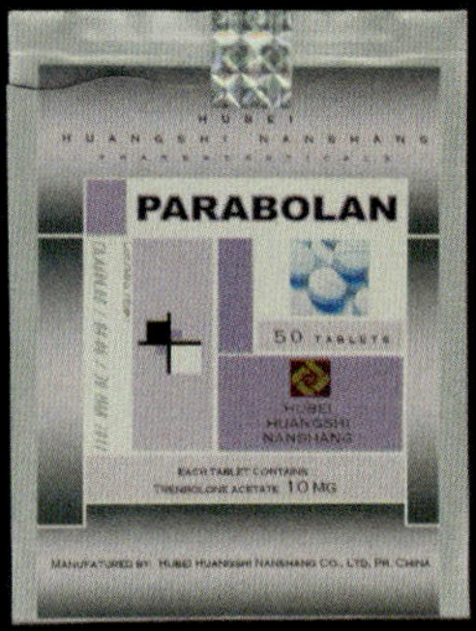

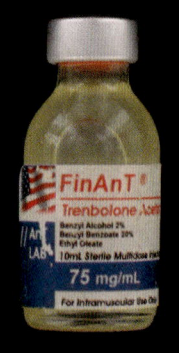

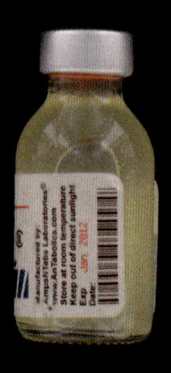

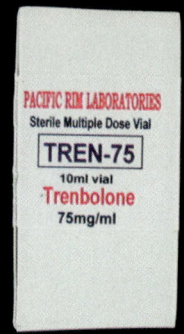

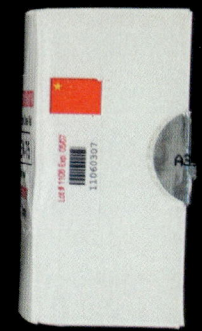

Underground products from Hubei, AnT Labs, and Pacific Rim

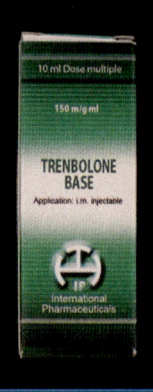

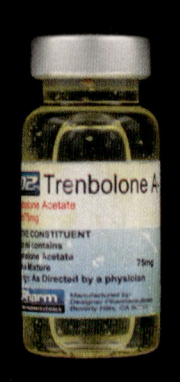

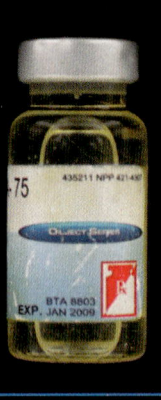

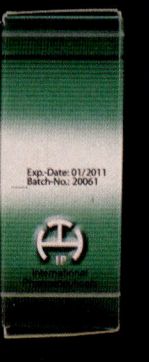

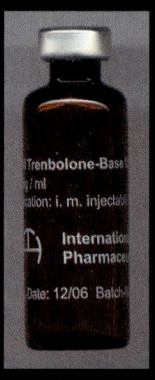

Designer (Underground) — International Pharmaceuticals (UG) 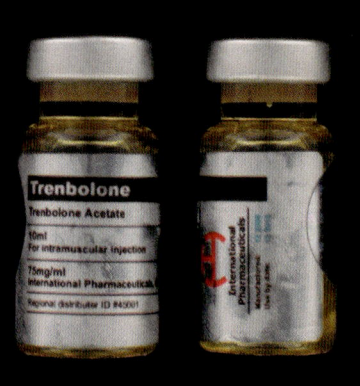 — Counterfeit IP vial

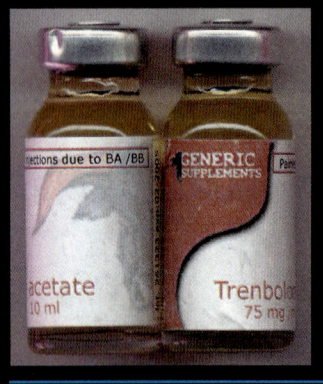

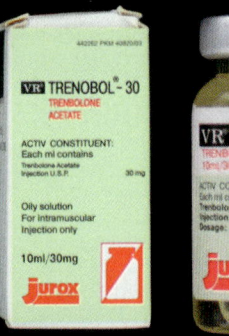

Generic Supplements vial (UG) 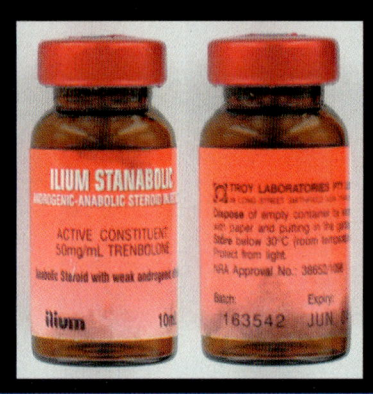 — Fake Ilium injectable (Australia) 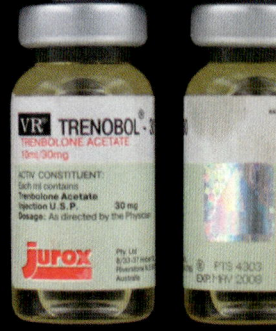 — Fake Jurox injectable (Australia)

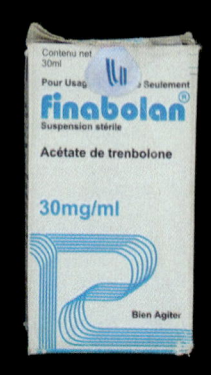

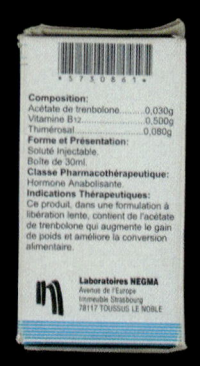

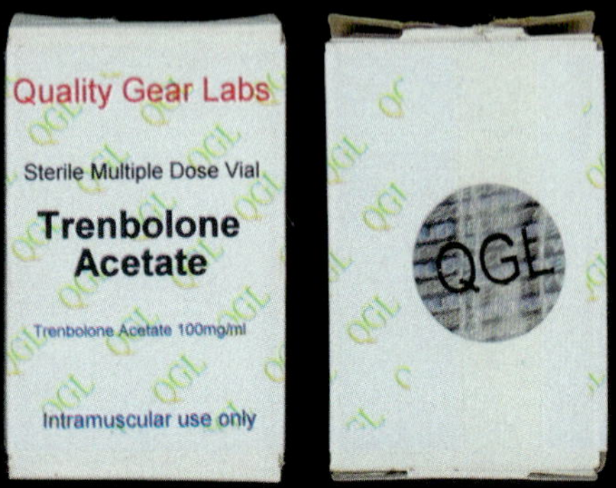

Generic from Quality Gear Labs (Underground) — Fake Finabolan (France) 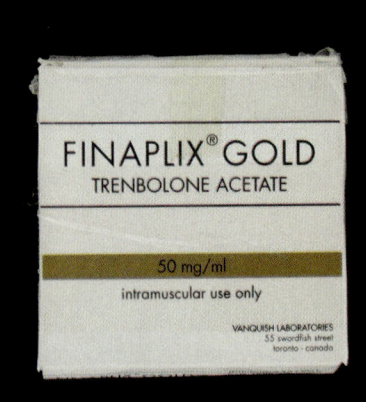 — Fake Finaplix Gold from Canada

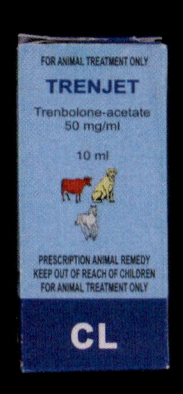

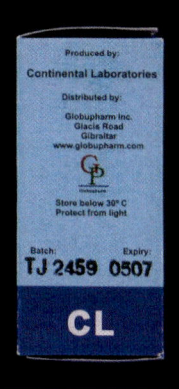

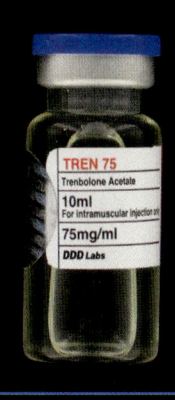

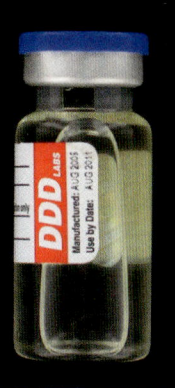

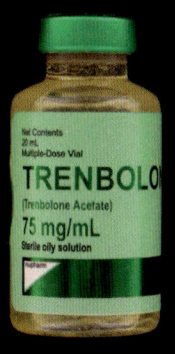

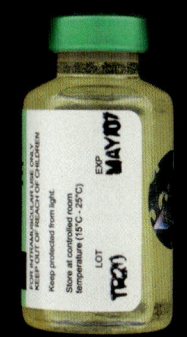

Underground products from Continental, DDD, and Nupharm

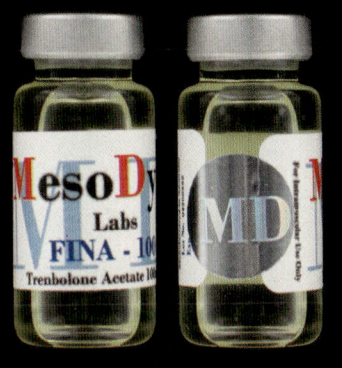

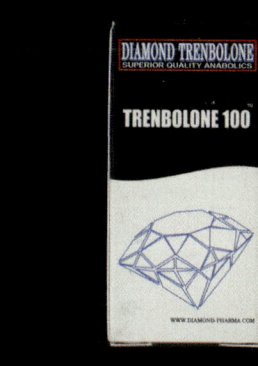

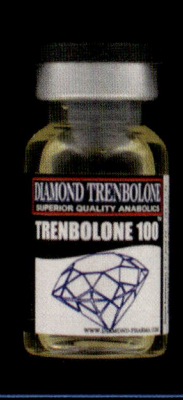

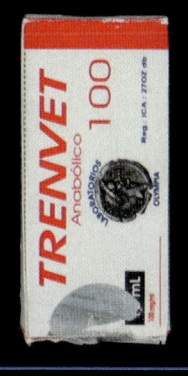

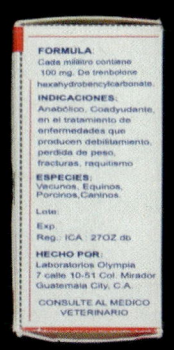

MesoDyne (Underground) Diamond (Underground) Fake Trenvet (Guatemala)

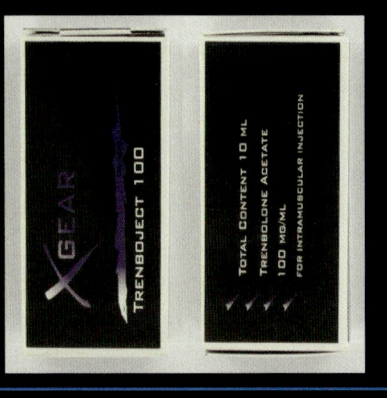

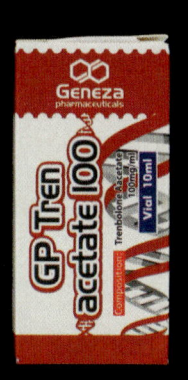

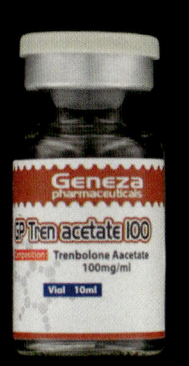

Trenbolone Enanthate

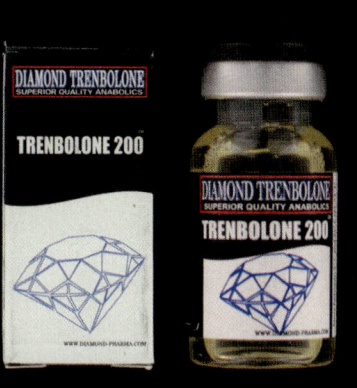

X Gear (Underground) Geneza (Underground) Diamond (Underground)

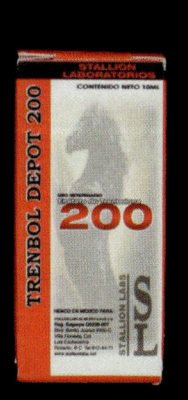

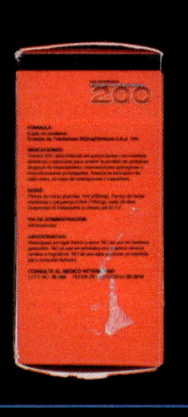

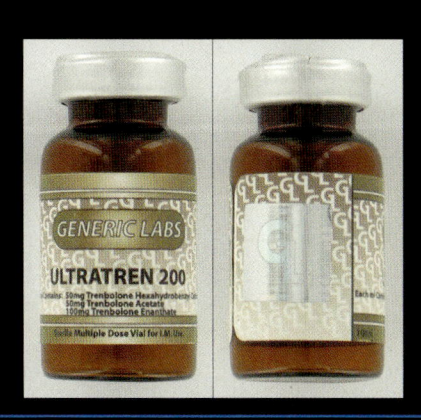

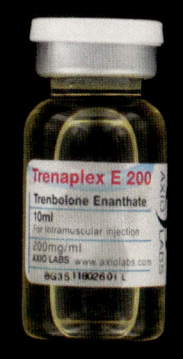

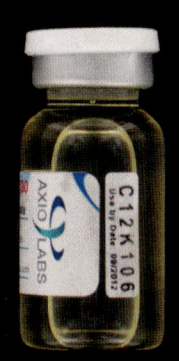

Trenabol from Stallion (Mexico, UG) NLM Generic Labs (Underground) Axio Labs (Underground)

Appendix B

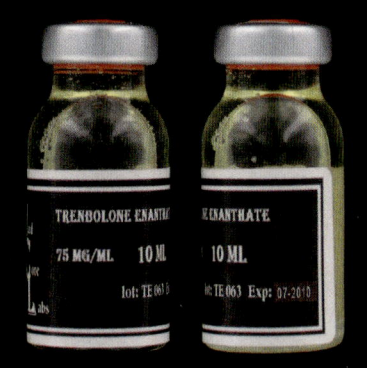

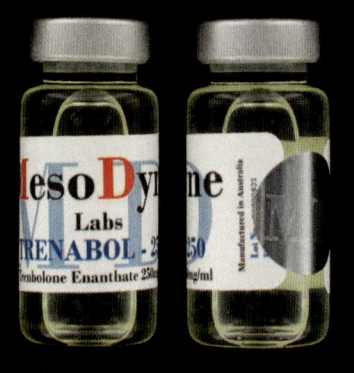

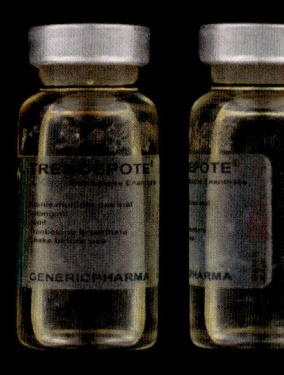

Underground products from Hardcore Labs, MesoDyne, and Generic

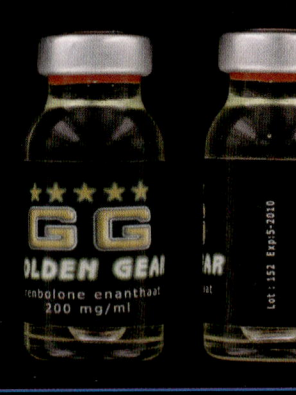

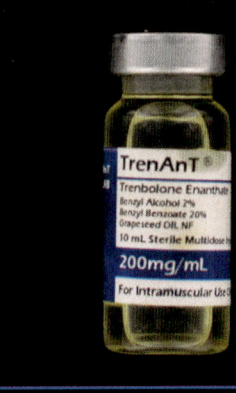

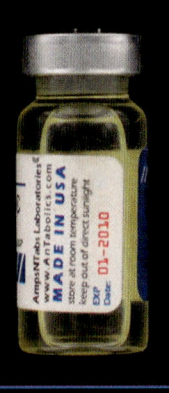

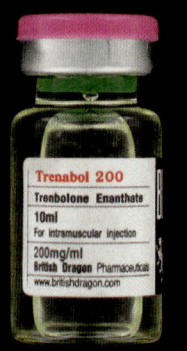

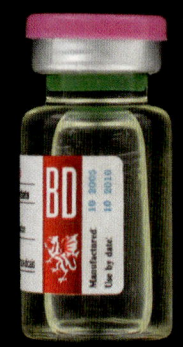

Golden Gear (Underground)   AnT Labs (Underground)   Trenabol from BD (UG) NLM

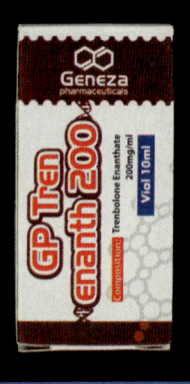

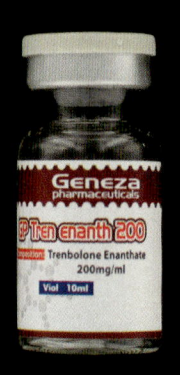

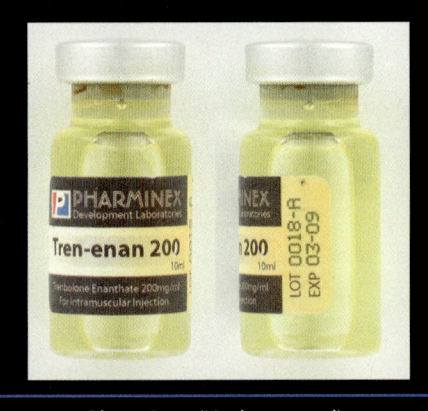

Geneza (Underground)   Pharminex (Underground)

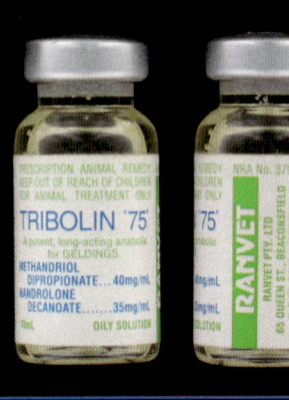

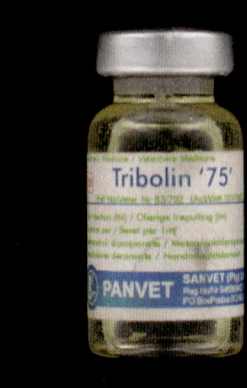

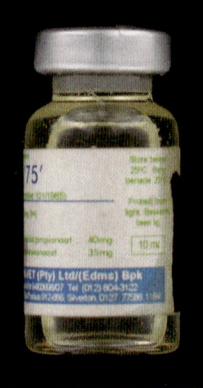

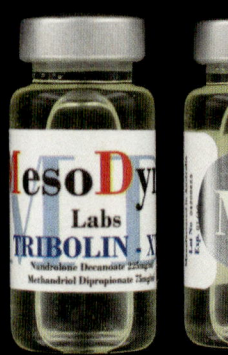

Tribolin

Tribolin from Ranvet (Australia)   Counterfeit "Panvet" (Australia)   MesoDyne (Underground)

B-116

Tri-Trenabol

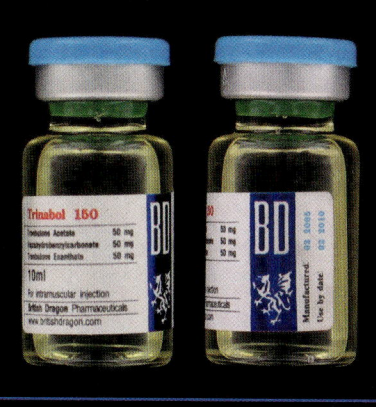

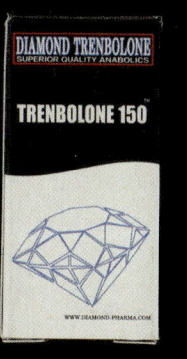

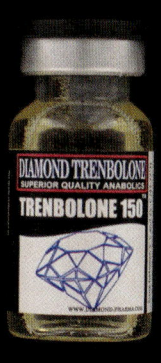

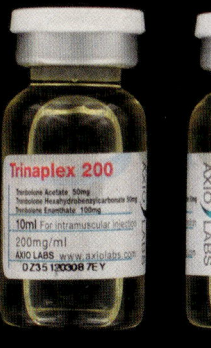

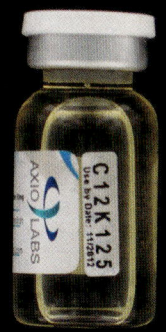

British Dragon (Thailand) NLM | Diamond (Underground) | Axio Labs (Underground)

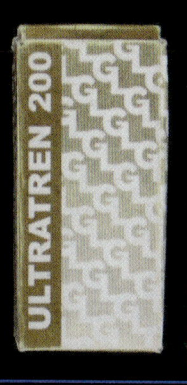

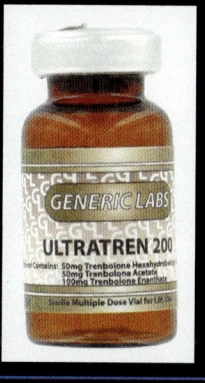

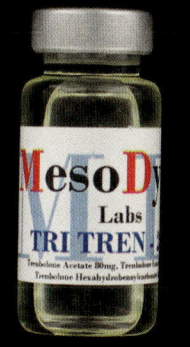

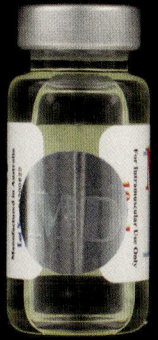

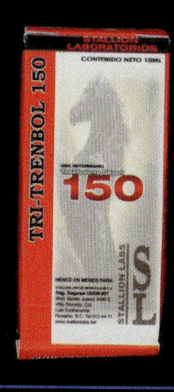

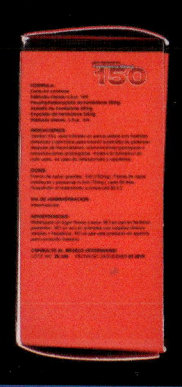

200 mg/mL clone from Generic Labs (UG) | MesoDyne (Underground) | Stallion (Mexico, UG) NLM

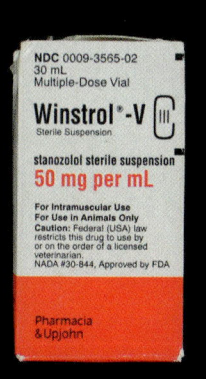

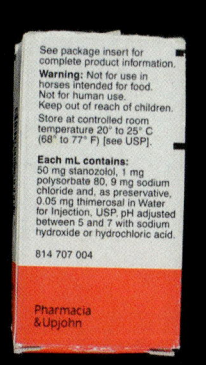

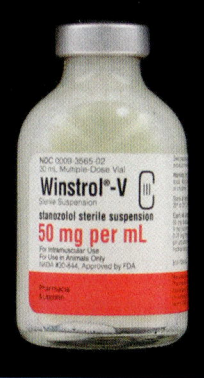

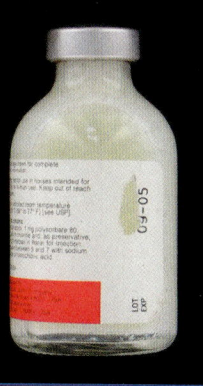

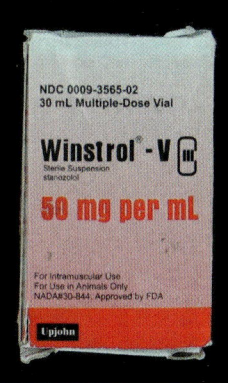

Winstrol

U.S. Winstrol-V from Pharmacia & Upjohn (NLM) | U.S. counterfeit

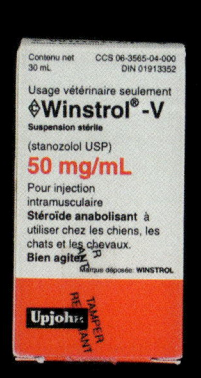

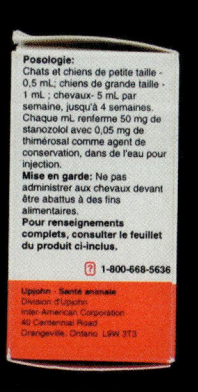

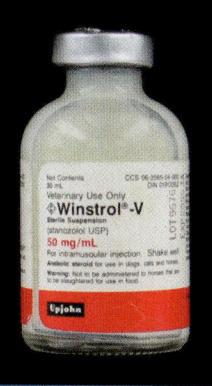

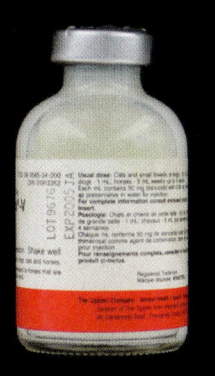

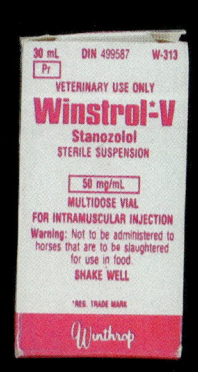

Canadian Winstrol from Upjohn (NLM) | Canadian counterfeit

Appendix B

B-117

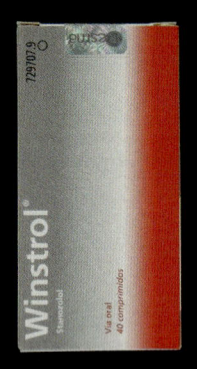

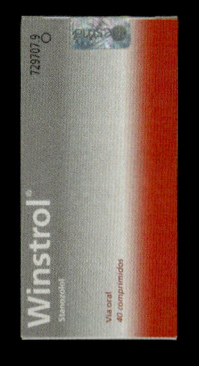

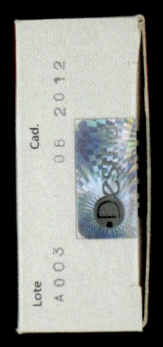

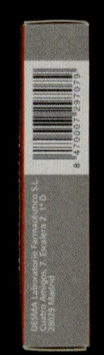

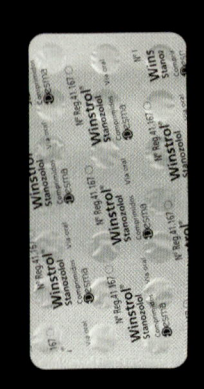

Winstrol tablets from Desma (Spain)

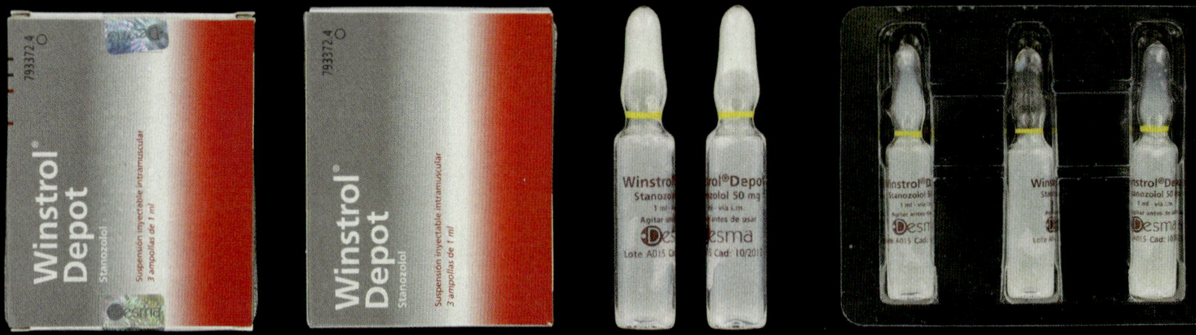

Winstrol Depot from Desma (Spain)

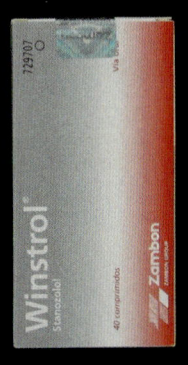

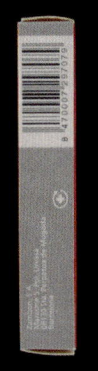

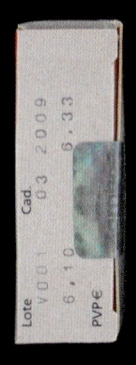

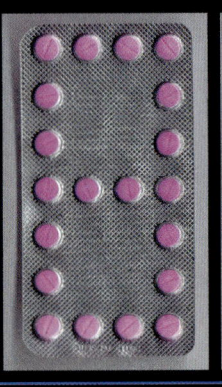

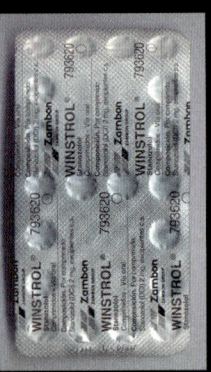

Zambon Winstrol tablets (Spain) NLM

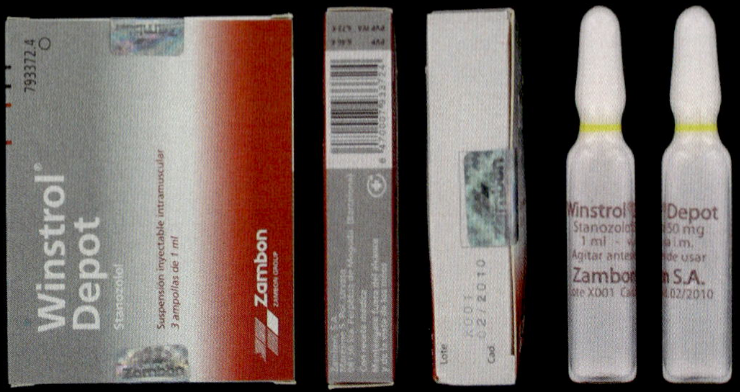

Winstrol Depot from Zambon (Spain) NLM 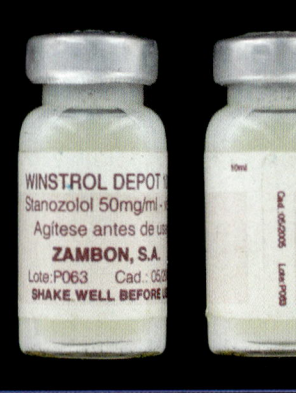   Counterfeit Zambon vial

B-118

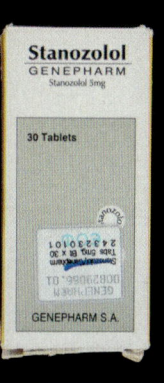

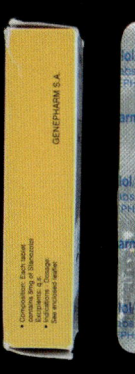

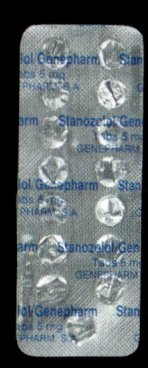

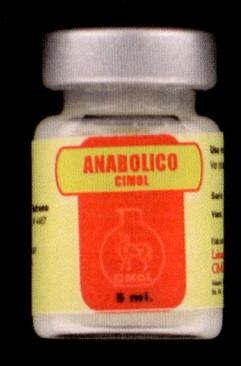

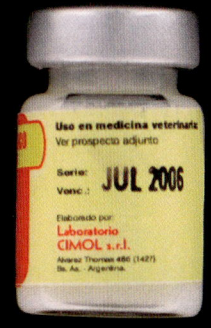

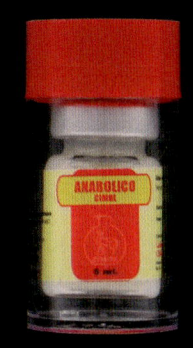

Genepharm tabs (Greece)

Anabolico Cimol (Argentina)

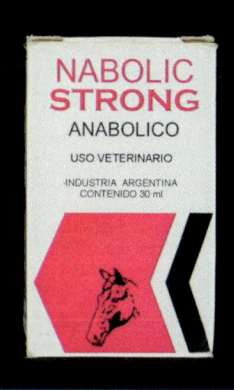

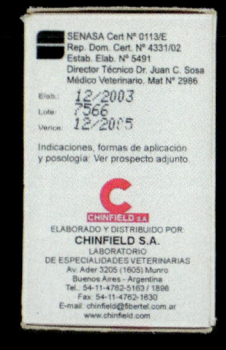

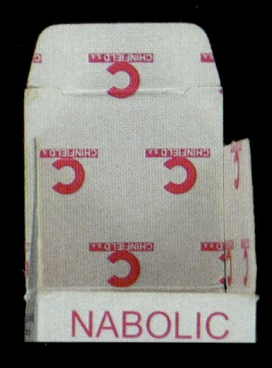

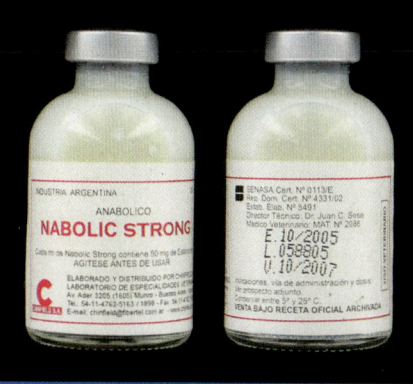

Nabolic Strong from Chinfield S.A. (Argentina)

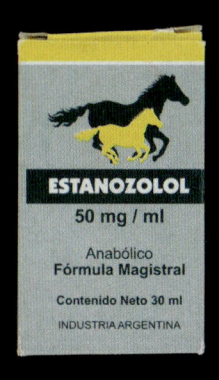

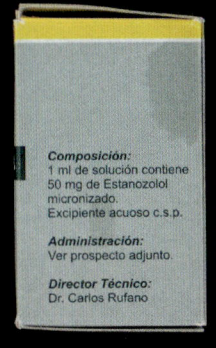

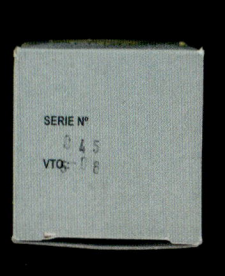

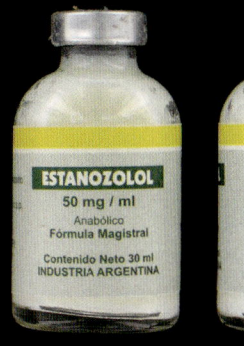

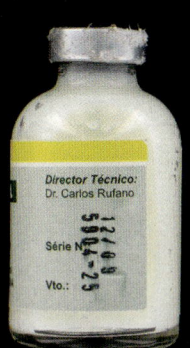

Estanozolol from Formula Magistral (Argentina)

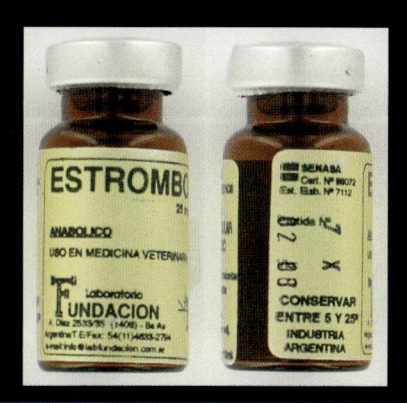

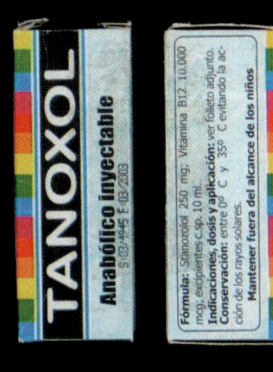

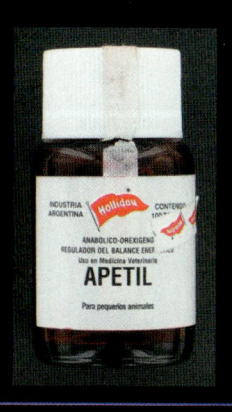

Estrombol (Argentina)

Tanoxol (Argentina)

Fake Apetil (Argentina)

Appendix B

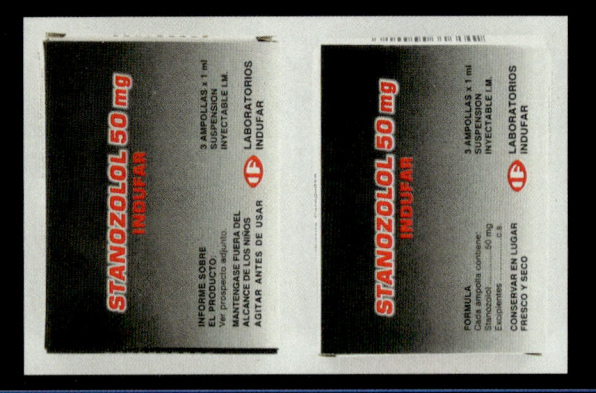

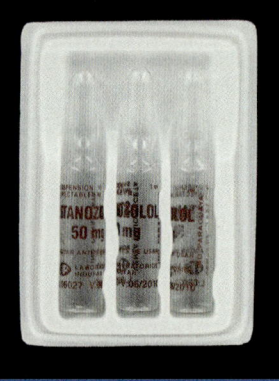

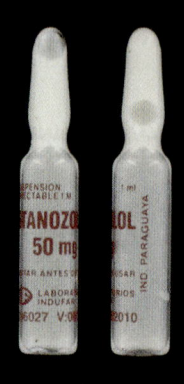

Stanozolol from Indufar (Paraguay)

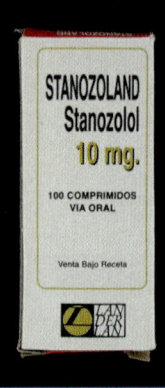

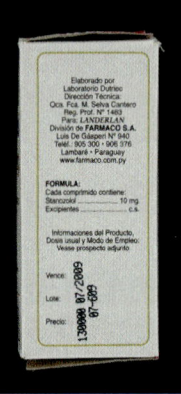

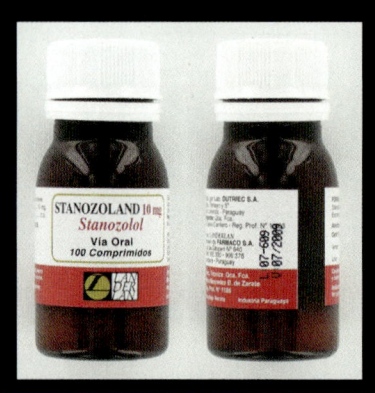

Stanozoland from Landerlan (Paraguay)

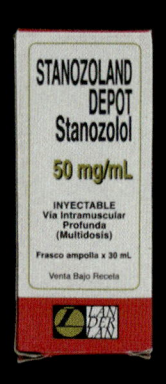

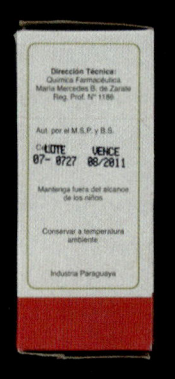

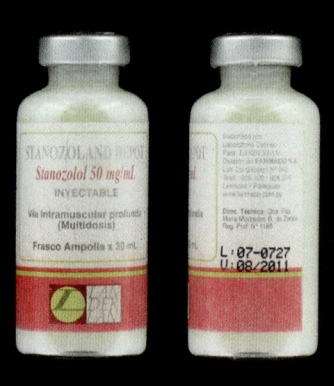

Stanozoland Depot from Landerlan (Paraguay)

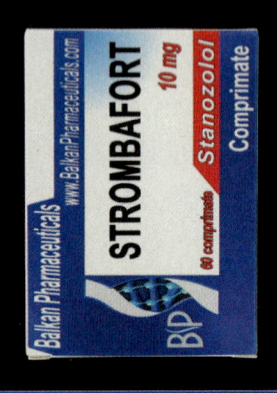

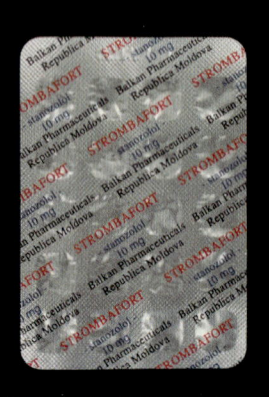

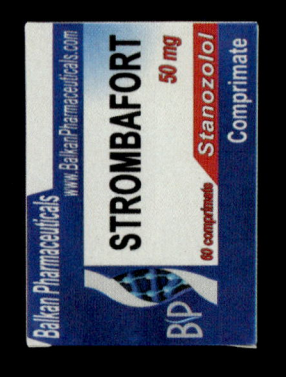

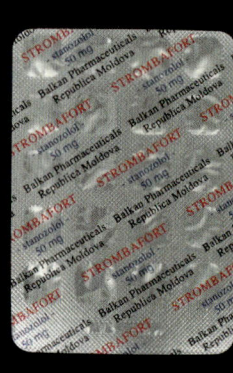

10mg and 50mg Strombafort from Balkan Pharmaceuticals (Moldova)

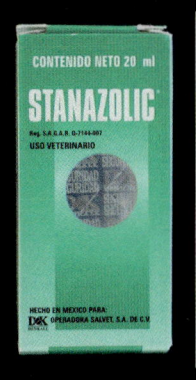

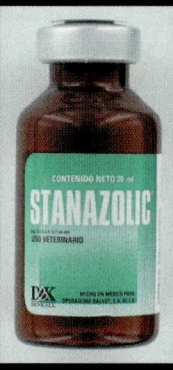

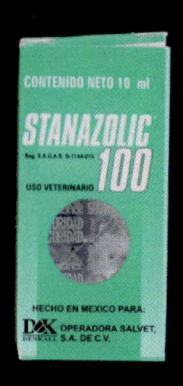

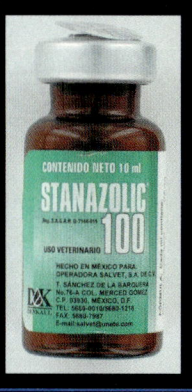

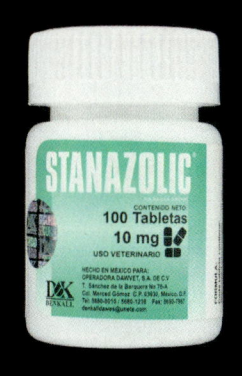

Stanazolic from Denkall (Mexico) NLM   Stanazolic 100 from Denkall (Mexico) NLM   Stanazolic tabs NLM

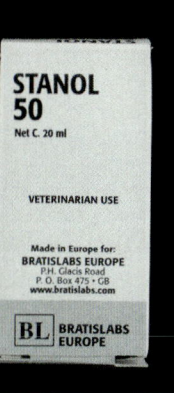

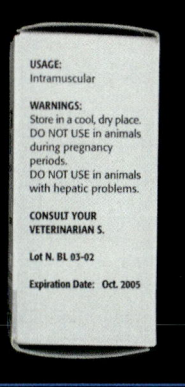

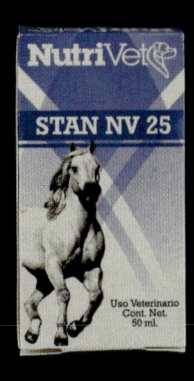

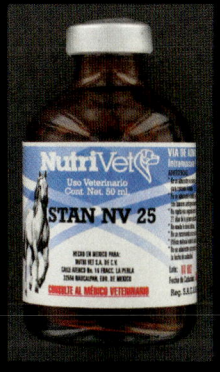

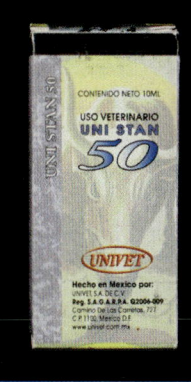

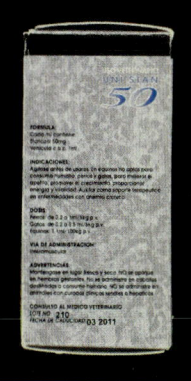

Bratis (Mexico, UG) NLM   NutriVet (Mexico, UG) NLM   Univet (Mexico, Underground)

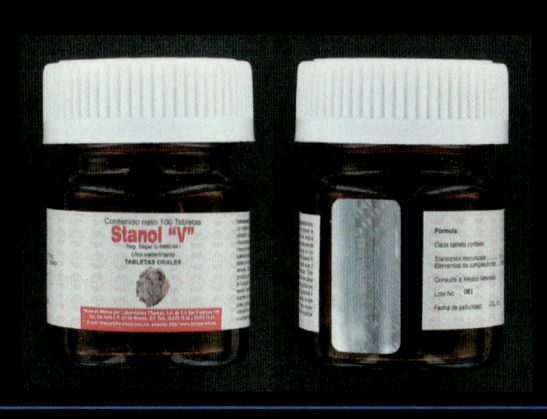

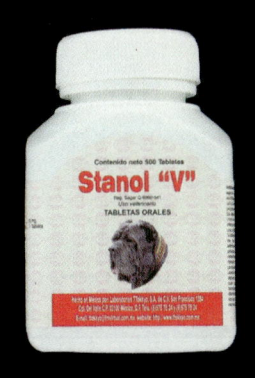

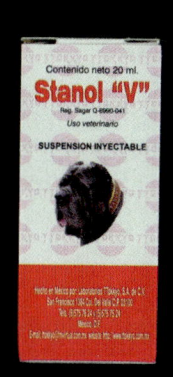

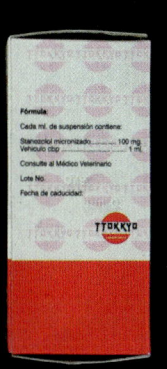

Orals and injectable from Ttokkyo Mexico (NLM)

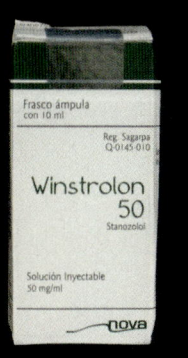

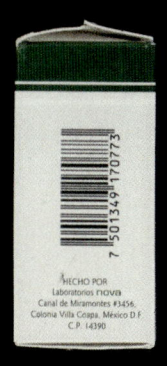

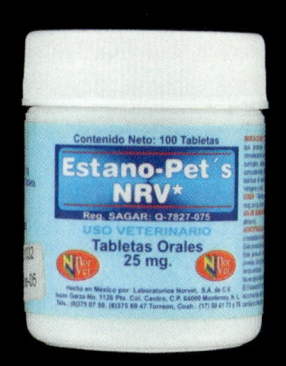

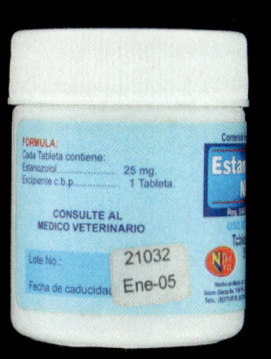

Nova (Mexico, Underground)   Norvet (Mexico) NLM

Appendix B

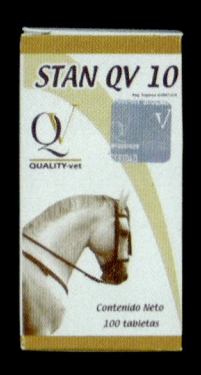

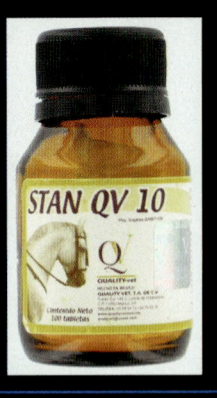

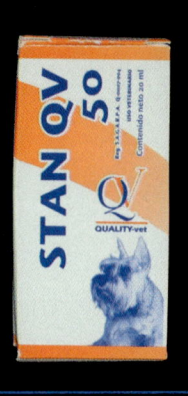

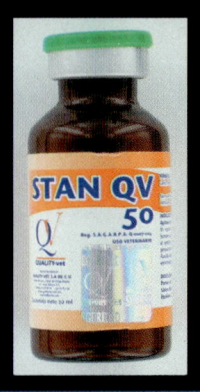

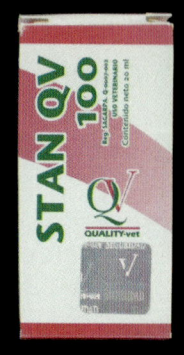

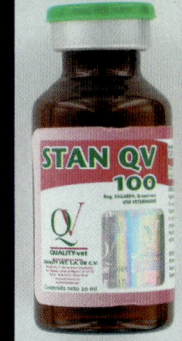

Stan QV tabs and 50mg/mL and 100mg/mL injectables from Quality Vet (Mexico) NLM

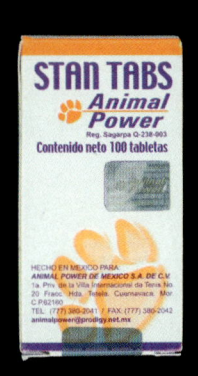

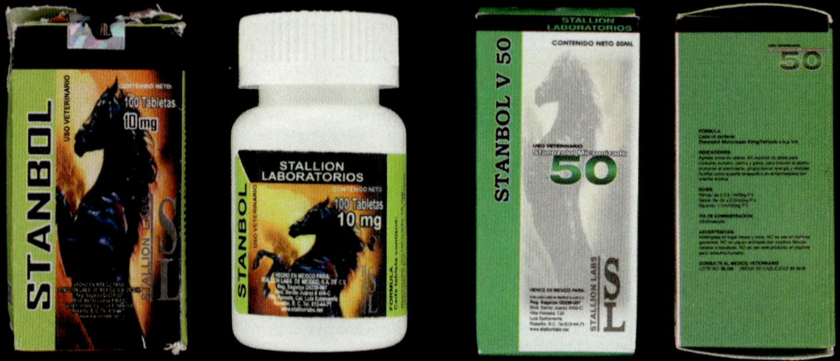

Stanbol oral and injectable from Stallion (Mexico, UG) NLM 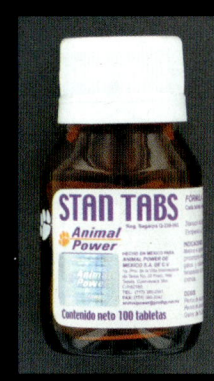   Animal Power (Mexico) NLM

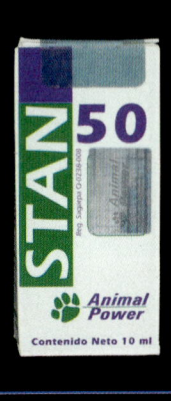

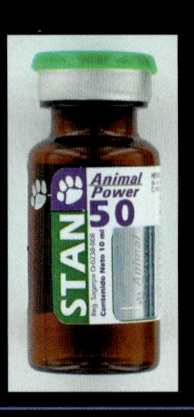

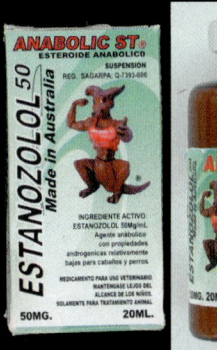

Animal Power (Mexico) NLM 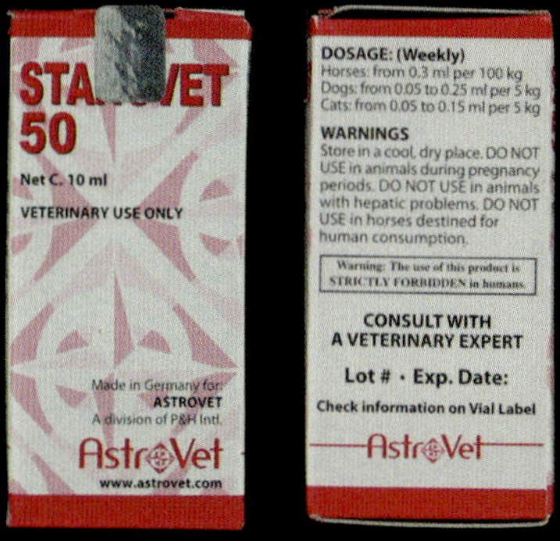   AstroVet (Mexico, Underground) 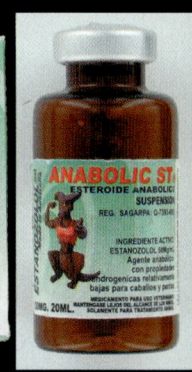   SYD Group (Mexico) NLM

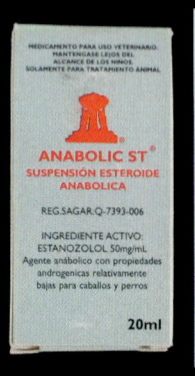

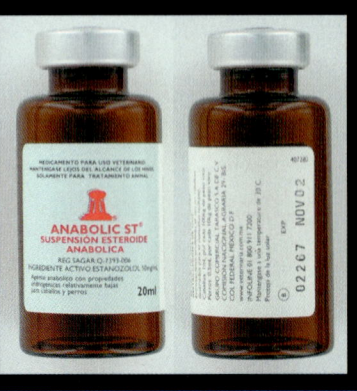

Grupo Tarasco (Mexico) NLM 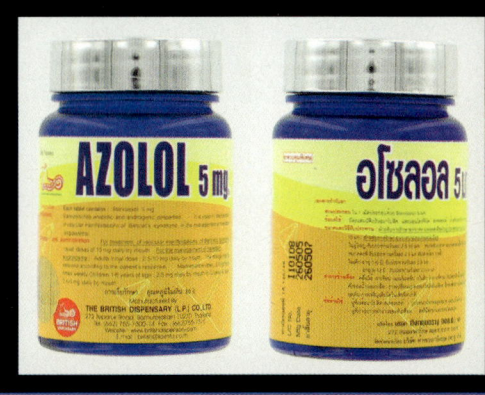   Azolol from British Dispensary (Thailand)

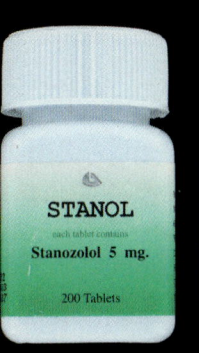

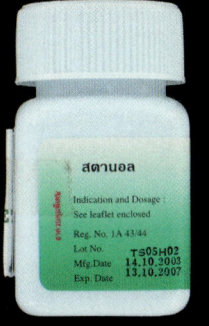

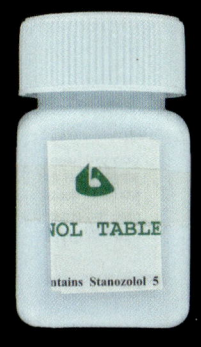

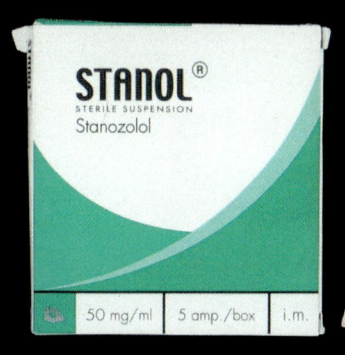

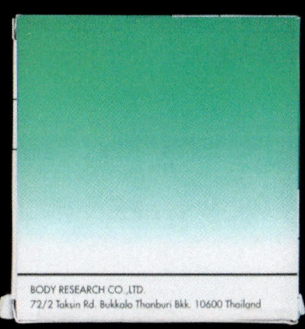

Stanol tabs from Body Research (Thailand)

Body Research Stanol injectable

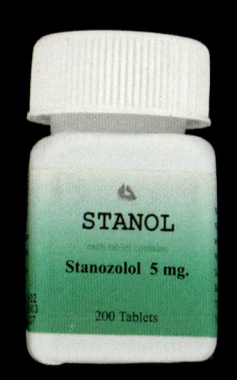

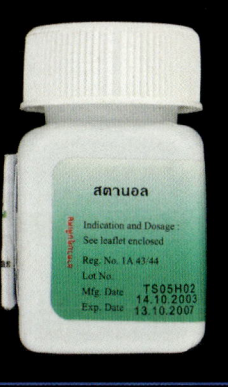

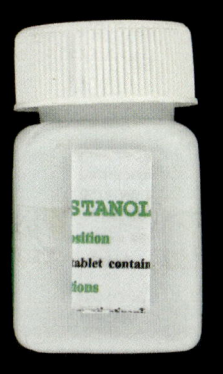

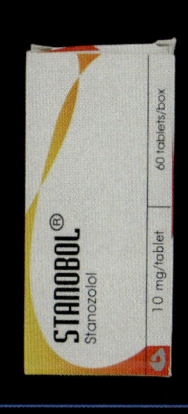

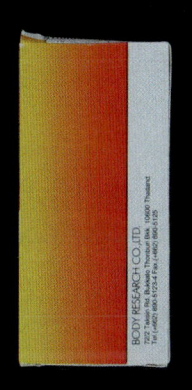

Counterfeit Stanol tabs

Counterfeit Body Research (Thailand)

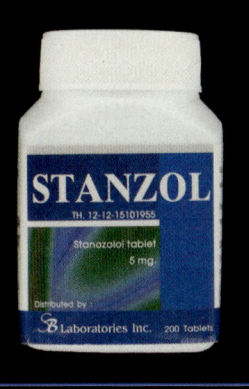

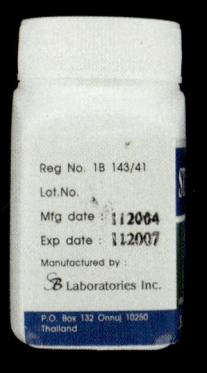

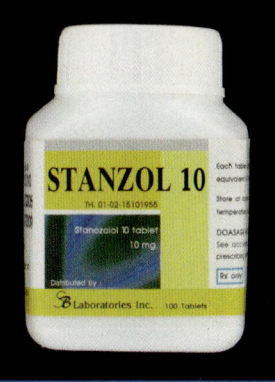

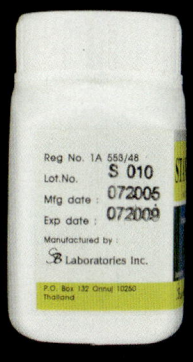

5mg and 10mg tabs from SB Laboratories (Thailand, Underground)

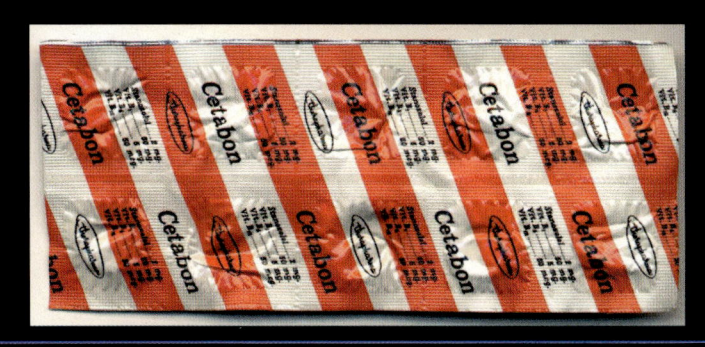

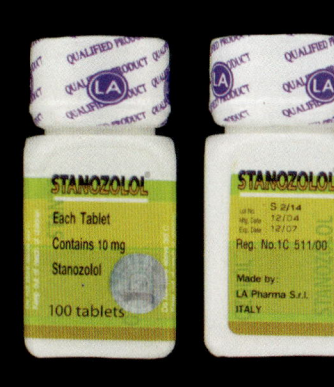

Thai Cetabon tablet strip

LA (Thailand, Underground)

Appendix B

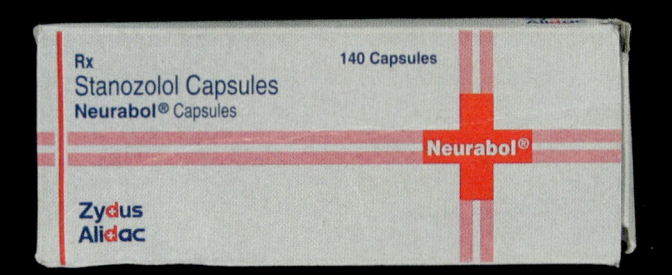

Neurabol tablets (India)

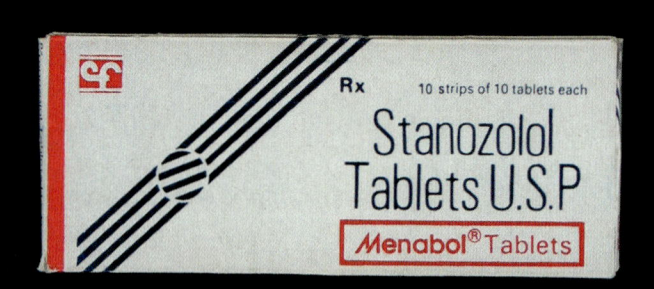

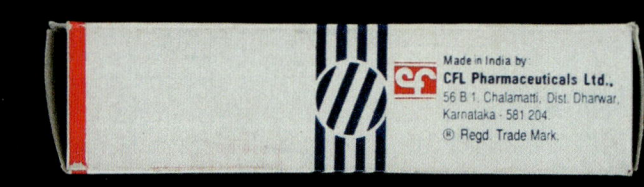

Menabol tablets (India)

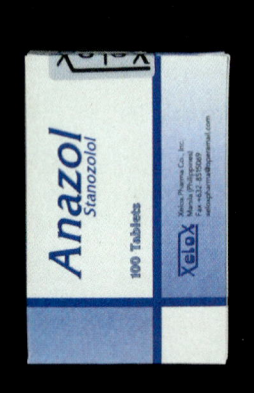

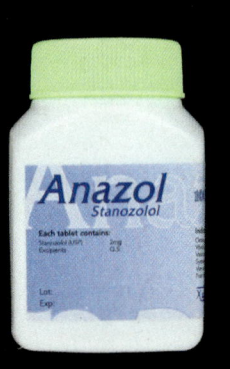

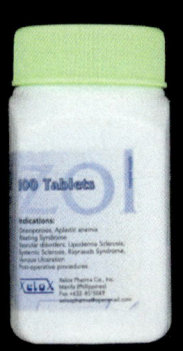

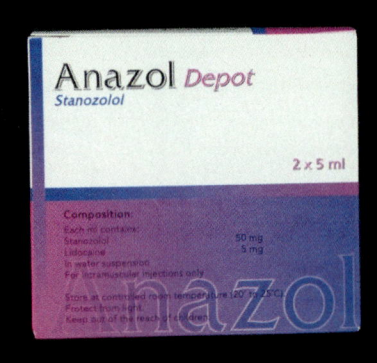

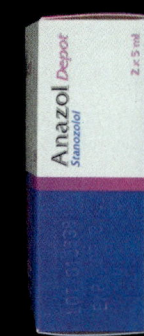

Anazol tablets and injection from Xelox (Philippines)

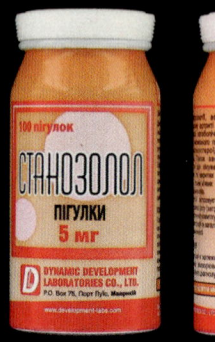

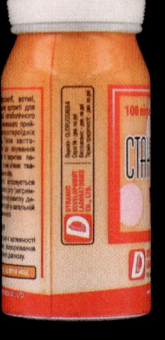

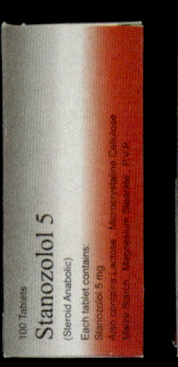

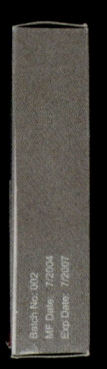

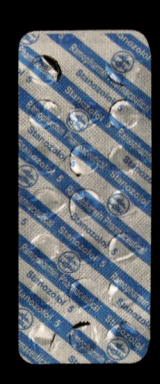

Development Labs (Mauritius, export)   Generic from Ramopharmin (Iran)

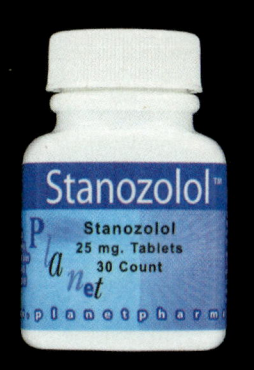

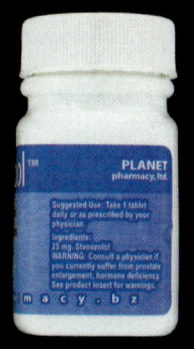

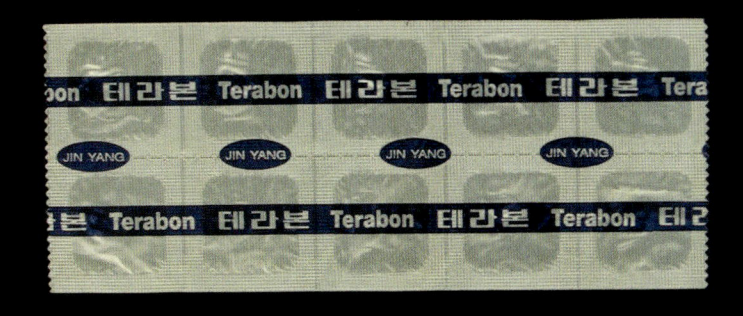

Generic from Planet Pharmacy (Belize) NLM

Terabon tablet strip (Korea)

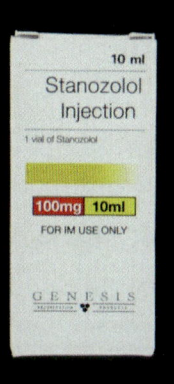

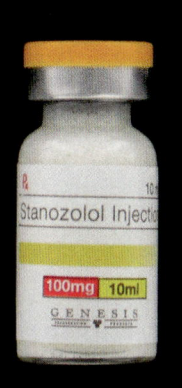

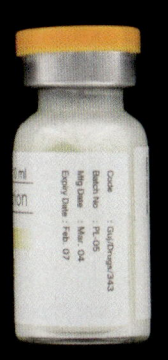

Genesis (Singapore, export) NLM

Ilium Stanabolic (Australia)

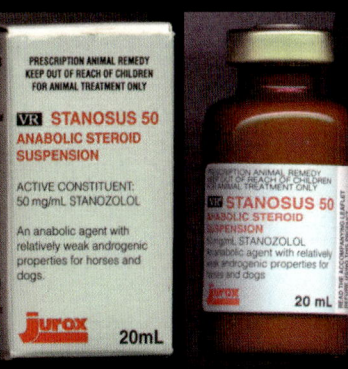

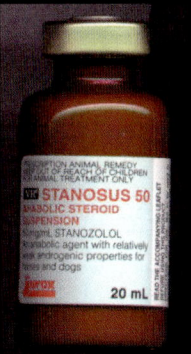

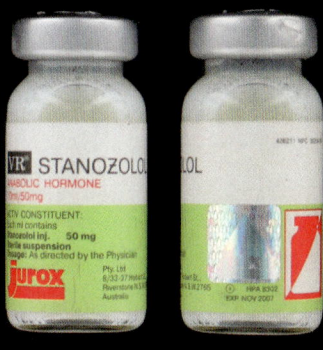

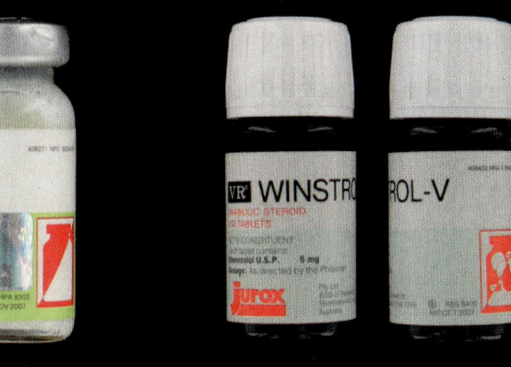

Stanosus from Jurox Australia (NLM)

Counterfeit Jurox stanozolol

Fake Jurox Winstrol tabs

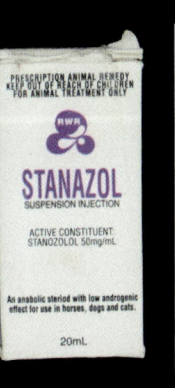

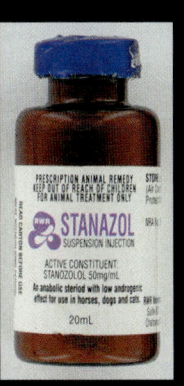

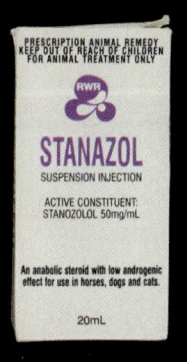

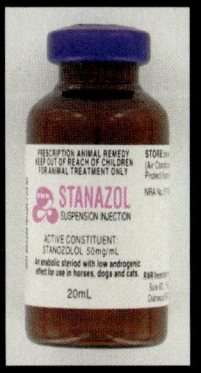

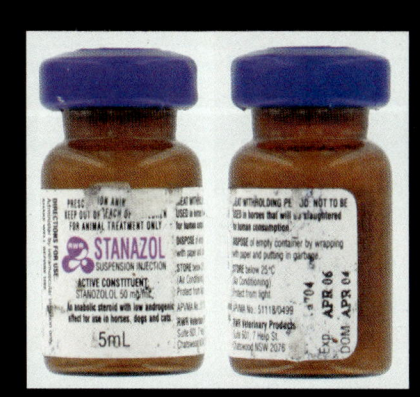

RWR Stanazol (Australia)

Counterfeit box and vial

Another RWR counterfeit

Appendix B

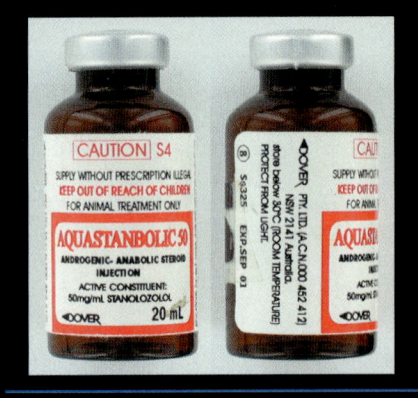

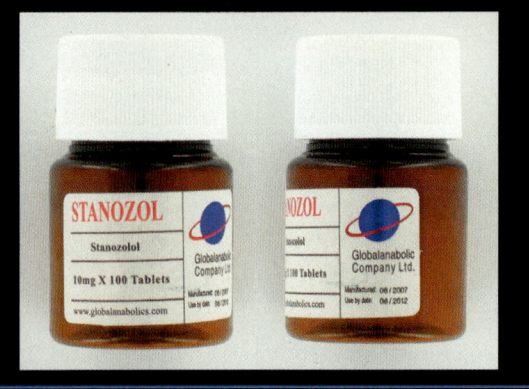

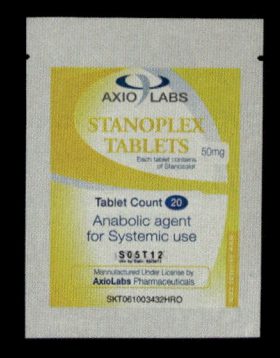

Fake Aquastanbolic (Australia)

Underground products from Global and Axio Labs

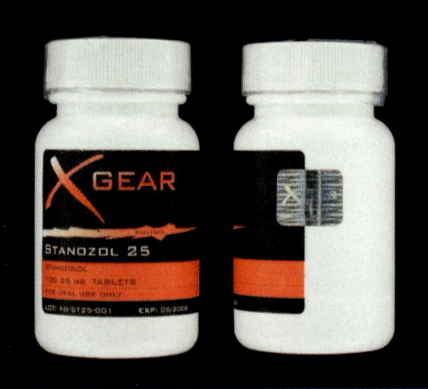

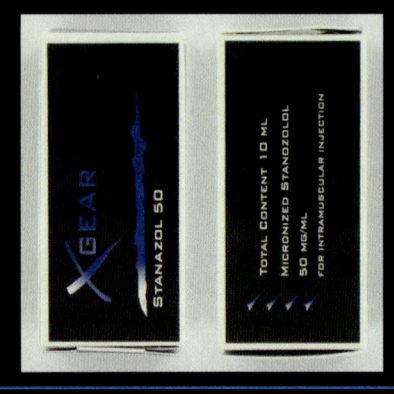

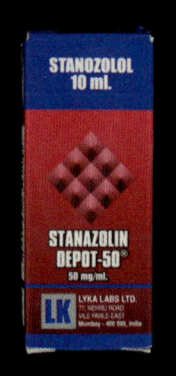

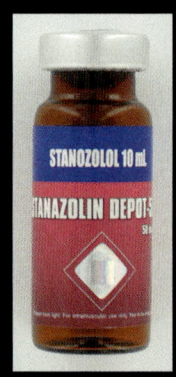

Underground products from X Gear (2) and Lyka

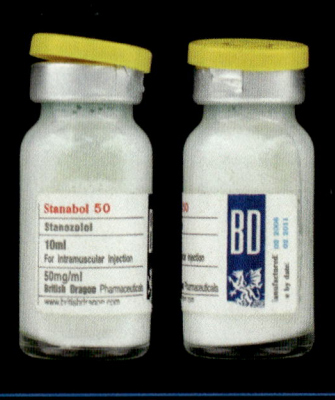

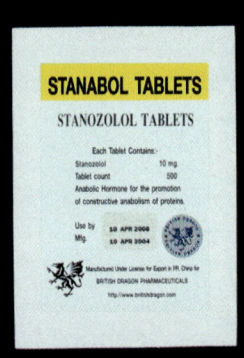

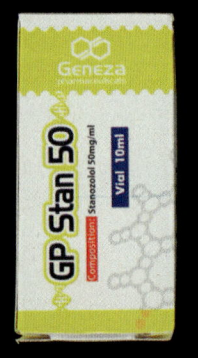

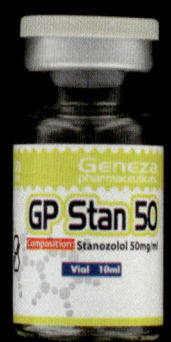

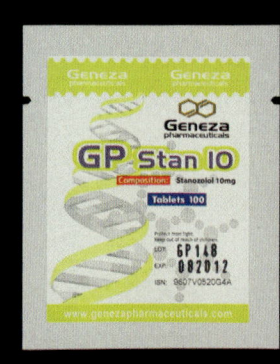

British Dragon Inj and Oral (Underground) NLM

Geneza Inj and Oral (Underground)

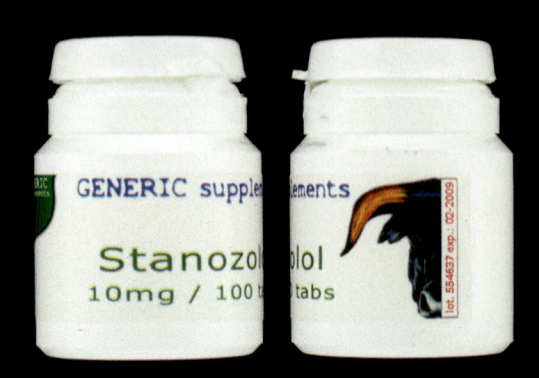

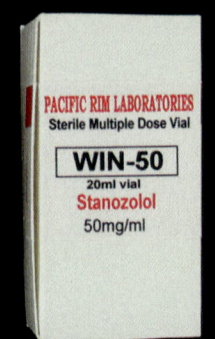

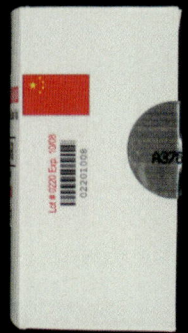

Generic Supplements tablets (Underground)

Win-50 from Pacific Rim (Underground)

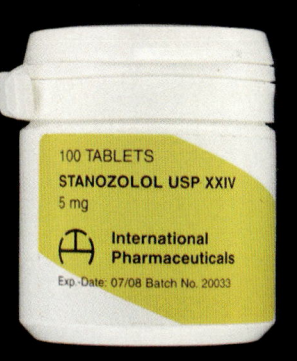

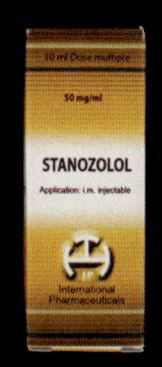

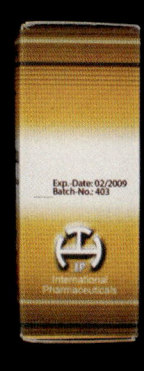

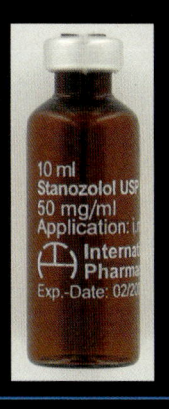

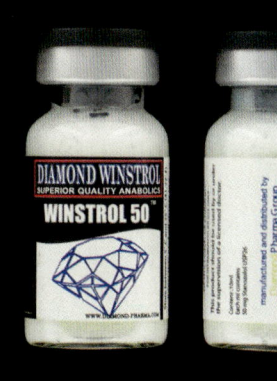

International Pharmaceuticals tabs and 10mL injectable (UG)　　　　Diamond (Underground)

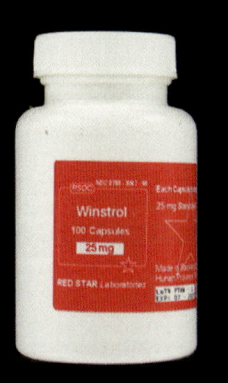

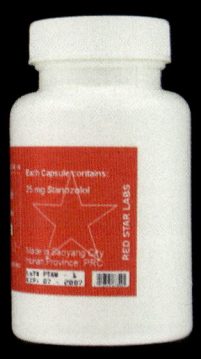

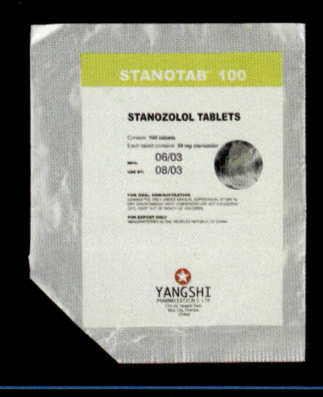

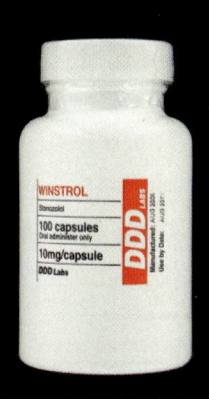

Underground products from Red Star (NLM), Yangshi, and DDD

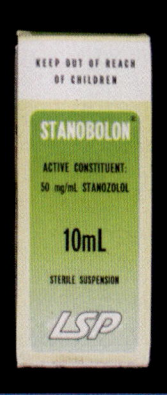

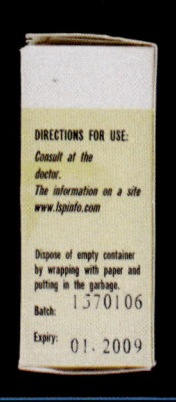

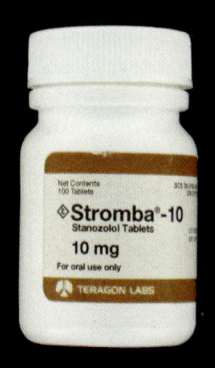

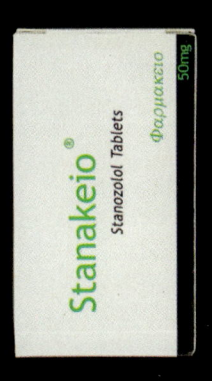

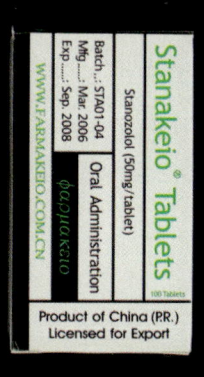

Underground products from LSP, Teragon, and Farmakeio

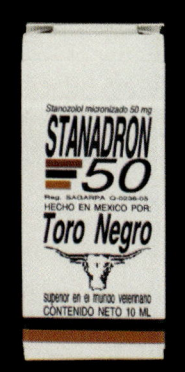

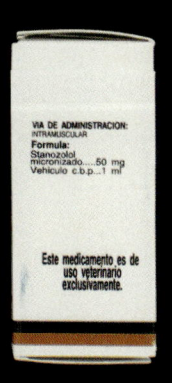

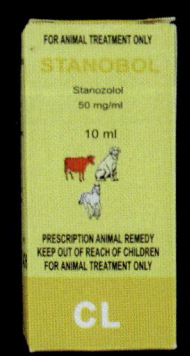

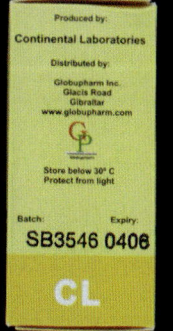

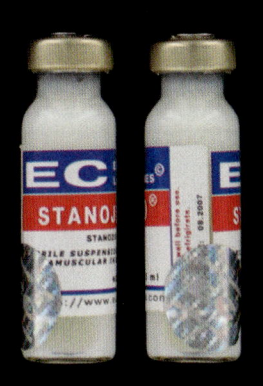

Toro Negro (Underground)　　　　Continental Labs Stanobol (UG)　　　　Eurochem vial (UG)

Appendix B

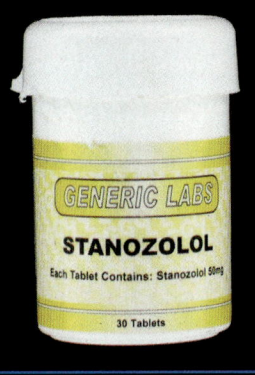

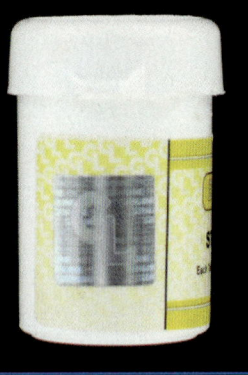

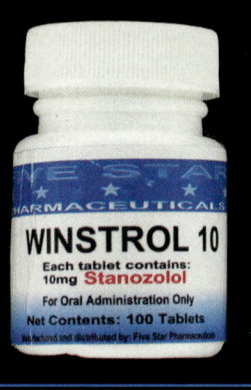

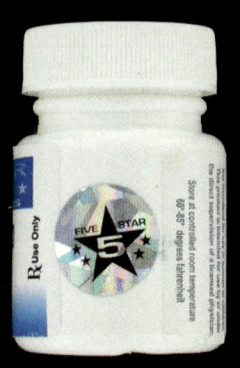

Generic Labs tablets (Underground)

Five Star (Underground)

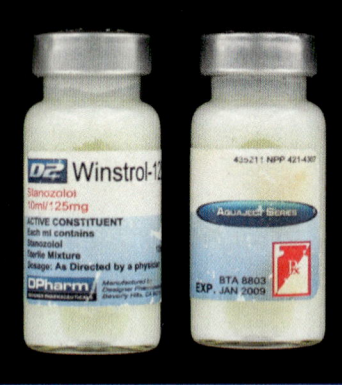

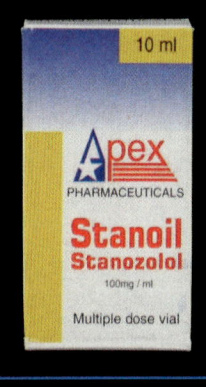

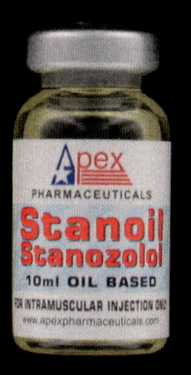

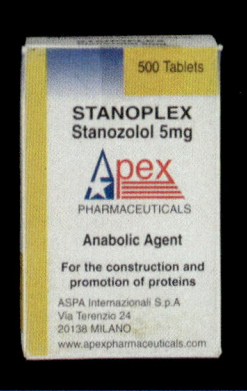

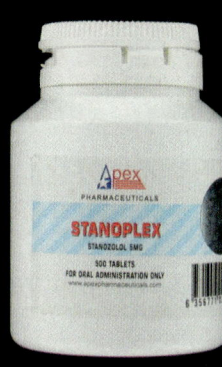

Designer (Underground)

Stanoil from Apex (Underground)

Stanoplex tablets by Apex

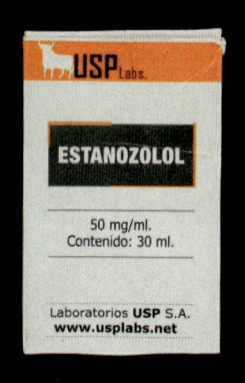

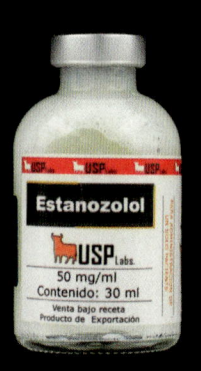

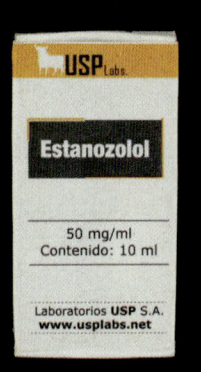

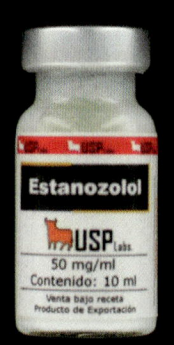

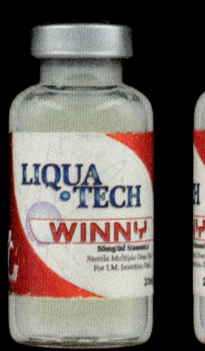

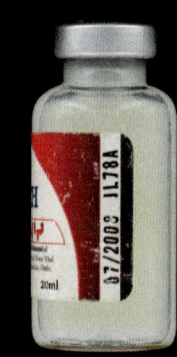

Underground products from USP Labs (2) and Liqui-Tech

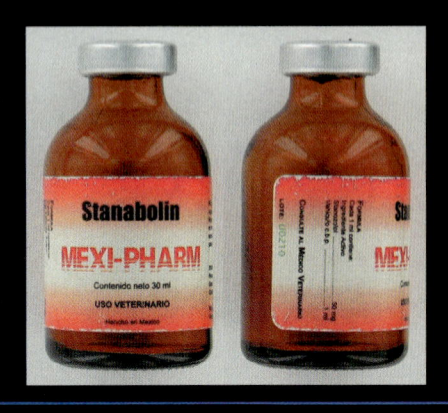

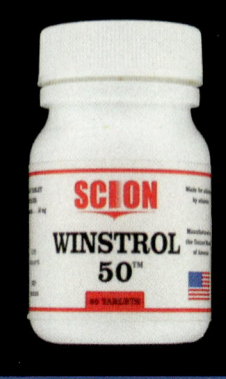

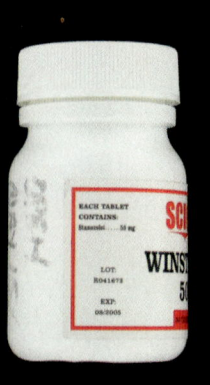

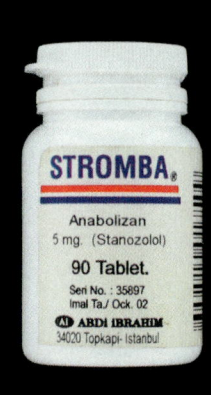

Mexi-Pharm injectable (UG)

Scion (Underground)

Fake Turkish bottle

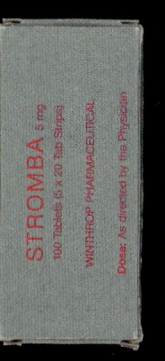

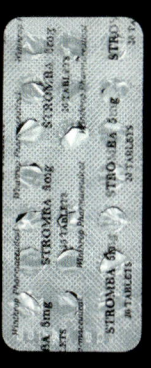

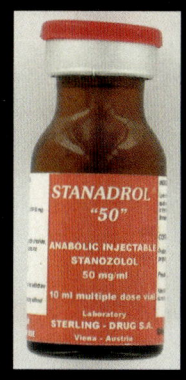

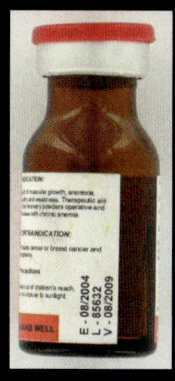

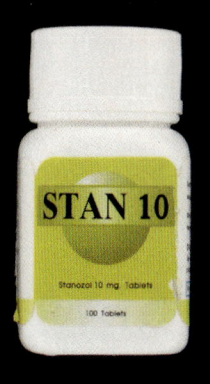

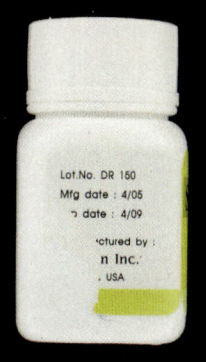

Counterfeit Stromba tabs

Two fake products from Austria and U.S.A.

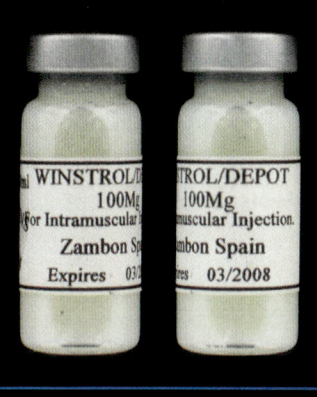

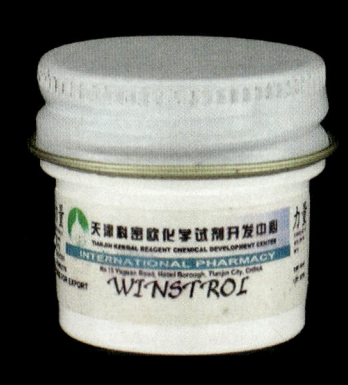

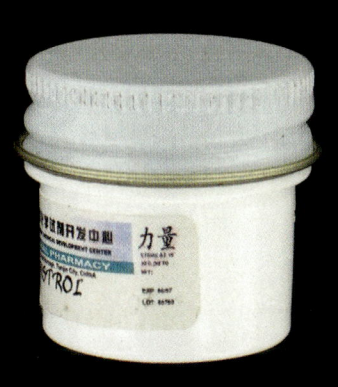

Counterfeit Zambon Winstrol

Int. Pharmacy Counterfeit (China)

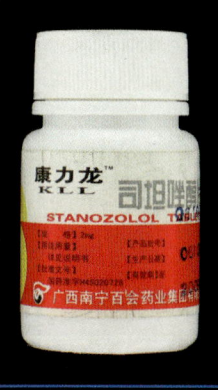

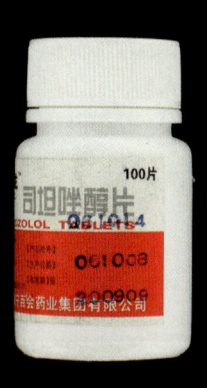

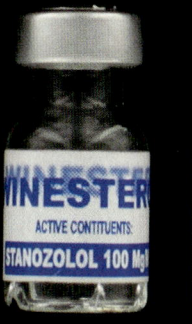

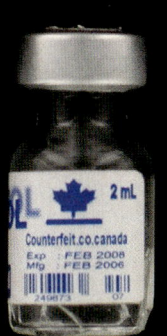

Counterfeit (China)

Fake Canadian "Winesterol"

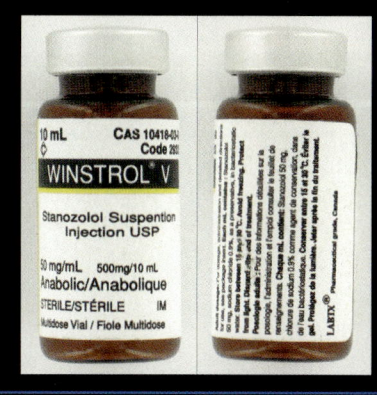

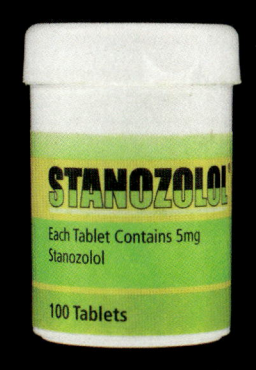

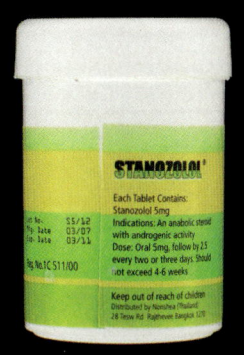

Fake Canadian LabTx Winstrol

Fake Thai generic

Appendix B

B-129

Aldactone

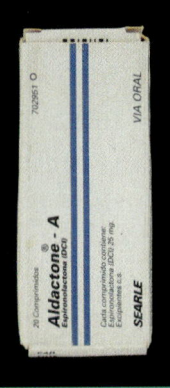

(Spain) 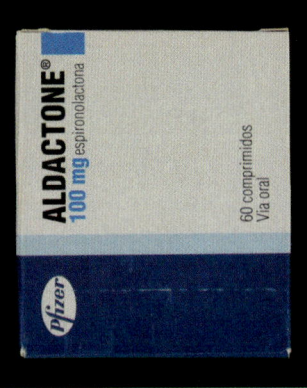 (Portugal) 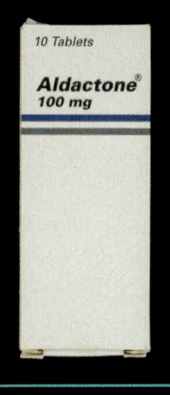 (U.K.) 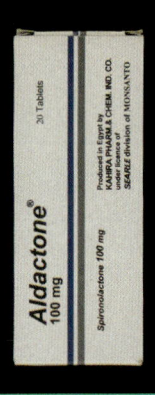 (Egypt)

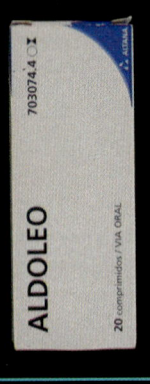

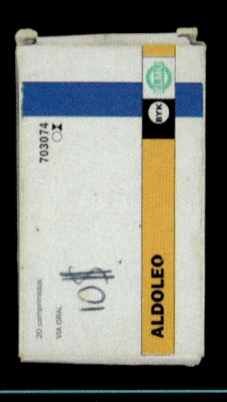

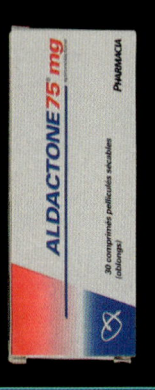

Aldoleo from Spain (old box on right) 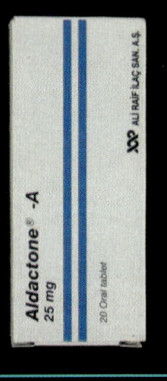 (Turkey) (France)

Arimidex

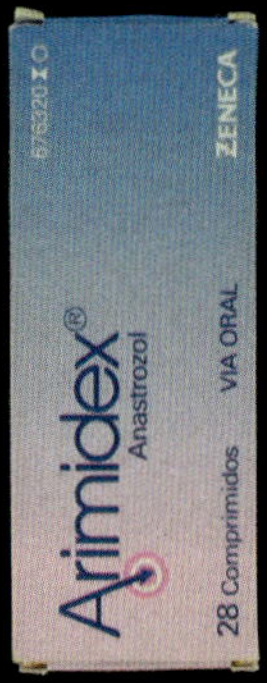

(Spain)

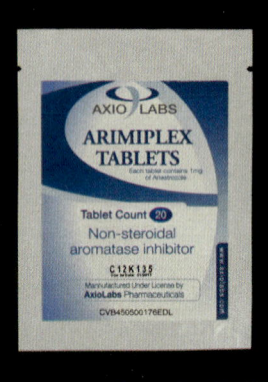

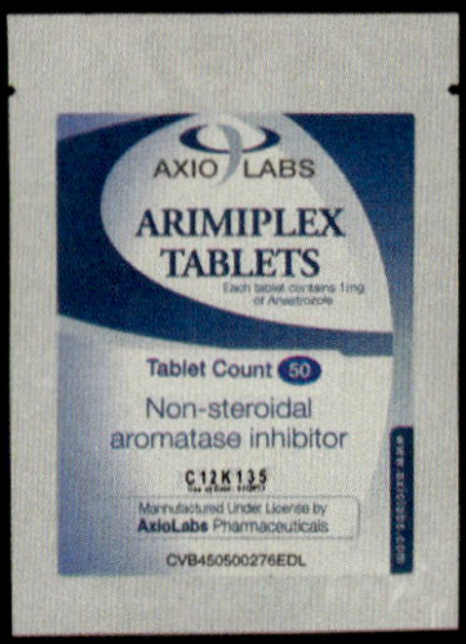

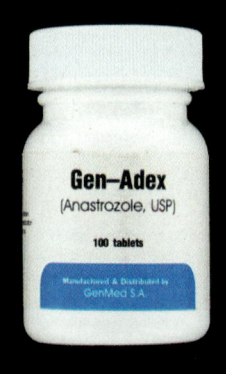

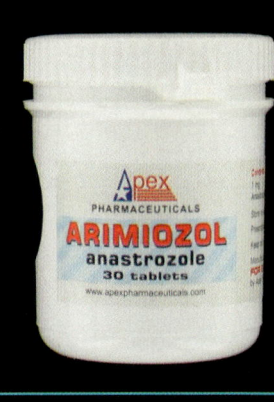

Four different underground preparations containing anastrozole

Avodart

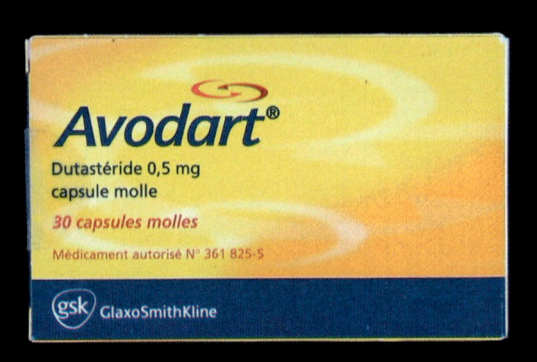

French Avodart

C-1

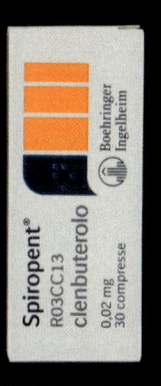

Clenbuterol

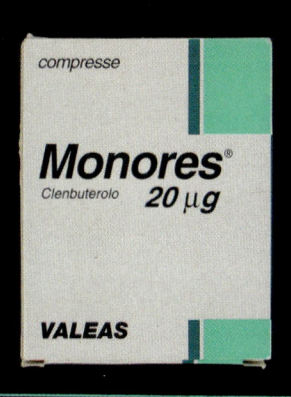

Monores and Spiropent from Italy 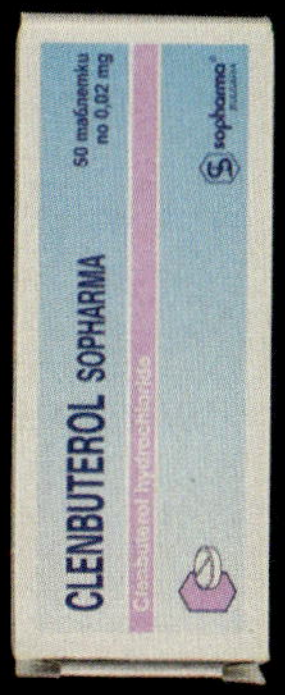   (Bulgaria) 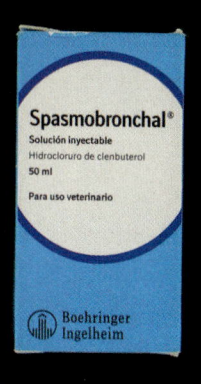   (Germany)

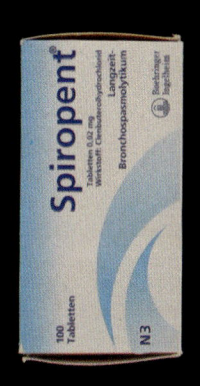

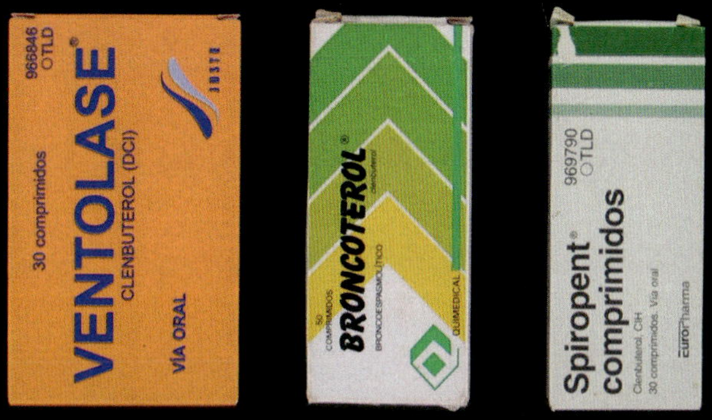

Ventolase, Broncoterol, and Spiropent (Spain) 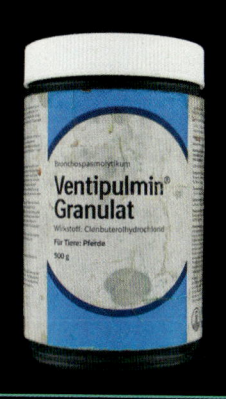   Ventipulmin and Spiropent from Germany

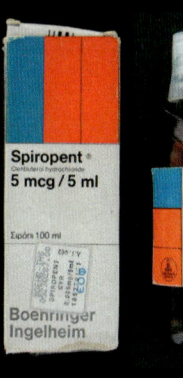

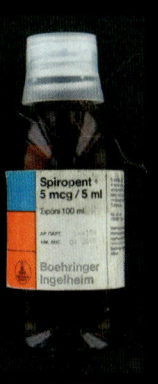

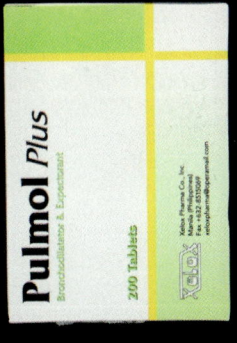

(Greece) 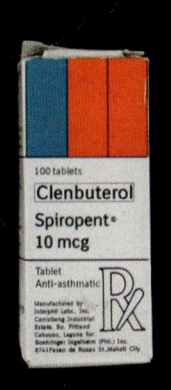   (Thailand) 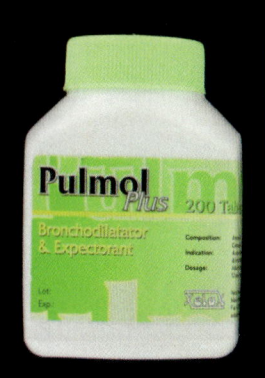   (Philippines) 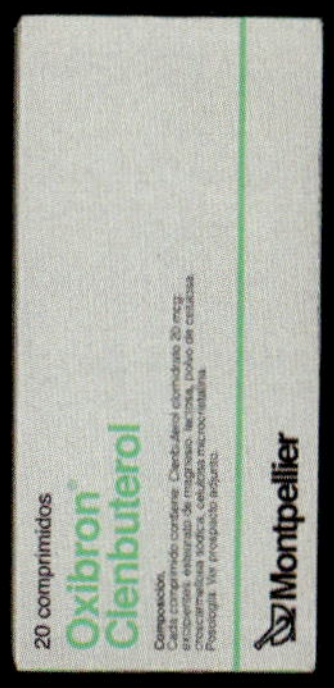   (Argentina)

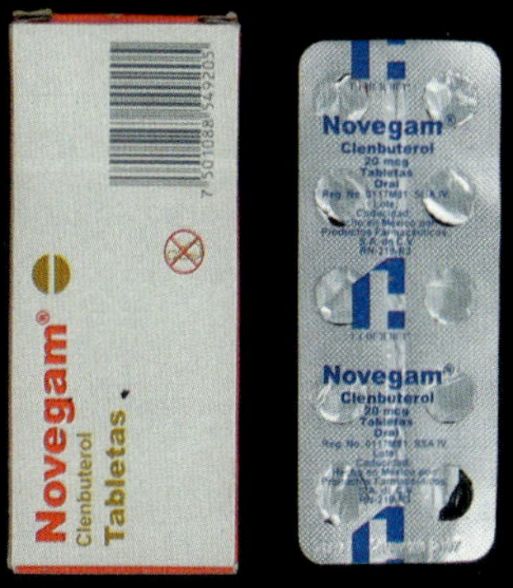

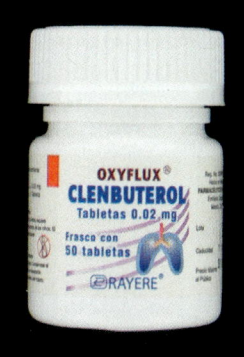

Novegam (Mexico) 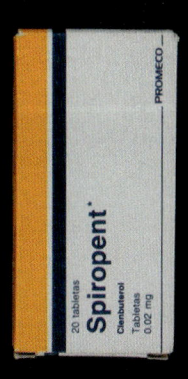   Mexican Spiropent 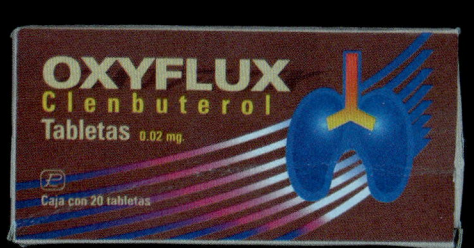   Mexican Oxyflux

Appendix C

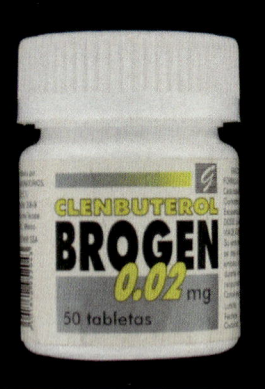

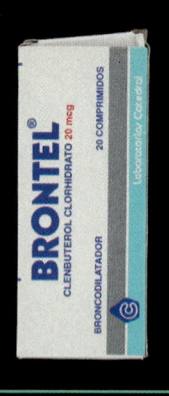

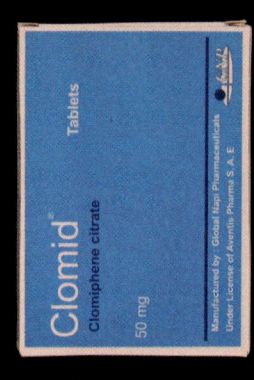

Brogen (Mexico) and Brontel (Brazil) 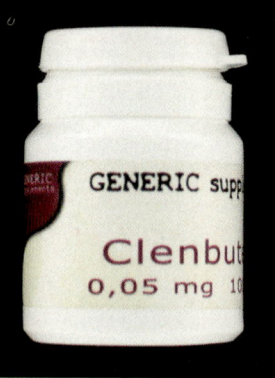 — Generic Supplements (UG) — Clomid from Egypt

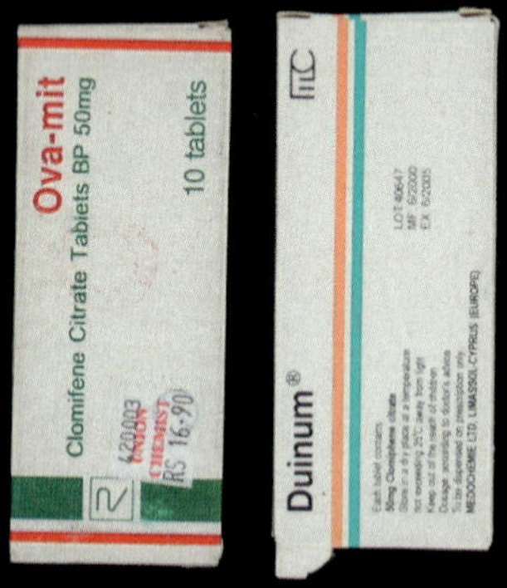

Ovamit and Duinum (Cyprus) 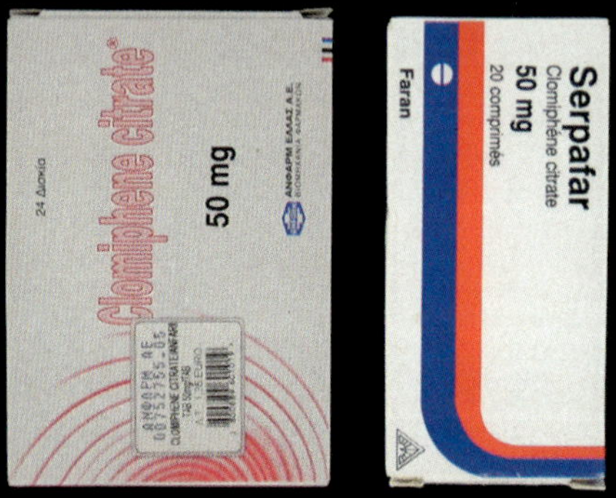 — Generic and Serpafar (Greece) 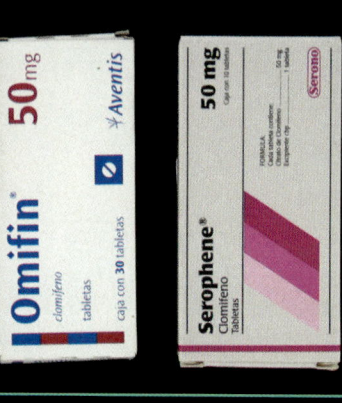 — Omifin and Serophene (Mexico)

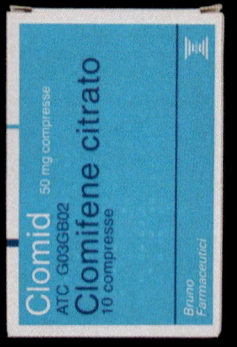

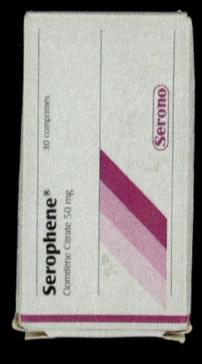

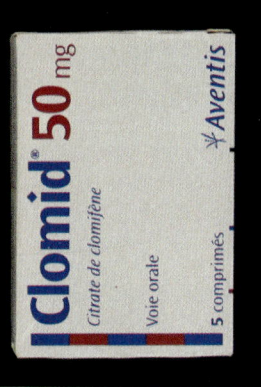

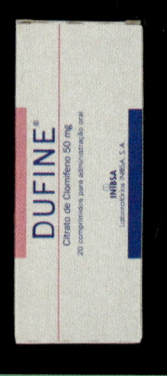

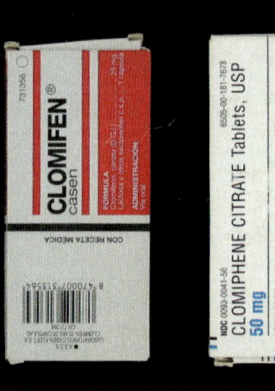

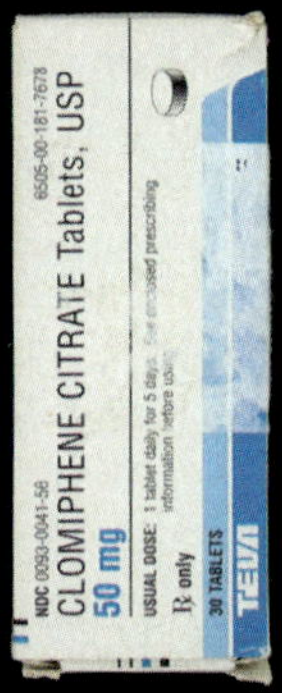

Italian Clomid and Serophene — Clomid and Dufine from Portugal — (Spain) — (Israel)

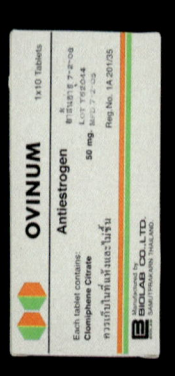

Cyclofenil

(Thailand) — (Turkey) — (Turkey) — (Sweden)

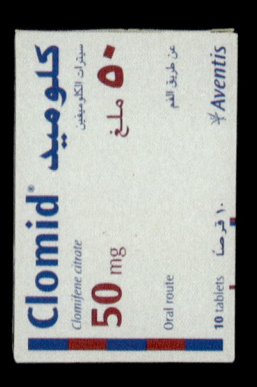

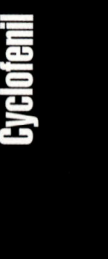

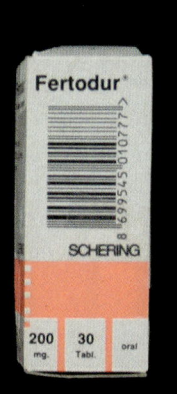

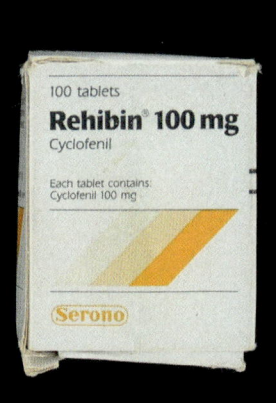

Cytadren

(Spain) (England)

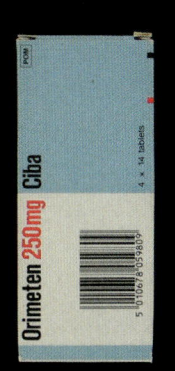

Cytomel

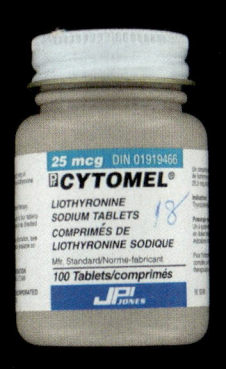

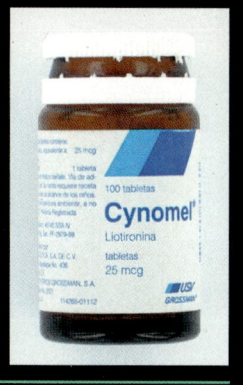

U.S. Cytomel Cynomel (Mexico)

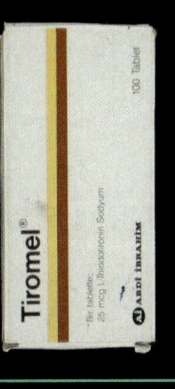

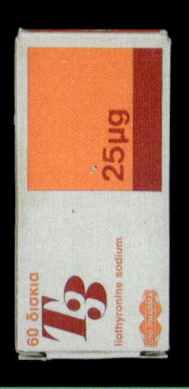

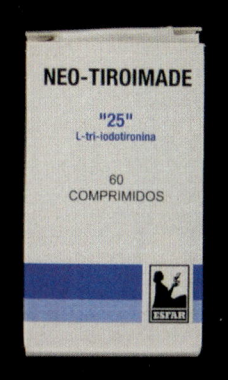

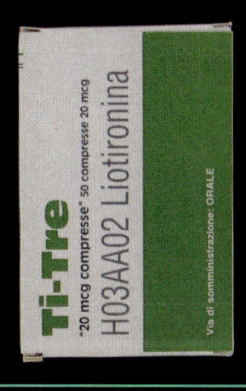

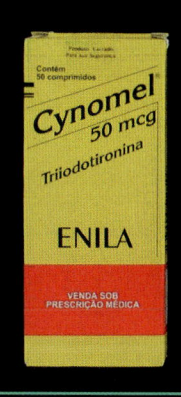

(Turkey) (Greece) (Portugal) (Italy) (Brazil)

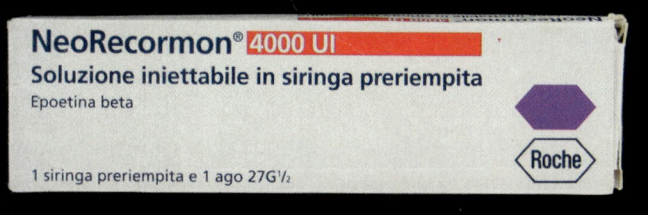

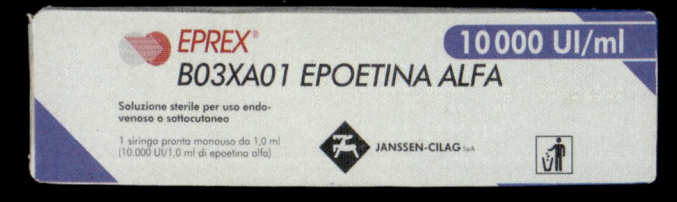

EPO

Two different brands of EPO from Italy

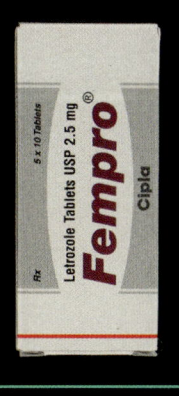

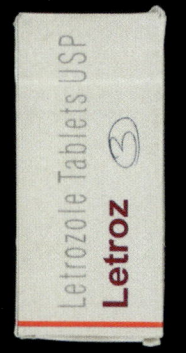

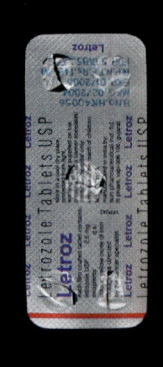

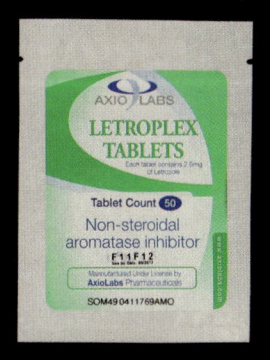

Femara

Fempro (India) Letroz (India) Axio Labs (Underground)

Appendix C

Growth Hormone

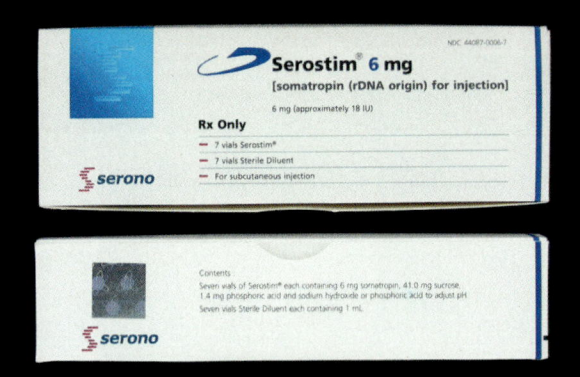

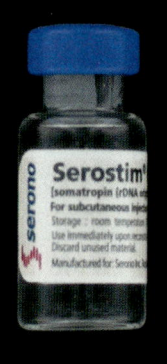

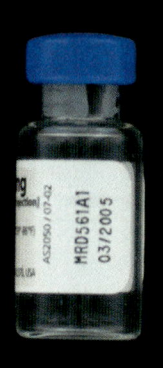

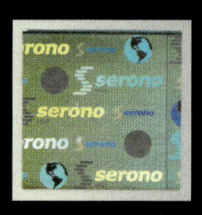

U.S. Serostim

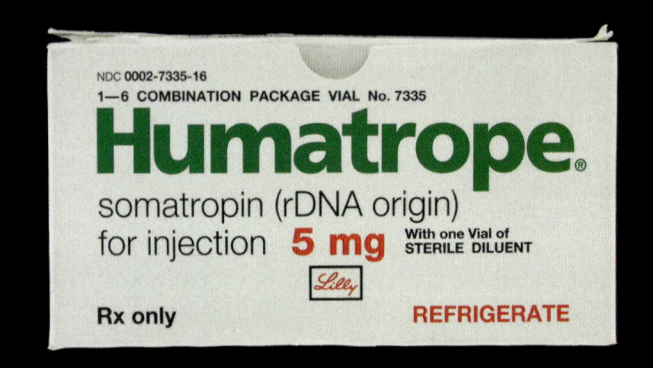

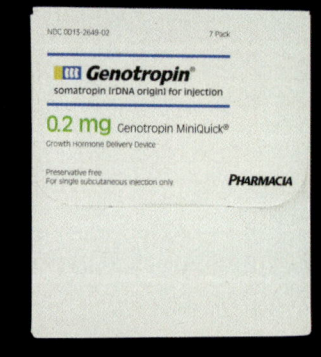

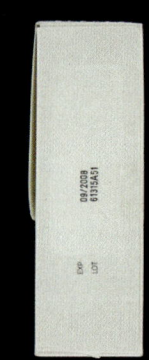

Humatrope (U.S.)

Genotropin (U.S.)

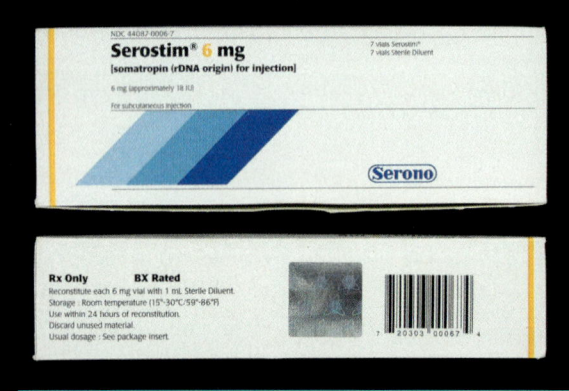

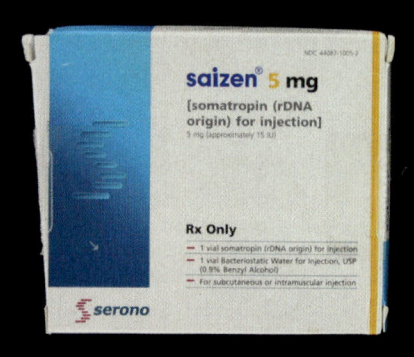

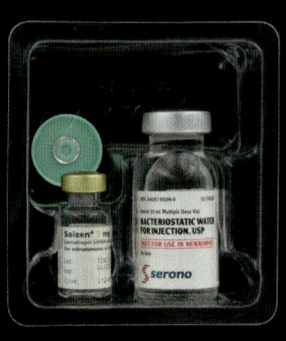

Older U.S. Serostim box

U.S. Saizen

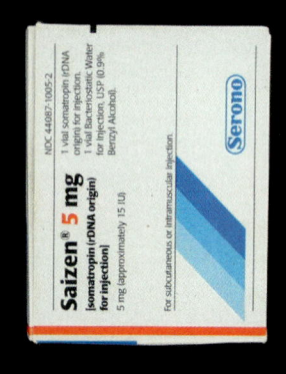

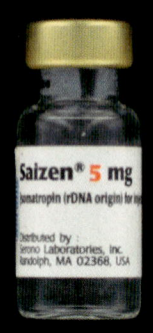

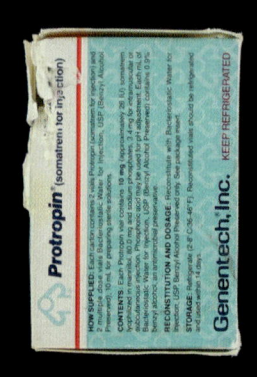

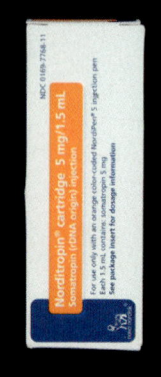

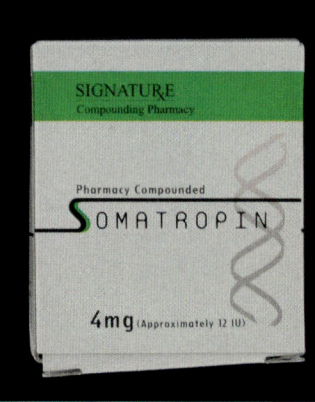

Old U.S. Saizen packaging   U.S. Protropin (somatrem)   (U.S.)   Signature (U.S.) NLM

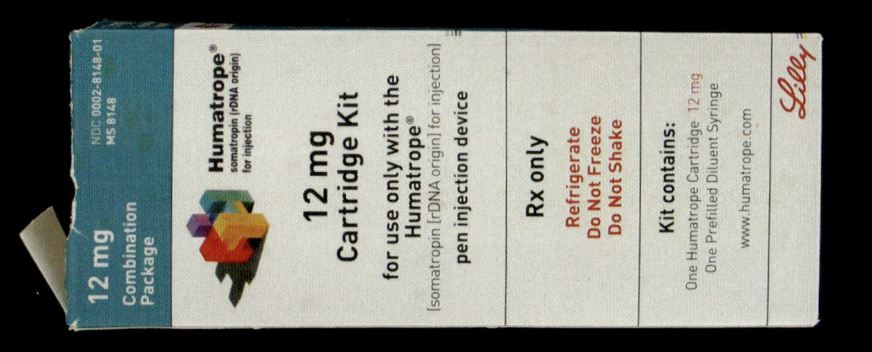

Humatrope 12mg kit (U.S.)

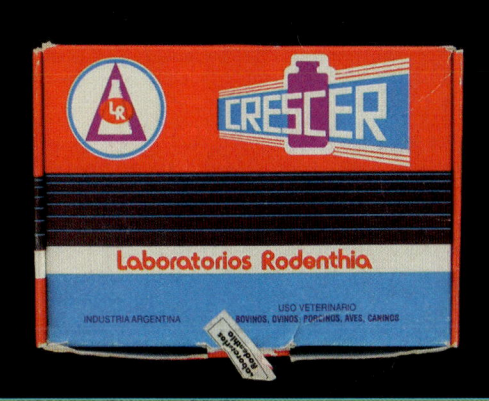

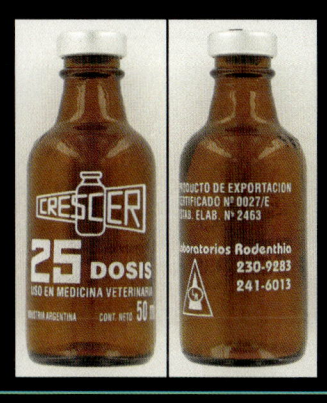

Veterinary GH (Argentina) - Not equivalent to human somatropin

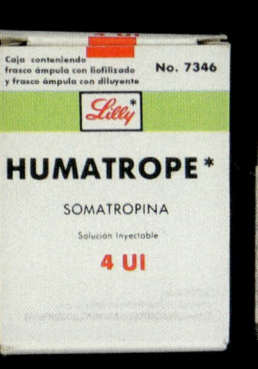

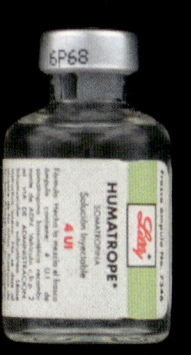

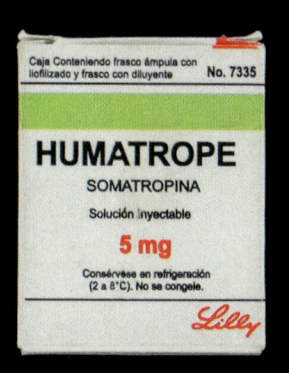

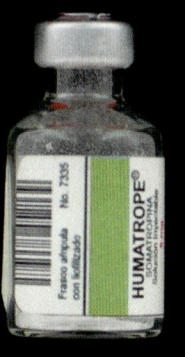

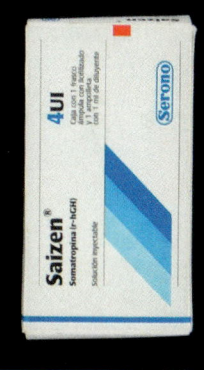

Humatrope (Mexico) · Counterfeit Mexican Humatrope · Saizen (Mexico)

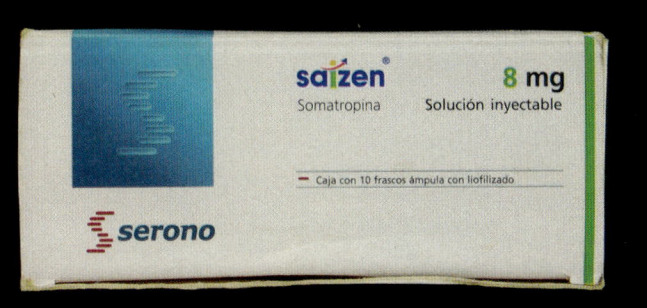

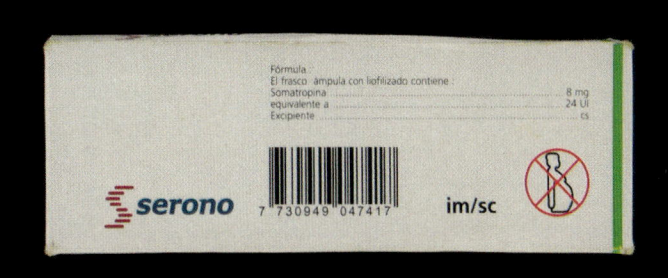

Serono Saizen 8mg (Mexico)

Appendix C

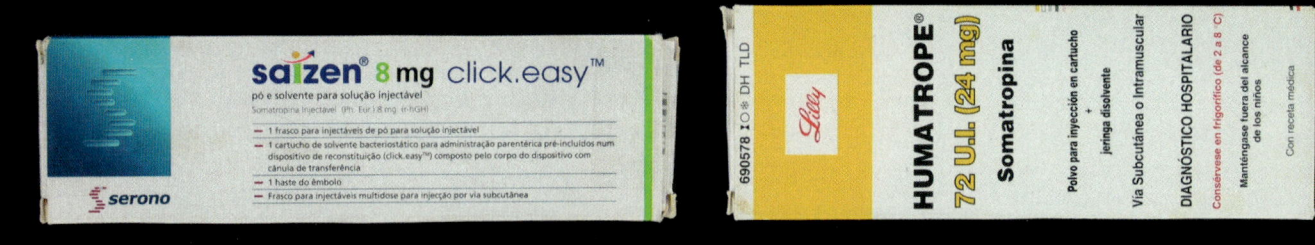

Saizen and Humatrope from Spain

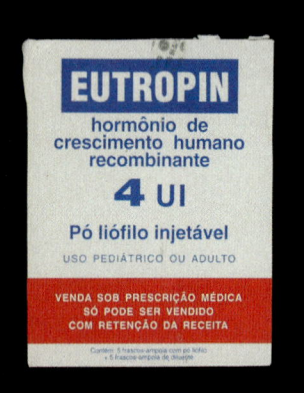

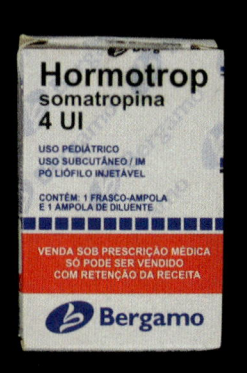

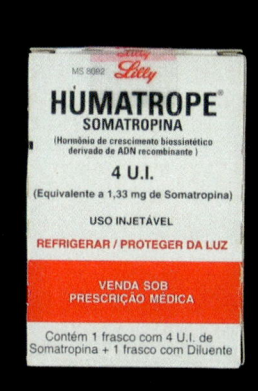

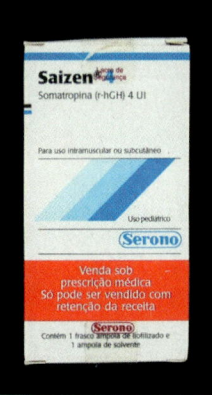

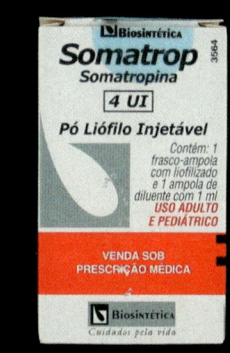

Eutropin, Hormotrop, Humatrope, Saizen, and Somatrop from Brazil

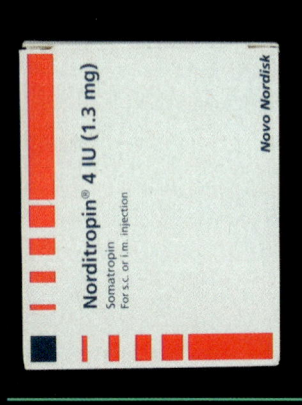

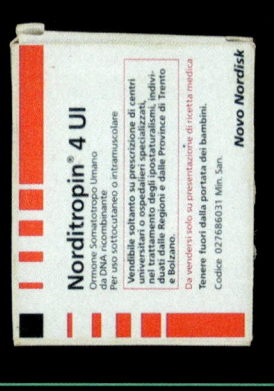

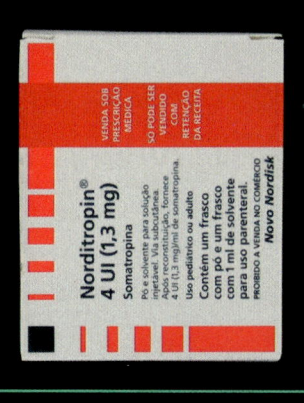

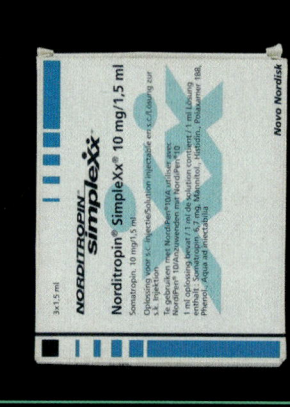

Norditropin from Iran, Italy, and Denmark   Norditropin SimpleXX

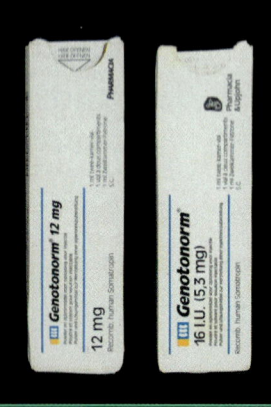

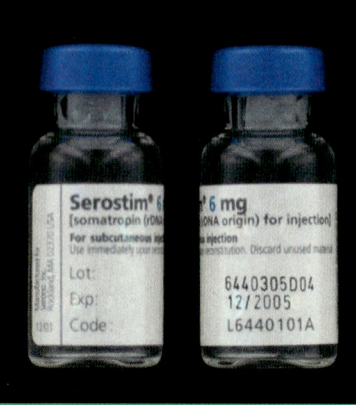

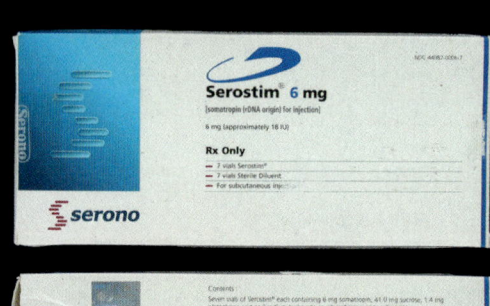

Genotonorm (Belgium)   Serostim from Switzerland

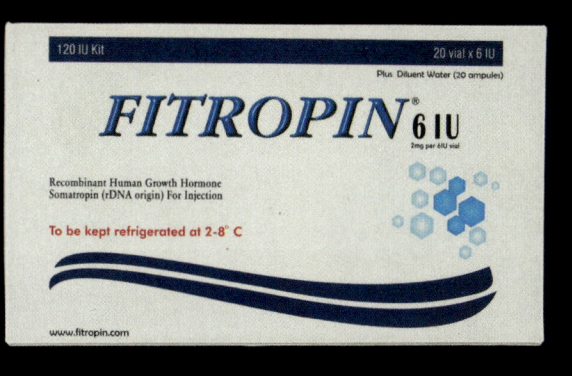

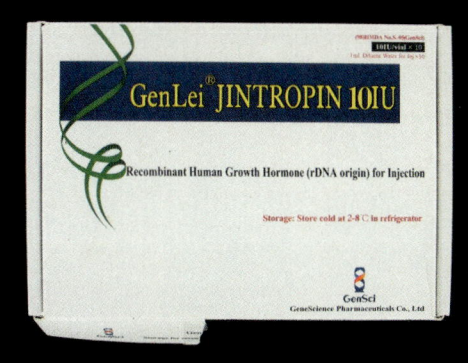

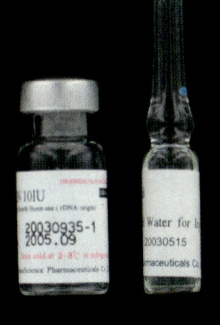

Chinese Fitropin

Jintropin from China (NLM)

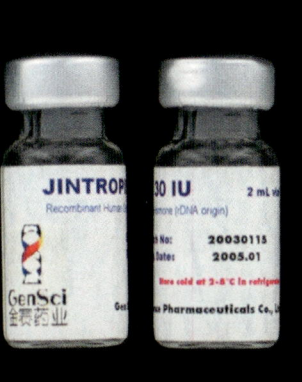

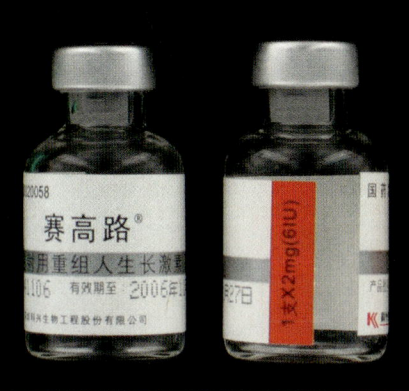

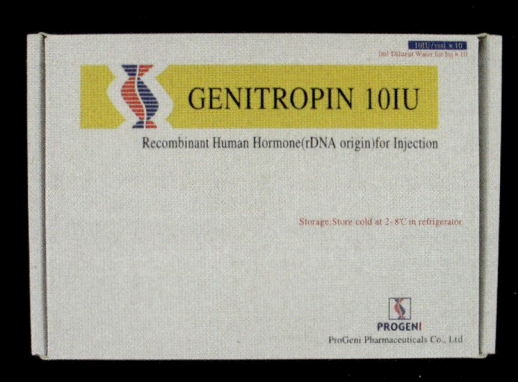

Counterfeit Jintropin

Kexing GH (China)

Genitropin (China)

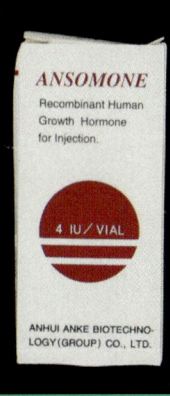

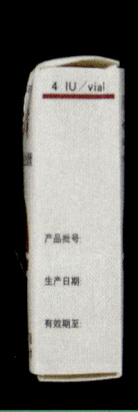

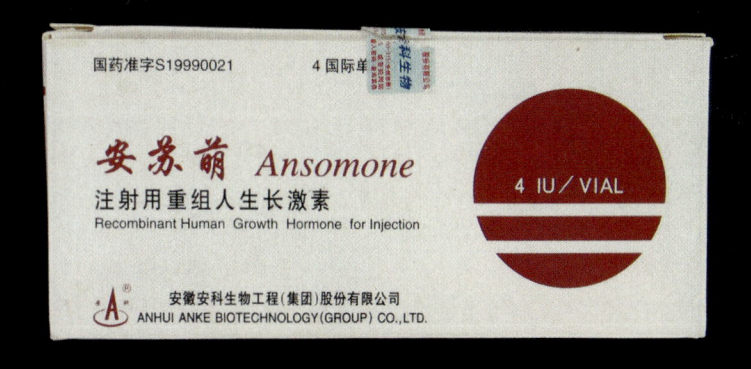

Ansomone (China)

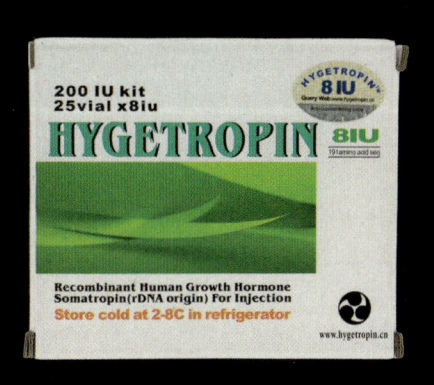

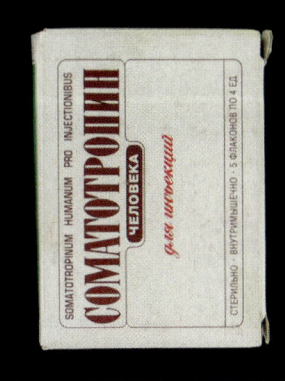

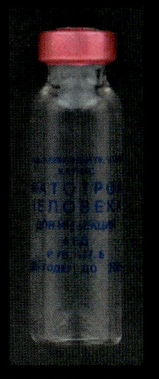

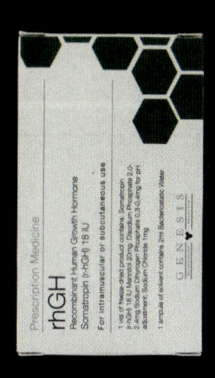

Hygetropin (China)

Russian GH

GH from Genesis (Singapore)

Appendix C

HCG

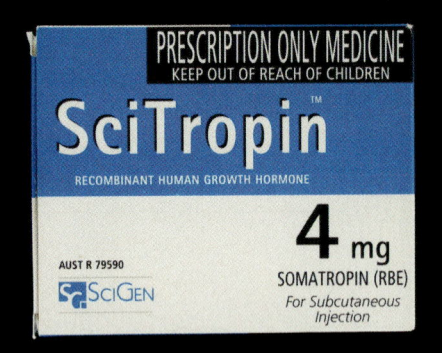

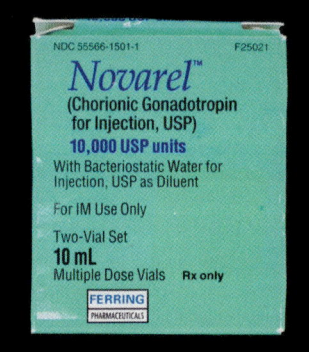

SciTropin (Australia)

U.S. Novarel

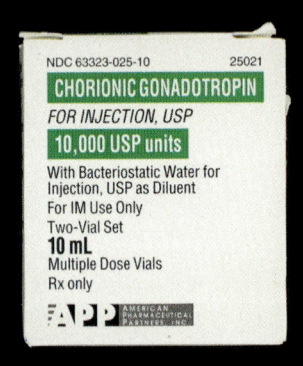

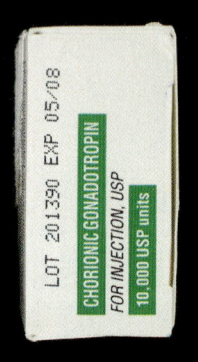

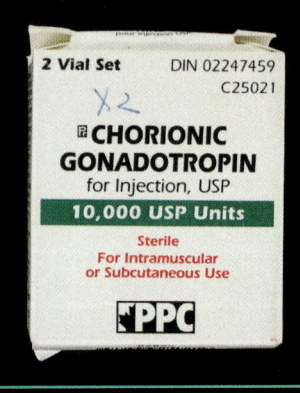

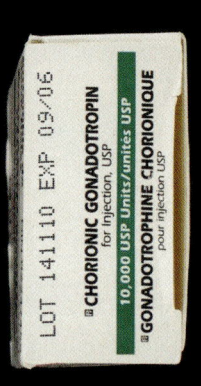

APP generic (U.S.)

PPC generic (Canada)

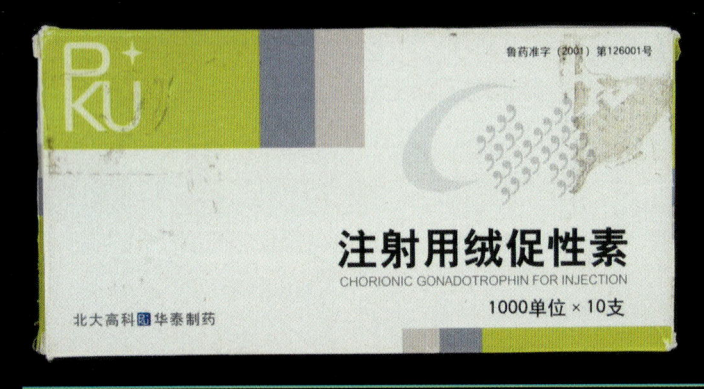

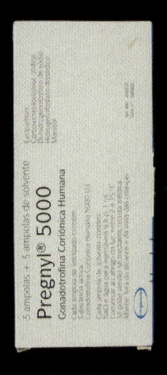

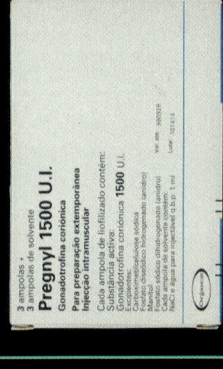

HCG from China

Two boxes from Portugal

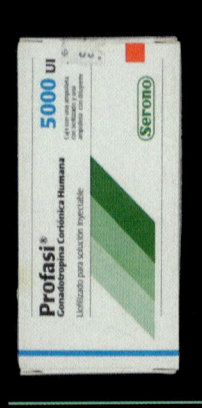

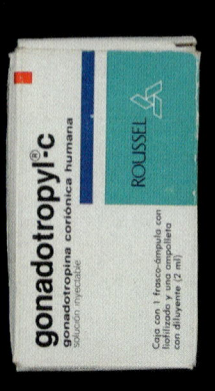

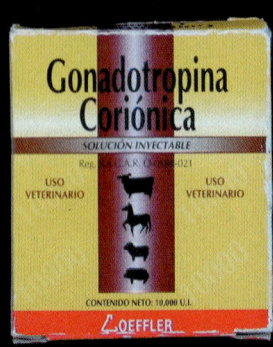

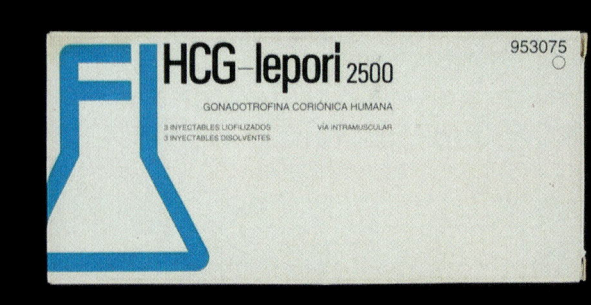

Three different brands from Mexico

HCG-Lepori (Spain)

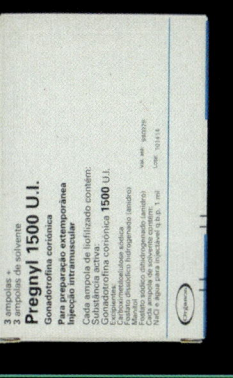

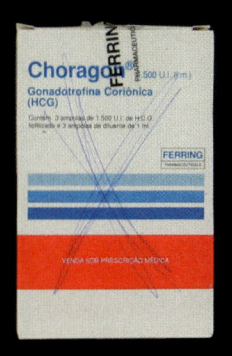

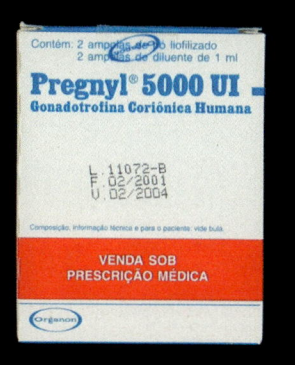

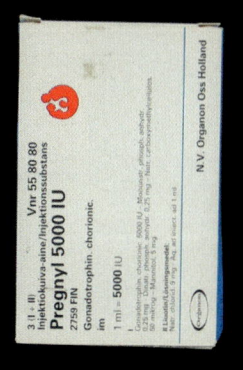

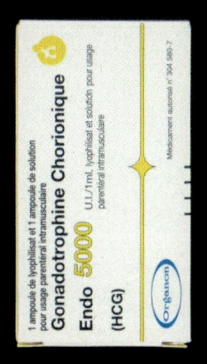

(Greece) — Choragon and Pregnyl from Brazil — (Estonia) — (France)

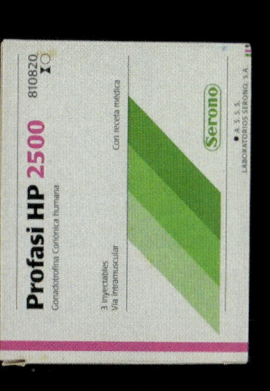

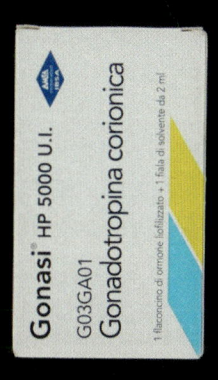

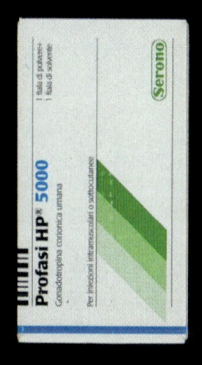

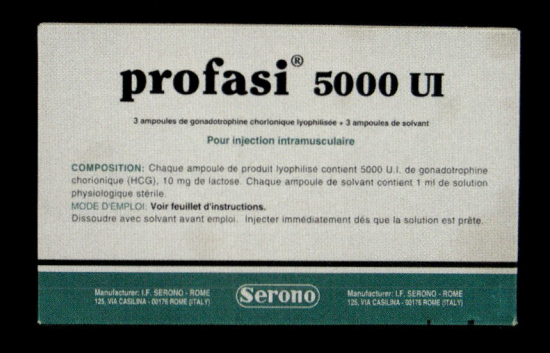

(Spain) — Gonasi, and two different boxes of Profasi from Italy

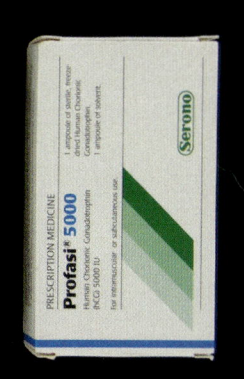

Insulin

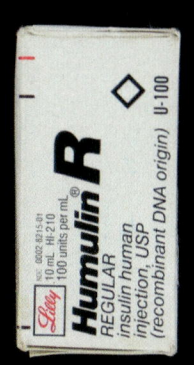

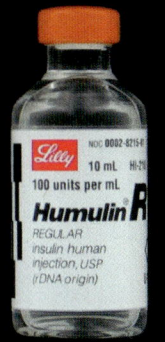

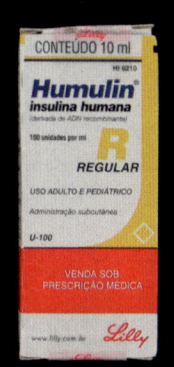

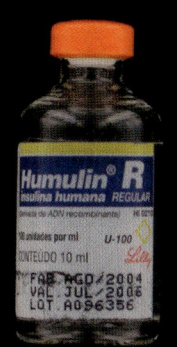

(Switzerland) — U.S. Humulin — Humulin from Brazil

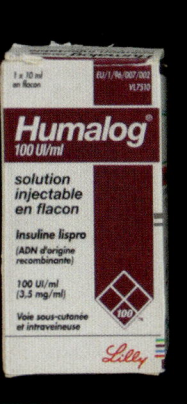

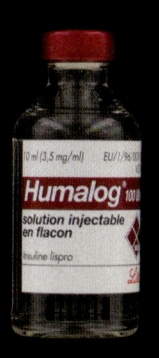

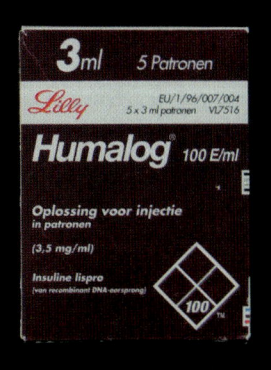

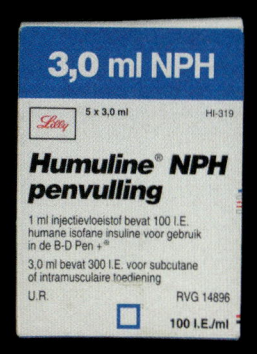

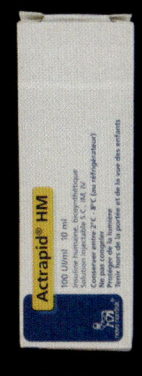

Humalog (France) — Humalog and Humuline from Lilly — (Tunisia)

Appendix C

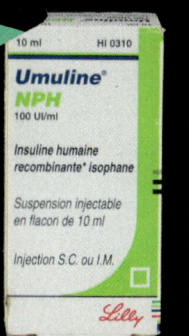

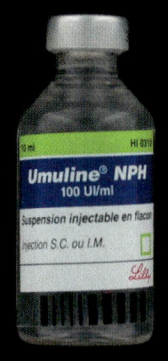

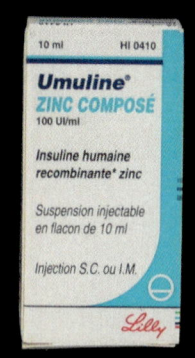

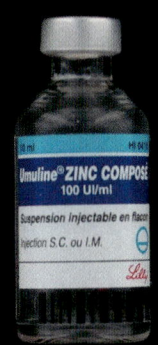

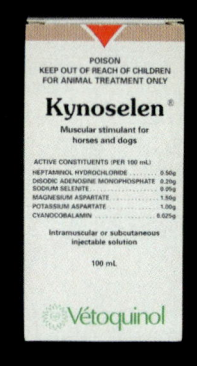

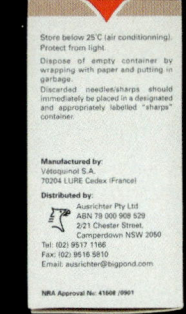

Two versions of French Humuline

Kynoselen (U.K.)

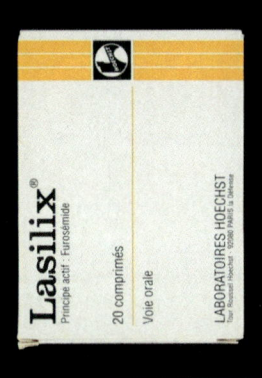

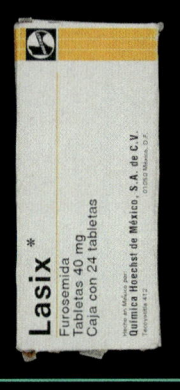

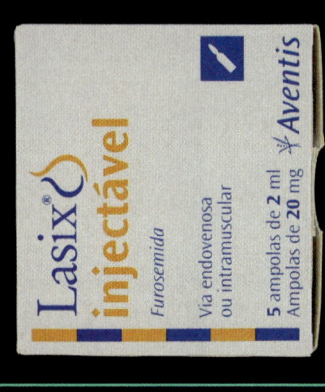

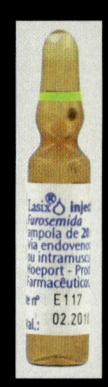

Lasix

(France)

(Mexico)

(Portugal)

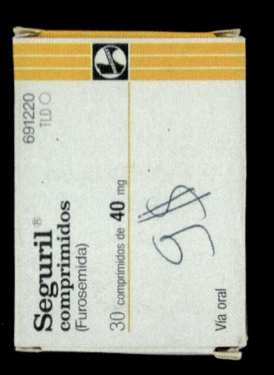

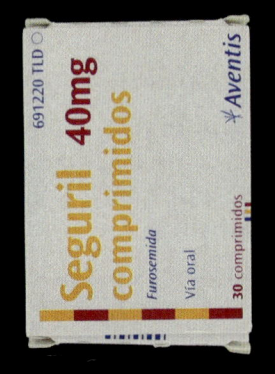

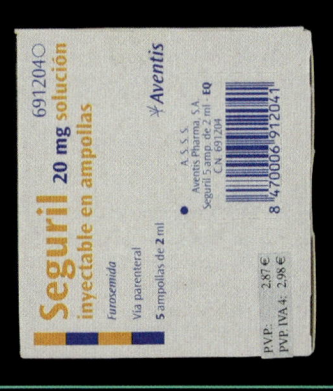

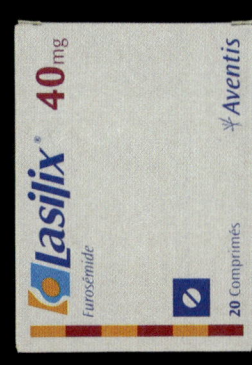

Three different boxes from Spain

Lasix from Tunisia

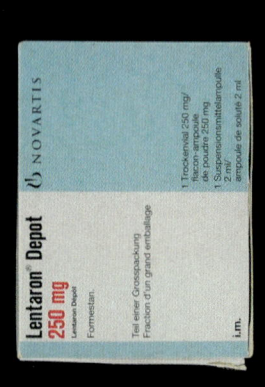

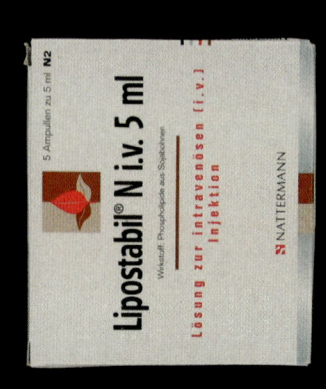

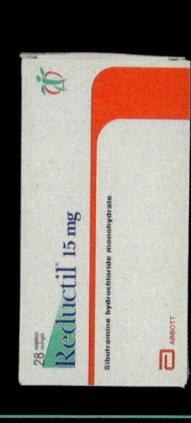

Lentaron

Lentaron Depot from Novartis

Lipostabil

Lipostabil N from Germany

Meridia

(Greece)

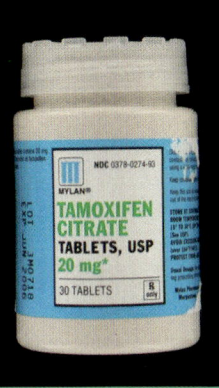

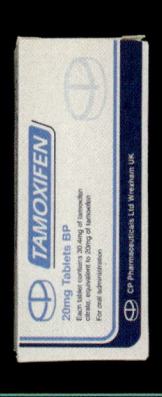

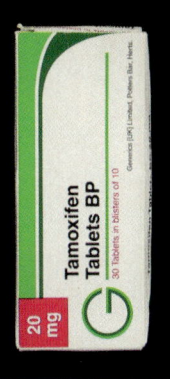

Nolvadex

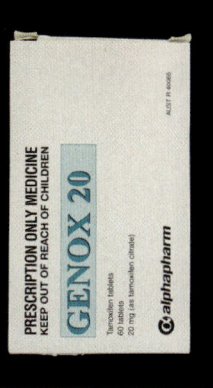

U.S. generic   (U.K.)   (Australia)   (U.K.)

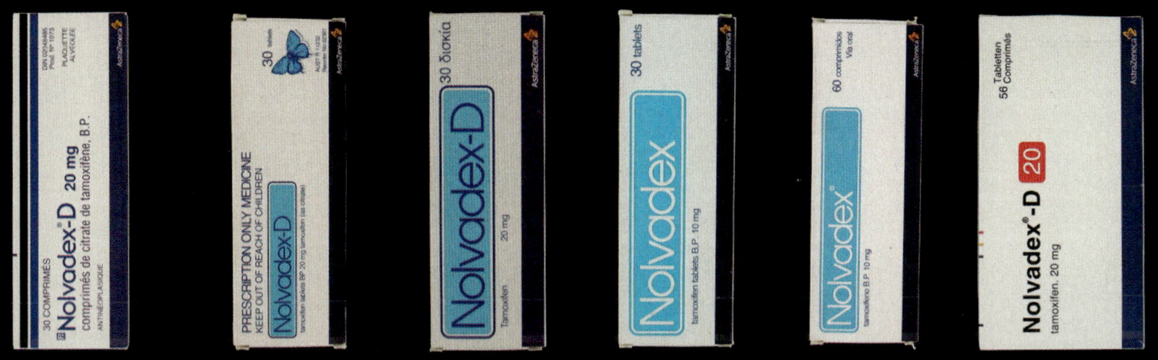

AstraZeneca Nolvadex from Canada, Australia, Greece, U.K., Portugal, and Belgium

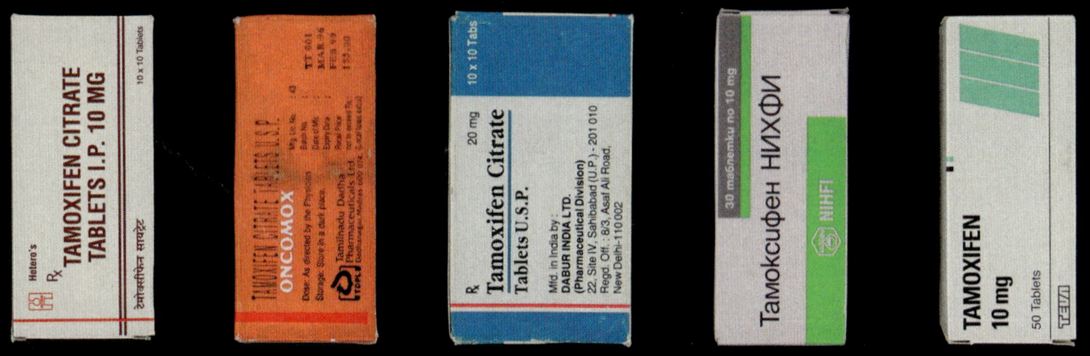

Three different brands from India   (Bulgaria)   (Israel)

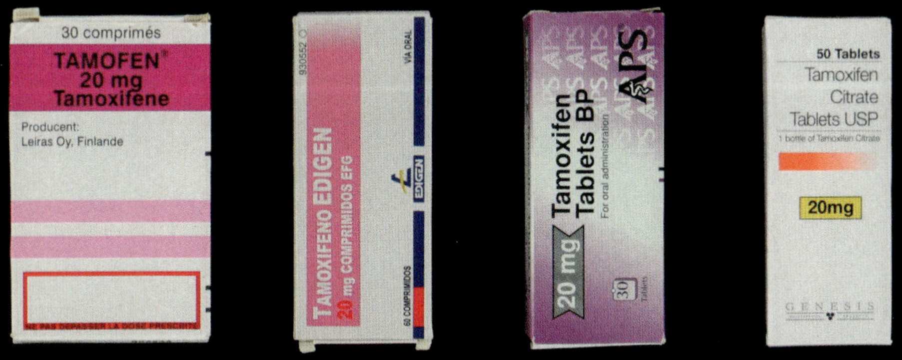

Tamofen from Finland, Tamoxifeno Edigen from Spain, APS Generic, and Genesis Generic (Singapore)

Appendix C

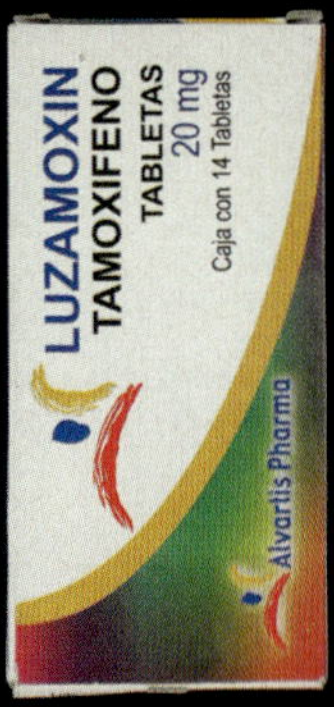

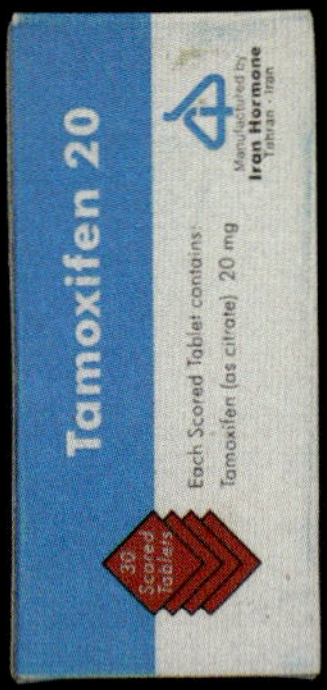

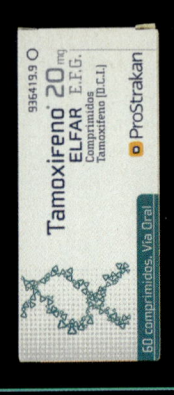

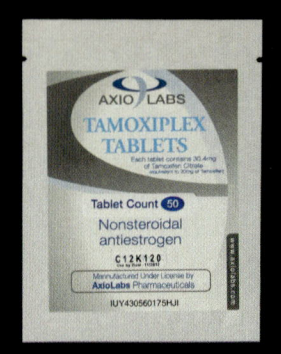

(Mexico) (Iran) (Spain) Axio Labs (Underground)

Parlodel

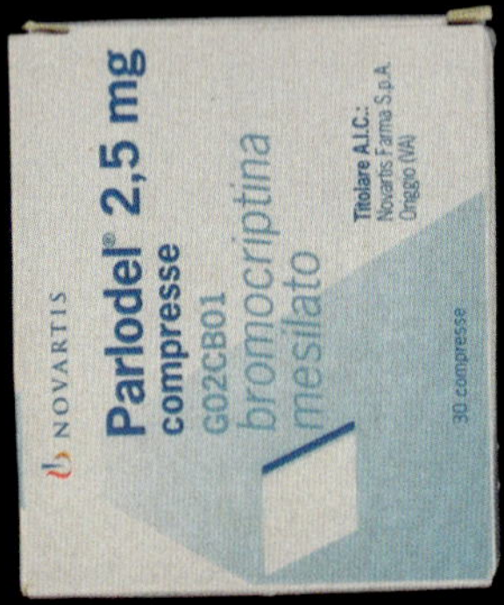

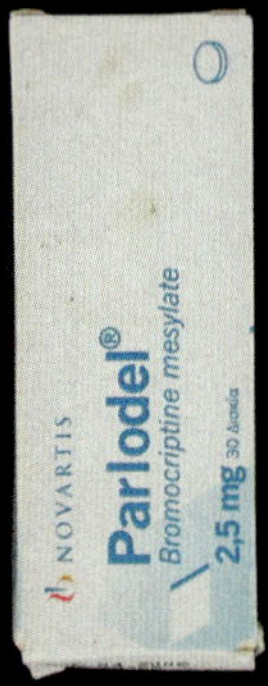

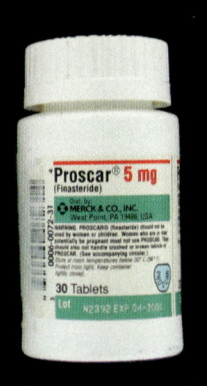

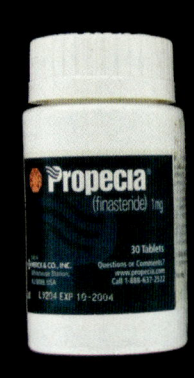

(Italy) (Greece) U.S. Proscar and Propecia

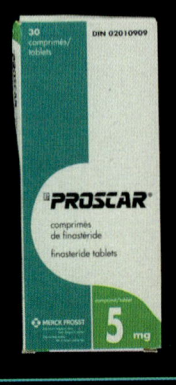

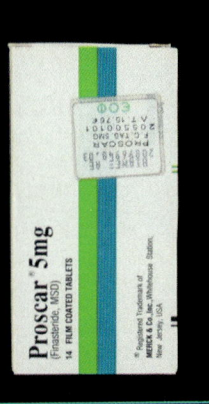

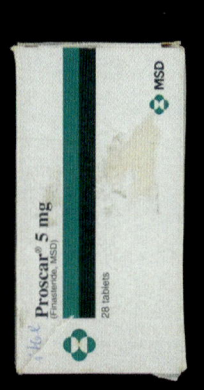

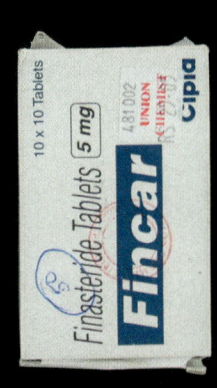

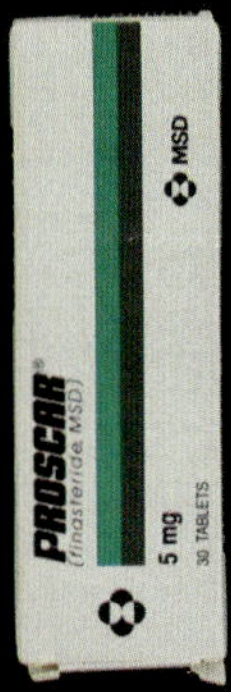

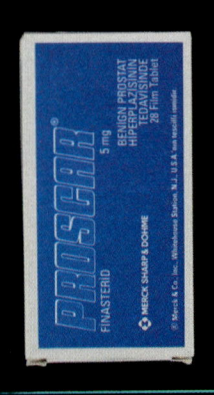

Proscar

(Canada) (Greece) (Holland) (Sri Lanka) (Thailand)

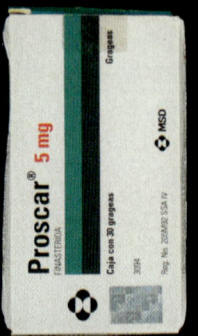

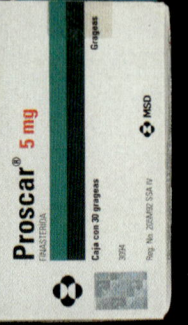

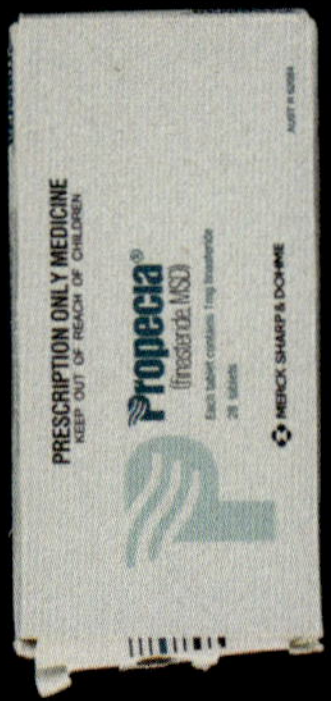

Synthroid

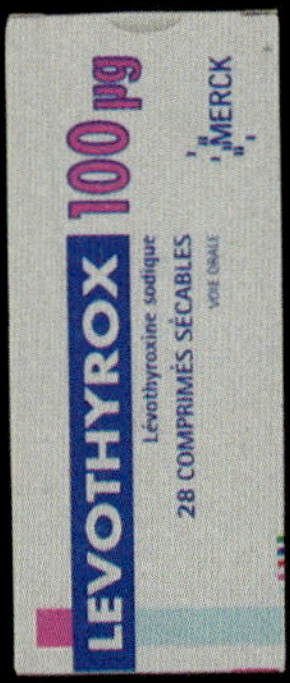

(Mexico) (Australia) (Turkey) (France)

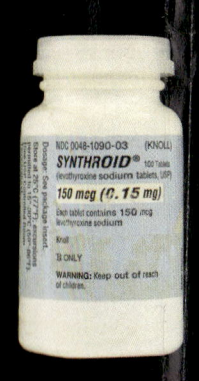

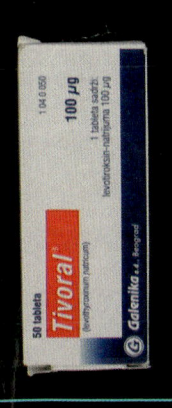

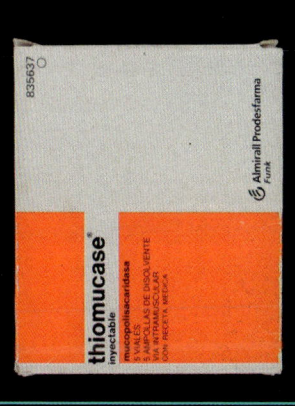

(U.S.) 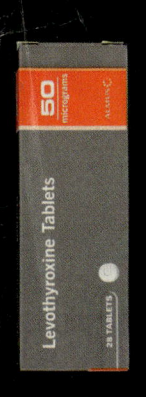 (U.K.) 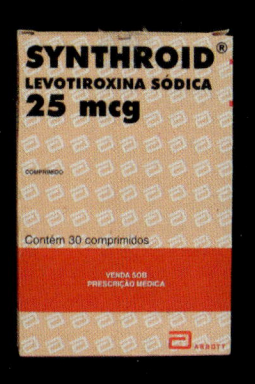 (Brazil) 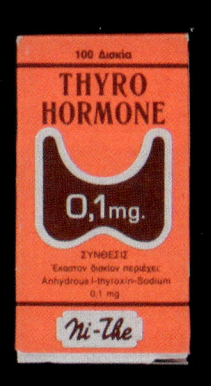 (Greece) 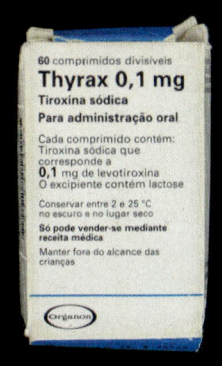 (Portugal)

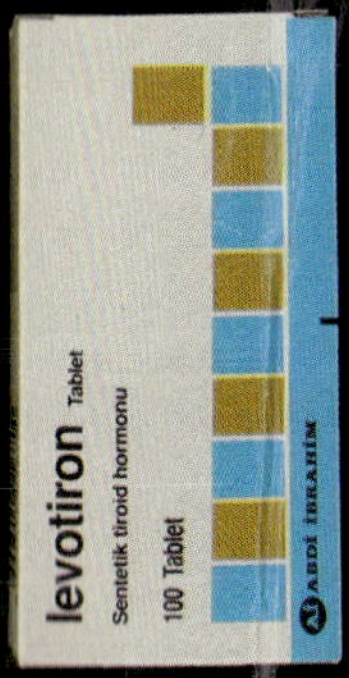

(Turkey) (Serbia) 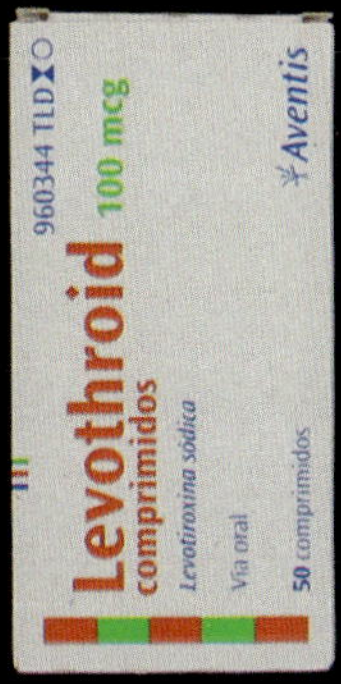 (Spain) Thiomucase Spanish injectable

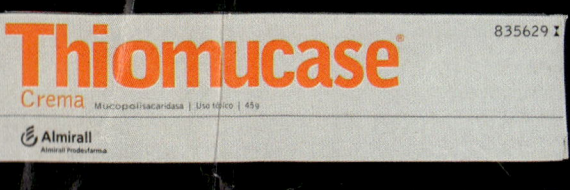

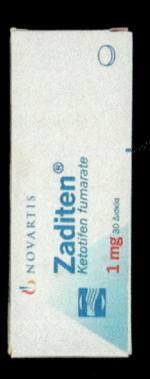

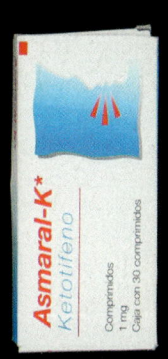

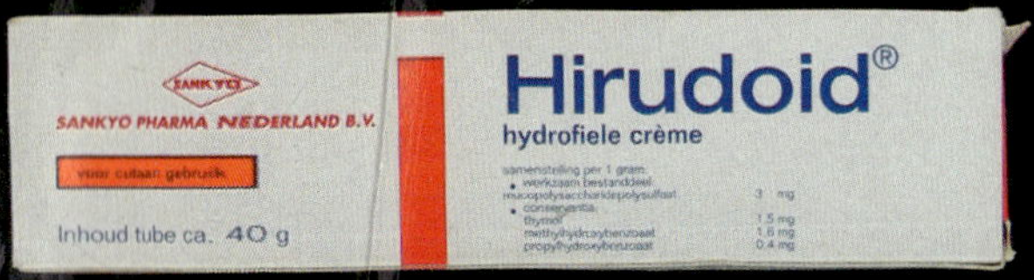

Thiomucase from Spain and Hirudoid from Holland Zaditen (Greece) (Mexico)

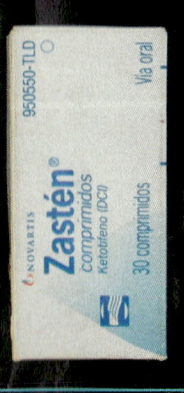

(Spain) (Turkey)

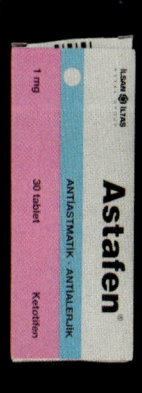

Appendix C

FREE ANABOLICS 10th Edition!

Do you have an empty steroid box, vial, ampule, bottle, or tablet strip you don't see in ANABOLICS 10th EDITION? Send it to Photography Department at the address below. If we use your sample, your copy of **ANABOLICS 10th EDITION** is **ABSOLUTELY FREE!**

ANABOLICS has become THE "standard-issue" global resource on performance-enhancing drugs because athletes know the information inside is the most recent and reliable! No other book of its type has ever been so comprehensive and up-to-date. The information in the latest update was aided in part by the efforts of readers all over the world, who share in William Llewellyn's thirst for knowledge. Bill receives thousands of letters every year containing empty steroid packaging samples for him to examine. This global web of supporters has helped make ANABOLICS the invaluable resource it is today. As a special thanks for the help, Llewellyn will send a free copy of the next book to anyone that submits an empty steroid packaging sample that he doesn't have. It helps other readers get the most current info, and helps you get your next copy **FIRST AND FREE**!

Send your CLEAN and EMPTY boxes, vials, or ampules to:

Photography Department
c/o Body of Science
5500 Military Trail
Ste. 22-318
Jupiter, FL 33458

Cleaning and Mailing Instructions:

Ampules/Vials: Empty contents completely. Flush with rubbing alcohol or water, if necessary, to remove residue. Mail all glass items in a box for protection.

Remember, EMPTY packaging samples only. Privacy protected.

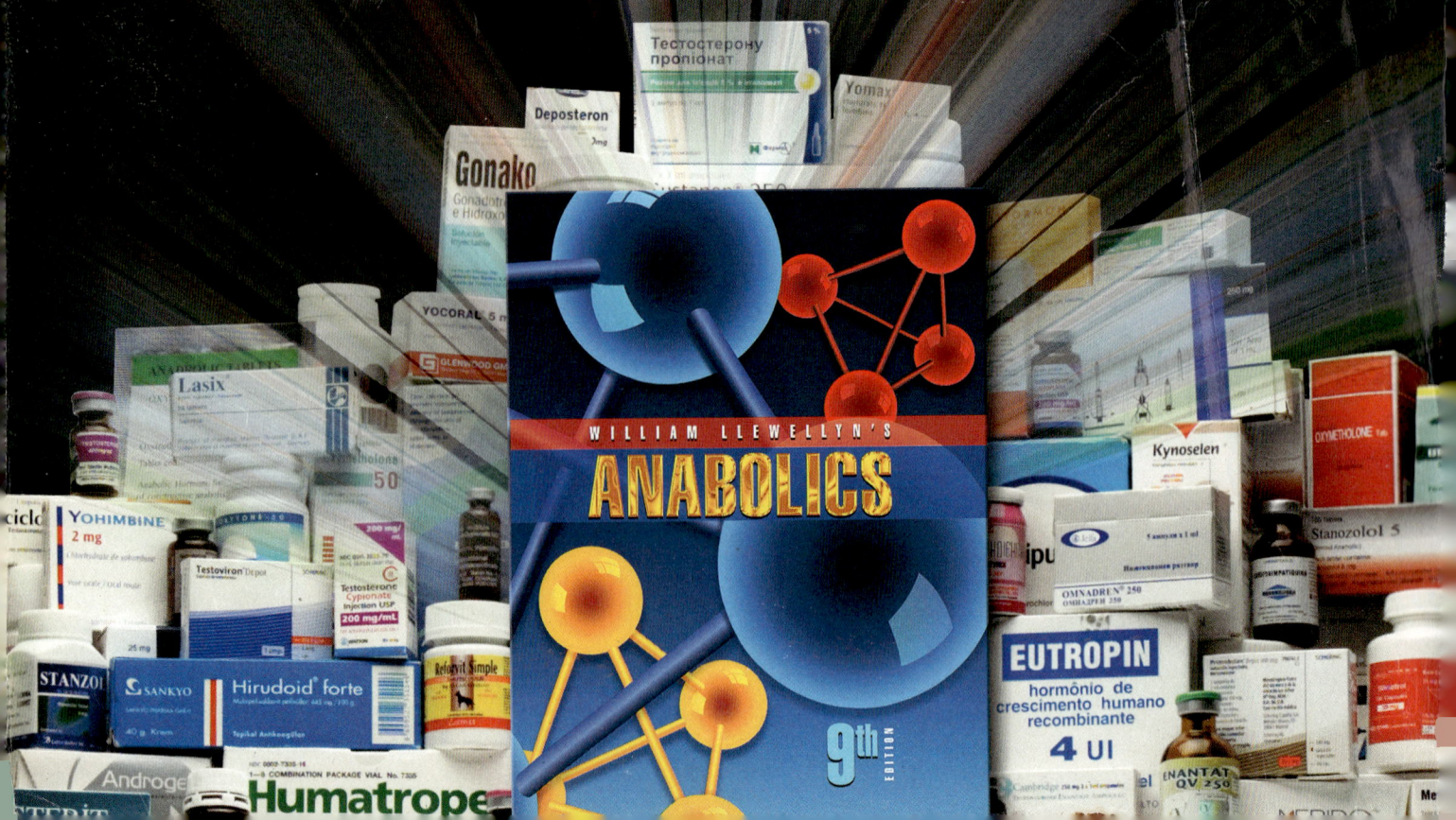